Principles and Practice of Head and Neck Oncology

Edited by

Peter H Rhys Evans DCC (Paris) FRCS
Consultant Otolaryngologist/Head & Neck Surgeon and
Honorary Senior Lecturer, Institute of Cancer Research
Royal Marsden Hospital
London
UK

Paul Q Montgomery BSc MB ChB FRCS(Eng) FRCS(ORL)
Director of The Norfolk and Waveney Head & Neck Cancer Centre
Norfolk & Norwich University Teaching Hospital
Honorary Research Fellow, The School of Biological Sciences
University of East Anglia
Norwich, Norfolk
UK

Patrick J Gullane MB FRCSC FACS
Otolaryngologist-in-Chief
University Health Network
Wharton Chair in Head and Neck Surgery
Princess Margaret Hospital
Professor and Chairman, Department of Otolaryngology, University of Toronto
Toronto, Ontario
Canada

MD Martin Dunitz
Taylor & Francis Group
LONDON AND NEW YORK

First published in the United Kingdom in 2003
by Martin Dunitz, an imprint of the Taylor & Francis Group, 11 New Fetter Lane, London EC4P 4EE

Tel.: +44 (0) 20 7583 9855
Fax.: +44 (0) 20 7842 2298
E-mail: info@dunitz.co.uk
Website: http://www.dunitz.co.uk

A CIP record for this book is available from the British Library.

ISBN 1 89906 606 3

Distributed in the USA by
Fulfilment Center
Taylor & Francis
10650 Tobben Drive
Independence, KY 41051, USA
Toll Free Tel.: +1 800 634 7064
E-mail: taylorandfrancis@thomsonlearning.com

Distributed in Canada by
Taylor & Francis
74 Rolark Drive
Scarborough, Ontario M1R 4G2, Canada
Toll Free Tel.: +1 877 226 2237
E-mail: tal_fran@istar.ca

Distributed in the rest of the world by
Thomson Publishing Services
Cheriton House
North Way
Andover, Hampshire SP10 5BE, UK
Tel.: +44 (0)1264 332424
E-mail: salesorder.tandf@thomsonpublishingservices.co.uk

Artwork by Adrian and Gudrun Cornford
Composition by Scribe Design, Gillingham, Kent
Printed and bound in Spain by Grafos S.A. Arte Sobre Papel

Contents

Contributors

David J Adelstein MD
Staff Physician
Department of Hematology and Medical Oncology
Cleveland Clinic, FNDTN
9500 Euclid Avenue
Cleveland, OH 44195-0001, USA

Daniel J Archer FRCS FDSRCS
Consultant Maxillofacial Surgeon
Royal Marsden Hospital
203 Fulham Road
London SW3 6JJ, UK

Nigel JP Beasley BSc MBBS FRCS(ORL-HNS)
Clinical Fellow in Head and Neck Surgery
Wharton Head and Neck Centre
Princess Margaret Hospital
610 University Avenue
Toronto, ONT M5G 2M9, Canada

Eric D Blom PhD
Speech Pathologist
Head and Neck Associates
Indianapolis, IN, USA

Karen E Broadley MBBS FRCP
Consultant in Palliative Medicine
Department of Palliative Medicine
Royal Marsden Hospital
203 Fulham Road
London SW3 6JJ, UK

Gary C Burget MD FACS
Clinical Associate Professor
Section of Plastic and Reconstructive Surgery
University of Chicago School of Medicine
Chicago, IL, USA

Camilla MA Carroll MB MS FRCSI
Previous Fellow, Department of
Otolaryngology/Head and Neck Surgery
Wharton Head and Neck Centre, 3rd Floor
Princess Margaret Hospital
610 University Avenue
Toronto, ONT M5G 2M9, Canada

Christopher P Cottrill BSc PhD MRCP FRCR
Consultant Clinical Oncologist
Clinical Oncology
Royal Hospital of St Bartholomew and The Royal
London Hospital
London, UK

Melville da Cruz FRACS
Fellow in Otoneurological and Skull Base Surgery
Addenbrooke's Cambridge University Teaching
Hospital Trust
Cambridge, UK

Aongus Curran MB ChB FRCSI
Consultant Otolaryngologist
Department of Otolaryngology
Consultant Ear, Nose & Throat/Head and Neck
St. James Hospital
James's Street
Dublin 8, Ireland

Carmel Ann Daly MB LRCP&SI FFRRCSI
Consultant Radiologist (locum)
Waterford Regional Hospital
Waterford, Ireland

David T Gault MB ChB FRCS
Consultant Plastic Surgeon
Department of Plastic Surgery
Mount Vernon Hospital
Rickmansworth Road
Northwood HA6 2RN, UK

Martin E Gore PhD FRCP
Professor of Cancer Medicine
Department of Medical Oncology
Royal Marsden Hospital
203 Fulham Road
London SW3 6JJ, UK

Patrick J Gullane MB FRCSC FACS
Otolaryngologist-in-Chief
University Health Network
Wharton Chair in Head and Neck Surgery
Princess Margaret Hospital
Department of Otolaryngology
University of Toronto
200 Elizabeth STreet, Suite 7EN-242
Toronto, ONT M5G 2C4, Canada

Clive L Harmer MB FRCP FRCR
Consultant Oncologist and Head of Thyroid Unit
Department of Radiotherapy
Royal Marsden Hospital
203 Fulham Road
London SW3 6JJ, UK

J Michael Henk MD FRCR
Honorary Consultant Clinical Oncologist
Royal Marsden Hospital
203 Fulham Road
London SW3 6JJ, UK

Jonathan C Irish MD MSc FRCSC FACS
Associate Professor, University of Toronto
Chief of Surgical Oncology/Department of Surgical Oncology
Wharton Head and Neck Centre
Princess Margaret Hospital
610 University Avenue, 3-952
Toronto, ONT M5G 2M9, Canada

Colm Irving MB BCh FRCA
Consultant Anaesthetist
Department of Anaesthesia
Royal Marsden Hospital
203 Fulham Road
London SW3 6JJ, UK

Nicholas K James MBBS FRCS(Plast)
Consultant Plastic Surgeon
The Lister Hospital
Stevenage
Herts, UK

John K Joe MD
Clinical Fellow
Head and Neck Service
Memorial Sloan-Kettering Cancer Center
1275 York Avenue
New York, NY 10021, USA

Suzanne Kamel-Reid PhD
Director Molecular Diagnostics
Associate Professor, University of Toronto
Princess Margaret Hospital
610 University Avenue, 9-622
Toronto, ONT M5G 2M9, Canada

D Michael King FRCR
Consultant Radiologist
Department of Diagnostic Imaging
Royal Marsden Hospital
203 Fulham Road
London SW3 6JJ, UK

Valerie J Lund MS FRCS FRCSEd
Professor in Rhinology and
Honorary Consultant Otorhinolaryngologist
Professorial Unit
Royal National Throat Nose and Ear Hospital
350-352 Gray's Inn Road
London WC1X 8DA, UK

Jeremy McMahon FRCS
Consultant Oral and Maxillofacial Surgeon
Monklands Hospital
Lanakshire, Glasgow, UK

David A Moffat BSc MA MB BS FRCS
Head, Department of Otoneurological and Skull Base Surgery
Addenbrooke's Cambridge University Teaching Hospital Trust
Associate Lecturer
University of Cambridge
Cambridge, UK

Paul Q Montgomery BSc MB ChB FRCS(Eng) FRCS(ORL)
Director, Norfolk and Waveney Head & Neck Cancer Centre
Norfolk and Norwich University Teaching Hospital
Honorary Research Fellow, The School of Biological Sciences
University of East Anglia
Norwich, Norfolk NR4 7UY, UK

Peter C Neligan MB FRCSI FRCSC FACS
Professor and Chairman
Division of Plastic Surgery
Wharton Chair in Reconstructive Plastic Surgery
University of Toronto
200 Elizabeth Street, EN7-228
Toronto, ONT M5G 2C4, Canada

Christopher M Nutting MRCP FRCR MD
Consultant and Senior Lecturer in Clinical Oncology
Head and Neck Unit
Royal Marsden Hospital
203 Fulham Road
London SW3 6JJ, UK

Christopher J O'Brien MS FRACS
Director, Sydney Head and Neck Cancer Institute
Royal Prince Alfred Hospital
Associate Professor of Surgery, Sydney University
Sydney, Australia

Pornchai O-charoenrat MD MSc PhD FRCS
Attending Surgeon and Lecturer
Division of Head and Neck Surgery
Department of Surgery
Siriraj Hospital Medical School
Mahidol University
Bangkok 10700, Thailand

Brian O'Sullivan MB FRCPC FRCPI
Bartley-Smith/Wharton Chair in Radiation Oncology
Professor, Department of Radiation Oncology, University of Toronto
Princess Margaret Hospital, 5th Floor
610 University Avenue
Toronto, ONT M5G 2M9, Canada

Snehal G Patel MD MS FRCS Glas
Consultant Head and Neck Surgeon
Royal Marsden Hospital
203 Fulham Road
London SW3 6JJ, UK

Irvin Pathak MD FRCSC
Head and Neck Surgeon
Royal Jubilee Hospital
Victoria, BC and
Clinical Instructor, University of British Columbia, Canada

Saurin R Popat MD FRCSC
Assistant Professor & Program Director
Department of Surgery, Division of Otolaryngology
School of Medicine and Dentistry
University of Rochester
601 Elmwood Avenue, Box 629
Rochester, NY 14642, USA

Frances Rhys Evans RGN ITUCert OncCert MSc
Clinical Nurse Specialist
106 Harley Street
London W1N 1AF, UK

Peter H Rhys Evans DCC (Paris) FRCS
Consultant Otolaryngologist/Head and Neck Surgeon
Royal Marsden Hospital
203 Fulham Road
London SW3 6JJ, UK

David Ross MD FRCS (Plast)
Consultant Plastic Surgeon
Department of Plastic Surgery
St Thomas' Hospital
Lambeth Palace Road
London SE1 7EH, UK

Asha Saini PhD MRCP
Consultant Medical Oncologist
Kent Cancer Centre
Maidstone, Kent, UK

Andrew See MMed(Surg) FRCSEd FRCSGlas
Senior Consultant Head & Neck Surgeon
Department of Surgery
Changi General Hospital
2 Simei Street 3
Singapore 529889, Singapore

Ashok R Shaha MD FACS
Professor of Surgery
Cornell University Medical College
Attending Surgeon
Memorial Sloan-Kettering Cancer Center
1275 York Avenue
New York, NY 10021, USA

Clare Shaw BSc SRD
Chief Dietitian
Royal Marsden Hospital
203 Fulham Road
London SW3 6JJ, UK

Jeffrey D Spiro MD FACS
Professor of Surgery
Division of Otolaryngology/Head and Neck Surgery
University of Connecticut School of Medicine
Farmington, CT 06030, USA

Ronald H Spiro MD
Attending Surgeon
Department of Surgery
Head and Neck Service
Memorial Sloan-Kettering Cancer Center
New York and
Professor of Clinical Surgery
Cornell Medical College
New York, NY, USA

John E Williams MBBS FRCA
Consultant in Anaesthetics and Pain Management
Department of Palliative Medicine
Royal Marsden Hospital
203 Fulham Road
London SW3 6JJ, UK

Robert E Wood DDS PhD FRCDC
Consultant Dentist
Department of Dental Oncology
University of Toronto
Princess Margaret Hospital
610 University Avenue
Toronto, ONT M5G 2M9, Canada

Foreword

At the time of my appointment in 1963 as Professor of Laryngology and Otology within the University of London and Consultant in Ear, Nose and Throat (ENT) Surgery at the Royal National Throat, Nose and Ear Hospital, London, most head and neck oncology was largely in the hands of a relatively small number of general and ENT surgeons. The emphasis in most patients was on control of primary lesion and lymphatic drainage, following the dictum of the late John Conley of New York.....the "big cut out". Although utilizing the increasing availability of radiotherapeutic expertise these patients were largely the responsibility of specific individuals, who consequently acquired considerable experience of many thousands of patients. In my own case I had the assistance of full-time academic staff, plentiful hospital beds, dedicated anaesthetists and pathologists supported by skilled nurses in both ward and operating theatre. Local control was limited by extension within the complex anatomy of the head and neck region, but over the next two decades technical advances enabled more successful extirpation of both primary lesion and draining lymphatics in many sites. Operative mortality and morbidity was reduced by better understanding of the physiological challenges of such major surgery and, of course, the technical skills gained by increased experience. However, better local control also brought increasing awareness of the need for effective rehabilitation and it was at this stage that the plastic surgeon played an important role, although frequently these procedures were provided by the head and neck team. Unfortunately, the consequent improvement, modest though it was in long term survival rates, was overshadowed by a concurrent increase in life expectancy in many countries, and the appearance of late metastasis or new tumours. The emergence of chemotherapy, although helpful in certain pathologies, proved disappointing, although initially utilized enthusiastically by surgeons and later the medical oncologist.

By the time of my retirement in 1990 the emergence of a truly multidisciplinary team had ensured that most patients should have received the best advice, particularly for the control of early lesions, together with realistic rehabilitation following major excisional surgery. However, failure to increase the frequency with which early tumours were diagnosed still resulted in low cure rates for many sites.

During these exciting years for those primarily interested in the technical challenges posed by radical excisions and effective rehabilitation, greater interest developed in sophisticated pathological examination of the surgical specimen in the hope of determining the causes for local failure. Coincidental with this came the possibility of combining radical excision of the neoplasm with the possibilities of preserving some residual function.

However, most of the major textbooks and publications at this time concentrated on surgical technique, with bigger and better procedures described by those whose experience and facilities had attracted large numbers of patients. The development of comprehensive multidisciplinary teams gradually added a wide variety of expertise, which now included not only those primarily concerned with tumour control but others skilled in nutrition and pain relief and so important for so many patients.......realistic palliation.

I have the good fortune to have known two of the editors of this new book for many years as well as many of the contributors. Their collective experience cannot be questioned and they are the products of the learning curve which I have briefly described. The principles of head and neck oncology have changed dramatically, although many of the problems remain. When considering these basic principles they have skillfully set the scene for all the complex sites within the head and neck. These are then considered in some detail followed by an important resume of the increasing improvements in rehabilitation and reconstruction, so vital if patients are to be returned to a meaningful life in society.

Perhaps the most challenging task in this book is to anticipate the future. Developments in molecular biology may eventually explain individual susceptibility although I have to confess to considerable doubt if this modality will ever feature largely in treatment. Surgical excisions may well become more organ sparing, although again these techniques rely on earlier diagnosis. Clearly the best management will depend on a team effort utilizing the many varied modalities now available.

This book is to my mind a most important and timely account of our present knowledge of both the principles and present day practice of the management of the varied neoplasms which affect the head and neck region. It reflects considerable personal experience combined with a deep concern for the welfare of these unfortunate people. Such a philosophy cannot be underestimated when it is remembered that with an aging population the number of potential sufferers is increasing. This brings a greater responsibility to cure those that are curable with as little disability as possible but also offers less favourable patients realistic palliation. The authors have clearly succeeded in translating such a philosophy to paper and are to be greatly commended.

Sir Donald Harrison MD MS PHD FRCS FRCOPHTH
HON. FRCSE FRACS FCM (SA) FACS FRCSI
Emeritus Professor of Laryngology and Otology
University of London
London, UK

Preface

Cancer of the head and neck accounts for under 10% of all malignant tumours and yet nowhere in the field of human oncology are the effects of progression of disease more readily apparent, more cosmetically deforming and more functionally and psychologically disturbing than in this region. Unlike cancer at other sites in the body it is not a disease of one organ but it includes a wide variety of tumours affecting not only the diversity of upper aerodigestive tract organs such as the tongue, the pharynx, the larynx, the nose and the ear, but also other related structures including the thyroid, salivary glands, and the skin and lymphatics of the head and neck.

During the last 20 years progress in head and neck cancer therapy has not only benefited from an increased understanding of the molecular genetics of tumour growth and lymphatic metastatic spread, but also from a better knowledge of epidemiological and aetiological factors. At the same time cohort and accurate population-based studies have helped to identify more precisely the incidence and changing trends in head and neck cancer. Great progress has also been made in the field of diagnosis with refinement of computerized tomography (CT), magnetic resonance imaging (MRI) and positron emission tomography (PET) as well as greater use of cytology and endoscopic techniques. A greater understanding of the clinico-pathological correlation of tumour types, tumour invasion and patterns of spread have allowed clinicians to plan combined management for each individual patient in a more practical and objective fashion.

We have also seen a fundamental change in attitude and philosophy of patient management in the last two decades from one of prescriptive tumour treatment to a much more considered and holistic approach taking greater account of quality of life issues. This has been made possible by increased use of conservation laser and other surgical techniques as well as chemo-radiotherapeutic regimes in appropriate settings. Early patient rehabilitation following surgery has been greatly enhanced by developments in one-stage reconstructive techniques and a better understanding of the functional requirements and limitations of speech and swallowing rehabilitation.

The majority of contributing authors in this book have worked or are currently on the staff of the Royal Marsden Hospital in London and Princess Margaret Hospital, University of Toronto. Their combined experience and multidisciplinary philosophy is hopefully reflected in giving a broad, comprehensive and balanced view of current approaches to management of tumours. We hope that the book will be of value not only to the trainee head and neck surgeons and oncologists but will provide a useful source of knowledge and references to the established specialist entrusted with the care of patients with head and neck cancer.

PRE
PQM
PJG

This book is dedicated to my wife Fran and our children Olivia, Sophie and James who have been a source of inspiration and whose patience, encouragement and support have been greatly appreciated. It is also dedicated to my father who first aroused my interest in otolaryngology and to my patients whose courage and determination in the face of adversity inspire us to achieve improved chances of cure and a better quality of life.

PRE

I would like to dedicate this book to my wife Katie and our children Isabelle, Harry and Jemima for their support and tolerance. I would also like to pay tribute to the courage and dignity of my patients.

PQM

I would like to dedicate this book to Bob and Gerardina Wharton for the generous support they provided us in establishing "The Wharton Head and Neck Centre" and the endowment of three Chairs within the Princess Margaret Hospital/University of Toronto. This contribution has helped enhance patient care, research and education.

My thanks also to my children, Kira and John for their patience, understanding and sacrifice of family time. To my sister Anna and brothers Eamon and Tomas for your friendship. Finally, to my colleagues for their support of my vision and to my patients for the confidence they have placed in me.

PJG

Acknowledgments

We would like to express our appreciation to Martin Dunitz and in particular Clive Lawson and Robert Peden who have overseen the final stages of production of this book. The artists have also made an invaluable contribution. We would also like to thank our secretarial help from Tracey Marshall, Kathryn Dilkes, Kathleen Nicholson & Stephanie Kandel for their support in preparing many of the manuscripts.

PRE
PQM
PJG

PART I

Basic principles of management

1 Introduction

Peter H Rhys Evans and Snehal G Patel

Introduction

Incidence

Head and neck cancer encompasses a wide range of malignant tumours arising from many diverse and complex structures in this region of the body, and which have major physiological and aesthetic importance. The incidence of these tumours varies considerably around the world and hence their impact on public health. In the United Kingdom and in America head and neck cancer is one of the more uncommon group of malignancies, constituting 5–10% of all tumours but in other countries such as the Indian subcontinent they account for up to 45% of all malignancies (Table 1.1).

About 90% of these tumours are squamous carcinomas arising from the surface epithelium and as such they do have many common features concerning their aetiology, natural history and classification.

Table 1.1 Global incidence of head and neck cancer

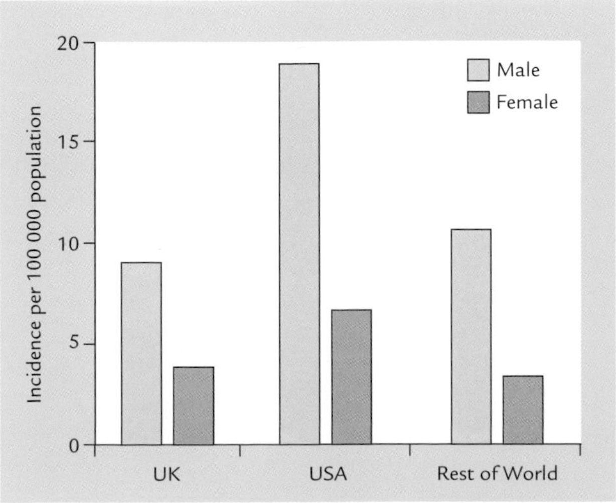

There are however great differences in modes of presentation and treatment depending on the individual sites within the head and neck and also wide variations in the incidence of individual tumours in each country and around the world.

Management

Management presents a major challenge and is determined by local expertise and regional resources. Ideally it should only be undertaken by an experienced multidisciplinary team with adequate resources for optimal investigation, treatment and rehabilitation. In many countries, however, resources are very limited and the possibility of curative radiotherapy or expert surgical treatment is only available to a small minority of patients. This is a serious global health-care problem but great strides have been made in the last few decades to disseminate knowledge and expertise through teaching and publications and from global health care initiatives.

Practical issues

Primary referral of head and neck cancer may be to one of a number of specialists (ear, nose and throat (ENT), oromaxillofacial (OMF), plastic or general surgeon, physician or medical oncologist) any of whom may take charge of management of the patient although few are head and neck cancer specialists. This dissemination of cases, coupled with the heterogeneous nature and relative rarity of tumours at each individual site means that cancer of the upper aerodigestive tract (UADT) invariably only forms a small portion of the workload of these disciplines, severely restricting the experience and expertise of the individual clinician.

In the United Kingdom 6500 new patients with UADT cancer are seen and treated each year by over

900 consultants, which averages at less than 10 cases per consultant, even allowing for joint management.[1] At present there are 57 trainees annually in ENT, OMF and plastic surgery receiving accreditation (including head and neck surgical oncology)[2] although it has been estimated that only a tenth of this number are required with specialist expertise in this field in order to avoid the problems of low volume caseload.[3,4] Clinicians subspecializing in the management of head and neck cancers readily acknowledge that optimal treatment, survival and rehabilitation can only be achieved with a detailed understanding of the anatomy, pathology and natural history of the disease, concentrated experience in its management and constant updating of knowledge from audit of results and published research.

Table 1.2 Site incidence of head and neck cancer[5]

Site	Number	Incidence/100 000
Larynx	2376	4.16
Oral cavity	2156	3.78
Pharynx	1241	2.17
Thyroid	979	1.72

Epidemiology

In 1988 there were 6752 new cases (4443 males, 2309 females) of head and neck cancer registered in the UK in a population of 57 million, giving an average incidence of 11.8 per 100 000. This combined rate for head and neck cancers (excluding thyroid and skin) is similar to that of the pancreas (12.3), leukaemia (10.2) and non-Hodgkin's lymphoma (12.2), and contrasts with the commoner cancers such as lung (76.7) and female breast (52.4). This makes it the eighth most common cancer in males and sixteenth most frequent in females (Table 1.2).[5]

The larynx remains the most common individual site in the head and neck for carcinoma with an incidence of about 4 per 100 000 p.a. and although the incidence is static in males, in females it is being seen more frequently. There has also been a worrying increase in incidence and mortality in oral cavity cancer over the past three decades in the young adult population, particularly in women, a trend which is not wholly explained by changing habits of smoking. Other aetiological agents such as drug abuse, genetic predisposition, nutritional and environmental factors may have increasing significance.

There may also be a wide variation in regional incidence of head and neck cancer within a particular country due to ethnic, industrial, environmental and social influences. In the United Kingdom for example, the incidence of head and neck cancer ranges from about 8 per 100 000 in the Thames and Oxford region, a relatively affluent area, to 13–15 in other regions (Wales 15.3, North Western 13.7, Scotland 12.9). The incidence and mortality rates from oral cancer are higher in Scotland than in the rest of the UK, and in England there is a distinct North–South gradient for males, with higher rates in the north of the country.[6] The annual incidence in the West Midlands, where there is a high registration rate of almost 100%, is given in Table 1.3. It also shows the incidence as a percentage of all cancers.[7]

Table 1.3 Incidence of cancer in major head and neck sites (rate per 100 000 population)[7]

	Males			Females		
Site	Number	Rate	All cancer (%)	Number	Rate	All cancer (%)
Skin	748	29.5	8.2	602	23.2	7.0
Oral cavity	59	2.3	0.6	30	1.2	0.3
Oropharynx	36	1.4	0.4	12	0.5	0.1
Nasopharynx	13	0.5	0.1	5	0.2	0.1
Hypopharynx	26	1.1	0.3	20	0.8	0.2
Nasal cavity/sinus	22	0.9	0.2	17	0.7	0.2
Larynx	118	4.8	1.3	16	0.7	0.2
Thyroid	21	0.9	0.2	50	1.9	0.6
Lymphoma	30	1.2	0.3	26	1.0	0.3
Sarcoma	5	0.2	0.1	5	0.2	0.1
Head and neck	1078	42.6	11.7	783	30.3	9.1

Table 1.4 Male incidence for selected head and neck cancers[10]

Site	Bas-Rhin (France)	Geneva (Switzerland)	Varese (Italy)	Sao Paulo (Brazil)	Bombay (India)	Birmingham (UK)
Lip	0.2	1.7	2.9	5.1	0.3	0.9
Tongue	7.4	3.2	3.8	5.4	10.2	0.8
Oral cavity	9.6	5.1	4.1	6.8	5.8	1.4
Oropharynx	11.6	5.7	4.1	3.8	4.7	0.7
Hypopharynx	10.2	4.2	3.2	1.6	8.0	0.7
Larynx	11.2	10.1	16.0	15.8	12.9	4.0
Head and neck	50.2	30.0	34.1	38.5	41.9	8.5

The incidence of head and neck cancer is increasing in most parts of the world, although the epidemiological profile of individual subsites tends to vary.[8,9] Compared to other more common cancers, it is a heterogeneous disease with behaviour patterns being histologically and site dependent (Table 1.4).[10,11]

In most regions the majority of cancers arises in the larynx but there is a clustering of buccopharyngeal carcinomas in the Latin European countries. The incidence in the Bas Rhin department of France, however, far exceeds that in any other Latin country and is more comparable with levels seen in Bombay where the high incidence is attributable to the habit of chewing betel nut and tobacco. The high rates of laryngeal cancer are also noted in Italy (Varese) and Brazil (Sao Paulo).

There has been an almost universal fall in the incidence of lip cancer to low levels (0.2–5.1) atttibutable to the decreasing incidence of clay pipe smoking and reduced agricultural exposure to carcinogens. Very high levels however are still seen in Newfoundland (22.8) assumed to be due to tar on nets used by the fishermen.[12]

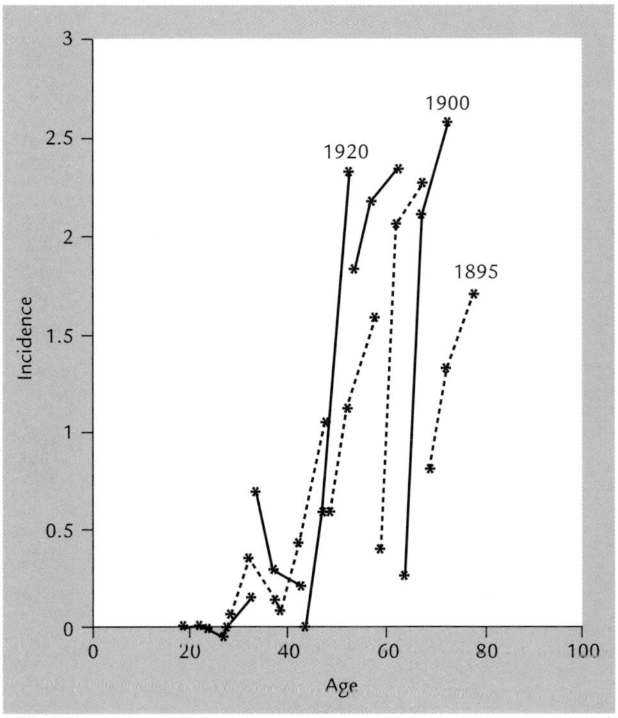

Figure 1.1 Incidence of laryngeal cancer in women for successive birth cohorts.[7]

The geographical differences in the rates of nasopharyngeal cancer are well recognized with exceptionally high numbers seen in South-East Asia. This is associated with Epstein–Barr virus and inhalation of carcinogens from cured fish and other aetiological agents.

With the exception of skin cancers, head and neck tumours are predominantly seen in males, particularly squamous carcinomas of the UADT, and in the sixth and seventh decades of life. The incidence of larygeal cancer in women is increasing for successive birth cohorts (Figure 1.1) consistent with increased female smoking habits[12] and there also appears to be a similar trend in buccopharyngeal carcinoma. For oral cavity cancer there is an unusual sex ratio amongst Singapore Indians, the rates being 8.6 in females and 8.8 in males, with similar rates being found in the migrant Indian population of Natal in South Africa.[12] The habit of reverse smoking in some Indian female populations results in high rates of palatal carcinoma and in Visakhapatnam three-quarters of oral and oropharyngeal cancers were at this site.

Time trends are difficult to interpret because the necessary systematic data is not readily available over 15–20 years. Increasing rates are seen in relation to smoking habits but there is also a disturbing increase in the incidence of malignant melanoma. An average annual increase of 5% in most fair-skinned populations has been noted with the implication of it doubling every 10–12 years.[13]

Aetiology

It has become increasingly apparent over recent years that the state of our health depends to a large extent on our environment and our personal habits, and in particular the risks of developing cancer. We are being constantly reminded of the deterioration of the world-wide environment which affects us all, and our daily exposure to a number of pollutants. The majority of these pollutants are either ingested or inhaled and initial exposure is therefore to the upper aerodigestive tract.[14] Smoking and drinking are understandably considered the most important aetiological agents[15,16] but less information is available on other factors such as pollutants, occupational agents, diet, viral infections and genetic influences (Table 1.5).[14,17–19] There is a great deal of statistical evidence supporting the major aetiological role of tobacco and alcohol but there are fewer case-controlled epidemiological studies on other agents.

Tobacco is by far the most important aetiological factor in UADT squamous carcinoma and in about 90% of patients there is a history of smoking or other forms of ingestion of tobacco such as chewing in some ethnic populations. The synergistic effect of alcohol in those exposed parts of the UADT (oral cavity, oropharynx, hypopharynx and supraglottic larynx) is due to increased mucosal absorption of the carcinogens

Table 1.5 Aetiological factors in head and neck cancer

	Agent	Site(s)
Social	Tobacco	Oral cavity, oropharynx, hypopharynx, larynx, cervical oesophagus[15]
	Alcohol	Oral cavity, oropharynx, hypopharynx, larynx (supraglottis), cervical oesophagus[16]
Occupational	Asbestos	Larynx[16,20–22]
	Man-made fibres	Larynx, pharynx, oral cavity[23]
	Textiles	Larynx, pharynx, oral cavity[24]
	Wood workers	Nasal cavity/sinuses,[25] larynx,[26] nasopharynx
	Plastics	Larynx (resins,[27] rubber[24])
		Oral cavity and pharynx (vinyl chloride[28])
	Mustard gas	Larynx[29]
	Naphthalene	Larynx (glottic)[30]
	CME and BCME	Larynx[31]
	Pesticides	Larynx[32]
	Alcohol manufacture	Larynx,[31] oral cavity and pharynx[34]
	Sulphuric acid	Larynx[34]
	Leatherworkers	Oral cavity, pharynx, larynx[35]
	Paint and print	Larynx,[36] oral cavity,[37] pharynx[36]
	Car mechanics	Larynx,[26,38] oral cavity[38]
	Nickel refiners	Larynx[16,39]
	Metal workers	Larynx[36,40]
		Tonsil, pharynx and alveolus[37]
	Coal and stone dust	Larynx[22,31]
	Cement and concrete	Larynx[40]
	Farmers	Larynx[31,40]
	Bartenders	Larynx[31,41]
Radiation	Accidental	
	Chernobyl	Paediatric thyroid[42]
	Occupational	
	Watch dial makers	Osteosarcoma of the jaw[43]
	Therapeutic	
	Acne, tinea etc	Sarcomas[44,45]
		Thyroid[46]
	Thorotrast	Larynx, non-Hodgkin's lymphoma[47]
Genetic predisposition		UADT cancer[14]
Viral agents		Pharynx, larynx[19]
Atmospheric pollution		Pharynx, larynx[48]

from chronic inflammation and hyperaemia, as well as increased solubility of the carcinogens in alcohol compared with aqueous saliva. The reviewed case-control studies provide substantial evidence for increased risk from a number of occupational agents[17] and radiation listed in Table 1.5. In most of these studies the increased risk remains high even after adjustment for tobacco and alcohol consumption.

There is also recent evidence of genetically based susceptibility and predisposition for the development of UADT cancer in patients without necessarily any history of tobacco or alcohol exposure.[14] Mutagen sensitivity, which is a measure of an individual's intrinsic DNA repair capacity against free radical damage, has been demonstrated as a risk factor in the disease. A low intake of vitamins C and E was also associated with an increased risk and when both factors were evident, patients were at greatest risk. This supports the concept that the risk of head and neck cancer is determined by a balance of factors that either enhance or protect against free radical oxygen damage, including innate capacities for DNA repair.[14]

The potential role of viral agents, particularly human papilloma virus (HPV) 16, in the pathogenesis of head and neck squamous carcinoma has also been extensively studied and there seems to be a definite association between the virus and tumour formation although this is not very consistent.[19]

The study by Wake[48] revealed interdistrict variation in the incidence of head and neck cancer in the West Midlands with a definite urban/rural divide. Atmospheric pollution data (mean sulphur dioxide and smoke concentrations) from a national survey are positively correlated with squamous carcinoma of the pharynx and larynx. Further epidemiological information is required on environmental and occupational agents since firm evidence can only be identified by prospective data collection.

Natural history

The natural history of the disease should provide the opportunity for successful intervention. The majority of head and neck cancers progress in a relatively orderly fashion, from a small primary tumour to a larger lesion and lymph node metastases. This direct size relationship generally holds true for sites such as the oral cavity and larynx but for other sites such as the nasopharynx, oropharynx and to a lesser extent the hypopharynx neck metastases are seen just as frequently with T1 as with T4 lesions. Indeed the nasopharynx and oropharynx are the commonest sites of origin of the apparent 'occult primary' (Table 1.6).

Table 1.6 Relationship of tumour size (T) and node metastases (N)

Direct size relation	
	Larynx
	Oral cavity
	Salivary glands
	Lip
	Nasal cavity and sinuses
No size relation	
	Oropharynx
	Nasopharynx
	Hypopharynx
	Thyroid

Distant metastases are nearly always a sequel to advanced nodal disease, and remain a relatively uncommon feature, although now occurring rather more frequently as local treatment becomes more successful, as are second UADT primaries. Although distant metastases have been found at autopsy in up to 40% of fatal cases[49] progressive local disease often dominates the clinical picture during the final stages of the illness. Uncontrolled disease in the head and neck is distressing for the patient and carers, so successful elimination of the primary tumour and neck node metastases is of paramount importance. This requires early diagnosis, accurate assessment of the extent of the tumour, and radical treatment. In this respect the skill of the treating clinicians can make the difference between success and failure.

However, successful curative treatment of more advanced head and neck cancers may involve severe disturbance of function and/or obvious deformity. Also, many head and neck cancer patients present in poor general health because of other smoking and alcohol-related problems, and may not be able to withstand very aggressive treatment. Therefore the choice of treatment must take all these factors into account together with the wishes of the patient and his family. It is for the patient to decide whether he wants the greatest possible chance of cure despite loss of his larynx, for example, or the possibility or organ preservation with a slightly lower chance of survival.

Treatment

Historical developments

Surgical excision of the tumour or cautery were historically the only effective methods of treatment

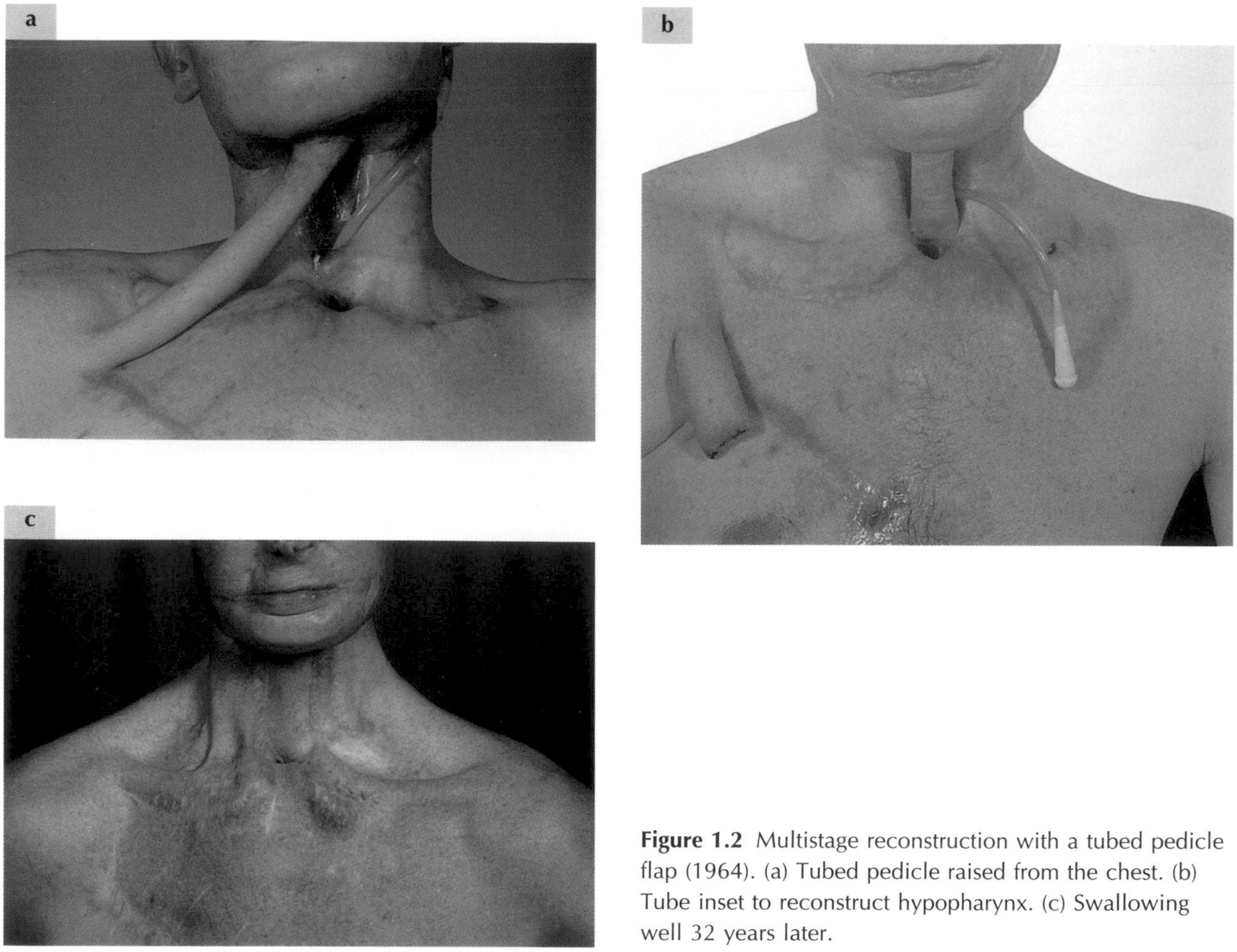

Figure 1.2 Multistage reconstruction with a tubed pedicle flap (1964). (a) Tubed pedicle raised from the chest. (b) Tube inset to reconstruct hypopharynx. (c) Swallowing well 32 years later.

until the early 1900s when the introduction of radium was shown to not only shrink tumours but to eliminate some completely. The concept of combining the curative effects of surgery and radiotherapy was a logical progression introduced in the 1920s. In 1929 a report from Sweden compared the results of treatment using either radiotherapy alone or preoperatively for oral cancers and cervical metastases.[50] None of the patients treated with radiotherapy alone was symptom-free at 5 years compared with 40% in the group treated with combined pre-operative radiation and surgery. Orthovoltage irradiation dominated treatment until the 1930s curing possibly 25% of oral, pharyngeal and laryngeal cancers.[51] It became employed more commonly postoperatively, although the long-term morbidity and skin damage caused by orthovoltage was becoming apparent. As a result many oncologists reserved radiotherapy for recurrence or for palliation.[52]

In the 1940s a resurgence of surgical treatment was pioneered by Hayes Martin who introduced the concept of radical excision of the primary tumour and neck disease where feasible. This was only made possible because of improvements made in anaesthesia and blood transfusion during the Second World War and the introduction of antibiotics. Although this improved locoregional control, the complications and mutilating effects from such radical surgery were considerable. Reconstruction was usually multistaged using tubed-pedicles (Figure 1.2) and many patients died before functional and aesthetic rehabilitation could be achieved.

By the 1950s megavoltage radiotherapy had been introduced with its skin-sparing effects and this renewed interest in combined therapy. Other improvements in dosimetry, fractionation and the use of electron beam therapy further reduced the limiting side effects of radiotherapy.

Head and neck surgery began to evolve as a subspecialty with the concept of combined clinics and otolaryngologists became predominantly involved with the help of plastic surgeons. The differentiation between random and axial pattern cutaneous flaps introduced by McGregor in 1972[53] heralded major advances in reconstructive surgery. Bakamjian's successful deltopectoral flap (1965)[54] had already gained widespread recognition and its axial pattern explained why it was so reliable. The ready availability and length of this and also McGregor's forehead flap permitted immediate and effective reconstruction of most defects in the head and neck. The only drawback was that most reconstructions required a second stage to divide and inset the pedicle.

The introduction in 1979 by Ariyan of myocutaneous flaps[55] allowed immediate one-stage reconstructions of large internal mucosal defects possible for the first time. Further technical and microvascular surgical advances since the 1980s have permitted widespread adoption of skin, visceral and complex free grafts, giving the surgeon a wide variety of options for optimum reconstruction and rehabilitation. During this period there have also been significant advances in voice rehabilitation since the introduction in 1979 of the tracheo-oesophageal speech valve by Eric Blom.

Single modality treatment is now well established in the management of early stage disease, whether surgery or radiotherapy, and combined therapy gives optimal chance of cure for advanced tumours. There have been high expectations that chemotherapy might provide an effective alternative treatment for squamous carcinoma or at least to reduce the morbidity of conventional therapy. At the moment its use is mainly for palliation, although there is evidence that chemotherapy may have a role in the neoadjuvant or concomitant setting combined with radiotherapy or surgery.

Principles of combined therapy

Surgery is used for benign tumours of the head and neck, and surgical excision remains the most dependable and effective method of eliminating gross malignant disease. There are exceptions, such as nasopharyngeal carcinoma which is very radiosensitive, which is fortunate for such a relatively inaccessible tumour. Radiotherapy is most effective in eradicating microscopic disease which is less amenable to surgery. It will help reduce tumour cell dissemination by sealing lymphatics, thus confining the tumour to the primary site, decreasing the potential for metastatic spread. It may also have an effect of enhancing the local immune reaction in irradiated tissue adjacent to the tumour.[56]

Multidisciplinary care

Head and neck cancer is primarily a mucosal disease of the upper aerodigestive tract with 90% of tumours arising as squamous carcinomas from epithelial membranes of the oral and nasal cavities, the pharynx and larynx. Common symptomatic presentation of cancers in this region is therefore mainly to ENT surgeons with hoarseness, oral ulceration, sore throat, earache, bleeding, nasal obstruction, dysphagia or cervical lymphadenopathy. Secondary symptoms such as deafness or middle ear symptoms due to secretory otitis media (SOM) or sinusitis due to osteomeatal obstruction also commonly present to otolaryngology departments and their significance to possible underlying malignant disease is generally well appreciated. The maxillofacial specialist diagnoses many cases of oral malignancies and contributes expertise in resection and restoration of the oral cavity. Needless to say, the radiotherapist will also be an essential lead clinician in the multidisciplinary team and input from a medical oncologist is required for inclusion of chemotherapeutic agents.

Optimal reconstruction following ablative head and neck surgery requires a specialist plastic and reconstructive surgeon as part of the surgical team with a broad knowledge of different free and pedicled flaps at their disposal. Also included in the multidisciplinary team are the nurse specialists, speech therapists, dietitians, dental hygienists and physiotherapists with specialized training and expertise in head and neck cancer.

Such expert teams can be developed only in units treating large numbers of patients. As head and neck cancer is relatively uncommon, it is essential to centralize its treatment into a relatively small number of large centres. This principle is embodied in the Calman–Hine report published by the Department of Health in 1995,[57] which recommends the setting up of accredited cancer centres. The report of the British Association of Head and Neck Oncologists[58] recommends that a centre treating head and neck cancer should treat at least 80 cases per year, but even this number is less than ideal. Any inconvenience to the patient from having to receive treatment some distance from home is far outweighed by the potential for improved chances of cure, and especially of a better functional outcome, provided by the expert multidisciplinary team.

Recent developments in diagnostic techniques

Endoscopy

The introduction of new fibreoptic and rigid endoscopic techniques with stroboscopy has greatly enhanced the diagnostic and dynamic assessment of tumours of the upper aerodigestive tract, particulary the pharynx and larynx. Postoperatively they have also significantly improved the ability and accuracy of follow-up of early recurrence and function in the outpatient/office setting. The recent development of contact endoscopy by Andrea is interesting but its practical value has yet to be established.

Radiology

Over the past 20 years improvements in computerized tomography (CT) and magnetic resonance imaging (MRI) have helped to increase diagnostic accuracy and detection of small volume and occult tumours. Staging is more accurate, especially in the neck, and these techniques have also greatly facilitated more accurate planning of operations. Positron emission tomography (PET) scanning is not widely available but has been shown to be particularly useful in detecting occult disease and residual tumour following radiation therapy. Ultrasound is well established as a simple diagnostic tool and has been used increasingly in conjunction with fine-needle aspiration cytology (FNAC).

Pathology

In recent years histological studies have given us a greater understanding of the process of invasion and metastatic spread. We are more aware of the true incidence of occult micrometastases in the neck from certain tumour sites allowing us to tailor elective neck treatment with surgery or radiotherapy more effectively to reduce the risk of recurrence. Advances in immunocytochemistry techniques have also improved accuracy of diagnosis and the field of molecular biology has opened up a whole new avenue of research which has given us a greater insight into the cellular processes involved in tumour genesis.This hopefully will in time be of therapeutic value using techniques of genetic engineering. The introduction of FNAC and true-cut biopsy have enabled rapid outpatient diagnosis with a high degree of accuracy particularly when used with ultrasound. Finally, the use of frozen section at operation has enabled us to verify margins of resection to give greater reliability in complete tumour excision and also in many instances will help to avoid a second operation by confirming histology on the spot so that the surgeon can proceed and complete the procedure (e.g. neck dissection, thyroidectomy).

Recent developments in surgical access and conservation

Oral cavity/oropharynx

One of the most effective operations to be developed in the 1950s was the 'Commando' procedure for access and resection of oral cavity and oropharyngeal tumours. The lower lip was split and the mandible routinely sacrificed to facilitate resection and also, in the absence of effective flap reconstruction, to enable direct closure of the mucosa. This resulted in the typical cosmetic deformity and mandibular swing (Figure 1.3) but the procedure was potentially curative. In the majority of cases, however, the mandible was not involved with tumour.

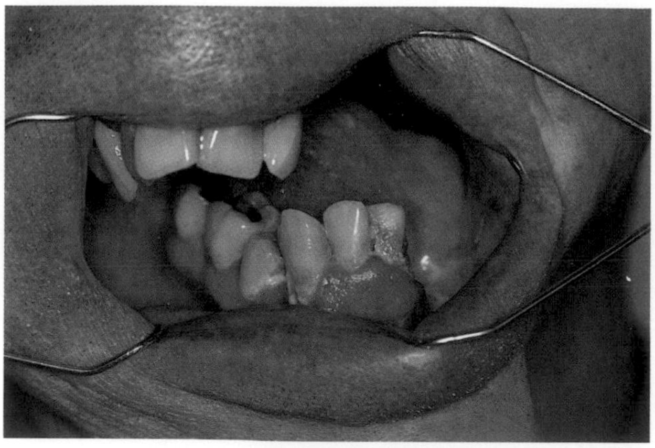

Figure 1.3 Mandibular swing following hemimandibulectomy.

With the advent of myocutaneous and free skin flap reconstruction that allowed immediate replacement of the mucosal defect a more conservative approach was possible with preservation of the unaffected mandible. There is still some controversy about the use of routine mandibulotomy and splitting the lower lip for access, which adds unnecessary time to the operation as well as increases morbidity. Head and neck surgeons should be well trained in peroral surgery of the oropharynx and most resections and reconstructions can be successfully carried out via that approach combined with access through the neck. We feel that mandibulotomy is only indicated in some difficult posterior lesions.

The free radial forearm flap is ideal for reconstruction of most defects and is much more pliable and mobile than pedicled myocutaneous flaps, which are more suitable for large defects where bulk is required.

Skull-base surgery

The skull base has traditionally been considered a natural frontier to the head and neck but increased co-operation with neurosurgical teams has allowed the development of complex craniofacial resections for tumours that do not respect such boundaries. Morbidity and mortality rates have been reduced to acceptable levels with increasing expertise, even for the most inaccessible tumours.

Superior mediastinal surgery

Malignant disease extending down into the superior mediastinum has generally been considered a contraindication to surgery and many patients have been considered inoperable and referred for palliative care. The combined thoracocervical approach[59] developed for resection of benign tumours is also appropriate for selected cases of thyroid and other malignancies of the superior mediastinum and is associated with minimal morbidity.

Neck dissection

The radical neck dissection introduced by Crile in 1906 has stood the test of time as the most effective treatment for malignant disease in the neck. For 60 years this was the 'all or nothing' surgical approach to treatment of the neck and even now it is still practised in its original form with routine sacrifice of the sternomastoid muscle, the accessory nerve and the internal jugular vein together with the lymphatic field in all situations, irrespective of the extent of neck involvement.

Conservation or 'functional' techniques have been introduced and, as many studies have shown, provided that they are carried out meticulously, they do not add any greater risk of recurrence. The unnecessary extra morbidity of a full radical neck dissection is not justified if these vascular and neuromuscular structures are not involved with tumour and some type of modified radical neck dissection is appropriate in most instances. Consideration should also be given to routine preservation of the great auricular nerve and other branches of the cervical sensory plexus as well as the ansa cervicalis if these stuctures are not directly involved.

In the management of N0 disease and some node-positive necks (e.g. thyroid) the use of selective neck dissections has combined the therapeutic value of neck dissection with minimal morbidity. The choice of neck incision is also important and most dissections can be carried out through some form of McFee skin crease incision which gives more reliable healing and gives a better cosmetic result than vertical incisions.

Tracheostomy and postoperative care

A temporary tracheostomy has been widely used to avoid potential postoperative airway problems of obstruction and bleeding particularly following oral cavity and oropharyngeal resections. It is usually removed after a few days but does add time to the operation, involves extra nursing care and has significant morbidity. These complications are rare and occur usually within 8 hours of the operation. Patients undergoing such surgery should be routinely monitored in a high dependency unit and we prefer to keep them ventilated overnight in a more controlled situation, extubating them after careful assessment the following morning thus avoiding a tracheostomy.

Lasers in head and neck surgery

The carbon dioxide laser was introduced into otolaryngology practice in 1976[60] and soon became established as an effective method of relatively bloodless resection of lesions in the upper aerodigestive tract, particularly for laryngeal microsurgery. Over recent years Steiner[61] and others have pioneered its extended use for endoscopic resection of more substantial tumours of the larynx and pharynx.

Photodynamic therapy is another form of laser treatment using selective photoactivation. Although Tappenier and Jesionek reported some good results from phototherapy in 1903[62] it was not until the 1970s that further progress[63] was made using haematoporphorin derivative (HPD). The principle of injecting a dye which is selectively taken up by tumours and then exposing the tumour to laser light causing destruction of the sensitized malignant cells is potentially very promising. Consistent results have not been achieved although newer agents such as Foscan and intralesional laser fibres may be more effective.

Combined salvage surgery with brachytherapy

Tumour recurrence following radiotherapy is a challenging problem especially when access is difficult such as in the nasopharynx or where vital structures (e.g. the carotid artery) may be adjacent to or involved by tumour in the neck. Reirradiation with external beam therapy may be possible and can be curative, but is associated with significant morbidity from radionecrosis of bone, skin or neural tissue. Patients may be offered chemotherapy but this is palliative and potential benefits and symptom control may only last an average of 6 months.

Neck

Accurate diagnosis and assessment of neck disease after radiotherapy is notoriously difficult and may be delayed because of clinical or radiological uncertainty or false negative cytology. By the time a diagnosis is reached many patients are genuinely incurable. Others, however, are wrongly considered inoperable and relegated to palliative care when they are potentially curable. This may be because of inexperience of the surgeon who is unwilling to tackle a difficult surgical problem or unwilling to

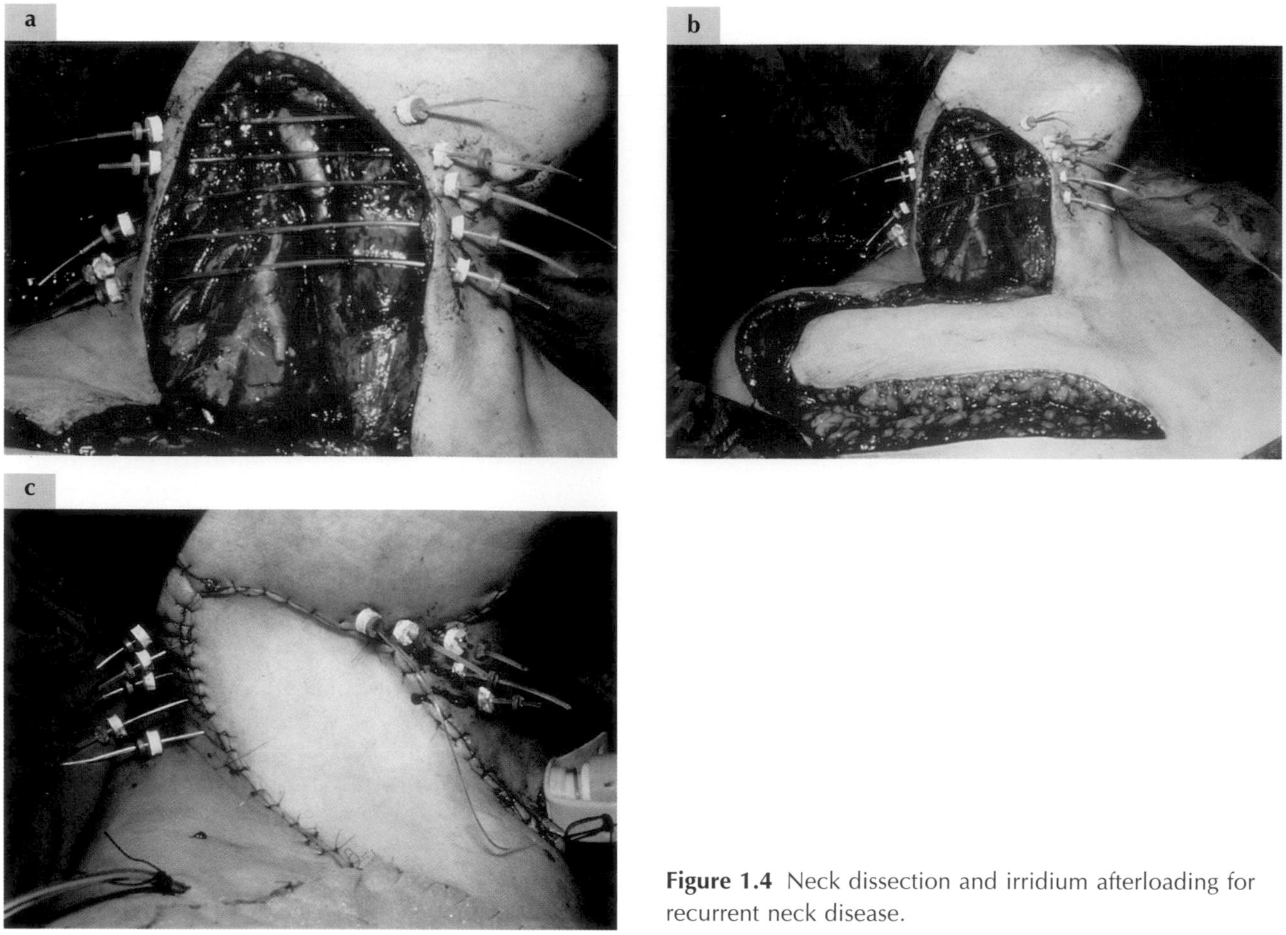

Figure 1.4 Neck dissection and irridium afterloading for recurrent neck disease.

seek more experienced advice elsewhere. The decision about operability is generally made on the basis of a CT scan but after radiotherapy it is very difficult to distinguish between tumour and post-radiation fibrosis, particularly around the carotid sheath. At surgery there is often a clear plane of dissection around the adventitia of the artery separating it from a fibrous capsule surrounding the tumour. Actual invasion of the artery is much less common than involvement of the internal jugular vein and in many cases it is possible to achieve complete or near complete excision.

With this limited margin of resection there is an almost certain risk of further recurrence but the combined use of surgical excision and afterloading irridium brachytherapy[64] (Figure 1.4) has achieved a 60% local control at 12 months and a significant number of long-term (> 5 year) survivors.

Nasopharynx

Local recurrence of nasopharyngeal carcinoma occurs in 10–50% of patients depending on the initial stage. Reirradiation with external beam

Table 1.7 Survival trends for head and neck cancer[66]

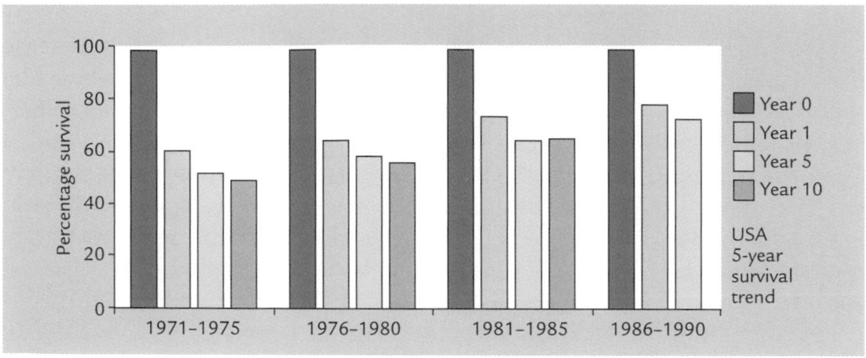

therapy is sometimes used to good effect but is associated with complications. Excision (or laser destruction) of the tumour is possible with appropriate access through a Le Fort osteotomy approach[65] combined with afterloading brachytherapy.

Reconstruction, rehabilitation and quality of life

Long-term cure rates for head and neck cancer have not changed appreciably over the past 40 years since ultimate long-term survival is limited by metastatic disease, the appearance of second primaries and other smoking-related conditions but there is good evidence that survival rates have improved steadily (Table 1.7). There has, however, during this period been a definite change of emphasis in treatment of patients, not only to cure them of cancer but to rapidly restore their quality of life and functional rehabilitation. This has been made possible by tremendous improvements in reconstruction, using a variety of free and pedicled reconstructions, and also rapid restoration of speech using tracheo-oesophageal silicone valves.

REFERENCES

1. Edwards DM, Johnson NW, Cooper D, Warnakulasuriya KAAS. A survey of consultants treating upper aerodigestive tract cancer in the UK. *Ann R Coll Surg* 1998; **80**: 283–287.
2. Birchall M. Head and neck cancer services in Avon and the south west: profile and proposals for development. Report to the Regional Health Authority, July 1995.
3. Lore JM. Dabbling in head and neck oncology. (A plea for added qualifications). *Arch Otolaryngol Head Neck Surg* 1987; **113**: 1165–1168.
4. Bradley PJ. Survey of current management of laryngeal and hypopharyngeal cancer. *J R Coll Surg Edinb* 1989; **34**: 197–200.
5. Rhys Evans PH. Provision and quality assurance of head and neck cancer care in the United Kingdom: a coordinated multidisciplinary approach. *Report for the British Association of Otolaryngologists/Head and Neck Surgeons.* March 1995.
6. Cancer Research Campaign Factsheet – Oral cavity 1993.
7. Powell J, Robin PE. Cancer of the head and neck: the present state. In: Rhys Evans PH, Robin PE, Fielding JWL (eds) *Head and Neck Cancer.* Tunbridge Wells: Castle House Publications, 1983; 3–16.
8. Tobias JS. Current issues in cancer: cancer of the head and neck. *Br Med J* 1994; **308**: 961–966.
9. Gile G. Thursfield V, Staples M. The bottom line: trends in cancer mortality, Australia 1950–1991. *Cancer Forum* 1994; **18**: 12–23.
10. Waterhouse J, Muir CS, Shanmugaratnam K, Powell J. *Cancer Incidence in Five Continents, Volume IV* IARC Scientific Publication No 42. Lyons, 1982.
11. McMichael AJ. Increases in laryngeal cancer in Britain and Australia in relation to alcohol and tobacco consumption trends. *Lancet* 1978; **i**: 1244–1247.
12. Muir CS, Nectoux J, Stukonis M. The changing incidence of head and neck cancers. In: Rhys Evans PH, Robin PE, Fielding JWL (eds.) *Head and Neck Cancer.* Tunbridge Wells: Castle House Publications, 1983; 17–28.
13. Muir CS, Nectoux J. Time trends: malignant melanoma of skin. In: Magnus K (ed.) *Trends in Cancer Incidence: Causes and Practical Implications.* Washington: Hemisphere Publishing Corporation, 1982; 365–385.
14. Maier H, De Vries N, Snow GB. Occupational factors in the aetiology of head and neck cancer. *Clin Otolaryngol* 1991; **16**: 406–412.
15. Khan HA. The Dorn study of smoking and mortality among US veterans: report on 8½ years of observation. *J Natl Cancer Inst* 1966; **19**: 1896–1906.
16. Burch JD, Howe GR, Miller AB, Semenciw R. Tobacco, alcohol, asbestos and nickel in the etiology of cancer of the larynx: a case-control study. *J Natl Cancer Inst* 1981; **67**: 1219–1224.
17. Schantz SP, Zhang ZF, Spitz MS et al. Genetic susceptibility to head and neck cancer: interaction between nutrition and mutagen sensitivity. *Laryngoscope* 1997; **107**: 765–781.
18. Jafek BW, Smith CM, Moran DT et al. Effects on the upper respiratory passages. *Otolaryngol Head Neck Surg* 1992; **106**: 720–729.
19. Brandsma JL, Abramson AL. Association of papillomavirus with cancers of the head and neck. *Arch Otolaryngol Head Neck Surg* 1989; **115**: 621–625.
20. Stell PM, McGill T. Asbestos and laryngeal carcinoma. *Lancet* 1973; **i**: 416–417.
21. Stell PM, McGill T. Exposure to asbestos and laryngeal carcinoma. *J Laryngol Otol* 1975; **89**: 513–517.
22. Zemla B, Wojcieszek Z. The epidemiological risk factors of the larynx cancer among the native and migrant male population. *Neoplasma* 1984; **31**: 465–474.
23. Moulin JJ, Mur JM, Wild P et al. Oral cavity and laryngeal cancers among man-made mineral fibre production workers. *Scand J Work Environ Health* 1986; **12**: 27–31.
24. Zagraniski RT, Kelsey JL, Walter SD. Occupational risk factors for laryngeal cancer: Connecticut, 1975–1980. *Am J Epidemiol* 1986; **124**: 167–176.
25. Acheson ED, Cowdell H, Hadfield E, Macbeth RG. Nasal cancer in woodworkers in the furniture industry. *Br Med J* 1970; **ii**: 587–596.
26. Wynder EL, Covey LS, Mabuchi K, Mushinski M. Environmental factors in cancer of the larynx. A second look. *Cancer* 1976; **38**: 1519–1601.
27. Gerosa A, Turrini O, Bottasso F. Laryngeal cancer in a factory molding thermoplastic resins. *Med Lav* 1986; **77**: 172–176.

28. Tabershaw IR, Gaffey WR. Mortality study of workers in the manufacture of vinyl chloride and its polymers. *J Occup Med* 1974; **16**: 509–518.
29. Manning KP, Skegg DCG, Stell PM, Doll R. Cancer of the larynx and other occupational hazards of mustard gas workers. *Clin Otolaryngol* 1981; **6**: 165–170.
30. Wolf O. Larynxkarzinome bei Naphtalinreinigern. *Z Gesamte Hyg* 1978; **24**: 737–739.
31. Alderson MR, Ratten NS. Mortality of workers on an isopropyl alcohol plant and two MEK dewaxing plants. *Br J Ind Med* 1980; **37**: 85–89.
32. Klayman MB. Exposure to insecticides. *Arch Otolaryngol* 1968; **88**: 116–117.
33. Lynch J, Hanis NM, Bird MG et al. An association of upper respiratory cancer with exposure to diethyl sulfate. *J Occup Med* 1979; **211**: 333–341.
34. Soskolne CL, Zeighami EA, Hanis NM et al. Laryngeal cancer and occupational exposure to sulfuric acid. *Am J Epidemiol* 1984; **120**: 358–369.
35. Decoufle P. Cancer risk associated with employment in the leather and leather products industry. *Arch Environ Health* 1979; **34**: 33–37.
36. Delager NA, Mason TJ, Fraumeni JF et al. Cancer mortality among workers exposed to zinc chromate paints. *J Occup Med* 1980; **22**: 25–29.
37. Wynder EL, Bross IJ, Feldman RM. A study in etiological factors in cancer of the mouth. *Cancer* 1957; **10**: 1300–1323.
38. Schwartz E. Proportionate mortality ratio analysis of auto mechanics and gasoline service station workers in New Hampshire. *Am J Ind Med* 1987; **12**: 91–99.
39. Pedersen E, Hogetveit AC, Andersen A. Cancer of the respiratory organs among workers at a nickel refinery in Norway. *Int J Cancer* 1982; **30**: 681–685.
40. Flanders WD, Rothman KJ. Occupational risk of laryngeal cancer. *Am J Public Health* 1982; **72**: 369–372.
41. Morris Brown L, Mason TJ et al. Occupational risk factors for laryngeal cancer on the Texas Gulf Coast. *Cancer Res* 1988; **48**: 1960–1964.
42. Nikiforov Y, Gnepp DR. Pediatric thyroid carcinoma after the Chernobyl disaster: pathomorphologic study of 84 cases (1991–1992) from the Republic of Belarus. *Cancer* 1994; **74**: 748–766.
43. Martland HS. Occurrence of malignancy in radioactive persons; a general review of data gathered in the study of radium dial painters, with special reference to the occurrence of osteogenic sarcoma and the inter-relationship of certain blood diseases. *Am J Cancer* 1931; **15**: 2435–2516.
44. Patel SG, See ACH, Rhys Evans PH et al. Radiation induced sarcomas of the head and neck. *Head Neck* 1999; **7**: 346–353.
45. Mark RJ, Bailet JW, Poen J et al. Post irradiation sarcoma of the head and neck. *Cancer* 1993; **72**: 887–893.
46. Hall P. Radiation-induced thyroid cancer. *Med Oncol Tumor Pharmacother* 1992; **9**: 183–184.
47. van Kaick G, Wesch H, Luhrs H et al. Neoplastic diseases induced by chronic alpha-irradiation – epidemiological, biophysical and clinical results of the German Thorotrast Study. *J Radiat Res (Tokyo)* 1991; **32**: 20–33.
48. Wake M. The urban/rural divide in head and neck cancer: the effect of atmospheric pollution. *Clin Otolaryngology*. 1993; **18**: 298–302.
49. O'Brien PH, Carlson R, Steubner EA. Distant metastases in epidermoid cell carcinoma of the head and neck. *Cancer* 1927; **304**: 1071.
50. Forssell G. Radiotherapy of malignant tumours in Sweden. *Br J Radiol* 1930; **3**: 198–234.
51. Harrison DFN. Multimodal treatment and new approaches to therapy. In: Rhys Evans PH, Robin PE, Fielding JWL (eds) *Head and Neck Cancer.* Tunbridge Wells: Castle House Publications, 1983; 233–246.
52. Fletcher GH. Combination of irradiation and surgery. In: Fletcher GH (ed.) *Textbook of Radiotherapy.* 3rd edn. Philadelphia: Lea and Febiger, 1980; 219–224.
53. McGregor IA. In: *Fundamental Techniques of Plastic Surgery.* 5th edn. Edinburgh: Churchill Livingstone, 1972.
54. Bakamjian VY. A two-stage method for pharyngoesophageal reconstruction with a primary pectoral skin flap. *Plast Reconstr Surg* 1965; **36**: 173–.
55. Ariyan S. The pectoralis major myocutaneous flap. A versatile flap for reconstruction in the head and neck. *Plast Reconstr Surg* 1979; **63**: 73.
56. Hewitt HB, Blake ER. The growth of transplanted murien tumours in pre-irradiated sites. *Br J Cancer* 1968; **22**: 808–824.
57. Calman KA. Policy Framework for Comissioning Cancer Services. *Department of Health Publication.* 1995.
58. British Association of Head and Neck Oncologists. Provision and quality assurance for head and neck care in the United Kingdom. 1998.
59. Ladas G, Rhys Evans PH, Goldstraw P. Anterior cervical transsternal approach for the resection of benign tumours of the thoracic inlet. *Ann Thorac Surg* 1999; **67**: 785–789.
60. Mihashi S, Jako GJ, Incze J. Laser surgery in otolaryngology: interaction of CO_2 laser and soft tissues. *Ann NY Acad Sci* 1976; **267**: 263–294.
61. Steiner W. Experience in endoscopic laser surgery of malignant tumours of the upper aero-digestive tract. *Adv Otorhinolaryngol* 1988; **39**: 135–144.
62. Tappenier H, Jesionek A. Therapeutische Versuche mit Fluoreszierenden Stoffe. *Munchen Med Wochschr* 1903; **1**: 2042–2044.
63. Diamond I, Granelli S, McDonagh AF et al. Photodynamic therapy of malignant tumours. *Lancet* 1972; **2**: 1175–1177.
64. Cornes PGS, Rhys Evans PH, Cox HJ et al. Salvage treatment for inoperable neck nodes in head and neck cancer using combined irridium 192 brachytherapy and surgical reconstruction. *Br J Surg* 1996; **83**: 1620–1622.
65. Pracy JP, Rhys Evans PH, Henk JM, Archer DJ. Treatment of recurrent nasopharyngeal carcinoma by combined surgery and brachytherapy. *Proceedings of the British Association of Head and Neck Oncologists Meeting,* London 1999.
66. Rhys Evans PH, Harmer CL. Head, neck and thyroid cancer. In: Gore M, Russell D (eds) *Cancer in Primary Care.* Oxford: Isis Medical Media, 2002 (in press).

2 Molecular biology

Jonathan C Irish, Suzanne Kamel-Reid, Patrick J Gullane, Pornchai O-charoenrat and Paul Q Montgomery

Introduction

Advances in the treatment of head and neck cancer in the last 15 years have been largely limited to those that impact on patient morbidity and quality of life, meanwhile, patient mortality statistics remain static. The application of new technologies in molecular biology and immunology may provide the head and neck oncologist with the tools to enhance patient survival.

To the clinician there appears to be an obvious qualitative 'black and white' difference between the patient with a cancer and one without. However, at the molecular level, the mechanisms which underlie the genesis of malignant or normal tissue are so intimately related that reported molecular differences are often found to be quantitative rather than qualitative. In addition, the significance of these differences is often uncertain in the complex chain of molecular events leading to cancer.

The focus of this chapter is to provide a brief simplified description of the basic science of molecular biology for the head and neck clinician and to outline potential applications and limitations of our current knowledge. A glossary is included for the clinician who is unfamiliar with the terminology of molecular biology.

DNA, genes and jargon

DNA

The DNA molecule is a replicating chemical information system, based on a quaternary code, whose essential property is to generate more DNA in an ever-changing environment.

The information is formatted as a sequence of any of four flat nitrogen-based molecules (the nucleotide bases adenine (A), thymine (T), cytosine (C), guanine (G)) with the sequence being held on a sugar-phosphate backbone. Every strand of DNA is attached to a 'complementary' DNA strand with each of the four bases being able to 'bond' only with its complement: A with T and C with G. The complementary nature of these nucleic acids is critical for replication.

It is worth discussing the nature of the 'bonds' between these bases, as this is very significant with respect to how DNA is studied. They are 'hydrogen' bonds; the same bonds that stick water molecules to each other. When water is heated to boiling point these bonds break and the water molecules separate from each other. The same process occurs with double-stranded DNA; heating (or bathing in an alkali environment) denatures or 'melts' these bonds resulting in two separate complementary single DNA strands. The effect of cooling reverses this process allowing the separated complementary DNA strands to line up and stick to each other, a process called annealing or hybridization or renaturing.

The 'central dogma'

The central dogma of molecular biology is that DNA makes RNA makes proteins and more specifically, DNA is transcribed to messenger RNA which is then translated into protein.

Genes

A gene is a stretch of DNA that codes for a protein. In the total human genetic complement, the genome, there are approximately 35 000 genes. Less than 5% of the genome appears to code proteins and regulatory sequences with the rest having no known function. Within a gene there are some sequences that code for amino acids (exons) and some sequences that do not (introns). In gene transcription both exon and intron sequences are transcribed to mRNA but the introns are subsequently excised.

Gene regulation

As cancer may be viewed as the deregulation of the growth control aspects of the genome it is useful to review how gene expression is controlled in the normal situation.

Gene regulation has been extensively studied in bacteria and we describe the function of a gene regulation system called an 'operon' as it demonstrates important regulatory concepts. The operon model described is based on the lactose operon of the bacteria *Escherichia coli*, which is used to produce enzymes to allow the bacteria to metabolize lactose when it is in high concentrations in its environment. It is important to note there are many other regulatory models both in prokaryocytes (e.g. bacteria) and eukaryocytes (e.g. human cells), with the latter being far less well characterized.

Operons

An operon is a sequential cluster of related genes, which are needed to generate a collection of enzymes required for the metabolism or production of a substance. The purpose of this linked production is to produce functional groupings of enzymes at the correct time for the cell to react efficiently to signals in its environment. To aid the efficiency of the cell it is also designed to minimize the production of enzymes when the need for them is absent.

Operon structure and function

At the start of an operon is a promoter region. It is at this site where the enzyme RNA polymerase attaches to the DNA so that it can transcribe the gene-bearing area into mRNA. The next segment of the sequence is called the operator region. This is the key controlling area as it is capable of binding a protein called the repressor. If the repressor binds to the operator region it stops the enzyme RNA polymerase from moving onto the gene-bearing area and so stopping transcription. If the operator site is unoccupied then the RNA polymerase transcribes the genes (Figure 2.1).

The repressor has a 'signal' receptor binding site and an 'operator' binding site. If the signal receptor site is occupied by the correct chemical signal then the operator binding site is distorted in such a manner as to prevent the repressor from binding to the operator, thus, transcription begins. If the signal receptor site is unoccupied then the binding site is capable of attaching to the operator so transcription is prevented.

It can be seen that an unregulated operon can occur if the repressor fails to bind to the operator. This may be due to:

1. A mutation in the repressor gene code so that repressor protein does not bind to the promoter region;
2. A mutation in the promoter region so that normal repressor protein cannot bind to it;
3. Mutations of the operon genes, and thus the gene products, which may affect the regulatory control of the operon by altering the signal to the repressor.

Thus, an unregulated cell growth operon could reveal both qualitative and quantitative differences, for example a mutant repressor protein and/or overexpression of normal growth enzymes.

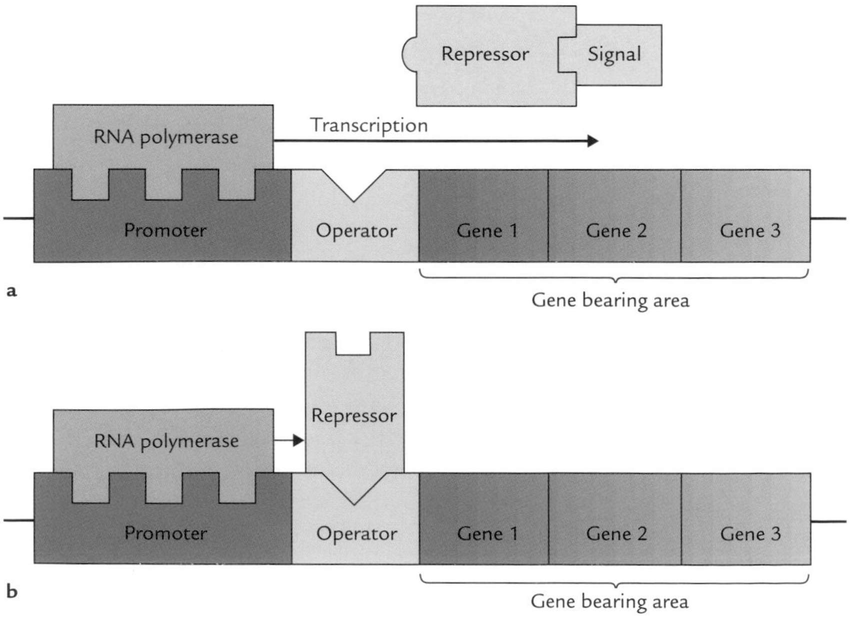

Figure 2.1 Operon structure and function. (a) The active state with transcription being possible due to the presence of the signal binding to the repressor. (b) The inactive state with transcription not being possible due to the absence of signal.

The conceptual basis of the molecular biology of cancer

Proto-oncogenes and oncogenes

Proto-oncogenes

Proto-oncogenes are normal cellular genes that are thought to be crucially involved in normal growth regulation and cell differentiation.[1] The signals for mitogenic stimulation of cells may come from different sources including growth factors, growth factor receptors, cytoplasmic signal transduction proteins and nuclear proteins (Figure 2.2).[2] Proto-oncogenes that function at each step of this pathway have been discovered and thus are thought to play an important role in a regulatory network that extends from the cell surface into the cell nucleus. When mutated or deregulated these genes attain the capacity to destabilize normal cell growth and regulation and, in this state, are referred to as oncogenes.[3]

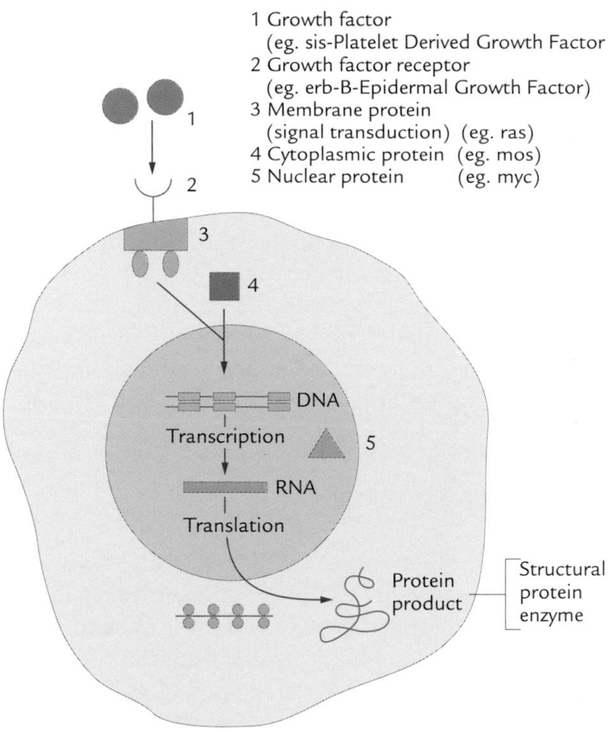

Figure 2.2 Signals of mitogenic stimulation of cells come from growth factors, with the information passed to growth factor receptors, signal transduction proteins and nuclear proteins. Proto-oncogene products function at each step of the regulatory pathway. Dysregulation results when these genes and their protein products are altered.

Oncogenes

The resultant oncogene is a gene that can contribute to malignant transformation of cells and cause tumours in animals and humans.[3] The protein product that they direct to be synthesized by the cell mediates the effect of oncogenes. The differences between the oncogene-directed protein product and that which would have been formed by the normal cellular gene can be qualitative (e.g. novel proteins secondary to mutations in the gene sequence) or quantitative (e.g. too many copies of a normal protein product).[3]

Oncogene activation

Oncogene activation is known to occur in at least four ways (Figure 2.3).

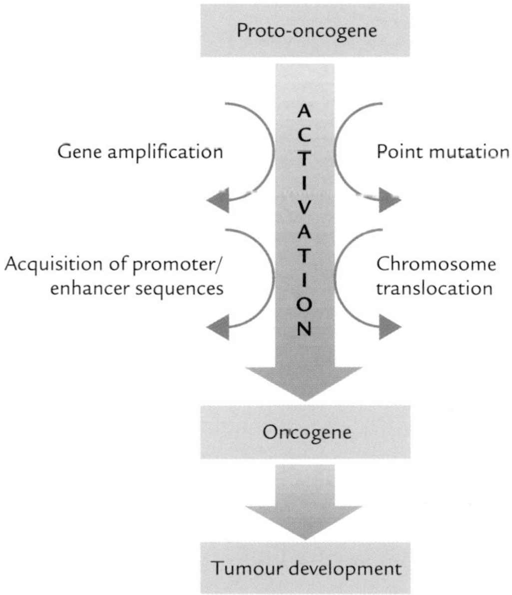

Figure 2.3 Mechanisms of proto-oncogene to oncogene activation.

1. Gene acquisition of a novel transcriptional promoter. This results in gene overexpression with resultant increased gene product.
2. Chromosome translocation with resultant deregulation of a proto-oncogene close to the chromosomal breakpoints. An example of this is the Philadelphia chromosome commonly found in chronic myelogenous leukaemia (CML). In CML, the *c-abl* proto-oncogene on chromosome 9 is moved (translocated) to a region on chromosome 22 called the breakpoint cluster region (*bcr*) as a result of a reciprocal chromosomal movement. The resultant *bcr-abl* combination codes for a novel protein product resulting in unregulated stimulation to growth and thus chronic myelogenous leukaemia.
3. Gene amplification due to increased gene copy number. This process, called gene amplification, has been implicated in playing a causative role in a number of malignancies. For example, amplification of the N-*Myc* proto-oncogene occurs in approximately 40% of human neuroblastomas.[4]

4. Point mutation in the gene resulting in an altered protein product. An oncogene may be formed by a single nucleotide base-pair substitution in a proto-oncogene, which can result in the production of a mutant protein with loss of normal cell regulation. Analysis of a series of human pancreas tumour biopsies demonstrated a 95% incidence of K-*ras*-2 codon 12 mutations.[5] Other members of the *ras* gene family, such as H-*Ras* and N-*ras*, have been implicated in a wide range of human malignancies. Mutagenic agents such as the components of tobacco smoke, alcohol and radiation appear to play an important role.

Tumour suppressor genes

There is another class of genes, called tumour suppressor genes, whose expression inhibits malignant transformation of cells. Mutation of such genes may lead to neoplastic transformation. Tumour suppressor genes were first recognized in the aetiology of the inherited forms of retinoblastomas and Wilm's tumours. It is now evident that mutation in the p53 tumour suppressor gene occurs in a wide variety of human cancers including lung, bone, colon, mammary and various haematological neoplasms.[6] Li-Fraumeni families, who have a germ line p53 mutation, can develop cancer at any of these sites emphasizing the role of p53 as the 'guardian of the genome'.

The multistage models of malignancy

Human cancers develop through a process involving several stages. The classical model is a successive passage of the cell through the three stages of initiation, promotion and progression.[7]

Tumour initiation

A rapid, irreversible process that presumably results from genetic changes within the cell as a result of the cell's interaction with a carcinogenic agent. Initiated cells may be thought of as being primed for the development of malignancy although they themselves do not express this neoplastic potential unless they undergo promotion.

Tumour promotion

Unlike initiation, the process of promotion is reversible with a prolonged latency period. Initiated cells develop into viable neoplastic lesions under the stimulus of the promoting agent. While the generation of a tumour cell appears to be a multistep event, the activation of a single oncogene by the various mechanisms described earlier is a single discrete event. This apparent discrepancy may be explained by the fact that activation of single oncogenes may only be one facet of a complex process leading to the eventual development of a fully malignant cell.

Tumour progression

Tumour progression is that characteristic of already established malignant tumours to successively acquire more aggressive grades of malignancy. These acquired qualities include such properties as propensity to tumour metastasis and development of radiation and chemotherapy resistance. Studies from in vitro models, experimental animals and studies of human cancer have strongly supported the concept that several molecular events must occur during carcinogenesis.

Investigational techniques in molecular biology

Southern blot

Southern blot technique is the analysis and comparison of the electrophoretic patterns of DNA fragments. It involves extracting DNA from a tumour sample and enzymatically digesting it into small fragments (Figure 2.4). Electrophoresis results in a size fractionation of the DNA fragments, with the larger segments remaining close to the well of origin and the smaller segments travelling farther down the gel. The DNA is then transferred, or blotted, onto nylon or other synthetic membrane. The membrane

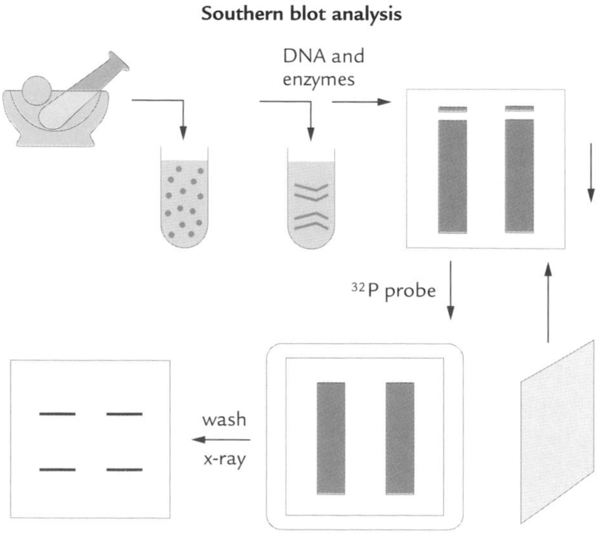

Figure 2.4 Steps involved in Southern blotting.

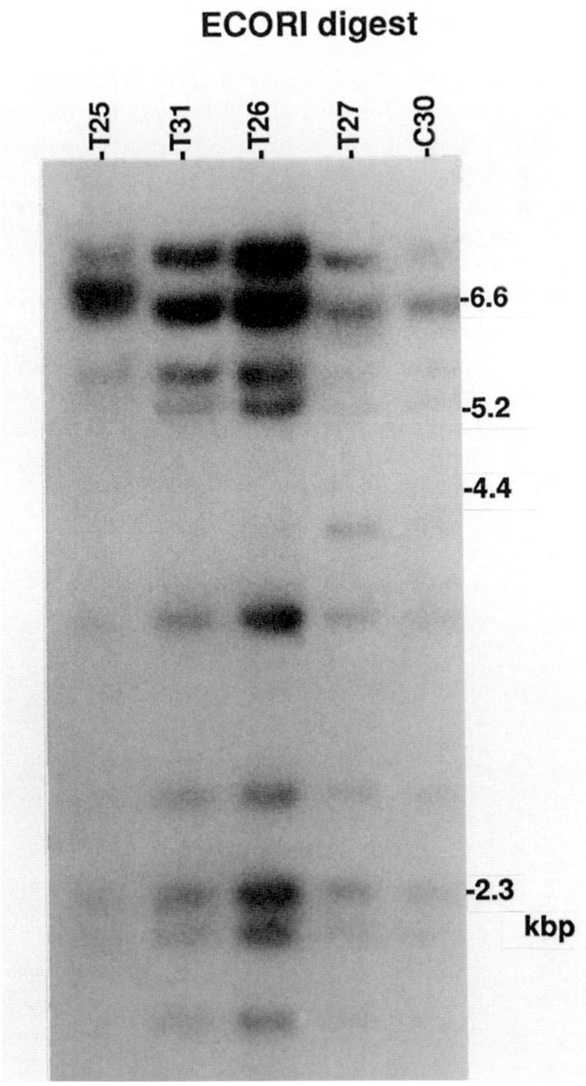

Figure 2.5 Southern blot of tumour DNA (T25, T31, T26, T27) and control DNA (C30). The DNA has been enzymatically digested resulting in characteristic DNA 'fingerprints' or restriction fragment length polymorphisms (RFLPs). Tumour T26 showed increased uptake of the radioactive probe (*erb*-B) compared to control DNA suggesting *erb*-B amplification.

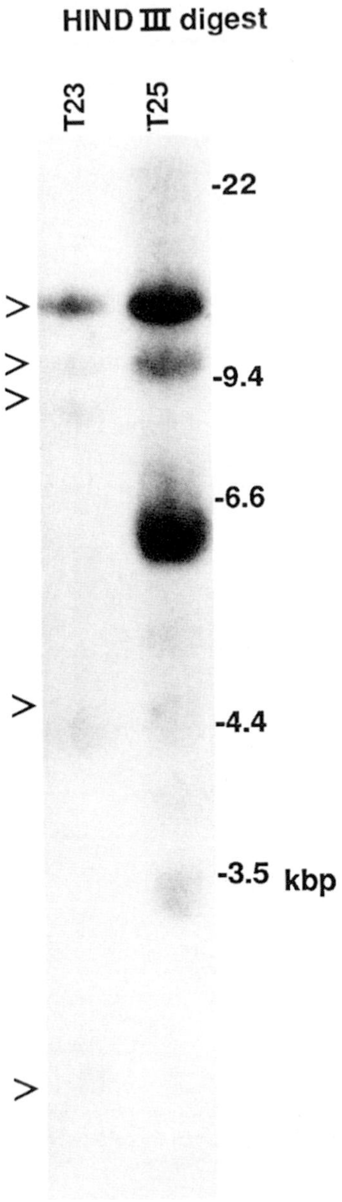

Figure 2.6 Southern blot of tumour DNA (T23, T25). In this case, the arrows mark the site of expected 'fingerprints' or RFLPs. Tumour T25 demonstrates alteration of the DNA RFLP pattern (a new band at 6.6 kbp) indicating gene deletion or point mutation.

can then be exposed ('hybridized') to radioactively labelled probes that are short DNA strands complementary to the known gene of interest. Radiolabelled probe, which has bound to homologous DNA sequence on the membrane, will result in a dark band on the X-ray film (Figure 2.5).

Those tumours with an increased gene DNA copy number (gene amplification) will take up more radioactively labelled probe and result in a more intense signal on the radiographic film. In addition to gene amplification the Southern blot technique allows tumours to be analysed for alterations in DNA structure. A gross deletion of a gene or point mutation at a restriction enzyme site will produce altered banding patterns (restriction fragment length polymorphisms; RFLPs) when tumour DNA is compared with normal DNA (Figure 2.6).

Northern blot

The northern blot technique is the analysis and comparison of the electrophoretic patterns of RNA fragments. It involves an analogous process to the Southern blot except that instead of tumour DNA being extracted and analysed, RNA is analysed. Whereas Southern blotting can yield information about the genomic structure and the number of gene copies, northern blotting allows the expression levels of a gene to be analysed.

Western blot

The western blot technique is the analysis and comparison of the electrophoretic patterns of proteins. It involves the extraction of tissue protein and electrophoresis on polyacrylamide gels. Protein is then transferred onto a membrane and treated with a blocking solution. Instead of hybridization to a complementary DNA probe as in Southern or northern blot techniques the western blot uses labelled antibody to detect the protein of interest.

Polymerase chain reaction

The polymerase chain reaction (PCR) technique creates multiple copies of a DNA segment, that is amplified biochemically from a very small quantity of DNA (Figure 2.7). The amplification involves a series of biochemical reactions consisting of three phases: denaturation, annealing and extension. The reaction consists of the DNA sample to be amplified (target), a thermostable enzyme (Taq polymerase) and two (forward and reverse) primers, which are small segments (usually 10–20 oligonucleotides long) of DNA complementary to each end of the target DNA fragment that is to be amplified. The mixture is heated to denature the DNA double-strand and then actively cooled to allow the two primers to

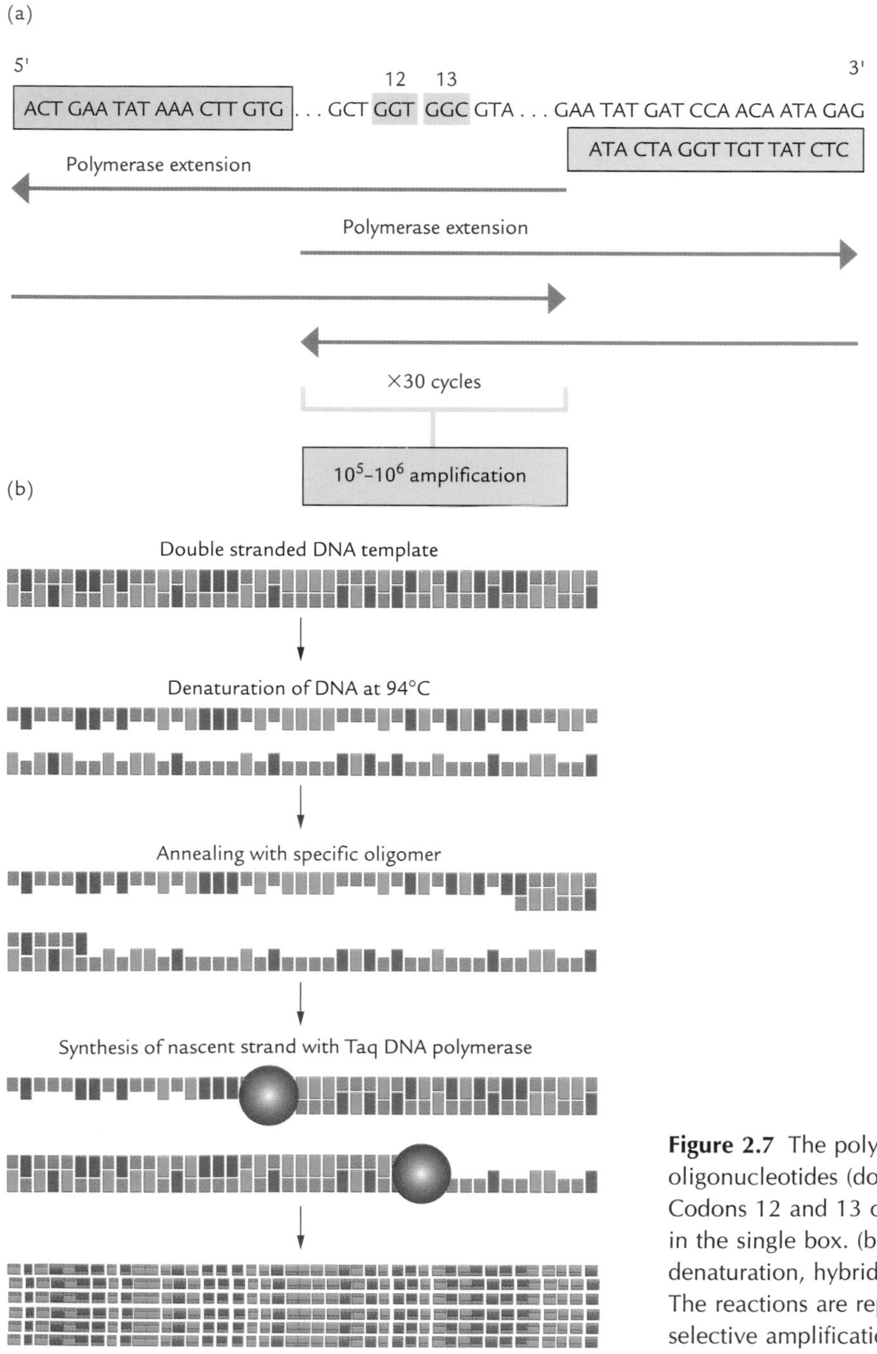

Figure 2.7 The polymerase chain reaction. (a) Two oligonucleotides (double box) flank a target gene segment. Codons 12 and 13 of the target gene segment are shown in the single box. (b) PCR consists of repeated denaturation, hybridization and polymerase extension. The reactions are repeated 25–30 times resulting in selective amplification of the desired gene segment.

anneal to the now single-stranded DNA target template. The primers should only anneal to the homologous DNA sequences flanking the target template. The forward and reverse primers then act as start sites for synthesis of a new DNA strand by Taq polymerase. With each cycle of denaturation, annealing and extension the amount of target DNA between the two primers is doubled. The products of one cycle serve as templates for the next cycle so that the PCR product accumulates exponentially. Theoretically, therefore, after 30 PCR cycles 2^{30} copies of target DNA are created allowing for visualization and subsequent analysis (Figure 2.8).

Quantitative 'real time' PCR analysis

Until recently it has been difficult to obtain reproducible quantitative PCR results. Quantitation necessitated the use of serial dilutions and the analysis of multiple replicates; these steps introduce variability and increase the potential for contamination. Recently, new technology has been developed that allows the quantitation of PCR products through the measurement of fluorescence using laser-based technology (Figure 2.9).

During PCR, a fluorogenic probe, consisting of an oligonucleotide with both a reporter and a quencher dye attached, anneals specifically between the forward and reverse primers in the region of interest. Owing to the 5' to 3' exonuclease activity of Taq polymerase, as it copies the DNA the reporter dye is cleaved from the quencher dye, and a sequence-specific signal is generated. With each cycle, additional reporter dye molecules are cleaved from their respective probes. To quantitate the amount of specific product the fluorescence intensity is measured during the PCR and compared to a standard curve that will determine absolute or relative amount of product generated. This technology has been used for many purposes, including the measurement and monitoring of disease specific transcripts.[8]

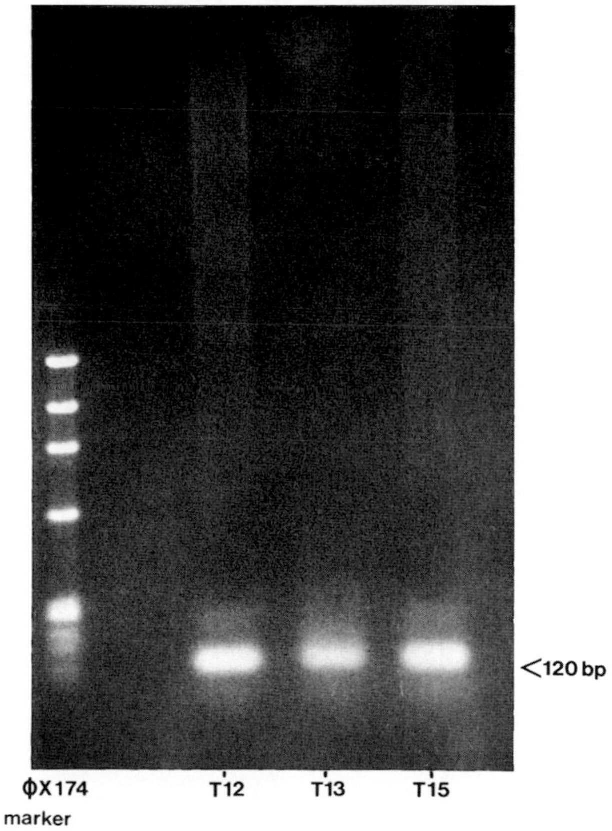

Figure 2.8 Stained gel of PCR-amplified products from three head and neck tumour specimens (T12, T13, T15). A 120-bp target of the *ras* gene from three head and neck tumours was amplified 10^6 times such that the product can be seen with the naked eye on this stained agarose gel. The PCR technique has allowed amplification of genetic segments of interest for further study.

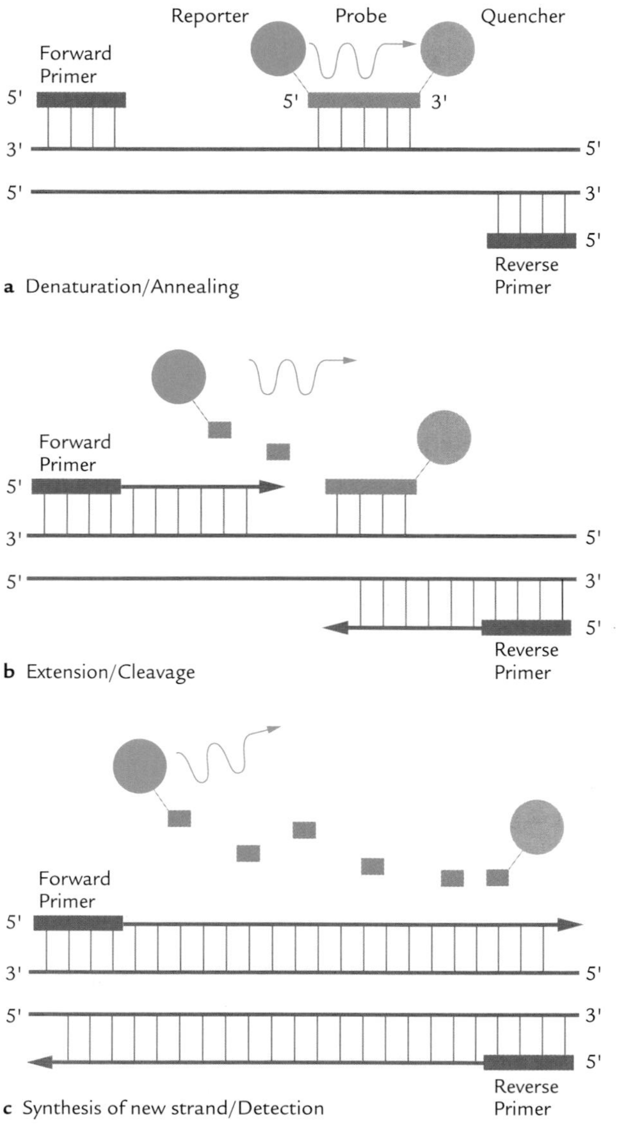

Figure 2.9 'Real time' PCR analysis. Schematic of sequence-specific annealing and 5'–3' exonuclease-based cleavage of the fluorescent dye-labelled probe.

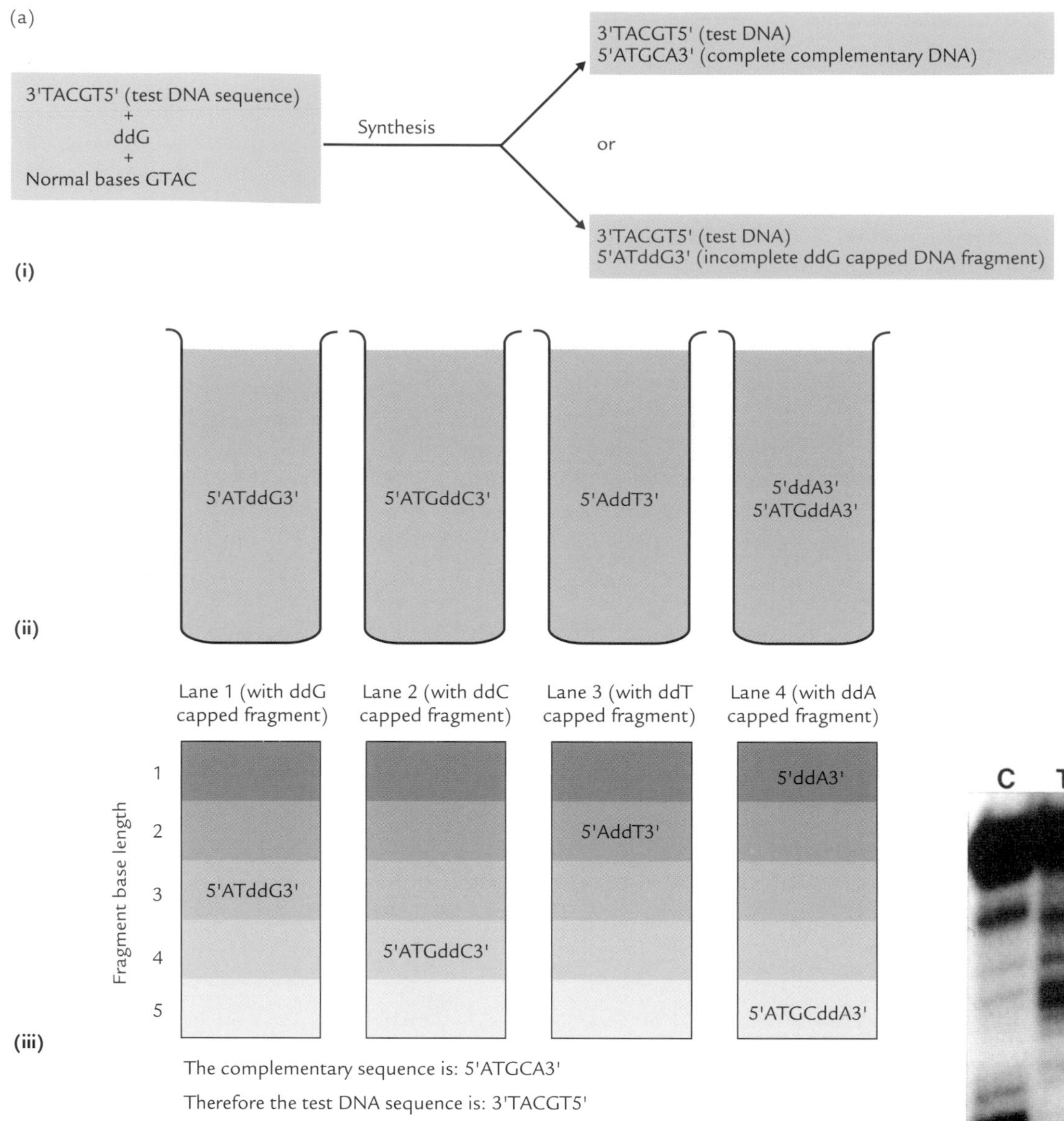

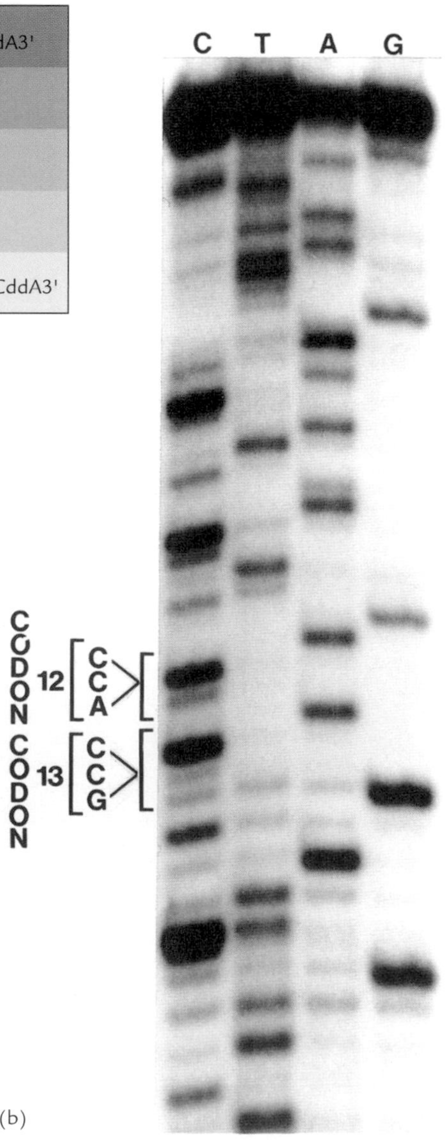

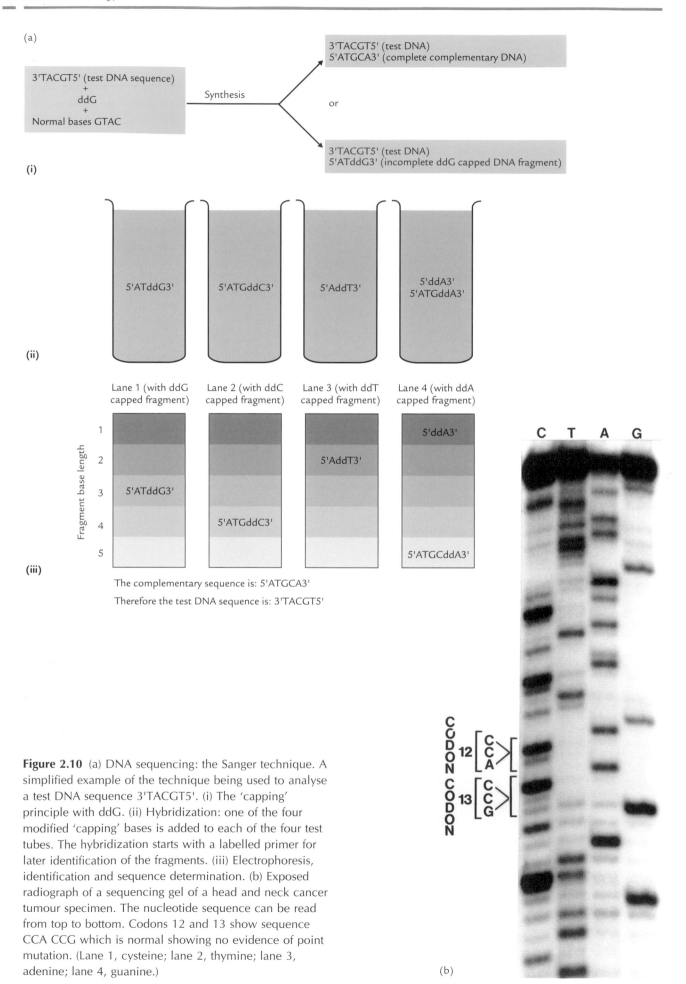

Figure 2.10 (a) DNA sequencing: the Sanger technique. A simplified example of the technique being used to analyse a test DNA sequence 3'TACGT5'. (i) The 'capping' principle with ddG. (ii) Hybridization: one of the four modified 'capping' bases is added to each of the four test tubes. The hybridization starts with a labelled primer for later identification of the fragments. (iii) Electrophoresis, identification and sequence determination. (b) Exposed radiograph of a sequencing gel of a head and neck cancer tumour specimen. The nucleotide sequence can be read from top to bottom. Codons 12 and 13 show sequence CCA CCG which is normal showing no evidence of point mutation. (Lane 1, cysteine; lane 2, thymine; lane 3, adenine; lane 4, guanine.)

DNA sequencing

The order of bases in a DNA sequence is of great value as it is the 'anatomy' of the genetic material and helps in understanding its 'physiology'. DNA sequencing using the Sanger and the Maxam–Gilbert sequencing techniques can determine the precise order of the nucleotide bases in a DNA strand.

The Sanger technique

This elegant technique is founded on the use of modified bases (dideoxynucleotides; ddN), which terminates further base additions to a DNA sequence. A pure sample of single stranded DNA of unknown base sequence is separated into four test tubes. Into each sample is added the ingredients required to generate a complementary DNA chain and small quantities of a single type of the modified bases that is incapable of allowing the polymerizing or hybridizing process to continue, thus 'capping' the sequence at that complementary base point. Some of the modified bases successfully compete with the normal bases and manage to be incorporated at various complementary points on the sequence. This results in each test tube containing fragments of various lengths of complementary DNA terminated with the modified base that was added. These samples are individually electrophoresed, identified (each fragment starts with a labelled primer) and lined up next to each other; then the sequence of the original strand can be determined (Figure 2.10) This technique can also be used to compare the bands produced from normal and tumour DNA and to allow determination of gene sequence and identification of point mutations (Figure 2.11).

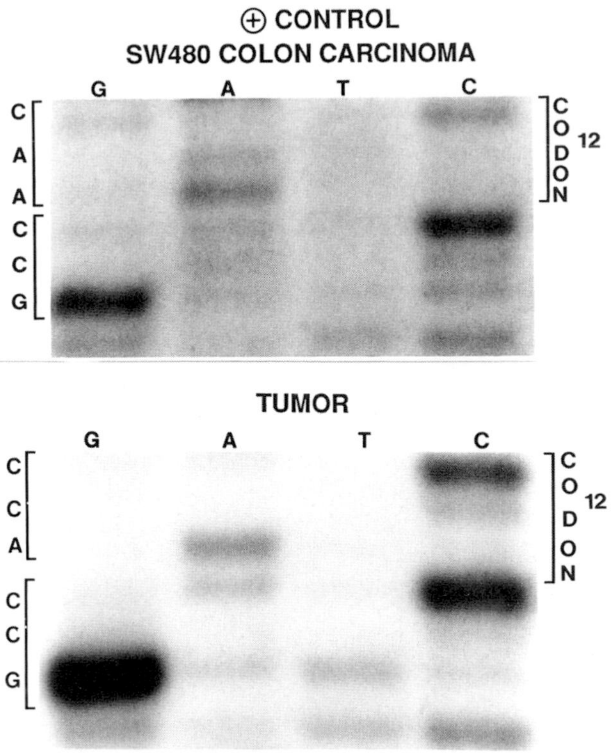

Figure 2.11 Close-up sequencing gel radiograph of codons 12 and 13 in a colon carcinoma (SW480, top) known to demonstrate a CAA nucleotide sequence at codon 12 instead of the normal CCA sequence of a head and neck tumour (T15, below). The SW480 cell line has a point mutation in codon 12 of the *ras* oncogene.

Fluorescence in situ hybridization

Cytogenetic analysis of head and neck tumours has improved dramatically in the past decade due to fluorescence in situ hybridization (FISH) technology with techniques such as colour karyotyping (multiplex FISH; M-FISH[9] and spectral karyotyping; SKY[10]) and comparative genomic hybridization (CGH).[11]

The traditional chromosomal banding techniques cannot define complex karyotypes with multiple marker chromosomes as well as translocations involving regions that are cytogenetically similar by G-banding. The advent of multicolour FISH techniques, known as M-FISH and SKY, using five fluorochromes allow the detection of several targets simultaneously. Sophisticated computer analysis is required to differentiate the colours and to identify the origin of every chromosome in a hybridized metaphase cell. CGH allows screening of the whole tumour genome for DNA sequence gains or losses in a single experiment. It is based on simultaneous in situ hybridization of equal amounts of differentially labelled tumour DNA and normal DNA to a normal metaphase chromosome preparation. Differences in the fluorescence ratio between the tumour and reference DNA implicate regions of abnormal DNA content in the tumour sample. Both multicolour karyotyping and CGH have limitations: neither can detect chromosomal inversions or point mutations, CGH cannot detect balanced chromosomal translocations and aberrations present in low frequency, and multicolour karyotyping cannot detect subtle deletions and duplications.

Microarray analysis

Traditional differential gene expression techniques examine single genes, by northern blot, or a limited number of genes through the use of nylon membrane-based 'slot blot' techniques. More recently, PCR-based methodologies, including reverse transcriptase (RT)-PCR and differential display, have been established that allow for the simultaneous evaluation of numerous genes under a variety of experimental conditions. While valuable, these methods are incapable of evaluating global gene expression in a comprehensive manner. Recent technological advances have addressed the limitations of these approaches and have revolutionized differential gene expression profiling. The availability of libraries of expressed sequence tagged (EST) cDNA, approaching the full complement of human genes, and the ability to immobilize thousands of these ESTs on solid supports has facilitated the development of microarrays for differential expression studies. There is increasing interest in the application of microarray analysis for gene expression profiling in human cancers to evaluate expression differences between normal and tumour tissue as well as following exposure of tumours to therapeutic agents.[12,13]

Molecular biology of head and neck cancer

Genetic susceptibility

Among genes that activate or eliminate tobacco carcinogens, the null genotypes of the carcinogen-metabolizing genes glutathione-S-transferase (GST)T1 and GSTM1, the GSTP1 (AG or GG) genotype have been shown to represent risk factors for head and neck squamous cell carcinoma (HNSCC) and markers for genetic susceptibility to tobacco-induced carcinogenesis.[14,15] Mutagen sensitivity (a higher rate of spontaneous chromosomal aberrations in lymphoblastoid cells) induced by tobacco-associated cancer mutagen, benzo[a]pyrene diol epoxide is also associated with risk of HNSCC development.[16]

Cytogenetic (chromosomal) changes

The most frequent chromosomal abnormalities in HNSCCs are unbalanced translocations leading to chromosomal deletions affecting 3p13-q24 (in > 60% of tumours), 4p (43%), 5q12-q23 (30%), 8p22-p23 (65%), 9p21-p24 (43%), 10p (39%), 13q12-q24 (30%), 18q22-23 (> 60%), and 21q (52%).[17] Loss of the inactive X and loss (or rearrangement) of Y occur in 70% of tumours from female and male patients respectively. Less common consistent changes found in 30–40% of tumours are gain affecting 3q21-qter, 5p, 7p, 8q, and 11q13-23.[18] Allelic losses at marker loci in specific genomic regions, indicating the inactivation of critical tumour suppressor genes within the regions, have been demonstrated at 3p, 5q, 9p, 11q, 13q, 18q, and 17p.[19,20] A genetic progression model for HNSCC has been postulated[21] with certain genetic events indicated as early (loss of heterozygosity (LOH) at 3p, 9p21, and 17p13), intermediate (11q, 13q11, and 14q), and late (6p, 4q, and 8). The accumulation of genetic events is associated with histopathological progression although there may be a prolonged latency period during which clonal genetic alterations may be present before an invasive phenotype is produced.[22] Some studies have correlated chromosome deletion or mutation with poor clinical outcome (LOH at 2q, 3p, 9p, 11q, 18q)[23] or biological behaviour such as radiation therapy resistance (1p, 3p, 8p 14q).[24] In nasopharyngeal cancer, comparative genomic hybridization (CGH) has identified the most common copy number increases on chromosome arms 12p, 1q, 17q, 11q, and 12q, whereas the most frequent losses were found at 3p, 9p, 13q, 14q, and 11q.[25]

Cellular oncogenes in head and neck cancer

Erb*B receptor proto-oncogenes*

The protein products of the *erb*B proto-oncogenes belong to the transmembrane type I receptor tyrosine kinase family.[26] The *erb*B receptors have four homologous members in the family: the epidermal growth factor receptor (EGFR or *erb*B-1 or HER-1 for human EGF receptor-1), *erb*B-2 (*neu* or HER-2), *erb*B-3 (HER-3) and *erb*B-4 (HER-4). Head and neck tumours analysed for RNA expression, gene amplification and structural alteration of the EGFR gene, *erb*B-1, showed that 13% displayed *erb*B-1 gene amplification and/or gene rearrangement.[27] Overexpression of the *erb*B-1 gene has been observed in 67% of the head and neck tumours studied whereas a stepwise increase of EGFR expression in histologically normal epithelium, premalignant and cancerous lesions has been observed following the histologic progression.[28] Those patients expressing high levels of EGFR or showing EGFR gene amplification had tumours that were clinically more advanced.[29] Although there is no evidence for gene amplification or increased RNA transcript of *erb*B-2 in HNSCC,[30–34] increased *erb*B-2 oncoprotein expression has been noted.[33,35–38] Overexpression of *erb*B-3 and *erb*B-4 mRNA and protein have been found in some HNSCC lines, whereas no gene amplification was detected.[32,33,39,40] In clinical settings, the roles of *erb*B-3 and *erb*B-4 in HNSCC progression are less clear.[34,38,41–45] However, their ability to form heterodimers among the *erb*B family members upon stimulation by their direct ligands, that is heregulins (HRG)-β1 has been shown to enhance the signalling pathways of EGFR or *erb*B-2 and the invasive properties in HNSCC cells.[46,47]

At least six distinct peptides can bind directly to EGFR including EGF, transforming growth factor-alpha (TGF-α), amphiregulin (AR), betacellulin (BTC), heparin-binding-EGF-like growth factor (HB-EGF), and epiregulin. The direct ligands of *erb*B-3 and *erb*B-4 are isoforms of the HRGs, and no exogenous ligand for *erb*B-2 has yet been characterized.[26] In HNSCC, the expression of multiple *erb*B ligands apart from EGF and TGF-α has only recently been described.[48,49] In addition, all *erb*B ligands can interact with each other by a mutual amplification mechanism as well as by autocrine induction.[49] *Erb*B ligand-receptor complex recruits a unique set of signalling proteins activating multiple distinct pathways that elicit specific biological responses associated with carcinogenesis and/or metastasis.[46–48]

Ras *proto-oncogene*

The *ras* family of oncogenes (N-*ras*, H-*ras*, K-*ras*) encode the membrane-associated G-proteins, guanosine triphosphatases (GTPases), that constitutively maintain an activated GTP-bound state and serve as signal transducers for cell surface growth factor receptors. Conflicting results have been reported regarding the importance of the *ras* family in HNSCC. NIH/3T3 transfection assay uncovered activated c-H-*ras-1* proto-oncogenes in two squamous cell carcinoma cell lines established from human oral carcinoma patients.[50] Anderson and Irish found that approximately 15% of oral and oropharyngeal malignancies demonstrate point mutations in the H-*ras* gene at codon 12 while K-*ras* mutations were rare.[29]

Raf *proto-oncogene*

The *raf* oncogene has been shown to be activated from a cell line (SQ2OB) derived from a human laryngeal squamous cell carcinoma.[51] Under in vitro conditions this cell line is resistant to the effects of ionizing radiation. However, demonstration of *raf* oncogene mutations in fresh uncultured head and neck tumour specimens has been variable. The failure to demonstrate *raf* gene alterations in fresh tumour specimens illustrates some of the problems introduced when studying cancer cells under *in vitro* conditions as artefactual changes can occur both during the DNA transfection process and in the milieu of cell culture.

CCND1 (PRAD1)

Transition from the Gl to the S phase (the DNA synthesis phase) and from the G2 to the M phase (the mitosis phase) are critical control points in the cycle of a growing cell. A group of proteins called cyclic-AMP-dependent protein kinases (cdks) participate in the regulation of these transitions. These cdks form complexes with proteins called cyclins, including cyclin D1. The *CCND1* gene that encodes the cyclin D1 protein is located on chromosome 11q13, and this locus is amplified in 20–52% of HNSCC. Overproduction of cyclin Dl may push a tumour cell through the G1/S transition, resulting in uncontrolled cell division and perpetuation of other genetic alterations. *CCND1* gene amplification and overexpression have been shown in HNSCC and premalignancy[52–54] and correlated with poor outcome.[55,56]

EMS1

The *EMS1* oncogene is located in the same region as the *CCND1* gene on chromosome 11q13. *EMS1* encodes a cytoskeletal protein homologous to the avian F actin-binding protein (cortactin), which is involved in regulating the interactions between components in the adherens junctions. *EMS1* amplification in tumours results in overexpression of cortactin leading to a redistribution of cortactin from the cytoplasm into cell-matrix contact sites. This might affect the functioning of cytoskeleton and cell-adhesion structures and contribute to the invasive behaviour of tumour cells. In HNSCC, *EMS1* amplification occurs in 20% and predicts early recurrence and reduced survival independent of other known risk factors.[57]

MPP11

Genetic high-copy amplification of the 7q22–31 genomic region has been recognized as an important event in the progression of HNSCC.[58] A novel human candidate oncogene, *MPP11*, encoding a phosphoantigen with a regulatory role in the mitotic phase of the cell cycle, has been mapped to the critical region of 7q22–31.1.[59] Increased copy number of *MPP11* and overexpression in the majority of primary HNSCC tissues and cell lines examined suggest that this gene is activated during malignant progression and may play an oncogenic role in HNSCC.

Tumour suppressor genes in head and neck cancer

p16

The most commonly deleted chromosome site in HNSCC is located at 9p21–p24, which is the locus for the *CDKN2/MTS1/INK4A* tumour suppressor gene.[20] The $p16^{INK4A}$ gene product is an inhibitor of the cyclin/cyclin-dependent kinase complex and inactivation of the *INK4A* gene leading to absence of the p16 protein is found in 80% of HNSCC.[60] The $p16^{INK4A}$ gene is proposed as the earliest known tumour suppressor gene to be inactivated in HNSCC, whereas deregulation of p53 and cyclin D1 occurs later.[21] Although only 10–15% of HNSCCs demonstrate point mutation at the p16 gene,[61] frequent homozygous deletion in this region[62] and transcriptional silencing through promoter methylation[60] are major inactivation mechanisms in these tumours. Recently, a significant relationship between loss of $p16^{INK4A}$ expression and an adverse disease outcome in HNSCC has been shown.[56]

p53

Loss of 17p13 occurs in up to 60% of invasive SCCs and is the locus of the p53 tumour suppressor gene.[63] Alterations of the p53 gene by allelic losses, point mutations, deletion, or inactivation disrupt its role as a guardian of the genome by impairing the cell's ability to repair and undergo apoptosis in response to DNA damage and thus leads to genomic instability. An overall p53 mutation incidence of 40–50% has been reported in a study of invasive tumours studied by direct sequencing of exons 5 through 8.[64] A higher incidence of p53 mutation has been found in the tumours of smokers and drinkers than in the tumours of patients who developed HNSCC without exposure to these agents.[65] It would appear that p53 gene mutation could be an early event in HNSCC carcinogenesis as it has been observed in premalignant lesions.[63] In addition, an increasing pattern of p53 alterations has been demonstrated in premalignant lesions following the histologic progression.[66] Overexpression of p53 in tumour-distant epithelia of HNSCC patients has been reported to correlate with an increased incidence of second primary tumour.[67] The findings of p53 mutations in histologically negative margins of completely resected tumours and the distinct p53 genotypes in synchronous primary tumours suggest that p53 can be used as a marker for molecular staging and fingerprinting in HNSCC.[64]

ING1

LOH at the chromosomal 13q33-34 region occurs in 68% of HNSCC,[68] where the *ING1* tumour suppressor gene is located. Inhibition of *ING1* expression promotes the transformation of epithelial cells and protects the cells from apoptosis. A considerable subset of HNSCCs has been shown to harbour inactivating mutations in the *ING1* gene accompanied by selective loss of another allele.[69] Recent evidence suggests that the *ING1* gene mutation may be restricted to only HNSCC although the clinical significance of this novel tumour suppressor gene is still largely unknown.

FHIT

The *FHIT* (fragile histidine triad) gene, located at 3p14, contains FRA3B, the most common fragile site in humans, and is frequently the target of allelic loss, homozygous deletions, and genetic rearrangement in many human tumour types. Alterations of *FHIT*, such as homozygous deletions of exons at the genomic level, insertions of intronic sequence and aberrant transcripts at the mRNA level, and lack of detectable protein can be found in up to 66–68% of patients with HNSCC[70,71] and the loss of *FHIT* has recently been shown to be an independent adverse prognostic factor for disease-free survival in oral tongue cancers.[71] Overexpression of the *FHIT* gene has been shown to induce cell apoptosis and altered cell cycle processes although the underlying mechanism is still not well understood.[72]

Evidence suggests that several additional putative tumour suppressor genes may reside at chromosomes 3p, 6p, 8p, 9p, 13q21, and 18q.[20,21,73–75] For example, there are at least two candidate tumour suppressor genes at 9p21-22 in addition to the p15/p16/p19 genes.[76] Further study is required to identify new markers and to find the possible candidate genes within the consistently lost regions.

Diagnostic and therapeutic applications of molecular biology

As discussed previously cellular oncogenes are cancer-causing genes that are formed when the function of a normal cellular gene is altered in some way. Like all genes the protein product that they code for mediates their effect. These proteins are usually, if not always, involved in signal transduction, which is how growth regulatory signals from outside the cell are directed to the nucleus of the cell. The differences between the oncogene-directed protein product and that, which would have been formed by the normal cellular gene, can be qualitative or quantitative. Activated oncogenes may differ substantively from the normal cellular gene so that its expression results in a truly novel protein specific only to the transformed cell. Alternatively, deregulation may result in a quantitative change in the levels of the gene product formed. In the second case, the protein product is not unique to the cancer cell, which limits the diagnostic and therapeutic impact of these tumour markers.

Diagnostic applications

Indentification of premalignant lesions at risk of progression

Identifying patients with lesions at risk of transformation or progression is important so that they can limit the exposure to risk factors and can be given more aggressive treatment strategies such as chemoprevention. Increased polysomies, defined as the presence of three or more copies of the chromosome, of chromosomes 7 and 17 were associated with progression from normal epithelium to dysplastic mucosae and with risk of development of oral cancer.[77] Using the technique of microsatellite assay, which provides information about the frequency of allelic imbalance (AI) at polymorphic markers within chromosomal regions that harbour the tumour suppressor genes, Mao et al[78] demonstrated that the presence of AI at 3p and 9p can identify patients with dysplastic lesions at risk of progression. Further studies incorporating markers at additional chromosomal arms revealed that patients with dysplastic lesions with AI at two or more of the key chromosomal loci have a 75% chance of developing an upper aerodigestive tract tumour in 5 years.[79] Identical allelic losses at 9p21, 11q13, 17p13, 3p, and 13q21 were identified in histologically benign mucosal specimens and cervical nodal metastases of patients with unknown primary HNSCC, suggesting the foci of clonal precancerous cells within these sites presumed to harbour the primary tumour.[80]

Cancer detection

Failure to diagnose HNSCC in its earliest stages is the most important factor contributing to the poor treatment outcome. Early detection is also crucial to effective surveillance after treatment of HNSCC. Head and neck cancers are among the most antigenic tumours and several potential tumour markers for HNSCC have been suggested such as squamous cell carcinoma antigen (SCCAg)[81] and cytokeratin fragment 19 (CYFRA 21-1).[82] High urinary levels of TGF-α have been detected in patients with advanced head and neck cancer and preliminary findings indicate that the quantity of marker detected is proportional to the clinical extent of the malignancy.[83] Standard cytological method has been shown to have potential value for the detection of second primary tumours in the oesophagus of head and neck cancer patients.[84] However, the lack of sensitivity and specificity remains the main problem. Using the PCR technique, Feinmeisser et al revealed that the detection of the Epstein-Barr virus (EBV) genome in fine needle aspirates of metastatic neck nodes was highly predictive of a nasopharyngeal primary.[85] These findings may carry important implications regarding the treatment of the unknown primary lesion and may result in earlier treatment of the unrecognized early nasopharyngeal carcinoma. Recent studies using quantitative real-time PCR have also shown that viral sequences of EBV[86] and human papillomavirus (HPV)[87] may be detectable in sera of patients with advanced HNSCC and may represent novel markers for disseminated disease. Microsatellite analysis of LOH or microsatellite instability demonstrated tumour-specific DNA alterations in the serum[88] and saliva[89] of a significant percentage of patients with HNSCC. No microsatellite alterations were detected in any of the samples from the healthy control subjects, indicating the very high specificity of the assay. Innovations in molecular technology such as microcapillary array may allow more rapid and efficient screening of large numbers of samples.[90]

Cancer localization

Tumour cells expressing oncogene products, which differ qualitatively from their normal counterparts, offer situations where it may be possible to perform new tests for cancer diagnosis and imaging. These proteins in turn have the potential to act as antigen targets that specifically designed antibodies can recognize. An oncoprotein must satisfy three criteria to be of maximal use for in vivo studies:

1. the protein must be easily accessible by the injected antibody (i.e. it must be expressed on the cell surface);
2. the protein target should be specific to the cancer cell;
3. the target protein should be significantly overexpressed relative to background levels.

In HNSCC, radioimmunoscintigraphy using indium–111-labelled antibodies directed against the EGFR[91] or ^{99m}technitium-labelled antibody against the keratinocyte-specific CD44 splice variant 6[92] have been evaluated in a phase I clinical trial. The techniques can be safely administered and seem to be useful in imaging patients due to high and selective tumour uptake.

Prognostic applications

Tumour stage associations

As our knowledge of oncogenes increases it seems apparent that some oncogene products are necessary at the earliest stages of carcinogenesis. However, other genes are turned on late in the malignant process and seem to be required to stimulate the cancer to advanced stages of malignancy. In addition, it appears that still other genes are necessary for the development of certain tumour characteristics such as angio-/lymphangiogenesis and propensity to metastases. Overexpression of EGFR seems to be an important marker in HNSCC. Advanced clinical lesions (T4 stage) had significantly different EGFR RNA levels from those lesions of the T3 or T1/2 stages. In addition, those tumours with nodal metastases have statistically significant EGFR overexpression levels compared with those with no evidence of nodal disease.[29] Another group has recently demonstrated in patients with oral SCCs that the expression of all four *erb*B receptors was significantly associated with shortened survival and the combination of *erb*B-2, B-3, and EGFR but not *erb*B-4 significantly improved the predicting power.[38] Telomerase is a reverse transcriptase enzyme that extends telomeric repeats and is involved in cellular immortality. Like EGFR, it is overexpressed in HNSCCs and also seems to predict advanced disease.[93] Telomerase activity increases with late stage carcinoma and is present at lower levels in all earlier stages. The finding of increased telomerase activity in histologically normal tissue suggests that the enzyme may be useful as a molecular marker of disease and may have a role in the molecular assessment of tumour margins. Overexpression of p53 in initial HNSCC predicts for increased incidence of second primary tumours and recurrences of the primary tumours.[94]

HNSCC is characterized by its capacity to invade adjacent tissues and metastasize loco-regionally. The co-operation of multiple proteolytic enzymes that are secreted by tumour cells and/or host cells and whose substrates include extracellular matrix (ECM) components is required for cancer cells to invade the ECM and penetrate the lymphatic or blood vessel wall where they may grow and metastasize to distant sites. ECM proteolysis is also involved in the angiogenesis necessary for the continued growth of solid tumours. Recent studies demonstrated that the expression of multiple key molecules involved in HNSCC invasion, angiogenesis and metastasis including matrix metalloproteinases (MMPs) and vascular endothelial growth factors (VEGFs) is a common feature in both experimental[47,95] and clinical models of HNSCC,[96,97] and that the analysis of specific MMPs and VEGFs may be useful to evaluate the malignant potential in individual HNSCCs.

Predictors of other aspects of tumour behaviour

In addition to being markers for tumour staging, oncogene expression is also a predictor of tumour behaviour. Activation of certain proto-oncogenes may predict radiation resistance and chemotherapy resistance. Radiation-resistant human laryngeal cancer cell lines showed evidence of altered *raf* proto-oncogenes.[98] The recent prospective studies reveal that p53 alterations can predict tumour response to neoadjuvant chemotherapy in HNSCC.[99]

Therapeutic applications

Anti-oncogene therapeutics

Anti-DNA/RNA therapeutics

Theoretically, by preventing the flow of abnormal cellular information from the oncogene DNA to RNA to protein, one could inhibit the expression of the malignant phenotype. Specific anti-sense molecules could be designed to block replication or expression of oncogene DNA.[100] Similarly, blocking molecules could be directed to prevent translation of the oncogene RNA into its abnormal oncoprotein. In vitro experiments have shown promising results. It can be difficult, however, to regulate the amount of blocking that occurs due to in vivo mechanisms such as feedback regulation.

Anti-oncoprotein therapeutics

Immunotherapy is one particular application of this technology that may be a promising approach to cancer therapy. The created monoclonal antibody is able to recognize a specific tumour target such as an oncogene protein product. Anti-EGFR monoclonal antibody (mAb) has been shown to be an effective antiproliferative agent for HNSCC via several mechanisms including induction of G1 cell cycle arrest and apoptosis,[101] direct terminal differentiation,[101] inhibition of production of proteolytic enzymes[95] and angiogenic factors,[47] and enhancement of antitumour activity of chemotherapeutic drugs[102] and radiation therapy.[103] Currently, phase III clinical trial evaluation of combining anti-EGFR mAb, C225, with radiation or chemotherapy for patients with advanced HNSCC is underway. Another approach using immunotoxin is composed of an antibody or a cytokine and a conjugated molecule capable of destroying the cancer cell such as a toxin, drug or radionucleotide. Based on the uniform expression of interleukin-4 (IL-4) receptor on HNSCC cells, a chimeric protein composed of circular permuted IL-4 and a truncated form of a bacterial toxin called *Pseudomonas* exotoxin was produced and found to be highly and specifically cytotoxic to HNSCC cells via induction of apoptosis.[104]

Gene therapy

The aim of gene therapy is to introduce new genetic material into cancer cells that will selectively kill cancer cells with no toxicity to the neighbouring non-malignant cells. Gene therapy uses a vector to deliver a DNA sequence into cells and then the DNA incorporates itself into the cellular genome and produces proteins that have a therapeutic effect. A variety of gene therapy approaches have been described as follows.

Replacing or compensating for tumour suppressor gene

Active tumour suppressor genes that are lost or altered through acquired genetic mutations can be reintroduced into tumour cells to control progression through the cell cycle. Transfection of human HNSCC cell lines with functional p53 temporarily arrested the growth of cells in tissue culture[105] and reduced tumour growth in nude mice.[106] A phase I study using human adenovirus/p53 gene transfer as a surgical adjuvant in advanced head and neck cancers has been completed and revealed a survival benefit compared with that reported in chemotherapy trials.[107] A phase II clinical trial for anti-tumour efficacy is currently underway.

Inserting genes that produce cytotoxic substances

'Suicide' gene therapy or genetic prodrug activation therapy inserts a gene into the tumour that encodes for a protein that will convert a non-toxic prodrug into a toxic substance. In HNSCC, the herpes simplex virus thymidine kinase (HSV-*tk*) gene therapy has been the most investigated.[108] Tumour cells are genetically modified with HSV-*tk* gene and are then treated with the prodrug ganciclovir. HSV-*tk* enzyme phosphorylates ganciclovir to ganciclovir monophosphate and then triphosphate. Ganciclovir triphosphate inhibits DNA synthesis and results in apoptosis (or programmed cell death).

Modulating the immune system

Tumour necrosis factor-α (TNF-α), interferon-γ (IFN-γ), IL-2 and IL-4 genes have each been transfected into tumour cells in tissue culture. When these transfected cells are then introduced into humans or mice, the host immune response is increased, and growth of the tumour is limited.[109] The effect of IL-2 and IL-4 transfection has been attributed to direct stimulation and proliferation of cytotoxic T-lymphocytes by tumour cells.

Future directions in gene therapy

Genes currently under investigation include suicide gene (HSV-*tk*-ganciclovir[108]), immune-modulatory cytokine genes (IL-2, GM-CSF, IL-12[110]) and tumour suppressor genes (p16,[111] p21,[112] p53,[113] FHIT[72]). Delivery vehicles under investigation include viral and non-viral systems.[23] Viral vector systems include those based on adenoviruses, retroviruses, defective adenoviruses, adeno-associated virus, and herpes virus. Various techniques are being developed to enhance the viral infection efficiency and selectivity of tumour cells such as using bispecific antibodies that recognize domains of viral vector as well as the EGFR[114] and using a modified viral vector that recognizes integrins of the $\alpha_2\beta_1$ and $\alpha_3\beta_1$ class frequently overexpressed in HNSCC.[115] Non-viral gene delivery systems include liposomes and naked DNA. Another modality is 'non-gene gene therapy' using agents to restore the DNA binding function of key growth-regulatory elements or to target pathways that affect the ability of p53 binding protein, Mdm2, to degrade p53.[116] Targets under investigation include the inhibition of tumour angiogenesis as this will decrease vascular support required for tumour growth and support.[96,117] A novel gene therapy approach uses an adenovirus called ONYX-015 that lacks the E1B region of the virus. The E1B region normally binds and inactivates p53 and is needed for viral replication in normal cells. The ONYX-015 lacks E1B and therefore only infects cells that lack functional p53 leading to apoptosis.[106,118]

The escape of malignant cells from the local host tissues, metastasis, penetration and then the successful acquisition of the distant host environment by sequential enzyme activation is also coded by specific proto-oncogene activation and tumour suppresser gene deactivation.[119] Overcoming extracellular barriers to tumour spread is fundamental to the definition and spread of malignancy.[119] These spreading factors are coded and can be detected at enzymatic, cytoplasmic mRNA and DNA levels. It is hoped that the 'profile' of spreading factors for a tumour[97] may provide an index to later prognosis and survival, and perhaps even provide therapeutic interventions with anti-metastatic factors to supplement the growing armamentarium available to the surgical oncologist.

Conclusion

The understanding of how cancer cells progress has increased substantially in the last two decades. With this increased understanding, our ability to apply new technologies to control and prohibit the growth of cancer is coming closer to reality.

REFERENCES

1. Weinberg R. The molecular basis of oncogenes and tumor suppressor genes. *Ann N Y Acad Sci* 1995; **758**: 331–338.
2. Hatakeyama M, Herrera R, Makela T et al. The cancer cell and the cell cycle clock. *Cold Spring Harb Symp Quant Biol* 1994; **59**: 1–10.
3. Budillon A. Molecular genetics of cancer. Oncogenes and tumor suppressor genes. *Cancer* 1995; **76**: 1869–1873.
4. Brodeur GM, Seeger RC, Schwab M et al. Amplification of N-myc in untreated human neuroblastomas correlates with advanced disease stage. *Science* 1984; **224**: 1121–1124.
5. Almoguera C, Shibata D, Forrester K et al. Most human carcinomas of the exocrine pancreas contain mutant c-K-ras genes. *Cell* 1988; **53**: 549–554.
6. Masuda H, Miller C, Koeffler HP et al. Rearrangement of the p53 gene in human osteogenic sarcoma. *Proc Natl Acad Sci USA* 1987; **84**: 7716–7719.
7. Fearon E, Hamilton S, Vogelstein B. Clonal analysis of human colorectal tumours. *Science* 1987; **238**: 193–197.
8. Pongers-Willemse M, Verhagen O, Tibbe G et al. Real time quantitative PCR for the detection of minimal residual disease in acute lymphoblastic leukemia using junctional region specific TaqMan probes. *Leukemia* 1998; **12**: 2006–2014.
9. Speicher M, Ballard S, Ward D. Karyotyping human chromosomes by combinatorial multi-color FISH. *Nat Genet* 1996; **12**: 368–375.
10. Schrock E, duManoir S, Veldman T et al. Multicolor spectral karyotyping of human chromosomes. *Science* 1996; **273**: 494–497.
11. Bergamo N, Rogatto S, Poli-Frederico R et al. Comparative genomic hybridization analysis detects frequent over-representation of DNA sequences at 3q, 7p, and 8q in head and neck carcinomas. *Cancer Genet Cytogenet* 2000; **119**: 48–55.
12. Kononen J, Bubendorf L, Kallioniemi A et al. Tissue microarrays for high-throughput molecular profiling of tumor specimens. *Nat Med* 1998; **4**: 844–847.
13. Golub TB, Slonim DK, Tamayo P et al. Molecular classification of cancer: class discovery and class prediction by gene expression monitoring. *Science* 1999; **286**: 531–537.
14. Cheng L, Sturgis E, Eicher S et al. Glutathione-S-transferase polymorphisms and risk of squamous-cell carcinoma of the head and neck. *Int J Cancer* 1999; **84**: 220–224.
15. Jourenkova-Mironova N, Voho A, Bouchardy C et al. Glutathione S-transferase GSTM1, GSTM3, GSTP1 and GSTT1 genotypes and the risk of smoking-related oral and pharyngeal cancers. *Int J Cancer* 1999; **81**: 44–48.
16. Wang L, Sturgis E, Eicher S et al. Mutagen sensitivity to benzo(a)pyrene diol epoxide and the risk of squamous cell carcinomas of the head and neck. *Clin Cancer Res* 1998; **4**: 1773–1778.
17. Van Dyke DL, Worsham MJ, Benninger MS et al. Recurrent cytogenic abnormalities in squamous cell carcinoma of the head and neck. *Genes Chromosomes Cancer* 1994; **9**: 192–206.
18. Carey T, Worsham M, Van Dyke D. Chromosomal biomarkers in the clonal evolution of head and neck squmaous neoplasia. *J Cell Biochem* 1993; **17F (Suppl)**: 213–222.
19. Ah-See K, Cooke T, Pickford I, Soutar D, Balmain A. An allelotype of squamous carcinoma of the head and neck using microsatellite markers. *Cancer Res* 1994; **54**: 1617–1621.
20. Nawroz H, van der Riet P, Hruban R et al. Allelotype of head and neck squamous cell carcinoma. *Cancer Res* 1994; **54**: 1152–1155.
21. Califano J, van der Riet P, Westra W et al. Genetic progression model for head and neck cancer: implications for field cancerization. *Cancer Res* 1996; **56**: 2488–2492.
22. Califano J, Westra W, Meininger G et al. Genetic progression and clonal relationship of recurrent premalignant head and neck lesions. *Clin Cancer Res* 2000; **6**: 347–352.
23. Partridge M. Current status of genetics for prediction, prognosis, and gene therapy. *Curr Opin Otolaryngol Head Neck Surgery* 2000; **8**: 69–79.
24. Cowan J, Beckett M, Weichselbaum R. Chromosome changes characterising in vitro response to radiation in human squamous cell carcinoma lines. *Cancer Res* 1993; **53**: 5542–5547.
25. Chen Y-J, Ko J-Y, Chen P-J et al. Chromosomal aberrations in nasopharyngeal carcinoma analyzed by comparative genomic hybridization. *Genes Chromosomes Cancer* 1999; **25**: 169–175.
26. Klapper LN, Kirschbaum MH, Sela M, Yarden Y. Biochemical and clinical implications of the ErbB/HER signalling network of growth factor receptors. *Adv Cancer Res* 2000; **77**: 25–79.
27. Irish J, Bernstein A. Oncogenes in head and neck cancer. *Laryngoscope* 1993; **103**: 42–53.
28. Grandis JR, Tweardy DJ. Elevated levels of transforming growth factor alpha and epidermal growth factor receptor messenger RNA are early markers of carcinogenesis in head and neck cancer. *Cancer Res* 1993; **53**: 3579–3584.
29. Anderson J, Irish J, Ngan B-Y. Prevalence of Ras oncogene mutations in head and neck carcinomas. *J Otolaryngology* 1992; **21**: 321–326.
30. Kearsley JH, Leonard JH, Walsh MD, Wright GR. A comparison of epidermal growth factor receptor (EGFR) and c-erbB-2 oncogene expression in head and neck squamous cell carcinomas. *Pathology* 1991; **23**: 189–194.
31. Riviere A, Becker J, Loning T. Comparative investigation of c-erbB2/neu expression in head and neck tumors and mammary cancer. *Cancer* 1991; **67**: 2142–2149.

32. Rodrigo JP, Ramos S, Lazo PS et al. Amplification of ERBB oncogenes in squamous cell carcinomas of the head and neck. *Eur J Cancer Part A* 1996; **32A**: 2004–2010.
33. O-charoenrat P, Rhys-Evans P, Eccles SA. Characterization of ten newly-derived human head and neck squamous carcinoma cell lines with special reference to c-*erb*B proto-oncogene expression. *Anticancer Res* 2001; **21**: 1953–1963.
34. O-charoenrat P, Rhys-Evans PH, Archer DJ, C-erbB receptors in squamous cell carcinomas of the head and neck: clinical significance and correlation with matrix metalloproteinases and vascular endothelial growth factors. *Oral Oncol* 2002; **38**: 73–80.
35. Craven JM, Pavelic ZP, Stambrook PJ et al. Expression of c-*erb*B2 gene in human head and neck carcinoma. *Anticancer Res* 1992; **12**: 2273–2276.
36. Field JK, Spandidos DA, Yiagnisis M et al. c-*erb*B2 expression in squamous cell carcinoma of the head and neck. *Anticancer Res* 1992; **12**: 613–620.
37. Hou L, Shi D, Tu SM et al. Oral cancer progression and c-erbB-2/neu proto-oncogene expression. *Cancer Lett* 1992; **65**: 215–220.
38. Xia W, Lau Y-K, Zhang H-Z et al. Combination of EGFR, HER-2/neu, and HER-3 is a stronger predictor for the outcome of oral squamous cell carcinoma than any individual family members. *Clin Cancer Res* 1999; **5**: 4164–4174.
39. Issing WJ, Heppt WJ, Kastenbauer ER. erbB-3, a third member of the erbB/epidermal growth factor receptor gene family: its expression in head and neck cancer cell lines. *Eur Arch Otorhinolaryngol* 1993; **250**: 392–395.
40. Funayama T, Nakanishi T, Takahashi K et al. Overexpression of c-*erb*B-3 in various stages of human squamous cell carcinomas. *Oncology* 1998; **55**: 161–167.
41. Shintani S, Funayama T, Yoshihama Y et al. Prognostic significance of ERBB3 overexpression in oral squamous cell carcinoma. *Cancer Lett* 1995; **95**: 79–83.
42. Werkmeister R, Brandt B, Joos U. The erbB oncogenes as prognostic markers in oral squamous cell carcinomas. *Am J Surg* 1996; **172**: 681–683.
43. Werkmeister R, Brandt B, Joos U. Clinical relevance of *erb*B-1 and -2 oncogenes in oral carcinomas. *Oral Oncol* 2000; **36**: 100–105.
44. Ibrahim SO, Vasstrand EN, Liavaag PG et al. Expression of c-erbB proto-oncogene family members in squamous cell carcinoma of the head and neck. *Anticancer Res* 1997; **17**: 4539–4546.
45. Srinivasan R, Poulsom R, Hurst HC, Gullick WJ. Expression of the c-erbB-4/HER4 protein and mRNA in normal human fetal and adult tissues and in a survey of nine solid tumour types. *J Pathol* 1998; **185**: 236–245.
46. O-charoenrat P, Rhys-Evans P, Court WJ et al. Differential modulation of proliferation, matrix metalloproteinase expression and invasion of human head and neck squamous carcinoma cells by c-*erb*B ligands. *Clin Exp Metastasis* 1999; **17**: 631–639.
47. O-charoenrat P, Rhys-Evans P, Modjtahedi H, Eccles SA. Vascular endothelial growth factor family members are differentially regulated by c-*erb*B signaling in head and neck squamous carcinoma cells. *Clin Exp Metastasis* 2000; **18**: 155–161.
48. O-charoenrat P, Modjtahedi H, Rhys-Evans P et al. Epidermal growth factor-like ligands differentially upregulate matrix metalloproteinase-9 in head and neck squamous carcinoma cells. *Cancer Res* 2000; **60**: 1121–1128.
49. O-charoenrat P, Rhys-Evans P, Eccles SA. Expression and regulation of c-*erb*B ligands in human head and neck squamous carcinoma cells. *Int J Cancer* 2000; **88**: 759–765.
50. Tadokoro K, Ueda M, Ohshima T et al. Activation of oncogenes in human oral cancer cells: a novel codon 13 mutation of c-H-ras-1 and concurrent amplification of c-erb-B-1 and c-myc. *Oncogene* 1989; **4**: 499–505.
51. Kasid U, Pfeifer A, Weichselbaum RR et al. The raf oncogene is associated with a radiation-resistant human laryngeal cancer. *Science* 1987; **237**: 1039–1041.
52. Berenson J, Yan J, Mickle R. Frequent amplification of the bcl-1 locus in head and neck squamous cell carcinomas. *Oncogene* 1989; **4**: 1111–1116.
53. Callender T, el-Naggar AK, Lee MS. PRAD-1 (CCND)/cyclin D1 gene amplification in primary head and neck squamous cell carcinoma. *Cancer* 1994; **74**: 152–158.
54. Izzo J, Papadimitrakopoulou V, Li X et al. Dysregulated cyclin D1 expression early in head and neck tumorigenesis: in vivo evidence for an association with subsequent gene amplification. *Oncogene* 1998; **17**: 2313–2322.
55. Michalides R, van Veelan N, Hart A et al. Overexpression of cyclin D1 correlates with recurrence in a group of forty-seven operable squamous cell carcinomas of the head and neck. *Cancer Res* 1995; **55**: 975–978.
56. Bova R, Quinn D, Nankervis J et al. Cyclin D1 and p16^{INK4A} expression predict reduced survival in carcinoma of the anterior tongue. *Clin Cancer Res* 1999; **5**: 2810–2819.
57. Rodrigo J, Garcia L, Ramos S. *EMS1* gene amplification correlates with poor prognosis in squamous cell carcinomas of the head and neck. *Clin Cancer Res* 2000; **6**: 3177–3182.
58. Bockmuhl U, Schwendel A, Dietel M, Petersen I. Distinct patterns of chromosomal alterations in high- and low-grade head and neck squamous cell carcinomas. *Cancer Res* 1996; **56**: 5325–5329.
59. Resto V, Caballero O, Buta M et al. A putative oncogenic role for MPP11 in head and neck squamous cell cancer. *Cancer Res* 2000; **60**: 5529–5535.
60. Reed A, Califano J, Cairns P et al. High frequency of p16 (CDKN2/MTS-1/INK4A) inactivation in head and neck squamous cell carcinoma. *Cancer Res* 1996; **56**: 3630–3633.
61. Cairns P, Mao L, Merlo A et al. Rates of p16 (MTS1) mutations in primary tumours with 9p loss. *Science* 1994; **265**: 415–417.
62. Wu C, Roz L, McKown S et al. DNA studies underestimate the major role of CDKN2A inactivation in oral and oropharyngeal squamous cell carcinomas. *Gene Chromosomes Cancer* 1999; **25**: 16–25.

63. Boyle J, Hakim J, Kock W et al. The incidence of p53 mutations increases with progression of head and neck cancer. *Cancer Res* 1993; **53**: 4477–4480.
64. Brennan JA, Mao L, Hruban RH et al. Molecular assessment of histopathological staging in squamous-cell carcinoma of the head and neck. *N Engl J Med* 1995; **332**: 429–435.
65. Brennan JA, Boyle JO, Koch WM et al. Association between cigarette smoking and mutation of the p53 gene in squamous-cell carcinoma of the head and neck. *N Engl J Med* 1995; **332**: 712–717.
66. Qin G-Z, Park J, Chen S-Y, Lazarus P. A high prevalence of p53 mutations in pre-malignant oral erythroplakia. *Int J Cancer* 1999; **80**: 345–348.
67. Homann N, Nees M, Conradt C et al. Overexpression of p53 in tumor-distant epithelia of head and neck cancer patients is associated with an increased incidence of second primary carcinoma. *Clin Cancer Res* 2001; **7**: 290–296.
68. Gupta V, Schmidt A, Pashia M, Sunwoo J, Scholnick S. Multiple regions of deletion on chromosome arm 13q in head-and-neck squamous cell carcinoma. *Int J Cancer* 1999; **84**: 453–457.
69. Gunduz M, Ouchida M, Fukushima K et al. Genomic structure of the human *ING1* gene and tumor-specific mutations detected in head and neck squamous cell carcinomas. *Cancer Res* 2000; **60**: 3143–3146.
70. Tanimoto K, Hayashi S, Tsuchiya E et al. Abnormalities of the *FHIT* gene in human oral carcinogenesis. *Br J Cancer* 2000; **82**: 838–843.
71. Lee J, Soria J-C, Hassan K et al. Loss of Fhit expression is a predictor of poor outcome in tongue cancer. *Cancer Res* 2001; **61**: 837–841.
72. Ji L, Fang B, Yen N et al. Induction of apoptosis and inhibition of tumorigenicity and tumor growth by adenovirus vector-mediated fragile histidine triad (*FHIT*) gene overexpression. *Cancer Res* 1999; **59**: 3333–3339.
73. Partridge M, Emillion G, Pateromichelakis S et al. The location of candidate tumour suppressor gene loci at chromosomes 3p, 8p and 9p for oral squamous cell carcinoma. *Int J Cancer* 1999; **83**: 318–326.
74. Ishwad C, Shuster M, Bockmuhl U et al. Frequent allelic loss and homozygous deletion in chromosome band 8p23 in oral cancer. *Int J Cancer* 1999; **80**: 25–31.
75. Takebayashi S, Ogawa T, Jung K-Y et al. Identification of new minimally lost regions on 18q in head and neck squamous cell carcinoma. *Cancer Res* 2000; **60**: 3397–3403.
76. Nakanishi H, Wang X-L, Imai F et al. Localization of a novel tumor suppressor gene loci on chromosome 9p21–22 in oral cancer. *Anticancer Res* 1999; **19**: 29–34.
77. Voravud N, Shin D, Ro J et al. Increased polysomies of chromosomes 7 and 17 during head and neck multistage tumorigenesis. *Cancer Res* 1993; **53**: 2874–2883.
78. Mao L, Lee J, Fan Y et al. Frequent microsatellite alterations at chromosomes 9p21 and 3p14 in oral premalignant lesions and their value in cancer risk assessment. *Nat Med* 1996; **2**: 682–685.
79. Partridge M, Emillion G, Pateromichelakis S et al. Allelic imbalance at chromosomal loci implicated in the pathogenesis of oral precancer; cumulative loss and its relationship with progression to cancer. *Oral Oncol Eur J Cancer* 1997; **34**: 77–83.
80. Califano J, Westra W, Koch W et al. Unknown primary head and neck squamous cell carcinoma: molecular identification of the site of origin. *J Natl Cancer Inst* 1999; **91**: 599–604.
81. Snyderman C, D'Amico F, Wagner R, Eibling D. A reappraisal of the squamous cell carcinoma antigen as a tumor marker in head and neck cancer. *Arch Otolaryngol Head Neck Surg* 1995; **121**: 1294–1297.
82. Yen T, Lin W, Kao C et al. A study of a new marker, CYFRA 21–1, in squamous cell carcinoma of the head and neck, and comparison with squamous cell carcinoma antigen. *Clin Otolaryngol* 1998; **23**: 82–86.
83. Fazekas-May M, Suen JY, Yeh YC et al. Investigation of urinary transforming growth factor alpha levels as tumor markers in patients with advanced squamous cell carcinoma of the head and neck. *Head Neck* 1990; **12**: 411–416.
84. Pellanda A, Grosjean P, Loeni S et al. Abrasive esophageal cytology for the oncological follow-up of patients with head and neck cancer. *Laryngoscope* 1999; **109**: 1703–1708.
85. Feinmesser R, Miyazaki I, Cheung R et al. Diagnosis of nasopharyngeal carcinoma by DNA amplification of tissue obtained by fine needle aspiration. *N Engl J Med* 1992; **326**: 17–21.
86. Lo Y, Chan L, Lo K et al. Quantitative analysis of cell-free Epstein-Barr virus DNA in plasma of patients with nasopharyngeal carcinoma. *Cancer Res* 1999; **59**: 1188–1191.
87. Capone R, Pai S, Koch W et al. Detection and quantitation of human papillomavirus (HPV) DNA in the sera of patients with HPV-associated head and neck squamous cell carcinoma. *Clin Cancer Res* 2000; **6**: 4171–4175.
88. Nawroz H, Koch W, Anker P. Microsatellite alterations in serum DNA of head and neck cancer patients. *Nat Med* 1996; **2**: 1035–1037.
89. Spafford M, Koch W, Reed A et al. Detection of head and neck squamous cell carcinoma among exfoliated oral mucosal cells by microsatellite analysis. *Clin Cancer Res* 2001; **7**: 607–612.
90. Wang Y, Hung S, Linn J et al. Microsatellite-based cancer detection using capillary array electrophoresis and energy-transfer fluorescent primers. *Electrophoresis* 1997; **18**: 1742–1748.
91. Soo KC, Ward M, Roberts KR et al. Radioimmunoscintigraphy of squamous carcinomas of head and neck. *Head Neck Surg* 1987; **9**: 349–352.
92. Stroomer J, Roos J, Sproll M et al. Safety and biodistribution of ^{99m}Technitium-labeled anti-CD44v6 monoclonal antibody BIWA 1 in head and neck cancer patients. *Clin Cancer Res* 2000; **6**: 3046–3055.
93. Mao L, El-Naggar AK, Fan YH et al. Telomerase activity in head and neck squamous cell carcinoma and adjacent

tissues. *Cancer Res* 1996; **56**: 5600–5604.

94. Shin DM, Lee JS, Lippman SM et al. p53 expression: predicting recurrence and second primary tumors in head and neck squamous cell carcinoma. *J Natl Cancer Inst* 1996; **88**: 519–529.
95. O-charoenrat P, Rhys-Evans P, Modjtahedi H et al. Over-expression of epidermal growth factor receptor in human head and neck squamous carcinoma cell lines correlates with matrix metalloproteinase-9 expression and in vitro invasion. *Int J Cancer* 2000; **86**: 307–317.
96. O-charoenrat P, Rhys-Evans P, Eccles SA. Expression of vascular endothelial growth factor family members in head and neck squamous cell carcinoma correlates with lymph node metastases. *Cancer* 2001; **92**: 556–568.
97. O-charoenrat P, Rhys-Evans P, Eccles SA. Expression of matrix metalloproteinases and their inhibitors correlates with invasion and metastasis in squamous cell carcinoma of the head and neck. *Arch Otolaryngol Head Neck Surg* 2001; **127**: 813–820.
98. Kasid U, Pfeifer A, Brennan T et al. Effect of antisense c-raf-1 on carcinogenicity and radiation sensitivity of a human squamous carcinoma. *Science* 1989; **243**: 1354–1356.
99. Cabelguenne A, Blons H, de Waziers I et al. p53 alterations predict tumor response to neoadjuvant chemotherapy in head and neck squamous cell carcinoma: a prospective series. *J Clin Oncol* 2000; **18**: 1465–1473.
100. Yuen A, Sikic B. Clinical studies of antisense therapy in cancer. *Front Biosci* 2000; **5**: 588–593.
101. Modjtahedi H, Affleck K, Stubberfield C, Dean C. EGFR blockade by tyrosine kinase inhibitor or monoclonal antibody inhibits growth, directs terminal differentiation and induces apoptosis in the human squamous cell carcinoma HN5. *Int J Oncol* 1998; **13**: 335–342.
102. Mendelsohn J, Fan Z. Epidermal growth factor receptor family and chemosensitization. *J Natl Cancer Inst* 1997; **89**: 341–343.
103. Huang S-M, Bock J, Harari P. Epidermal growth factor receptor blockade with C225 modulates proliferation, apoptosis, and radiosensitivity in squamous cell carcinomas of the head and neck. *Cancer Res* 1999; **59**: 1935–1940.
104. Kawakami K, Leland P, Puri R. Structure, function, and targeting of interleukin 4 receptors on human head and neck cancer cells. *Cancer Res* 2000; **60**: 2981–2987.
105. Braun-Falco M, Doenecke A, Smola H, Hallek M. Efficient gene transfer into human keratinocytes with recombinant adeno-associated virus vectors. *Gene Ther* 1999; **6**: 432–441.
106. Heise C, Williams A, Xue S. Intravenous administration of ONYX-015, a selectively replicating adenovirus, induces antitumoral efficacy. *Cancer Res* 1999; **59**: 2623–2628.
107. Clayman G, Frank D, Bruso P, Goepfert H. Adenovirus-mediated wild-type p53 gene transfer as a surgical adjuvant in advanced head and neck cancers. *Clin Cancer Res* 1999; **5**: 1715–1722.
108. Goebel E, Davidson B, Graham S, Kem J. Tumor reduction in vivo after adenoviral mediated gene transfer of the herpes simplex virus thymidine kinase gene and ganciclovir treatment in human head and neck squamous cell carcinoma. *Otolaryngol Head Neck Surg* 1998; **119**: 331–336.
109. Liu TJ, Zhang WW, Taylor DL et al. Growth suppression of human head and neck cancer cells by the introduction of a wild-type p53 gene via a recombinant adenovirus. *Cancer Res* 1994; **54**: 3662–3667.
110. Li D, Jiang W, Bishop J et al. Combination surgery and nonviral interleukin 2 gene therapy for head and neck cancer. *Clin Cancer Res* 1999; **5**: 1551–1556.
111. Rocco J, Li D, Liggett WJ et al. p16INK4A adenovirus-mediated gene therapy for human head and neck squamous cell cancer. *Clin Cancer Res* 1998; **4**: 1697–1704.
112. Mobley SR, Liu TJ, Hudson JM, Clayman GL. In vitro growth suppression by adenoviral transduction of p21 and p16 in squamous cell carcinoma of the head and neck. *Arch Otolaryngol Head Neck Surg* 1998; **124**: 88–92.
113. Clayman G, El-Naggar A, Lippman S et al. Adenovirus-mediated p53 gene transfer in patients with advanced recurrent head and neck squamous cell carcinoma. *J Clin Oncol* 1998; **16**: 2221–2232.
114. Blackwell J, Miller C, Douglas J et al. Retargeting to EGFR enhances adenovirus infection efficiency of squamous cell carcinoma. *Arch Otolaryngol Head Neck Surg* 1999; **125**: 856–863.
115. Kasono K, Blackwell J, Douglas J et al. Selective gene delivery to head and neck cancer cells via an integrin targeted adenoviral vector. *Clin Cancer Res* 1999; **5**: 2571–2579.
116. Selivanova G, Iotsova V, Okan I et al. (1997) Restoration of the growth suppression function of mutant p53 by a synthetic peptide derived from the p53 C-terminal domain. *Nat Med* 1997; **3**: 632–638.
117. Homer J, Greenman J, Stafford N. Angiogenesis in head and neck squamous cell carcinoma. *Clin Otolaryngol* 2000; **25**: 169–180.
118. Heise C, Sampson-Johannes A, Williams A et al. ONYX-015, an E1B gene-attenuated adenovirus, causes cytolysis and antitumoral efficacy that can be augmented by standard chemotherapeutic agents. *Nat Med* 1997; **3**: 639–645.
119. Vassalli J, Pepper M. Membrane proteases in focus. *Nat Med* 1994; **370**: 14–15.

Glossary

Alleles: alternative forms of a gene at a specific chromosomal location (locus).

Allelic imbalance: a situation where one member (allele) of a gene pair is lost (loss of heterozygosity) or amplified.

Amplification: the production of many DNA copies from one or a few copies.

Aneuploidy: a chromosome profile with fewer or greater than a normal (diploid) number. This phenomenon is an index of the deregulation of the genome and is associated with carcinogenesis.

Anneal: the joining of complementary base pairs to from a double-stranded DNA molecule.

Anti-parallel: the opposite orientations of the two strands of a DNA double helix; the 5' end of one strand aligns with the 3' end of the other strand.

Antisense: the complementary DNA or RNA sequence that does not code for the gene and is not transcribed. It is only important for maintaining the structure and integrity of the double helix and allows replication and transcription.

cDNA: synthetic complementary (c) DNA produced in vitro from an mRNA template and the initial product is double-stranded and complementary to the mRNA (it contains no introns).

Chromosomes: separate aggregates of the genome that allow cell division. The arms are classified into short arm (p) and long arm (q).

Chromosome transposition: an alteration in the structure of a chromosome by the movement of genetic material from one site in the (homologous) chromosome to another, that is the intra-homologous chromosome genetic movement. This may deregulate proto-oncogenes or tumour suppressor genes resulting in carcinogenesis.

Chromosome translocation: an alteration in the structure of a chromosome by movement of part or whole of a chromosome (genetic material) to another non-homologous chromosome, that is the inter-non-homologous chromosome genetic movement. This may deregulate proto-oncogenes or tumour suppressor genes resulting in carcinogenesis.

Codon: a triplet of bases which may code for an amino acid or the end of transcription.

Cytogenetics: the study of human chromosomes, their structure and transmission.

Deletion: loss of genetic material.

Disease transcripts: disease-associated mRNA sequences.

Diploid: two sets of genes, one from each parent.

*erb*B proto-oncogene: this has been implicated in carcinogenesis by two mechanisms. (i) An altered version of the epidermal growth factor (EGF)-receptor gene whose mutant EGF-receptor protein product sends growth signals into the cell in the absence of bound epithelial growth factor; (ii) the EGF-receptor protein product may be normal but overexpressed as seen in breast and ovarian carcinomas.

Eukaryocyte: a cell with a nucleus.

Exon: a coding fragment in a gene.

Extension: during the PCR process the thermostable enzyme copies the single-stranded DNA template.

Gene: an area of DNA coding for a polypeptide.

Gene amplification: an increase in the number of copies of a gene.

Gene rearrangement: the reordering of a gene sequence within a genome.

GTL-banding or 'G-banding' (giemsa/trypsin/leishman banding): chromosomes are G-banded to facilitate the identification of structural abnormalities. Slides are dehydrated, treated with the enzyme trypsin, and then stained.

Haploid: a cell (typically a gamete) with only a single copy of each chromosome.

HNSCC: head and neck squamous cell carcinoma.

Homozygous deletion: a deletion of both copies of the gene. Such deletions can be small such as a single gene or can stretch up to 10 million base pairs and delete several genes.

Hybridize: anneal.

Karyotype: the chromosome content of a cell.

Li-Fraumeni syndrome: a cancer predisposition syndrome associated with soft-tissue sarcoma, breast cancer, leukaemia, osteosarcoma, melanoma, and cancer of the colon, pancreas, adrenal cortex and brain. LFS is an autosomal dominant disorder with children of an affected individual having a 50% chance of inheriting the disease-causing mutation. About 70% of patients diagnosed clinically have an identifiable disease-causing mutation in the *TP53* gene (chromosomal locus 17p13).

L-*myc*: a related gene to *c-myc* (see below) which is amplified in small cell carcinoma.

Locus: a unique area of the chromosome where a gene or DNA sequence lies.

Loss of heterozygosity (LOH): the loss of one allele at a specific locus, caused by a deletion mutation; or loss of a chromosome from a chromosome pair. It is detected when heterozygous markers for a locus appear monomorphic because one of the alleles was deleted. When this occurs at a tumour suppressor gene locus where one of the alleles is already abnormal, it can result in neoplastic transformation.

Meiosis: the process of halving of the amount of DNA in a cell, which is seen in the generation of germ cells (gametes) with only a haploid set of chromosomes. Crossing over of homologous chromosomal elements, originally from both parents, is involved to aid gene shuffling (sexual reproduction).

Mitogenic: the promotion of mitosis.

Mitosis: the process of duplication of DNA seen in cell division producing a diploid set of chromosomes. There is no crossing over of gene sequences and it is thus asexual; the production of identical copies.

Mutagenic: promotes malignant progression by a change in the DNA sequence.

c-myc protein: a nuclear protein which activates other genes that are responsible for cell proliferation. Thus, although the protein is normal in structure it is carcinogenic due to being overexpressed.

*Neu/erb*B-2: a gene that specifies a cell surface mitogen receptor. It is amplified in breast and ovarian cancer. It is also termed HER-2/*neu*.

N-*myc*: a related gene to *myc* (see above) that is amplified in childhood neuroblastoma.

Nucleotide: the monomeric unit linked by 3' and 5' positions of each pentose (ribose) sugar component to form polynucleotide polymers called nucleic acids (DNA, RNA). These polynucleotide chains (DNA or RNA) have polarity (i.e. they are not the same in each direction), and are read in the 5' to 3' direction.

Null genotype: a mutated gene that is not transcribed into RNA and/or translated into a functional protein product.

Oncogene: an *unregulated* gene sequence whose product in the host presents a continuous growth stimulus by intervening in the normal growth mechanism in an unregulated manner causing carcinogenesis. (i) Viral oncogenes: a parasitic viral gene sequence, denoted v-onc; (ii) cellular oncogene: a cellular gene sequence, denoted c-onc, derived from the deregulation or mutated normal cellular proto-oncogene (see below).

Over-expression: the increased production by a cell of an RNA or protein product.

Paracrine: the release of a chemical substance by a cell having a local effect on adjacent cells (c.f the distant actions of hormones in the endocrine system).

Plasmids: circular double-stranded extrachromosomal DNA capable of autonomous replication. It can be used as a vector to introduce new DNA into a cell.

Point mutation: a single change in the sequence of base pairs which may result in a different amino acid or protein product.

Polymorphisms: differences in DNA sequences.

Prokaryocytes: organisms without a nucleus.

Properties of malignancy: (i) The proliferation of a cell outside the normal control mechanisms; (ii) invasion of the basement membrane in epithelial tumours; (iii) metastasis to aberrant sites within the body.

Proto-oncogene: a normal gene found in normal tissue, highly conserved in evolution and has central roles in signal transduction pathways that control cell growth and differentiation. If deregulated or mutated they may be carcinogenic and thus a deregulated or mutated proto-oncogene that is carcinogenic is referred to as a cellular oncogene.

Raf proteins: growth-related proteins in the cytoplasm.

Ras protein: a cytoplasmic protein involved in signal transduction. If mutated it remains in an excited, cell growth signal-emitting mode and consequently is carcinogenic.

Recombinant DNA technology: the modification of gene sequences.

Restriction enzyme: an enzyme that breaks double-stranded DNA into fragments at sequence specific points. These enzymes work by recognizing a specific base sequence and cleave the DNA molecule at that point. This property has provided geneticists with a powerful tool for analysis and gene manipulation.

Restriction fragment length polymorphism (RFLP) analysis: this is a technique in which organisms may be differentiated by analysis of patterns derived from cleavage of their DNA. If two organisms differ in the distance between sites of cleavage of a particular restriction endonuclease, the length of the fragments produced will differ when the DNA is digested with a restriction enzyme. The similarity of the patterns generated can be used to differentiate species (and even strains) from one another.

Sense: the gene bearing DNA or RNA is called the sense strand, that is it directly contains the genetic information.

Southern blot: the analysis and comparison of the electrophoretic patterns of DNA fragments using radioactive probes.

Telomerase: an enzyme that synthesizes the telomere, which is composed of tandem repeats of the sequence TTTAGG. This is significant as chromosome replication requires the telomere. If lost, replication ceases; if overactive then replication and cell division may continue unchecked.

Transcriptional promoter: an agent that enhances gene copying.

Transfection: the infection of a cell with isolated DNA or RNA by a viral vector.

Tumour suppressor gene: genetic elements whose loss or mutational inactivation allows cells to display one or more phenotypes of neoplastic growth.

Tyrosine kinase activity: a large number of regulatory pathways rely on enzymes that have tyrosine residues which, if phosphorylated by oncoproteins with tyrosine kinase activity, can be changed in functionality. The effect is to disrupt many regulatory pathways at the same time: a property that aids the multiplicity of effects from one change (see the section on multistage models of malignancy).

Western blot: the analysis and comparison of the electrophoretic patterns of proteins using labelled antibodies.

Wild type genes: the normal genes found in normal tissue.

3 Imaging in head and neck cancer

Carmel Ann Daly and D Michael King

Introduction

Imaging techniques used in the investigation of patients with head and neck cancer have become increasingly valuable in patient management by providing the following:

1. Display of direct tumour extent (T staging), nodal involvement (N staging) and evaluation for distant spread (M staging). These applications therefore play a critical role in the UICC/AJC staging systems and in so doing help to define management protocols.
2. Diagnostic information on patients who are difficult to examine clinically or in whom clinical examination is unrewarding. These may be cases of occult primary malignancy when subtle anatomical displacement or submucosal changes in the upper aerodigestive tract may be impossible to detect clinically, or in cases of trismus or obesity where the primary tumour or neck may be difficult to access.
3. Evaluation of changes resulting from treatment.
4. The detection of recurrent disease.
5. Imaging interrogation for the synchronous or metachronous primary. Synchronous tumour rates of 5–15% have been recorded in patients with head and neck cancer and metachronous tumour rates of 3–7% per annum contribute greatly to overall mortality. Most are squamous and most commonly involve the lung or oesophagus.[1,2]

Imaging techniques

Plain radiography

Plain radiography in the assessment of tumours of the neck and aerodigestive tract remains valuable as a rapid, easily acquired, readily available, low radiation dose screening technique. Its fundamental restriction is its lack of sensitivity and specificity for anything other than major structural abnormalities. Soft tissue anatomical display on plain films is, at best, limited.

Plain radiography of the chest, however, is an essential early part of the assessment algorithm in patients with head and neck tumours. Rapidly acquired with negligible radiation dose and very little cost, it provides an excellent first-line screening tool for the assessment of pulmonary and mediastinal metastatic disease. Synchronous bronchogenic primary carcinoma is of increased incidence in these patients and should be excluded by the chest film.

Facial and sinus films may provide valuable diagnostic clues by allowing display of bony destruction or sinus opacification. The orthopantomograph remains of particular value in the display of delicate dental and mandibular architecture and is generally superior to other plain radiographs. It frequently enables display of bony erosion by oral cavity or glossal tumours and the technique should be available in all head and neck units.

Contrast radiography and video fluoroscopy

Contrast media studies have a particular application in the evaluation of oropharyngeal tumours when the barium swallow examination may provide an excellent demonstration of not only tumour intrusion into and distortion of the food channel but often also mucosal disruption. Functional complications such as aspiration still justify the dynamics of barium swallow, in its most simple form of screening radiography and static radiographs. Cine type studies using 100 mm cameras acquiring small images at rates of up to six frames per second have largely been replaced by real-time video fluoroscopy. Dynamic contrast studies after surgery provide an important objective assessment of anastomotic integrity but more particularly, when combined with video, form a vital part of the re-education and training of the postoperative patient in the new methods of swallowing and speech. At a later stage, a barium swallow or video should be requested when complications or poor healing are suspected. Recurrence may be apparent as a new mass, ulceration, stricture or fistula.

Computerized tomography and magnetic resonance imaging

Computerized tomography (CT) and magnetic resonance imaging (MRI) have become the predominant methods of choice for imaging in cases of suspected or proven head and neck malignancies as they provide detailed anatomicopathological data. The choice of which technique to use is based on an understanding of the relative advantages and disadvantages of each system (see Tables 3.1 and 3.2) as well as their availability. Today they are often complementary investigative techniques but it appears likely that in the future, MRI will become the predominant tool for the display of tumours in the head and neck.

CT and MRI imaging technique

Most commonly, CT images are acquired in the axial plane. For this, the patient lies supine with the head in the neutral position and sections or slices are produced parallel to the body of the mandible. This accurately reproduces the anatomic relationships and helps minimize dental amalgam artefacts. Maximum image quality is delivered by using thin slices (3–5 mm) and contiguous acquisition, from the mastoid process (to include the skull base) to the manubrium sterni. Direct coronal CT scans are obtained by positioning the patient prone with the chin extended in order to produce images at 90 degrees to the axial plane. Both MRI and CT can display the anatomy of the neck in these two planes but the acquisition of the coronal plane by CT is dependent on the patient's ability to tolerate marked extension of the neck. An additional sagittal plane is easily available with MRI. With helical or volume CT scanners rapid reconstruction software allows reformation of multiplanar or 3D images providing the data were acquired on the initial scan with thin contiguous slices.

The use of intravenous iodinated contrast medium in CT increases delineation of soft tissue tumours most of which show more enhancement than surrounding normal soft tissue. Contrast enhancement also accurately highlights vascular structures allowing differentiation from tumour or lymphadenopathy and confirmation of vessel patency is clearly of strategic importance when planning excision. Accurate display of the extent of involvement by enveloping tumour may define inoperability and well-timed vascular opacification on CT accurately

Table 3.1 Relative advantages of CT

Widely available and relatively cheap
Rapid image acquisition times, particularly with helical scanners when the whole neck can be examined in 20–25 seconds. (cf. MRI make take 15–25 minutes)
Excellent delineation of bony and cartilage detail
Currently superior to MR in the assessment of metastatic adenopathy particularly extracapsular tumour extension
Less affected by motion artefact than MR due to short image acquisition time, which may be as short as 0.6 second per image with helical CT scanners. This is particularly advantageous in patients who find it difficult to keep still or who constantly need to swallow as a result of their disease
For patients in whom MRI is not appropriate (e.g. patients with pacemakers, ferrous or paramagnetic aneurysm clips or claustrophobics)

Table 3.2 Relative advantages of MRI

No ionizing radiation dose as the received imaging signal is induced by magnetic fields
Superior multiplanar reconstruction capability
Soft tissue contrast display is superior to that of CT hence more sensitive and accurate T staging of inaccessible tumour extension (e.g. lateral spread of nasopharyngeal tumours)
Superior sensitivity for assessment of extent of bone marrow involvement
Superior sensitivity for assessment of perineural infiltration
Less image degradation than CT resulting from dental repair material
MR uses gadolinium-DTPA contrast agent which is associated with a lower adverse reaction rate than iodinated agents employed in CT
Use in thyroid carcinoma where iodine CT contrast is contraindicated

provides that information. In MRI, gadolinium DTPA compounds can be used intravenously in the same way to assess tumour enhancement and improve soft tissue contrast.

Ultrasound

Diagnostic ultrasound employs a high frequency pulse-echo sound technique to allow the real-time display of slice images under the transducer. Frequencies employed in the neck may be high, in the order of 7.5–10 MHz, as deep tissue imaging is not needed in the neck and this use of high frequency results in very high spatial resolution images. The technique is harmless, painless, quick and cheap. Unfortunately, diagnostic ultrasound is rendered useless by gas and bone hence its application in the neck is concerned with the characterization of palpable masses, the examination of the thyroid gland and evaluation of cervical lymph nodes. It may also be employed in the evaluation of parotid or submandibular gland masses. In this respect it achieves high sensitivity and specificity and has the additional attribute of allowing guidance for needle biopsy.

Radioisotope imaging

Other than for the investigation of thyroid masses and the detection of parathyroid adenomas in hyperparathyroidism, imaging using radioisotopes is seldom part of the diagnostic algorithm. The increasing use of positron emission tomography (PET) in the management of suspected recurrence is, however, achieving considerable significance as by this technique small foci of recurrent active tumour may be distinguished from fibrosis (see PET scanning).

Cancer types and patterns of distribution

The majority of primary tumours involving the pharynx, oral cavity, and larynx are squamous cell carcinomas (SCC). They have a propensity for cervical nodal metastasis, which on CT characteristically exhibit ring enhancement around a low density centre sometimes showing necrosis. The principal sites of distant metastases for SCC are the lungs, bones and occasionally liver. Chest radiographs (CXR) detect most metastases greater than 1 cm but CT has greater sensitivity for detection of smaller nodules. The greater sensitivity for smaller nodules is at the expense of decreased specificity as tiny postinflammatory granulomata are frequently present in normal subjects. Thoracic CT is, however, recommended for all head and neck cancer patients with N2 and N3 lymph node disease because in patients with a known primary tumour, the sensitivity of CT for lung nodules is reported to be in the order of 54–91% compared with plain CXR[3,4] and isolated pulmonary metastases from head and neck cancer are potentially curable by surgical resection.[5] Synchronous bronchogenic primaries are also more common in patients with head and neck cancer.

After squamous cell carcinoma, the second most common head and neck malignancy is lymphoma. This diagnosis should be considered when multiple, non-necrotic lymph nodes are demonstrated in the deep lymphatic chains, especially if large and bilateral. Similarly when both superficial and deep lymph node chains are involved simultaneously and no mucosal abnormality of the aerodigestive tract is seen, lymphoma should be considered. Hodgkin's disease tends to remain nodal and is often associated with contiguous disease in the mediastinum. Patients with bulky supraclavicular adenopathy or bilateral neck disease have a higher incidence of disease below the diaphragm. Lymphoma should also be considered when multiple sites of disease are identified in an extranodal site. Extranodal disease is a common presentation of non-Hodgkin's lymphoma (NHL). The single most common site for extranodal disease is the tonsillar bed in Waldeyer's ring and this may be indistinguishable from SCC. Extranodal NHL is commonly associated with acquired immunodeficiency syndrome (AIDS) and may be the first manifestation of the condition.[6] Bone involvement may also occur also in lymphoma but is typically not the aggressive lytic destruction seen more commonly in association with SCC.

The nasopharynx

Anatomy

This site extends from the base of skull to the superior surface of soft palate, and includes the posterior margins of the choanal orifices and the posterior margin of the nasal septum. In the nasopharynx, the soft tissues of the posterior wall are thinnest in the midline with the prevertebral muscles causing symmetrical thickening 1–2 cm on either side of the midline.

Clinicoradiological correlations

Nasopharyngeal carcinomas typically arise posterosuperiorly in the nasopharynx in the region of the lateral pharyngeal recess (fossa of Rosenmuller), which then appears blunted on axial CT scanning.

However airway asymmetry is not specific as it may also be seen as a normal variant especially with lymphoid hyperplasia.[7] The complex anatomy of this region predisposes for early spread into the base of skull and paranasal sinuses via multiple foramina (Figures 3.1 and 3.2). A particular feature of nasopharyngeal carcinomas is their tendency for submucosal spread. Consequently ulceration or fungation into the nasopharyngeal lumen is rare and presents late in the course of the disease. Conversely, infiltration of underlying muscles develops early and MRI and CT techniques require optimization for the demonstration of this local infiltration, making maximal use of appropriately timed contrast enhancement. In this respect MRI, with its much higher soft tissue contrast display, more readily separates tumour from normal soft tissue. Since these muscles border the Eustachian tube orifice a serous otitis media is a frequent complication, demonstrated as opacification of the middle ear and mastoid air cells. There may be inferior extension into the oropharynx and soft palate or anterior extension along the levator palatini muscle. Extension of the tumour into the osteomeatal complex causes outlet obstruction and opacification of the sinuses. Infiltration of the posterior musculature of the nasopharynx can be due to direct extension of the tumour into the prevertebral muscles through the retropharyngeal section of the paralaryngeal space; metastatic involvement of nodes in this space may lead to destruction of the vertebral bodies and invasion of the carotid sheath.

All squamous cell carcinomas have intermediate signal intensity on T2-weighted images. Inflammatory disease, in contrast, has bright signal intensity on T2-weighted images. This signal difference can therefore delineate tumour margins whenever there is associated inflammatory disease. Malignancy often masquerades as benign inflammatory disease and because MR imaging can more accurately differentiate tumour from inflammatory changes on T2-weighted sequences, this modality is more accurate in determining the true extent of the disease than CT.

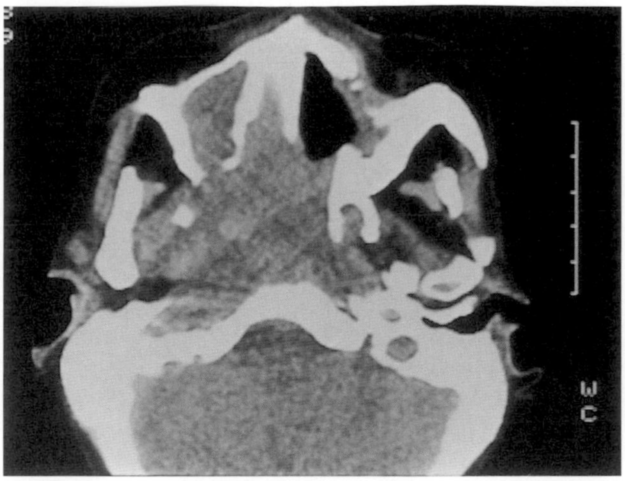

Figure 3.1 Unenhanced axial CT demonstrating a soft mass filling the postnasal space, with extensive bony destruction affecting the pterygoid plates and the apex of petrous temporal bone together with invasion of the right maxillary sinus.

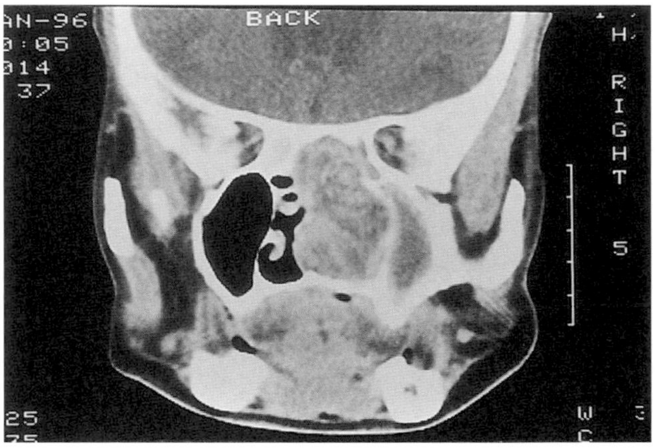

Figure 3.2 Coronal enhanced CT section showing tumour filling the right nasal cavity, displacing the nasal septum medially and displacing the lateral nasal wall laterally. The obstructed right maxillary sinus is filled with low-density fluid (darker grey) in contrast to tumour, which is of soft tissue density (lighter grey).

Parapharyngeal space

The parapharyngeal space is visible as a fat density plane just deep to the tonsillar pillars which merges posterolaterally with the carotid sheath running through the space. Inferiorly it terminates at the level of the hyoid bone. The parapharyngeal space can also appear asymmetric, but it should always be visualized and its obliteration or narrowing on one side should stimulate suspicion even in the absence of an obvious mass lesion. Once tumour invades this space, extension along a craniocaudal direction occurs very readily and this conduit provides an oropharyngeal tumour ready access to the skull base with consequent bony destruction.

Displacement, compression or invasion of the parapharyngeal space is a sensitive indicator of a malignant soft tissue mass. Nasopharyngeal tumours arise medial to this space but frequently spread laterally infiltrating the space and eventually the pterygoid muscles. The fat of the parapharyngeal space provides a low resistance path for descent of tumours that invade it. Interfaces between soft tissue tumour and normal surrounding structures as well as tumour–marrow interfaces are better demonstrated on MR imaging.[8] Thus MR can differentiate normal muscle from tumour and this is a particular advantage when combined with the multiplanar capabilities of MRI in defining T staging. Sagittal and coronal projections are particularly useful in displaying intracranial extension. By using the intracranial contour of the masses, one can differentiate malignant and benign lesions using MR imaging.[9]

Skull base erosion

Skull base erosion is common in nasopharyngeal carcinomas and may be seen in 31% of patients (Figure 3.3).[10] It is generally accepted that CT is superior to MRI in identifying bone destruction or cortical erosion as bone does not return a signal on MRI and is consequently seen as a black signal void. Invasion of the skull base can be identified as thinning or absence of the normal cortical bone (Figure 3.4.) However the diagnostic capability of MRI may be underestimated as MRI is superior when the bone marrow is infiltrated rather than destroyed.

On MRI, absence of the signal void that represents cortical bone or the replacement of high signal fatty marrow on T1-weighted images with intermediate signal identifies invasion of the skull base. Small areas of bony destruction however may be missed on MRI and a complementary CT may demonstrate this with increased confidence. In the nasopharynx, the bony septae are lined with mucosa that gives a bright signal on MRI, with the bony septum being visualized as a negative shadow or absent signal between the layers of soft tissue[11] thus loss of this signal void can be interpreted as bony invasion.

Direct superior extension into the skull base is easily visualized on high resolution, thin section (2–3 mm) bone algorithm CT. The route of extension is usually through the lateral pharyngeal wall to gain access to the prestyloid parapharyngeal space and thence to the foramina ovale, spinosum and lacerum and into the cavernous sinus and middle cranial fossa. Invasion of the poststyloid space or its compression by cervical adenopathy may produce signs referable to the cranial nerves IX, X, XI, XII and the sympathetic plexus. Tumour extension anteriorly into the pterygoid canal and into the middle cranial fossa via the inferior orbital fissure and cavernous sinus can also occur.

Perineural extension

Perineural extension of tumour is a particular feature of adenoid cystic carcinomas (an aggressive tumour of minor salivary glands found throughout the nasopharynx, oropharynx and paranasal sinuses) but squamous cell carcinoma and non-Hodgkin's lymphoma may also spread via perineural infiltration.

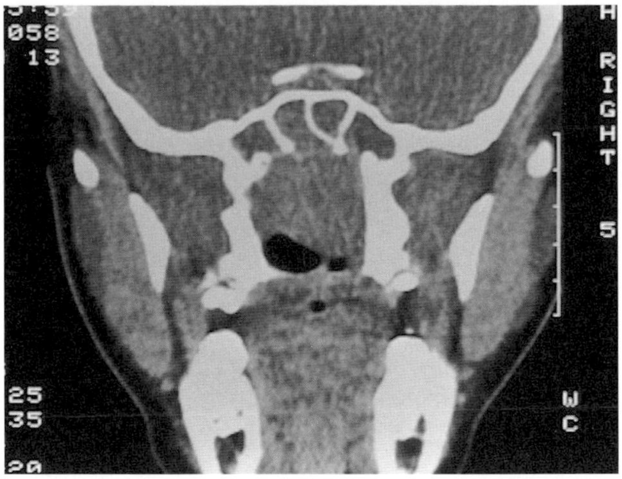

Figure 3.3 A coronal non-contrast CT section showing superior extension of a nasopharyngeal tumour into the sphenoid sinus.

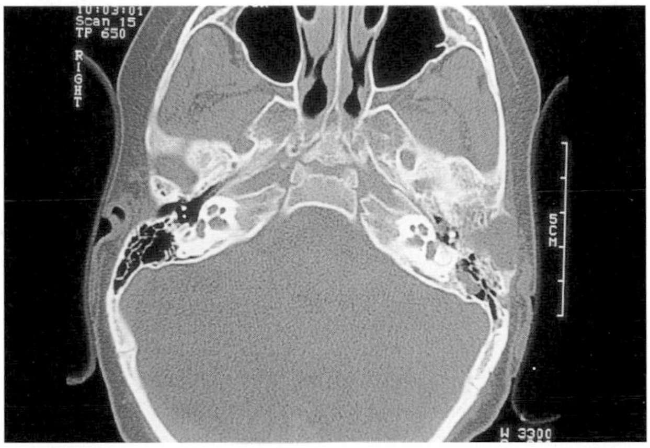

Figure 3.4 Axial CT on bony settings showing filling of the middle ear by soft tissue tumour, invasion of the petrous bone and obstruction of the mastoid air cells on the left due to rhabdosarcoma.

Pain and anaesthesia denoting trigeminal nerve involvement is frequently an early symptom of nasopharyngeal carcinoma, and motor involvement of the nerve can be confirmed when the ipsilateral laterally placed muscles of mastication become atrophied. They will show smaller muscle bulk and increased fat content (dark on CT and bright on T1- and T2-weighted MRI images). Most commonly the third division of the trigeminal nerve is involved and evidence of enlargement of the foramen ovale by a mass of intermediate signal on MRI that extends towards the nasopharynx should be sought. On MRI, neural tumour extension may be determined as diseased nerve sheaths may be enhanced after intravenous gadolinium injection. Skull base erosion

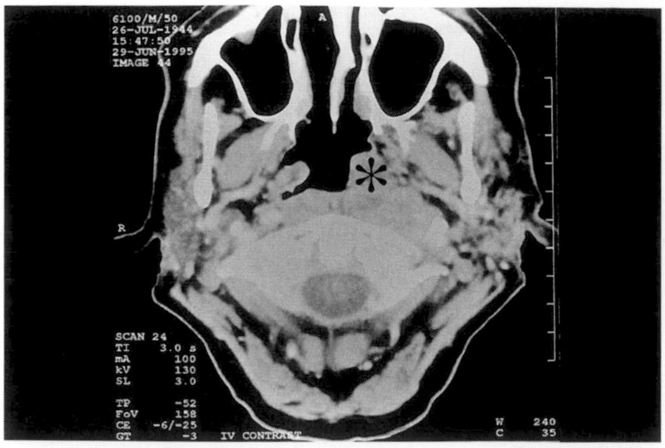

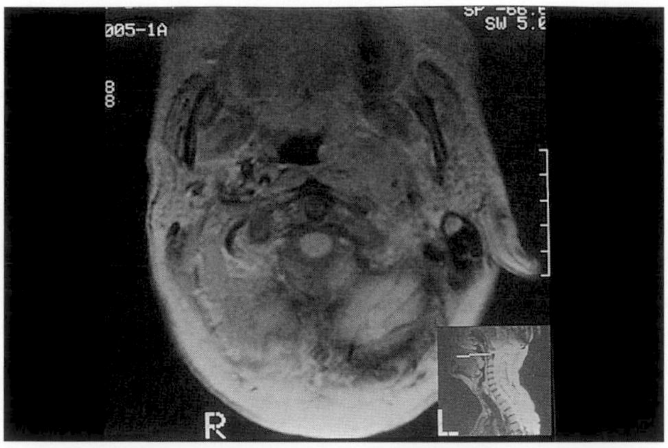

Figures 3.5 and 3.6 Axial CT and axial T2-weighted MRI on the same patient. The MRI section is at a lower level than the CT image. This patient was staged as T3 N2 and although the carcinoma in the left posterior oropharyngeal wall is not large, it has obliterated the fossa of Rosenmuller (asterisk) and invaded the carotid artery (note its normal opacification on the contralateral side). The deep lateral extension is more clearly demonstrated on MRI.

with or without cavernous sinus involvement or cranial nerve palsy is stage IV disease. However, skull base erosion as such does not carry as ominous a prognosis as cranial nerve palsy secondary to cavernous sinus involvement.[10] Although perineural tumour involvement is often seen, neural fibres themselves are relatively resistant to infiltration and this may explain the relatively low incidence of cranial nerve palsy in patients with cavernous sinus involvement.

Cervical lymphadenopathy is common in nasopharyngeal carcinoma and 86–90% have enlarged nodes at presentation.[12] Encasement of the internal carotid artery by a primary tumour or by adjacent lymph nodes is a poor prognostic indicator and a potential contraindication to resection (Figures 3.5 and 3.6). Youssem et al found on CT that tumour, which encompasses more than 270 degrees of the carotid artery diameter, probably cannot be removed from the artery. Tumour that involves 270 degrees or less can be removed.[13] Gritzman et al showed on ultrasound that when malignant adenopathy is in contact with a 4-cm or greater length of carotid artery, the wall is invaded in 80% of cases.[14] However problems arise with ultrasound as it is an operator-dependent modality and invasion of the carotid vessels above the mandible at the skull base cannot be visualized. Arteriography is less helpful than CT or US because of high false negative rates.[15]

Differential diagnosis

On MRI, focal areas of signal void suggest flow voids within vessels. If this occurs within soft tissue of intermediate signal on T1 and high signal intensity on T2, a hypervascular lesion occurring in the parapharyngeal space such as a paraganglionoma or haemangioma, should be considered. Capillary haemangiomas however do not have these serpiginous signal voids. Such signal voids could also be caused by bone fragments or dystrophic calcification.[9] CT could corroborate this as it is the superior modality in detection of calcification.

The nasopharynx is the second most common site for extranodal lymphoma in the head and neck. Lymphomas appear smooth, exophytic, submucosal, non-ulcerative and enhance homogeneously. Lymphoma occurring in the nasopharynx is usually detected earlier here than anywhere else as early occlusion of the adjacent Eustachian tube results in serous middle ear disease.

The differential diagnosis of tumours involving the skull base includes maxillary sinus tumours (which are usually large when involving the skull base and show extensive destruction of the pterygoid plates), chordomas (these usually have a bulky intracranial component, mainly involve the sphenoid, contain irregular calcification and can involve the retropharyngeal tissues), rhabdomyosarcomas (these are tumours of children and skull base invasion occurs in over a third of patients, and frequently involves the cavernous sinus) and adenoid cystic carcinomas.

The oral cavity and oropharynx

Anatomy

The oral cavity extends from the posterior or vermilion border of the lips to the anterior pillar of the tonsils. The oropharynx is a cuboidal space extending from the anterior pillar of the tonsil to the posterior pharyngeal wall.[16]

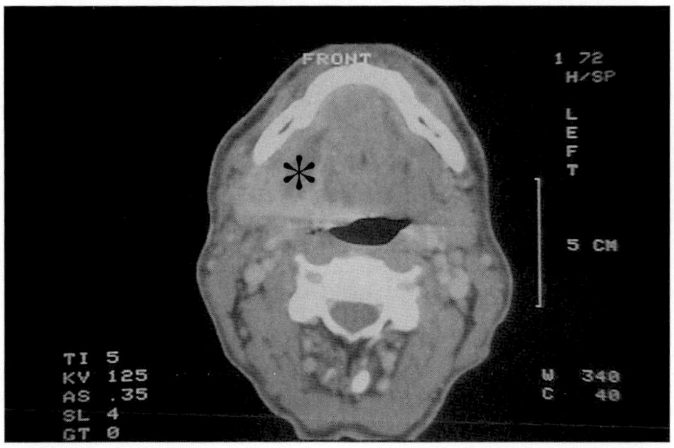

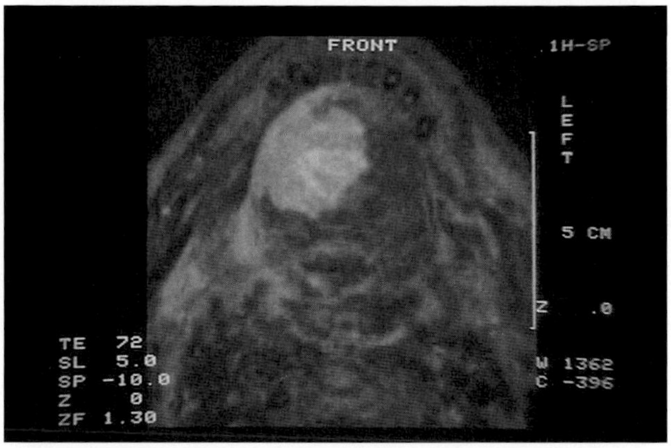

Figures 3.7 and 3.8 Axial postcontrast CT and axial T2-weighted MRI of the same patient at a similar level. A soft tissue mass with central necrosis arises in the right side of tongue (asterisk). Although part of the lingual septum is apparent on CT, the full extent of soft tissue spread is more clearly delineated by the MRI. On this imaging the bright signal mass clearly crosses the midline.

Clinicoradiological correlation

The tongue

The extrinsic muscles of the tongue and floor of the mouth should normally be symmetrical unless involved by tumour. Artefactual distortions can occur in patients whose heads are slightly tilted and these can be evaluated by assessing symmetry of the mandible. The intrinsic muscle mass of the tongue can be readily displayed and is generally of lower density (10–20 Hounsfield units) on CT, that is slightly darker than the density of the extrinsic muscles. The tongue mucosa cannot be identified separately as it is adherent to underlying muscle.

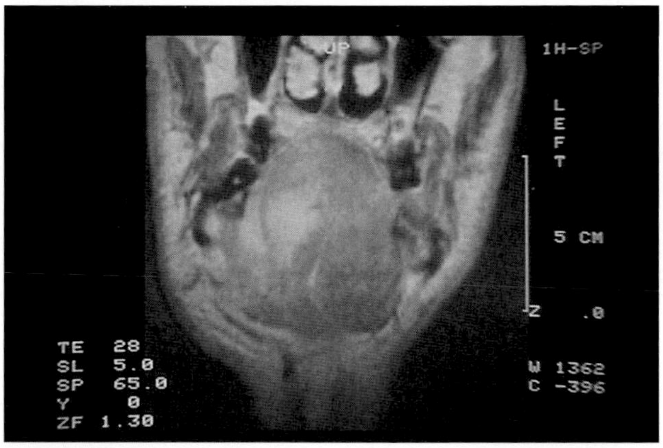

Figure 3.9 Coronal MRI on the same patient demonstrates the deep extension of this tongue tumour and confirms midline infiltration.

The pattern of spread of oral cavity and oropharyngeal tumours is mainly along muscle fibres, which may be associated with displacement, infiltration or obliteration of fatty fascial planes and interfaces, with later involvement of neurovascular bundles and periosteal surfaces as the tumour enlarges. Subsequently a soft tissue mass may be detectable as it enlarges, and it may show added enhancement with the administration of intravenous contrast, that is become brighter than the surrounding normal muscle density. In tongue tumours enhancement may be homogeneous or heterogeneous.

Obliteration or deviation of the normal midline lingual septum, which is a linear area of fat-density should be sought as it may be the most obvious sign of an adjacent mass. Subsequently extension of tumour across the midline may be demonstrated and this may have a major impact on surgical planning. Information on the midline of the tongue may be delineated by CT but this relies on obliteration of fat planes whereas MRI is more sensitive for earlier, smaller lesions (Figures 3.7, 3.8 and 3.9). Contrast enhancement of the lingual vessels will display their relationship to a tumour. The deep tissues of the tongue, tongue root and muscles of the floor of the mouth are normally symmetrical and any asymmetry of muscle size or loss of definition of the muscle bundles should be regarded with suspicion.

Tumour can grow beneath intact mucosa[17] and this is especially important in the oropharynx where tumours may begin in the tonsillar crypts and grow until they ulcerate rather than growing in an exophytic fashion (Figure 3.10). Ulceration on the dorsum of the tongue may be demonstrated if outlined by air (Figure 3.11) and reactive hyperaemia in the margin of the mass may show rim enhancement after intravenous contrast.

On MRI, squamous carcinoma in this area tends to show a low to intermediate signal on T1-weighted images similar to surrounding muscle and this contrasts with the high signal from adjacent fat. On

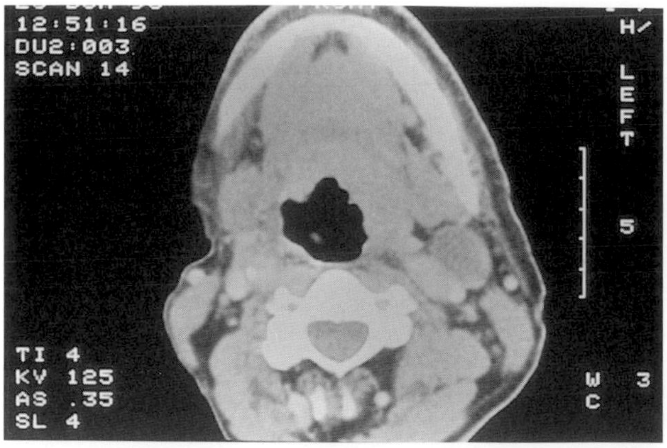

Figure 3.10 The scan shows asymmetry in the oropharynx as a carcinoma causes thickening of the left side wall of the oropharynx with extension across the midline. A low-density involved node is shown on the left. The patient has also had a previous right parotidectomy.

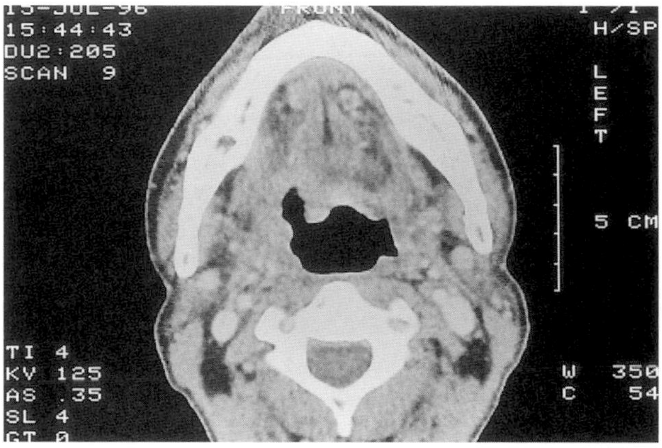

Figure 3.11 Ulcerating carcinoma of the right side of the tongue (arrow) on axial postcontrast CT.

T2–weighted images, the tumour may exhibit varying degrees of high signal intensity thereby contrasting and differentiating it from muscle. Normal lymphoid tissue of the lingual tonsil will also display increased signal on T2-weighted images and as the lingual tonsils hypertrophy they can appear to project into the intrinsic muscle mass of the tongue. When greatly enlarged and nodular or asymmetric this may be indistinguishable from tumour, however the lack of deep infiltration should suggest that this appearance is due to benign lymphoid hypertrophy.[18] Therefore signal intensity alone cannot accurately diagnose malignancy in the tonsillar region. The thickness of lymphoid tissue in the Waldeyer ring at this level tends to be variable and asymmetric[19] hence soft tissue asymmetry alone should not be viewed as a definitive indication of tumour. The anterior soft palate may have increased signal on T2-weighted MR images due to a concentration of normal minor salivary glands, which is therefore not necessarily pathological.[20] The pharyngoepiglottic folds more commonly appear asymmetric than symmetric.[21]

Neither CT nor MRI are tissue specific. Lymphoma may resemble carcinoma in signal/density characteristics on imaging but necrotic foci within lymph nodes (i.e. low density, resembling fluid) are more commonly seen with squamous carcinoma.[20]

The retropharyngeal space

The retropharyngeal space is a space along the midline of the extracranial portion of the head and neck posterior to the pharynx, which extends from the skull base to the superior mediastinum. It is bounded by the deep layers of the deep cervical fascia, which fuse inferiorly. Both fat and lymph nodes are found in the suprahyoid portion of the retropharyngeal space while only fat is present in the infrahyoid portion. In a feature similar to that of the parapharyngeal space, the retropharyngeal space also provides a conduit for the spread of infection or tumour between the neck and mediastinum.

Mandibular invasion

CT is more sensitive than plain radiography for the detection of mandibular invasion but both these are less sensitive than nuclear bone scanning.[22] Bony invasion of the mandible is best identified on CT when the image is presented with particular bone settings. Attention to precise positioning will ensure that if the change is subtle, the appearances may be compared with the symmetrical opposite side (Figure 3.12). MRI has usurped this role slightly as it has the particular property of detection of bone marrow infiltration although it remains inferior to CT for the detection of cortical bone destruction.

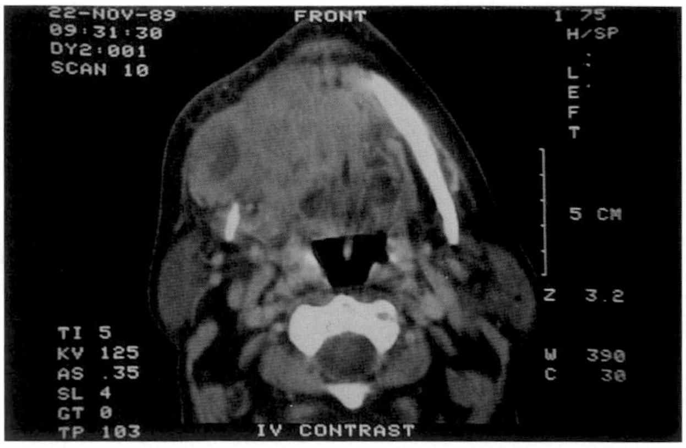

Figure 3.12 A large squamous cell carcinoma extending from the right side of the tongue, through destroyed mandible to involve the skin.

The hypopharynx

Anatomy

The hypopharynx links the oropharynx superiorly to the larynx and oesophagus below. Its boundaries are roughly the hyoid and valleculae above and the cricoid below. Common sites for squamous cell cancers here are the pyriform sinuses, the posterior pharyngeal wall and the postcricoid space. The normal pyriform sinuses are frequently asymmetric both in width and depth

Clinicoradiological correlation

Hypopharyngeal cancer is a disease of the elderly, often presenting in the seventh decade. Presentation is usually late with advanced disease and generally hypopharyngeal tumours have a poor prognosis. Pyriform fossa and postcricoid tumours are equally common but carcinoma of the posterior pharyngeal wall is relatively unusual. Carcinoma of pyriform fossa has the same aetiology as squamous cell carcinomas elsewhere in the head and neck but cancer of the postcricoid region does not. One specific factor associated with postcricoid malignancy is Patterson–Brown–Kelly syndrome of iron-deficiency anaemia, postcricoid web and upper oesophageal stricture. The risk of developing cancer in this condition is 10–30% and malignancy may develop decades after the anaemia has been treated.

Unilateral sore throat, odynophagia and otalgia are early symptoms of hypopharyngeal cancer. True dysphagia and hoarseness tend to develop late. The area of the hypopharynx affected influences the presenting symptoms, for example postcricoid tumours result in early dysphagia whereas this is a late symptom in pyriform fossa cancer.

Submucosal spread is the rule in hypopharyngeal tumours. Pyriform fossa tumours arising from the medial wall may spread into the larynx or may extend superiorly as far as base of tongue (Figure 3.13). Tumours arising from the lateral wall can breach the thyroid cartilage and may invade the thyroid gland. Large pyriform sinus squamous cell tumours often contain areas of decreased density due to necrosis. Postcricoid tumours may extend into the trachea resulting in airway narrowing. The proximity of these lesions to the cervical oesophagus and rich submucosal lymphatic plexus, ensures that skip lesions within the cervical oesophagus are not uncommon and lymph nodes along the internal jugular vein tend to be involved.

Posterior pharyngeal wall tumours are usually large and exophytic by the time of diagnosis (Figure 3.14),

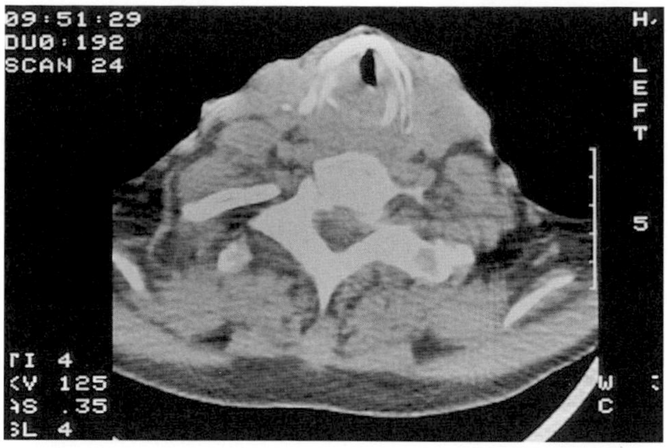

Figure 3.13 Axial CT of squamous cell carcinoma arising in the right pyriform sinus, extending anteriorly to destroy cartilaginous framework.

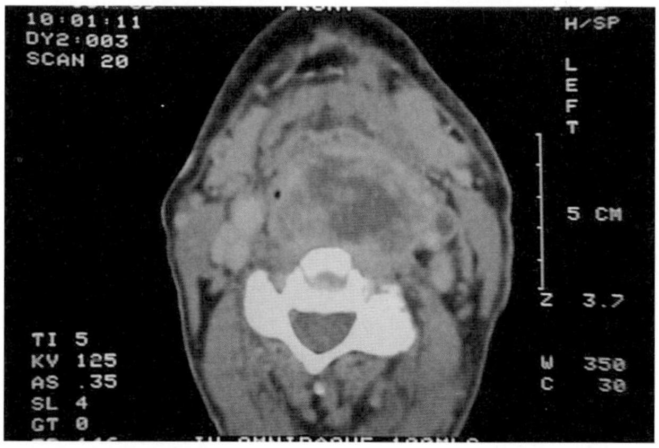

Figure 3.14 Late presentation of a huge locally infiltrative tumour arising in the posterior hypopharynx, shown on axial enhanced CT.

and almost always involve the posterior wall of the oropharynx at diagnosis. As the tumour is so large it tends to ulcerate, typically in a linear pattern.

There is a high incidence of involved lymph nodes in pyriform and posterior pharyngeal wall cancers of approximately 80% but postcricoid tumours have a lower incidence of lymph node involvement. Sites for distant metastatic spread are lung, liver and bone where deposits are usually osteolytic.

The larynx

Anatomy

The larynx communicates with the oropharynx above and the trachea below. Posteriorly it is partly surrounded by the hypopharynx. It may be functionally divided into three important areas. The supraglottis contains epiglottis, aryepiglottic folds, arytenoids, false cords and includes the laryngeal ventricle. The glottis includes the vocal cords and anterior commissure and posterior commissure. The subglottis is limited by the undersurface of the true cords to the inferior margin of the cricoid cartilage.

Clinicoradiological correlations

On imaging, the normal epiglottis is bilaterally symmetrical in thickness and the median glossoepiglottic fold runs forward to the tongue. At this level, the submandibular gland can be recognized laterally as well as the vascular bundle posterolateral to the hyoid bone. The epiglottic fibrocartilage is of soft tissue density, but at the infrahyoid epiglottic level, the pre-epiglottic fat is seen as a low density structure on CT. It is larger above than below and is contiguous laterally with the paraglottic space. This extends inferiorly medial to the thyroid laminae and is therefore related to the aryepiglottic folds and both false and true cords.

The aryepiglottic folds are of equal thickness as they pass inferoposteriorly from the lateral epiglottic margin and merge inferiorly with the false cords to insert at the muscular process of the arytenoid cartilage. Abnormalities of the aryepiglottic folds may be easily identified as they are outlined by air and any asymmetry can be assessed.

The pyriform sinuses form immediate lateral relationships to the aryepiglottic folds. The junction of the false cords anteriorly is much wider and at a more obtuse angle than that of the true cords and this provides a discriminatory feature. The anterior commisure at the true cord level is acutely angled and is composed of soft tissue of minimal thickness and the posterior commisure too, is composed of a thin rim of soft tissue. Normal true vocal cords are symmetrically triangular and of soft tissue density. Mucosa in this area cannot be detected separately from underlying soft tissue and muscle. It should be noted that the laryngeal ventricle lying between the true and false cords may be recognized in only 10% of patients on an axial CT scan.[23] Tumour at this level is detected by enlargement of the cord, irregularity of its margins, and obliteration or replacement of the paraglottic space. This is normally fatty, hence low density or dark on CT and high signal intensity or bright on MR. The true cords are symmetric and of intermediate intensity on MRI but the false cords are slightly more intense on T1-weighted sequences because of the increased loose areolar tissue and extensive mucosal glands.[24] The most consistent feature for identifying the true vocal cord is to identify the forward projection of the arytenoid cartilage.

Virtually all tumours in this area are squamous cell carcinomas of which 30% are supraglottic and virtually all the remainder are glottic (Figures 3.15 and 3.16). Tumour involvement of the pre-epiglottic space requires tumour breaching the fibrocartilage and therefore, when this occurs, the chance of cure by radiotherapy is decreased. Most glottic cancers involve the anterior cord and about one-quarter will be associated with perineural or vascular infiltration. This is poorly detected by CT but may be delineated by MRI.

The arytenoid cartilages are usually homogeneously and symmetrically dense but may appear unequal due to unequal calcification. When tumour involves the arytenoid cartilage, it most commonly causes displacement but sclerosis and erosion have also been known to occur (Figure 3.17).[25] Intravenous contrast medium does not

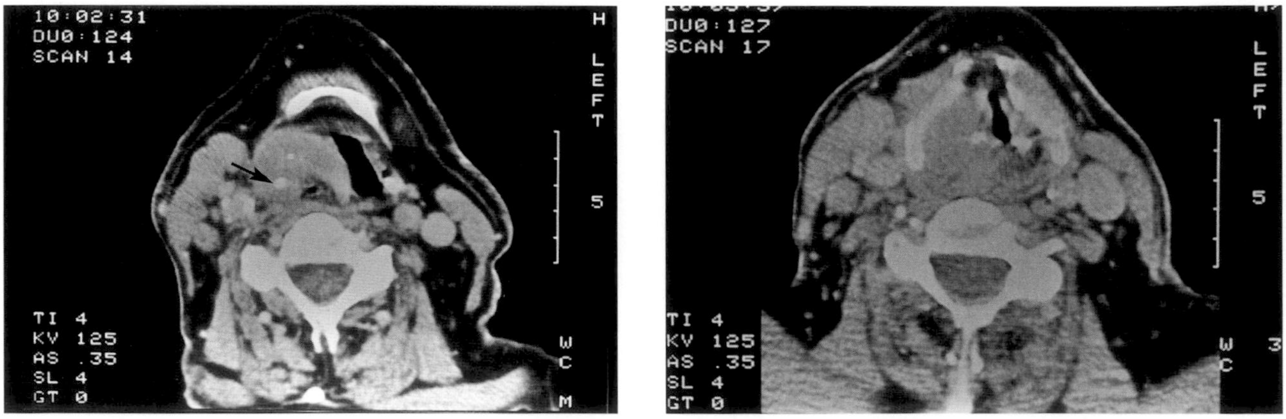

Figures 3.15 and 3.16 Two axial postenhancement CT sections of the same patient show a large supraglottic soft-tissue mass extending from the level of the true cord to the pyriform fossa causing marked airway narrowing. Invasion posterolaterally to the right adjacent to the enhanced vessels (arrow) should be noted.

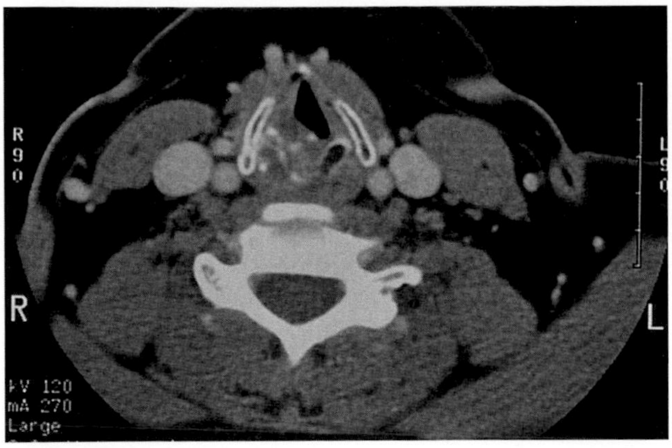

Figure 3.17 CT scan after enhancement showing a bulky tumour centred on the right cord, posteriorly, destroying the adjacent arytenoid.

produce useful enhancement of laryngeal tumours on CT or MRI but its major use is in differentiating lymph nodes from vessels in the neck on CT, especially when their proximity to the carotid sheath suggests pathological adherence. However special vascular imaging sequences in MRI can also perform this function without the requirement for intravenous contrast.

Cartilage invasion

The thyroid cartilages comprise inner and outer layers of cortex with an intervening marrow space. Cartilage sclerosis has been described in normal patients and is also frequently seen after radiotherapy, but normally, the thyroid cartilage will calcify or ossify patchily. This may cause confusion and limit sensitivity when assessing for cartilage destruction by tumour as the inner surfaces may appear irregular in the normal patient because of this patchy calcification (Figure 3.18). The normal thyroid notch anteriorly should not be mistaken for cartilage destruction.

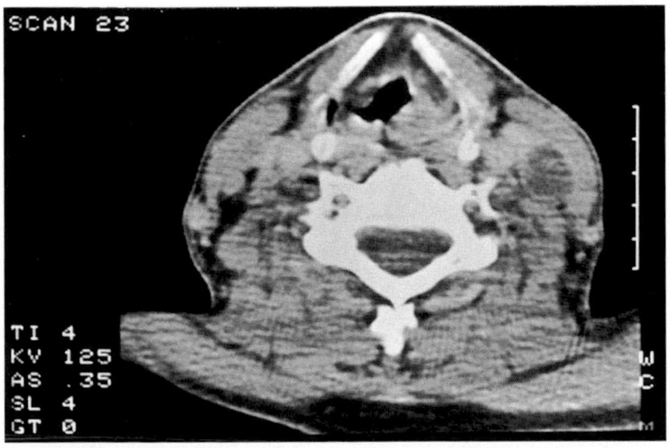

Figure 3.18 An axial CT showing a laryngeal squamous cell carcinoma on the left side posteriorly with an involved ipsilateral low-density lymph node. The cortex of the left thyroid cartilage shows subtle destruction.

Detection of cartilage invasion is important as subsequent radiotherapy seldom eliminates tumour and may secondarily produce perichondritis or even cartilage necrosis. Tumour lying against cartilage is not, in itself, evidence of invasion as the cartilage margin may not be visible if it is not calcified. On MRI, calcification is seen as a signal void and the appearances of cartilage vary with the degree of ossification and marrow deposition within the marrow cavity. Ossified cartilage is low in signal on all sequences and unossified hyaline cartilage is intermediate in signal intensity on T1 and of low intensity on T2. Fatty marrow within ossified hyaline cartilage is high in intensity on T1 and slightly lower intensity on T2 (but still greater than that of muscle) (Figures 3.19, 3.20 and 3.21). In contrast, on CT, fatty marrow is low in density relative to soft tissue and unossified cartilage is relatively high in density. The mucosal surface of the endolarynx is intermediate to high on all MR imaging sequences.[24] On MRI, the muscles are low in intensity on all sequences and the fine intralaryngeal muscles are better seen on MRI than CT.

Ligaments are important barriers to the extension of laryngeal carcinoma and the thyrohyoid, cricothyroid and quadrangular membranes are low in intensity on both T1- and T2-weighted sequences, but cannot be individually demonstrated on CT.[25] Improvement of the MR image after injection of gadolinium may be achieved as tumours are better delineated and there is enhancement of the mucosa. However unenhanced T1-weighted images should be obtained before injection of contrast in order to differentiate between tumour and fat. Comparison between T1-weighted images with and without gadolinium administration appears to be sensitive for detection of cartilage invasion and this technique is also useful in the detection of metastatic lymph nodes.[26] Other authors have argued for the accuracy of other techniques.

The subglottis

The subglottis can be identified by recognizing the cricoid cartilage, which is larger posteriorly, and a medullary cavity can be identified. The anterior part of the cricoid ring slopes downward so the entire cricoid may not be seen in a single slice. The subglottic submucosal space is extremely thin so that any soft tissue recognizable in this area is suggestive of subglottic extension. Primary tumours here are rare but the subglottis should be scrutinized for inferior extension of glottic primaries.

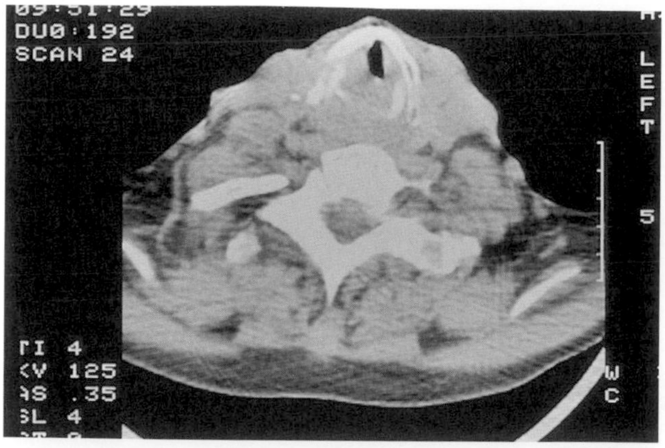

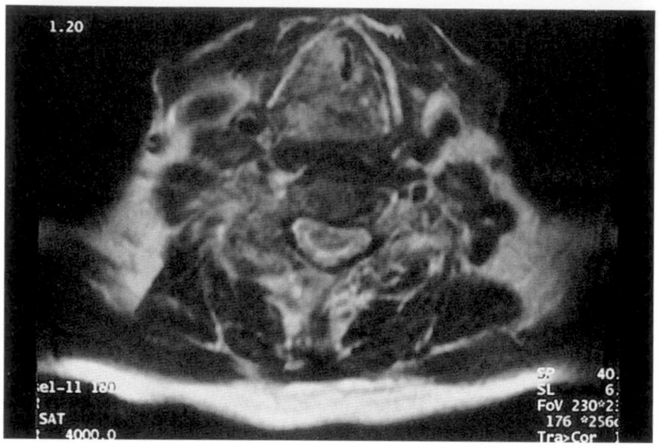

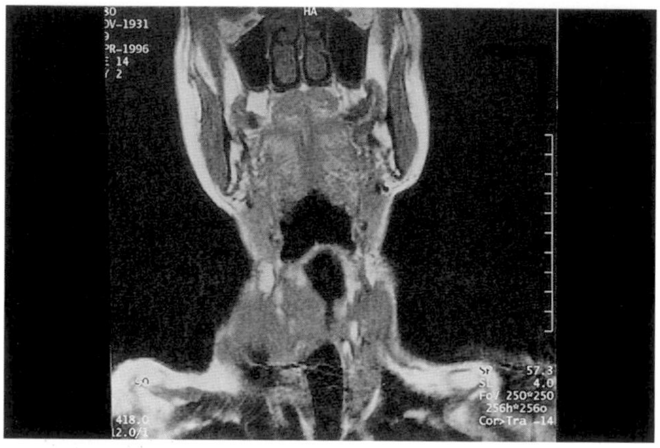

Figures 3.19, 3.20 and 3.21 Axial CT, axial T2- and coronal T1-weighted MRI, demonstrating a transglottic squamous cell carcinoma extending superiorly towards the pyriform sinus. The axial MRI shows that the high signal intensity of marrow within the thyroid cartilage is maintained but delineation of the low signal inner cortex is not as clear on the right as on the left.

The paranasal sinuses

Anatomy: the maxillary antra, ethmoid sinuses and frontal sinuses

The adult ethmoid sinus is narrowest anteriorly in a section known as the osteomeatal complex and this is the site of drainage of the maxillary and frontal sinuses. The lateral margin is the medial orbital wall, which is paper-thin especially anteriorly and is called the lamina papyracea. The posterior wall separates the ethmoids from the sphenoid sinus and superiorly the roof slopes upward to form the cribriform plate.

Frontal sinus pneumatization and size varies considerably in adults. Asymmetry is the norm and frontal sinus floor and posterior walls are thin but anterior walls are rather thicker. The maxillary sinuses or antra lie within the maxillary bone and extend between zygoma and orbital floor. The upper molars and premolars usually form a noticeable bulge into the floor of the sinus.

Clinicoradiological correlation

Occupational hazards for paranasal tumours are exposure to wood and leather dust. Exposure to hardwood dust increases the risk of adenocarcinoma especially of the ethmoid sinus. Softwood woodworkers are also at increased risk of squamous cell carcinoma but outside occupational exposure, the predominant influence on the development of sinus tumours remains smoking.

Common symptoms are unilateral nasal obstruction and rhinorrhoea. Epistaxis is especially associated with lymphoma, malignant melanoma (Figures 3.22 and 3.23) and angiofibroma. Orbital symptoms may be the presenting problem resulting from local invasion, that is proptosis and occasionally diplopia. Dental symptoms are also common and toothache may be the first feature of maxillary or ethmoid carcinoma together with oroantral fistula. Intracranial invasion may be intimated by anosmia

The maxillary sinus is the most common site for paranasal sinus tumours and most arise from the nasal wall (Figures 3.24, 3.25 and 3.26). Tumours are usually squamous cell, adenocarcinoma and adenoid cystic in type in order of frequency. The ethmoid sinuses are occasionally the primary site for malignant disease (Figures 3.22 and 3.23) but frontal and sphenoid sinuses are rarely primarily involved. CT and MRI show opacification of the involved sinus often associated with bone destruction. However, abnormal sclerotic bone may well reflect chronic inflammatory disease rather than malignancy. Imaging is vital for T-staging these tumours whose boundaries are rarely clinically ascertainable and should surgery be precluded the imaging data will be applicable for planning radiation therapy. CT elegantly displays bony involvement and evaluate cervical lymphadenopathy. MRI provides a very sensitive method of evaluating involvement of the dura as well as submucosal spread.

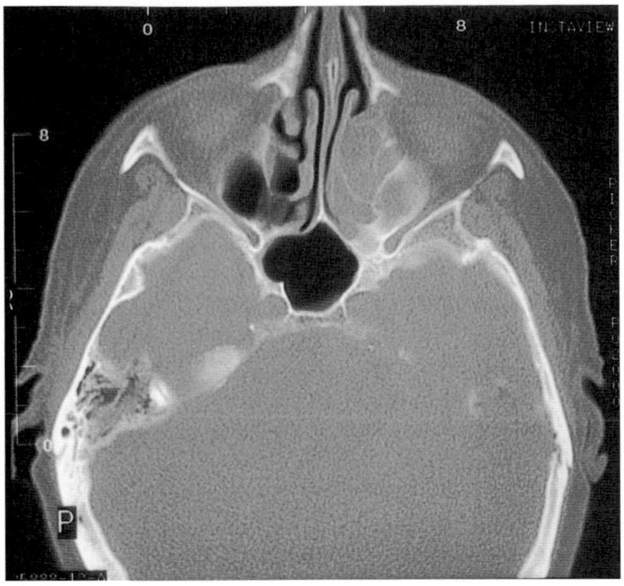

Figure 3.22 Axial unenhanced CT showing a soft tissue polyp arising from the left posterior ethmoids. Note the elegant display of preserved fine bony architecture.

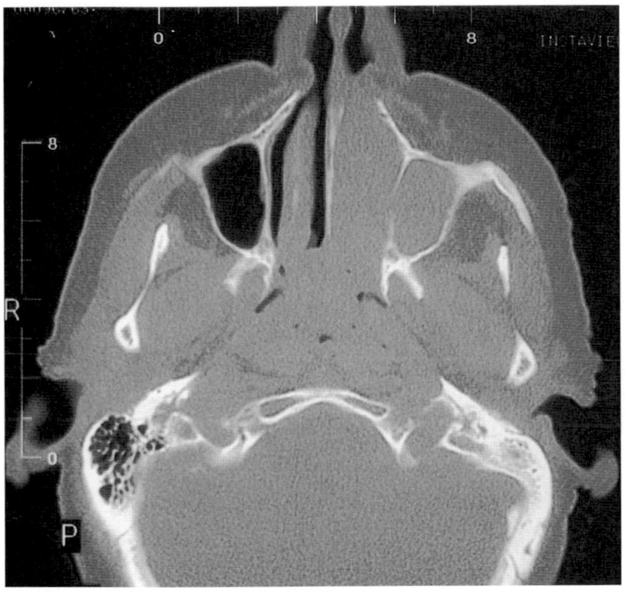

Figure 3.23 At a lower level, the tumour, which proved to be melanoma, fills the left nasal cavity. Opacification of the antrum was due to inspissated mucus indistinguishable on CT from low-density tumour. MRI would more accurately differentiate between the two.

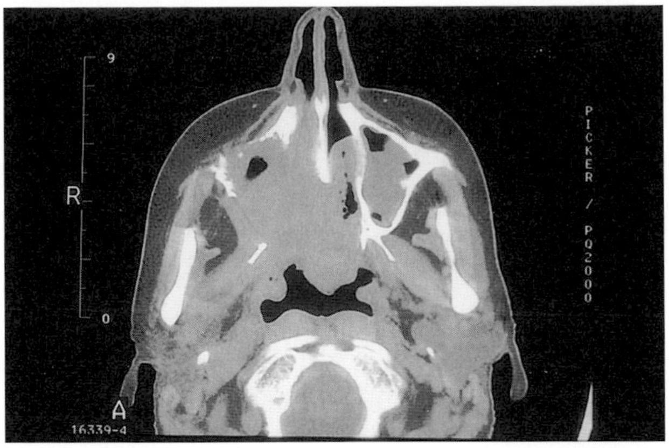

Figure 3.24 Axial CT of extensive squamous cell carcinoma centred on the right maxillary antrum filling its base, breaching medial and posterolateral walls and extension into the nasal cavity.

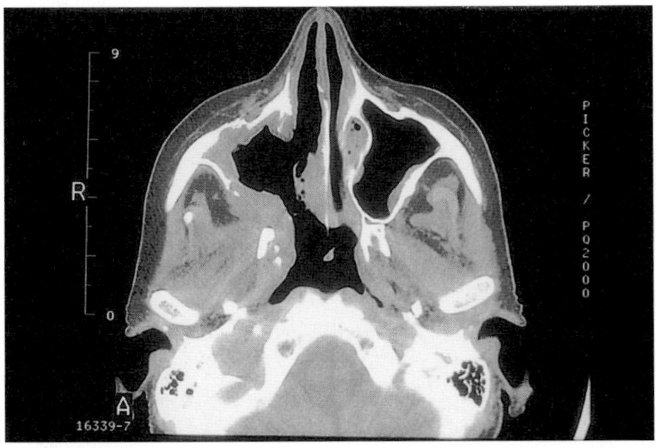

Figure 3.25 Diffuse lateral invasion of right infratemporal fossa more superiorly.

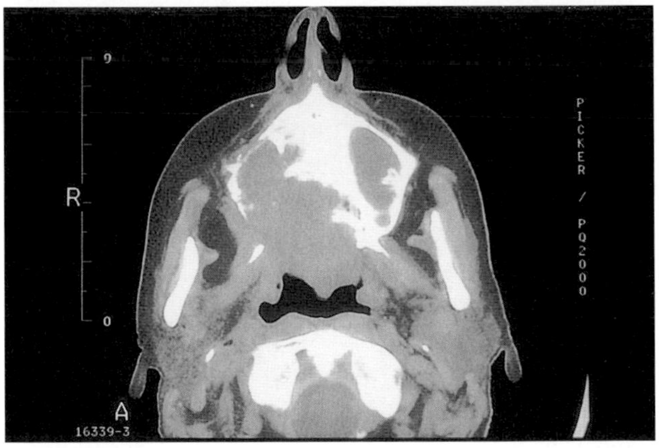

Figure 3.26 Inferior descent of maxillary sinus tumour with destruction of antral floor and hard palate and tumour encroachment into the oral cavity.

Both MR and CT examinations should include coronal views as well as conventional axial sections. MRI, especially T2-weighted studies, is superior to CT with respect to distinction between tumour, normal mucosa and entrapped secretions. Bone destruction is usually evident on CT, but may be simulated by non-ossified parts of the medial wall of the maxillary sinus. These studies will display any tumour spread to pterygopalatine fossa, the orbit (via the infraorbital fissure), the middle cranial fossa (via foramen rotundum), the palate and through the ethmoid sinus to the anterior cranial fossa.

Paranasal cancers involve regional lymph nodes in 25–35% of cases. Distant spread occurs occasionally, usually to the lungs and rarely to bone. Thus chest radiography should form part of the routine imaging algorithm, supplemented where necessary by targeted bone films or isotope bone scanning.

Thyroid and parathyroid glands

Thyroid: clinicoradiological correlations

The incidence of thyroid nodules at autopsy is reported as high as 50% although the incidence of palpable thyroid nodules is estimated at only 4–7% of the general adult population, and occurring more frequently in women and increasing with increasing age.[27,28] Slightly less than 5% of thyroid nodules are found to be malignant.[29]

Four procedures commonly used for the evaluation of thyroid nodules are: ultrasound; radionuclide imaging; CT; and fine-needle aspiration biopsy (FNAB). Thyroid scintigraphy can be performed using the radioisotopes technetium-99m or ^{123}I. Thyroid gland imaging for head and neck surgery is mainly concerned with establishing the function and morphology of clinically detected thyroid nodules.

High-resolution ultrasound employing high-frequency transducers of 5–10 MHz detects many impalpable nodules and seeks to tissue characterize them. Although certain appearances suggest a benign aetiology, such as uniform echogenicity and well-defined margins or a malignant aetiology with complex masses, irregular outline and posterior acoustic shadowing, ultrasound appearances alone are not specific enough for the characterization of thyroid nodules and this test should not therefore be used as the sole imaging method in the evaluation of a clinically suspicious nodule. The ultrasound test may be supplemented by guided fine-needle biopsy so that cells may be retrieved from the most suspicious area shown on imaging.

Alternatively, ultrasound may be combined with radionuclide imaging, which provides a functional as well as a morphological imaging method. Iodine-123 is trapped and organified, has a high target to background ratio but is not readily available and consequently very expensive. In contrast, technetium-99m is trapped but not organified, is more readily available, is easily administered intravenously and useful images are produced within 20–30 minutes of injection. Consequently it remains the most commonly used thyroid imaging agent. Radionuclide imaging provides anatomical information and can detect physiological information. This is not an imaging modality for precise anatomic imaging as the resolution is generally in the order of 0.5–1 cm.[30] Although less specific than conventional imaging and a focus of high activity can be due to both tumour and infection, nonetheless nuclear medicine is highly sensitive to abnormalities usually secondary to an alteration in function.

An ultrasound will rapidly differentiate innocent cystic masses from solid nodules. The complementary radionuclide test will differentiate active, benign thyroid solid nodules from inactive, that is 'cold' solid lesions, which are thus suspicious. Innocent cysts will also be cold but these will have been demonstrated on ultrasound.

The patient is imaged by means of an array of radioactivity detectors, which are interfaced with a computer. When the computer is combined with a camera that can rotate 360 degrees around the body, reconstructed tomographic images in any plane may be achieved by the use of emitted gamma rays (single-photon emission computed tomography or SPECT) or positrons (positron emission tomography or PET). The latter technique utilizes specially labelled short lived tracers, for example fluorinated glucose, which necessitate access to a cyclotron. Although this is therefore expensive and not widely available it is producing outstanding results in identifying active small-volume recurrent cancer, which may be hidden in innocent postoperative scarring.

Thyroid nodules shown on radionuclide imaging are classified according to the amount of activity present. Hyperfunctional or 'hot' nodules concentrate more radionuclide than the normal areas of the gland and hypofunctional or 'cold' lesions show little or no concentration of radiopharmaceutical by the nodule and are suspicious if ultrasound shows them to be solid. Thyroid scintigraphy will therefore determine which nodules should have FNAC or excision. The vast majority of hot nodules are autonomous functioning thyroid adenomas and show preferential suppression of function of extra-nodular tissue. These should be correlated with thyroid function tests in which enough thyroid hormone should be produced to suppress pituitary TSH production. They are generally benign, although carcinoma has been described in a small percentage.[31]

About 85–90% of solitary nodules are cold, but only 6–10% of cold nodules are malignant.[32] Indeterminate nodules comprise approximately 4–7% of solitary nodules and, as with cold nodules, require biopsy. It is also wise to biopsy dominant cold nodules when part of a multinodular goitre as similar rates of malignancy in both solitary and multiple cold nodules were found in a recent review of 5637 patients.[33]

Isotope tests can also be used for identification of thyroid tissue in ectopic sites when iodine-123, which is a longer lasting agent with better signal characteristics, is a superior agent. This can also be used to detect metastases of thyroid carcinoma after total thyroidectomy, and is more sensitive for bony thyroid metastases than conventional bone scanning using technetium-99m. Thallium-201 labelled agent, which acts as a potassium analogue, has been recommended for routine follow-up of thyroid cancer patients[34] as it is known to accumulate in metastatic foci of differentiated thyroid carcinoma. It has been suggested by Charkes et al that thallium imaging can be improved by combining with SPECT imaging.[35] CT and MRI are useful for the evaluation of extension of malignancy beyond the margins of the thyroid (Figure 3.27).

Parathyroid: clinicoradiological correlations

The parathyroid glands and thyroid gland may be imaged using thallium-201 or Tc-99m sestamibi. Technetium-99m pertechnetate images the thyroid but not parathyroid thus when both are administered the respective images may be digitally subtracted by computer, one from another, and abnormalities such as adenomas, hyperplasia or carcinoma may be localized within one of the parathyroid glands. Frequently these tests are combined with ultrasound, CT or MR but the whole subject of imaging in hyperparathyroidism is controversial and some advocate the use of imaging in the investigation of recurrent disease only.

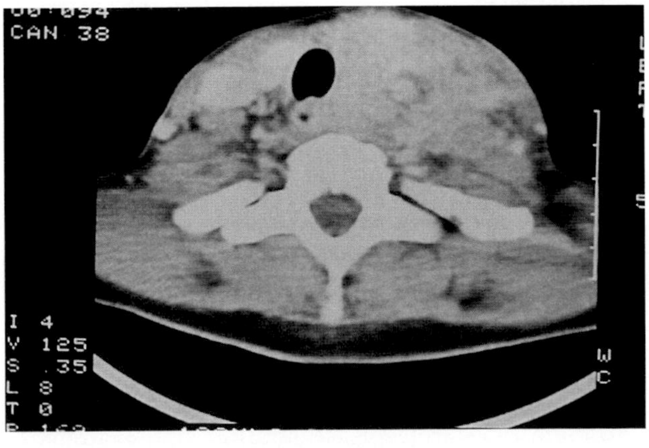

Figure 3.27 Enhanced axial CT showing expansion of the left lobe of thyroid due to medullary carcinoma with invasion of the tumour into the prevertebral muscles and deviation of the trachea from the midline.

Salivary glands

Parotid, submandibular, sublingual and minor salivary glands: clinicoradiological correlations

Specific methods for imaging the salivary glands include sialography, which involves the direct injection of radiopaque contrast into the relevant duct followed by the acquisition of radiographic or CT images, and ultrasound, CT or MRI. Sialography is an invasive and unpleasant examination that is of benefit in diagnosing ductal abnormalities such as sialectasis but it does not make significant contribution in the detection of masses and, even when combined with CT, does not provide significant added information over that provided by a conventional enhanced CT.

Ultrasound is very useful in the primary examination for parotid and submandibular tumours. Ultrasound is, however, limited by its inability to interrogate the deeper aspects of the gland and its quality and value is related to the experience of the operator. Contrast-enhanced CT provides better evaluation of extension into the deep lobe of the parotid and provides evaluation of surrounding structures. Survey for enlarged cervical lymph nodes, evaluation of anatomical relationships and tumour calcification are more readily demonstrated by CT.[36] The US and CT features of parotid and submandibular malignancies are generally an irregular parenchyma and an ill-defined border, a markedly inhomogenous internal structure, lymph node metastases, and invasion of the surrounding structures.

On ultrasound the echogenicities of both the parotid and submandibular glands are similarly homogeneous and higher than that of surrounding muscles and fatty tissue. Malignancies appear as poorly echogenic masses relative to the surrounding parenchyma but tissue differentiation on tissue echogenicity alone is not possible. On CT, the parotid gland is usually shown to be of much lower density than adjacent muscles and greater in density than the surrounding fat and is thus usually easily demonstrated. Following intravenous contrast, the salivary glands take up iodine avidly so that their density increases substantially rendering them more visible but also delineating the relationship of the enhanced adjacent great vessels. Unlike the parotid gland, the submandibular gland rarely contains fat and therefore the parenchyma is more radiodense than the parotid gland on unenhanced CT. It is not surprising, therefore, that submandibular tumours are often isodense with the gland parenchyma and parotid tumours appearing to be relatively radiodense.

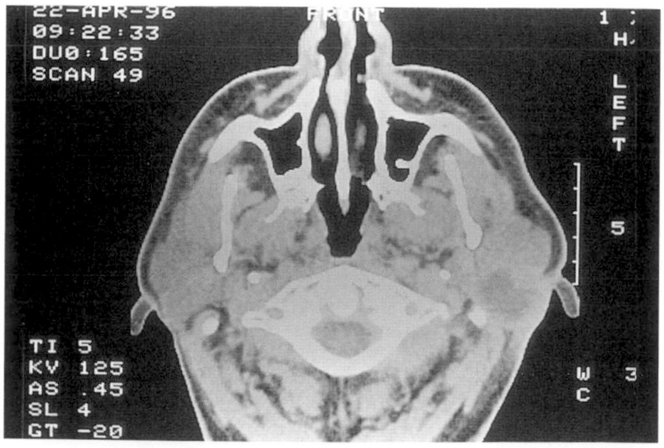

Figure 3.28 The low-density area within the enhanced left parotid gland on this axial CT was confirmed as carcinoma on biopsy.

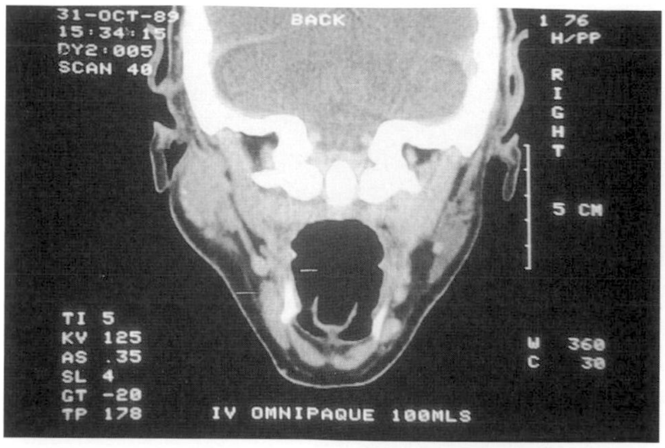

Figure 3.29 Coronal postcontrast CT demonstrates enlargement of the left parotid gland secondary to lymphoma.

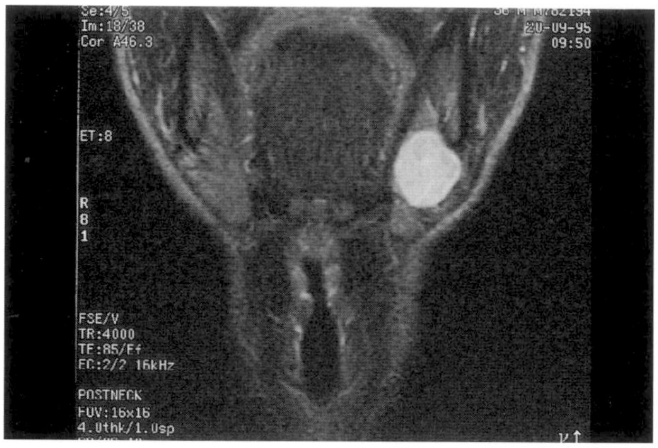

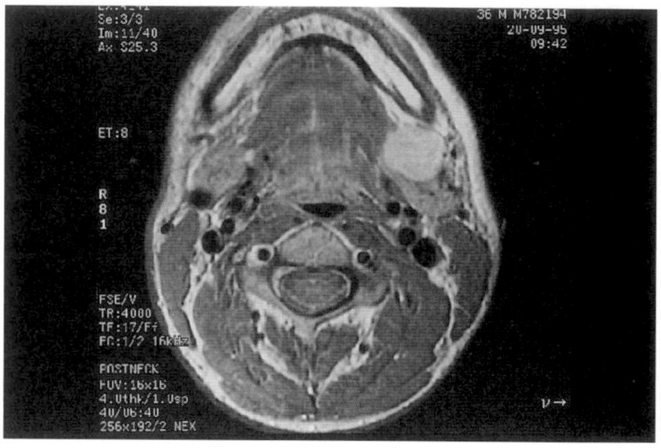

Figures 3.30 and 31 Coronal and axial T2-weighted MRI demonstrating the characteristic high signal of a well-defined rounded pleomorphic adenoma in the left submandibular gland.

Bryan et al found on CT that benign salivary tumours were discrete, sharply marginated and of relatively high density embedded in an otherwise normal gland, but invasive malignant tumours were poorly defined, relatively radiodense lesions that obliterated or transgressed adjacent fat and fascial planes (Figures 3.28 and 3.29).[37] The incidence of malignancy is much higher for submandibular tumours than for parotid tumours, that is 47% and 25% respectively of all salivary gland tumours.[38] However, adenoid cystic carcinoma has a particular propensity to involve the submandibular gland, unlike the parotid, and is manifest as a well-defined mass within the affected gland.

Lymphoma affects the lymph nodes within the parotid gland, but importantly there are no nodes inside the submandibular gland and lymphoma of the submandibular gland is most unusual. A quarter of all pleomorphic adenomas (Figures 3.30 and 3.31) eventually undergo malignant change, if left in situ[39] and the presence of focal calcification within a parotid mass suggests an old pleomorphic adenoma and thus an increased risk of developing carcinoma. The delineation of the facial nerve, lateral to the styloid process and posterolateral to the retromandibular vein, can aid surgical planning as tumours, if small enough, may be localized as deep to or superficial to the facial nerve.

Fine-needle aspiration biopsy of a mass under ultrasound control can be performed for tissue characterization.

On MRI parotid glandular parenchyma has a higher signal intensity compared with muscle and lower than that of fat on T1- and T2-weighted images. A disadvantage of MR is, however, the poor sensitivity for calculi within the gland. The facial nerve and main duct are seen as medium signal intensity on all sequences but the nerve running through the gland cannot be distinguished on CT. As elsewhere, MRI is unable to reliably differentiate benign from malignant tumours except in the case of vascular

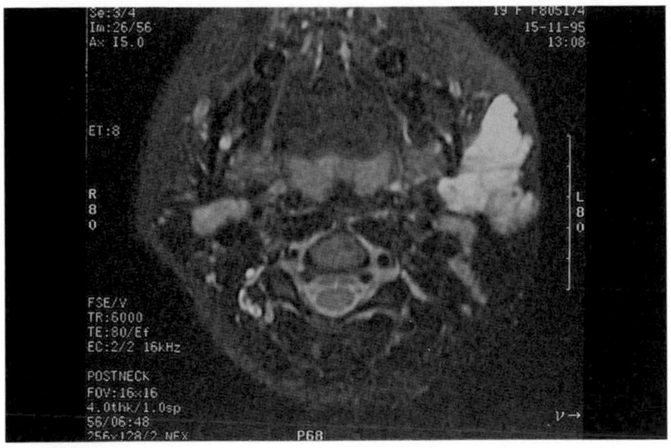

Figure 3.32 This left parotid haemangioma is less well defined than the adenoma, has a more amorphous pattern and characteristically shows increased signal with increasing T2 weighting, exhibiting similar signal characteristics to fluid on this heavily T2-weighted image.

malformations (Figure 3.32) although with gadolinium enhancement irregular margins can suggest the presence of an infiltrating tumour. Smoothly marginated masses may be either benign or malignant but precise differentiation of malignant tumours is also not possible on MRI.[40]

Enlargement of a nerve in association with a salivary gland neoplasm is strongly suspicious for malignant perineural spread and this is a particular characteristic of adenoid cystic carcinoma. Perineural extension along the facial nerve will obliterate the normal fat beneath the stylomastoid foramen and may ultimately expand the foramen.

Salivary gland scintigraphy may be employed and this technique utilizes technetium-99m pertechnetate. The parotid and submandibular glands may be identified but not usually the sublingual glands. The major application of radionuclide imaging is in the assessment of function in salivary gland masses. Whether the lesion is 'hot' or 'cold' is nonspecific but, the incidence of malignancy in hot salivary masses, as in hot thyroid nodules, is extremely rare.

Lymph node disease

Anatomy

The classification of cervical lymph nodes is in transition from the classic anatomical system of Rouviere, described in 1934 and based in part on the surface triangles of the neck to the simpler numerical or level system (Table 3.3).[41]

Table 3.3 Lymph node levels

Level I	Submandibular and submental triangle (above the posterior belly of digastric)
Level II	Deep to sternomastoid and posteroinferior to the posterior belly of digastric extending from the base of skull to hyoid
Level III	Deep to sternomastoid extending from the hyoid to cricoid
Level IV	Deep to sternomastoid extending from the cricoid to the clavicle
Level V	The posterior triangle (anterior to trapezius and posterior to the sternomastoid)
Level VI	Anterior compartment including the thyroid, paratracheal and paraoesophageal areas

Clinicoradiological correlations

The clinical asymmetrical enlargement of one or more cervical lymph nodes in an adult has at least an 85% chance of being the result of malignant disease.[42] Lymphoma should be considered when multiple, non-necrotic, well-defined nodes with intact capsules are present or multiple sites of disease are identified in extranodal tissue (Figure 3.33).

CT is more accurate than palpation in determination of size and number of pathologically involved nodes. The literature is in agreement regarding the ability of CT to upstage clinically negative necks. The accuracy of nodal staging with CT (90–95%) has been shown to be superior to the accuracy obtained by clinical nodal staging (75–80%).[43,44] There is a predominance of metastatic lymph node involvement in levels II, III and IV, and levels I and V tend not to be involved without involvement of the other levels.[45]

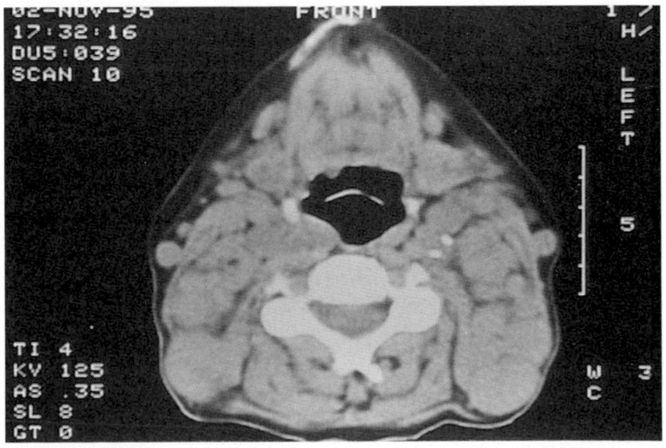

Figure 3.33 This non-contrast CT shows extensive bilateral cervical lymph node enlargement. The nodes are well defined, with intact capsules, typical of lymphoma.

Criteria for malignancy

Van den Breckel et al[43] determined that lymph node size and shape varied among different regions of the neck and formulated different criteria for their consequent staging. Lymph nodes to be considered metastatic are:

1. Nodes with a minimum axial diameter of 11 mm or more in the subdigastric region or 10 mm or more in other lymph node regions;
2. Groups of three or more lymph nodes of borderline size (9–10 mm in the subdigastric area and 8–9 mm in other lymph node areas);
3. All nodes that on CT show irregular enhancement or are surrounded by a rim of enhancing material.

The presence of an ipsilateral nodal metastasis reduces survival by 50% and contralateral nodal disease is said to reduce life expectancy by a further 25%. Thus, its demonstration on imaging has a crucial impact on management and survival. Central low-density ring enhancement 'necrosis' has been found to be 100% specific in the radiologic diagnosis for the presence of metastatic squamous cell lymphadenopathy but only 74% sensitive.[43,46] Radiographically, central necrosis refers to nodes demonstrating central low-density on CT (Figures 3.34 and 3.35), but the low-density centre is recognized by virtue of the enhancing rim on CT, or central low intensity on fat suppressed, contrast-enhanced T1-weighted MR sequences. The central component may actually represent true necrosis, particularly when large masses are present, but viable, but less-well enhancing tumour is often found on histological examination.

Pitfalls in diagnosing low density nodes may however occur. Ring nodal contrast enhancement may represent central tumour necrosis, cystic tumour growth or keratinization within a node.[12] Necrosis can be simulated by cysts, abscesses, spontaneous lymph node necrosis or adipose metaplasia. Occasionally thrombus within the jugular vein will show ring enhancement around the central clot and may thus simulate a nodal metastasis. When the latter occurs centrally, it may mimic necrosis within a contrast-enhanced node. However MRI may help distinguish between the two as fat has a characteristically high signal on both T1- and T2-weighted images whereas the high water content associated with necrosis follows the signal of water, that is low (dark) on T1- and high (bright) on T2-weighted images. Lymph nodes, however, enhance following contrast administration and may be therefore less conspicuous against a background of high signal intensity fat. It follows therefore that a fat suppression technique to eliminate the fat tissue signal should be employed.[47]

Munck et al have found nodal necrosis appears to be a predictive factor for the efficacy of chemotherapy. The greater the degree of necrosis, the poorer the response to chemotherapy.[48]

Comparisons between T1-weighted images with and without gadolinium administration seem to be very sensitive for the detection of metastatic lymph nodes,[26] but the accuracy of MRI is felt presently to be inferior in identifying central necrosis although gadolinium enhancement may be helpful for extranodal tumour spread.[44,46] T2-weighted imaging[49] and T1- and T2-weighted gradient echo imaging are sequences of choice for other authors for detection of lymph node metastases.[50] Currently, CT is far superior to MR in the demonstration of extranodal disease extension, which in itself decreases by a further 50% the outcome expectancy.

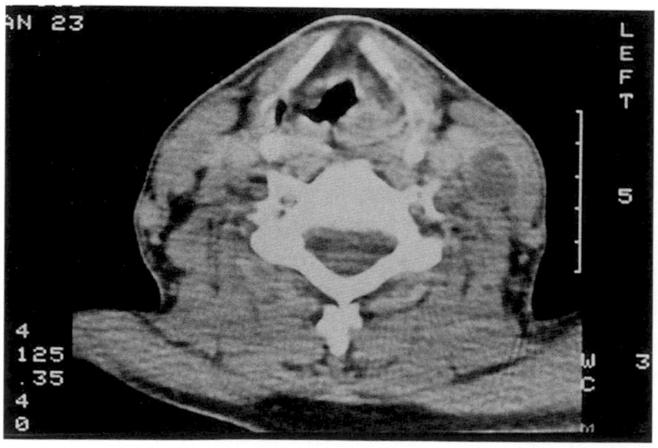

Figure 3.34 A 1.5-cm metastasis in a left-sided node deep to sternocleidomastoid, showing typical rim enhancement. The adjacent supraglottic carcinoma is also evident on this enhanced CT scan.

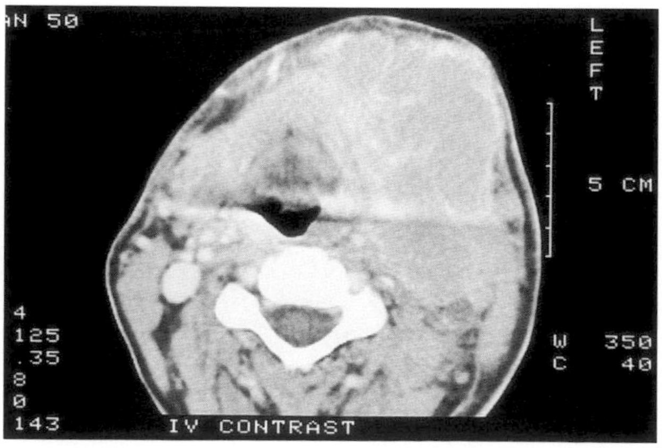

Figure 3.35 Axial contrast enhanced CT showing a large left anterolateral composite lymph node mass with areas of low density as well as peripheral enhancement. The demonstration of extracapsular extension defines poor prognostic implication.

Extranodal spread

Extranodal spread of tumour is diagnosed whenever the lymph node exhibits capsular enhancement, ill-defined margins and apparent involvement of adjacent tissues. The frequency of extranodal disease is greatest in larger malignant nodes but extranodal extension in CT-pathological studies has been found in almost a quarter of nodes which are 1 cm or smaller.[46] There is a very high likelihood of fixation and invasion if tumour involves three quarters or more of the circumference of the carotid and if there is evidence of capsular penetration and surgical cure is severely compromised in this circumstance.[51]

Ultrasound

The normal lymph node on ultrasound is an ovoid low echogenic structure with an echogenic fatty hilus. Patterns of infiltration are not specific enough to enable a confident diagnosis; however, replacement of the fatty hilus and change in morphology of the node such as enlargement or change in shape is suspicious. High-frequency ultrasound is useful in assessing nodal disease in the neck and a sensitivity rate of 92.6% has been recorded versus a 78% sensitivity rate for clinical examination in similar circumstances.[52] Ultrasound-guided FNAC is valuable in assessment of possible metastatic or recurrent disease. The use of this technique may well invalidate the need for open biopsy in the initial assessment of a metastatic lymph node deposit prior to search for a primary. Open biopsy has been documented as increasing the incidence of recurrence at the biopsy site and distant metastasis.[53]

Fine-needle aspiration cytology

FNAC of a suspected malignant neck lump when the primary remains occult will diagnose as many as 95% of cervical metastatic squamous cell carcinomas but is much less accurate for other tumour types.[54] Ultrasound will differentiate between vessel thrombosis and severe compression by the use of dynamic colour flow or doppler technique after performing a Valsalva manoeuvre. Whereas CT can readily detect thrombosis but may miss vascular compression, extracapsular extension cannot be determined by ultrasound.[52]

All imaging modalities suffer from limited sensitivity for lymph node disease when the tissue planes have been destroyed by previous radical neck dissection or by radiotherapy.

Microscopic metastases within lymph nodes of normal size go undetected on CT and with MRI. Abnormal lymph nodes have to be identified on these imaging tests by the presence of mass effect or by characteristics of location. Van den Breckel et al did not find any combination of lymph node shape with the minimal axial diameter as valid a criterion for accuracy as the minimal axial diameter alone.[55]

2-Deoxy-2-[fluorine-18] fluoro-D-glucose (FDG) PET imaging may be applicable as a functional tumour detection alternative to anatomic imaging techniques.

Post-treatment radiological changes

Resection

Surgery in the neck is applied to the resection of the primary tumour, regional lymph node dissection, reconstruction and revision after recurrence. A number of studies has shown a predictable involvement of certain lymph node groups (see above), and disease is less likely in other nodal groups. Therefore the concept of removing only the high-risk nodes and leaving the low-risk nodes has arisen[56,57] and differing surgical approaches to neck dissections all have differing appearances on imaging. Assessment by means of identifying the symmetry between tissues in patients in whom a major resection, combined with a neck dissection and possibly a reconstruction has been performed without adequate clinical information is, therefore, unwise. Precise surgical information on the extent of surgical resection and the type of flap used for repair is needed if correct assessment of the postsurgical changes is to be made.[58]

A radical neck dissection removes all lymph nodes from level I to V, the ipsilateral submandibular gland, the internal jugular vein, the sternocleidomastoid muscle and the spinal accessory nerve. This can be recognized on a plain chest X-ray or CT with time as the denervated trapezius muscle causes a progressive ipsilateral shoulder drop. The appearances on CT or MRI show a noticeable flattening of the ipsilateral neck, absence of the internal jugular vein and sternocleidomastoid muscle, blurring of local tissue planes and the demonstration of the common carotid artery lying immediately deep to the skin (Figures 5.36 and 5.37). An extended radical neck dissection results from the inclusion in the resection of additional lymph node groups and/or non-lymphatic structures not automatically included in a radical neck dissection and produces further anatomical distortion.

A modified radical neck dissection refers to the preservation of non-lymphatic structures normally removed in a radical neck dissection (Figure 3.38)

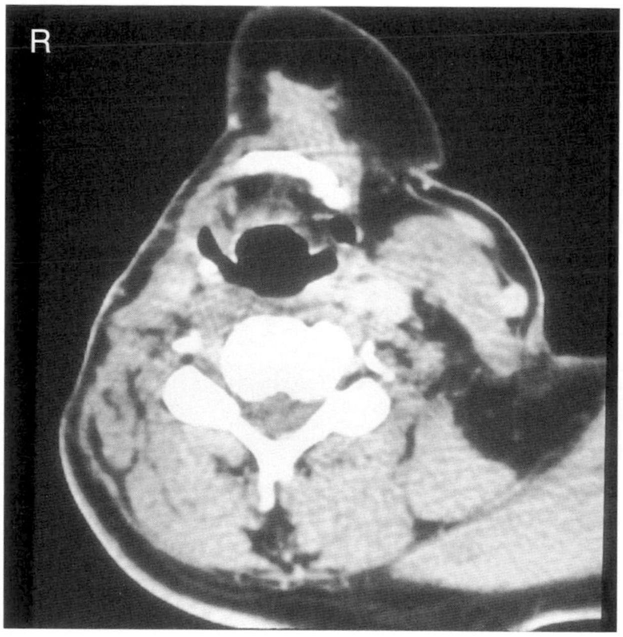

Figure 3.36 Right-sided radical neck dissection at the level of the hyoid bone shown on axial CT.

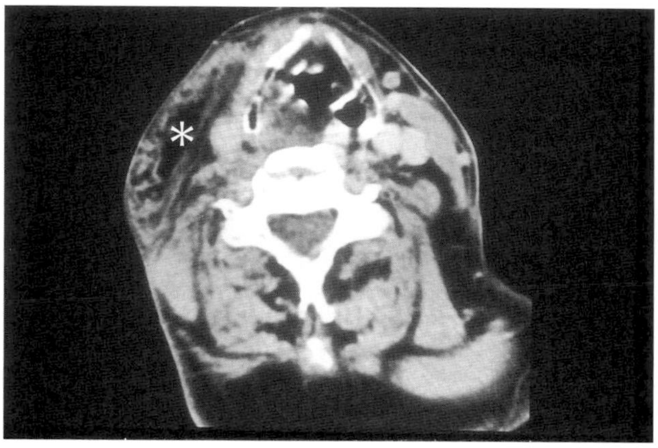

Figure 3.37 Right-sided neck dissection with the formation of a trapezius muscle flap (*). As it is denervated, the muscle has wasted and become fatty.

but when there is preservation of one or more lymph node groups, normally removed in a radical neck dissection, the operation is termed a selective neck dissection. These may be a supraomohyoid neck dissection, a posterolateral neck dissection, a lateral neck dissection, or an anterior compartment neck dissection. When a limited neck dissection has been performed the postsurgical appearances may be almost normal in radiological appearance and the only radiological finding may be skin thickening at the operative site. As in the radical neck dissection whenever level I nodes are removed (the submandibular lymph nodes), the submandibular gland is also removed to aid in controlling tumour spread.

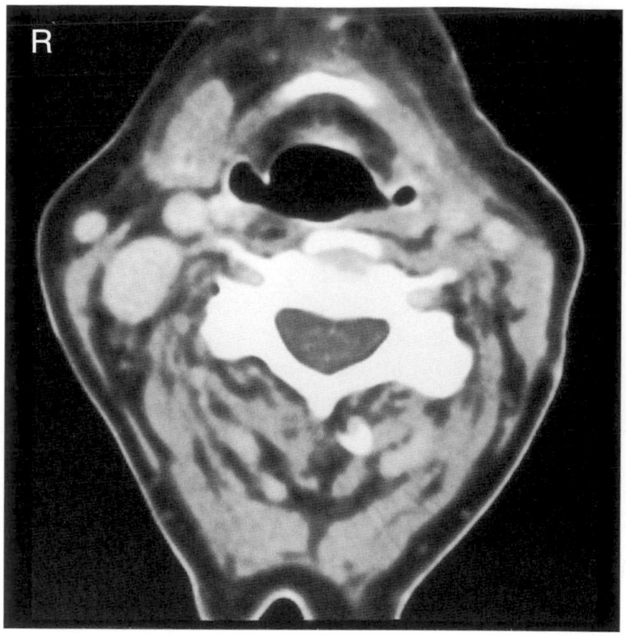

Figure 3.38 This is an example of a modified left-sided neck dissection at the hyoid bone level. The submandibular gland and upper levels of lymph nodes have been removed on the left but the sternocleidomastoid muscle and internal jugular vein are preserved.

The supraomohyoid neck dissection is used in patients with oral cavity and oropharyngeal tumours with stage N0 or N1 neck disease and removes the nodes in levels I, II and III but leaves nodes in levels IV and V.[59]

A posterolateral neck dissection is associated with the surgical treatment of cutaneous malignancies in the posterior portion of the scalp and the neck and refers to removal of the suboccipital and retroauricular lymph nodes in addition to removal of lymph nodes from level II to V. A lateral neck dissection is used for stage T1 glottic carcinomas and stage N0 neck disease and removes level II to IV lymph nodes.[60] An anterior compartment neck dissection is used most in treatment of thyroid cancer and extends from the hyoid bone to the suprasternal notch between the common carotid arteries. It involves removal of midline visceral neck structures including level VI nodes.

Immediately postoperatively, neck dissection causes local trauma resulting in localized haemorrhage and oedema. This can obscure anatomical detail; thus the timing of any routine baseline postoperative scan should be at least 4–6 weeks after the operation. This allows healing and resolution of oedema and haemorrhage to occur, enabling a better assessment of the postoperative prognostic status. This healing process is prolonged if postoperative radiotherapy

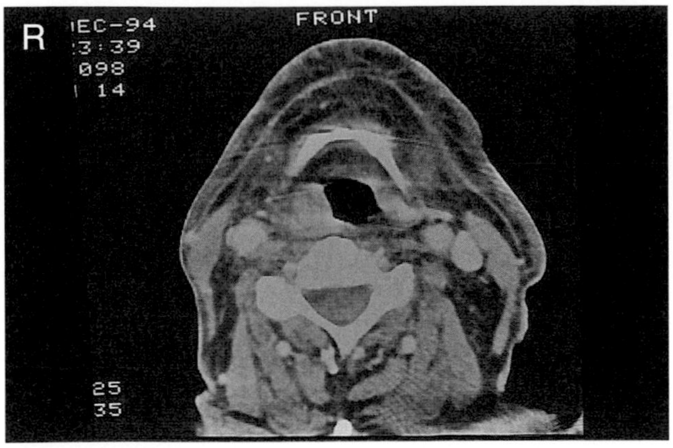

Figure 3.39 Enhanced axial CT of the neck following recent radiotherapy for a right pyriform fossa tumour. The low-density fat is interspersed with fine reticulations and lines consistent with acute radiation change.

has been given. In the immediate postoperative period, residual haemorrhage will initially be slightly irregular and appear infiltrative of the fatty and soft tissue planes. This may mimic an infiltrating tumour and appropriate clinical information is, again, vital. Further follow-up scans will demonstrate shrinkage and its margins will become more sharply defined and undergo fibrous replacement. Although most purely oedematous changes eventually resolve, there is usually a persistent thickening of the skin and the subcutaneous fat may have a lace like pattern of stranding structures that represent obstructed venules and lymphatics. These features may persist for years (Figure 3.39).[61]

On MR imaging, haemorrhage may have a high signal on both T1- and T2-weighted images due to its methaomoglobin content. Over time this signal decreases to a low/intermediate signal on T1- and bright (to muscle) on T2-weighted images. This indicates a transition to a vascular scar. Eventually haemosiderin is deposited which causes low/absent signal intensity on all sequences signalling inactive scar.

Repair and reconstruction

In the oral cavity a partial glossectomy may be recognized on imaging by loss of symmetry of the extrinsic muscles and a decrease in the volume of intrinsic musculature. The defect is replaced by low density fat within the muscle used for repair and this may subsequently atrophy (Figure 3.40 and 3.41).

Surgical defects may be repaired with cutaneous, myocutaneous or free flaps. Cutaneous flaps include skin and subcutaneous tissue. Myocutaneous flaps are composed of muscle, skin and subcutaneous

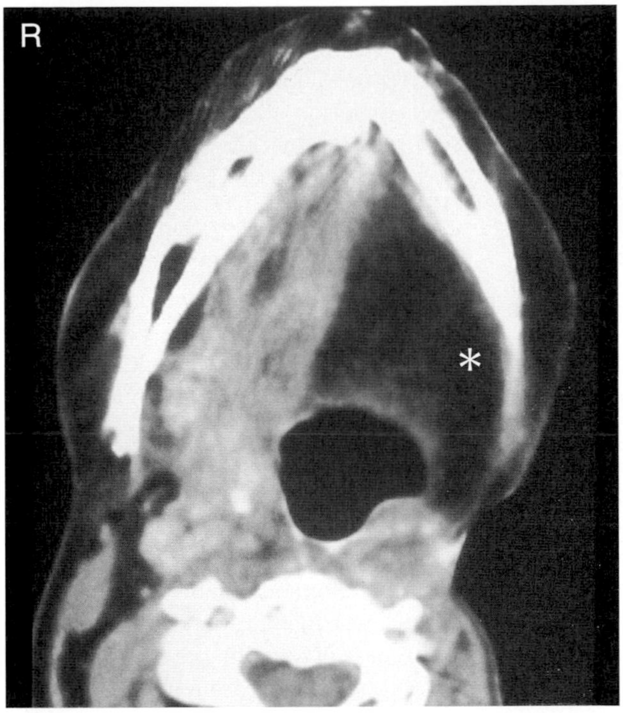

Figure 3.40 A hemiglossectomy and reconstruction with myocutaneous flap has been performed here for a glossal cancer, that has not crossed the median raphe. The preserved muscle on the right is of normal soft-tissue density whilst the inserted flap has become fatty and low in density (*).

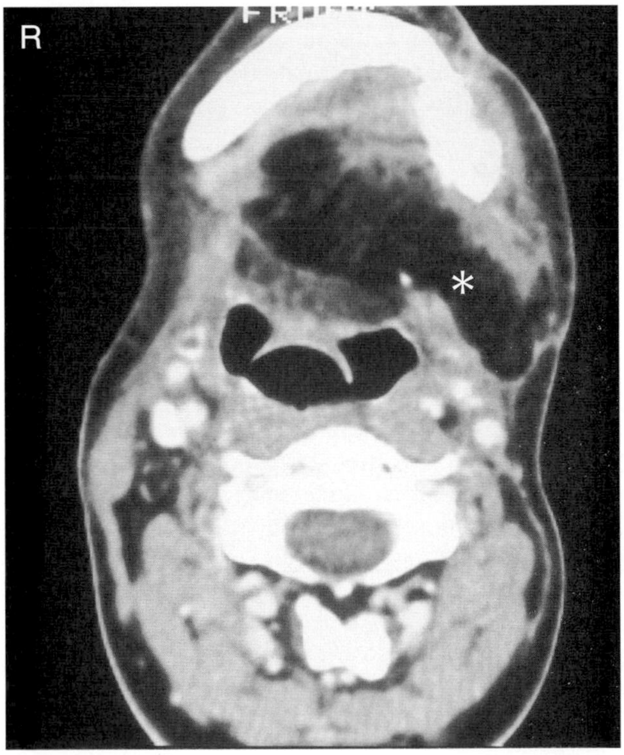

Figure 3.41 Replacement of the tongue musculature by a myocutaneous flap after total glossectomy, shown on axial CT (*).

tissue. Osteocutaneous or osteomyocutaneous flaps contain vascularized bone and skin alone or bone and skin with muscle. These are most commonly used in the reconstruction of mandibular defects. The bone is fixed to the remaining bone by metallic internal fixation, which will produce imaging artefacts on both CT and MR.

Flaps may be local and arise in the head and neck region and may be raised on a pedicle from the forehead, nasolabial or deltopectoral areas and rotated to the relevant area. Regional flaps are muscles with their own neurovascular bundles and with a covering of skin to cover the surgical defect. These utilize chest and back muscles that may be latissimus dorsi, pectoralis major or trapezius in order to protect the underlying vessels and provide skin cover. The commonest regional flap seen on imaging is the pectoralis major myocutaneous flap. Both regional and local flaps have a vascular supply that is not interfered with in the process of creating the flap, thus they may be differentiated on imaging from free flaps as the course of the nutrient muscle can usually be traced.

Free flaps have a transected vascular pedicle and by using microvascular anastomoses the flap vessels are grafted to similar sized vessels at the surgical resection site. On cross-sectional imaging, a myocutaneous flap will show the bulk of the muscle mass nearest the origin of the muscle. The overlying skin of the flap is slightly thicker than the remaining skin of the neck and the main substance of the flap is fatty in appearance, due to fatty denervated muscle fibres and subcutaneous tissue[62,63] and often the only reason it is recognized is that the normal structures are replaced with a soft tissue mass composed primarily of fat.

Changes after radiotherapy

Radiation therapy in the neck causes reactive changes within the skin and platysma as well as reticulation (lace-like pattern) of the subcutaneous and deep fat and these changes may be demonstrated radiologically (Figure 3.39). These are chronic changes seen several months after radiotherapy. Resolution of these features usually occurs in approximately 50% of patients by the first anniversary after treatment.[64] Increased enhancement of the pharyngeal mucosa after radiation therapy occurs in 55% of patients, perhaps due to neovascularization arising as a consequence of radiation-induced mucositis.[65] CT and MRI studies may show obliteration of pre-epiglottic fat occurring in one-third of patients treated with radiation therapy alone, but this feature by itself is not indicative of treatment failure.

Radiation therapy in the neck may also lead to premature atherosclerosis and adventitial fibrosis thereby predisposing or accentuating cerebral ischaemia. Radiotherapy has also been recorded as precipitating carotid artery wall necrosis with subsequent carotid blow-out.

Symmetrical thickening of the aryepiglottic folds and false vocal cords, laryngeal mucosa and subglottis occurs in the vast majority of postlaryngeal irradiation patients and these changes may be seen for years.[62] Laryngeal cartilages are relatively unaltered by acute radiation damage due to their poor cellularity but damage to the overlying nutrient perichondrium can result in perichondritis, which if severe can eventually lead to frank laryngeal necrosis and eventual laryngeal collapse.[65] Perichondritis or chondronecrosis can resemble a progressively enlarging mass and may be mistaken for local recurrence. Changes in cartilage sclerosis can be an important predictor of outcome in patients after laryngeal radiotherapy. Mukherji et al have found that new or progressive cartilage sclerosis appears to be a poor prognostic factor, and in their study this feature was associated with treatment failure in 50% of patients. Progressive cartilage sclerosis may occur in the absence of an associated mass and it may well be that this subgroup requires closer surveillance.[66]

Imaging of post-treatment complications

There are a varied number of non-malignant complications of the treatment of head and neck cancer including vascular occlusion, carotid blow-out, pharyngocutaneous fistula, flap necrosis, lymphocoeles, abscess and neo-oesophageal stenosis. Cerebrospinal fluid (CSF) rhinorrhoea may complicate sinus or nasopharyngeal surgery. The use of contrast especially intravenously is of particular use in highlighting tumour recurrences, abscesses and new improvement of lymph nodes.

Internal jugular occlusion

Non-opacification of the internal jugular vein on imaging may be due to its removal at the time of radical neck dissection, or to compression of the vein by a recurrent mass or because of thrombosis.

Irradiation effects on the carotid tree

Therapeutic irradiation may accelerate atherosclerosis increasing to vascular stenosis or occlusion that may give rise to neurological symptoms due to carotid artery intimal damage following irradiation.[67] Carotid blow-out may occur also at any time also

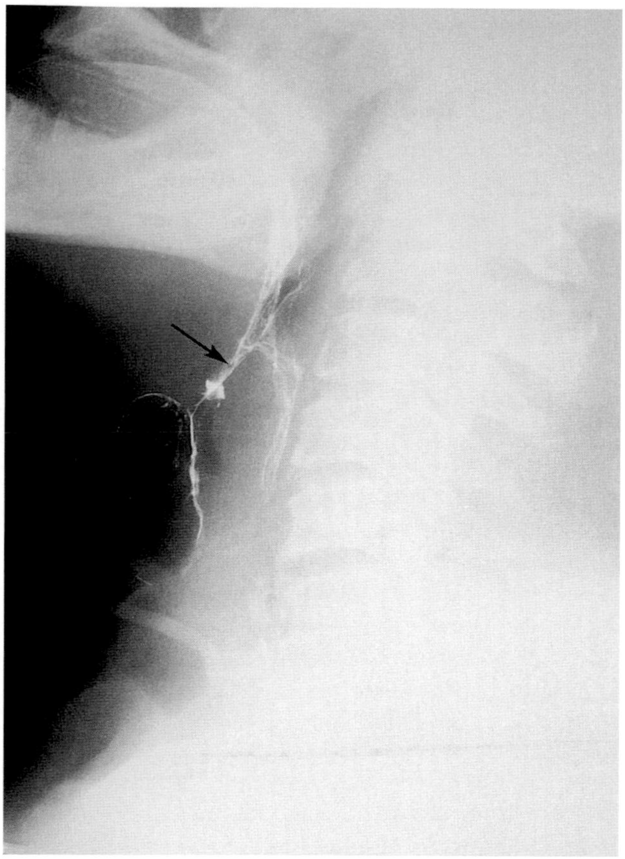

Figure 3.42 A non-barium contrast swallow radiograph delineating a sinus into the soft tissues of the neck post laryngectomy.

secondary to radiation damage. There is no radiological predictor of this; it can only be anticipated on clinical grounds.

Fistulae

Pharyngocutaneous fistulae are a not uncommon complication following pharyngolaryngectomy (Figure 3.42). Two factors that have been found to significantly affect the incidence of fistulae are prior radiation and the need for flap reconstruction of the pharynx.[68]

Flap necrosis

Flap necrosis is an early surgical complication of failed or impaired microanastomoses. It is usually diagnosed clinically and imaging examinations do not contribute.

Lymphocoeles

Lymphocoeles that are irregularly shaped with thick enhanced walls may mimic recurrent tumour but most lymphocoeles are isodense with water on CT, are thin walled and unilocular and these masses tend to appear soon after surgery.

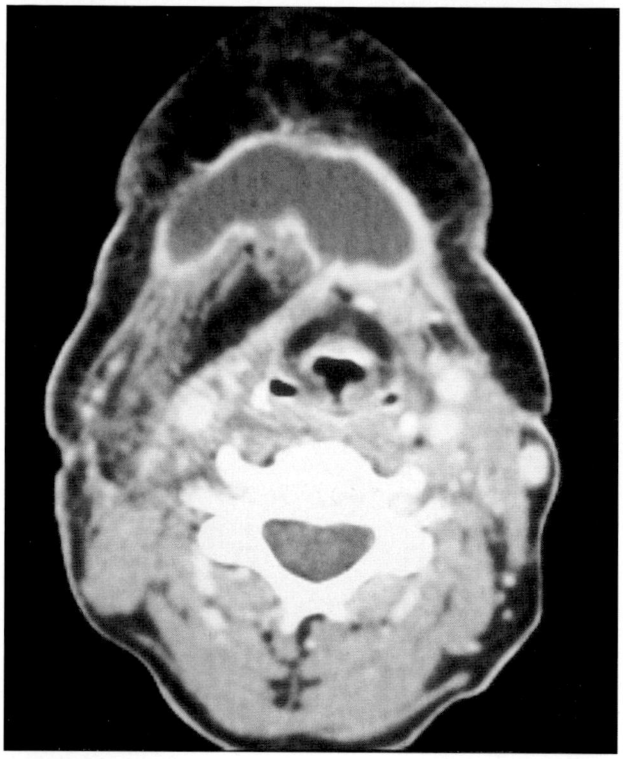

Figure 3.43 This axial postcontrast CT shows a postoperative low-density lesion with an enhancing margin proven to be postsurgical abscess.

Abscesses

Abscesses have been described as difficult to distinguish from recurrent tumour on radiographic appearance alone and there is a very great overlap in their imaging features (Figure 3.43).[63] They are frequently displayed as thick-walled rim-enhancing low-density masses. Correlation with the clinical features will often point towards abscess as the cause of the mass, but if doubt persists, then image-guided aspiration should provide the answer.

Neo-oesophageal stenosis

Neo-oesophageal stenosis is a complication of radiotherapy and presenting with dysphagia which can be acute secondary to oedema or chronic due to fibrosis.

CSF Leakage

At tumour resection the dura may be breached, and a leak of CSF ensues. CSF rhinorrhoea may be demonstrated by CT cisternography or radionuclide cisternography by intrathecal injection of contrast agent or radionuclide.[69] An active leak may be seen if coronal CT sections are taken with the patient prone. Using radioisotope injection radioactivity may be detectable on cotton nose pledgets 4–6 hours later.

Imaging of recurrent disease

Locally recurrent disease usually develops at the margins of surgical resection. If abnormal soft tissue, seen on the baseline postoperative examination, is seen to progressively decrease in size on subsequent examinations it should be regarded as innocent continued healing. New masses or baseline soft tissue masses that progressively increase in size clearly should be presumed to be recurrence until proven otherwise (Figures 3.44 and 3.45). If tumour-free margins are achieved at the time of resection, it is rare for a recurrence to develop within the postoperative 4–8 weeks,[63] before the establishment of the baseline postoperative study.

The majority of nodal recurrences occur within 2 years of diagnosis and most deaths from head and neck cancer occur within the first 3 years following treatment.[70] Close imaging follow-up within the first 3 postoperative years would therefore appear sensible and this might take the format of 4–6 monthly CT scans. Change on imaging has been shown to be more reliable than clinical examination alone and when suspected the requirement is for identification of the margins of this recurrence, including invasion of local structures such as blood vessels, nerves, cartilage and bone. In addition, the remainder of the neck should be assessed, especially the contralateral neck to detect any subclinical disease.

Active scar or granulation tissue may mimic recurrent or residual tumour on CT scan, but on MR images, a scar has a much lower signal intensity than tumour and may therefore be differentiated from tumour.[62] However, since both tumour recurrence and vascularized scar enhance to variable degrees with both MR and CT, enhancement with contrast agents does not allow distinction between these two types of tissue with any confidence. In general, the progressive decrease in size of a soft tissue mass indicates that it is not a tumour. A mature scar has low signal intensity or a signal void on both T1- and T2-weighted MR images.[71]

Tumour recurrence occurring around the carotid sheath is quite common and can be seen as increased soft tissue surrounding the neurovascular bundle, eliminating the fat planes in the neck. The tumour may also use the graft as a conduit as well as a site for recurrence (Figures 3.46 and 3.47). A thin rim of tissue adjacent to the carotid sheath is compatible with postsurgical change but greater than this would be suspicious of recurrence of disease.

Positron emission tomography

In those patients in whom tumour markers are rising but in whom no radiological evidence of recurrence has been found a PET scan should be considered.[72] With administration of intravenous 2-deoxy-2-[fluorine-18] fluoro-D-glucose (FDG), PET imaging is used to non-invasively estimate tissue glucose metabolism in vivo. As malignant tissues often have a glucose metabolism that is increased compared with that of normal tissues,[73] FDG PET imaging can be used as a functional tumour detection alternative to anatomic imaging techniques (Figures 3.48 and 3.49).

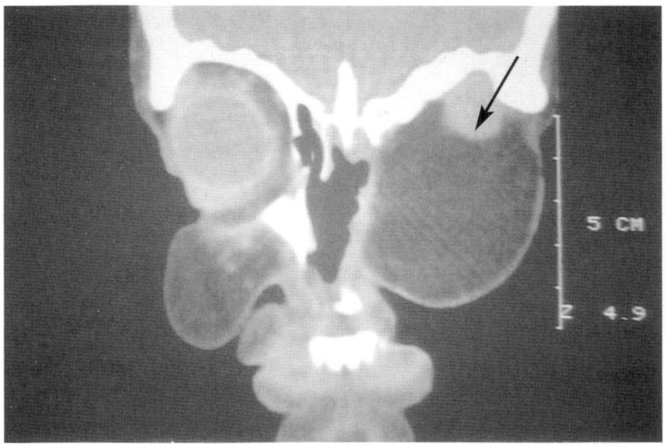

Figure 3.44 Coronal CT demonstrating recurrence of squamous cell carcinoma of the maxillary sinus occurring within a flap in the orbital remnant at the skull base (arrow).

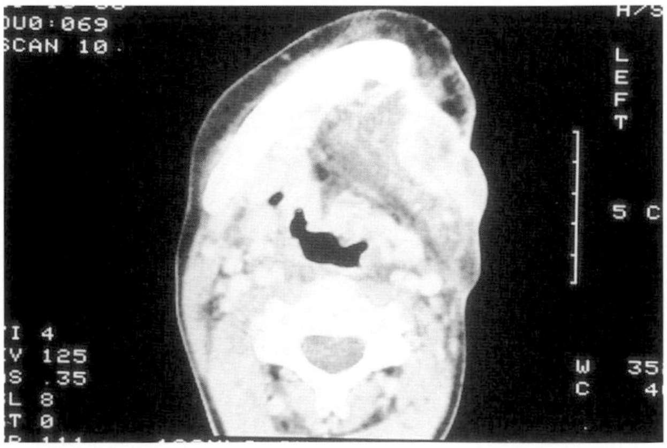

Figure 3.45 This axial post-contrast CT performed 10 weeks after a left hemiglossectomy for a squamous cell carcinoma of the tongue shows an enhancing recurrence in the flap.

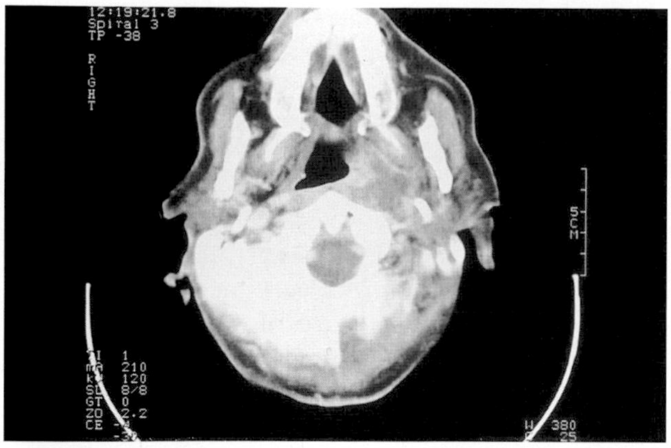

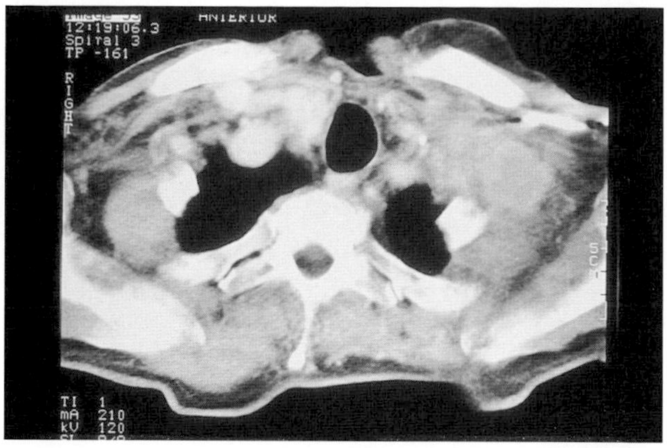

Figures 3.46 and 3.47 Post-contrast CT sections at the top and bottom of a pectoralis major flap demonstrate enhancing soft tissue recurrences at the flap margins superiorly in the region of the left tonsillar fossa and inferiorly at the lung apex.

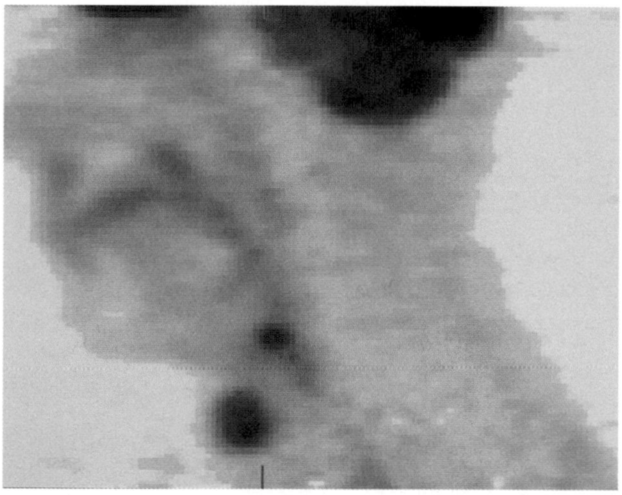

Figure 3.48 This patient had a resection for laryngeal cancer and baseline and follow-up scans were normal yet tumour markers were rising. The lateral view of the PET scan shows two hot spots, one anterior and one posterior to the airway.

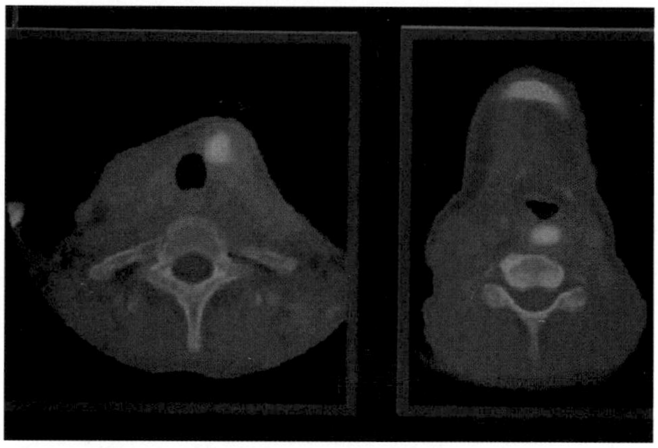

Figure 3.49 Conformal superimposition on the axial CT scans and with colour rendering demonstrates the anatomical site. At operation, recurrence was confirmed in the anterior lesion (a) but no abnormality was determined in respect of the posterior lesion (b).

Precise coregistration between anatomic and functional images is required because functional images alone often do not provide the sufficiently detailed anatomic display of surrounding anatomy that is necessary for surgical and/or radiation therapy planning. Image coregistration needs modification of the standard contour methods, because the shape and outline of the neck is much affected by patient positioning.[74] Lapela et al have reported that the sensitivity and specificity in the detection of recurrent head and neck cancers were 88% and 86% for PET and 92% and 50% for CT.[75] Inflammatory tissue will also show some accumulation.

REFERENCES

1. Dhooge IJ, De-Vos M, Albers FW, Van-Cauwenberge PB. Panendoscopy as a screening procedure for simultaneous primary tumours in head and neck cancer. *Eur Arch Otorhinolaryngol* 1996; **253**: 319–334.
2. Stack BC, Ridley MB, Endicott JN. Simultaneous squamous cell carcinoma of the head and neck and reticuloendothelial malignancies. *Am J Otolaryngol* 1996; **17**: 178–183.
3. Schaner EG, Chang AE, Doppman JL et al. Comparison of computed and conventional whole lung tomography in detecting pulmonary nodules; a prospective radiologic–pathologic study. *Am J Roentgenol* 1978; **131**: 51–54.

4. Lund G, Heilo A. Computed tomography of pulmonary metastases. *Acta Radiol Diagn* 1982; **23**: 617–620.
5. Wedman J, Balm AJ, Hart AA et al. Value of resection of pulmonary metastases in head and neck patients. *Head Neck* 1996; **18**: 311–316.
6. Zapeter E, Bagan JV, Campos A et al. Non-Hodgkin's lymphoma of the head and neck in association with HIV infection. *Ann Otolaryngol Chir Cervicofac* 1996; **113**: 69–72.
7. Silver AJ, Mawad ME, Hilal SK et al. Computed tomography of the nasopharynx and related spaces. Part II: pathology. *Radiology* 1983; **147**: 733–738.
8. Vogl TJ, Dresel SHJ. Diagnostic procedures in nasopharyngeal illness. *Curr Opin Radiol* 1992; **4**: 127–135.
9. Som PM, Braun IF, Shapiro MD et al. Tumours of the parapharyngeal space and upper neck: MR imaging characteristics. *Radiology* 1987; **164**: 823–829.
10. Sham JSY, Cheung YK, Choy D, Leong L. Cranial nerve involvement and base of skull erosion in nasopharyngeal carcinoma. *Cancer* 1991; **68**: 422–426.
11. Som PM, Sacher M, Stollman AL et al. Common tumours of the parapharyngeal space: refined imaging diagnosis. *Radiology* 1988, **169**: 81–86.
12. Som PM. Lymph nodes of the neck. *Radiology* 1987; **165**: 593–600.
13. Youssem DM, Hatabu H, Hurst RW et al. Carotid artery invasion by head and neck masses: prediction with MR imaging. *Radiology* 1995; **195**: 715–720.
14. Gritzman N, Grasl MC, Helmer M, Steiner E. Invasion of the carotid artery and jugular vein by lymph node metastases: detection with sonography. *Am J Roentgenol* 1990; **154**: 411–414.
15. Reilly MK, Perry MO, Netterville JL, Meacham PW. Carotid replacement in conjunction with resection of squamous cell carcinoma of the neck: preliminary results. *J Vasc Surg* 1992; **15**: 324–329.
16. Muraki AS, Mancuso AA, Harnsberger HR et al. CT of the oropharynx, tongue base, and floor of the mouth: normal anatomy and variations, and applications in staging carcinoma. *Radiology* 1983; **148**: 725–731.
17. Mancuso AA, Hanafee WN. Elusive head and neck carcinomas beneath intact mucosa. *Laryngoscope* 1983; **93**: 133–139.
18. Gromet M, Homer MJ, Carter BL. Lymphoid hyperplasia at the base of the tongue. *Radiology* 1982; **144**: 825–828.
19. Abemayor E, Dennis MM, Hanson DG. Identification of synchronous tumours in patients with head and neck cancer. *J Surg Oncol* 1988; **38**: 94–96.
20. Kassel EE, Keller MA, Kucharczyk W. MRI of the floor of the mouth, tongue and oropharynx. *Radiol Clin North Am* 1989; **27**: 331–351.
21. Cooke J, Parsons C. Computed scanning in patients with carcinoma of the tongue. *Clin Radiol* 1989; **40**: 254–256.
22. Alazraki NP, Mishkin FS. *Fundamentals of Nuclear Medicine.* 2nd edn. New York: Society of Nuclear Medicine, 1988.
23. Parsons C. Computed tomography of laryngeal tumours. *J Belge Radiol* 1983; **66**: 343–349.
24. Sakai F, Gamsu G, Dillon WP et al. MR imaging of the larynx at 1.5T. *J Comput Assist Tomogr* 1990; **14**: 60–71.
25. Lloyd GAS, Michaels L, Phelps PD. The demonstration of cartilaginous involvement in laryngeal carcinoma by computerised tomography. *Clin Otolaryngol* 1981; **6**: 171–177.
26. Vogl T, Teger W, Grevers G et al. MRI with Gd-DTPA in tumours of larynx and hypopharynx. *Eur Radiol* 1991; **1**: 58–64.
27. Vander JB, Gaston EA, Dawber TR. The significance of nontoxic thyroid nodules: final report of a 15–year study of the incidence of thyroid malignancy. *Ann Intern Med* 1968; **69**: 537–540.
28. Mazzaferri EL, de los Santos ET, Rofagha-Keyhani S. Solitary thyroid nodule: diagnosis and management. *Med Clin North Am* 1988; **72**: 1177–1211.
29. Gharib H, Goellner JR. Fine needle aspiration biopsy of the thyroid: an appraisal. *Ann Intern Med* 1993; **118**: 282–289.
30. Noyek AM, Witterick IJ, Kirsch JC. Radionuclide imaging in head and neck surgery. *Arch Otolaryngol Head Neck Surg* 1991; **117**: 372–378.
31. Sandler MP, Fellmeth B, Salhany KE, Patton JA. Thyroid carcinoma masquerading as a solitary benign hyperfunctioning nodule. *J Nucl Med* 1987: **28**; 122–129.
32. Freitas JE, Freitas AE. Thyroid and parathyroid imaging. *Semin Nucl Med* 1994; **24**: 234–245.
33. Belfiore A, LaRose GL, LaPorta GA et al. Cancer risk in patients with cold thyroid nodules: relevance of iodine intake, sex, age and multinodularity. *Am J Med* 1992; **93**: 363–369.
34. Hoefnagel CA, Delprat CC, Marcuse HR, de Vijlder JJM. Role of thallium-201 in total-body scintigraphy in follow-up of thyroid carcinoma. *J Nucl Med* 1986; **27**: 1854–1857.
35. Charkes ND, Vitti RA, Brooks K. Thallium-201 SPECT increases detectability of thyroid cancer metastases. *J Nucl Med* 1990; **31**: 147–153.
36. Yasumoto M, Shibuya H, Suzuki S et al. Computed tomography and ultrasonography in submandibular tumours. *Clin Rad* 1992; **46**: 114–120.
37. Bryan RN, Miller RH, Ferreyro RI, Sessions RB. Computed tomography of the major salivary glands. *Am J Roentgenol* 1982; **139**: 547–554.
38. Rabinov K. Salivary glands: pathology. In: Taveras JM (ed.) *Radiology*, Vol. 3. Philadelphia: J.B. Lippincott Company, 1986; (95) 1–8.
39. Thackray AC, Lucas RB. Tumours of the major salivary glands. In: *Atlas of Tumour Pathology*, 2nd series, Fasicle 10. Washington DC: Armed Forces Institute of Pathology, 1974; 1–144.
40. Gademann G, Haels J, Semmler W, van Kaick G. MRI of the parotid gland. *Laryngol Rhinol Otol* 1988; **67**: 211–216.
41. Robbins KT, Medina JE, Wolfe GT et al. Standardising neck dissection terminology. Official report of the Academy's Committee for Head and Neck Surgery and Oncology. *Arch Otolaryngol Head Neck Surg* 1991; **117**: 601–605.

42. Jacques DA. Management of metastatic lymph nodes in the neck from an unknown primary. In: Paperella MM and Shumrick DA (eds) *Otolaryngology*. Philadelphia: WB Saunders, 1980; 2998–3003.
43. van den Brekel MWM, Stel HV, Castelijins JA. et al. Cervical lymph node metastases: assessment of radiologic criteria. *Radiology* 1990; **177**: 379–384.
44. Close LG, Merkel M, Vuitch MF et al. Computed tomographic evaluation of regional lymph node involvement in cancer of the oral cavity and oropharynx. *Head Neck* **11**: 1989; 309–317.
45. Candela FC, Kothari K, Shah JP. Patterns of cervical node metastases from squamous carcinoma of the oropharynx and hypopharynx. *Head Neck* 1990; **12** : 197–203.
46. Som PM. Detection of metastasis in cervical lymph nodes: CT and MR criteria and differential diagnosis. *Am J Roentgenol* 1992; **158**: 961–969.
47. Panush D, Fulbright R, Sze G et al. Inversion recovery fast spin echo MR imaging: efficacy in the evaluation of head and neck lesions. *Radiology* 1993; **187**: 421–426.
48. Munck JN, Cvitkovic E, Piekarski JD et al. Computed tomographic density of metastatic lymph nodes as a treatment related prognostic factor in advanced head and neck cancer. *J Natl Cancer Inst* 1991; **83**: 569–575.
49. Phillips CD, Spencer B, Newton RL, Levene PA. Gadolinium enhanced MRI tumours of the head and neck. *Head Neck* 1990; **12**: 308–315.
50. Youssem DM, Som PM, Hackney DB. et al. Central nodal necrosis and extracapsular neoplastic spread in cervical lymph nodes: MR imaging versus CT. *Radiology* 1992; **182**: 753–759.
51. Mancuso AA, Harnsberger HR, Muraki AS et al. Computed tomography of cervical and retropharyngeal lymph nodes: normal anatomy, variants of normal and applications in staging head and neck cancer. Parts I and II. *Radiology* 1983; **148**: 709–714.
52. Brunton JN, Roux P, Caramella E et al. Ear, nose, and throat cancer: ultrasound diagnosis of metastasis to cervical lymph nodes. *Radiology* 1984; **152**: 771–773.
53. McGuirt WF, McCabe BF. Significance of node biopsy before definitive treatment of cervical metastatic carcinoma. *Laryngoscope* 1978; **88**: 594–597.
54. Young JEM, Archibald SD, Shier KJ. Needle aspiration cytologic biopsy in head and neck masses. *Am J Surg* 1981; **142**: 484–489.
55. Van den Breckel MWM, Castelijins JA, Stel HV et al. Detection and characterization of metastatic cervical adenopathy by MR imaging: comparison of different MR techniques. *J Comput Assist Tomogr* 1990; **14**: 581–589.
56. Lindberg R. Distribution of cervical lymph node metastases from squamous cell carcinoma of the upper respiratory and digestive tracts. *Cancer* 1972; **29**: 1446–1449.
57. Spiro RH. The management of neck nodes in head and neck cancer: a surgeon's view. *Bull NY Acad Med* 1985; **61**: 629–637.
58. Cooke J, Morrison G, Keyserlingk J, Parsons C. CT scanning in patients following surgery on the tongue and floor of the mouth. *Clin Radiol* 1990, **41**; 306–311.
59. Medina JE, Byers RM. Supraomohyoid neck dissection: rationale, indications and surgical technique. *Head Neck* 1989; **11**: 111–122.
60. Davis WL, Harnsberger HR, Smoker WRK, Watanabe AS. Retropharyngeal space: evalaution of normal anatomy and diseases with CT and MR imaging. *Radiology* 1990; **174**: 59–64.
61. Som PM, Urken ML, Biller H, Lidov M. Imaging the postoperative neck. *Radiology* 1993; **187**: 593–603.
62. Glazer HS, Niemeyer JH, Balfe DM et al. Neck neoplasms: MR imaging. II. Post-treatment evaluation. *Radiology* 1986; **160**: 349–354.
63. Som PM, Biller HF. Computed tomography of the neck in the postoperative patient: radical neck dissection and the myocutaneous flap. *Radiology* 1983; **148**: 157–160.
64. Mukherji SK, Mancuso AA, Kotzur IM. Radiologic appearance of the irradiated larynx. Part I. Expected changes. *Radiology* 1994; **193**: 141–148.
65. Ward PH, Calceterre TC, Kagen AR. The enigma of post-radiation edema and recurrence or residual carcinoma of the larynx. *Laryngoscope* 1974; **85**; 522–529.
66. Mukherji SK, Mancuso AA, Kotzur IM et al. Radiologic appearance of the irradiated larynx. Part II. Primary Site Response. *Radiology* 1994; **193**: 149–154.
67. Call GK, Bray PF, Smoker WR et al. Carotid thrombosis following neck irradiation. *Int J Radiat Oncol Biol Phys* 1990; **18**: 635–640.
68. Sarkar S, Mehta SA, Tiwari J, Mehta AR, Mehta MS. Complications following surgery for cancer of the larynx and pyriform fossa. *J Surg Oncol* 1990; **43**: 245–249.
69. Park JL, Strelzow VV, Friedman WH. Current management of cerebrospinal fluid rhinorrhoea. *Laryngoscope* 1983; **93**: 1294–1300.
70. Baker SR. Malignant neoplasms of the oral cavity. In: Cummings CW, Frederickson JM, Harker LA, Krause CJ, Schuller DE (eds). *Otolaryngology: Head and Neck Surgery*. Vol 2. St. Louis, Mo: Mosby, 1986; 1281–1343.
71. Hudgins PA, Burson JG, Guack GS, Grist WJ. CT and MR appearance of recurrent malignant head and neck neoplasm after resection and flap reconstruction. *Am J Neuroradiol* 1994; **15**: 1689–1694.
72. Anzai Y, Carroll WM, Quint DJ et al. Recurrence of head and neck cancer after surgery or irradiation: prospective comparison of 2-deoxy-2-[F-18]fluoro-D-glucose PET and MR imaging diagnoses. *Radiology* 1996; **200**: 135–141.
73. Di Chiro G, De la Paz RL, Brooks RA et al. Glucose utilization of cerebral gliomas measured by 18F-fluorodeoxyglucose and PET. *Neurology* 1982; **32**: 1323–1329.
74. Wahl RL, Quint LE, Cieslak RD et al. 'Anatometabolic' tumour imaging: fusion of FDG PET with CT or MRI to localise foci of increased activity. *J Nucl Med* 1993; **34**: 1190–1197.
75. Lapela M, Grenman R, Kurki T et al. Head and neck cancer: detection of recurrence with PET and 2-[F-18]fluoro-2-deoxy-D-glucose. *Radiology* 1995; **197**: 205–211.

4 Principles of head and neck radiotherapy

J Michael Henk

Introduction

Radiotherapy (radiation therapy) is defined as the use of ionizing radiation and comprises both external beam therapy and brachytherapy (see below). The use of radiotherapy in head and neck cancer was established between 1920 and 1940 by the pioneering work of Coutard in Paris and Paterson in Manchester UK, among others. Subsequently, opinions on its merits have fluctuated from time to time and from country to country, but radiotherapy retains an important place in the management of head and neck cancer, either as the sole treatment or in combination with other modalities.

Physical and biological basis

Physical effects of radiation

The term 'radiotherapy' refers to treatment using ionizing radiation, which interacts with fluids to produce free ions. The source of the ionizing radiation may be from a machine, for example a deep X-ray set or a linear accelerator, or from decay of a radioactive isotope.

Radiotherapy dosage is expressed in terms of absorbed dose. This is the quantity of ionizing radiation energy absorbed per unit mass of tissue. It is therefore a measurement of radiation effect, rather than a quantity of energy given. The SI unit of absorbed dose is the gray (Gy), defined as an energy absorption of 1 joule/kg. In some older publications quoted in this chapter absorbed doses are expressed in rads (100 rads = 1 Gy).

Biological action

The most important mechanism of the observed effects of radiotherapy on tumours and normal tissues is mitotic death, whereby an irradiated cell survives functionally intact until such time as it subsequently attempts to divide, when the DNA damage renders it unable to go through normal mitosis and death ensues. The first attempt at mitosis may be as short as a few minutes or as long as 20 years after irradiation, hence the varied time-scale of postradiotherapy events.

Tumour effects

Because of mitotic death the interval between irradiation and shrinkage of a tumour depends on the rate of cell proliferation in the tumour. In the case of a rapidly proliferating tumour, for example squamous cell carcinoma, cell death and lysis is often seen within a few days. On the other hand, a very slowly proliferating tumour, for example a pleomorphic adenoma, may not manifest radiation changes for many months or even years.

The chance of a given dose of radiation sterilizing all tumour cells depends on four factors:

1. Radiosensitivity. This is an inherent biological property of a cell type; it is determined by biochemical factors such as the ability of the cell to repair DNA damage. It is expressed as the proportion of a population of cells sterilized by a given dose of radiation: the higher the radiosensitivity the greater is the proportion of cells killed.
2. Oxygenation. The greater the concentration of oxygen present in the cell at the instant of radiation, the more likely is a free radical to cause a

lethal event. Some tumours, including squamous carcinoma, have an inadequate vasculature, so that a proportion of their cells are hypoxic and therefore relatively radioresistant.

3. Growth rate. During a course of radiotherapy surviving tumour cells are able to divide and generate more cells. This phenomenon of repopulation occurs in more rapidly growing tumours. Some tumours respond to cell killing by accelerated repopulation, probably because of better availability of oxygen and nutrients and the production of growth factors. Accelerated repopulation is a special property of well-differentiated squamous carcinoma.
4. Tumour size. This is probably the most important factor determining radiocurability. The dose-response relation of the effect of radiotherapy can be described as an exponential or logarithmic function. A constant increment of dose kills a constant fraction of cells. A simple example would be that if a unit of absorbed radiation kills 90% of cells, and if there were originally 100 cells, the effect of the first unit of absorbed radiation would be to leave only 10 viable cells; an additional 1 unit of radiation absorbed would leave only one viable cell. To kill the last remaining cell an additional 1 unit would have to be absorbed.

   Thus for a given amount of radiation it can be seen that the fewer the number of cells present initially the greater the probability of killing them all.

If a tumour is relatively radioresistant, for example an adenocarcinoma of the mucus or salivary glands, radiotherapy can usually effect a cure only if there is a very small population of tumour cells present, such as immediately after near-total surgical removal. With more radiosensitive tumours, for example squamous cell carcinoma, there is a fair chance of success of curing macroscopic disease, which diminishes with increasing tumour size. However, there is a wide variation in radiocurability between individual squamous carcinomas that may appear clinically and histologically identical, because of differences in oxygenation, proliferation kinetics and intrinsic radiosensitivity.

Normal tissue effects

The effects of radiotherapy on normal tissues are classified as acute, occurring during or immediately after a course of treatment, or late, occurring months or years later. Mitotic death is the major mechanism of normal tissue effects. Rapidly proliferating tissues manifest radiation changes quickly; mucosa after about 12 days and the skin after about 21 days following the start of a course of radiotherapy. These acute reactions normally heal completely as rapid cell repopulation takes place.

Mitotic death of vascular endothelial cells accounts for most of the delayed normal tissue effects. Endothelial cells have a turnover time of several months. Consequently, devascularization of irradiated tissues does not begin until at least 3 months after radiotherapy and tends to progress for several years with little or no recovery. Tissue changes occurring as a result of devascularization are generally irreversible.

Some normal cells do not usually undergo mitosis unless stimulated to do so. An example is the osteoblast, which may be stimulated to divide in order to remodel bone after trauma. Bone is largely unaffected by radiotherapy, unless trauma such as dental extraction provides a mitotic stimulus, in which case osteoblasts undergo mitotic death and bone necrosis may ensue.

Normal tissue tolerance

The concept of normal tissue tolerance to radiotherapy has developed from many years of observation of late normal tissue effects. The tolerance dose is defined as the maximum dose of irradiation that can be given to the volume of tissue being treated without producing an unacceptable incidence of late damage.

Radiation tolerance depends on tissue type. It is low in the lens of the eye and gonads, intermediate in liver, lung and kidney and high in bone and cartilage. It may also depend on the volume of tissue being irradiated. For instance, in the case of liver, kidney or lung, the tolerance dose depends on the proportion of the whole organ being irradiated. On the other hand the length of the spinal cord irradiated is less important because an overdose at any level may result in paraplegia. It also depends on the volume of tissue being irradiated; the larger the volume, the lower the tolerance dose.

Techniques of radiotherapy

There are two fundamentally different methods of administering radiotherapy. Teletherapy, or external beam irradiation, uses a machine to deliver beams of irradiation directed at the tumour from outside the patient. In brachytherapy the source of radiation is placed within, or in close proximity to, the tumour.

External beam therapy

External beam, or teletherapy, is the form of radiotherapy most widely used in treatment of head and neck cancer. It is usual to employ two or more beams of supervoltage radiation converging on the tumour volume, so that the latter is irradiated homogeneously to the required dose. Conventional radiotherapy will deliver a high dose to a cuboid volume, with neighbouring tissues receiving a lower dose. However, tumours do not normally have cuboid, but more complex, shapes. Accurate shaping of the beam to conform to the precise volume of tumour, with a small margin, can be achieved using multiple 'leaves' known as multi-leaf collimators (conformal therapy). Even more precise beam shaping can be realized by varying the beam intensity across the beam profile (intensity modulated radiotherapy or IMRT). Such techniques have the potential to increase the differential between tumour dose and normal tissue dose, thus greatly improving the therapeutic ratio, but it is essential to realize that these techniques are only as good as: (a) the imaging used; and (b) the immobilization system used. Highly accurate conformal therapy or IMRT in the presence of poor imaging quality or unsatisfactory immobilization is actually more dangerous than, and inferior to, conventional radiotherapy.

A course of external beam radiotherapy is fractionated, that is the total dose is divided into a number of smaller doses delivered over a period of several weeks. The larger the number of fractions, the greater the total dose required to produce the same effect (for example 50 Gy in 15 treatments over 3 weeks is roughly equivalent to 65 Gy in 30 treatments over 6 weeks).

The aim of fractionation is to increase the differential effect of the radiation on the tumour compared with the normal tissues. There are several mechanisms contributing to the beneficial effects of fractionation. Normal cells have a higher capacity than tumour cells to repair damage to DNA after exposure to small doses of radiation. The tumour response is enhanced by reoxygenation of hypoxic cells as the tumour regresses and there is the opportunity to irradiate tumour cells as they pass through more sensitive phases of the cell cycle. On the other hand accelerated repopulation of tumour cells constitutes a disadvantage of fractionation.

Conventional standard fractionation consists of delivering 2 Gy per day, 5 days per week to a total dose of 66–70 Gy. This is a compromise between convenience and biology and is not ideal. The optimum treatment time and number of fractions remains the subject of both research and controversy. Some radiotherapists have preferred 3-week schedules, based on the large study by Paterson of results at the Christie Hospital, Manchester.[1] There has been only one large prospective controlled trial comparing short and long courses of radiotherapy, a multicentre trial in carcinoma of the larynx conducted by the British Institute of Radiology.[2] This trial failed to show any difference in tumour control but there was a suggestion of less severe late morbidity from the shorter treatment. Recent studies show that there is an advantage to using more and smaller fractions over a shorter time than with standard fractionation (see Altered fractionation below).

Methods of improving results of external beam therapy

Better results from radiotherapy can be achieved only by increasing the differential effect of the radiation on the tumour compared with the normal tissues. Two possible exploitable differences between tumour cells and normal cells are the oxygen effect and cell proliferation kinetics.

Hypoxia

The presence of viable hypoxic cells in tumours but not in normal tissues is believed to be one of the major causes of radiotherapy failure, thus many of the efforts to improve the results of radiotherapy in the past 25 years have been directed towards overcoming this so-called 'oxygen effect.' An overview of all clinical trials of methods to overcome the oxygen effect in radiotherapy of head and neck cancer showed a small but significant benefit.[3] The various methods tried are shown in Table 4.1.

Hyperbaric oxygen proved moderately effective, but too time-consuming and hazardous for routine use.[10] Neutron therapy gave rise to unacceptable late normal tissue damage, but still has its advocates for inoperable salivary gland carcinoma.[11] Most trials of hypoxic-cell sensitizers have been negative, although meta-analysis of these studies does show a small effect.[7] The major problem with these agents is their

Table 4.1 Methods of tackling the oxygen effect in radiotherapy of head and neck cancer

1. Breathing oxygen and carbon dioxide (carbogen)[4]
2. Hyperbaric oxygen[5]
3. Neutron therapy[6]
4. Hypoxic-cell sensitizing drugs[7]
5. Raising haemoglobin level[8]
6. Carbogen plus a vasodilator ('ARCON'; accelerated radiotherapy carbogen and nicotinamide)[9]

neurotoxicity, which prevents their being given in effective doses. An exception is nimorazole, a drug similar to metronidazole, which was originally introduced as an antibiotic. In a large controlled trial conducted in Denmark, nimorazole improved long-term local control of oropharyngeal and supraglottic carcinoma significantly by 16%.[12] The other approaches have yet to be tested in prospective controlled trials.

Altered fractionation

There is some evidence that the effect of radiotherapy on late reacting normal tissues can be reduced relative to tumour effect by the use of small fraction sizes. Hence, a higher total dose can be given more safely if fraction sizes are reduced below the conventional 2 Gy. Inevitably, the total number of fractions must be increased. This increase in number and reduction in size of fractions is known as hyperfractionation. There is also evidence that shortening the overall treatment can minimize the effect of accelerated repopulation (accelerated fractionation). The various altered fractionation schemes used in head and neck cancer treatment are shown in Table 4.2.

Table 4.2 Altered fractionation regimens
Hyperfractionation without acceleration: 76–81 Gy in 6.5–7 weeks[13,14]
Hyperfractionated and accelerated split course[15,16]
CHART (continuous hyperfractionated accelerated radiotherapy): three fractions per day on 12 consecutive days, 54 Gy[17]
Conventional radiotherapy using six fractions per week: 68 Gy[18]
Concomitant boost: two fractions per day during the final 2 weeks[19]

All the schemes listed in Table 4.2 have proved superior to standard fractionation in controlled trials, although in the case of CHART the only advantage was a reduction in late morbidity. In all cases there is an increase in the severity of acute radiation mucositis, while the split course also caused increased late morbidity. A four-arm trial in the USA compared simple hyperfractionation, concomitant boost, split course, and standard fractionation: concomitant boost and hyperfractionation proved the most effective.[20]

Combined chemotherapy and radiotherapy

Combined treatment with radiotherapy and cytotoxic drugs is currently very popular for advanced and inoperable head and neck cancer. The drugs may be given before radiotherapy ('neoadjuvant' or 'induction' chemotherapy) or during radiotherapy ('synchronous' or 'concomitant' chemotherapy).

Neoadjuvant chemotherapy

Most head and neck squamous carcinomas respond at least to some extent to chemotherapy. The most effective drug combination, namely cisplatin and infusional fluorouracil, has been reported to produce some 40% of complete, and 90% partial responses when given as neoadjuvant therapy.[21] However, a so-called complete response may represent a reduction in tumour cell population of a factor of only 10^{-2} or 10^{-3}, whereas 10^{-11} at least is needed for cure. Nevertheless, tumour shrinkage before radiotherapy may reasonably be expected to improve cure probability, because of the lower cell number and possibly better oxygenation of the smaller tumours.

In practice, neoadjuvant chemotherapy has proved disappointing. Tumours that respond well to chemotherapy are more likely to be cured by subsequent radiotherapy (this is the basis of the use of neoadjuvant chemotherapy for 'organ preservation'), but survival rates are not increased. Overviews of a large number of controlled trials of neoadjuvant radiotherapy suggest a negligible survival benefit.[22]

There are several reasons for the failure of neoadjuvant chemotherapy. Chemotherapy may selectively destroy only the most radiosensitive proportion of the tumour ('killing the same cells twice'), or the partially shrunk tumour may have a faster repopulation rate[23] ('the leaner meaner tumour' phenomenon[24]). Also, the prognosis of a tumour that responds poorly to chemotherapy may be worsened by the delay in starting radiotherapy.

We use neoadjuvant chemotherapy only in the rare instance of a very advanced tumour to determine whether or not radical local treatment should be attempted. In the doubtful case, a good chemotherapy response may indicate that surgery and/or radiotherapy is worthwhile.

Synchronous chemotherapy

Administration of cytotoxic drugs during radiotherapy is a popular treatment option. A variety of drugs have been used, especially fluorouracil, bleomycin, cisplatin, mitomycin and hydroxyurea. Improvement in local control of head and neck cancer has been claimed for all these agents. Overviews of controlled clinical trials have revealed a highly significant improvement in survival from the use of synchronous chemotherapy,[22] but at the expense of increased acute and late radiation complications.[25] In most of these trials the same dose of radiotherapy was given to both the chemotherapy- and the radiotherapy-only arms; trials in which a higher radiation dose was given to the radiotherapy-only groups failed to show any survival difference. The effect of chemotherapy may be merely additive to radiotherapy on both tumour and normal tissues equally, and it remains an open question whether the administration of a cytotoxic drug or drugs concomitantly with radiotherapy is any different in effect from a higher dose of radiation.[26]

Brachytherapy

Brachytherapy (literally: short-distance treatment) is a general term applied to radiotherapy delivered from a source of radiation placed very close to the tumour. The principle of brachytherapy depends on the law of inverse squares, which states that the intensity of dosage of radiation at a point is inversely proportional to the square of the distance of that point from the source of the radiation. There are two methods: interstitial implants and surface/intracavitary moulds.

In interstitial treatment, solid sources of radiation are implanted directly into the tumour, producing a high intensity of radiation in the immediate vicinity of the sources, while the dose to surrounding normal tissues is low because of rapid fall-off. For interstitial treatment to be successful the whole visible and palpable tumour plus a margin of safety of at least 1 cm must receive an adequate dose of radiation delivered as homogeneously as possible, avoiding underdosed areas where disease may survive and overdosed areas where necrosis may ensue. In practice, this usually means that the radiation sources must encompass the whole lesion; therefore interstitial irradiation is generally applicable only to tumours confined to the soft tissue.

In those situations where it can be used, brachytherapy gives higher primary tumour control rates than external beam therapy.[27] This is mainly because a higher effective radiation dose can be delivered to the tumour with less irradiation of normal tissues. The treatment times are short, usually 3–8 days, so repopulation is not a problem. Also there may be less oxygen effect with low dose-rate continuous irradiation compared with external beam.[28]

Radiation sources

In the early days of radiotherapy radium was the only radioactive material available. It was enclosed in platinum needles 2.5 mm in diameter and 1.5–6 cm in length. Radium has now been superseded by artificially produced isotopes, which are safer to handle.

The most popular radioactive material for interstitial and intracavitary irradiation of head and neck cancer is now iridium-192. This is produced in the form of fine wire, which is inserted into the tissues using either slotted-guide needles or plastic tubing. The slotted-guide needle technique is used for intraoral insertion of 'hairpins' or single pins of iridium wire of 0.6-mm diameter. This method is applicable to smaller tumours of the tongue, floor of the mouth and buccal mucosa where the introducers can be inserted intraorally, that is the same types of lesions that were previously treated by radium needles (Figures 4.1 and 4.2). In this method, the positioning of sources does not involve handling of a radioactive material. The operator does not feel obliged to hurry and can take great care to ensure that the introducers

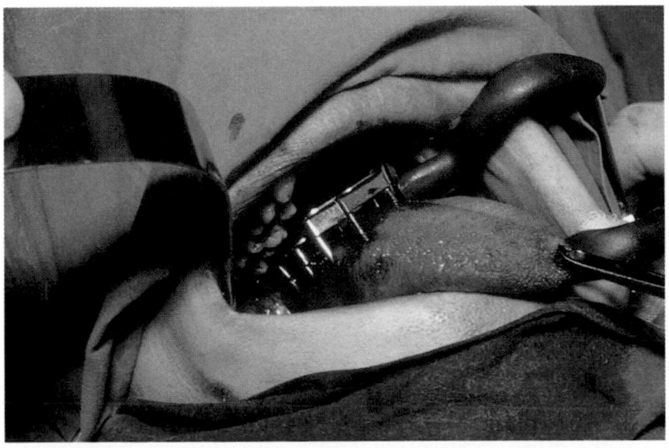

Figure 4.1 Slotted guide needles in position for iridium-192 implant to a carcinoma of the lateral border of the tongue.

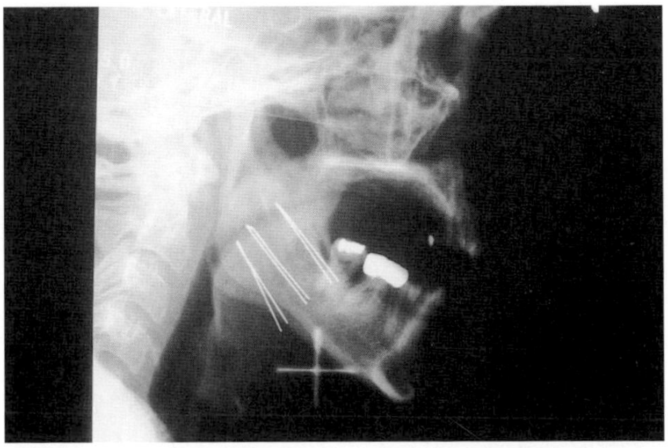

Figure 4.2 Radiograph of the radioactive hairpins in position.

are correctly positioned to give the desired dose and distribution of radiation. The position of the guide needles can be checked radiographically on the operating table before they are loaded with radioactive material. The only radiation exposure to the operating theatre staff occurs during the last few minutes of the procedure when the iridium is inserted into the guide needles and the latter removed. The flexible and thinner wires cause less discomfort to the patient than the thick rigid radium needles. They permit easier feeding and oral hygiene. In France the change from radium needles to iridium hairpins was reported to bring about improved results in the treatment of tongue and floor of mouth cancer.[29] This is probably because it is possible to take more time over the procedure and check the position of the sources when using iridium.

Another technique using iridium-192 involves the introduction of finer iridium wire of diameter 0.3 mm via plastic tubing The tubing is inserted by means of hollow guide needles inserted through the skin (Figure 4.3). With this technique, there is true afterloading, that is the tubes are positioned under general anaesthesia but not loaded with radioactive wire until the patient is returned to the ward. In this way radiation exposure to the operator and operating theatre staff is completely eliminated. This technique is useful for the cheek, and also for the posterior third of the tongue where the needles can be inserted between the mandible and the hyoid bone. It can also be used in the neck as an adjuvant to salvage neck dissection.

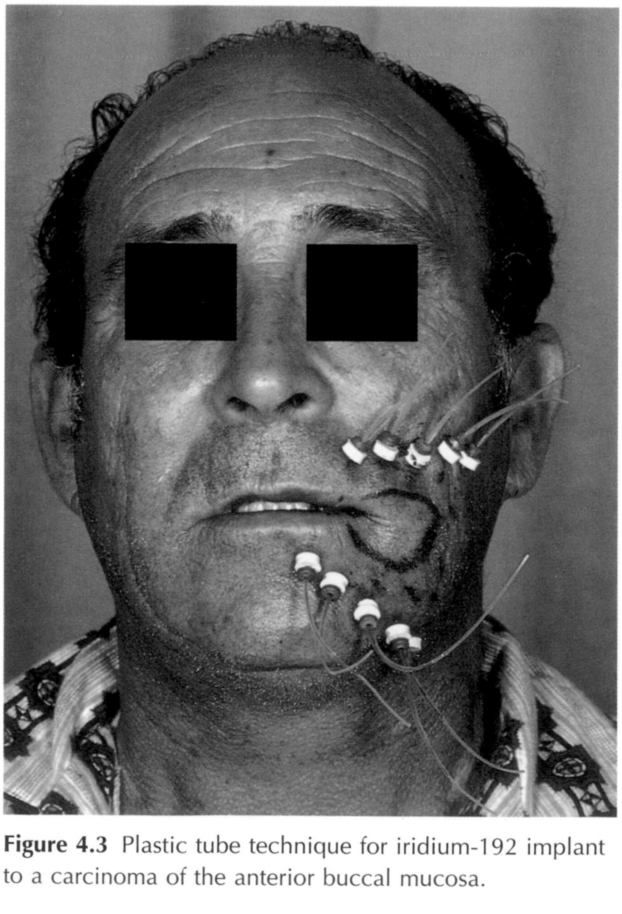

Figure 4.3 Plastic tube technique for iridium-192 implant to a carcinoma of the anterior buccal mucosa.

Dosage

If an oral cancer is treated by brachytherapy alone, a dose of 65–70 Gy is given over a time ranging between 5.5 and 8 days at a dose rate of 0.3–0.5 Gy per hour. It is believed that shorter times at a higher dose rate increase the risk of necrosis without improving the chances of tumour control.

External radiotherapy and brachytherapy can be used in combination, in which case the external beam is usually given first to a dose of 40 Gy over 4 weeks, followed by an implant as soon as possible giving a further 35–40 Gy, using the same dose rate as above. It is important that the total treatment time should not exceed 6 weeks because of the risk of failure due to tumour cell repopulation.[30]

The role of radiotherapy in the integrated management of head and neck cancer

Radical radiotherapy

The term radical refers to radiotherapy given with the objective of complete elimination of all tumour cells. To give the best chance of success a dose close to the maximum that can be tolerated by the normal tissues is administered. The aim of radical radiotherapy is to avoid surgery if possible. The patient is followed closely after radiotherapy, and surgery used only in the event of residual or recurrent disease. This strategy should be distinguished from planned preoperative radiotherapy (see below).

Radical radiotherapy is applicable in the following clinical situations:

- Radiosensitive tumours: some tumour types are very radiosensitive, so that local control by radiotherapy is achieved in nearly all cases with examples being lymphoma and undifferentiated carcinoma of nasopharyngeal type.
- Unresectable tumours: Some head and neck cancers are unsuitable for surgery by reason of site, for example nasopharynx, or extent, in which case radiotherapy offers the only hope of cure.

- Function or cosmesis: There are many sites and stages of squamous cell carcinoma of the head and neck in which radical radiotherapy and elective surgery are alternative strategies that lead to little or no difference in survival rates. Radical radiotherapy may be preferred to surgery because of the prospect of a better functional outcome, for example laryngeal cancer, or better appearance, for example carcinoma of the nasal columella.

Salvage surgery

Where radical radiotherapy fails and there is residual or recurrent tumour, surgical cure may yet be possible. Surgery performed after failure of radical radiotherapy is termed 'salvage' surgery. After radical radiotherapy the heavily irradiated tissues tend to have an impaired blood supply and poor healing properties. Consequently, salvage surgery carries a higher risk than elective surgery of complications such as delayed wound healing, fistula formation, wound breakdown and carotid artery rupture. The hazards of salvage surgery tend to increase with time after irradiation, as delayed radiation changes progress in the vasculoconnective tissues. The complication rate is lowest when surgery is performed within 3 months of completion of radiotherapy. Unfortunately it is not often possible to know whether or not radiotherapy has been successful within that period. Some tumours regress slowly after radiotherapy although completely sterilized, especially those with a low rate of cell turnover, such as many types of salivary gland tumours. Tissue abnormalities such as induration and ulceration may persist for several weeks after completion of the radiotherapy. During this period recognizable tumour cells may be found on biopsy and it is impossible to assess their viability. Sobel and Rubin found from their own experience, and after reviewing the literature, that an accurate clinical and histological assessment of tumour persistence after radical radiotherapy could not be made until 90 days had elapsed from the date of starting the treatment.[31] Consequently clinicians must beware of being too hasty in diagnosing residual tumour and proceeding to salvage surgery.

The same considerations apply to attempts to predict the radiation response during a course of radiotherapy. A policy sometimes adopted consists of assessing the response of the tumour two-thirds of the way through a course of radical radiotherapy, usually after 40 Gy has been given over 4 weeks. If the tumour seems to be regressing well it is regarded as radioresponsive and further radiotherapy is given to a full radical dose. If there is little or no regression surgery is performed. We do not adopt this policy because the correlation between the early tumour regression and cure is not sufficiently close for a reliable decision to be made. The rate of tumour shrinkage depends not only on radiosensitivity but also on the cell turnover rate, the rate at which dead tumour cells lyse, the rate of removal by phagocytic activity and does not necessarily indicate ultimate radiocurability. We therefore do not consider it logical or justifiable to abandon a radical course of radiotherapy two-thirds of the way through because of apparent poor response, except perhaps in the very rare instance where the tumour continues to grow during radiotherapy.

Elective combined surgery and radiotherapy

Preoperative radiotherapy

This term should be reserved for radiotherapy given to a patient for whom a decision to treat by elective surgery has been made. The aim of preoperative radiotherapy is to increase the chance of surgical cure, based on the assumption that local recurrence or metastases result from dissemination at operation of cells derived from the actively growing periphery of the tumour. These cells have a good blood supply, are well oxygenated, and are therefore radiosensitive. A moderate dose of radiotherapy insufficient to cause severe acute reaction or to delay wound healing can eliminate the majority of these well oxygenated peripheral cells. The more radioresistant, poorly oxygenated cells, which can be sterilized only by much larger doses of irradiation, are situated towards the centre of the tumour and are therefore most likely to be removed at operation without risk of dissemination.

Preoperative radiotherapy became very popular in the 1960s following demonstration of its effectiveness in animal tumours.[32] However it proved disappointing in clinical practice in head and neck cancer, and has now been largely abandoned following the demonstration of the superiority of postoperative radiotherapy.[33]

Postoperative radiotherapy

The rationale of postoperative radiotherapy is that a small number of malignant cells may be left behind after a radical operation, either implanted into the operative field or left at the deep margin of an excision, and postoperative recurrences subsequently develop from such cells left behind. Immediately after operation the residual cells should be few in number and therefore likely to be eliminated by a dose of radiation that would not have been sufficient to cure the original tumour.

Theoretically postoperative radiotherapy might be expected to be less effective than preoperative radiotherapy. It can affect only those tumour cells left in or adjacent to the operation field; such cells are likely to be poorly vascularized and therefore relatively radioresistant. Animal experiments tended to support this idea, showing that preoperative radiotherapy was more effective in increasing survival rates than postoperative radiotherapy.[33] Clinical studies nevertheless suggest that in head and neck cancer postoperative radiotherapy can prevent local recurrence in a proportion of patients with definite or probable microscopic residual disease after surgery. In a retrospective review from the Memorial Sloan-Kettering Cancer Centre, patients receiving postoperative radiotherapy had a much lower rate of local recurrence, both at the primary site and in the neck, compared with historical controls who received no radiotherapy. The largest effect was at the primary site where surgical margins were considered unsatisfactory: the local recurrence rate was reported as 73% without postoperative radiotherapy, and 10.5% with postoperative radiotherapy.[34]

A multicentre prospective randomized controlled trial in the USA compared 50 Gy pre-operatively with 60 Gy postoperatively.[35] All head and neck sites were included; the largest group was hypopharyngeal cancer with only 15% of the patients having oral cancer. The number of patients included in the trial was 277. Local regional control was significantly better in the postoperative radiotherapy group (70%, $P = 0.04$). However, there was no significant difference in survival.

There now seems little doubt that despite the theoretical considerations and animal experiments favouring preoperative radiotherapy, postoperative radiotherapy is preferable in clinical practice. Postoperative radiotherapy is indicated whenever there is a histological appearance of aggressive disease, close or involved surgical margins, or lymph node involvement with extracapsular spread.

The sooner radiotherapy can be started after surgery the better the prospect of success.[36] In the series reported from Sloan-Kettering the recurrence rate was higher in those patients in whom the interval was more than 6 weeks, but the negative effect of delay could be somewhat mitigated by a higher dose of radiation.[37]

Palliative radiotherapy

The aim of palliative radiotherapy is to relieve the symptoms of the disease, without attempting to cure the patient or causing new symptoms from acute normal tissue reaction. Palliative radiotherapy is only appropriate for patients with incurable disease and a short life expectancy. It is useful for relieving bleeding or pressure symptoms such as pain or obstruction caused by the bulk of the tumour.

A moderate dose of radiation is administered over a short time, for example, 20 Gy over 5 days. This dose is sufficient to kill a substantial proportion of the malignant cells, but not to effect a cure. As a result some tumour shrinkage is achieved with relief of symptoms.

This approach is useful for palliation of metastases, especially in bone, brain or skin. With advanced primary disease or nodal metastases palliative radiotherapy is of little benefit to the patient, as a brief period of regression of the tumour and amelioration of symptoms is followed by regrowth and a rapid return of symptoms before death ensues. Nothing short of complete control of the local disease can provide really worthwhile palliation.

Side-effects of radiotherapy

Acute effects

Mucositis

The acute mucosal reaction to radiotherapy results from mitotic death of cells in the epithelium lining the oral cavity and pharynx. The cell cycle time of the basal epithelial cells is about 4 days, and the epithelium is three or four cells thick. Hence radiation changes begin to appear at about 12 days after the start of irradiation. The time of onset is almost independent of the dose, fractionation or radiation technique. Initially there is erythema of the mucosa followed after a few days by the appearance of a patchy fibrinous exudate (Figure 4.4). If a high dose of radiation is given over a short time, ulceration may supervene with a thick fibrinous membrane covering the denuded surface.

Mucositis is painful and interferes with nutrition. It should be treated conservatively, to avoid damaging the few remaining cells from which the epithelium

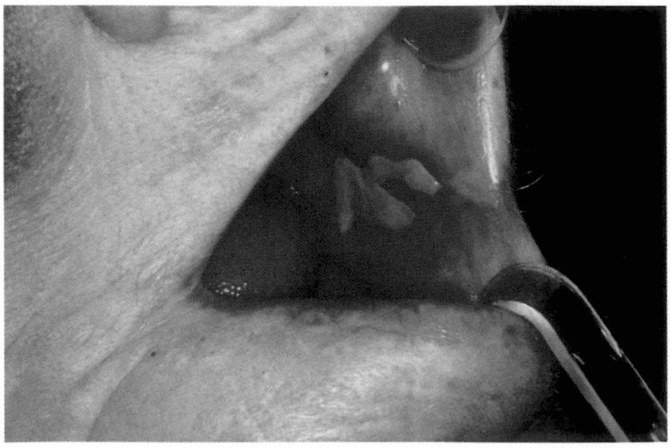

Figure 4.4 Radiation mucositis.

will regenerate. The patient should be advised to take a soft bland diet, avoiding irritants such as smoking, spirits or spicy foods. The mouth should be kept clean using saline mouthwashes. Sodium bicarbonate mouthwash is useful if there is sticky mucus or slough in the mouth. Proprietary mouthwashes, especially those containing alcohol are best avoided. Aspirin, as a gargle or mouthwash, or mixed with lemon mucilage is a useful local analgesic for the oral cavity and hypopharynx respectively. Local anaesthetics, such as mucaine for the hypopharynx and lignocaine for the mouth, may also be tried. The role of bacterial and fungal infection in the pathogenesis of mucositis is not clear; it is probably only a secondary effect, although a reduction in severity of mucositis has been reported from the use of combined anti-fungal and antibiotic pastilles.[38] Surviving epithelial cells respond to radiation damage by dividing more rapidly, so that complete healing is the rule. The length of time mucositis takes to heal depends on the dose intensity of the radiotherapy, but is usually complete within 3 weeks after the end of treatment. Cytotoxic drugs which have a selective action on cells in the mitotic cycle kill regenerating epithelial cells, so that the simultaneous use of chemotherapy and radiotherapy results in more severe and prolonged mucosal toxicity.

Skin reaction

The cell turnover in the skin is a little slower than in the mucosa, so skin changes take longer to appear. Erythema usually appears during the third week of treatment and may progress to a dry and then a moist desquamation according to the dose delivered. Most radiotherapy for oral cancer is given using supervoltage beams, which have a surface sparing effect, so that skin changes are usually mild. Healing is normally complete within 3 weeks of finishing treatment.

Epilation

Hair loss occurs with quite small doses of radiation, so it is seen at both the entrance and the exit of radiation beams. Skin close to the tumour being treated usually receives a dose sufficient to cause permanent epilation, but elsewhere the hair regrows after a few months.

Loss of taste sensation

Patients receiving radiotherapy to the oral cavity, oropharynx or salivary glands invariably experience some disturbance or loss of taste sensation. This is mainly due to a direct effect of radiation on taste receptor cells, but changes in the composition of saliva also play a part.[39] Taste loss can be a distressing symptom, and contributes to poor nutrition in patients receiving radiotherapy. Taste function usually recovers slowly within a few months after the end of radiotherapy, but in some patients the changes are permanent.

Xerostomia

Salivary and mucous glands are especially vulnerable to radiation damage. Loss of secretory cells occurs as an acute effect and the acini are incapable of regenerating and recovering their function. The vulnerability of salivary tissue is both age and dose dependent; as little as 20 Gy in adults can cause permanent cessation of salivary flow, so that glands in both the entry and exit path of radiation beams are at risk. Salivary flow diminishes within a few days of the start of radiotherapy. After 5 weeks, the flow from irradiated salivary glands falls to zero and never recovers. However, in most patients the sensation of dryness of the mouth tends to diminish after a few months. This may be partly subjective as they adjust to their diminished salivary flow, but also results from compensatory hypertrophy of unirradiated glandular tissue. Xerostomia is especially severe after radiotherapy to the nasopharynx as the treatment beams inevitably pass through both parotid glands.

Dryness of the mouth is a distressing symptom, and carries an increased risk of dental decay. Oral administration of pilocarpine may help to stimulate residual salivary tissue, but is rarely very successful. Many patients find a saliva substitute solution helpful. Several proprietary 'artificial salivas' are now available.

Infection

Acute bacterial infection during radiotherapy is uncommon. However, as a course of treatment progresses with increasing mucositis and xerostomia secondary superinfection with *Candida* often occurs. This may present as increased pain and widespread fiery erythema of the mucosa or as discrete white plaques. Candidal infections are treated as and when they occur using specific antifungal agents. In practice, miconazole gel, 10 ml used four times daily, is effective and well tolerated. Severe infections require systemic treatment with fluconazole.

Late effects

Ischaemia and fibrosis

Vascular endothelial cells are slowly replicating, with a turnover time of several months. Poststenotic dilatation of venules also occurs, which appears on skin and mucosal surfaces as telangiectasia. This process begins several months after irradiation and may progress for several years. The extent of devascularization depends on the dose of radiation administered and the volume of tissue irradiated. After excessive doses of radiation, tissue necrosis may supervene. Cell death in connective tissues attracts migrating fibroblasts, leading to excess deposition of collagen, which appears clinically as fibrosis.

Soft tissue necrosis

Acute mucositis normally heals within a few weeks of the end of radiotherapy. Over a period beginning within a few months and extending to several years, vascular changes in the submucosa lead to varying degrees of atrophy, telangiectasia, dryness and fragility of the mucosa. The mucosa can then be damaged by quite minor trauma, leading to ulceration that is slow to heal because of the impaired blood supply. The higher the radiation dose and the larger the volume irradiated, the more marked are the mucosal changes and the greater the risk of ulceration. Brachytherapy gives a higher but more localized mucosal dose, and tends to carry a higher risk of radionecrotic ulceration compared with external beam, although necrosis from the latter is more difficult to treat because of the larger area of devascularized mucosa.

A radionecrotic ulcer is typically flat with little surrounding induration. In some cases there may be associated fibrosis, giving the ulcer a leathery feel. Occasionally, when there is thickening at the edges of the ulcer, it is difficult to distinguish from recurrent carcinoma. A clinical diagnosis should be made if possible, trying to avoid biopsy, which may make the radionecrosis worse. A useful distinguishing feature is the character of pain. A deep boring pain, especially if referred to the ear, is suggestive of carcinoma. The pain of radionecrosis is usually more superficial, often with local tenderness. Treatment consists of scrupulous oral hygiene, irrigation of the ulcer to keep it free of food debris and a course of antibiotics. Most radionecrotic ulcers, especially those following brachytherapy, heal with conservative treatment. If there is no improvement after 2 weeks of treatment, recurrent carcinoma must be suspected and a biopsy performed.

A small minority of radionecrotic ulcers fails to heal and requires surgery. Local diathermy excision is usually adequate. It is very rare for a major excision and repair procedure to be required.

The radiovulnerable cells in bone are the vascular endothelium and the osteocytes. There is relatively little mitotic activity in the latter in the adult, so bone necrosis normally occurs only when there has been a high dose of radiation and a mitotic stimulus such as trauma (see below).

Osteoradionecrosis: definition

Osteoradionecrosis literally means death of irradiated bone. In clinical practice, the term is normally used to define the condition in which dead bone in an irradiated volume loses its mucosal covering, so becoming exposed.

Biological basis of osteoradionecrosis

In normal healthy adult bone, most cells are in the resting phase of the mitotic cycle. However, there is a slow but constant cell turnover accompanied by remodelling of the bone structure. Osteoclasts proliferate, resorb bone and disappear; osteoblasts proliferate to reconstruct the bone. This process continues throughout life. Trauma stimulates proliferation of osteoblasts mainly from the periosteum to repair the damage to the bone.

Irradiation lethally damages some osteoclasts and osteoblasts, which continue to survive and perform their vegetative functions until they attempt to divide, when mitotic death occurs and they disintegrate. An individual bone cell may undergo mitotic death at an interval of months or years after irradiation, or it may never in fact divide unless stimulated by trauma. There is therefore a slow loss of bone cells over a long period after radiotherapy with a consequent slowing down of the remodelling process, which may eventually lead to thinning and reduced strength of the bone, that is a radiation-induced osteoporosis. There is also diminished vascularity of the periosteum as a late effect of radiation on endothelial cells, which may also contribute to bone damage. The direct effect on the bone cells is probably the more important, as histological changes in bone after irradiation have been observed in the absence of any visible changes in the vasculature.

The mandible is affected much more commonly than the maxilla. The mandible consists of more compact bone with a higher density and therefore greater radiation absorption. Its blood supply in the age group who develop cancer is poor, being almost entirely via the periosteum. The maxilla with its lower density and rich vasculature is rarely the site of osteoradionecrosis.

Aetiological factors in osteoradionecrosis

The high absorbed dose from orthovoltage radiation was associated with a high incidence of necrosis.[40] With modern supervoltage radiation, the incidence is lower and markedly dose-dependent. Bedwinek et al[41] reported the incidence of necrosis of the healthy, uninvolved mandible at varying dose levels of supervoltage irradiation using daily fractions of 2 Gy. No cases of osteoradionecrosis were recorded with doses below 60 Gy, up to 70 Gy the incidence was 1.8%, and above 70 Gy was 9%.

The incidence of osteoradionecrosis is at least three times higher in dentate than in edentulous patients as a result of infection from periodontal disease and trauma from tooth extraction.[42] An extraction increases the demand on the remodelling process. If dental extraction is performed at an interval after radiotherapy when there is devascularization in addition to lethal damage to osteoblasts, there is a particularly high risk of bone necrosis. The risk of necrosis is less if dental extraction is performed before radiotherapy, but is still present as a consequence of the enhanced remodelling of bone, which proceeds for some months after the extraction.[43] Improvement in dental management of patients receiving radiotherapy is now tending to reduce the difference in incidence of necrosis between dentate and edentulous patients.

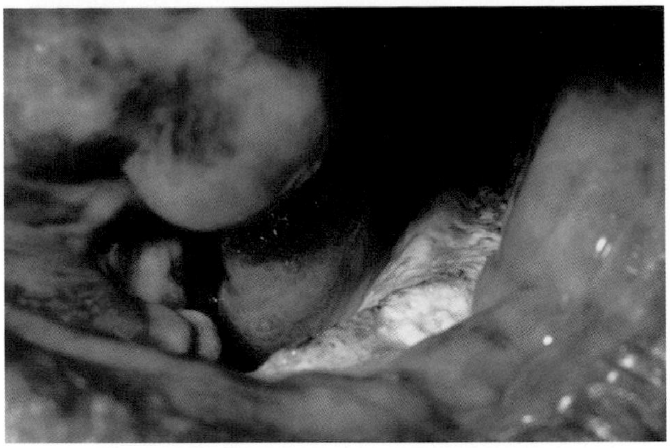

Figure 4.5 Osteoradionecrosis.

Infection can gain entry to the bone via traumatic injuries, tooth extractions, pulpal infection, periodontal infection or radionecrotic ulceration of the overlying mucosa.[44] In some cases the mucosal necrosis is the precipitating factor, and in others the mucosal necrosis is secondary to necrosis of the underlying bone.

Invading tumour suppresses osteoblastic remodelling, but if the malignant cells are killed by treatment the bone will attempt to regenerate so that mitotic death of osteoblasts occurs. Consequently, successful treatment by radiotherapy of a carcinoma invading the bone is almost inevitably followed by osteoradionecrosis.

Many patients with mouth cancer are alcoholic and in poor general condition. In these patients poor nutritional status and lack of oral hygiene make them particularly prone to mucosal ulceration and consequent osteoradionecrosis.

Diagnosis of osteoradionecrosis

If a segment of mandible undergoes necrosis, the process starts on the alveolar margin and is accompanied by ulceration of the alveolar mucosa. This gives a characteristic appearance of a flat ulcer with the brownish-looking dead bone at its base (Figure 4.5). Pain is not normally a feature of osteoradionecrosis per se, and even a pathological fracture due to this cause may be completely painless. However, the necrosis is often complicated by secondary infection, in which case there may be severe pain with trismus, fetor and general ill health. As in the case of soft tissue necrosis, bone necrosis must be distinguished from tumour recurrence.

Treatment of osteoradionecrosis

A conservative approach should be adopted for medical treatment of osteoradionecrosis. Meticulous oral hygiene is essential, including the use of 0.01% chlorhexidine mouthwash after every meal. Loss of the mucosa usually results in a cavity in the gum over the necrotic bone; this cavity should be regularly irrigated to dislodge any food debris and necrotic tissue. The patient should be instructed to do this themselves wherever possible. It is unimportant what solution is used for irrigation as it is the mechanical removal of debris that is important; possibly hydrogen peroxide or chlorhexidine solution may help to destroy anaerobic organisms.

Sequestra should be allowed to separate spontaneously. Any surgical interference only encourages extension of the necrotic process. When a sequestrum becomes loose, it should be removed gently and any sharp edges or spicules of bone smoothed off with bone rongeurs to prevent irritation of the tongue. Osteoblastic activity and reabsorption of non-vital bone may take many months or even years, because of the relatively avascular nature of irradiated bone. Therefore, great patience is required to resist the temptation to intervene surgically, even when a pathological fracture occurs. Pain, when present, usually indicates secondary infection. Attempts should be made to control the infection by the local measures outlined above and administration of systemic antibiotics. Antibiotics are not very effective because of the avascularity of the tissues, so prolonged treatment is necessary. The tetracyclines are the most useful antibiotics because of their selective bone uptake; a dosage of 250 mg four times a day for 10 days is recommended, followed by 250 mg twice daily continued for several months. Metronidazole, 200 mg three times a day, should be added in cases of severe infection in an attempt to combat anaerobic organisms. There are advocates of long-term low-dose tetracycline for all cases of osteoradionecrosis, but the value of this is difficult to assess because healing is always slow with or without treatment and no controlled study has been done.

Hyperbaric oxygen therapy has been shown to promote healing.[45] Best results have been obtained[46] using 2 atmospheres pressure for 2 hours per day for 60 days, that is a total of 120 hours in the chamber. This method of treatment is undoubtedly effective, but is cumbersome and time-consuming for both patients and hospital staff, and there are risks in subjecting patients with cardiovascular or respiratory disease to raised pressures. Consequently, hyperbaric oxygen cannot be recommended for routine use, but may have a place for the younger, fitter patient treated in a centre where the resources are available.

A simpler method, which has been claimed to promote cell growth, is ultrasound. Harris[47] recommends therapeutic ultrasound at a frequency of 3 mHz pulsed one in four at an intensity of 1 W/cm^2 applied to the mandible for 10 minutes daily for 50 days. Spontaneous healing occurs in about 50 per cent of cases using the conservative measures described. Failure of healing may be due to excessive radiation dosage, uncontrollable infection or the presence of persistent tumour. In those cases with persistent symptoms in whom there is no improvement after a few months of conservative therapy, surgical treatment should be considered.

The key to successful surgical management is the introduction of new vascularized soft tissue to cover the irradiated bone. The necrotic bone must be trimmed back until all obviously infected tissue is removed. The overlying soft tissue is then resected until viable non-friable margins are seen. A muscle flap is used to cover all exposed bone. Temporalis, trapezium, pectoralis major and latissimus dorsi flaps are all suitable, the choice being based on the size of the defect and any previous surgical intervention. Theoretically, all bone within the high-dose irradiated volume should be resected so that the bone margins are well vascularized. However, in some cases this would lead to massive defects, and in practice may not be necessary.

In most circumstances, it is better to avoid bone grafting even when a pathological fracture is present. If bone reconstruction is essential, then conventional bone grafting techniques combined with a course of hyperbaric oxygen pre- and postoperatively give the most reliable results.[48] Vascularized free flaps are rarely indicated in these circumstances as suitable recipient vessels are not usually available in the heavily irradiated patient.

REFERENCES

1. Paterson R. Studies in optimum dosage. *Br J Radiol* 1952; **25**: 505–516.
2. Wiernik G, Alcock CJ, Bates TD et al. Final report on the second British Institute of Radiology fractionation study: short versus long overall treatment times for radiotherapy of carcinoma of the laryngo-pharynx. *Br J Radiol* 1991; **64**: 232–241.
3. Overgaard J, Horsman MR. Modification of hypoxia-induced radio-resistance in tumours by the use of oxygen and sensitizers. *Semin Radiat Oncol* 1996; **6**: 10–21.
4. Rubin P, Hanley J, Keys HM et al. Carbogen breathing during radiation therapy. *Int J Radiat Oncol Biol Phys* 1979; **5**: 1963–1970.
5. Churchill-Davidson I. Oxygen therapy: clinical considerations. In: Deeley TJ (ed.) *Modern Trends in Radiotherapy*. London: Butterworths, 1967; 73–91.
6. Wells G, Koh W, Pelton J et al. Fast neutron teletherapy in advanced epidermoid head and neck cancer: a review. *Am J Clin Oncol* 1989; **12**: 293–300.
7. Overgaard J. Clinical evaluation of nitroimidazoles as modifiers of hypoxia in solid tumours. *Oncol Res* 1994; **6**: 509–518.
8. Fromhold H, Guttenberger R, Henke M. The impact of blood haemoglobin content on the outcome of radiotherapy: the Freiburg experience. *Strahlentherapie Onkologie* 1998; **4**: 31–34.
9. Rojas A, Hirst VK, Calvert AS, Johns H. Carbogen and nicotinamide as radiosensitizers in a murine mammary carcinoma using conventional and accelerated radiotherapy. *Int J Radiat Oncol Biol Phys* 1986; **34**: 357–365.
10. Henk JM. Does hyperbaric oxygen have a future in radiotherapy? *Int J Radiat Oncol Biol Phys* 1981; **7**: 1125–1128.
11. Griffin TW, Paiak TF, Laramore GE et al. Neutron vs photon irradiation of inoperable salivary gland tumours. *Int J Radiat Oncol Biol Phys* 1989; **15**: 1085–1090.
12. Overgaard J, Hansen HS, Overgaard M et al. A randomized double-blind phase III study of nimorazole as a hypoxic radiosensitizer of primary radiotherapy in supraglottic larynx and pharynx carcinoma. Results of the Danish Head and Neck Cancer Study (DAHANCA) protocol 5–85. *Radiother Oncol* 1998; **46**: 135–146
13. Horiot JC, le Fur T, N'Guyen C et al. Hyperfractionation compared with conventional radiotherapy in oropharyngeal carcinoma. *Eur J Cancer* 1990; **26**: 779–780.

14. Parsons JT, Mendenhall WM, Cassisi NJ et al. Hyperfractionation for head and neck cancer. *Int J Radiat Oncol Biol Phys* 1988; **14**: 649–658.
15. Wang CC, Blitzer PH, Suit HD. Twice-a-day radiation therapy for cancer of the head and neck. *Cancer* 1985; **55**: 2100–2104.
16. Horiot JC, Bontemps P, van den Bogaert W et al. Accelerated fractionation compared to conventional fractionation improves loco-regional control in the radiotherapy of advanced head and neck cancers: results of the EORTC 22851 randomized trial. *Radiother Oncol* 1997; **44**: 111–121.
17. Dische S, Saunders M, Barrett A et al. A randomised multicentre trial of CHART versus conventional radiotherapy in head and neck cancer. *Radiother Oncol* 1997; **44**: 123–137.
18. Overgaard J, Saad Hansen H, Sapne W et al. Conventional radiotherapy in the primary treatment of squamous cell carcinoma of the head and neck. A randomized multicentre study of 5 versus 6 fractions per week – preliminary report of the DAHANCA 6 and 7 trials. *Radiother Oncol* 1996; **40 (Suppl 1)**: 853.
19. Knee R, Fields RS, Peters LJ. Concomitant boost radiotherapy for advanced squamous cell carcinoma of the head and neck. *Radiother Oncol* 1985; **4**: 1–7.
20. Fu KK, Pajak TF, Trotti A et al. A radiation therapy oncology group phase III randomized study to compare hyperfractionation and two variants of accelerated fractionation to standard fractionation radiotherapy for head and neck squamous carcinomas: first report of RTOG 9003. *Int J Radiat Oncol Biol Phys* 2000; **48**: 7–16.
21. Vokes EE, Mick R, Lester EP et al. Cisplatin and fluorouracil chemotherapy does not yield long-term benefit in locally advanced head and neck cancer: results from one institution. *J Clin Oncol* 1991; **9**: 1376–1384.
22. Pignon JP, Bourhis J, Domenge C et al. Chemotherapy added to locoregional treatment for head and neck squamous-cell carcinoma: three meta-analyses of updated individual data. *Lancet* 2000; **335**: 949–955.
23. Bourhis J, Wilson G, Wibault P et al. Rapid tumour cell proliferation after induction chemotherapy in oropharyngeal cancer. *Laryngoscope* 1994; **104**: 468–472.
24. Rosenthal DI, Pistenmaa DA, Glatstein E. A review of neoadjuvant chemotherapy for head and neck cancer: partially shrunk tumours may be both leaner and meaner. *Int J Radiat Oncol Biol Phys* 1993; **28**: 315–320.
25. Henk JM. Controlled trials of synchronous chemotherapy with radiotherapy: overview of radiation morbidity. *Clin Oncol* 1997; **9**: 308–312.
26. Tannock IF. Chemotherapy in conjunction with radiotherapy and/or surgery in head and neck cancers. In: Peckham MJ, Pinedo HM, Veronesi U (eds) *Oxford Textbook of Oncology.* Oxford: Oxford University Press, 1995; 1083–1094.
27. Wallner PE, Hanks GE, Kramer S, McLean CT. Patterns of care study: analysis of outcome survey data – anterior two-thirds of tongue and floor of mouth. *Am J Clin Oncol* 1986; **9**: 50–57.
28. Hall EJ, Lam YM. Renaissance of interstitial brachytherapy. In: Vaeth JM (ed.) *Frontiers of Radiation Theapy and Oncology.* Basel: Karger, 1978; 12.
29. Pierquin B, Chassagne D, Cachin Y. Carcinomes epidermoides de la langue mobile et du plancher buccal. *Acta Radiol* 1970; **9**: 465–480.
30. Pernot M, Malissard L, Hofstetter S et al. The study of tumoral, radiobiological, and general health factors that influence results and complications in a series of 448 oral tongue carcinomas treated exclusively by irradiation. *Int J Radiat Oncol Biol Phys* 1994; **29**: 673–679.
31. Sobel S, Rubin P. Tumour persistence as a predictor of outcome after radiation therapy of head and neck cancers. *Int J Radiat Oncol Biol Phys* 1976; **1**: 873–877.
32. Powers WE, Palmer LA. Biologic basis of pre-operative radiation treatment. *Am J Roentgenol* 1968; **102**: 176–192.
33. Tupchong L, Scott CB, Blixter PH et al. Randomized study of pre-operative vs post-operative radiation therapy in advanced head and neck carcinoma: long-term follow-up of RTOG study 73–03. *Int J Radiat Oncol Biol Phys* 1990; **20**: 21–28.
34. Perez CA, Olsen J. Pre-operative vs post-operative irradiation: comparison in an experimental animal tumour system. *Am J Roentgenol* 1970; **108**: 396–404.
35. Vikram B, Strong EW, Shah J, Spiro RH. Elective post-operative radiation therapy in stages III and IV epidermoid carcinoma of the head and neck. *Am J Surg* 1980; **140**: 580–584.
36. Peters LJ, Goepfert H, Ang KK et al. Evaluation of the dose for postoperative radiation therapy of head and neck cancer: first report of a prospective randomized trial. *Int J Radiat Oncol Biol Phys* 1993; **26**: 3–11.
37. Vikram B. Post-operative irradiation for squamous cell carcinoma of the head and neck. *Int J Radiat Oncol Biol Phys* 1990; **18**: 267–272.
38. Symonds RP, McIlroy P, Khorrami J et al. The reduction of radiation mucositis by selective decontamination antibiotic pastilles: a placebo-controlled double-blind trial. *Br J Cancer* 1996; **74**: 312–317.
39. Fernando I, Patel T, Billingham L et al. The effect of head and neck irradiation on taste dysfunction: a prospective study. *Clin Oncol* 1995; **7**: 173–178.
40. Watson WL Scarborough JE. Osteoradionecrosis in intra-oral cancer. *Am J Roentgenol* 1938; **40**: 524–528.
41. Bedwinek JM, Shukovsky LJ, Fletcher GH, Daly TE. Osteoradionecrosis in patients treated with definitive radiotherapy for squamous cell carcinoma of the oral cavity and naso and oropharynx. *Radiology* 1976; **119**: 665–667.
42. Murray CG, Herson J, Daly TE, Zimmerman S. Radiation necrosis of the mandible: a 10-year study. *Int J Radiat Oncol Biol Phys* 1980; **6**: 543–548.
43. Hinds EC. Dental care and oral hygiene before and after treatment. *JAMA* 1971; **215**: 964–966.
44. Bragg DG, Shidnia H, Chu F, Higginbotham NL. Clinical and radiographic aspects of radiation osteitis. *Radiology* 1970; **97**: 103–111.
45. Ketchum SA, Thomas AM, Hall AD. Angiographic studies of the effect of hyperbaric oxygen on burn wound

vascularization. In: Wada J, Ina T (eds) *Proceedings of the 4th International Congress on Hyperbaric Medicine.* Baltimore: Williams and Wilkins, 1970; 380.
46. Hart GB, Mainous EG. The treatment of radiation necrosis with hyperbaric oxygen. *Cancer* 1976; **37**: 2580–2585.
47. Harris M. The conservative management of osteoradionecrosis of the mandible with ultrasound therapy. *Br J Oral Maxillofac Surg* 1992; **30**: 313–318.
48. Marx RE, Ames JR. The use of hyperbaric oxygen in bony reconstruction of the irradiated and tissue-deficient patient. *J Oral Maxillofac Surg* 1982; **40**: 412–420.

5 Chemotherapy for head and neck cancer

Asha Saini, Martin E Gore and David J Adelstein

Introduction

The role of chemotherapy in head and neck squamous cell cancer (HNSCC) remains controversial despite many years of intensive investigation. This chapter focuses on chemotherapy for squamous cell cancers of the head and neck region, including tumours of the oral cavity, oropharynx, larynx and hypopharynx. Squamous cell cancers account for over 90% of tumours arising in this region. Other epithelial malignancies including adenocarcinomas and neuroendocrine cancers as well as non-epithelial lesions such as sarcomas, have distinct biological features and are beyond the scope of this discussion.

Despite anatomic heterogeneity, HNSCC can be treated by the medical oncologist as essentially one disease entity. The optimal use of chemotherapy in this disease is as yet undefined, and until recently, the standard treatment modality in HNSCC was either surgery, radiotherapy or a combination of the two. Chemotherapy was reserved for the setting of recurrent, usually metastatic disease, providing short-lived palliation of symptoms, but no improvement in survival for this group of patients. Over the last two decades, the role of chemotherapy has gradually evolved away from use in the palliative setting alone. There are now randomized data supporting the use of chemotherapy in the context of combined modalities treatment to cure patients with unresectable disease, as well as in a neoadjuvant approach to downstage disease in patients. Moreover, the use of concomitant chemotherapy and radiotherapy in advanced disease has been shown to provide a statistically significant survival benefit in selected studies.

In the setting of advanced, unresectable local disease, primary chemotherapy is increasingly being used as an adjunct to standard primary treatment (surgery and/or radiotherapy) where one of the main aims of treatment is preservation of organ function as well as improving disease-free and overall survival. Despite the emergence of promising results, which are discussed in this chapter, the precise role of chemotherapy and the optimal treatment regimen is still not clearly established and currently its use should remain within the context of clinical trials.

The main focus of current research in recurrent or metastatic disease is phase I and phase II trials of new drugs and novel combinations. At the time of writing, despite the existence of many drugs giving high response rates, both as single agents and in combination, in this treatment setting, no chemotherapy trials have shown an improvement in patient survival. However, it is important to note that objective tumour response and overall survival may be inadequate as measures of the success of palliative treatment[1] and the value of chemotherapy can be debated around other aspects of disease control that make a significant contribution to a patient's quality of life. Such positive outcomes arising as a result of chemotherapy include locoregional tumour control, improvement in disease-free survival, control of pain, restoration of swallowing and appetite, improvement of weight loss and fatigue (Table 5.1). It must also be realized that the influence of treatment on overall survival may be obscured in this particular group of patients since there is typically a prolonged history of alcohol and tobacco abuse, social deprivation and concomitant cardiopulmonary morbidity all of which carry a high risk of death from unrelated causes (Table 5.2). Furthermore, there is a high incidence of second malignancies even in patients who have may have been cured of their primary cancers.

Table 5.1 Benefits of chemotherapy in advanced disease

Locoregional tumour control
Control of pain
Restoration of swallowing and appetite
Improvement of weight loss and fatigue
Increased disease-free survival

Table 5.2 Failure of chemotherapy to impact on survival in HNSCC patients

Alcohol and tobacco abuse
Comorbid conditions
Advanced age at diagnosis
Risk of second primaries
Risk of metastatic disease
Death from unrelated causes
Social deprivation

Table 5.3 Difficulties in assessment of objective response in HNSCC

Anatomic complexity
Coexisting ulceration
Coexisting bacterial infection
Treatment related oedema

Table 5.4 Toxicity of cytotoxic drugs used in treatment of HNSCC

Mucositis/ulceration
Nausea/vomiting
Anorexia
Myelosuppression (risk of infection/haemorrhage)
Pulmonary fibrosis
Nephrotoxicity
Neurotoxicity
Ototoxicity
Lethargy

Specific problems of chemotherapy for HNSCC

Measurement of objective response

Measurement of objective response, which is one of the most important means of evaluating the success of treatment, is difficult in HNSCC. Assessment by conventional radiological methods or direct vision is hampered by the anatomic complexity of the region, the presence of ulceration, treatment-related oedema and the frequent occurrence of bacterial superinfection (Table 5.3). Early evidence of response, within the first two cycles of treatment, is generally required in order to justify the continuation of treatment in patients with recurrent or metastatic disease. Histopathological evaluation is one way to circumvent this problem, but even with this approach there is scope for error. The use of novel imaging techniques may prove to be of use in the future. Interesting results have recently been reported using the technique of F_2-18 fluorodeoxyglucose positron emission tomography (FDG-PET). This technique provides tumour imaging by measuring metabolic activity of tissues and, by identifying changes in their metabolism after a course of chemotherapy, possibly predicting for response.[2] One recent study correlated the findings of serial PET scans with serial tissue biopsy findings in a small study of patients receiving primary chemotherapy for locally advanced HNSCC and found the sensitivity of PET scanning to be 90% and the specificity to be 83%.[3] This is a relatively new area of research and these interesting results warrant further investigation. At the present time, for patients with incurable disease, a judgement of response is perhaps best made in terms of symptom palliation and restoration of quality of life rather than in terms of actual tumour shrinkage.

Toxicity

Toxicity of chemotherapy is another important consideration in the treatment of HNSCC. Exacerbation of local symptoms by treatment-related mucositis, dermatitis, dysphagia, nausea and vomiting add considerably to patient morbidity and may outweigh any therapeutic advantage (Table 5.4). These problems are especially severe when combined modality treatments are used and frequently lead to a requirement for enteral feeding. In addition, relatively minor side-effects such as alopecia can add considerably to the disfigurement caused by the primary disease, while myelosuppression, which is almost universal with chemotherapeutic drugs, results in a higher incidence of life-threatening neutropenic sepsis than seen in other malignancies. This may be explained in part by the portal of entry for bacteria provided by areas of extensive dermatitis, mucositis and ulceration.

Table 5.5 Control and prevention of cytotoxic drug-induced toxicities

Neutropenia	G-CSF
Anaemia	Red cell transfusion, erythropoietin
Thrombocytopenia	Platelet transfusion, thrombopoietin
Mucositis	Sucralfate, GM-CSF, amifostine

While control of myelosuppression is currently within sight with the increasing use of haemopoietic growth factors such as granulocyte-colony stimulating factors, erythropoietin and thrombopoietin, mucositis remains a major dose-limiting toxicity of both chemotherapy and radiotherapy in HNSCC. In the past, manoeuvres to decrease the incidence and severity of mucositis have included use of sucralfate mouthwashes[4] and mouthwashes containing mixtures of antibacterial and antifungal components,[5] which were reported to decrease mucositis associated with cisplatin and 5-fluorouracil chemotherapy and radiotherapy respectively. However, the results obtained with these treatments were less than satisfactory and new ways of circumventing mucosal toxicity are currently under evaluation (Table 5.5).

Interesting recent evidence that colony-stimulating factors may have a role in reducing mucositis was derived from randomized trials in lymphoma patients treated with or without granulocyte-macrophage colony stimulating factor (GM-CSF) that documented fewer cases of mucositis in treated patients.[6] In a randomized study of 20 patients with advanced HNSCC treated with cisplatin and 5-fluorouracil, patients were randomized to receive subcutaneous injections of GM-CSF on days 5–14 either on the first or the second cycle of chemotherapy. Those patients who received it on the first cycle were found to have less severe mucositis, and those who received it on the second course had less mucositis on the second cycle. The chemotherapy regimen that was used in this study was relatively non-myelotoxic and oral mucositis was not influenced by the level of neutropenia. This suggests that GM-CSF may have a direct effect on the oral mucosa.[7] These results were obtained from a very small study and confirmatory studies are in progress at the time of writing. Trials are also being conducted to look at the use of GM-CSF mouthwashes in the treatment of chemotherapy and radiation-induced mucositis.[8,9]

Randomized studies using amifostine, an organic thiophosphate that acts as a free-radical scavenger, protecting normal tissues from the cytotoxic effects of radiation are currently under way to evaluate whether this can reduce the acute mucositis associated with radical radiotherapy. Preliminary results indicate that severity and duration of mucositis induced by radiotherapy is reduced when amifostine is used at a daily dose of 150–200 mg/m^2 but the drug is poorly tolerated with nausea, cutaneous eruptions and hepatic dysfunction.[10]

Many other specific drug-related toxicities exist and are discussed below in relation to each drug.

Unpredictable delivery of drugs to tumour tissue

Drug delivery to the tumour mass depends on intact vasculature, which is rarely present in this group of tumours as a result of necrosis, previous surgery and radiotherapy.

Chemotherapy for recurrent or metastatic disease

The aim of chemotherapy for patients with relapsed local disease after surgery or radiotherapy or those with distant metastatic disease is always palliative. Whilst expectation of cure remains unrealistic in this situation, palliation of tumour-related symptoms is an important goal that can frequently be achieved providing significant improvements in quality of life in the terminal stages. Tumour-related symptoms that may respond to chemotherapy include pain, discomfort, dysphagia, reduced appetite, weight loss and fatigue.[1] Only some of these symptomatic benefits are achieved by measurable tumour responses, and since this is usually the only outcome that is consistently and accurately reported in most randomized controlled trials, the results of such trials are often reported in an unnecessarily negative fashion. If symptom palliation, drug toxicity, convenience of administration and cost as well as the more formal standpoint of tumour measurement were reported, the palliative benefits of chemotherapeutic regimens may become apparent. Palliative treatment may lead to small improvements in patient survival in the advanced disease setting, but with presently available drugs, the survival benefit is likely to be obtained at the expense of severe toxicity.

Single agent chemotherapy

Many different cytotoxic drugs have been identified as having activity in recurrent or metastatic HNSCC, giving single agent response rates of up to 30%. The most active agents are listed in Table 5.6. Responses achieved in recurrent or metastatic disease are generally short-lived and the median survival of treated patients remains unaltered at 6–12 months.[11] Cisplatin, methotrexate, 5-fluorouracil, hydroxyurea,

Table 5.6 Single-agent chemotherapy for HNSCC

Drug	Response rate (%)	Reference
Methotrexate	31	Mitchell et al[18]
Cisplatin	28	Al-Sarraf[15]
Carboplatin	22	Al-Sarraf[15]
Bleomycin	21	Al-Sarraf[12]
5-Fluorouracil	15	Al-Sarraf[12]
Ifosfamide	26	Martin et al[59]
Paclitaxel	38	Forastiere et al[28]
Docetaxel	38	Dreyfuss et al[33]
Gemcitabine	13	Catimel et al[36]

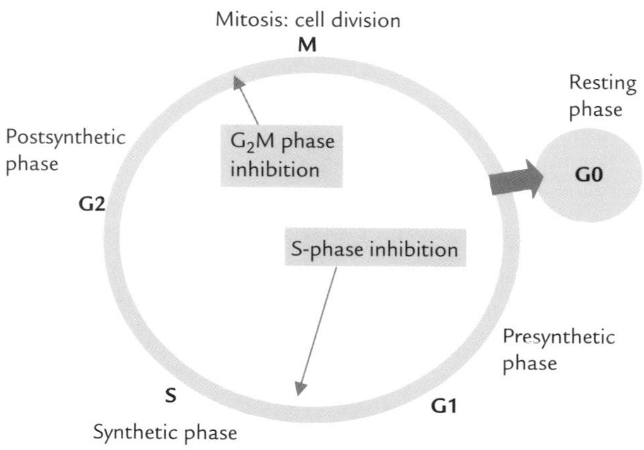

Drug	Mode of Action
Cisplatin, carboplatin	Formation of DNA crosslinks Cell cycle non-specific
5-Fluorouracil	Inhibition of DNA synthesis by mimicking pyrimidine metabolites Maximal effect in S-phase
Methotrexate	Inhibition of dihydrofolate reductase S-phase specific
Doxorubicin	Intercalation between base-pairs Cell cycle non-specific
Hydroxyurea	Inhibits ribonucleotide diphosphate reductase Maximal effect in S-phase
Bleomycin	Formation of DNA strand breaks Arrests cell division in G2 and M phases
Paclitaxel, Docetaxel	Irreversible stabilization of microtubules, prevents formation of mitotic spindle Cell arrest at G2/M
Gemcitabine	Antimetabolite S-phase specific

Figure 5.1 The cell cycle and mechanisms of action of anti-cancer drugs.

bleomycin and more recently, drugs such as irinotecan, gemcitabine and the taxanes have been found to be active in this disease (Figure 5.1). Some of the drugs commonly used in the treatment of HNSCC are discussed below.

Cisplatin

Cisplatin inhibits DNA synthesis by forming intrastrand and interstrand crosslinks between guanine–guanine pairs of DNA (Figure 5.2). It is currently regarded as the most active agent in HNSCC giving response rates of approximately 20–50% in phase II trials.[12] The dose range most often used is 80–120 mg/m^2 every 3–4 weeks. Comparison of standard and higher doses has not demonstrated any advantage to use of higher doses in terms of response or survival.[12] This finding was confirmed in a randomized study comparing 60 mg/m^2 and 120 mg/m^2.[13] Although pilot studies evaluating the use of very high doses (200 mg/m^2) as a single agent demonstrated higher response rates for the higher dose, use of this dose level carried a considerable risk of irreversible toxicity.[14]

Toxicities associated with use of conventional-dose cisplatin are considerable and include effects on

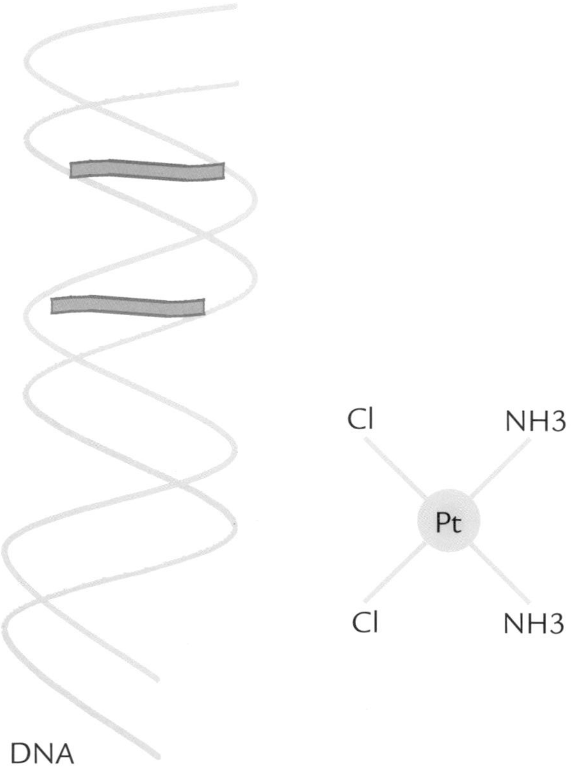

Figure 5.2 Structure of cisplatin and interstrand crosslinking of DNA

Table 5.7 Toxicity associated with cisplatin

Emesis
Nephrotoxicity
Cumulative ototoxicity
Late chronic neuropathy (up to 40% of patients)
Myelosuppression (nadir after approximately 10 days)
Electrolyte wasting (K^+, Mg^{2+}, Ca^{2+})

the kidney, bone marrow, gut and peripheral nervous system (Table 5.7). This makes the drug difficult to use in patients with poor performance status or with coexisting disease. Cisplatin analogues have been widely tested in HNSCC with the aim of maintaining efficacy with less toxicity. The most succesful is carboplatin, which has less renal, neurologic, otologic and gastrointestinal toxicity, but is dose-limited by myelosuppression. The response rate in HNSCC is slightly lower than cisplatin at 14–30% with a pooled average from single agent studies of 22%.[15] The lower efficacy of carboplatin compared to cisplatin has been confirmed in a randomized trial evaluating its use in combination with 5-fluorouracil.[16] Carboplatin therefore cannot be regarded as a substitute for cisplatin in HNSCC, but in clinical practice may be a reserve option in patients with peripheral neuropathy or renal impairment in whom cisplatin may be contraindicated. Studies evaluating iproplatinin, an alternative cisplatin analogue in the context of HNSCC have demonstrated an inferior response rate as well as worse toxicity.[17] Cisplatin therefore remains one of the reference agents in the treatment of HNSCC.

Methotrexate

Methotrexate is the 4-amino 10-methyl analogue of folic acid. It binds and inhibits dihydrofolate reductase (DHFR) which is a critical enzyme in the maintenance of intracellular folates in their reduced form as tetrahydrofolates. These reduced folates are vital for the synthesis of nucleic acids and their depletion interferes with cellular capacity to repair DNA, resulting in DNA strand breaks. The mode of action of methotrexate is extremely complex and drug-mediated inhibition of DHFR is only one of several mechanisms of its action (Figure 5.3). It also acts by direct inhibition of folate-dependent enzymes and by incorporating aberrant nucleotides into DNA, resulting in inhibition of DNA synthesis. In palliative therapy for recurrent or metastatic HNSCC, single agent methotrexate has been regarded as the least toxic drug and has been widely used for many years (Table 5.8).

Table 5.8 Toxicity associated with methotrexate

Renal toxicity
Gingivitis, stomatitis, mouth ulceration
Mild nausea
Bone marrow depression
Photosensitivity
Hepatotoxicity
Renal failure
Cystitis
Pulmonary changes

Many different doses and schedules have been tested, but the most commonly used schedule is weekly intravenous bolus treatment, using a dose of 40–60 mg/m², tailored according to the dose-limiting toxicities of mucositis, bone marrow depression and renal impairment. The objective response rate to methotrexate given in this dose range is 10–30%. A degree of dose-dependence is apparent from several non-randomized studies in the literature in which doses up to 500 mg/m² have

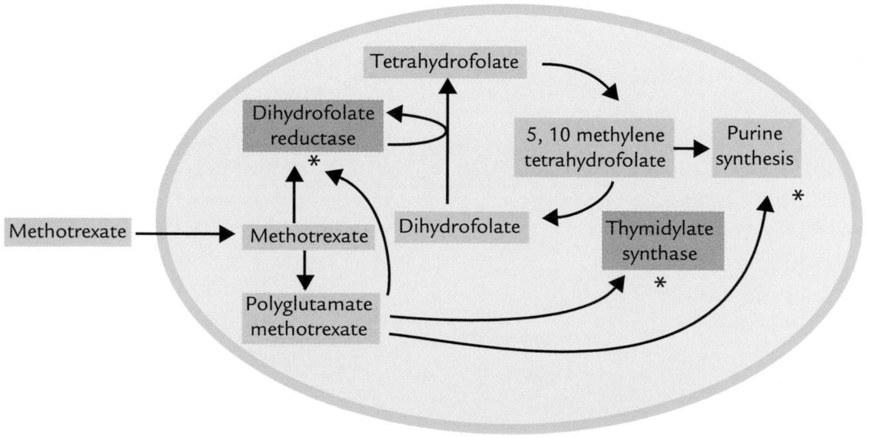

Figure 5.3 Mechanism of action of methotrexate (* site of inhibition)

been used.[18,19] However, the toxicity of higher doses is considerable, negating any benefit in the palliative setting. Moreover, doses greater than 70 mg/m^2 require specific hydration and urine alkalinization regimes, making administration more cumbersome.

Use of folinic acid (leucovorin) can reverse many of the cytotoxic effects of methotrexate on both normal and malignant cells and this drug, used appropriately, can enhance the therapeutic index of methotrexate by limiting the toxicity of higher doses of methotrexate. Doses greater than 70 mg/m^2 require folinic acid rescue. Randomized trials comparing high-dose methotrexate with folinic acid rescue with standard dose methotrexate have, however, failed to show any survival advantage to the higher doses.[20,21] Over the last decade, a number of methotrexate analogues have been evaluated including trimetrexate,[22] edatrexate[23] and piritrexin.[24] To date, these have not been shown to have any advantage over methotrexate and edatrexate in particular has a worse toxicity profile.

Bleomycin

This drug was originally derived from glycopeptides produced by a strain of streptomyces found in soil. Bleomycin intercalates between opposing strands of DNA, generating free radicals that produce single- and double-stranded DNA breaks. Cells in the G2 and M phases of the cell cycle are most sensitive, with cells in the G1 phase showing least sensitivity (Figure 5.1).

Bleomycin has been extensively evaluated in HNSCC; single-agent response rates are of the order of approximately 21%. One of the advantages of bleomycin is that it is not associated with myelosuppression and thus can be given at full doses in combination with other drugs. Other toxicities, however, are considerable and include a risk of hypersensitivity resulting in urticaria, periorbital oedema and bronchospasm (Table 5.9). Pulmonary fibrosis occurs in approximately 10% of patients and is associated with administration of cumulative doses above 400 units, elderly patients and patients with a previous history of radiotherapy to the chest. It manifests as insidious dyspnoea and the onset of patchy reticulonodular infiltrates on chest X-ray. Fibrotic changes in the lungs can partially regress with cessation of treatment and steroids, but in some cases this pulmonary toxicity can be fatal. The many other toxic effects include fevers, mucositis, alopecia, hyperpigmentation and hyperkeratosis of hands, joints and previously irradiated areas of skin.

Table 5.9 Toxicity associated with bleomycin

Tumour pain
Allergic reaction 3–5 hours after administration
Fever
Chills
Skin reactions, rash, striae, erythema, inflammation of hands
Stomatitis
Pulmonary fibrosis
Pnemonitis
Nail ridging

5-Fluorouracil

5-Fluorouracil is an antimetabolite that exerts its cytotoxic effects in several different ways. The predominant effect is thought to be through the inhibition of thymidine synthase, leading to depleton of nucleotides required for DNA synthesis and repair. Early studies with 5-fluorouracil in patients with advanced, multiply relapsed HNSCC indicated a single agent response rate of 15%. Randomized trials have demonstrated that higher response rates are obtained when 5-fluorouracil is given by continuous infusion over 96 or 120 hours and when its effect is modulated by the use of modulators such as leucovorin. Delivery of 5-fluorouracil by continuous infusion may be associated with a different spectrum of toxicity with mucositis and diarrhoea gaining predominance over myelosuppression (Table 5.10).[25]

5-Fluorouracil assumed increasing importance in the management of HNSCC following the discovery of synergy with cisplatin, which was shown to result in an increase in objective response rates up to 70% including a reported complete remission rate of up to 27% in recurrent HNSCC in the original study.[26]

Table 5.10 Toxicity of 5-fluorouracil

Diarrhoea
Stomatitis
Palmar-plantar erythema
Bone marrow suppression
Hyperpigmentation
Nausea

Taxanes

Paclitaxel and its semisynthetic derivative, docetaxel, are drugs with broad anti-cancer activity that have a novel mechanism of action. They act by promoting the formation of tubulin dimers, stabilizing microtubules during cell division and thereby leading to arrest of cells in the G2/M phase of the cell cycle (Figure 5.1). Docetaxel is twice as active as paclitaxel in promoting tubular polymerization. This greater cytotoxicity may be related to its higher affinity for microtubules or to greater intracellular accumulation.[26,27]

The optimal dosage and schedule for use of paclitaxel in HNSCC has not yet been determined. The original studies used a 3-hour infusion, but there is evidence that paclitaxel is schedule dependent, with greater activity seen with use of prolonged treatments. Delivery by 24-hour infusion may be more effective but the incremental benefit of higher doses or longer schedules needs to be further evaluated in HNSCC particularly in relation to greater toxicity and higher cost. The preliminary results of a phase II trial carried out by the Eastern Cooperative Oncology Group to evaluate the activity of single agent paclitaxel reported a 37% overall response rate in 19 patients with relapsed HNSCC[28] making it one of the most effective single agents in this disease. Early trials of paclitaxel adminstered by different schedules in combination with irradiation are currently ongoing in head and neck cancer (SWOG, unpublished data) as are trials of its use in combination with other active agents such as cisplatin and ifosfamide.[29]

In contrast to paclitaxel, the activity of docetaxel appears to be schedule independent.[30] Significant anti-tumour activity was originally found in human HNSCC tumour xenografts in nude mice.[31] Interestingly, cell lines with acquired resistance to cisplatin were shown to maintain sensitivity to docetaxel,[32] indicating lack of cross-resistance.

Clinically, use of docetaxel in recurrent/metastatic HNSCC results in objective responses in 22–45% of patients, with a median duration of response of 5 months, which compares favourably with currently used combination treatments. The major toxicities of docetaxel are neutropenia, mucositis and fluid retention (Table 5.11), which can be prevented by premedicating patients with corticosteroids and diphenhydramine.[33]

Taxanes are also potent radiosensitizers since G2/M is the cellular phase at which cells exhibit greatest radiosensitivity. Data derived from Tishler and colleagues showed that paclitaxel potentiated the effect of radiation in vitro in many cell lines at clinically achievable paclitaxel concentrations (< 10 nmol/l), indicating potential for developing a chemoradiation regimen simultaneously utilizing paclitaxel.[34,35]

Table 5.11 Toxicity associated with taxanes

Paclitaxel
Myelosuppression (dose-limiting)
Hypersensitivity (hypotension, bronchospasm, urticaria–abrogated by premedication)
Peripheral neuropathy
Myalgia/arthralgia
Docetaxel
Myelosuppression (dose-limiting)
Hypersensitivity
Capillary leak syndrome (ascites, pleural effusion, oedema)

Gemcitabine

Gemcitabine was initially synthesized as an antiviral agent with the ability to inhibit both RNA and DNA viruses. Structurally, it is a pyrimidine molecule resembling the endogenous nucleoside, deoxycytidine and inhibits DNA synthesis by competing with deoxycytidine during synthesis of the DNA strand. The toxicity is mild and consists of myelosuppression, lethargy, flu-like symptoms and proteinuria. Phase II studies of single-agent gemcitabine in patients with advanced HNSCC have shown response rates of 13–22%.[36]

Gemcitabine is also a radiosensitizer and low doses (200 mg/m^2 intravenously weekly) combined with radiotherapy gave a response rate of 70% with low toxicity in untreated patients with HNSCC in a small preliminary study.[37] Its future role in combination treatments is currently under evaluation.

Combination chemotherapy in recurrent and metastatic disease

The rationale for using multiple drugs in combination is to develop regimens that produce higher response rates and increase overall survival (Table 5.12). There are many comparative studies in the literature showing that responses using combinations of agents are higher in HNSCC compared with single agents. This difference is especially marked when cisplatin-containing regimens are compared with single agents.[38–41] In a study by Jacobs and

Table 5.12 Rationale for use of combination chemotherapy

Use of single drugs is not curative
Maximal cell kill within toxic range for each drug
Less likelihood of resistance

colleagues,[40] response rates were higher for cisplatin in combination with 5-fluorouracil compared with either single agent (32% versus 17% and 13% for cisplatin and 5-fluorouracil respectively). In a study comparing single-agent methotrexate with cisplatin/5-fluorouracil and carboplatin/5-fluorouracil,[42] the superior response rate of the combination treatments was clear (30% overall response rate for cisplatin/5-fluorouracil, 18% for carboplatin/5-fluorouracil versus 11% for methotrexate), but increased toxicity was observed for the combinations. Moreover, overall survival was not different between the three treatment arms.

Many other randomized studies of single agents versus combination chemotherapy in recurrent or metastatic HNSCC confirm the findings of higher response rate without impact on survival. Table 5.13 outlines the principles used in the selection of drugs in the most successful combinations.

The published randomized trials of different combination regimens were evaluated in a meta-analysis by Browman and Cronin in 1994.[43] They concluded that single agent cisplatin was superior to single agent methotrexate, and the combination of cisplatin and 5-fluorouracil was the most effective regimen in recurrent head and neck cancer, giving response rates varying from 72% in the original reports[26] to 24% reported in 1990 by the Liverpool Head and Neck Oncology Group.[44]

Table 5.13 Optimizing drug combinations

Drugs with known single-agent efficacy
Drugs known to produce complete remissions as single agents
Non-overlapping toxicity
Each drug within its optimal dose and schedule
Drug combinations should be given at consistent intervals. The treatment-free intervals should be the shortest time for recovery from toxicity (usually bone marrow)

Overall, in this disease setting, the response rate for cisplatin and 5-fluorouracil is approximately 32% and the median survival of treated patients is approximately 6 months (Table 5.14). Addition of other agents to this combination (vindesine, vincristine, bleomycin) has failed to improve the response rate achieved by the two agents.[45] Addition of interferon, which in the preclinical setting has been shown to increase the anti-tumour effect of both cisplatin and 5-fluorouracil has been evaluated in a phase III trial by the Head and Neck Interferon Cooperative Study Group.[46] In this study 244 patients with recurrent or metastatic HNSCC were randomized to receive cisplatin (100 mg/m^2) on day 1 and 5-fluorouracil 1g/m^2/day for 96 hours by continuous infusion every 21 days with or without

Table 5.14 Landmark studies in chemotherapy for metastatic disease

Reference	No. of patients	Regimen	Response rate (%)
Jacobs et al[88]	79	Cis (100 mg/m^2) d1 + 5FU 1g/m^2 d1–4	32
	83	Cis (100 mg/m^2) d1	17
	83	5FU 1 g/m^2 d1–4	15
Kish et al[91]	18	Cis (100 mg/m^2) + 5FU 600 mg/m^2 d1 + d8	20
		Cis (100 mg/m^2) d1 + 5FU 1 g/m^2 d1–4	72
Forastiere et al[16]	87	Cis (100 mg/m^2) d1 + 5FU 1 g/m^2 d1–4	32
	86	Carbo (300 mg/m^2) d1 + 5FU 1 g/m^2 d1–4	21
	88	Methotrexate 40 mg/m^2 iv weekly	10
Vokes et al[92]	25	Cis (100 mg/m^2) d1 + 5FU 0.8 g/m^2 d1–5 + leucovorin 50 mg/m^2 po 6 hourly	56

Cis: cisplatin; 5FU: 5-fluorouracil; carbo: carboplatin; d: day; iv: intravenously; po: per os.

Table 5.15 Novel combinations currently under evaluation

Regimen	Response rate (%)	Reference
Cisplatin, docetaxel, 5FU, leucovorin	100	Colevas et al[52]
Paclitaxel, carboplatin, ifosfamide (TIC)	55	Shin et al[89]
Vinorelbine, cisplatin, 5FU	55	Gaspar et al[90]

5FU: 5-fluorouracil.

interferon at a dose of 3 × 10^6 U/day subcutaneously over days 1–5. The response rate without interferon was 47% and with interferon was 38.4% ($P < 0.5$), with no difference in overall survival (approximately 6 months) between the two study arms.

The poor prognosis of this category of patients indicates the need for novel therapies (Table 5.15). Interesting results have been obtained with novel drug combinations such as the combination of cisplatin, 5-fluorouracil, leucovorin and docetaxel, which was tested recently in 23 patients with locally advanced HNSCC, giving an overall response rate of 100% with 14 patients (61%) achieving clinical complete remission. Such a regimen may improve outlook in advanced HNSCC, but the toxicity issues remain of paramount importance in the metastatic disease setting.

Since currently used 'standard' chemotherapy options in HNSCC are all palliative and both single agents and combinations of drugs may be appropriate, the choice of treatment should depend on the balance between efficacy and toxicity (Table 5.16). Patients with adequate performance status should recieve cisplatin and 5-fluorouracil or be entered into investigational protocols of new drugs or combinations. For patients with poorer performance status consideration can still be given to the use of single-agents such as taxanes, gematabine or methotrexate, but referral to a palliative care unit remains the main option.

Table 5.16 'Standard' therapies for recurrent or metastatic disease

Methotrexate 40–60 mg/m^2 iv weekly
Cisplatin 100 mg/m^2 every 3–4 weeks
Cisplatin 100 mg/m^2 and 5FU 800–1000 mg/m^2 continuously for 4–5 days every 3–4 weeks

5FU: 5-fluorouracil.

Table 5.17 Chemotherapy in the primary management of HNSCC

Neoadjuvant	Chemotherapy prior to loco-regional treatment where the aim is to reduce tumour burden prior to definitive local control
Adjuvant	Chemotherapy following local treatment designed to eradicate micrometastases following local therapy
Concomitant	Simultaneous administration of chemotherapy and radiotherapy
Rapidly alternating	Combined radiotherapy and chemotherapy schedule designed to minimize tissue toxicity and increase tumour kill

Primary chemotherapy in head and neck cancer

Whilst no improvements in patient survival have resulted from the use of chemotherapy in patients with recurrent or metastatic HNSCC, promising results have emerged from studies of primary chemotherapy in patients with advanced or extensive locoregional disease.

There are four ways in which chemotherapy has been incorporated into the initial management of HNSCC (Table 5.17).

Neoadjuvant chemotherapy

Neoadjuvant chemotherapy has been evaluated in the context of the primary management of HNSCC because the standard management of advanced disease involving surgery followed by radiotherapy

Table 5.18 Rationale for neoadjuvant chemotherapy

Potential advantages
Intact vascular bed, therefore better drug delivery
Reduced bulk results in less extensive surgery, or conversion of unresectable tumour into resectable status
Identify chemosensitive tumours, thus better prognosis, organ preservation surgery and adjuvant chemotherapy
Identify poor prognosis patients for intensified therapy
Better performance status, better tolerance of chemotherapy
Early therapy for micrometastatic disease
Potential disadvantages
Delay of potentially curative surgery
Noncompliance after a complete response (refusing potentially curative surgery)
Morbidity of therapy
Increased cost of therapy

can result in mutilation and considerable loss of function. In addition locoregional and distant relapse occurs in 60–70% of patients. Approximately one-third of patients with HNSCC have locally advanced disease at presentation.[11] The potential advantages of giving chemotherapy before definitive local treatment (Table 5.18) are that the patient's performance status, a major factor influencing response, is often better at this stage, the response to treatment can be easily assessed and, since tumour vasculature is relatively undisturbed, delivery of drugs to the tumour may be less impaired than after local treatment (surgery or radiotherapy). The main drawbacks of this approach are the possibilities of delaying and thereby compromising definitive local therapy, the possibility of inducing tumour resistance because of the phenomenon of repopulation. Furthermore, responding patients may refuse local treatment, particularly after chemotherapy-induced complete remissions. Finally, prolongation of treatment, which inevitably occurs with chemotherapy, has significant cost implications.

Numerous non-randomized studies carried out in the 1970s explored the use of drugs in the neoadjuvant setting. Use of single agents such as methotrexate, bleomycin and cisplatin gave disappointingly low response rates, but greater success was achieved with use of combination chemotherapy. The feasibility of the neoadjuvant approach in terms of toxicity and patient compliance was clearly demonstrated and induction chemotherapy was shown not to preclude subsequent surgery or radiotherapy.[47] Phase II trials showed that cisplatin was an important component of combination regimens. In 1979, Randolph and colleagues[48] reported the high efficacy of a combination of cisplatin and continuous infusion bleomycin, which gave a 71% overall response rate with 20% complete responses in 21 patients. In 1982, Kish and colleagues[49] originally reported the success of cisplatin used in combination with 5-fluorouracil. In this study, administration of three courses of chemotherapy resulted in an overall response rate of 93% with 54% of patients achieving clinically complete remission. The high activity of this regimen was subsequently confirmed in many other trials[50,51] and it became widely accepted as the standard regimen for neoadjuvant treatment. Modifications of the cisplatin/5-fluorouracil regimen have been made in an attempt to improve the rate of complete remission; these include addition of leucovorin, methotrexate and interferon, but have failed to confer any significant benefit. More recently, Colevas and colleagues[52] published the results of a small study in which docetaxel was added to the standard cisplatin and 5-fluorouracil schedule. Although 100% of patients responded and 61% of these were reported as having clinically complete responses, the toxicity was extremely high. A randomized comparison with the standard treatment is required before the value of such novel combinations is accepted.

Many of the studies of neoadjuvant chemotherapy report rates of pathologically confirmed complete remission of up to 60%; despite this, all patients tend to relapse unless further definitive local treatment is carried out.

The use of randomized phase III studies evaluating the overall benefits of neoadjuvant chemotherapy in the treatment of locally advanced HNSCC falls into two distinct historical phases. The original trials were conceived with the aim of improving locoregional control rates, decreasing the rate of distant recurrence and improving overall survival (Table 5.19). These studies randomized patients to immediate surgery followed by radiotherapy or induction chemotherapy followed by definitive local therapy for responding patients (Figure 5.4). One of the largest studies, conducted by the Department of Veterans Affairs Laryngeal Cancer Study Group,[53] showed similiar 2-, 3- and 4-year survival rates for patients randomized to either conventional surgery (laryngectomy) and radiotherapy or to induction chemotherapy followed by radiotherapy, which was only given to complete or partial responders to chemotherapy. In the chemotherapy arm, laryngectomy was only performed in patients not responding to the first two cycles of chemotherapy or in those with residual disease or recurrence following radiotherapy. An important finding was that the incidence of local failure was higher in the chemother-

Table 5.19 Neoadjuvant chemotherapy in head and neck cancer

Reference	No. of patients	Regimen	Response (%)	Local therapy	1-year disease-free survival (%)		Comment	Survival benefit
					Control	Chemotherapy and radiotherapy		
Toohill et al[93]	60	PF × 3	85 (19% CR)	S+R	70	70		No
Schuller et al[61]	158	PMBV × 3	70	S+R	23	23	Decrease in distant metastases	No
Richard et al[94]	222	VcB	48 (6% CR)	S+/-R	–	–		Reduction in locoregional recurrence with chemotherapy
DVALCSG[53]	332	PF × 2	98 (49%)	R+S	–	–	66% larynx preservation; decrease in distant metastases	No
Depondt et al[63]	324	CbF	57					No
Paccagnella et al[62]	237	PF × 4	70 (29% CR)	S+R	58	62	Decrease in distant metastases	Advantage for inoperable patients
Fonseca et al[95]	79	PF × 4	49	S+R				No
Lefebvre et al[64]	202	PF		S			Decrease in distant metastases; 28% alive at 3 years with larynx preserved	No

D: doxorubicin; P: cisplatin; F: 5-fluorouracil; M: methotrexate; Vc: vincristine; B: bleomycin; Epi: epirubicin; Cb: carboplatin; S: surgery; R: radiotherapy; CR: complete remission.

apy arm (Table 5.20). This may indicate the need for more thorough histopathological confirmation of complete response before treating patients with radiotherapy alone. As far as the impact of primary chemotherapy on distant metastases was concerned, although use of chemotherapy led to a lower rate of distant metastasis as a site of first relapse, there were no differences between the two groups with respect to eventual distant metastatic disease.

Patients achieving histologic complete response were found in this study to have improved disease-free and

Table 5.20 Sites of recurrence after neoadjuvant chemotherapy: DVALCSG[53]

	Surgery arm	CT arm
Primary disease	2%	12%
Regional disease	5%	8%
Distant metastasis	7%	11%

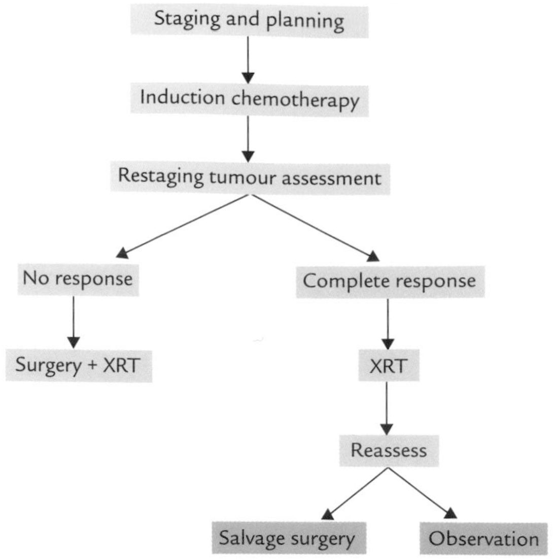

Figure 5.4 Randomization schema for preoperative chemotherapy.

overall survival compared to partial or clinically defined complete responders. Similiar observations have been made by other workers.[54–56] Chemotherapy response may select out a prognostically favourable group of patients whose tumours are biologically less aggressive. In addition, response to drugs is predictive for response to radiotherapy[57,58] and therefore may be selecting out those patients who can avoid surgery without impairing their chances of survival.

Factors predicting for a more favourable outcome with neoadjuvant chemotherapy are the T and N status of the tumour, primary site in the oral cavity and nasopharynx and patient performance status (Table 5.21). Future trials may identify further predictive factors for response to chemotherapy to enable this type of treatment to be delivered more selectively and new drugs, with higher activity against distant metastases and better radiosensitization potential may improve outlook.

In retrospect, many of the neoadjuvant chemotherapy studies detailed in Table 5.19 may have used suboptimal drug combinations, included heterogeneous tumour types and included too few patients. However, even those using the optimal cisplatin/5-fluorouracil regimen, while showing a trend towards reducing distant metastases (Table 5.19), failed to show any survival advantage to the addition of chemotherapy. In some reports there was a trend towards improved survival in a small subset of patients with improved locoregional control rate and improved distant failure rate.[62] This may represent a subgroup of patients with chemosensitive disease in whom surgery can be avoided without compromising long-term survival.

Table 5.21 Factors predicting favourable outcome with neoadjuvant chemotherapy

Primary site in the oral cavity or nasopharynx
T and N status of the tumour
Patient performance status
Use of combination chemotherapy

With dramatic response failing to translate into improved locoregional control or survival, the focus for neoadjuvant therapy since the mid-1980s has been within the context of using laryngeal preservation rates and quality of life as parameters to evaluate the success of treatment (Table 5.22). In the report from the DVALCSG study outlined above, of 166 patients randomized to receive neoadjuvant chemotherapy, only 38% required subsequent laryngectomy, indicating the benefit of this treatment as a laryngeal preservation approach.[53] However, since laryngeal preservation can be achieved in many patients with radiotherapy alone, it was not possible from this study to determine whether induction chemotherapy added any benefit over radiation alone in terms of organ preservation.

In a second study patients were randomized to either three cycles of carboplatin and 5-fluorouracil or no chemotherapy prior to locoregional treatment. Conservation of the larynx was possible in 57% of patients in the chemotherapy arm and in 24% of patients in the control arm.[63] A recent randomized phase III EORTC trial included 194 eligible patients with advanced hypopharyngeal cancer randomized between a conventional approach and induction chemotherapy with cisplatin and 5-fluorouracil.[64] This large study indicated that by utilizing induction chemotherapy, the probability of retaining a functional larynx at 3 years was 42% and at 5 years was 35%. Locoregional failure rates were equivalent in the two treatment arms and no differences in survival were noted, indicating the success of this approach in the context of preservation of function. As none of these studies included a radiotherapy-only treatment arm, the extent to which induction chemotherapy contributed to organ preservation could not be clearly defined. There are clinical data suggesting that laryngeal preservation may be achieved in a similiar proportion of patients treated with radiotherapy alone[65] and the application of' hyperfractionation techniques[66] may further improve the results of radiotherapy. The relative contribution of the two treatment modalities is a question that is currently being addressed in the Intergroup Laryngeal Preservation Study which has a radiation-only arm.[67]

Table 5.22 Larynx preservation trials

Reference	No. of patients	Regimen	3 year estimate of retaining larynx (%)
DVALCSG[53]	332	Chemo+XRT vs Surg +XRT	33
Lefebvre et al[64]	202	Chemo+XRT vs Surg + XRT	42

In conclusion, despite the high response rates achieved, neoadjuvant chemotherapy has failed to impact on patient survival and locoregional control rates. However, neoadjuvant chemotherapy may have a place as a standard approach in the management of very large tumours to reduce the size of the radiation field. It can also be considered as an alternative treatment option for patients with advanced disease who are otherwise facing laryngectomy, and laryngeal preservation is an option. Finally, it is unclear whether newer radiation rechniques or strategies involving neoadjuvant chemotherapy are the current standards of care.

Adjuvant chemotherapy

Despite surgery and postoperative radiotherapy, only 30% of patients with locally advanced, resectable HNSCC survive for 5 years. Approximately 20% of patients with advanced HNSCC eventually develop metastatic disease and a further 10–20% develop a second primary tumour. The goal of postoperative adjuvant chemotherapy following primary treatment is to eradicate sites of microscopic distant disease as well as to reduce the risk of locoregional recurrence. It has the advantage of not delaying definitive surgery and of not blurring the tumour–normal tissue interface for surgery. This approach has improved survival in other solid tumours, notably breast carcinoma, osteosarcoma and colorectal carcinoma. In HNSCC, there are very few published phase III randomized trials exploring this approach (Table 5.23) and only a limited subgroup of patients has been shown to benefit from adjuvant chemotherapy.

Laramore and colleagues randomized 499 patients with completely resected HNSCC to immediate

Table 5.23 Randomized trials of adjuvant chemotherapy in HNSCC

Reference	Regimen	No. of patients	Locoregional benefit	Survival benefit
Domenge et al[68]	CMB vs XRT alone	287	Yes	Worse in CT group
Laramore et al[67]	C + F + XRT vs XRT	499	No (trend towards benefit in CT group for high-risk patients)	No (trend towards improved survival in CT patients with high-risk disease)
Head and Neck contracts[60]	No CT vs neoadjuvant C vs neoadjuvant C + adjuvant C	462	No	No (but fewer distant metastases in adjuvant CT group)
Huang et al[102]	MBVL	126	?	No
Taylor et al[86]	MC +XRT	95	?	No
Ervin et al[97]	CMB (neoadjuvant +/- adjuvant)	114	?	No

C: cisplatin; M: methotrexate; B: bleomycin; F: 5-fluorouracil; V: vinblastine; L: leucovorin; P: platinum; FA: folinic acid; Vc: vincristine; XRT: radiotherapy; CT: chemotherapy.

postoperative radiotherapy or three cycles of cisplatin/5-fluorouracil followed by radiotherapy.[67] Overall, they found no effect on overall survival or time to locoregional failure, but in a specific high-risk group of patients with close resection margins (less than 5 mm) or extracapsular nodal extension, there was a trend towards improved survival. In a second study reported by Domenge and colleagues,[68] patients with extracapsular nodal extension were randomized to either radiotherapy alone or radiotherapy followed by bleomycin, cisplatin and methotrexate. These investigators reported improved locoregional control, but worse overall survival and distant metastatic rate in the chemotherapy group.

Factors relating to this negative outcome may be a result of the patient population studied or may be specific to this disease. Many of the trials of adjuvant chemotherapy have reported poor patient compliance, in particular, in two trials less than 10% of the patients in the adjuvant arm were able to complete planned treatment. Furthermore, in the patient population under study, the high death rate from other health problems related to old age or sequelae of cigarette or alcohol abuse may obscure any possible survival benefit arising from the use of chemotherapy.

Use of postoperative chemotherapy combined with radiation, compared with radiation alone was recently explored in a large phase III randomized trial and shown to confer a possible survival benefit,[69] but this finding requires confirmation and the benefit obtained has to be balanced against the high level of acute toxicity observed with such intensive treatments.

A meta-analysis of the results of 54 randomized trials of adjuvant chemotherapy in HNSCC suggested that use of chemotherapy may increase absolute survival by 6.5%. Furthermore, in those trials in which chemotherapy was given synchronously with radiotherapy, the increase in absolute survival was 12.1%, suggesting that this approach warrants further investigation in the adjuvant setting.[70] A second meta-analysis examined all those trials in which chemotherapy was added to local treatment. For a total of 25 trials examined, the addition of chemotherapy reduced mortality by 11%. Interestingly, use of concurrent chemoradiotherapy was found to reduce the mortality of HNSCC patients by 22%. Morbidity of treatment, however, was increased with the combined treatment[71] and the role of adjuvant chemoradiotherapy in resected HNSCC was not clear from this analysis. A third analysis using pooled patient data from eight clinical trials incorporating 1854 patients has failed to confirm any advantage to the use of adjuvant chemotherapy in HNSCC (Table 5.24).[72]

Table 5.24 Meta-analyses of effects of adjuvant chemotherapy

Munro[70]	6.5% absolute increase in survival
El-Sayed and Nelson[71]	11% reduction of mortality
Bourhis et al[72]	No advantage to adjuvant chemotherapy

Concomitant chemoradiotherapy

In the treatment of advanced, unresectable HNSCC, use of concomitant chemoradiotherapy has emerged as one of the most promising advances. The rationale for this approach is based on exploiting different toxicities and mechanisms of action of the two treatment modalities resulting in greater killing of tumour cells compared with surrounding normal tissue. Some drugs may also selectively enhance the effect of radiotherapy by acting as radiosensitizers (e.g. bleomycin, paclitaxel), whilst others inhibit enzymes involved in DNA damage repair after radiotherapy.

Early randomized trials of simultaneous single-agent chemotherapy combined with radiotherapy in the 1960s, while not providing any definitive results, provided essential information on treatment toxicity. For example, when hydroxyurea was used simultaneously with radiotherapy, the result was simply an enhancement in toxicity, without any increase in locoregional control.[73] Almost all single agents tested, including mitomycin C, bleomycin and 5-fluorouracil cause unacceptable increases in normal tissue toxicity and in some cases enhancement of late radiation damage. A trial in which methotrexate was combined with radiotherapy gave a marginal benefit in survival compared with radiotherapy alone, but the increase in mucosal toxicity tended to negate any benefits achieved by this approach.[74] Toxicity with use of concomitant chemoradiotherapy has proved to be a major problem. Despite this, data from phase II clinical trials using combinations of drugs have indicated that combining radiotherapy with chemotherapy is a feasible approach in HNSCC, giving excellent results in terms of complete response rates and disease-free survival.[75,76]

There are now several randomized trials comparing concomitant chemoradiotherapy with either radiotherapy alone[76,77] or with sequential schedules in which chemotherapy is given first and is followed by radiotherapy (Table 5.25).[78,79] Many of these trials have shown that concomitant chemoradiotherapy can improve disease-free survival and locoregional

Table 5.25 Randomised trials of combination chemotherapy and concurrent radiotherapy

Reference	Regimen	No. of patients	Survival benefit
Keane et al[76]	MF + XRT vs XRT alone	209	No
Smid et al[77]	MB + XRT vs XRT alone	49	Yes
Adelstein et al[79]	PF + concurrent XRT vs PF + sequential XRT	100	No, but improved DFS and locoregional control with concurrent radiotherapy
Wendt et al[98]	F/FA + P + XRT vs XRT alone	270	Yes and locoregional control benefit
Brizel et al[99]	PF + XRT vs XRT alone	116	Trend towards improved survival and locoregional benefit
Calais et al[100]	CbF + XRT vs XRT alone	226	Yes
SECOG[101]	VMB+/-F + concurrent XRT vs VMB+/-F + sequential XRT	267	No, but DFS improved with concurrent radiotherapy

C: cisplatin; M: methotrexate; B: bleomycin; F: 5-fluorouracil; V: vincristine; Cb: carboplatin; FA: folinic acid; XRT: radiotherapy; DFS: disease-free survival.

control rates, with a survival advantage observed in a subset of patients with unresectable disease. Encouraging results from a meta-analysis evaluating 3727 patients included in 26 randomized trials has shown an 8% survival benefit in favour of concomitant chemotherapy compared with locoregional treatment alone.[72] Toxicity with concomitant treatment is universally higher.

A recent study from the Intergroup investigators evaluating postoperative cisplatin delivered concurrently with radiotherapy in nasopharyngeal cancers showed the superiority of chemoradiotherapy compared with radiotherapy alone in terms of both progression-free survival and overall survival (3-year progression-free survival 69 versus 24% and 3-year overall survival 78 versus 47% in the chemoradiotherapy group and radiotherapy alone groups, respectively) and in this distinct tumour type, this is now the standard of care.[80]

Rapidly alternating chemoradiotherapy

In view of the heightened toxicity associated with simultaneous chemoradiotherapy, which leads to dose reductions, treatment delays and enhanced patient morbidity, Looney and Hopkins[81] proposed the use of alternating courses of radiotherapy and chemotherapy.

This schedule of treatment has been evaluated in unresectable HNSCC with great success. Use of rapidly alternating chemotherapy and radiotherapy was originally compared to neoadjuvant chemotherapy followed by definitive radiotherapy. This study revealed a survival advantage in favour of the alternating treatment.[82] The same authors recently published the results of their second phase III trial comparing alternating treatment against radiotherapy alone, reporting the superiority of the alternating approach over conventional radiotherapy.[83] The regimen used in this latter study was cisplatin 20 mg/m^2 and bolus 5-fluorouracil 200 mg/m^2 daily for 5 days. The frequency of complete response was 43% for the combined treatment arm compared with 22% for the radiotherapy only group ($P = 0.037$). Overall survival at 5 years was estimated at 24% (95% CI 14–40%) for the combined treatment group against 10% (95% CI 4–24%) for the radiotherapy-only group. The improved survival appeared to be related to improved locoregional control, which is in keeping with the findings of earlier investigators.[84–86] Interestingly, the incidence and intensity of mucositis was reported as being identical in the two treatment groups.

In the control arm of the Merlano study,[83] the patients had unexpectedly low rates of local tumour control and survival for reasons that are not immediately clear. Current overall survival rates for similiar stage patients treated by radiotherapy alone are 33%

compared with the 10% reported in this study. Similar discrepancies exist for disease-free survival.[87] Therefore, although this was a well-conducted trial, confirmatory studies are required before this approach becomes considered standard therapy for locally advanced unresectable HNSCC. If the success of alternating chemoradiation is confirmed, then the doubling of 5-year survival represents a significant treatment advance in the treatment of unresectable HNSCC.

Conclusions

The role of chemotherapy in the treatment of HNSCC has undergone intensive study over the past 20 years. Neoadjuvant chemotherapy, while not offering significant survival advantage, can be used in combination with radiotherapy for patients suitable for organ preservation. It may also have a place in the treatment of very large primary tumours that may otherwise be difficult to irradiate. Randomized studies of simultaneous chemoradiation suggest high local control rates and a possible impact on overall survival in advanced/unresectable disease. Schedules using new radiosensitizing drugs (taxanes, gemcitabine) need to be evaluated against the standard drug regimens currently used. The interesting results obtained with rapidly alternating chemoradiation schedules in the treatment of unresectable disease, if confirmed, may have an important role in organ preservation, combining the advantages of chemoradiation while reducing its toxicity.

Postoperative adjuvant chemotherapy may benefit selected patients identified at high risk of relapse.

For nasopharyngeal carcinoma, which is a distinct disease entity, randomized data unequivocally suggests an advantage to use of concomitant chemoradiation over radiotherapy alone.

REFERENCES

1. Constela DO, Hill ME, Ahern RP et al. Chemotherapy for symptom control on recurrent squamous cell carcinoma of the head and neck. *Ann Oncol* 1997; **97**: 445–449.
2. Brun E, Ohlsson T, Eriandsson K et al. Early prediction of treatment outcome in head and neck cancer with 2-18FDG-PET. *Acta Oncol* 1997; **36**: 741–747.
3. Lowe VJ, Dunphy FR, Varvares M et al. Evaluation of chemotherapy response in patients with advanced head and neck cancer using [F-18] fluorodeoxyglucose positron emission tomography. *Head Neck* 1997; **19**: 666–674.
4. Pfeiffer P, Madsen EL, Hansen O, May O. Effect of prophylactic sucralfate suspension on stomatitis induced by cancer chemotherapy. A randomized double-blind crossover study. *Acta Oncol* 1990; **29**: 171.
5. Spijkervert FKL, van Saene HKF, Panders AK et al. Mucositis prevented by selective elimination of oral flora in irradiated head and neck cancer patients. *J Oral Pathol Med* 1991; **19**: 486–489.
6. Nemunaitis J, Rosenfeld CS, Ash R et al. Phase III double-blind placebo controlled trial of rhGM-CSF following allogencie bone marrow transplant. *Bone Marrow Transplant* 1995; **15**: 949–954.
7. Chi KIH, Chen CH, Chan WK et al. Effect of granulocyte-macrophage colony stimulating factor on oral mucositis in head and neck cancer patients after cisplatin, fluorouracil and leucovorin chemotherapy. *J Clin Oncol* 1995; **13**: 2620–2628.
8. Wardley AM, Scarffe JH. Role of granulocyte-macrophage colony stimulating factor in chemoradiotherapy induced oral mucositis. *J Clin Oncol* 1996; **14**: 1741–1742.
9. Throuvalas N, Antonadou D, Pulizzi M et al. Evaluation of the efficacy and safety of GM-CSF in the prophylaxis of mucositis in head and neck cancer patients treated by radiotherapy. *Proc ECCO* 1995; **43**: 1 [abstract].
10. Bourhis J, Wibault B, Luboinski F et al. A randomized phase II study of very accelerated radiotherapy with and without amifostine in advanced head and neck cancer. *Proc Am Soc Oncol* 1999; **18**: 393a.
11. Vokes EE, Weichselbaum RR, Lippman SM, Hong WK. Medical progress: head and neck cancer. *N Engl J Med* 1993; **328**: 184–194.
12. Al-Sarraf M. Chemotherapeutic management of head and neck cancer. *Cancer Metast Rev* 1987; **6**: 191.
13. Veronesi A, Zagonel V, Rirelli U et al. High dose versus low dose cisplatin in advanced head and neck squamous carcinoma; a randomized study. *J Clin Oncol* 1985; **3**: 1105.
14. Forastiere AA, Takasugi BJ, Baker SR et al. High dose cisplatin in metastatic head and neck cancer. *Cancer Chemother Pharmacol* 1989; **19**: 155.
15. Al-Sarraf M. New approaches to the management of head and neck cancer. The role of chemotherapy. *Adv Oncol* 1990; **6**: 11–14.
16. Forastiere AA, Metch B, Schuller DE et al. Randomized comparison of cisplatin plus fluorouracil and carboplatin plus fluorouracil versus methotrexate in

advanced squamous-cell carcinoma of the head and neck: a Southwest Oncology Group study. *J Clin Oncol* 1992; **10**: 1245–1251.

17. Abele R, Clavel M, Rossi A et al. Iproplatin(JM-9) in advanced squamous cell carcinoma of the head and neck. A phase II study of the EORTC clinical trials group. *Proc ASCO* 1986; **5**: 147.
18. Mitchell MS, Wawro NW, DeConti RC et al. Effectiveness of high-dose infusions of methotrexate followed by leucovorin in carcinoma of the head and neck. *Cancer Res* 1968; **28**: 1088–1094.
19. Kirkwood JM, Canellos GP, Ervin TJ et al. Increased therapeutic index using moderate dose methotrexate and leucovorin twice weekly vs. weekly high dose methotrexate-leucovorin in patients with advanced squamous carcinoma of the head and neck. A safe new regimen. *Cancer* 1978; **47**: 2414.
20. Taylor SG, McGuire WP, Hauck WW et al. A randomized comparison of high dose infusion methotrexate versus standard dose weekly therapy in head and neck squamous cell carcinoma. *J Clin Oncol* 1984; **2**: 1006.
21. Woods RL, Fox RM, Tattersall MHN. Methotrexate treatment of squamous cell head and neck cancers: a dose response evaluation. *Br Med J* 1984; **282**: 600.
22. Robert F. Trimetrexate as a single agent in patients with advanced head and neck cancer. *Semin Oncol* 1988; **15**: 22.
23. Schornagel JH, Verweij J, DeMulder PHM et al. Randomised phase III trial of edatrexate versus methotrexate in patients with metastatic or recurrent HNSCC. *J Clin Oncol* 1995; **13**: 1649.
24. Degardin M, Demonge C, Copperleare P et al. Phase II piritrexim study. *Clin Oncol* 1992; **11**: 244.
25. Tapazoglu E, Kish J, Ensley J, Al-Sarraff M. The activity of single agent 5-fluorouracil infusion in advanced and recurrent head and neck cancer. *Cancer* 1986; **57**: 1105.
26. Kish JA, Weaver A, Jacobs J et al. Cisplatin and 5-fluorouracil infusion in patients with recurrent and disseminated epidermoid cancer of the head and neck. *Cancer* 1984; **53**: 1819.
27. Ringel I, Horwitz SB. Studies with RPS6976 (Taxotere): a semisynthetic analog of taxol. *J Natl Cancer Ins* 1991; **83**: 288.
28. Forastiere AA. Use of paclitaxel in squamous cell carcinoma of the head and neck. *Semin Oncol* 1993; **20**: 56–60.
29. Forastiere AA, Urba SG. Single agent paclitaxel and paclitaxel plus ifosfamide in the treatment of head and neck cancer. *Semin Oncol* 1995; **22**: 24–27.
30. Bissery MC, Guenard D, Gueritte-Voegelain F et al. Experimental antitumour activity of taxotere (RP56976) a Taxol analogue. *Cancer Res* 1991; **5**: 4845.
31. Braakhuus BJM, Kegel A, Welters MJP. The growth inhibiting effects of docetaxel in head and neck squamous cell carcinoma xenografts. *Cancer Lett* 1994; **81**: 151.
32. Hill BT, Whelan R, Shellard SA. Differential cytotoxic efects of docetaxel in a range of mammalian tumour cell lines and certain drug resistant sublines in vitro. *New Drugs* 1994; **12**: 169.
33. Dreyfuss AI, Clark JR, Norris CM et al. Docetaxel (taxotere): an active drug for squamous cell carcinoma of the head and neck. *J Clin Oncol* 1996; **14**: 1672–8.
34. Tischler RB, Schiff PB, Geard RM et al. Taxol: a novel radiosensitiser. *Int J Radiat Oncol Biol Phys* 1992; **22**: 613.
35. Tischler RB, Geard RM, Hall EJ et al. Taxol sensitises human astrocytoma cells to radiation. *Cancer Res* 1992; **52**: 3459.
36. Catimel G, Verrnorken JB, Clavel M et al. A phase II study of gemcitabine in patients with advanced squamous cell carcinoma of the head and neck. *Ann Oncol* 1994; **5**: 543.
37. Wildfang I, Raub M, Semet A. Low dose gemcitabine with radiotherapy in advanced head and neck cancer. A phase II study. *Proc Am Soc Clin Onc* 1999; **18**: 401a.
38. Clavel M, Vermorken JB, Cognetti F et al. Combination chemotherapy with methotrexate, bleomycin and vincristine with or without cisplatin in advanced squamous cell carcinoma of the head and neck. *Cancer* 1987; **60**: 1173.
39. Morton PP, Rugrnan F, Dorman EB et al. Cisplatin and bleomycin for advanced or recurrent squamous cell carcinoma of the head and neck: a randomized factorial phase III controlled trial. *Cancer Chemother Pharmacol* 1985; **15**: 283.
40. Jacobs C, Meyers F, Hendrickson C et al. A randomized phase III study of cisplatin with or without methotrexate for recurrent squamous cell carcinoma of the head and neck. *Cancer* 1983; **52**: 399.
41. Chauvergne J, Cappelaere P, Fargeot P et al. Randomised study with cisplatin alone or in combination for palliative chemotherapy in head and neck carcinoma of 209 patients. *Bull Cancer* 1988; **75**: 9.
42. Forastiere A, Metch B, Keppen M et al. Randomised comparison of cisplatin + 5-FU vs carboplatin + 5-FU vs methotrexate in advanced squamous cell carcinoma of the head and neck (abstract 421). *Proc Am Soc Clin Onc* 1989; **8**: 168.
43. Browman GP, Cronin L. Standard chemotherapy in advanced or recurrent squamous cell carcinoma of the head and neck. *Cancer* 1994; **60**: 2609.
44. Liverpool Head and Neck Oncology Group. A phase III randomized trial of cisplatinum, methotrexate, cisplatinum + methotrexate and cisplatinum + 5FU in end stage squamous carcinoma of the head and neck. *Br J Cancer* 1990; **61**: 311.
45. Armand JP, Cvitoyik E, Recondo G. Salvage chemotherapy in recurrent head and neck cancer. The Institut Gustav-Roussy experience. *Am J Oncol* 1993; **14**: 301.
46. Schrijvers D, Johnson J, Jiminez U et al. Phase III trial of modulation of cisplatin/fluorouracil chemotherapy by interferon alfa-2b in patients with recurrent or metastatic head and neck cancer. Head and Neck Interferon Cooperative Study Group. *J Clin Oncol* 1998; **16**: 1054–9.

47. Posner MR, Weichselbaum RR, Fitzgerald TJ. Treatment complications after sequential combination chemotherapy and radiotherapy with or without surgery in previously untreated squamous cell head and neck cancer. *Int J Radiat Oncol Biol Phys* 1985; **11**: 1887.
48. Randolph VL, Vallejo A, Spiro RH et al. Combination therapy of advanced head and neck cancer. Induction of remissions with cisplatin, bleomycin and radiation therapy. *Cancer* 1979; **41**: 460.
49. Kish JA, Dreligman A, Jacobs J et al. Clinical trial of cisplatin and 5FU as initial treatment for advanced squamous cell carcinoma of the head and neck. *Cancer Treat Rep* 1982; **66**: 471.
50. Weaver A, Fleming S, Ensley J et al. Superior clinical response and survival rates with initial bolus of cisplatin and 120 hour infusion of 5-fluorouracil before definitive therapy for locally advanced head and neck cancer. *Am J Surg* 1984; **148**: 525.
51. Rooney M, Kish J, Jacobs J et al. Improved complete response rate and survival in advanced head and neck cancer after three-course induction therapy with 120-hr 5-FU infusion and cisplatin. *Cancer* 1985; **55**: 1123–1128.
52. Colevas AD, Busse PM, Norris PM et al. Induction chemotherapy with docetaxel, cisplatin, fluorouracil and leucovorin for squamous cell carcinoma of the head and neck; a phase I/II trial. *J Clin Oncol* 1998; **16**: 1331–1339.
53. Department of Veterans Affairs Laryngeal Study Group. Induction chemotherapy plus radiation compared with surgery plus radiation in patients with advanced laryngeal cancer. *N Engl J Med* 1991; **324**: 1685–1690.
54. Cognetti F, Pinarro P, Carlini P, Ruggicri EM. Neoadjuvant chemotherapy in previously untreated patients with advanced head and neck cancer. *Cancer* 1988; **59**: 251.
55. Pennacchio JL, Hong WK, Shapshay S et al. Combination of cisplatin and bleomycin prior to surgery and or radiotherapy compared with radiotherapy alone for the treatment of advanced squamous cell carcinoma of the head and neck. *Cancer* 1982; **50**: 2795.
56. Spaulding MB, Lore JM, Sundquist N. Long term follow up of chemotherapy in advanced head and neck cancer. *Arch Otolaryngol Head Neck Surg* 1989; **115**: 68.
57. Ensley JF, Jacobs JR, Weaver A et al. Correlation between response to cisplatinum-combination chemotherapy and subsequent radiotherapy in previously untreated patients with advanced squamous cell cancers of the head and neck. *Cancer* 1984; **54**: 811–814.
58. Hong W, O'Donohue G, Sheetz S. Sequential response patterns to chemotherapy and radiotherapy in head and neck cancer. In: Wagener D, Bligham G, Sweets V, Wils J (eds) *Primary Chemotherapy in Cancer Medicine*. Vol. 201. New York: Alan Liss, 1985;191.
59. Martin M, Diaz-Rubio E, Gonzalez Larriba JL et al. Ifosfamide in advanced epidermoid head and neck cancer. *Cancer Chemother Pharmacol* 1993; **31**: 340–42.
60. Head and Neck Contracts Program. Adjuvant chemotherapy for advanced head and neck squamous carcinoma. Final report of the Head and Neck Contracts Program. *Cancer* 1987; **60**: 301–311.
61. Schuller DE, Metch B, Stein DW. Postoperative chemotherapy in advanced resectable head and neck cancer. Final report of the Southwest Oncology study group. *Laryngoscope* 1988; **98**: 1205.
62. Paccagnella A, Orlando A, Marchiori C et al. Phase III trial of initial chemotherapy in stage III or IV head and neck cancers: a study by the Gruppo di Studio sui Tumori della Testa c del Collo. *J Natl Cancer Inst* 1994; **86**: 265–272.
63. Depondt J, Gchanno P, Martin M et al. Neoadjuvant chemotherapy with carboplatin/5-fluorouracil in head and neck cancer. *Oncology* 1993; **50 (Suppl 2)**: 2327.
64. Lefebvre JL, Chevalier D, Luboinski B, Kirkpatrick A et al. Larynx preservation in piriform sinus cancer: preliminary results of a EORTC phase III trial. *J Natl Cancer Inst* 1990; **88**: 855–856.
65. Harwood AR, Hawkins NV, Rider WD, Bryce DP. Radiation therapy of early glottic cancer. *Int J Radiat Oncol Biol Phys* 1979; **5**: 473.
66. Horiot JC, LeFur R, N'Guyen T et al. Hyperfractionated compared with conventional radiotherapy in oropharyngeal carcinoma: an EORTC randomized trial. *Eur J Cancer* 1990; **26**: 779–780.
67. Laramore G, Scott C, Al-Sarraf M et al. Adjuvant chemotherapy for resectable squamous cell carcinomas of the head and neck. A report on Intergroup 0034. *Int J Radiat Oncol Biol Phys* 1992; **23**: 705.
68. Domenge C, Marandas P, Vignoud J et al. Post-surgical adjuvant chemotherapy in extracapsular spread invaded lymph node (N+ R+) epidermoid carcinoma of the head and neck. *Second International Conference on Head and Neck Cancer*. Boston, 1988.
69. Bachaud JM, Cohen JE, Alzeiu C et al. Combined postoperative radiotherapy and weekly cisplatin infusion for locally advanced head and neck carcinoma: final report of a randomized trial. *Int J Radiat Oncol Biol Phys* 1997; **36**: 999–1004.
70. Munro AJ. An overview of randomized controlled trials of adjuvant chemotherapy in head and neck cancer. *Br J Cancer* 1995; **71**: 83–91.
71. El-Sayed S, Nelson N. Adjuvant and adjunctive chemotherapy in the management of squamous cell carcinoma of the head and neck region: a meta-analysis of prospective and randomized trials. *J Clin Oncol* 1996; **14**: 838–847.
72. Pignon JP, Bourhis J, Domenge C, Designe L. Chemotherapy added to locoregional treatment for head and neck squamous-cell carcinoma: three meta-analyses of updated individual data. MACH-NC Collaborative Group. Meta-Analysis of Chemotherapy on Head and Neck Cancer. *Lancet* 2000; **355**: 949–55.
73. Richards GJ, Chambers RG. Combined therapy in the treatment of carcinomas of the head and neck. Cancer of the head and neck. Amsterdam, Excerpta Medica. W3 EX89. No 365. 1973.

74. Gupta NK, Pointon RCS, Wilkinson PM. A randomized clinical trial to compare radiotherapy with radiotherapy and methotrexate given simultaneously in head and neck cancer. *Clin Radiol* 1987; **38**: 575.
75. Taylor SG, Murthy AK, Vennetzel JM et al. Randomized comparison of neoadjuvant cisplatin and fluorouracil infusion followed by radiation versus concomitant treatment in advanced head and neck cancer. *J Clin Oncol* 1991; **12**: 385–395.
76. Keane TJ, Cummings BJ, O'Sullivan B et al. A randomized trial of radiation therapy compared to split course radiation therapy combined with mitomycin C and 5-fluorouracil as initial treatment for advanced laryngeal and hypopharyngeal squamous carcinoma. *Int J Radiat Oncol Biol Phys* 1993; **25**: 613–618.
77. Smid L, Lesnicar H, Zakotnik B et al. Radiotherapy, combined with simultaneous chemotherapy with mitomycin C and bleomycin for inoperable head and neck cancer – preliminary report. *Int J Radiat Oncol Biol Phys* 1995; **32**: 769–775.
78. Adelstein DJ, Sharan VM, Earle AS et al. Long-term follow-up of a prospective randomized trial comparing simultaneous and sequential chemoradiotherapy for squamous cell head and neck cancer. In: Salmon SE (ed.) *Adjuvant Therapy of Cancer Vl.* Philadelphia: JB Lippincott, 1993; 82–91.
79. Adelstein DJ, Saxton JP, Lavertu P et al. A phase III randomized trial comparing concurrent chemotherapy and radiotherapy with radiotherapy alone in resectable stage III and IV squamous cell head and neck cancer: preliminary results. *Head Neck* 1997; **19**: 567–575.
80. Al-Sarraf M, LeBlanc M, Shanker Giri PG et al. Chemoradiotherapy versus radiotherapy in patients with advanced nasopharyngeal cancer: phase III randomized Intergroup Study 0099. *J Clin Oncol* 1998; **16**: 1310–1317.
81. Looney WB, Hopkins HA. Solid tumour models for the assessment of different treatment modalities: comparison of one radiation fraction per day with multiple fractions given either continuously or intermittently on tumour response and normal tissie reaction. *Int J Radiat Oncol Biol Phys* 1986; **12**: 203–210.
82. Merlano M, Corvo R, Margarino G et al. Combined chemotherapy and radiotherapy in advanced inoperable squamous cell carcinoma of the head and neck. The final report of a randomized trial. *Cancer* 1991; **67**: 915–921.
83. Merlano M, Benasso M, Corvo R, Vitale V et al. Five year update of a randomized trial of alternating radiotherapy and chemotherapy compared with radiotherapy alone in treatment of unresectable squamous cell carcinoma of the head and neck. *J Natl Cancer Inst* 1996; **88**: 583–589.
84. Fu KK, Phillips TL, Silverberg IJ et al. Combined radiotherapy and chemotherapy with bleomycin and methotrexate for advanced inoperable head and neck cancer: update of a Northern California Oncology Group randomized trial. *J Clin Oncol* 1987; **5**: 1410–1418.
85. Lo TCM, Wiley AL Jr, Ansficid FJ et al. Combined radiation therapy and 5-fluorouracil for advanced squamous cell carcinoma of the oral cavity and oropharynx: a randomized study. *Am J Roentgenol* 1976; **126**: 229–235.
86. Magno L, Terranco F, Bertoni et al. Double blind randomized study of lonidamine and radiotherapy in head and neck cancer. *Int J Radiat Oncol Phys* 1994; **29**: 45–55.
87. Parsons JT, Mendenhall WM, Stringer SP et al. Twice a day radiotherapy for squamous cell carcinoma of the head and neck: the University of Florida experience. *Head Neck* 1993; **15**: 87–96.
88. Jacobs C, Lyman G, Velez-Garcia E et al. A phase III randomized study comparing cisplatin and fluorouracil as single agents and in combination for advanced squamous cell carcinoma of the head and neck. *J Clin Oncol* 1992;**10**: 257–63.
89. Shin DM, Khuri FR, Glisson BS. Phase II study of paclitaxel, ifosfamide and carboplatin in patients with recurrent squamous cell carcinoma of the head and neck. *Proc Am Soc Oncol* 1999; **1521**: 18 (abstr).
90. Gaspar C, Munoz MA, Yaya R. A phase II study of vinorelbine, cisplatin and 5FU in patients with locally advanced recurrent and/or metastatic squamous cell carcinoma of the head and neck. *Proc Am Soc Oncol* 1999; **1568**: 18 (abstr).
91. Kish JA, Ensley JF, Jacobs J et al. A randomized trial of cisplatin (CACP) + 5-fluorouracil (5-FU) infusion and CACP + 5-FU bolus for recurrent and advanced squamous cell carcinoma of the head and neck. *Cancer* 1985; **56**: 2740–4.
92. Vokes EE, Choi KE, Schilsky RL et al. Cisplatin, fluorouracil, and high-dose leucovorin for recurrent or metastatic head and neck cancer. *J Clin Oncol* 1988; **6**: 618–26.
93. Toohill RJ, Anderson T, Byhardt RW et al. Cisplatin and fluorouracil as neoadjuvant therapy in head and neck cancer. A preliminary report. *Arch Otolaryngol Head Neck Surg* 1987; **113**: 758–61.
94. Richard JM, Kramar A, Molinari R et al. Randomised EORTC head and neck cooperative group trial of preoperative intra-arterial chemotherapy in oral cavity and oropharynx carcinoma. *Eur J Cancer* 1991; **27**: 821–7.
95. Fonseca E, Cruz JJ, Gomez A et al. Neoadjuvant chemotherapy with cisplatin and 5-fluorouracil, both in continuous 96-hour infusion, in the treatment of locally advanced head and neck cancer. *Am J Clin Oncol* 1994; **17**: 6–9.
96. Taylor SG 4th, Applebaum E, Showel JL et al. A randomized trial of adjuvant chemotherapy in head and neck cancer. *J Clin Oncol* 1985; **3**: 672–9.
97. Ervin TJ, Clark JR, Weichselbaum RR et al. An analysis of induction and adjuvant chemotherapy in the multidisciplinary treatment of squamous-cell carcinoma of the head and neck. *J Clin Oncol* 1987; **5**: 10–20.
98. Wendt TG, Grabenbauer GG, Rodel CM et al. Simultaneous radiochemotherapy versus radiotherapy

alone in advanced head and neck cancer: a randomized multicenter study. *J Clin Oncol* 1998; **16**: 1318–24.
99. Brizel DM, Albers ME, Fisher SR et al. Hyperfractionated irradiation with or without concurrent chemotherapy for locally advanced head and neck cancer. *N Engl J Med* 1998; **338**: 1798–804.
100. Calais G, Alfonsi M, Bardet E et al. Randomized trial of radiation therapy versus concomitant chemotherapy and radiation therapy for advanced-stage oropharynx carcinoma. *J Natl Cancer Inst* 1999; **91**: 2081–6.
101. South-East Co-operative Oncology Group. A randomized trial of combined multidrug chemotherapy and radiotherapy in advanced squamous cell carcinoma of the head and neck. An interim report from the SECOG participants. *Eur J Surg Oncol* 1986; **12**: 289–95.
102. Huang AT, Cole TB, Fishburn R, Jelovsek SB. Adjuvant chemotherapy after surgery and radiation for stage III and IV head and neck cancer. *Ann Surg* 1984; **200**: 195–9.

6 Anaesthesia for head and neck tumour surgery

Colm Irving

Introduction

The perioperative anaesthetic management of patients undergoing resection of tumours of the head and neck presents the anaesthetist with a unique set of challenges.[1,2] They can be grouped into the following main categories: (a) preoperative assessment; (b) the difficult airway; (c) the shared airway; (d) pharyngolaryngo-oesophagectomy; (e) anaesthetic complications peculiar to head and neck surgery; (f) management of the free flap; and (g) postoperative high-dependency care.

The goal of this chapter is to give the surgeon a basic knowledge of those aspects of anaesthetic management that have either a direct bearing on surgical access and technique or contribute overall to a good outcome.

Preoperative assessment

Concurrent disease

The vast majority of patients will be in their sixth or seventh decade, many with a history of smoking and heavy alcohol intake and are therefore likely to have significant concurrent disease, which will require evaluation and possible remedial treatment as for other major surgery within the time available.[3] It is beyond the scope of this chapter to discuss individual conditions but certain key factors should be taken into account when considering the extent of preoperative preparation and investigation (Tables 6.1 and 6.2).

Table 6.1 Key factors in preoperative assessment

Tumour progression with or without encroachment into the airway may limit the time available for medical improvement
Surgery confined to the head and neck, even that involving major reconstruction, is generally speaking less likely to interfere with postoperative respiratory function than surgery to the chest and abdomen and therefore the potential for postoperative cardiorespiratory complications is less. Surgery involving the chest or abdomen carries a higher risk
Patients with a history of alcohol abuse may have alcoholic liver disease or alcoholic cardiomyopathy which will require further investigation prior to surgery
If the patient has had chemotherapy certain agents possess specific organ toxicities, for example bleomycin can cause lung fibrosis and daunorubicin and adriamycin are cardiotoxic[1]
Poor preoperative nutritional status is thought to contribute to a high incidence of postoperative anastomotic leakage and therefore nutritional support may be given prior to surgery.[4] The enteral route is preferred if the patient has a functioning and accessible gastrointestinal tract[5]

Airway assessment

A detailed assessment of the airway is mandatory in this population of patients in order to detect difficult intubations. The essence of the dilemma that faces the anaesthetist is that many patients who are difficult to intubate may be impossible to ventilate by any other means following the induction of general anaesthesia due to the attendant loss of supportive muscle tone in an already partially obstructed airway. The induction of general anaesthesia in this

Table 6.2 Preoperative investigations

FBC	All patients for general anaesthesia
Sickle screen	All patients of African descent. (A positive sickle test must be followed up with haemoglobin electrophoresis)
U&E	All patients for intermediate/major surgery All patients on diuretics All patients with a history of renal impairment
Calcium	Any patient with a history of thyroid or parathyroid surgery or undergoing laryngectomy/pharyngolaryngectomy
ECG	All patients with a history of cardiovascular disease As a baseline investigation in all patients over 40 years old for general anaesthesia
LFTs	Patients with a history of heavy alcohol consumption
Clotting screen	All patients on anticoagulants All patients with abnormal LFTs
Chest X-ray	If this has not been ordered as part of the surgical work-up it is indicated in All patients with acute respiratory symptoms or suspected TB All patients with chronic cardiorespiratory disorders who have not been X-rayed in the last 6 months[6]
Pulmonary function tests	All patients for oesophagectomy All patients with chronic airways disease
Echocardiography	At the request of the anaesthetist in patients with a history of heart failure or ischaemic heart disease.

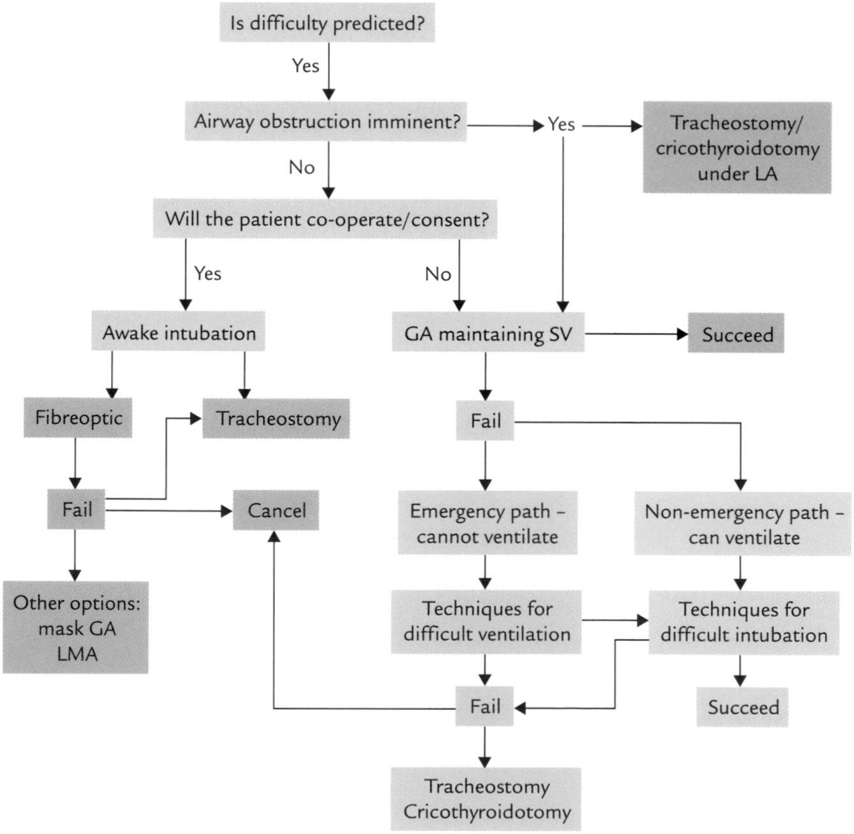

Figure 6.1 Algorithm for airway management. LMA: laryngeal mask airway; GA: general anaesthesia; LA: local anaesthesia; SV: spontaneous ventilation.

subgroup of patients is therefore potentially hazardous and the airway should be secured using an awake technique where possible in any patient predicted to be difficult (Figure 6.1).

History

The anaesthetic record of any preliminary endoscopy will give valuable information about the ease or difficulty of airway management. Previous resection may distort and scar normal anatomy and previous irradiation of the head and neck can cause fibrosis. All of these factors will render tissues inflexible and difficult to displace during direct laryngoscopy. The presence of a tracheostomy will naturally simplify airway management but it is advisable to ascertain whether the tracheostomy tube may be attached directly to the anaesthetic circuit or require replacement.

Examination and predictive tests

Conventional methods of tracheal intubation are dependent on the ability of the anaesthetist to view the glottis directly under general anaesthesia with a rigid laryngoscope. The glottis can only be visualized directly if the patient can open their mouth sufficiently wide, there is enough mandibular space into which the soft tissues may be displaced anteriorly by the instrument and they can extend the head on the neck in order to line up the mouth with the glottis. Several simple methods have been devised that test for these factors and therefore may be used to predict the likelihood of a difficult intubation (Table 6.3). More elaborate tests involving a combination of risk factors are generally not practical enough to perform routinely.

A problem common to all of these predictive tests used either alone or in combination[12] is that sensitivity tends to be of the order of 50–60%. In other words 40–50% of difficult intubations are not predicted. In addition the positive predictive value is poor, many patients predicted to be difficult will in fact be easy.[13] Another fundamental problem with

Table 6.3 Predictive tests of the airway

Mallampati[7] described a test, subsequently modified,[8] which grades the visibility of pharyngeal structures (Figure 6.2), a high grade suggests a lack of mandibular space and a potentially difficult intubation. Certain patients will be unable to open their mouths wide enough to view any pharyngeal structures and mouth opening should then be recorded in centimetres
The Patil test[9] measures both the mandibular space and the ability to extend the head (Figure 6.3). The thyromental distance is the distance from the inside of the mentum to the thyroid cartilage with the head fully extended on the neck. A distance of less than 6.5cm is predictive of a difficult intubation
Mandibular protrusion is a useful indicator of mandibular mobility, class C protrusion, the inability to protrude the lower incisors beyond the upper, being associated with a high incidence of difficult laryngoscopy.[10]
Wilson test[11]
Radiological assessment of the mandible or the cervical spine

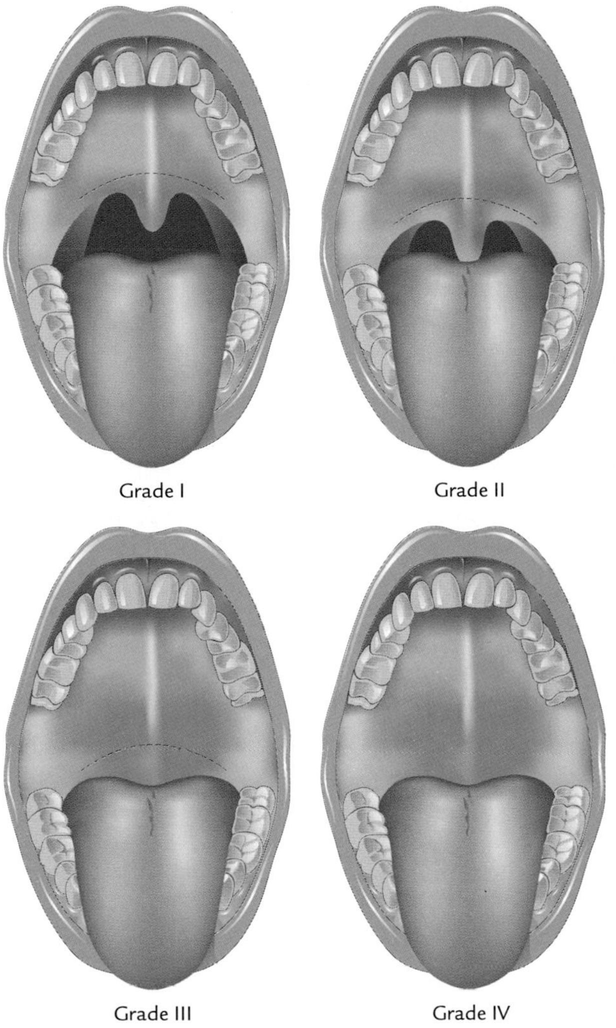

Figure 6.2 Mallampati grading of visibility of pharyngeal structures.[8] The posterior pharyngeal wall is visible below the soft palate in grades I and II, posterior pharyngeal wall not visible in grades III and IV.

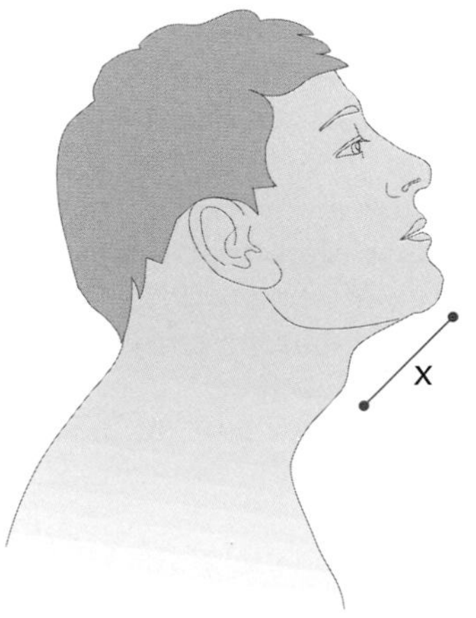

Figure 6.3 The Patil test of thyromental distance.[9]

these tests in this group of patients is that they cannot give any indication of potential obstruction from tongue base or supraglottic tumours that can block the airway when pharyngeal tone is lost on induction of anaesthesia.[14]

Investigations

These tests are therefore at best useful indicators and a true picture of the airway can only be built up by combining their results with the results of laryngoscopic examination and CT or MRI imaging (Table 6.4). Cervical spine flexion and extension views are indicated in rheumatoid arthritis to assess the stability of the atlantoaxial joint.

Table 6.4 Summary of preoperative airway assessment

History
Recent anaesthetic record
Previous surgery/tracheostomy
Previous irradiation
Examination:
Neck extension
Mallampati test
Patil test
Mouth opening
Mandibular protrusion
Wilson scoring
Investigation:
Direct/fibreoptic laryngoscopy
CT/MRI
Cervical spine Xray in rheumatoid arthritis

The difficult airway

Management of the difficult airway is a complex area that many authors have attempted to rationalize in the form of a management algorithm.[15] These algorithms are useful in that they outline the general principles involved around which the individual anaesthetist must formulate a plan for each particular patient in cooperation with the surgical team. A simplified airway management algorithm is shown (Figure 6.1).

Table 6.5 Potentially difficult intubation: an awake fibreoptic technique should be employed in these patients

Trismus
Mallampati class 3 or 4
Tongue base or supraglottic masses
A thyromental distance of less than 6.5 cm
Cervical or tongue immobility due to previous surgery/irradiation

Potentially hazardous intubation

The first step in this algorithm is to predict the difficulty of intubation. Taking into account the shortcomings of our present methods it is possible to construct a list of fairly reliable predictors (Table 6.5). For the majority of these patients awake intubation using a fibreoptic intubating bronchoscope is the technique of choice.

Awake intubation ensures the maintenance of airway tone and self ventilation of the patient's lungs and thus oxygenation in the event that oro- or nasotracheal intubation cannot be achieved. While many patients falling into these categories would have been easy asleep intubations, awake fibreoptic intubation in skilled hands is not an unpleasant experience and is associated with cardiovascular stability and good oxygen saturation.[16] It is preferable to subject a number of patients to an unnecessary awake intubation than to subject others to the potential morbidity and mortality of a failed intubation under general anaesthesia. Table 6.6 outlines a simple technique for awake fibreoptic intubation.

Tracheostomy under local anaesthetic is the recommended technique in cases of severe acute upper airway obstruction[17] because of the risk of precipitating complete obstruction using the fibreoptic technique as a result of irritation of the airway, bleeding or dislodging friable tumour.

Lesser degrees of predicted difficulty or in the unco-operative patient

For these patients conventional asleep intubation is indicated. Anaesthesia should be induced either with a slow intravenous injection or with an inhalational agent in an attempt to preserve airway tone and spontaneous breathing until adequate mask ventilation can be established at which point the patient can be paralysed or anaesthesia deepened to facilitate intubation. If intubation proves difficult but the lungs can still be ventilated endotracheal intubation will be achieved in the majority of cases using one of the following techniques for difficult asleep intubation (Table 6.7).

If one finds that the lungs cannot be ventilated nor the trachea intubated there are several techniques (Table 6.8) that may achieve adequate ventilation of the lungs. If the lungs cannot be ventilated or intubated one may elect to wake the patient up and

Table 6.6 Technique for awake intubation using the intubating bronchoscope

Always give a drying agent (hyoscine or glycopyrronium) to reduce secretions
Secure intravenous access
Otrivine (xylometazoline) drops to nose if nasal intubation planned
Anaesthetize the airway Lignocaine 2% gel to the nose 10% Lignocaine spray to the oropharynx 'Spray as you go' with 4% lignocaine
Oxygen supply via Nasal specs Oxygen mask Oxygen administered down suction channel of bronchoscope
Sedation with intravenous increments of 1 mg midazolam. Have flumazenil available
Mount a size 6.0 cuffed reinforced endotracheal tube onto the bronchoscope
Insert the scope to the oropharynx and visualize the epiglottis and vocal cords. The nasal route provides a better angle of access and produces less gagging
Lignocaine 4% to the vocal cords. Wait 2–3 minutes
Pass the scope through the cords. Spray the trachea with 4% lignocaine and wait a further 2–3 minutes
Pass the tube with a continuously rotating motion to avoid catching the bevel on vocal cords or tumour
After visually confirming correct positioning of the tube with the bronchoscope induce general anaesthesia

Table 6.7 Techniques for difficult asleep intubation: where the lungs can be ventilated but intubation is difficult

Bougie: passing a gum elastic bougie through the vocal cords and railroading the endotracheal tube over the bougie
Alternative laryngoscope blades: using a straight blade, anterior commisure or McCoy laryngoscope to elevate the epiglottis
Fibreoptic intubating bronchoscope
Blind intubation: attempting to pass the endotracheal tube through the cords without direct visualization
Retrograde intubation: passing a guide-wire or catheter retrograde through the cricothyroid membrane and through the vocal cords and then railroading the endotracheal tube over the guide

Table 6.8 Techniques for difficult lung ventilation: when the lungs cannot be ventilated using a face mask and the trachea cannot be intubated

Laryngeal mask airway
Oral/nasopharyngeal airways
Rigid bronchoscopy and jet ventilation
Two-person mask ventilation

then either cancel the procedure or attempt an awake intubation if it is judged that there is sufficient time for the patient to wake before hypoxia or hypercarbia cause a cardiac arrest. If there is insufficient time one must proceed immediately to a surgical airway.

Emergency intubation

In an emergency where complete airway obstruction is imminent awake fibreoptic intubation is not a recommended option. In this situation the safest options are as follows.

1. Tracheostomy under local anaesthetic.
2. Cricothyroidotomy under local anaesthetic using a large gauge cannula and Venturi or jet ventilation with general anaesthesia provided via the intravenous route. A 13- or 14-gauge cannula will allow sufficient flow rates to adequately oxygenate the lungs and there are several custom-made cannulae (for example Ravussin needle). This method of ventilating the lungs is essentially a short-term measure that buys time to establish a more secure airway, such as endotracheal intubation or tracheostomy. Although good oxygenation is usually achieved, adequate carbon dioxide elimination cannot be guaranteed. In order to avoid barotrauma always ensure that there is egress for the expired gas either through the glottis or through another cannula inserted through the cricothyroid membrane.
3. With the surgeon scrubbed ready to perform an emergency tracheostomy the anaesthetist may attempt an inhalational induction if the patient is judged unlikely to tolerate the above.

The shared airway

Tracheostomy

Where surgery involves the fashioning of a permanent or temporary tracheostomy a reinforced

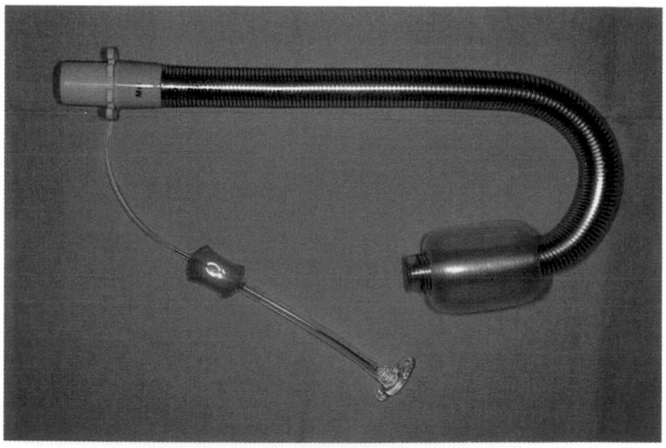

Figure 6.4 The Rusch laryngoflex tracheostomy tube. The curvature and length of the tube allow the breathing circuit and attachments to be kept away from the surgical field.

tracheostomy tube (Rusch laryngoflex; Figure 6.4) is used to maintain the airway and facilitate ventilation during surgery while ensuring as little encroachment as possible into the surgical field.

Tracheostomy is a procedure that requires close co-operation between surgeon and anaesthetist and one should never remove an endotracheal tube until one is satisfied that the tracheostomy tube is correctly positioned. Once the anterior tracheal wall is exposed by the surgeon, preferably after division of the thyroid isthmus, a stay silk safety suture is placed through the trachea ring below the intended tracheostomy site and the long suture ends are brought out onto the the chest skin where they are taped. The tracheal opening is then made and the tracheostomy tube is carefully inserted taking care not to rupture the tube cuff.

The purpose of the stay suture is to help find the tracheal opening again if the tube becomes dislodged. This is a particularly hazardous situation if it occurs on the ward, but by gently pulling on the long stay suture the tracheal opening above it will be more easily identified.

To allow insertion of the tracheostomy tube, the endotracheal tube should be withdrawn so that its tip lies just proximal to the tracheostome and only when correct positioning of the tracheostomy tube is confirmed should it be withdrawn completely. Incorrect placement of the tracheostomy tube will be detected first by the anaesthetist and potential hazards include extratracheal placement, endobronchial intubation and herniation of the cuff.

To prevent extratracheal placement, following insertion of the tube, first and foremost ensure that it is positioned within the airway. Failure to inflate the lungs, the absence of an end-tidal carbon dioxide trace and a gross elevation of airway pressure all indicate that the tube is either not positioned within the airway or that its lumen is obstructed. A fall in oxygen saturation is a relatively late sign. If positioning outside the airway is suspected, stop ventilation, remove the tracheostomy tube and regain control of the airway by advancing the endotracheal tube so that its cuff lies distal to the tracheostome.

Endobronchial intubation is a potential hazard because of the shorter tracheal length compared to the non-tracheostomized patient. Endobronchial intubation is detected by observing unequal ventilation of the lungs, a fall in end-tidal carbon dioxide, a rise in airway pressure and a late fall in oxygen saturation. This situation is easily rectified by withdrawing the tube slightly until equal ventilation of the lungs is observed and suturing the tube securely in place.

Herniation of the cuff over the end of the tube or abutment of the tip of the tube against the tracheal mucosa can partially or completely occlude the lumen. The picture produced is one of inadequate or absent lung inflation, failure to detect end-tidal carbon dioxide, elevation of airway pressure and again a late fall in oxygen saturation. This can be remedied by deflating and then gently reinflating the cuff with only as much air as is needed to achieve an airtight seal. Overinflation of the cuff not only predisposes to cuff herniation but will damage tracheal mucosa leading to either perforation of the back wall or necrosis and later stenosis.

At the end of the operation the reinforced tracheostomy tube should be replaced with a standard cuffed tracheostomy tube.

Endoscopy and microsurgery

Endoscopy of the aerodigestive tract and microsurgery of the larynx require the least possible obstruction of the surgical view by the endotracheal tube. This can be achieved in one of two ways.

First, small-bore microlaryngoscopy endotracheal tubes with an internal diameter of 4–5 mm can be used. These can be passed orally or nasally depending on the site of the lesion and anaesthetic preference. These tubes are suitable only for short-term anaesthesia as their narrow bore predisposes them to blocking and kinking during more prolonged procedures.

Secondly, where a completely unimpeded view is required as for laser microsurgery, and in particular for posterior commisure lesions, ventilation is achieved using a Venturi needle attached to a

Table 6.9 The advantages and disadvantages of jet ventilation

Advantages
- Much better surgical access especially postcommisure lesions
- Ideal for laser microsurgery

Disadvantages
- Not suitable for obese patients
- CO_2 elimination and tidal volume difficult to monitor
- Increased risk of barotrauma
- Suitable only for short-term procedures
- Airway not protected from soiling

suspension laryngoscope which in turn is attached to a jet ventilator or injector device (e.g. Sanders injector). This is an elegant technique in that it provides optimal access for the surgeon but requires greater vigilance than standard endotracheal anaesthesia (Figure 6.5).

There are severeal points to note. The scope and needle must be in line with the airway or ventilation will be inadequate and there is a risk of damage to paralaryngeal tissues. Obese patients are not suitable for this technique as ventilation is invariably inadequate due to the excessive weight of the chest wall and pressure from abdominal contents. Barotrauma, that is pneumothorax and pneumomediastinum are constant risks. Anaesthesia must be maintained via the intravenous route.

Although ventilation and carbon dioxide elimination are usually adequate, tidal volume is impossible to measure because of the open nature of the system and during prolonged procedures arterial blood gas sampling, or gas sampling through a separate sampling tube, is required to determine carbon dioxide levels.

Laser surgery

The carbon dioxide laser offers several advantages over conventional surgical methods in the treatment of certain lesions of the oral cavity, pharynx and larynx.[18,19] The less precise Nd YAG laser is more suitable for lower airway lesions. Their use poses certain problems for the anaesthetist[20] that can be grouped into two main categories: competition for the airway and fire hazards.

Competition for the airway: endotracheal tubes and jet ventilation

Lesions of the oral cavity and pharynx can be managed with a laser-proof endotracheal tube in situ. The advantages of a tube are that it ensures adequate ventilation at all times and protects the lower airway from blood, smoke and debris. The disadvantages are the possibility of tube ignition and a partially impeded surgical access.

If a completely unimpeded view of the vocal cords is required as for posterior laryngeal lesions the ideal method is jet ventilation through a Venturi needle mounted on the suspension laryngoscope (Figure 6.5). In addition to the usual precautions that must be taken with this technique it is necessary to remove smoke with an adequate suction system (Figure 6.6) during breaks in ventilation in order to avoid contamination of the lower airways and the theatre atmosphere.

Fire hazards: anaesthetic agents and tracheal tube ignition

Nitrous oxide supports combustion and should be avoided in laser surgery and replaced with air.

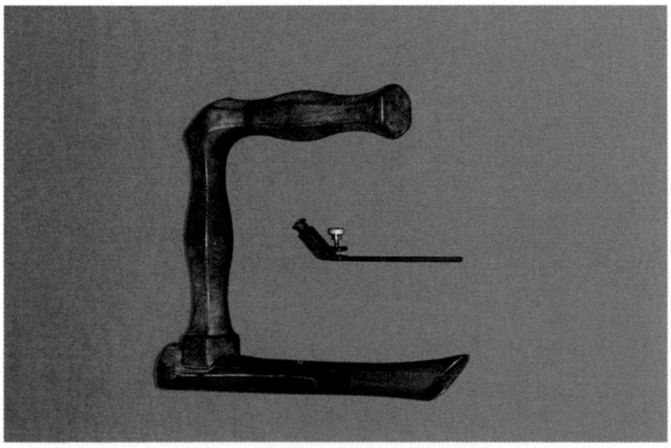

Figure 6.5 Venturi needle for jet ventilation and a Downs (Rhys Evans) microlaryngoscope.

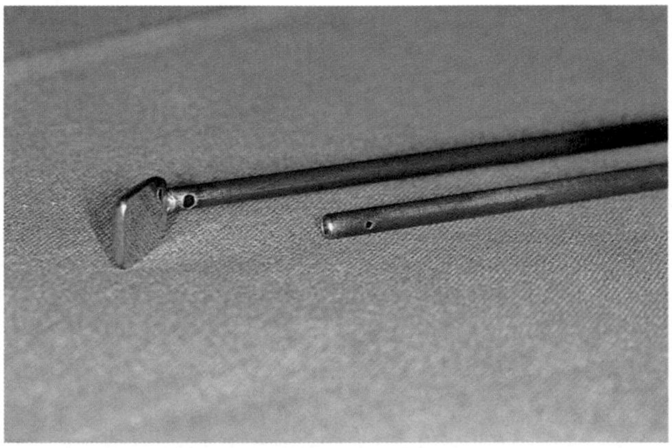

Figure 6.6 Downs (Rhys Evans) laser gas-aspirating sucker and mirrors.

Oxygen, naturally, cannot be avoided but the inspired concentration should be kept as low as possible while maintaining an adequate oxygen saturation. It should be noted that when using the Venturi attachment attached to a Sanders injector the device is driven by compressed oxygen at a concentration of 100% and although tube ignition (see below) is not a problem, any other material ignited in the airway will have a rich supply of oxygen. Modern volatile anaesthetic agents are not flammable at the concentrations likely to be found in clinical practice.

Laser radiation will ignite most non-glass and non-metal material and standard endotracheal tubes made of PVC or rubber will readily ignite when exposed to a laser beam and should never be used for laser surgery. Several methods of providing a laser-proof tube have been devised. These range from the protection of standard red rubber and PVC tubes with aluminium tape[18] to the use of all-metal flexible tubes (e.g. Mallinkrodt laserflex; Figure 6.7). Perhaps the most satisfactory solution is the use of a cuffed tracheal tube made of silicone, which is less flammable than rubber or PVC amd which possesses an outer metallic coating, for example Xomed lasershield (Figure 6.8). The thin-walled cuffs of these tubes are unprotected and the subglottis must be packed off with saline soaked gauze to protect them from the laser beam. The cuff should be inflated with saline so that if it is penetrated the saline will act as a heat sink and lessen the likelihood of ignition. Some tubes have a double cuff so that if the upper cuff is penetrated an airtight seal is still provided by the lower cuff. A further refinement is to add methylene blue to the saline so that a cuff penetration is more readily detected.

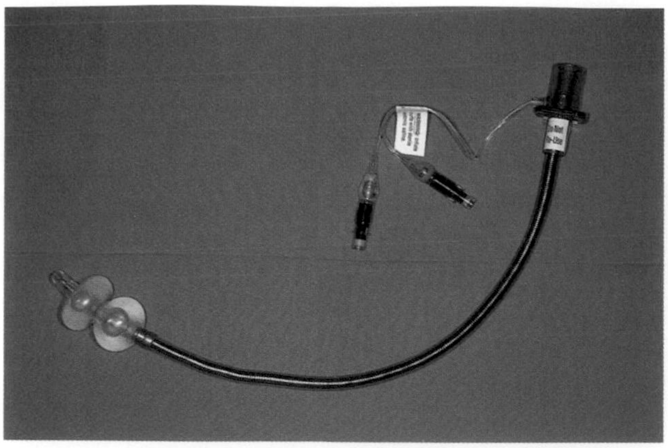

Figure 6.7 The Mallinkrodt laserflex tube. A metal tube with a non-reflective matt surface. Note the double cuff inflated with saline.

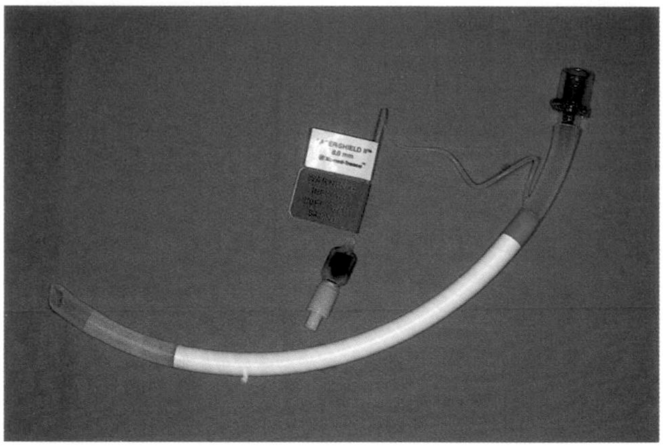

Figure 6.8 The Xomed Lasershield. A silicone tube with an outer metallic coating. Note the methylene blue in the pilot balloon.

Indications for elective tracheostomy

There are certain absolute indications for the provision of a temporary tracheostomy following head and neck surgery (Table 6.10); these are operations following which postoperative swelling, haemorrhage or secretions in the upper airway will almost certainly lead to respiratory obstruction or soiling of the lower airway.[1,2]

There are other situations (Table 6.11) where the indication is not clear-cut but where a tracheostomy would have certain advantages such as the facilitation of postoperative ventilation and airway toilet and the maximization of oxygen delivery to free flaps and tissue devitalized following radiotherapy. The decision to perform a tracheostomy in these cases is a balance between the potential for present or future airway obstruction or soiling and the potential morbidity of the procedure and will depend largely on the postoperative care facilities available. An acceptable alternative in many cases is to leave the endotracheal

Table 6.10 Absolute indications for elective tracheostomy
Partial laryngectomy
Total glossectomy
Disrupted mandible
Bilateral radical neck dissection

Table 6.11 Relative indications for elective tracheostomy
Total or partial pharyngectomy
Partial glossectomy
Any operation on the palate or oral cavity
Patient likely to need prolonged postoperative respiratory support
Difficult intubation, patient likely to need further anaesthesia in the near future

tube in place for 24–48 hours and extubate when the swelling has subsided but only where facilities for mechanical ventilation are available and the expertise exists for immediate reintubation.

Operations on the trachea

Greatest competition for the airway undoubtedly occurs during operations for resection and reconstruction of the trachea and for surgery on an end tracheostome.

Endotracheal intubation

It is possible for the surgeon to operate around a tube placed in the trachea with its cuff distal to the site of surgery provided it is of a small diameter. It is even feasible for the tube to be removed from the airway for short periods provided the patient remains well oxygenated, there is no soiling of the airway with blood or debris and the tube is reinserted before arterial desaturation begins. The disadvantage to this technique is that ventilation is necessarily interrupted, the lower airway is not protected and it is not possible to monitor end-tidal carbon dioxide.

Jet ventilation

Perhaps the most satisfactory method of providing adequate ventilation while allowing optimal surgical access is to ventilate the patient using high-frequency jet ventilation (HFJV) through a small-diameter catheter or jet ventilation tube placed with its tip distal to the site of surgery. The problems associated with jet ventilation have been discussed previously.

Intraoperative tracheal injury

The management of intraoperative tracheal injury depends on the level of the tear. A tear proximal to the endotracheal tube cuff can be repaired with the endotracheal tube in situ. However if the surgeon requires more complete access or if the tear extends distal to the endotracheal tube the situation is best managed with HFJV using a suitable catheter such as the Cook airway exchange catheter, which may be passed down an existing endotracheal tube.[21] In very low tracheal tears individual intubation of the bronchi may be necessary.

Pharyngolaryngo-oesophagectomy

Continuity of the gastrointestinal tract following circumferential excision of the pharynx or upper oesophagus can be restored using a jejunal free flap, pedicled flap or gastric transposition. The latter procedure, because of the encroachment into the abdomen and thorax, represents a greater physiological insult than other head and neck procedures with greater potential for postoperative cardiorespiratory complications[22,23] and a mortality in the region of 5–10%[23] and therefore deserves separate discussion.

Patient assesment

Most patients with carcinoma of the hypopharynx/cervical oeophagus are elderly and there is a high incidence of coexisting illness. A study of 107 Japanese patients[24] who underwent oesophagectomy for carcinoma of the oesophagus divided them into low-, medium- and high-risk groups on the basis of a score allocated to various preoperative risk factors (Table 6.12). Of those in the high-risk group (4 points or greater) the overall mortality was 40% but those high-risk patients who underwent a transhiatal rather than a transthoracic approach had significantly fewer pulmonary complications (25% and 64%, respectively) and a lower hospital mortality rate (13% and 57%). A review of 120 patients who underwent gastric ‘transposition’ showed that whereas overall mortality was 11%, patients over 60 years of age had a rate of 14% compared with a rate of 4% in those less than 60.[23] These findings suggest that while the transhiatal approach of the gastric ‘transposition’ would appear to be an intrinsically safe procedure offering better short term survival than thoracoabdominal oesophagectomy, mortality is still high for elderly patients and those with cardiac, pulmonary or renal disease. Careful preoperative assesment is necessary to detect these high-risk patients who may then be offered an alternative treatment.

Other studies have confirmed that pre-existing pulmonary disease predisposes to the development of postoperative pulmonary complications.[4] Those with a preoperative%FVC (measured/predicted FVC) of less than 90%, an FEV_1 of less than 70% or a low preoperative PaO_2 are more likely to develop pulmonary complications.[4,25] Preoperative irradiation is thought to contribute to the risk of developing postoperative lung complications.

Intraoperative management

Factors that have been shown to or are likely to decrease the incidence of postoperative cardiorespiratory complications include epidural analgesia, fluid administration and chest drains.

Epidural analgesia

Thoracic epidural analgesia, used in conjunction with general anaesthesia as part of the anaesthetic

Table 6.12 Risk factors in pharyngolaryngo-oesophagectomy. A score of 4 or more points is associated with a mortality rate of 40%. The phenolsulfonphthalein test is obsolete but any abnormality of renal function could be assigned a score of 1.[24]

Risk factor			Risk score
Age	Age < 70		0
	Age > 70		1
Heart	Normal		0
	Sinus arrhythmia, left ventricular hypertrophy, right bundle branch block		1
	Atrial fibrillation, atrioventricular block, heart failure, ischaemic heart disease		2
Lung	Normal		0
	70% < % FVC < 80%	60% < FEV_1 > 70%	1
	% FVC < 70%	FEV_1 < 60%	2
Kidney	Normal		0
	Phenolsulfonphthalein test 15 min < 25%		1
Protein	Albumin > 35 g/litre		0
	30 g/l < albumin < 35 g/litre		1
	Albumin < 30 g/litre		2

technique and continued into the postoperative period, has been shown to decrease the incidence of respiratory complications after thoracoabdominal oesophagectomy (Table 6.13).[26] It would be reasonable to assume that the transhiatal approach would benefit from a similar reduction.

Fluid administration

Limiting intraoperative fluids to 5–6 ml/kg/hour is associated with a decrease in the incidence of respiratory complications when compared to rates of 10–11 ml/kg/hour.[23] However, there is a unique feature of the transhiatal procedure that may limit the degree to which fluids may be restricted.[27,28] Digital dissection of the oesophagus and transfer of the stomach to the neck interferes with venous return, which may lead to gross hypotension and initiates ventricular dysrhythmias as a result of direct mechanical stimulation of the myocardium. Ensuring adequate hydration and short-term inotropic support can attenuate the fall in blood pressure but only a pause in surgical manipulation can fully restore cardiac output and blood pressure. Similarly prolonged dysrhythmias can only be terminated by a surgical pause.

Table 6.13 The advantages of epidural analgesia in oesophagectomy

- Provides good quality postoperative analgesia
- Facilitates coughing, spontaneous breathing and chest physiotherapy
- Minimizes opioid and sedative requirements
- Need for postoperative ventilation is reduced
- Facilitates early mobilization
- Reduced ITU and hospital stay

Chest drains

Although the pleural cavity is not deliberately entered during the transhiatal approach trauma to the pleura during blind digital dissection of the oesophagus may lead to pneumothorax or the accumulation of large pleural effusions that will interfere with postoperative pulmonary function. It is therefore advisable to place prophylactic bilateral chest drains at operation.

Postoperative management

The continuance of epidural analgesia into the postoperative period is associated with a reduction in postoperative pulmonary complications following thoracoabdominal oesophagectomy.[24] The total amount of opiate administered is reduced, the need for postoperative ventilation is reduced, physiotherapy and mobilization are facilitated (Table 6.13). Length of stay in the intensive care unit and total hospital stay were reduced in patients receiving epidural analgesia following oesophagectomy compared to a group receiving intravenous morphine.[29]

Fluid restriction at a rate of approximately 1.5–2 ml/kg per hour is also associated with fewer respiratory complications[4,25,29] and this is achievable in the majority of patients but there are occasions when it can prove difficult in practice to limit fluid intake so strictly. There exists the potential for major fluid shifts that can lead to loss of fluid from the intravascular space, which cannot be measured directly. There are four sources of such occult loss.

The first is so-called third space loss, that is fluid lost into oedematous tissue at the surgical site; secondly considerable amounts of fluid can accumulate in the pleural cavity after chest drains have been removed or are less than optimally positioned; thirdly, fluid can sequester in the bowel lumen during periods of ileus; and lastly insensible losses can be as much as 0.5 ml/kg per hour.[30] These shifts can be aggravated by a low serum albumin in preoperatively malnourished patients with a consequent reduction in plasma oncotic pressure.

The classical clinical picture is one of a hypovolaemic patient who is in positive fluid balance and with an increased body weight.[30] When this situation arises the priority is to restore the intravascular volume with colloid or blood rather than crystalloids thereby retaining as much fluid in the intravascular space as possible: the patient in effect is further fluid overloaded but with more fluid in the correct compartment.

An early return of spontaneous breathing and early extubation are desirable as the longer the duration of intubation and ventilation the greater the risk of iatrogenic pulmonary complications.[31] Extubation should not take place until an adequate cough can be demonstrated, for example the generation of more than four coughs upon the installation of saline into the endotracheal tube.[22] Oesophagectomy can interfere with the cough reflex as a result of injury to the bronchial branch of the vagus and oedema secondary to interference with lymph flow after extensive lymphadenectomy.

When total thyroidectomy is performed serum calcium should be frequently checked every 4 hours postoperatively and any deficiency corrected (see below).

Enteral nutrition via jejunostomy begun on the first postoperative day helps to maintain serum albumin levels thus attenuating any fluid shifts from the intravascular space and promotes anastomotic integrity.[4]

Anaesthetic complications peculiar to head and neck surgery

In addition to the complications common to all major surgery there are particular hazards in head and neck surgery.

Air embolism

The head-up position is employed in head and neck surgery to reduce bleeding in the surgical field. In this position the veins of the head and neck are above the level of the right atrium and if the difference is greater than the central venous pressure, air will enter the venous circulation if a vein is breached. The danger from venous air embolism lies not just in its obstructive effects on the right side of the circulation with a reduction in cardiac output and resulting hypotension but in the possibility of air entering the arterial side of the circulation via a patent foramen ovale or right to left shunt and embolizing a coronary or cerebral artery (so called paradoxical embolism). Up to 30% of the population have a probe patent foramen ovale at postmortem.[32]

The precordial Doppler is a highly sensitive ultrasonic probe that is used in neurosurgery to detect air emboli as small as 0.12 ml; however, it is prone to interference from surgical diathermy and is highly dependent on operator experience. The most sensitive clinical sign is a fall in end-tidal carbon dioxide as detected by the capnograph (Table 6.14), the other signs depend on the presence of large volumes of air or occur relatively late. Management (Table 6.14) is directed at preventing the ingress of further air and aspirating or minimizing the effects of air already embolized. Nitrous oxide replaces nitrogen in air-containing spaces and diffuses in 35 times more rapidly than nitrogen diffuses out causing the embolus to expand. The administration of 100% oxygen not only improves oxygen saturation but has the effect of decreasing the embolus size.

Table 6.14 The detection and management of air embolism

Detection
Fall in end tidal CO_2
Hypotension
Fall in oxygen saturation
Elevation of central venous pressure
Millwheel murmur
ECG evidence of right heart strain
Management
Flood the area with saline
Head-down position
Discontinue nitrous oxide
100% O_2
Aspirate air from right heart via central line with patient in left lateral position

Carotid sinus reflex

Surgical manipulation of the carotid sinus can lead to profound bradycardia and hypotension. This is most likely to occur in hypertensive men over the age of 50 and while the above response is the most common, hypotension alone, bradycardia alone or even hypotension and tachycardia can occur.[2] The anaesthetist should immediately inform the surgeon who can then stop temporarily while either an anticholinergic such as atropine or glycopyrrolate is administered to restore the heart rate and/or a vasopressor is given to restore the blood pressure or local anaesthetic is applied directly onto the sinus thus blocking the afferent limb of the reflex.

Cerebral oedema

The internal jugular veins constitute the major venous drainage from the head and these vessels are commonly subjected to manipulation and temporary occlusion if not sacrifice, as in radical neck dissection. The resultant interference with venous drainage in addition to the hypotension and reduction in cerebral perfusion pressure caused by anaesthesia and the head-up position can lead to cerebral oedema.[33]

Cerebral oedema can be difficult to detect under the masking effect of general anaesthesia but unexplained changes in pulmonary and cardiac function should alert one to the possibility of raised intracranial pressure. Neurogenic pulmonary oedema and the neurogenic myocardial damage syndrome may account for these changes. The latter is thought to be due to hypothalamic sympathetic discharge causing focal coronary artery spasms leading in turn to areas of myocardial ischaemia.

For these reasons it is recommended that a bilateral radical neck dissection be undertaken as a staged procedure with an interval of at least 3 weeks between each operation. If a staged procedure is not possible or if a radical neck dissection is carried out in a patient known to have an absent or thrombosed internal jugular vein on the opposite side, a tracheostomy should be performed or overnight intubation and ventilation be considered to prevent airway obstruction until the vertebral veins accommodate.

Postoperative facial oedema or haemorrhage not directly related to the surgery, cyanosis and airway obstruction are all signs of raised intracranial pressure. The management of cerebral oedema is outlined in Table 6.15.

Table 6.15 The management of cerebral oedema

Head up position 20–30°
Increase blood pressure to elevate cerebral perfusion pressure
Mannitol or frusemide to reduce oedema
If ventilated, hyperventilate to PCO_2 of 3.5–4.5 kPa.
If not ventilated, consider ventilation if no response to above measures.

Management of the free flap

The general principles that govern the anaesthetic management of free flap surgery are neatly encapsulated in the Poiseuille–Hagen formula.

$$\text{Flow} = \frac{\text{Pressure} \times \text{Radius}^4 \times \pi}{\text{Length} \times \text{Viscosity} \times 8}$$

Although this formula describes laminar flow in a Newtonian fluid (blood is not a Newtonian Fluid as its viscosity changes with flow) it usefully relates the factors that will determine flow to a transplanted flap, that is maximum flow is achieved with blood of low viscosity under a high perfusing pressure through non-constricted vessels. (Note how flow is related to the fourth power of the radius.)

The goal of the anaesthetic technique is to maintain a flow of oxygenated blood to the flap by achieving a state of hyperdynamic circulation, that is a state of high cardiac output and vasodilatation, by the avoidance of myocardial depression, hypovolaemia, vasoconstriction and hypothermia (Table 6.16).[34] There are however some areas of controversy.

Vasodilators

Several workers have advocated the use of systemic vasodilators to prevent vasospasm in the vessels feeding the flap.[35] However, there is the risk that their use may steal flow from the flap, in which the vessels are maximally dilated, rather than improve it. In addition the use of sodium nitroprusside can lead to a reflex vasoconstriction on cessation due to an increase in plasma renin and angiotensin II levels.

The use of nitroprusside has been shown to reduce the incidence of intraoperative vasospasm in one series[35] but the overall flap success rate was no better than a similar series in which vasodilators were not used.[36]

Table 6.16 Principles of anaesthesia for free flap surgery

Maintain blood pressure
Maintain isovolaemic or slightly hypervolaemic circulation
Use inodilating agents e.g. dopexamine or dobutamine
Avoid vasoconstriction
Keep patient warm in warm theatre, use warm fluids and a warming blanket
Keep well hydrated
Avoid hypocarbia
Avoid acidosis
Vasodilators e.g. sodium nitropusside
Maximize oxygen delivery
Haemodilution
Avoid acidosis
Maintain good oxygen saturation

Dexamethasone and mannitol can be given postanastomosis to decrease oedema and swelling in the graft but again the success rate was no better than that of a similar group not given these agents.[35,36]

Haemodilution

It is common practice to replace blood loss during the operation with crystalloid and colloid until an haematocrit of 30–35% is achieved (normovolaemic haemodilution), the aim being to reduce viscosity and hence improve blood flow in small vessels. Some workers have recommended the employment of hypervolaemic haemodilution, that is the administration of fluids at a greater rate than blood loss to elevate the central venous pressure to greater than 10 cmH_2O.[29] There is no evidence to suggest that either approach is more beneficial than the other and it would seem prudent, in a population of patients likely to have concurrent cardiac or pulmonary disease, to adopt the normovolaemic approach and maintain central venous pressure at normal levels (5–10 cmH_2O).

Inodilation

There are theoretical advantages in the use of agents such as dopexamine or dobutamine that improve cardiac output by simultaneously improving myocardial contractility and vasodilatation. As with all inotropic agents a state of adequate hydration must exist before they are employed and they are most useful in those situations where blood pressure and graft perfusion are inadequate despite adequate volume replacement.

Postoperative high dependency care

Fluid and electrolyte management

The fluid management of patients undergoing pharyngolaryngo–oesophagectomy has already been discussed. Fluid management in surgery confined to the head and neck is much simpler as there will be no occult or third space losses, the site is relatively superficial, haemostasis and drainage are given a high priority and any losses of blood or fluid will be readily apparent. Hence in this group it is acceptable to prescribe maintenance fluids only for the first 24 hours and replace any drain losses as they occur with colloid. A range of 1–1.5 ml/kg per hour of normal saline should ensure adequate hydration without the risk of fluid overload.

In free flaps and major pedicle flaps, in addition to maintenance requirements as above, colloid should be administered to keep the central venous pressure within the normal range (5–10 cmH_2O) in order to ensure adequate perfusion of the graft.

Enteral feeding should commence on the first postoperative day unless there is an ileus or lower gastrointestinal anastomosis. Once absorption of feed is confirmed intravenous fluid intake should be reduced to prevent fluid overload.

Following total thyroidectomy it is essential to monitor calcium levels (it is best to request ionized levels, the active moiety) 4 hourly and maintain a level above 1.1 mmol/litre with boluses of 10 ml 10% calcium gluconate or an infusion of 40 ml in 500 ml saline over 2–8 hours. If the total serum calcium is measured, correct for serum albumin: for every 1 g/litre difference between the patient's serum albumin and a figure of 40 g/litre add 0.02 mmol/litre to the patient's serum calcium to arrive at the corrected value.

The free flap

In addition to the fluid management outlined above it is important to keep the patient warm, well oxygenated and pain free and the haematocrit in the range 30–35% to maximize oxygen delivery to the flap.

Pain relief

Pain is not a major problem in surgery confined to the head and neck. The intravenous or intramuscular administration of opiate will provide adequate pain relief for the first 24 hours, thereafter enteral analgesia in the form of codeine, non-steroidal anti-inflammatories or paracetamol is usually adequate. The advantages of epidural analgesia for chest wall and abdominal surgery have already been discussed.

Conclusion

Head and neck surgery is unique in that the surgeon and anaesthetist share a common pathway, it is not so much that they compete for the airway but that they co-operate closely to maintain it and both should respect the other's role in airway management. The flexible fibreoptic intubating bronchoscope has revolutionized the management of difficult intubation in anaesthesia for head and neck surgery and many patients are now intubated using this technique who formerly would have required a tracheostomy either awake or asleep after failed attempts at intubation. It is not, however, the answer in all situations and the anaesthetist must know when to request a surgical airway: a bad situation can be made worse by repeated attempts at securing an airway via the supraglottic route when a tracheostomy under local anaesthetic would have saved the day, and the patient. The role of the anaesthetist is not confined to the airway; involving them early in the assessment and preparation of patients for major head and neck surgery will help to minimize perioperative morbidity and mortality and good anaesthetic technique and postoperative high-dependency care leads to good surgical outcome.

REFERENCES

1. Robbie DS. Anaesthesia for surgery in malignant disease of the head and neck. In: Filshie J, Robbie D (eds). *Anaesthesia and Malignant Disease.* London: Edward Arnold, 1989; 135–149.
2. Howland WS, Rooney SM, Goldiner PL.*Manual of Anaesthesia in Cancer Care.* New York: Churchill Livingstone, 1986.
3. Fee JPH, McCaughey W. Preoperative preparation, premedication and concurrent drug therapy. In: Nimmo WS, Rowbotham DJ, Smith G (eds). Oxford: Blackwell, 1989; 677–703.
4. Nishi M, Hiramatsu Y, Hioki K et al. Risk factors in relation to postoperative complications in patients undergoing esophagectomy or gastrectomy for cancer. *Ann Surg* 1988; **207**: 148–154.
5. Ziegler T. New developments in specialised nutritional support. *Curr Topics Intens Care* 1995; **2**: 144–174.
6. *Guidelines for Doctors.* London: The Royal College of Radiologists, 1995.
7. Mallampati SR, Gatt SP, Gugino LD et al. A new sign for predicting difficult intubation. *Can Anaesth Soc J* 1985; **32**: 429–434.
8. Samsoon JLT, Young JRB. Difficult tracheal intubation; a retrospective study. *Anaesthesia* 1987; **42**: 487–490.
9. Patil V, Stehling LC, Zaunder HL. *Fiberoptic Endoscopy in Anaesthesia.* Chicago: Year Book Medical Publishers, 1983.
10. Calder I. Predicting difficult intubation. *Anaesthesia* 1992; **47**: 528–529.
11. Wilson ME, Speighalter D, Robertson JA, Lesser P. Predicting difficult intubation. *Br J Anaesth* 1988; **61**: 211–216.
12. Lewis M, Keramati S, Benumof JL, Berry CC. What is the best way to predict oropharyngeal classification and mandibular space length to predict difficult laryngoscopy. *Anesthesiology* 1994; **81**: 69–75.
13. Calder I, Calder J, Crockard HA. Difficult direct laryngoscopy in patients with cervical spine disease. *Anaesthesia* 1995; **50**: 756–763.
14. Editorial. *Br J Anaesth* 1996; **77**: 309–311.
15. American Society of Anaesthesiologists Task Force on Management of the Difficult Airway. Practice guidelines for management of the difficult airway. *Anaesthesiology* 1993; **78**: 597–602.
16. Sidhu VS, Whitehead EM, Ainsworth QP et al. A technique of awake fibreoptic intubation. Experience in patients with cervical spine disease. *Anaesthesia* 1993; **48**: 910–914.
17. Mason RA. Learning fibreoptic intubation: fundamental problems. *Anaesthesia* 1992; **47**: 729–731.
18. Rhys Evans PH, Frame JW, Brandrick J. A review of carbon dioxide laser surgery in the oral cavity and pharynx. *J Laryngol Otol* 1986; **100**: 69–77.
19. Frame JW, Das Gupta AR, Dalton GA, Rhys Evans PH. Use of the carbon dioxide laser in the management of premalignant lesions of the oral mucosa. *J Laryngol Otol* 1984; **98**: 1251–1260.
20. Paes ML. General anaesthesia for carbon dioxide laser surgery within the airway: a review. *Br J Anaesth* 1987; **59**: 1610–1620.
21. Montgomery PQ, Mochloulis G, Sidhu VS. A Cook airway exchange catheter in the management of intraoperative tracheal injury*Anaesth Intensive Care* 1996; **24**: 617.

22. Byth P. Perioperative care for oesophagectomy patients. *Aust Clin Rev* 1991; **11**: 45–50.
23. Spiro RH, Bains MS, Shah JP, Strong EW. Gastric transposition for head and neck cancer: a critical update. *Am J Surg* 1991; **162**: 348–352.
24. Yamanaka H, Hiramatsu Y, Kawaguchi Y et al. Surgical treatment for poor risk patients with carcinoma of the oesophagus. *Jpn J Surg* 1991; **21**: 178–182.
25. Nishi M, Hiramatsu Y, Hioki K et al. Pulmonary complications after subtotal oesophagectomy. *Br J Surg* 1998; **75**: 527–530.
26. Watson A. Influence of thoracic epidural analgesia on outcome after resection for oesophageal cancer. *Surgery* 1994; **115**: 429–432.
27. Plant M. Anaesthesia for pharyngolaryngectomy with extrathoracic oesophagectomy and gastric transposition. *Anaesthesia* 1982; **37**: 1211–1213.
28. Condon HA. Anaesthesia for pharyngo-laryngo-oesophagectomy with pharyngo-gastrostomy. *Br J Anaesth* 1971; **43**: 1061–1065.
29. Smedstad KG, Beattie WS, Blair WS, Buckley DN. Postoperative pain relief and hospital stay after total esophagectomy. *Clin J Pain* 1992; **8**: 149–153.
30. Izumi K, Abo S, Kitamura M et al. The significance of body weight measurement of oesophageal cancer patients in intra- and postoperative fluid management. *Nippon Kyobu Geka Gakkai Zasshi* 1993; **41**: 234–237.
31. Blass J, Staender S, Moerlen J, Tondeli P. Early extubation without complications after thoraco–abdominal esophagectomy. *Anaesthetist* 1991; **40**: 315–323.
32. Hagen PT, Scholtz DG, Edwards WD. Incidence and size of patent foramen ovale during the first 10 decades of life: an autopsy study of 965 normal hearts. *Mayo Clin Proc* 1984; **59**: 17–20.
33. Donham RT. Complications of anaesthesia. In Johns ME (ed.) *Complications in Otolaryngology. Vol. 2. Head and Neck Surgery*. London: BC Decker, 1986
34. McDonald DJF. Anaesthesia for microvascular surgery: a physiological approach. *Br J Anaes* 1985; **57**: 904–912.
35. Aps C, Cox RG, Mayou BJ, Sengupta P. The role of anaesthetic management in enhancing peripheral blood flow in patients undergoing free flap transfer. *Ann R Coll Surg* 1985; **67**: 177–179.
36. Inglis M, Robbie DS, Edwards J, Breach NM. The anaesthetic management of patients undergoing free-flap reconstructive surgery following resection of head and neck neoplasms: a review of 64 patients. *Ann R Coll Surg* 1988; **70**: 235–238.

7 Nursing care of head and neck cancer patients

Frances Rhys Evans

Introduction

The head and neck is perhaps one of the most complex sites for cancer treatment, not only because of the difficult management problems, but also because of the many physical and psychological traumas potentially affecting the patient. Nowhere else in the body does an area have tissue with such diversity of function. Disease and its progression can dramatically alter the patient's appearance, as well as their basic functions, such as breathing, eating, speaking, hearing and sight. With such physical and functional changes comes the emotional trauma of reintegrating back into society as an independent and autonomous member.

It is vital that nurses working within this demanding specialty have sound theoretical knowledge of the anatomy and physiology of the area, the disease process and treatment options. Complex surgical reconstruction procedures are necessary to restore appearance and function and a comprehensive rehabilitation service to support this work is essential for the smooth reintegration of the patient into every day life.

Nursing care

Caring for the head and neck cancer patient is one of the most challenging and exciting areas for nurses. Owing to the multifaceted nature of the work, one is constantly reviewing and learning to try to improve the delivery of care. A multidisciplinary approach is necessary to provide quality care throughout the course of treatment, as well as during the rehabilitation period. Members of the supporting multidisciplinary care team should include those listed in Table 7.1.

Table 7.1 The supporting multidisciplinary care team

Clinical nurse specialist	Nursing staff
Dietitian	Speech and language therapist
Physiotherapist	Pain management specialist
Pharmacist	Dentist
Dental hygienist	Maxillofacial prosthedontist
Occupational therapist	Community liaison nurse
Social worker	Psychotherapist
Palliative care team	Chaplain

The relevant core members of the team should meet the patient and family prior to treatment so that introductions can be made and needs assessed for the course of care, thus facilitating a cohesive approach.

Preadmission clinic

This is where the concept of a supporting multidisciplinary care team is formalized and brought together to offer a tailored plan of care for the patient's individual needs. The patient will have been seen by the consultants in charge of their overall care and the course of treatment discussed and agreed with them in the multisciplinary clinic. We fail ourselves and the patient if we do not remember that the patient will be shocked, frightened and unable to concentrate to some degree on all that has been said since the potentially life-threatening diagnosis of cancer.

At the subsequent preadmission consultation, it is imperative that all aspects of care are reviewed with the patient and family so that they are informed as fully as possible.

Physical aspects of treatment can be reinforced, and more readily understood with the use of diagrams, illustrations, anatomical models and equipment. The patient will be able to visualize the normal, and then altered and reconstructed anatomical changes in a more logical and sequential way.

Specific issues of care

Nutrition

The dietitian will assess the patient's nutritional status, and may prescribe a tailored regime straight away, especially if the patient has been experiencing dysphagia or is otherwise nutritionally debilitated. A nasogastric tube or percutaneous gastrostomy may be required prior to commencement of definitive treatment.

Oral care

Good oral hygiene is essential for any head and neck treatment. The dentist and dental hygienist will see the patient and diagnose and treat any dental or periodontal disease. A maxillofacial prosthodontist should also be available to take any intraoral and facial impressions.

Speech therapy

The speech therapist will meet any patient who has or may have any speech or hearing impairment. It is vital that they see the speech therapist while they are still able to communicate freely in order to get to know each other, make assessments and discuss the rehabilitation programme. Audiological evaluation is a valuable base line, and assists in comparing changes that may occur following treatment, either surgery, radiotherapy or chemotherapy.

Social worker

The social worker can meet the patient and make an assessment and advise and help with any necessary documentation and employment benefits.

Physiotherapy

Those patients with pulmonary problems or due to undergo a radical neck dissection can be seen by the physiotherapist for preoperative assessment of muscle strength and range of movement. Exercises can be given and an explanation of a postoperative exercise programme to decrease the degree of shoulder drop and limitation of movement following a radical neck dissection.

Clinical nurse specialist

The clinical nurse specialist should also meet the patient and family to discuss the rationale for postoperative nursing interventions and the equipment used. This would be at the depth and pace that the patient demanded and would also be supported with illustrations, models, patient booklets and other written materials. The patient may like to tour the head and neck unit or ward at this stage and see where they would be nursed. The clinical nurse specialist could also offer advice on any psychological or clinical problems.

Summary

The aim of the preadmission clinic is for the patient and family to feel that the whole team is working together for the patient's physical, psychological and social well-being and optimum quality of life, and to facilitate the smooth transition back into society.

Nursing interventions

In view of the multiple aspects of care that may be required for each individual patient, the main nursing interventions have been subdivided for clarity.

Airway management

Airway management and tracheostomy maintenance are some of the most demanding and anxious aspects of any nursing care. This mostly stems from fear of potentially acute and life threatening situations, particularly in head and neck oncology because of the complex surgery involved and the unpredictable nature of any possible emergency.

For this reason it is imperative that nurses caring for this group of patients have a thorough clinical and theoretical knowledge of airway management. The patient and family will experience feelings of apprehension and uncertainty over an altered airway. Therefore it is vital that the nursing staff manage and teach the patient and family how to care for the airway in a calm, sensible and logical way. By sharing one's knowledge and adopting this manner, it will reduce anxiety and build confidence and trust for the patient and family.

Those patients who are temporarily stridulous or who have a compromised airway, not necessitating a tracheostomy, can gain respiratory relief from humidified oxygen or from heliox (helium and oxygen). The helium gas in heliox has a lower viscosity than normal air and therefore produces less airway resistance so that the patient can ventilate more easily.

Tracheostomies are of two fundamental types: 'end' or 'side'. An end tracheostomy is seen in a total laryngectomy where the trachea is diverted to come out of the neck above the suprasternal notch. A side tracheostomy is where a passageway is made through the tissues of the neck into the side wall of the trachea. It may be a permanent or, more likely, temporary procedure to provide and maintain a patient's airway. In the latter situation obstruction such as tumour or oedema caused by surgery or radiotherapy are bypassed. A side tracheostomy can also be performed to enable the removal of tracheobronchial secretions when the patient is too weak to expectorate independently. Many patients with head and neck cancer do also have chronic obstructive airway disease or chronic bronchitis and may benefit from a tracheostomy to assist in reducing dead space and removal of secretions.

Tracheostomy care

Equipment

It is essential that a patient who has a tracheostomy should always have at their bedside (or easily accessible if the patient is self caring or ambulant) the items mentioned in Table 7.2 and Figure 7.1.

Specific management issues

Expectoration

The airway should be kept free of secretions at all times and this is most effectively accomplished by encouraging the patient to cough. Not only is the airway cleared but the lungs expand to prevent atelectasis and pneumonia.

Table 7.2 Essential equipment for tracheostomy care

Humidified oxygen with tracheostomy mask
Suction unit with a selection of suction catheters
Bowl of water and sodium bicarbonate to clear suction tubing of secretions following suctioning
Clean disposable gloves
Two cuffed tracheostomy tubes, one the same size as worn by the patient, the other a size smaller in the event of an emergency tracheostomy tube change
One 10-ml syringe to inflate the cuff on the tracheostomy tube
A tube of lubricating jelly to facilitate tube insertion
Tracheal dilators for the situation where the tracheostomy tube falls out or where it has been removed and where insertion of another tube is difficult. The tracheal dilators can be used to keep the stoma patent until medical assistance arrives[1]

Suctioning

With a newly formed tracheostomy or if the patient is too weak to cough, the secretions must be suctioned from the trachea. This is a clean procedure and sterilized equipment must be used. The catheter should not be inserted further than the carina and suction should only be applied upon withdrawal of the catheter in a gentle rotating movement. The whole procedure should not take longer than 10 seconds.

Type of tube

Various types of tracheostomy tube are available but for safety it is essential to use one that has a separate inner tube and one which is comfortable for the patient. These are available in cuffed, non-cuffed, fenestrated and non-fenestrated forms in different sizes, the use of each of them being indicated in different clinical situations.

Montgomery T-tube

These are used following operations for laryngotracheal stenosis (Figure 7.2) and crusting may be a problem at the junction of the horizontal and vertical

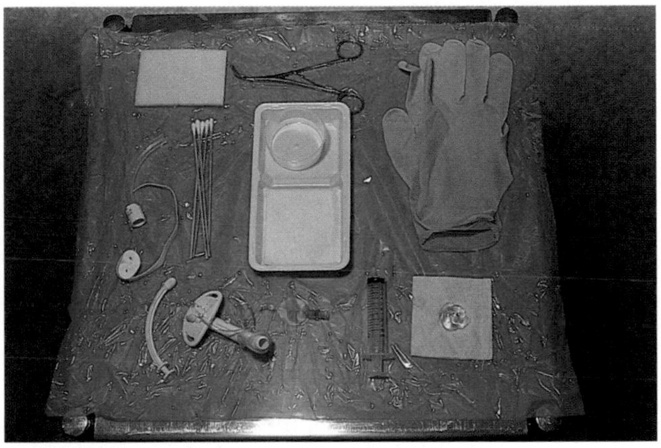

Figure 7.1 Equipment for tracheostomy care.

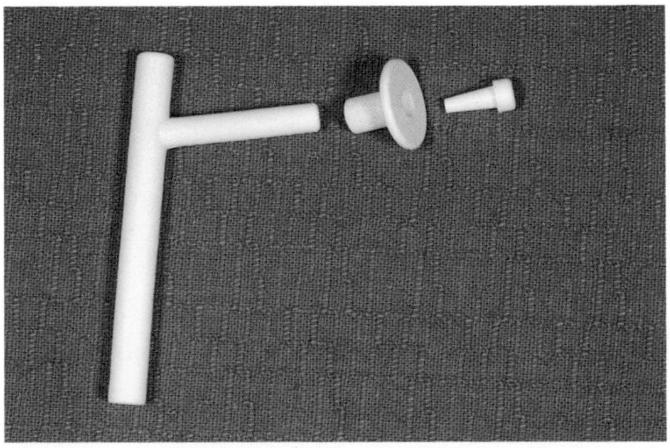

Figure 7.2 Montgomery T-tube.

limbs. The attending nurse must have a clear understanding of the slightly different suctioning and cleaning techniques.

Tube changes

The frequency of tracheostomy tube changes is mostly dependent on the type of secretion. The inner tube may initially have to be changed every half an hour but every patient should be carefully assessed on a continual basis. Any nurse who is starting a span of duty should always do a baseline assessment of the airway and tube to check on the type and amount of secretions and the need for humidification or nebulizing spray. Listening to the breathing is vital for early signs of obstruction.

The outer tube needs changing less frequently but a patient with copious tenacious secretions will need a daily or twice daily tube change, as this is the only way of ensuring that the stoma and tube are free from secretions. It is not uncommon for acute airway obstruction to occur because of a build-up of crusts at the bottom end of a tracheostomy tube, which is not recognized unless the whole tube is changed. If the patient has minimal secretions they may only need a weekly tube change.

Laryngectomy tubes or stoma buttons

Some of these do not have an inner tube and therefore will need to be changed frequently especially when they are first used. Whenever the tube is removed it is essential that the airway is checked with a torch to make sure that there are no crusts building up below the tube. These can be removed carefully with angled forceps.

Peristomal wounds

Those patients with wounds in or around the stoma (Figure 7.3) will need to have their tube removed in order to get good visualization of the wound and access for toileting.

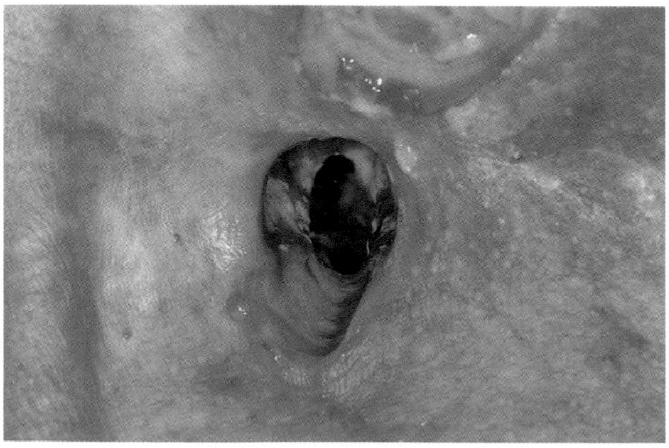

Figure 7.3 Large stomal tracheo-oesophageal fistula.

Tracheostomy dressing

The tracheostomy dressing should be renewed and the circumference of the stoma cleaned and dried at least once, if not twice a day or more frequently depending on mucus production, to ensure secretions are cleared and do not lie wet against the skin causing excoriation. The dressing procedure can be done without removing the tube if appropriate.

Self care

Gradually as the patient and family members feel ready, tracheostomy care can be taught to them. The main focus is to help the patient feel confident in keeping their tracheostomy tube patent by themselves by teaching the three basic aspects of tracheostomy care: changing the inner tubes of their tracheostomy tube, humidifying with a nebulizing spray; and expectorating secretions. This is obviously the patient's main priority and they must be supported and encouraged. It must be recognized that each patient and their circumstances are different: some patients feel ready to learn all aspects of care from changing the tracheostomy dressing to doing a complete tube change, whereas others need considerable support.

Laryngectomy

The laryngectomy patient will need to learn all aspects of stomal toilet care and what to do in the event of an emergency. The permanency of their condition makes a laryngectomy patient realize that their freedom, independence and survival depends on their knowledge and practical care. However, this type of permanent stoma (an 'end' stoma) is easier to manage and laryngectomy tubes are very rarely needed in the long term. Stoma buttons or stoma vents[2] are much easier to use but may not be necessary for permanent use.

Wound care

Astute and skilled nursing intervention is necessary for care of head and neck wounds, which often involve intricate reconstructive techniques. It is essential that specialist head and neck nursing attention is available throughout the wound healing process, to deal with these complex wounds that are at a high-risk of developing serious complications.

In the first 24 hours the patient will be nursed on a one to one basis for close observation and monitoring, sometimes in a high dependency unit, particularly if they have a flap repair. The patient needs to be nursed in a semi-sitting position since gravity will help to reduce oedema. Basic wound observation remains the same but specific observations are necessary for skin flaps.

Skin flaps

General issues

A skin flap is composed of skin and subcutaneous tissue and survives provided that it continues to have an intact and functioning arterial and venous circulation. There are two main types of skin flap:

1 Free flap: bowel, skin, subcutaneous tissue and sometimes muscle/bone with a main artery and vein, which is separated and then transferred from one area of the body to another. Using microvascular techniques, the artery and vein are anastomosed to a recipient artery and vein in the neck.
2. Pedicle flap: skin, subcutaneous tissue and muscle are transferred from one area to another but the base or pedicle remains attached to its original blood supply.

The aim of nursing care of any type of flap is to ensure flap viability. Frequent and thorough observation, at least every 15–30 minutes in the immediate postoperative period for the first 24 hours is essential. Circulation is paramount to the flap's survival. Blood flow into the flap must be adequate and blood draining from the flap must also be unobstructed. The skin flap should be pink, warm and blanch, showing brisk capillary return when touched.

Flap monitoring

A white discoloration indicates a dearterialized flap where the blood supply is inadequate. When pricked the flap should bleed if the circulation is adequate but not if the arterial supply is compromised. It must be remembered however that the normal colour for the flap is the same as its original donor site, which is often paler than mucosal areas within the mouth (Figure 7.4). Arterial devascularization is more commonly seen in the first 24 hours after operation. A blue or dusky discoloration indicates venous congestion and this may occur later, after several days.

Tapes and dressings

There must be no kinking, tension or pressure on the flap. Vigilant attention must be given to ensure that tracheostomy tapes, dressing tapes and bandages are not tied too tightly around the flap or wound. Care should also be taken with Hudson or tracheostomy mask tapes that they are not too tight around the neck thus impeding blood flow. Oxygen tubing and other lines should not lie over the wound or flap site causing pressure.

Observation of mottling, duskiness or sudden tightness of the neck dressing can be indicative of haematoma formation and possibly impending flap failure. Bandages used around the neck can also have the disadvantage of preventing visualization of important signs of skin changes and are generally not needed when suction drainage is used. Fans should also be used with caution as they can cause a vasoconstriction of the flap and subsequent failure. The patient should be kept warm to avoid vasoconstriction.

Drainage bottles

All drainage bottles must be patent and checked regularly because a devacuumed or clamped bottle can cause flap failure. If the Redivac tubing is temporarily clamped for movement of the patient, it is essential that it is reopened.

Fluid balance

The patient must have an adequate fluid balance. The haemoglobin should be ideally over 10 grammes and if below this, the patient should be transfused to ensure that sufficient oxygen is perfusing all wound areas. When a flap is being used, the haemoglobin should not be too high as the blood circulation may become more sluggish and this may jeopardize the circulation particularly in the first few days after operation.

Flap failure

The medical team must be notified immediately if the flap is showing any signs of failure. Flaps can tolerate approximately 4 hours of ischaemia before irreversible tissue necrosis occurs. The team will assess the situation and start medical intervention to

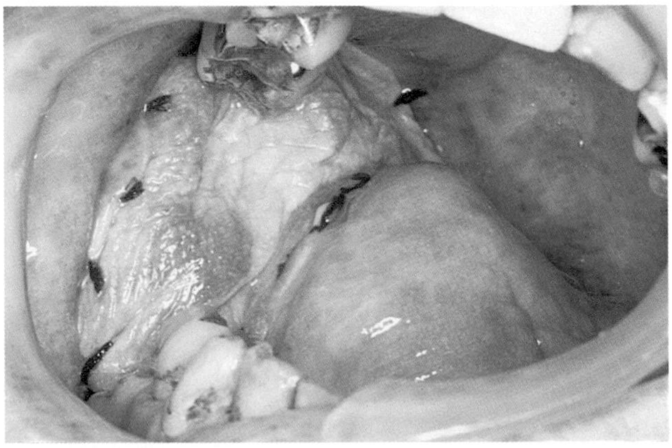

Figure 7.4 Free radial forearm flap in the oral cavity.

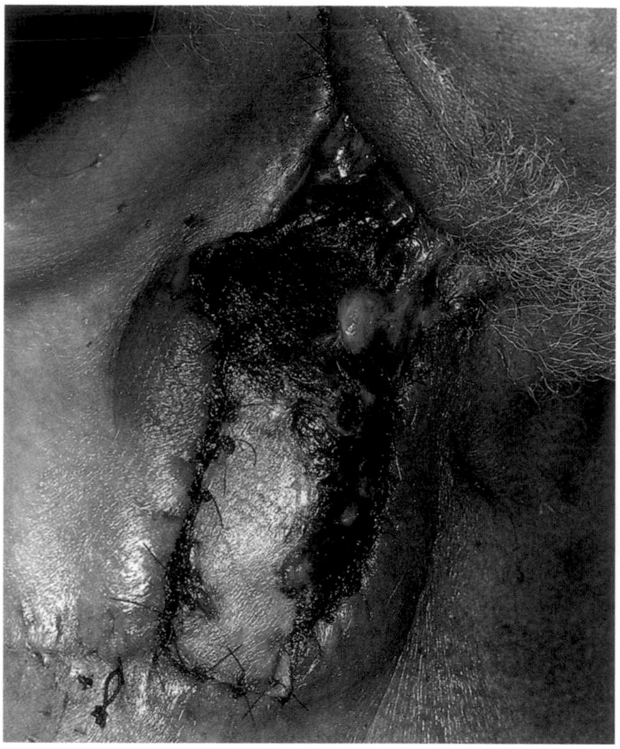

Figure 7.5 Partial loss of a latissimus dorsi flap.

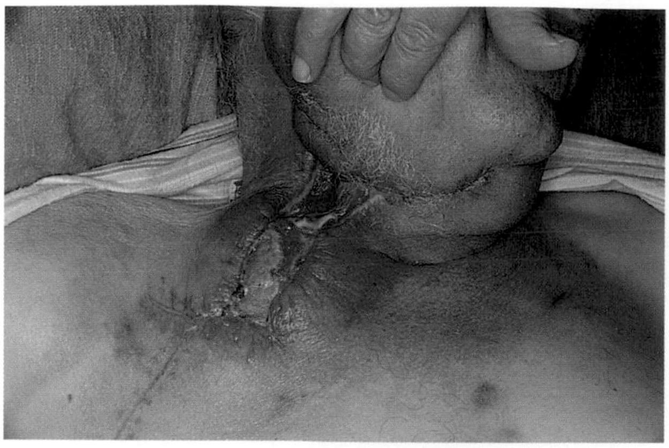

Figure 7.6 Satisfactory healing after 2 weeks.

save the flap if necessary. Such measures may include releasing one or two vital sutures to ease pressure or tension, evacuating a haematoma, which can be done either on the ward or may necessitate the patient going back to theatre. Pedicled latissimus dorsi flaps sometimes can suffer circulation problems if the axilla is compressed but this can be relieved if the arm is abducted and supported.

In general the survival of free flaps is an 'all or nothing' phenomenon because the circulation failure is usually in the main artery or vein. Salvage of a compromised flap is an emergency procedure to evacuate the clot and/or redo the anastomosis. For pedicled cutaneous or myocutaneous flaps, tissue loss is usually partial and a 'wait and see' policy is adopted to allow demarcation. The underlying muscle is normally viable and will eventually granulate well (Figures 7.5 and 7.6).

Leeches

Another simple, non-invasive and painless measure to reduce congestion in a flap is by the application of leeches. Each leech can remove approximately 10 ml of blood. Three or four leeches can be applied as necessary in the acute situation to the congested area and may be all that is necessary to ease the tension and improve blood flow (Figures 7.7 and 7.8). Improvements in the skin colour are noticed almost immediately. With a skilled, professional and empathetic approach, patients will understand and comply especially as the alternative could be a lengthy surgical procedure.

In summary the early detection of a compromised flap combined with prompt expert management can prevent putting the patient through further surgery and disfigurement that would occur if a replacement flap had to be harvested.

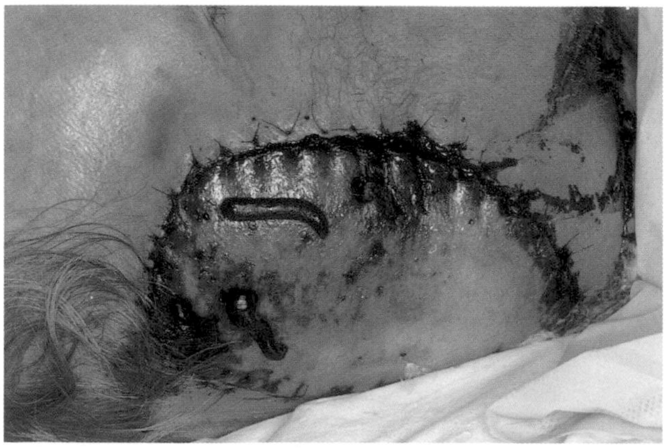

Figure 7.7 Leeches on a congested flap.

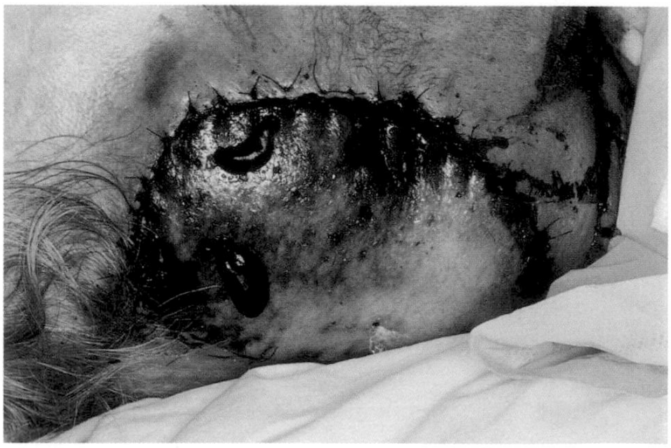

Figure 7.8 After 30 minutes.

Skin grafts

Skin grafts are composed of epidermal tissue and a thin layer of dermis. Skin grafts vary in thickness dependent on the recipient area to be covered. It may be a full thickness (Wolfe) graft, which is often taken from the postauricular sulcus or the inguinal region. The most commonly used type of skin graft is a split thickness (Thiersh) graft, which may be taken from the upper arm or from the thigh. The skin graft is removed from the donor site and sutured or laid on the recipient area. It acts as a dressing to cover the wound site and eventually becomes incorporated as skin epidermis. A Thiersh graft may also be taken from the buttocks as this is a useful area especially if the patient is worried about the potential scarring and disfigurements at the donor site. Even with the smallest amount of clothing cover such as bikini bottoms, trunks or underwear, the graft area would be covered.

Nursing observation and care will include both the donor site and the recipient site. The protective covering of the donor site will depend on the surgeon's preference. Commonly tulle gras with cotton wool with crepe bandage pressure dressing is used. Transparent dressings such as Opsite or an alginate such as Keltostat can also be used. The cotton wool pressure dressing remains in situ for approximately 14 days. Alginate can be removed at an earlier time of 5 to 7 days.

If the wound leaks excessive exudate the top dressing can be taken down and rebandaged. However if the exudate looks or smells infected the dressing should be soaked off and assessed.

When it is time for the dressing to be removed it should be gently soaked off in the bath or shower. Re-epithelialization occurs in the donor site area as the healing process takes place. For this reason the dressing must never be forced off as the granulation tissue will be damaged.

Patients often complain of most of their pain being in the donor site area postoperatively. Some anaesthetists give a regional nerve block to ease the pain on the donor limb particularly if it has been bilateral. A local injection of Marcain can also dull the pain in the early postoperative period. The pain is due to exposure of nerve endings. Regular analgesia and avoidance of friction from night clothes and bedding is essential.

The donor site is often exposed to air whilst healing occurs. If this is too painful in the early days, a non-adherent dressing such as mepital or geliperm can be used. It is essential that the area is reassessed every day with a view to exposing it to the air to dry as soon as the patient can tolerate this. If it is covered for too long, the area becomes wet and infected. Once the area has begun to dry, moisturizing cream can be applied to prevent crust formation and to ease any discomfort. The massaging effects of the moisturizing are very beneficial in preventing taught scar tissue and facilitating a smooth supple skin. Fragrance-free homeopathic creams are ideal such as calendula or aloe vera, but any non-perfumed cream will suffice. Arnica cream is helpful to ease discomfort where there is excessive bruising and can be used as long as the skin is intact.

Wound complications

A wound complication is not only distressing and discouraging for the patient and medical staff but it also invariably means a prolonged stay in hospital.

Fistulas

These require patience and perseverance and will often gradually close spontaneously but if larger may need surgical intervention. Keeping the fistula clean, free from infection and as dry as possible may at times be very demanding but will encourage healing (Figures 7.9 and 7.10).

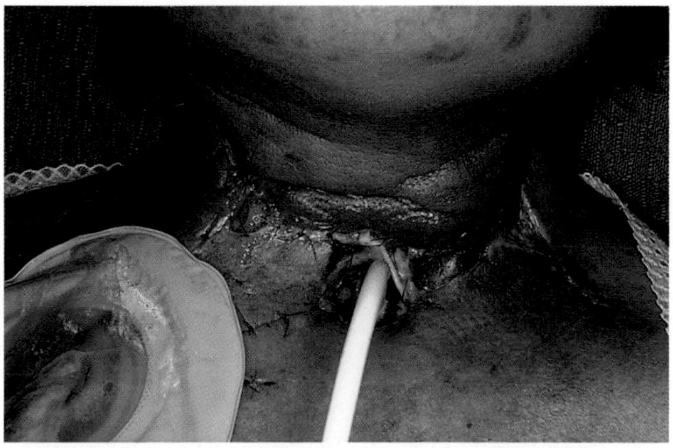

Figure 7.9 Pharyngocutaneous fistula postjejunum anastomosis requiring stoma bag for secretions.

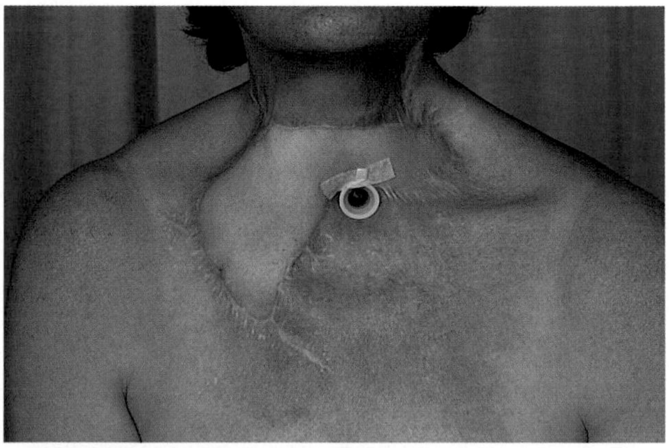

Figure 7.10 Six months later after complete healing using a latissimus dorsi flap.

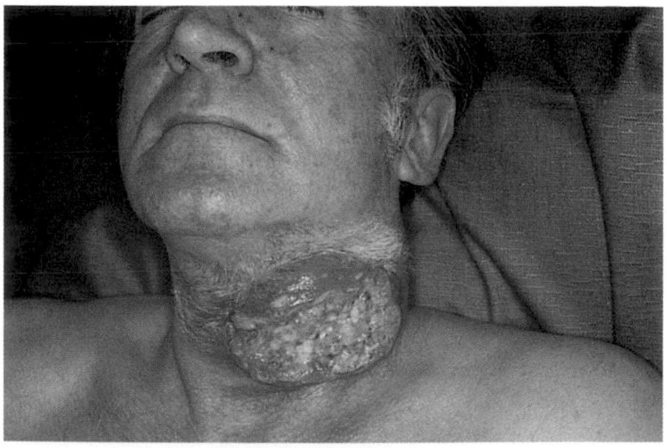

Figure 7.11 Fungating neck wound.

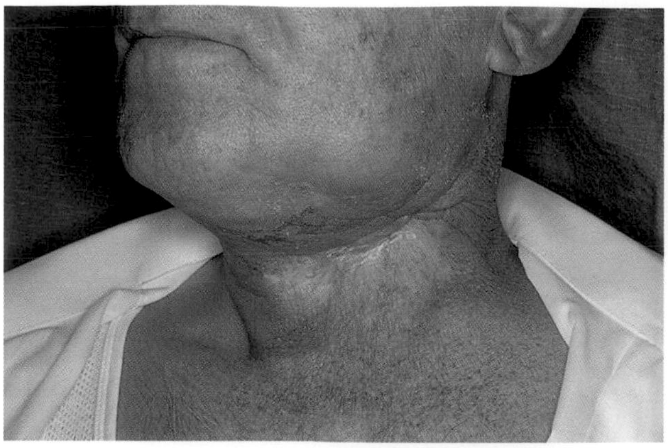

Figure 7.12 Eight months later after chemoradiation.

Sloughing wounds

These may require surgical debridement and/or the use of a topical desloughing agent.

Fungating and malodorous wounds

These can be covered with carbon-impregnated dressings and topical antibiotics can be applied such as metronidazole which is an excellent deodorizer. Metronidazole taken systemically is also most effective for malodorous wounds (Figure 7.11 and 7.12).

Vascular wounds

These can be dressed with alginate products such as Keltostat.

Intraoral bleeding

Minor bleeding can be controlled by rinsing with tranexamic acid.

Major arterial bleeds

These are potentially fatal for some patients but even minor bleeds can be very distressing. A massive haemorrhage is usually heralded over preceding hours by more minor episodes of bleeding and the source of any minor bleeding must be very carefully investigated. Patients with a previous history of radiation therapy and who have had a fistula or infection are most at risk if the wound has broken down. The patient should be cannulated for administering volume expanders and blood if the patient is for resuscitation. The nurse must wear gloves and apply firm pressure with large pads and call for emergency assistance. The rest of the team can administer artificial resuscitation and co-ordinate theatre staff if appropriate.[2]

If the patient is terminally ill with massive untreatable recurrent disease intravenous access can be used to deliver diamorphine or hyponoval to relieve the severe pain, anxiety and fear induced by the sudden hypovolaemia associated with a carotid blowout.

Pain management

Pain is experienced by 40–80% of patients suffering from head and neck cancer[3] in all different phases of the disease and its treatment. It is often difficult to assess and not always easy to elicit the exact cause due to the complex structure of the head and neck and diverse sensory innervation. Medical expertise from a specialist in pain management, who has a good understanding of head and neck disease and treatment, is imperative in helping to control this symptom. Access for administration of analgesia is an important issue for the head and neck patient because swallowing is often difficult or inadvisable during the early postoperative phase. A nasogastric tube or gastrostomy is the preferred option. Aspirin-based products should not be used preoperatively and postoperatively with great caution as they interfere with haemostasis in surgery and may predispose to postoperative haematoma formation.[2]

Complementary methods are also of value in pain management such as acupuncture, diversional therapy, massage, aromatherapy as well as the prescribed regular analgesic medication. Monitoring the effectiveness and evaluating the pain management regimen should be continued throughout the patient's course of treatment and at follow-up appointments.

Mouth care

The aim of comprehensive mouth care is to maintain good oral hygiene, to prevent plaque build-up, dental decay and infection. It also is essential to keep the oral mucosa moist and intact and to promote patient comfort and well-being. To help achieve good oral status, the patient must be adequately hydrated and the appropriate instruments, solutions and methods used.

Incapacitated patients and those unable to perform their own oral toilet are most at risk for developing mouth-care problems. It is essential that the nurse makes a thorough assessment of the patient's oral status and assists them in the most appropriate regimen. Irrigation of the oral cavity is very beneficial when the patient has an intraoral lesion or surgical site. Irrigation helps to keep the mouth or any cavities fresh and clean. It stimulates blood supply, reduces oedema, helps to alleviate pain and discomfort, controls odour and helps to prevent and clear debris and infection. When the patient is learning to irrigate, the nurse assists by offering support and advice. The patient is guided and helped to avoid trauma to exposed tissues, flaps or grafts.

If the oral cleaning is painful or uncomfortable, the patient must be offered analgesia half an hour prior to their oral hygiene regimen.

There will be periods when the patient feels inundated and overwhelmed at the many aspects of their care rehabilitation that they are trying to manage, such as tracheostomy care and enteral feeding. It is therefore both practical and sensible to keep all of these regimens as simple and as logical as possible for optimum patient compliance, especially if they are going to be long term.

Communication

Most patients at some stage in their course of treatment have their ability to communicate interrupted. This can be temporary due to a side tracheostomy, to laryngeal oedema from radiotherapy or tumour or to severe stomatitis. Speech will also be affected following laryngectomy, glossectomy and other oral and pharyngeal reconstructions for varying periods of time.

To help the patient, the nurse may ask questions in such a way that a 'yes' or 'no' or 'nod' of the head would suffice in the initial postoperative period. Written communication is always made available such as pen and paper or a magic slate. Flash cards depicting areas of care are also useful as a temporary measure or for the illiterate patient. Attempting to communicate will be extremely frustrating at times for the patient especially if they are feeling depressed or unwell and it is vital that the nurse is gentle, encouraging and patient in helping the person to communicate so that they do not regress or become mute.

Often conversation has to be repeated several times before it is understood but practice at communication must be encouraged in a safe and private environment, especially in the early postoperative period where the patient may be upset at the sound of their initial voice. Nothing irritates a patient more than if the rushed nurse, doctor or frustrated family member finishes the patient's sentence for them in their desire to be helpful, particularly if it has been interpreted incorrectly. Family and friends should be reassured and educated on these points.

Tracheostomy tubes should be fitted with speaking valves as soon as possible to help ease feelings of isolation for the patient and facilitate practice of speech. Laryngectomy patients may have had a tracheo-oesophageal puncture performed either as a primary or secondary procedure. They will wear a Foley catheter in the puncture site until they are ready to be fitted with the surgical voice prosthesis. If this is done primarily at the time of laryngectomy, the valve is usually fitted after normal swallowing has been started after 7–10 days. As a secondary procedure the valve can usually be fitted within 2–3 days.

Psychological support

When a patient is first diagnosed as having cancer, a potentially life-threatening disease, the initial shock, anger, sense of loss, lack of control and grief are virtually the same feelings one experiences after bereavement. It is therefore important to recognize that the patient will be in need of the appropriate support. They are grieving the loss of part of themselves and their life as they once had, which will never be quite the same again.

Feelings of anger and spiritual questioning 'why did God allow this to happen to me?', 'why me, what have I done to deserve this?' are common and entirely normal. It is a rare person who can live contentedly with an uncertain and unpredictable life. The patient and family will be desperate to alleviate that uncertainty and in doing so will cling to the medical staff's every verbal and non-verbal response to elicit a hint or shred of reassurance for the future.

It is best to give clear and honest answers to questions asked by the patient concerning their future survival and quality of life. However, it should be sensitively done as maintaining hope can give the patient a sense of strength and security. Often the patient will give a direct or indirect indication of how much information they want to be told. For some, the prospect that they will still be able to enjoy some quality of life, pursue a hobby, travel, be free from pain and so forth is tremendously reassuring. If the patient's symptoms are controlled and are minimal then hopefully a relatively normal lifestyle can be resumed. Various studies have found that patients who maintain close relationships with their family and friends are more likely to cope with the course of their treatment and rehabilitation.[4]

Patients will experience a degree of depression at some stage in their illness and this too must be recognized as a normal response to the threat of disfigurement, dysfunction and possibly death. The patient and family must be given the opportunity, time and privacy to express their anxiety and fears.

Once the period of grieving has begun, the diagnosis of cancer can also precipitate the onset of the patient's coping mechanisms as recognized by Caplan.[5] Most patients demonstrate an extraordinarily brave determination to get on with their life, whatever their dysfunction and/or disfigurement, especially if the alternative is death.[6] Most patients employ a coping mechanism, which we all practise to some extent in our lives, that of social comparison. They frequently compare themselves to others, with the subconscious intent to be in a stronger, more positive position. By comparing their handicaps with others, they will reason that to lose their ear or voice or part of their tongue for example is better than to lose an eye or to be confined to a wheelchair for life. By making these comparisons, the patient tries to relieve some of their fate and enhance the value and quality of their life.

Helping patients and their families to express themselves, and feel comfortable to interact with the staff involved with their care, will foster trust and reassurance with the knowledge that everyone is seen to be working together to achieve an acceptable quality of life.

Some patients and families may want to talk to someone who is not involved in their immediate care. Often referral to a mental health professional or support group can be helpful.

Sexual health

Sexual health must be addressed if the head and neck cancer patients' care is to be covered in its entirety. Whether in health or sickness, we are all sexual beings with the fundamental needs of being loved, desired and finding comfort in another person.

Sexual expression

The need to support sexual expression in patients with cancer, or any illness for that matter, confirms their vitality and being able to talk about it gives confidence in their survival.[2] It may not be appropriate to discuss sexual health problems with all patients. One may not feel comfortable in doing so, but in these cases it does not mean that the situation should be overlooked. The patient should be referred to someone who is more comfortable and qualified in discussing sexual health issues such as the clinical nurse specialist or another member of the team.

When is the best time?

The patient needs to know that they have permission to broach the subject and that it will not be a matter of shock or embarrassment. Preoperatively, a gentle way of initiating the subject of appearance and attractiveness may be when the operative procedure is discussed. For example, if the patient is going to have a split skin graft taken and they have a choice of where the donor site can be, the patient can be asked for their preference. It can be suggested that some people like to wear shorts or sleeveless shirts if they feel they have nice legs or attractive arms. Does the patient have a personal preference? The skin can alternatively be taken from the buttocks so that the area would be covered in most situations.

If the patient is to have a myocutaneous flap, in a female the latissimus dorsi flap is cosmetically much more acceptable than a pectoralis major flap. It might be possible to make the incision in a more horizontal fashion so that the scar can be covered by a bra or bikini top.

By adopting this approach, the patient will recognize that it is accepted as normal that they will be concerned about their appearance. We all have aspects of our body that we prefer and it is important that the patient recognizes that the head and neck surgical team is aware of these potential sources of concern and that they will take these personal factors into consideration.

Oral expression

Many head and neck surgical procedures involve breaching the integrity of the oral cavity. Research has shown that sexual adjustment is a common concern for the patient, especially if the mouth is affected, as this plays an important role in oral stimulation and expression.[6] Most patients complain that they cannot enjoy a proper kiss or cuddle with their partner or kiss their children properly and long for the warmth, intimacy and reassurance this provides.

Facial expression

Limitations in spontaneous facial expressions are also frustrating and inhibiting for sexual expression and these concerns should be addressed if there is likely to be potential weakness of the facial nerve or facial muscles.

Sputum

Sputum production, particularly if copious from the oral cavity or uncontrollable from a stoma is another major concern. The patient worries that they appear dirty as well as unattractive. Agents that help dry up the secretions can be a useful temporary measure. For stoma patients, in the early days of their sexual rehabilitation or until their confidence increases with their new stoma, practical suggestions can be made such as filling a bathroom with steam from the bath or shower, which will in turn humidify the patient's stoma. Bathing together can be incorporated as foreplay with their partner. Alternative positions for love making can also be suggested if the patient is anxious about coughing over their partner.

With sensitivity, ingenuity and appropriate humour, most patients' anxiety can be relieved. It is imperative however that the patient and family feel reassured of complete trust and confidentiality.

Cosmetic camouflage

A cosmetic camouflage service and a good prosthetics departments are also vital for some patients in helping them to regain their identity and confidence in facing their partner, family and the public.

Continuing support

Information on support services and groups must also be made available for those patients who would like to attend. It is important to continue to inquire in the follow-up clinics how the patient is coping at home and if they have any relationship or personal worries as many problems sometimes manifest only when the patient is back at home. It may be appropriate for the patient to be followed up in the clinical nurse specialist (or equivalent) led clinic for ongoing psychological, social or sexual health support, which also ensures continuity for the patient. In the general follow-up clinic where the patient may meet a new or different member of the medical team it is often difficult or inappropriate to discuss personal matters. The patient is usually only concerned with one vital medical issue: that they are still free of cancer.

Conclusion

Intensive and comprehensive nursing and a unified approach to care with the medical staff and multidisciplinary team, offers the patient an optimum opportunity to regain, in their perception, a quality of life that is acceptable after the impact of head and neck cancer and its treatment. The delivery of this care should be with total empathy and consideration at all times.

REFERENCES

1 Rhys Evans F. Tracheostomy care and laryngectomy voice rehabilitation. In: Mallett J, Bailey C (eds) *The Royal Marsden NHS Trust, Manual of Clinical Nursing Procedures*. London: Blackwell Science, 1996; 550–565.

2. Rhys Evans F. Tumours of the head and neck. In: Tshudin V (ed.) *Nursing the Patient with Cancer*. London: Prentice Hall, 1996; 178–201.

3. Bonica JJ. Treatment of cancer pain: current status and future needs. In: Fields HL (ed.) *Advances in Pain and Therapy*. Vol 9. New York: Raven Press, 1985; 589–617.

4. Wortman CB, Dunkel-Schetter C. Interpersonal relationships and cancer: a theoretical analysis. *J Clin Issues* 1979; **39**: 120–155.

5. Caplan G. *Principles of Preventative Psychiatry*. London: Basic Books, 1966.

6. Rhys Evans F. An investigation into functional problems following major oral surgery in head and neck cancer patients, and coping mechanisms employed by the patient. MSc Thesis, University of Surrey 1993.

FURTHER READING

Drettner B, Ahlbom A. Quality of life and state of health for patients with cancer in the head and neck. *Acta Otolaryngolog* 1983; **96**: 307–314.

Bowlby J. *Attachment and Loss*. Vol. 3, 2nd edn. London: Penguin Books, 1998.

Rhys Evans PH. *Provision and Quality Assurance for Head and Neck Cancer Care in the United Kingdom. A Nationally Coordinated Multidisciplinary Approach.* London: Royal Marsden Hospital, 1995.

8 Nutritional support of head and neck cancer patients

Clare Shaw

Introduction

Up to 60% of head and neck cancer patients may be malnourished at diagnosis.[1] Weight loss and malnutrition in head and neck cancer patients are primarily caused by a reduced food intake that may be due to both physical or psychological factors. Metabolic changes due to malignant disease may also contribute to the development of malnutrition. Treatment of head and neck cancer may further exacerbate a poor dietary intake thereby increasing the risk of complications during treatment.[2]

Causes of poor dietary intake and weight loss

The causes of a poor diet and weight loss are complex (see Table 8.1) and are exacerbated by the metabolic effects of the tumour. These include increased glucose–carbon cycling, elevated protein turnover and possibly increased fat oxidation.[5] These metabolic changes may be mediated by cytokines including interleukin-1, interleukin-6 and tumour necrosis factor.[6] Surgery, trauma and sepsis cause an elevation in metabolic rate, increased protein breakdown and nitrogen excretion resulting in a loss of lean body mass.

Benefits of nutritional support

Whilst nutritional support may be able to maintain or improve body weight, body fat and lean body mass, the effect may not be as great as in those who do not have underlying malignant disease.[7] Nevertheless, nutritional support has been shown to be of benefit in several ways.

Table 8.1 Causes of poor dietary intake and weight loss

Anorexia	Cytokines produced by the body in response to the presence of a tumour, such as interleukin and tumour necrosis factor, may depress appetite[3]
Psychological factors	Depression and anxiety
Excessive alcohol intake	Depression of appetite
	Displacement of foods from the diet
	Thiamin deficiency and Wernicke–Korsakoff syndrome may occur in chronic alcoholics
Dysphagia and/or trismus	Dietary deficiency of all nutrients particularly energy
Poor oral hygiene and oral infection	Tumour burden and opportunistic infection
Taste changes	May occur in up to 70% of patients and can be due to tumour, radiotherapy or chemotherapy[4]
Stomatitis or mucositis	Caused by radiotherapy or chemotherapy[4]
Pain on chewing or swallowing	Caused by presence of tumour, treatment or infection
Xerostomia	Often occurs after radiotherapy to salivary gland[4]

Perioperative nutritional support

Perioperative nutritional support may reduce both morbidity and mortality.[8] Studies that have failed to show the benefit of perioperative nutritional support have often not distinguished between patients with a good nutritional status and those who are malnourished. It is likely that severely malnourished patients benefit more from nutritional support than those patients who are already well nourished. For preoperative nutritional support to be effective in influencing clinical outcome it should be given to malnourished patients for 7–15 days before surgery.[9] Preoperative enteral nutrition is as effective as parenteral nutrition and should always be the method of choice when there is a functioning gastrointestinal tract. Postoperative parenteral nutrition, enteral nutrition or adequate oral nutrition are equally effective in reducing nutrition-related postoperative complications.

Tolerance to treatment

Studies of the nutritional support of patients undergoing treatment have provided varying results. Some studies, but not all, have shown the benefits of nutritional support with respect to chemotherapy or radiotherapy toxicity in patients.[7] The benefits included a decrease in medications given for symptom control, a reduction in the duration of chemotherapy-induced nausea and vomiting, better tolerance of chemotherapy and fewer treatment delays. This may have an impact in terms of control of disease as it is recognized that delays in treatment may contribute to a poorer outcome for the patient.

Malnutrition in head and neck cancer patients has been shown to be associated with immunoincompetence although studies have failed to show a significant improvement in immune function on feeding such patients.[10]

Intensive nutritional support of head and neck patients undergoing radiotherapy treatment, in the form of gastrostomy feeding, helps patients maintain their nutritional status and quality of life during treatment.[11]

Nutritional assessment

All patients with head and neck cancer must undergo a nutritional assessment at first contact with the hospital. All patients who are assessed as being malnourished or at risk of developing malnutrition must be referred to a dietitian. It is likely that nearly all head and neck cancer patients will require dietary advice during the course of their disease and treatment.

Nutritional assessment and early identification of problems can be quick and easy to perform. The dietitian will then undertake a more detailed assessment. The following questions may be used for a rapid assessment of whether a dietetic referral is required.

Have you lost weight?

An unintentional weight loss of 10% of normal body weight should be regarded as being clinically significant and requires nutritional input. It may be obvious on examination that the patient exhibits muscle wasting and depletion of fat stores but it should also be remembered that patients who are overweight but who are losing weight may still becoming malnourished if they are not given sufficient support.

Do you have any eating difficulties?

Difficulties with eating may include loss of appetite or difficulty with chewing or swallowing. A good guide is to ask patients whether they can eat food of a normal consistency and how much of their usual portions they can manage. Patients who have not eaten for more than 24 hours require an urgent referral to a dietitian.

Patients should be reassessed on a weekly basis as nutritional status and ability to eat can change rapidly. Additional methods of assessing nutritional status are available such as calculation of body mass index, triceps skinfold thickness, mid-arm muscle circumference and measurements of muscle function but these are often time consuming and not necessary to identify patients who need a referral to a dietitian. Patients must have their nutritional status monitored, preferably by a dietitian, throughout the course of their disease and treatment. Nutritional intake and changes in nutritional status can occur rapidly in this group of patients and appropriate intervention must be implemented quickly to avoid weight loss. Frequency of monitoring will depend on the patient's clinical condition, treatment and frequency of hospital visits. The parameters that should be monitored are shown in Table 8.2.

Nutritional requirements

Cancer patients may have elevated energy requirements due to the metabolic changes that occur in cancer cachexia, surgery, trauma and sepsis.[5,6]

Table 8.2 Nutritional parameters

Appearance
Weight and height
Difficulties with eating and drinking
Nutritional intake
Fluid intake
Biochemistry: urea and electrolytes, liver function tests, blood glucose, urinalysis, vitamin and mineral status

Energy requirements

Energy requirements may range from 30 kcal/kg to 40 kcal/kg although requirements may exceed this range for patients who are particularly cachectic.[7] To determine initial energy requirements a figure of 35 kcal/kg may be used or basal requirements may be calculated using the Schofield equation.[12] The dietitian may carry out a detailed assessment of requirements.

Nitrogen requirements

Adequate dietary nitrogen and energy are required for patients to maintain nitrogen balance. Immediately postoperatively patients may be unable to maintain nitrogen balance due to the metabolic effects of trauma. Nitrogen requirements range from 0.16 g/kg to 0.3 g/kg per day (1 g protein per kg body weight to 1.9 g protein per kg body weight). Hypoalbuminaemia may arise as a result of the metabolic response to injury and infection and therefore may not respond to an increase in dietary protein.[13] A decrease in plasma albumin due to trauma is associated with a rise in acute phase proteins such as C-reactive protein. Measurement of acute phase proteins may give an indication of the distinction between hypoalbuminaemia due to trauma or that due to malnutrition.

Fluid requirements

Normal fluid requirements may range from 20–50 ml/kg per day. Requirements may be increased in patients requiring ventilation, during sepsis or where output is high, for example, in diarrhoea.

Vitamins and minerals

Dietary intake should aim to meet the daily requirements for all vitamins and minerals.[14] Vitamin and mineral supplementation may be indicated in a number of patients where dietary intake is poor or requirements for particular nutrients may be increased. Head and neck cancer patients may require a liquid preparation. Some studies have shown the benefit of additional vitamin C and zinc in the healing of pressure sores and leg ulcers in nutritionally depleted non-cancer patients.[15,16] The potential benefit in cancer patients has been more difficult to demonstrate due to the lack of studies and evidence that cancer patients may have abnormally low plasma levels of some vitamins and minerals.[17] Supplementation with individual vitamins or minerals at high doses may affect the metabolism of other nutrients, for example supplementation with high doses of zinc may cause alterations in copper metabolism.[18] It is often more appropriate to ensure an adequate supply of vitamins and minerals with diet and enteral feeds and use a multivitamin and mineral preparation when intake continues to be inadequate. Parenteral thiamin (vitamin B1) may be required for patients with thiamin deficiency due to a high alcohol intake.

Methods of nutritional support

Oral nutrition

Patients who can swallow sufficient food and fluids safely may be able to meet their requirements orally. Patients who are at risk of aspiration should be referred to a speech and language therapist to assess swallowing and whether it is safe to proceed with oral intake. The dietitian may advise the patient on the following:

1. Suitability and consistency of food;
2. Fortification of food to increase energy and/or protein;
3. Adequacy of energy intake;
4. Adequacy of fluid intake;
5. Vitamin and mineral supplementation where appropriate;
6. Use of nutritional supplements where appropriate.

Dietary management of eating difficulties and nutritional supplement strategies are listed in Tables 8.3 and 8.4. Patients who are particularly anorexic may benefit from an appetite stimulant such as medroxyprogesterone acetate or megestrol acetate.[19]

Enteral tube feeding

Enteral tube feeding may need to be considered for the following situations:

Table 8.3 Dietary management of eating difficulties

Symptom	Dietary management
Anorexia	Small portions Increase frequency of eating Encourage foods that are enjoyed Make use of best meal of the day e.g. this may be breakfast Encourage high-energy foods Fortify food to increase energy intake e.g. use full cream milk, use extra butter, cheese, cream Use alcohol as an appetite stimulant (in moderation) Medroxyprogesterone acetate or megestrol acetate as appetite stimulant
Dysphagia	Small frequent meals Modify consistency of food so all food is soft. Food may need to be pureed or liquidized Fortify food to increase energy intake May require additional nutritional supplements May need to use commercial thickening agent for thin liquids if risk of aspiration (needs assessment from speech and language therapist)
Mucositis	Modify consistency of food so all food is soft Avoid rough, coarse or dry food Avoid acidic, salty or highly spiced food Avoid alcohol Avoid hot food, foods that are cold or at room temperature may be better tolerated May require additional nutritional supplements Take food after taking analgesia
Xerostomia	Moist foods, use sauces, gravies, butter, custard, cream and milk to make food moist Food may need to be soft or pureed May require additional nutritional supplements Take frequent small sips of water Try sour or tart foods e.g. lemon, acid drops, pineapple (only if no stomatitis) Try sugar free chewing gum to stimulate saliva Avoid dry or crisp foods e.g. bread, nuts, crackers Try artificial saliva Refer to a dental hygienist

1. Patients with dysphagia;
2. Patients with severe mucositis;
3. Patients who are at risk of aspiration;
4. Patients who are required to be nil by mouth e.g. postoperatively;
5. Patients who can swallow but are unable to take sufficient to meet their nutritional requirements.

Methods of tube feeding

Nasogastric feeding

Nasogastric feeding may be the route of choice for patients requiring relatively short-term feeding such as for periods of less than 4 weeks. Fine bore tubes made from soft polyurethane or silicone are less likely to cause complications such as rhinitis, oesphageal irritation and gastritis.[20] Weighted nasogastric tubes may be preferable in patients who require tracheal suctioning.[21] The position of the nasogastric tube must be checked before feeding is started to avoid accidental intrapulmonary aspiration in accordance with local guidelines. It may be advisable to radiograph all nasogastric tubes in patients who have altered anatomy of the head and neck or have altered swallowing or gag reflex. Radiographs may also be used to assist with the difficult insertion of nasogastric tubes. All tubes should be secured to the nose and face with adhesive tape to help prevent accidental removal.

Patients who may require periods of nasogastric feeding include those having undergone surgery such as a partial glossectomy, mandibulectomy or maxillectomy. Patients receiving brachytherapy or conventional radiotherapy where there have not been swallowing problems prior to treatment may also require periods of nasogastric feeding. Patients who

Table 8.4 Nutritional supplements suitable for head and neck patients

Type of supplement	Nutritional value and use of supplement
Nutritionally complete	Designed to replace all food if sufficient volume is consumed, usually 1.5–2 litres depending on energy density Contains protein, fat, carbohydrate, vitamins and minerals in a liquid form May be used as a supplement to food when total food intake is poor. Available in a variety of flavours both sweet and savoury Often based on milk protein Usually provide 1–1.5 kcal/ml Some may contain dietary fibre
Energy and protein supplements	Often available as milk protein-based drinks or fruit juice-flavoured drinks Provide protein and energy but may not meet vitamin and mineral requirements Used as a supplement to a poor food intake Usually provide 1–2 kcal/ml
Carbohydrate supplement	Available as a powder or liquid Provides 3.75 kcal/g for powder and up to 2.25 kcal/ml for liquid Can be added to ordinary food and drinks Provides energy but no vitamins and minerals
Protein supplement	Available as a powder Can be added to ordinary food to increase protein content Rarely used in isolation in cancer patients who often require energy, vitamins and minerals in addition to protein

undergo surgery followed by a course of radiotherapy may require a gastrostomy inserted at the time of their initial surgery. This would be appropriate for patients who may have a number of short periods of time when they require enteral tube feeding. This avoids the patient undergoing multiple insertions of a nasogastric tube and avoids delay in being able to feed the patient when side-effects develop.

Tracheo-oesophageal catheter feeding

Patients who have a tracheo-oesohageal puncture as a primary procedure for the fitting of a voice valve may be fed immediately postoperatively via a catheter inserted through the puncture site. It has been proposed that this method of feeding with the catheter placed in the oesophagus may reduce the likelihood of gastric acid and bacteria tracking up the tube towards the site of surgery. The tip of the catheter is in the lower oesophagus not the stomach. The gastro-oesophageal sphincter is not compromised and can close properly thereby reducing the chance of reflux. In addition this method of feeding avoids the feeding tube irritating the site of surgery as the catheter is inserted below the pharyngeal repair. This route for feeding would include patients who had undergone a laryngectomy or pharyngolaryngectomy. The catheter would be expected to be used for feeding for approximately 7 days in patients who had not undergone previous radiotherapy and approximately 10 days in patient who had undergone previous radiotherapy treatment. Once swallowing and oral intake has been established postoperatively the catheter is removed and replaced with a voice prosthesis, for example a Blom–Singer valve.

Gastrostomy feeding

Gastrostomy feeding may be appropriate for patients requiring enteral feeding for periods of longer than 3–4 weeks (see Table 8.5). Patients who

Table 8.5 Indications for insertion of PEG

- Poor nutritional intake and deteriorating nutritional status despite dietary advice on fortifying foods and dietary supplements
- Dysphagia – unable to take adequate oral nutrition
- Aspiration of food or fluids
- Fistulae where patient is required to be nil by mouth for a period of greater than 3–4 weeks
- Enteral tube feeding required for period of longer than 3–4 weeks
- At the time of surgery where resumption of oral intake is anticipated to be slow, e.g. total glossectomy
- At the time of oropharyngeal resection to avoid irritation by nasogastric tube
- Prior to hyperfractionated radiotherapy

are at high risk of having a prolonged period of establishing oral intake should be considered for insertion of a gastrostomy tube at the time of their initial surgery.[11] Examples include total glossectomy, hemilaryngectomy or patients having extensive or hyperfractionated radiotherapy. It may also be preferable for patients who have undergone oropharyngeal resection and repair as this avoids a nasogastric tube causing irritation to the site of repair. Gastrostomy tubes are cosmetically more acceptable to patients and avoid some of the complications that may arise with the long-term use of nasogastric tubes.

Gastrostomy tubes may be inserted surgically, radiologically or more commonly via endoscopy. Tubes inserted via endoscopy are percutaneous endoscopic gastrostomy tubes and are commonly known as a PEG. Tubes may vary in size from 9 French to 22 French and are retained within the stomach with a flange or balloon. This procedure may be difficult in patients with extensive disease or a stricture that prevents the passage of an endoscope. In such patients a tube may be placed radiologically or as an open gastrostomy. Radiologically placed tubes require the insertion of a nasogastric tube to inflate the stomach with air prior to the tube placement. This may be difficult in some patients due to the presence of tumour or fibrotic tissue.

Morbidity associated with PEG insertion is usually less than 10% with the most common complications including local site infection, leakage or bleeding although some centres have identified that complication rates may be higher in head and neck cancer patients.[22,23] Major complications that can occur include necrotizing fasciitis and intra-abdominal wall abscesses. Once the gastrostomy tract has become established it may be replaced with a 'button'. This serves the same purpose as a gastrostomy but lies flush with the patient's abdomen. Care of the gastrostomy site is important in maintaining the tract and reducing the risk of infection (see Table 8.6).

Jejunostomy feeding

Fine-bore feeding jejunostomy tubes may be inserted with a fine catheter to access the jejunum through the anterior abdominal wall. Jejunostomy tubes may be used in patients who have had upper gastrointestinal surgery making the use of a gastrostomy tube inappropriate or where gastric emptying is severely compromised. Such patients would include those who have undergone a stomach pull up. Jejunostomy feeding often requires the use of a feeding pump for continuous feeding.

Table 8.6 Care of the PEG site

PEG tube and retention device should be left in position for 24 hours postinsertion
Commence care of PEG site 24–48 hours postinsertion
Note the position of external fixation device on PEG tube
Release exterior retention device and clean skin with sterile saline
Rotate PEG tube through 360° to maintain stoma tract
Dry skin surrounding PEG tube
Replace external fixation device to usual position; the position of the external fixation device may change if the patient gains weight
Seven days postinsertion it is no longer necessary to use sterile saline and a clean technique may be used to care for the skin

Enteral feeds

Commercially prepared enteral feeds should be used for nasogastric, gastrostomy or jejunostomy feeding as they are sterile when packaged and are of known nutritional composition (see Table 8.7).

Details of the exact composition of commercially produced enteral feeds can be obtained from the manufacturers. For the vast majority of head and neck cancer patients a whole protein polymeric feed can be used. Energy dense feeds may be required for patients with increased energy requirements.

Feeding regimens

Enteral feeding regimens must be devised to fit in with the patient's lifestyle and tolerance to feed. Various regimens may be used (see Table 8.8).

During the postoperative period feed may be started at full strength and in a small volume such as 50 ml/hour. The rate of feed can gradually be increased according to tolerance with the aim of meeting nutritional requirements within 24–48 hours. During this period additional intravenous fluid may be required to meet the patient's fluid requirements. As enteral feeding is established the intravenous fluids must be decreased. It is rare for patients to require greater than 2–2.5 litres daily. Where feed tolerance appears to be poor, gastric emptying may be assessed by gastric aspiration. Gastric stasis may require the use of drugs that encourage gastric emptying such as metoclopramide. The incidence of pharyngocutaneous fistula after laryngectomy may be reduced with the use of a gastro-oesophageal reflux prophylaxis regimen based on metoclopramide and ranitidine.[24]

Table 8.7 Enteral feeds

Type of feed	Features of feed
Whole protein/polymeric containing protein, hydrolysed fat and carbohydrate	Requires digestion Generally provides 1–1.5 kcal/ml feed Usually adequate intake of vitamins and minerals when 1000–1500 ml taken May contain dietary fibre
Isotonic whole protein but containing protein, hydrolysed fat, medium chain triglycerides and maltodextrins	Requires digestion Suitable for patients with suspected gastrointestinal intolerance May contain dietary fibre
Chemically defined peptide or elemental	Does not require digestion, may be absorbed directly into bloodstream May be low in fat or contain medium chain triglycerides Suitable for patients with impaired gastrointestinal function Hyperosmolar and low in residue
Special application feeds May have altered levels of energy, protein, electrolytes, vitamins and minerals to suit particular conditions such as renal failure	Require digestion as for whole protein/polymeric feeds Rarely required in head and neck cancer patients The value of glutamine, arginine, omega-3 fatty acid enriched feeds to promote immune function has yet to be demonstrated

Table 8.8 Feeding regimens

Feeding regimen	Advantages	Disadvantages
Continous feeding via a pump	Easily controlled rate Reduction of gastrointestinal complications Minimizes stress on cardiac, respiratory and renal function	Patient connected to feeding pump for majority of day
Intermittent feeding via a pump or gravity drip	Patient has periods of time free of feeding Some patients may find gravity feeding easier than managing a pump Some feed may be given overnight	May have an increased risk of gastrointestinal symptoms e.g. early satiety Overnight feeding may not be suitable for those at high-risk of aspiration
Bolus feeding	May reduce time connected to feed	Increased risk of gastrointestinal side-effects Administration of feeds time consuming

Patients with dysphagia, aspiration or mucositis who require enteral tube feeding may be able to tolerate their full nutritional requirements within the first 24 hours.

Complications of enteral tube feeding

(See Table 8.9.)

Monitoring of enteral tube feeding

Patients on enteral tube feeds should be monitored regularly (see Table 8.10). Changes in nutritional status may require nutritional requirements to be recalculated and the feeding regimen changed. The frequency of monitoring will decrease with time but should continue with patients after discharge from hospital.

Table 8.9 Complications of enteral tube feeding

Complication	Possible cause	Suggested management
Diarrhoea	Antibiotics Bacterial infection Hypoalbuminaemia Hyperosmolar feed Impaired intestinal function Drugs e.g. magnesium salts, chemotherapy Overuse of laxatives Use of sorbitol-based drugs	Review antibiotic administration Stool culture if persistent Reduce rate of feed Reduce osmolarity of feed Use fibre containing feed Anti-diarrhoea medication
Constipation	Opioid drugs Lack of dietary fibre Lack of fluid	Laxatives or enema Use fibre-containing feed Increase fluid intake
Nausea	Drugs Rapid administration of feed Hyperosmolar feed	Anti-emetics Reduce rate of feed Use isotonic feed
Aspiration	Patient unconscious Displacement of nasogastric tube	4-hourly aspiration Postpyloric feeding e.g. nasoduodenal or jejunal feeding Drugs to encourage gastric emptying, e.g. metoclopramide Prop patient's head so there is a minimum 45° elevation between head and neck and thorax

Table 8.10 Monitoring of enteral tube feeding

- Body weight
- Urea and electrolytes
- Full blood count
- Tolerance to feed e.g. nausea, fullness, bowels
- Quantity of feed taken
- Care of tube
- Stoma site (in case of PEG and jejunostomy)

Withdrawal of enteral tube feeding

Enteral tube feeding should only be stopped when sufficient oral diet and fluids are being taken. There may need to be a weaning period during which enteral feeding is reduced and oral intake is increased. The dietitian should assess oral intake during this period and the enteral tube feed stopped only when oral intake is considered to be adequate. Method of removal of PEG tubes depends on the type of tube used and may require a repeat endoscopy. It is necessary to refer to the manufacturer's guidelines.

Home enteral feeding

Patients who are unable to resume an adequate oral intake can be taught to manage enteral tube feeding at home.[25] Adequate time should be allowed in the hospital setting for patients to become fully accustomed to the techniques of administration of feed and care of the gastrostomy tube prior to discharge home. The feeding regimen should be planned to fit into the home circumstances, feed tolerance and patient choice (see Table 8.8).

Home support in the form of the general practitioner, community nursing and community dietetic services should be established although the amount of support may vary depending on local resources. Patients at home should be monitored from a nutritional perspective. Patients with a PEG should have the site monitored regularly by the community nurse and by the doctor at outpatient appointments.

Many of the enteral feed manufacture companies have a home delivery service that may be of help to patients as this avoids having to carry heavy feed and bulky equipment. The hospital or community dietitian can arrange this.

Management of a chylous fistula

A chylous fistula as a complication of a neck dissection may be treated conservatively if the output remains below 600 ml.[26] Some clinicians have advocated the use of a low fat diet, use of medium-chain triglycerides or the use of parenteral nutrition in supporting patients with this complication.[27,28] The use of strict diets, on which patients find it difficult to maintain an adequate nutritional intake, or intravenous feeding, with its associated risks, may not be absolutely necessary. Nutritional and electrolyte support is essential in the conservative management of low-volume chylous fistulae and this may be achieved with the administration of an isomolar enteral feed over 24 hours.[29]

Parenteral nutrition

Parenteral nutrition should only be used when it is not possible to feed patients via the enteral route. Its use carries the risk of life-threatening complications, such as sepsis and metabolic disorders, and therefore it must be administered and monitored correctly. It is rarely used in head and neck cancer patients as the gastrointestinal tract is usually accessible.

It may be considered for the following patients:[30]

1. When all methods and routes of enteral nutrition have been considered but are not deemed appropriate;
2. When the gastrointestinal tract is inaccessible and it is not possible to insert an enteral feeding tube;
3. When complete rest of the gastrointestinal tract is required.

REFERENCES

1. Guo C-B, Ma D-Q, Zhang K-H. Nutritional status of patients with oral and maxillofacial malignancies. *J Oral Maxillofac Surg* 1994; **52**: 559–562.
2. Lopez MJ, Robinson P, Madden T, Highbarger T. Nutritional support and prognosis in patients with head and neck cancer. *J Surg Oncol* 1994; **55**: 33–36.
3. von Meyenfeldt MF, Fredrix EWHM, Haagh WAJJM, Van der Aalst ACMJ, Soeters PB. The aetiology and management of weight loss and malnutrition in cancer patients. *Bailliere's Clin Gastroenterol* 1988; **2**: 869–885.
4. Thiel H-J, Fietkau R, Sauer R. Malnutrition and the role of nutritional support for radiation therapy patients. *Recent Results Cancer Res* 1988; **108**: 203–226.
5. Hyltander A, Drott C, Korner U et al. Elevated energy expenditure in cancer patients with solid tumours. *Eur J Cancer* 1991; **27**: 9–15.
6. Espat NJ, Moldawaer LL, Copeland EM. Cytokine-mediated alterations in host metabolism prevent nutritional repletion in cachetic cancer patients. *J Surg Oncol* 1995; **58**: 77–82.
7. Bozzetti F. Nutrition support in patients with cancer. In: Payne-James J, Grimble G, Silk D (eds). *Artificial Nutrition Support in Clinical Practice.* London: Edward Arnold, 1995; 511–533.
8. Heys SD, Park KGM, Garlick PJ, Eremin O. Nutrition and malignant disease: implications for surgical practice. *Br J Surg* 1992; **79**: 614–623.
9. Campos ACL, Meguid MM. A critical appraisal of the usefulness of perioperative nutritional support. *Am J Clin Nutr* 1992; **55**: 117–130.
10. Brookes GB, Clifford P. Nutritional status and general immune competence in patients with head and neck cancer. *J R Soc Med* 1981; **74**: 132–139.
11. Fietkau R, Iro H, Sailer D, Sauer R. Percutaneous endoscopically guided gastrostomy in patients with head and neck cancer. *Recent Results Cancer Res* 1991; **121**: 269–282.
12. Schofield WN, Schofield C, James WPT. Basal metabolic rate: review and prediction. *Hum Nutr Clin Nutr* 1985; **39c** (Suppl 1): 5–96.
13. Rothschild MA, Oratz M, Schreiber SS. Serum albumin. *Hepatology* 1988; **8**: 385–401.
14. Dietary Reference Values for Food Energy and Nutrients in the United Kingdom. *Department of Health Report on Health and Social Subjects.* City: Publisher 1991; Report No. 41. London: HMSO.
15. Taylor TV, Rimmer S, Day B et al. Ascorbic acid supplementation in the treatment of presssure sores. *Lancet* 1974; **ii**: 544–546.
16. Hallbook T, Lanner E. Serum zinc and healing of venous leg ulcers. *Lancet* 1972; **ii**: 780–782.
17. Doerr TD, Prasad AS, Marks SC et al. Zinc deficiency in head and neck cancer patients. *J Am Coll Nutr* 1997; **16**: 418–422.
18. Walsh CT, Sandstead HH, Prasad AS et al. Zinc: health effects and research priorities for the 1990s. *Environ Health Perspect* 1994; **102** (Suppl 2): 4–46.
19. Tchekmedyian NS, Hickman M, Siau J et al. Megestrol acetate in cancer anorexia and weight loss. *Cancer* 1992; **69**: 1268–1274.
20. Payne-James J. Enteral nutrition: tubes and techniques of delivery. In: Payne-James J, Grimble G, Silk D (eds). *Artificial Nutrition Support in Clinical Practice.* London: Edward Arnold, 1995; 197–213.
21. Metheny NA, Spies M, Eisenberg P. Frequency of nasoenteral tube displacement and associated risk factors. *Res Nurs Health* 1986; **9**: 241–247.

22. Bailey CE, Lucas CE, Ledgerwood AM, Jacobs JR. A comparison of gastrostomy techniques in patients with advanced head and neck cancer. *Arch Otolaryngol Head Neck Surg* 1992; **118**: 124–126.
23. Walton GM. Complications of percutaneous gastrostomy in patients with head and neck cancer: an analysis of 42 consecutive patients. *Ann R Coll Surg Engl* 1999; **81**: 272–276.
24. Seikaly H, Park P. Gastroesophageal reflux prophylaxis decreases the incidence of pharyngocutaneous fistula after total laryngectomy. *Laryngoscope* 1995; **105**: 1220–1222.
25. Campos ACL, Butters M, Meguid MM. Home enteral nutrition via gastrostomy in advanced head and neck cancer patients. *Head Neck* 1990; **12**: 137–142.
26. Spiro JD, Spiro RH, Strong EW. The management of chyle fistula. *Laryngoscope* 1990; **100**: 771–774.
27. Martin IC, Marinho LH, Brown AE, McRobbie D. Medium chain triglycerides in the management of chylous fistulae following neck dissection. *Br J Oral Maxillofac Surg* 1993; **31**: 236–238.
28. Younus M, Chang RWS. Chyle fistulae. Treatment with total parenteral nutrition. *J Laryngol Otol* 1988; **102**: 384.
29. Al-Khayat M, Kenyon GS, Fawcett HV, Powell-Tuck J. Nutritional support in patients with low volume chylous fistula following radical neck dissection. *J Laryngol Otol* 1991; **105**: 1052–1056.
30. Collins C. Parenteral nutrition. In: Thomas B (ed.) *Manual of Dietetic Practice*. Oxford: Blackwell Scientific, 2001; 100–107.

9 Dental management of the head and neck cancer patient

Robert E Wood

Integration of dental treatment with medical and surgical treatment

The goal of dental management of the head and neck oncology patient is to ensure the patient enters their active treatment phase without delay and in possession of a healthy, functional, and well-maintained dentition. If possible, all potential sources of infection should be removed prior to oncologic treatment. The dental treatment plan will be decided with consideration given to the types of anti-cancer treatment, the patient's wishes and the dentist's experience and knowledge in the management of other similar patients. Close co-operation between the dental team and the responsible physician is imperative.

Pretreatment assessment

The dental assessment of the head and neck cancer patient commences in the same manner as the conventional dental patient. A myriad of intercurrent disorders may affect both the type and the method of dental service delivery. Concomitant serious systemic disease may ultimately alter the oncologic treatment plan. Part of the medical history should include inquiries as to the value the patient places on their teeth, how well they care for their teeth, whether they have, and wear dental protheses, and whether they are under the regular care of a dentist. If a patient is under the care of a family dentist it is likely that they will overestimate the frequency of their routine visits. Further, many conditions that may be observed and followed in a general dental practice, without intervention, must be dealt with in the oncology patient.

Following review of the medical history it is imperative that a thorough clinical examination of the teeth, their supporting structures and the remainder of the oral cavity be completed. This assessment includes charting of the patient's teeth, measurement of the quantity of saliva, evaluation of temporomandibular joint function, description of the periodontal status. Biopsy of any oral sites suspicious of malignancy is necessary as upper aerodigestive tract malignancies may be multiple in nature i.e. field cancerization.[1] An objective assessment of oral hygiene level and the presence of plaque and calculus deposits should also be undertaken.

As part of the overall assessment a dental radiographic examination must be completed.[2] At the author's institution this is composed minimally of a pantomographic examination supplemented with intraoral bite-wing and periapical radiographs as clinically indicated. Frequently, a full mouth series of sixteen or more intraoral radiographs is exposed. This is done to afford both the dental surgeon and the oncologist as much information as possible on the health of the dentition (Figure 9.1). The amount of radiation received in this procedure is trivial when compared to the prescribed dose.

Preradiation treatment

The twin primary goals of dental care for radiation patients are the prevention of postradiation caries and avoidance of osteoradionecrosis. A secondary goal is communicating to the patient the complications of radiation therapy treatment of the head and neck, which may include: mucositis, xerostomia, trismus, dysgeusia, dysphagia, pain, and susceptibility to both fungal infection and postradiation caries. After consultation with the radiation oncologist

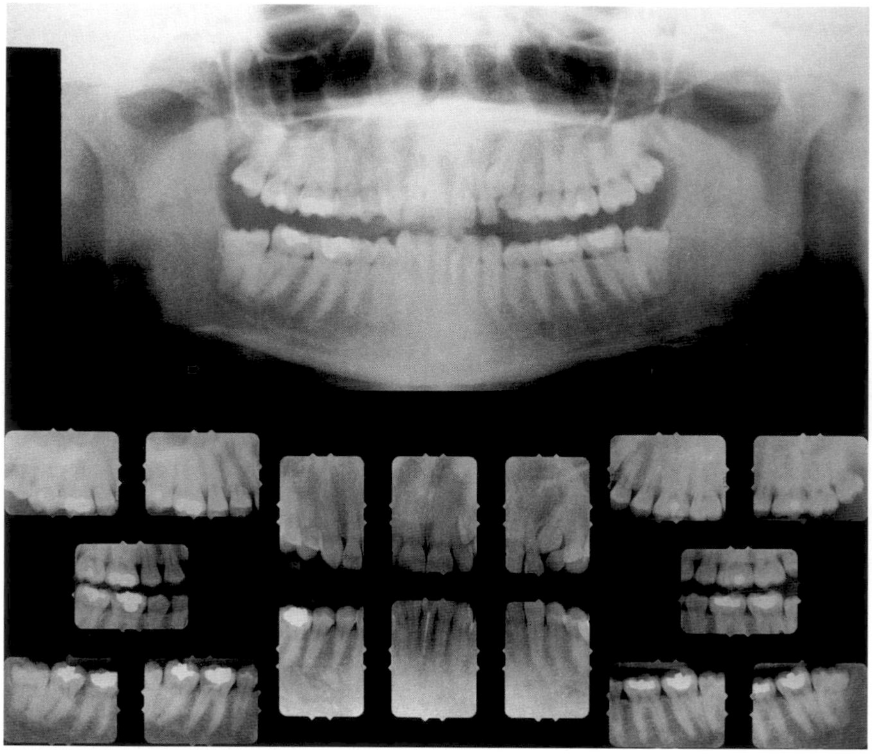

Figure 9.1 Panoramic radiograph of jaws with 4 bitewings supplies the dentist and the surgeon with more information on which to base a treatment decision.

concerning field sizes and prescribed doses of radiation, an adequate amount of time should be spent with each patient discussing how their individualized radiation treatment will affect their mouth.

Dental extractions should be done as soon as possible in those patients that require them. Teeth may be extracted because they: are decayed and unrestorable; lack opposing teeth; are prosthetically useless; are likely to be lost during the course of treatment; or in patients who are unwilling to carry out the rigorous oral hygiene regimen required. In addition, partly erupted third molar teeth and teeth with severe periodontal disease should be removed to prevent pericorinitis or other infections. Teeth with periapical inflammatory disease or non-vital teeth may be kept if the patient is willing to undergo root canal treatment. The author is generally more aggressive with respect to extractions 'in the field' and in the posterior mandible. If a large number of teeth are to be removed it is important for the dentist to liaise with the radiation oncologist to ensure that any such extractions do not interfere with the final mask or treatment planning.

Restorative dentistry should, if possible, be completed prior to radiation treatment; however, it may be delayed until after cancer treatment since it is imperative that the dental treatment be completed in as short a time window as possible. Dentistry should not delay radiation treatment. If this is to occur, patients should be referred immediately after their first hospital consultation so that their dental work may be done while the radiation planning, mask, and simulator appointments are being done. Ill-fitting dentures may be adjusted or adapted but new prostheses are generally not fitted until well after the completion of radiation.

Sanative periodontal treatment and institution of appropriate oral hygiene care are pivotal and may involve the services of the dental hygienist. The patient's teeth are cleaned thoroughly and oral hygiene instruction is given. Fluoride trays are made for most patients. This is done by fabricating dental stone models and making vinyl athletic mouth guards. When the mouth guards are finished they are delivered to the patient along with a prescription for neutral sodium fluoride gel, written instructions for their correct use, and a clear warning that they must be used as directed for life. An example of fluoride instructions is provided in Table 9.1. The use of topical fluoride has been proven to markedly reduce the incidence of postradiation caries.[3] The fluoride tray has an additional use in the patient with fixed cast metal bridgework in that it may be placed in the mouth during the radiation treatment. When this is done it displaces the adjacent soft tissue off the bridgework and avoids radiation 'hotspots' thereby preventing undue radiation mucositis.

Periradiation treatment

Patients should be seen as required but minimally at least once by the dental team during the course of

Table 9.1 Oral hygiene recommendations

The life-long daily application of the topical neutral sodium fluoride gel is mandatory if you wish to keep your teeth and prevent serious health consequences. Use only the fluoride gel prescribed by your dentist or physician. Make sure that before you leave the cancer centre that you are shown how to use the trays and you understand that this is a life-long commitment. Never discontinue its use unless advised by your doctor or physician at the cancer centre.

Daily procedure
Select a time of day when you will not need to rinse, eat or drink for a minimum of 1 hour. Many people apply the fluoride before retiring to bed.

Brush and floss your teeth thoroughly. If you are having problems mechanically removing the plaque from your teeth ask the advice of your dental hygienist.

Using the custom trays provided to you by your dentist, place a small quantity of fluoride gel in each of the upper and lower trays. The trays are custom made for you so there is no need to 'fill them up'.

Using a cotton swab distribute the gel throughout the tray so all teeth will be covered with a thin film of fluoride when the tray is placed on the teeth.

Place one, if possible both trays on the upper and lower arches and leave in place for 5 minutes. The 5 minutes must be rigidly adhered to.

After 5 minutes has elapsed remove the trays and spit out the excess.

Do not rinse, eat or drink for 1 hour.

Rinse the trays out with cool water and let them dry. Do not store them on the stone models and do not clean them with denture cleaners or subject them to heat.

If you have any questions about their correct use contact your dentist or physician at the cancer centre.

their radiation treatment. This visit serves to assess the presence of radiation-related side-effects and provides an opportunity to ameliorate or remove them.

The patient will undoubtedly experience some degree of radiation mucositis (Figure 9.2). This is part of the treatment and is troublesome because it is painful and prevents patients from maintaining adequate nutrition.[4] It may be managed through use of topical anaesthetic agents, ice chips, rinsing with cool, weak, sodium bicarbonate and water rinses and

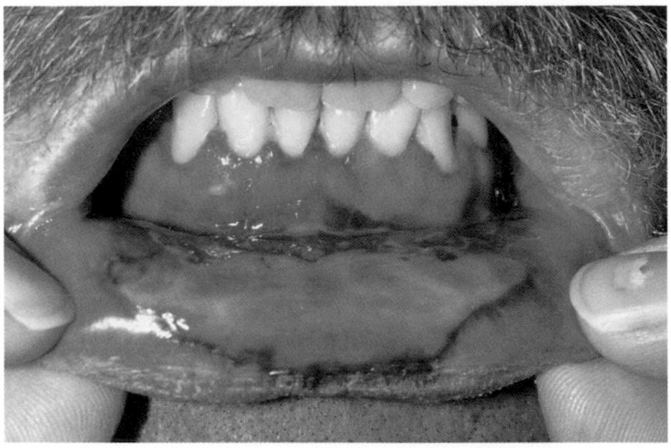

Figure 9.2 Typical appearance of intraoral radiation mucositis.

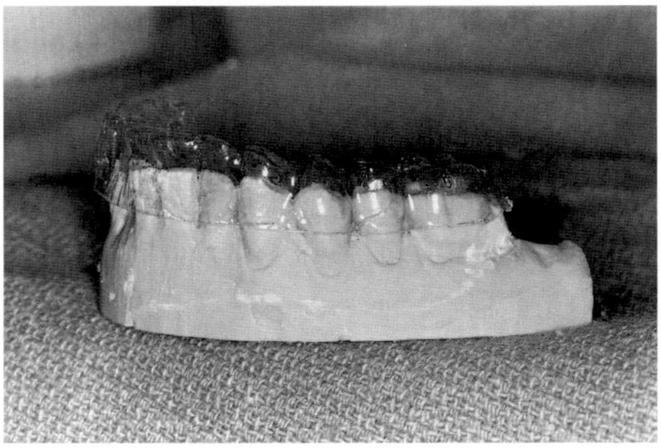

Figure 9.3 Acetate dental splint allows smooth movement of buccal mucosa and tongue across dental surfaces. It may be fabricated from study models or fluoride tray models.

by using systemic analgesics. The type of anti-mucositis therapy may range from simple bicarbonate of soda and water rinses, to topical anaesthetics and systemic analgesics. The occasional patient will complain that the vestibular and lingual soft tissues are sore as a result of roughened or sharp tooth edges. These teeth may be smoothed using a dental hand piece or they can be covered with a thin form-fitting acetate layer (Figure 9.3), which provides a smooth contacting surface and allows the soft tissues to glide across the teeth.

Candidiasis occurs in most radiation patients some time during the course of their treatment (Figure 9.4). It presents clinically as a whitish plaque present on the oral mucosa that may be removed with gentle pressure on a wet gauze. In some cases the oral mucosa may appear red and atrophic. Most cases of candidiasis can be managed by the judicious use of topical, or more rarely systemic anti-fungal agents. Topically applied mycostatin ointment, rinses, or

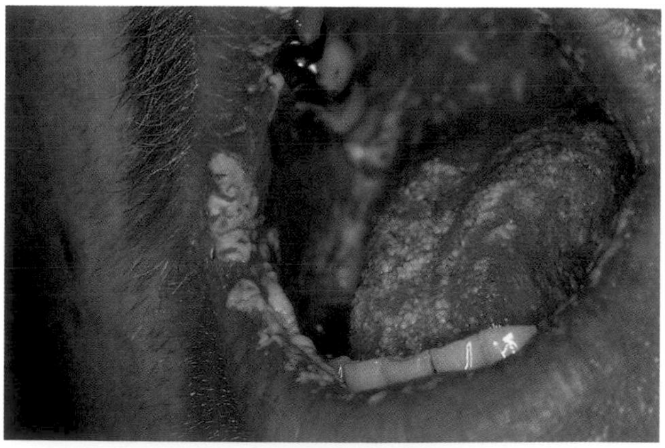

Figure 9.4 Intraoral candidiasis as seen here is a common occurrence in the mouths of head and neck cancer patients.

troches can be used directly or on the tissue surface of dentures according to manufacturers[1] instructions for the particular agent chosen.

Mastication and swallowing may be altered or hindered during radiation treatment. Patients should be encouraged to follow a soft diet and the services of a clinical dietician should be employed to ensure that the patient is receiving an adequate caloric and nutrient intake. For patients in whom the tongue is involved, dysgeusia may occur making the motivation to eat less. This lack of taste will resolve itself given time but is troubling to the patient. The patient should be reassured that they will regain their sense of taste; however, it may be a period of months before their foods taste as they should.

Xerostomia is the side-effect of radiation treatment that patients find most troubling. Whilst saliva substitutes are helpful most patients tend to carry a small supply of water with them. Patients should be firmly discouraged from relying on sugar-containing sweets/candies or chewing gum to stimulate salivary flow since these substances will markedly hasten the caries process.[5] Salivary stimulants such as pilocarpine may stimulate salivary flow and are suitable in selected patients.[6]

In a few patients dental sensitivity occurs. This manifests as marked tooth sensitivity to cold, and occasionally hot. The daily topical fluoride applications help to lessen this but some patients may benefit from desensitizing dentifrices, alteration in the temperature of their fluids and, in many cases, professional application of desensitizing agents.

Finally denture prostheses may become loose when body weight is lost. They may also become irritating. If this occurs, temporary soft-tissue conditioning relines may be used to temporarily alter the fit of the denture. Permanent changes to the dentures should be avoided until well after the radiation has ended. Inevitably patients will regain their body weight and the dentures will no longer fit.

Postradiation treatment

It is anticipated in most cases that the head and neck cancer patient will have a long life following completion of the radiation treatment. For this reason it is important to liaise with the family dentist and provide either an information package or a list of references, which he/she may consult. The cancer centre dental unit should see the patient annually to see that they are compliant with respect to their oral hygiene measures and to see that they are free of postradiation caries and are receiving the appropriate level of care. Teeth affected by postradiation caries (Figure 9.5) are difficult to restore. In the author's institution direct restorative materials such as amalgam and resin-modified glass ionomer are used to treat postradiation caries.[7,8]

Teeth, which are unrestorable due to postradiation caries, may require extraction. Alternatively they may be treated with root canal therapy and then allowed to exfoliate on their own. If extractions are required it is important to discuss the location of the teeth with respect to the radiation fields with the radiation oncologist. Teeth that are well outside the field do not require any special handling. Teeth within the field should be extracted without raising a surgical flap. In addition the use of a low epinephrine-containing local anaesthetic and systemic antibiotics are recommended.[9] Very few patients, in

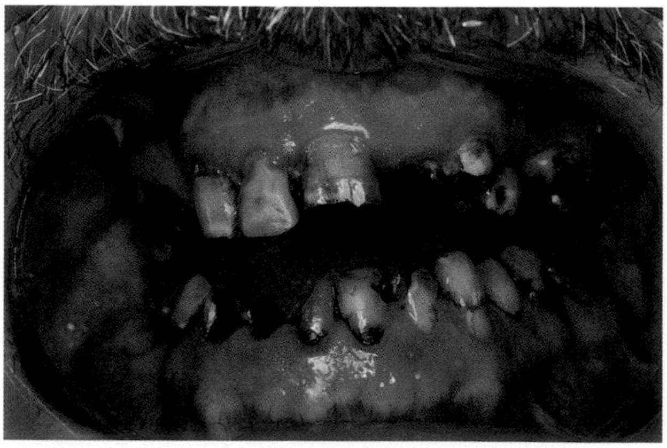

Figure 9.5 Rampant post-radiation caries as pictured here almost always occurs in those patients who are xerostomic, have poor oral hygiene and neglect to use daily sodium fluoride gel as directed.

the author's experience, require prophylactic hyperbaric oxygen unless there is pre-existing osteoradionecrosis or the radiation dose is high. Generally the mandible is more susceptible to osteoradionecrosis than the maxilla. Minor cases of osteoradionecrosis can be handled by the dental team.[10] The determination of what constitutes a minor case of osteoradionecrosis rests in the hands of the surgeon.

Postradiation trismus and lack of biting power has been seen in many patients and is likely to be a problem in the future as radiation doses escalate. Current therapy is not satisfactory in preventing or altering these sequelae although physiotherapy may assist in diminishing the symptoms.

Implications of chemotherapy

It is likely that chemotherapy in adjuvant form may play a larger role in the management of head and neck malignancy in the future.[11] The same general rules of management as seen in the head and neck radiation patients apply to the patient receiving chemotherapy. It is known that dental sepsis is responsible for many febrile episodes[12] and may be entirely avoided by implementing the same general treatment planning principles described above. An additional consideration with the chemotherapy candidate is the concept of zero tolerance for sources of infection, the requisite need to know current blood count values and the use of prophylactic antibiotic coverage.

Prosthetic rehabilitation for surgical oncology patients

The dental management of the prosthetic patient includes the general principles of diagnosis and treatment detailed above. The dentition should be in a good state of repair and the patient must be motivated to care for it.

Prosthetic rehabilitation should begin prior to the cancer surgery. It is pivotal that the treating dentist or prosthodontist assess the patient prior to surgery and devise the appropriate prostheses to suit both the individual patient and the surgeon. In addition a thorough physical record of what was present prior to the surgery will allow a better result postsurgery. The initial appointment also serves as an opportunity to develop a working rapport with the patient and allows determination of what they want as an end result. The dentist can communicate to the patient what can realistically be expected from each appliance. Surgeons should be cautioned with respect to promising the patient that the dentist will replace and relieve all their symptoms with a prosthetic device. This sets the patient, the dentist and the surgeon up for certain failure. If patients' expectations are at the same level as what can be delivered postoperatively and if they understand when each event is likely to occur there is a greater likelihood of clinical success.

Maxillectomy candidate

The candidate for maxillectomy should be assessed with the surgeon. The surgeon should indicate the proposed limits of the surgery and what structures are to be removed and which are to remain. If possible the surgery should take into account three important principles, which ultimately govern the success or failure of prosthetic rehabilitation namely: support, stability and retention. Support is the feature of the denture base, which contributes the resistance to intrusion of the denture. Leaving horizontal bony areas on which the denture sits, if this does not compromise the surgical/oncological result, maximizes support. Stability is that feature of the denture base that makes the denture resistant to side-to-side and front-to-back movement. Teeth and vertical bony elements with suitable mucosal coverage contribute to the stability of the denture. Retention of a denture is that property of the denture that keeps the denture affixed to the supporting structures. It is derived in the partially edentulous patient by placing clasp elements about the residual teeth. In both partially and completely edentulous patients the patient's ability to mechanically adapt and learn to wear their prostheses may be the biggest contributing factor to the denture's overall stability

At the time of the presurgical planning session it is impossible to give the exact location of the surgical margins to the dentist; however, a best estimate should be provided after physical examination and assessment of the diagnostic images. Immediately subsequent to this, the patient should be brought to the dental suite and be assessed. The usual history and conservative dental treatment should be done as outlined above and the patient should know in as much detail as possible, what the dentist is going to do and when it is going to be done. The dentist should deduce how much the patient expects from the prostheses with respect to speech, mastication and cosmetics.

In most instances irreversible hydrocolloid impressions (Figure 9.6) should be taken of the upper and lower jaws. In the maxillectomy patient the standard impression material may need to be extended posteriorly to allow a wide impression of the posterior hard and soft palate. This is uncomfortable for most

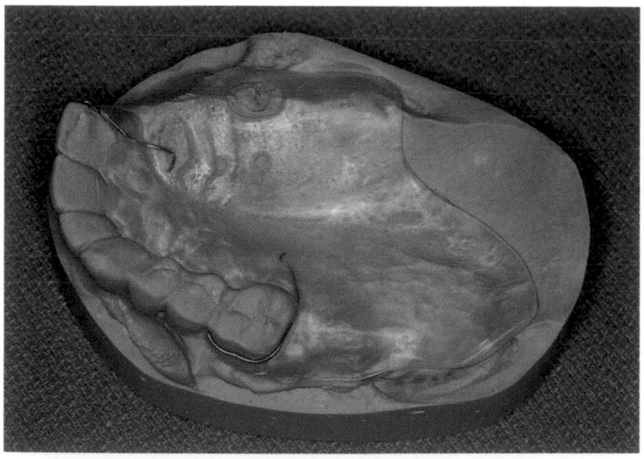

Figure 9.6 Irreversible hydrocolloid impression made prior to excision of a palatal tumour. Note the posterior extent of the impression onto the soft palate. In addition to these impressions a vinyl polysiloxane bite registration is often taken to orient the upper and lower jaws.

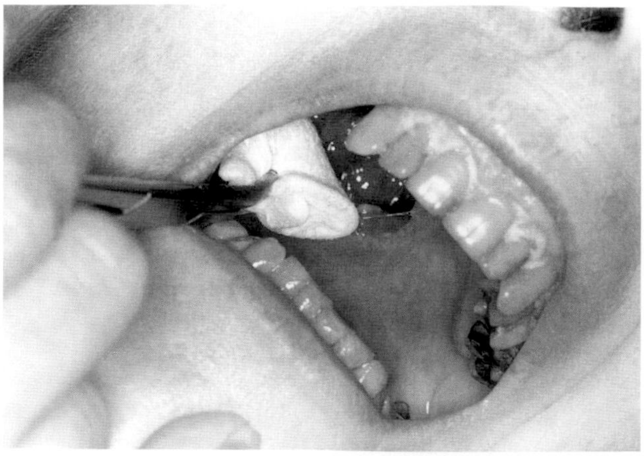

Figure 9.7 Figure depicting a gauze positioned in a hemostat or snap for use in cleaning the intra-oral defect of a maxllectomy patient. Patients must be encouraged to commence cleaning and looking after their defect to allow proper healing and general wound cleanliness.

patients and the purpose of the procedure, if properly explained, will be accepted. If teeth are to form part of the appliance a shade and mould should be selected and recorded and a bite registration should be obtained in a permanent material such as polyvinyl siloxane. If soft palate is to be resected, allowances may be made in the appliance to prevent velopharyngeal insufficiency.

In some instances it is wise to pour the impressions twice in crown and bridge stone reserving a duplicate set of models for use at a later date. The patient's models are then brought back to the surgeon and the margins of the excision are scribed on the cast. The surgical splint obturator is then fabricated out of clear acrylic with the bulb portion slightly shy of the surgeon's margins. After a surgeon and a dentist have worked together for some time the latter will have a greater appreciation of the slight variations in surgical techniques of the former. The appliance must be ready for the date of surgery, which should be noted in the chart. In the author's institution the prosthodontist or dentist attends the latter portion of the operation and adapts the borders of the surgical splint with one of the cold-cure soft-tissue conditioning materials, after the surgeon has completed his resection. When the dentist has positioned the device in its appropriate final position the surgeon fixes the appliance in place over the packing.[13] The prosthesis may be self-retentive in patients with a large number of teeth but more likely needs to be fixed with circumzygomatic wiring, wiring into pre-prepared holes or held in place with a lag screw directly into the palate. If a lag screw is used it is important to ensure that the screw is readily removable via the oral aperture postoperatively. It must be positioned and angled in a manner that allows placement of the screw-driver head for removal. The patient is then taken to the recovery room and is seen by the dentist and surgeon about 1–2 weeks postoperatively. The purpose of the surgical splint is to allow the patient to take oral sustenance quickly, facilitate speech and provide a matrix for healing. The splint minimizes the length of the hospital stay and allows the patient to function well during the immediate postoperative period.

At the first postoperative appointment it is prudent to provide an appropriate level of systemic analgesia for the patient. This should be given about 1 hour prior to the contemplated removal of the appliance. It is preferable to have the surgeon that placed the fixation devices remove them as well as the packing. The appliance and the patient are then brought to the dental suite where the defect is debrided gently with moistened gauze. At this time the dentist explains to both the patient and the caregiver the method of cleaning the defect and the importance of keeping the surgical site clean. At the author's institution this is done with hemostats and 2 × 2 moist gauze. The gauze is folded in half and fixed in the end of the hemostat. It is then rolled against the outer border of the defect to remove the hardened nasal secretions and clotted blood (Figure 9.7). The appliance and the cavity are both cleaned thoroughly and then the appliance is adapted to the developing scar band using cold-cure soft-tissue conditioning material. Many choices of material are available depending on the geographic location of the dentist as well as the dentist's personal preference. Patients may be expected to be seen on a weekly to bi-weekly basis for about 8–10 weeks. At each appointment the bulb of the appliance is cleaned and re-adapted to the changing defect. Patients are then seen monthly for another 2–3 months at which time an interim or in some cases final appliance is fabricated. The time line for implementation of each stage of treatment varies drastically from patient to patient.

After 4 months and in some cases before, the surgical splint outlives its usefulness. The soft-tissue conditioning material has started to deteriorate and the porous nature of the adapted appliance becomes inadequate from both a fit and an olfactory standpoint. At this time an interim appliance can be fabricated. The interim appliance is designed to improve cosmetics and address the masticatory as well as the speech concerns of the patient. It is generally made of tissue-coloured acrylic with wrought wire clasps and appropriately coloured and shaped denture teeth. It may be made from irreversible hydrocolloid impressions or with polyvinyl siloxane impressions made using custom impression trays from the reserved presurgical casts. A number of things need to be assessed at this point including: the lip position and height, phonetics, the location of the denture neutral zone and the degree of healing. The neutral zone is the three-dimensional space in between the tongue and the cheeks and lips in which one can place the teeth without fear that the patient will bite their cheek or lips. On occasion the interim appliance will serve as a final prosthesis whereas in other cases it allows completion of healing for another 6–8 months until the denture base is ready to accept a final prosthesis. The hard, non-porous surface of the interim appliance bulb allows for a cleaner oral environment. In addition the revised appliance is made to more closely approximate the defect as well as the surrounding structures. It may, for this reason be thinner, smaller and slightly lighter in weight than the surgical splint. The general rules of denture construction for the normal patient can be adapted to prosthesis fabrication for this group of patients.

If the interim appliance is satisfactory for the long-term (greater than 1 year) cancer survivor there is no need to fabricate a 'final' prosthesis. If a patient has adapted well to the interim appliance and is pleased with chewing ability, cosmetics and speech it may not be advisable to place a new, now foreign appliance and require another period of adaptation. After a prolonged period of healing and assurances that no further surgery is planned for the near future the final prosthesis can be fabricated. An assessment of the patient's desires with respect to cosmetics, chewing, and speech is then undertaken with recommendations by the patient with respect to which is most important to them. The dentist, while doing the physical intraoral examination again evaluates the areas of the denture base that will afford stability, support and retention.

The final appliance: timing and function

When the final appliance is being planned the patient will hopefully be capable of cleaning and caring for their oral defect (Figure 9.8). In addition they will be used to having an appliance present in their mouth and be ready for fabrication of a final appliance. If the patient is dentate it is very important to ensure that the abutment teeth are healthy, vital and have good periodontal support. Teeth requiring root canal treatment and restorations

(a)

(b)

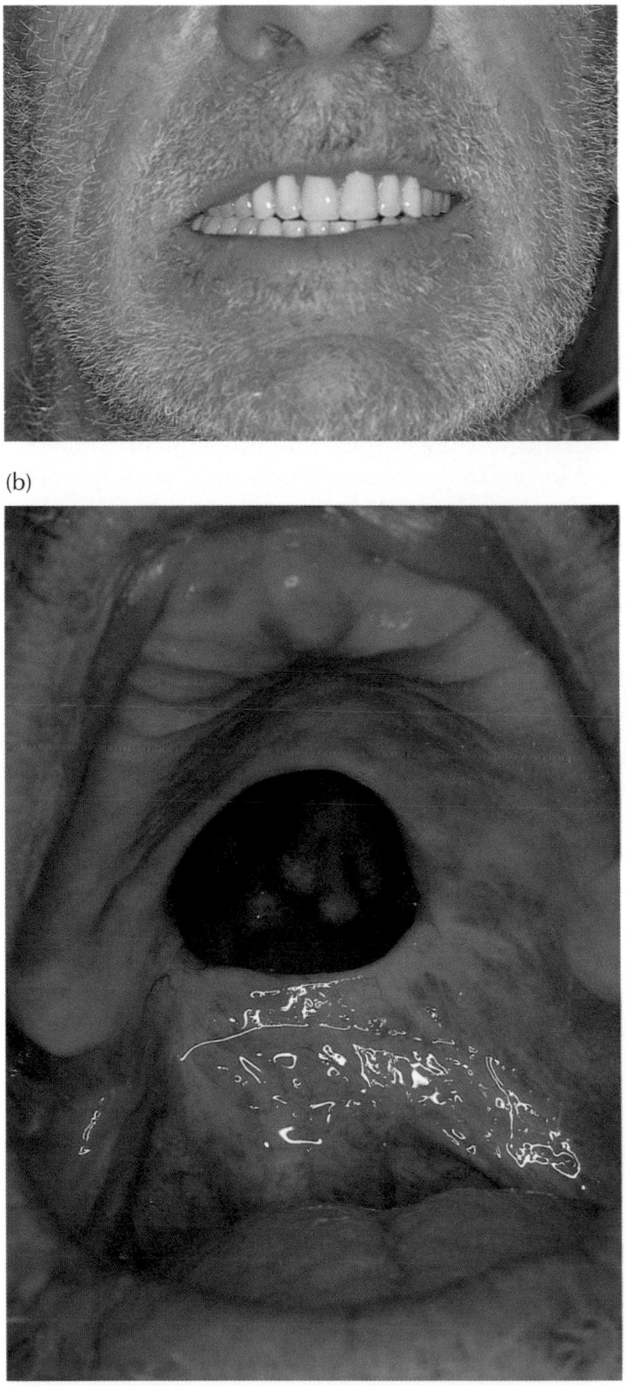

Figure 9.8 Example of a final obturator appliance in situ (a) and removed to show the defect (b).

should be managed during the phase the patient is wearing their interim appliance. Often teeth that would normally be extracted in a conventional patient will be retained in the oncology patient if they are, at all, prosthetically useful from the standpoint of offering stability, support or retention. Once the patient's dentition is appropriately restored and they are demonstrating good oral hygiene practice they are ready for the final appliance. All soft tissues visible to the dentist should be examined for any sign of mucosal abnormality, which, if present should be brought to the surgeon's attention.

At this time the patient should be questioned with respect to what they expect and want from their new appliance. There should be a firm and frank discussion with the patient to explain, once again what may be accomplished and what may not be feasible. This discussion should be done with the dentist sitting in front of the patient and taking an adequate amount of time to listen to the patient's concern and be assured that the patient fully comprehends what the dentist can do. The results of this conversation should be recorded in the chart and the dentist may elect to read them back to the patient. Taking an adequate amount of time at this appointment avoids the possibility of failure later, assures the patient that the dentist is genuinely interested in the outcome and lowers the patient's expectations to an appropriate level.

In the partly dentate patient the final appliance is frequently made of a combination of cast chrome-cobalt with cast or wrought wire clasps, rests and an acrylic bulb with teeth of appropriate shade and a soft tissue-coloured denture acrylic base. The bulb and the periphery of the denture must extend to the margin of the scar band and put slight pressure on this band. This gentle pressure will form a seal when the patient swallows and will prevent nasal regurgitation. The amount of pressure varies but an obturator bulb that is too large will cause ulceration and pain. An obturator bulb that is inadequate in size will not prevent nasal escape of fluids. The nasal aspect of the obturator bulb may be made hollow from above or be entirely hollow to lighten the weight of the appliance. Alternatively it may be made entirely of acrylic. The nasal portion should avoid contact with any nasal bones left by the surgeon since they will invariably be irritated and haemorrhage. If the entire nasal and sinus contents are removed at surgery the bulb may be extended upwards to allow more normal sounding speech with the caveat that the bulb can only be extended as far as the mouth will allow entrance. Occasionally a two-part appliance may be used with an upper portion fitted to the nasal/sinus cavity and extending up to the orbital floor and a lower denture portion which keys into this. The oral portion of the obturator should allow placement of the teeth in the prosthetic neutral zone, which may be altered by surgery. Additionally it should extend as far as possible for support but should not cause ulceration nor interfere with normal occlusion or mastication. The vestibular surface and palatal surfaces should be shaped in a manner that allows the oral musculature to assist in holding the appliance in place. In a posterior appliance this may mean having a concave vestibular surface (Figure 9.9). The oral surfaces should also be highly polished to allow the soft tissues to glide across them.

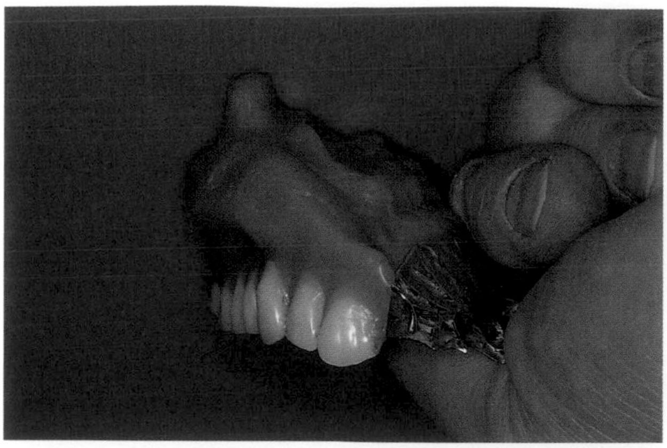

Figure 9.9 Vestibular concavity of the obturator allows, in some patients, the buccinator muscle to assist in keeping the denture in place.

The spectrum of appliances for rehabilitation of maxillary defects is huge and for more comprehensive information in treating this group of patients the reader is referred to the following references articles.[14,15]

Mandibulotomy candidate

The mandibulotomy splint is used in instances where a mandibular 'swing' approach is used to gain access to upper aerodigestive tract malignancies. It is an alternative to a mandibular resection and is usually used in cases where there is no underlying bony involvement of the mandible.[16] During the course of the procedure an osseous cut is made, usually in the anterior, and preferably through either an edentulous area or an extraction socket. The distal ends of the right and left sides of the mandible are then rotated outwards allowing direct view of the tongue and adjacent structures.

Following removal of the tumour the mandibular segments are reapproximated and plated with rigid fixation devices. The mandibulotomy splint is used to orient the teeth in three planes (coronal, axial, and mediolateral) so that when the segments are realigned the teeth and the temporomandibular joints are in virtually the same position they were in prior to the splitting of the mandible. If the mandible is re-approximated in the absence of an appropriate splint, joint pain and malocclusion may result and expensive fixed prosthetic or removable appliances may be required to alleviate what is an essentially iatrogenic condition. The competent surgeon should not underestimate the degree of discomfort associated with what are seemingly trivial changes in the position of the teeth. In addition to occlusal disharmony, teeth may become non-vital if not loaded properly and some patients will suffer significant impairment to the function of their temporomandibular apparatus. Whilst it is best if both dentate and edentulous patients are managed with the use of a splint it is particularly important in the former.

Mandibulotomy splints require about 5 working days to complete. At the first appointment the status of the dentition is assessed and irreversible hydrocolloid impressions are made from which dental stone models are poured. Impressions of both the upper and lower arches are done and kept for occlusal analysis postoperatively. The lower model is used to fabricate the mandibulotomy splint. The splint may be made of either orthodontic wire embedded in acrylic resin or alternatively it may be cast from chrome-cobalt alloy. In the author's experience the latter are difficult to adjust and less forgiving than the acrylic ones. Prior to the mandibulotomy operation the splint is tried in clinically (Figure 9.10) to make sure it fits the lower teeth and is not causing occlusal disharmony with the upper teeth. At the time of operation the surgeon makes the osseous cut and removes the tumour. The right and left mandibular segments are swung back into position and the splint is applied. If necessary it may be cemented or bonded to the teeth temporarily using zinc phosphate cement or light-cured acrylic resin. When it is firmly in place, the right and left mandibular segments are plated with the surgeon's preferred plating system. Compression plating will tend to move the segments closer together disrupting occlusion whereas passive plating may leave a saw-cut width gap of bone between the segments. The splint may then be removed or left for removal at a later date. The attending dentist may do this postoperatively.

Mandibulectomy/glossectomy patient

In general mandibular appliances are less well tolerated than upper ones. This is most likely due to the presence of the tongue and paramandibular musculature, which makes prosthetic restoration of the lower jaw a functional challenge. Following tongue or mandibulectomy surgery this challenge is heightened.

Patients with uncomplicated marginal mandibulectomy may be treated using variations of partial or complete lower dentures. Remembering the trinity of support, stability and retention the surgeon should plan ahead to leave as much horizontal bony surface as possible for denture support. Stability can be improved by assuring that the buccal and lingual vestibules are not obliterated but are deep. Both stability and support are highly dependent on the surgeon's ability to provide the dentist with tissue that is firmly bound down to bone. Large bulky grafts are not amenable to prosthetic rehabilitation. Retention is improved by ensuring that as many dental units are kept as possible and that they are well cared for. Seemingly hopeless teeth can be used

(a) (b)

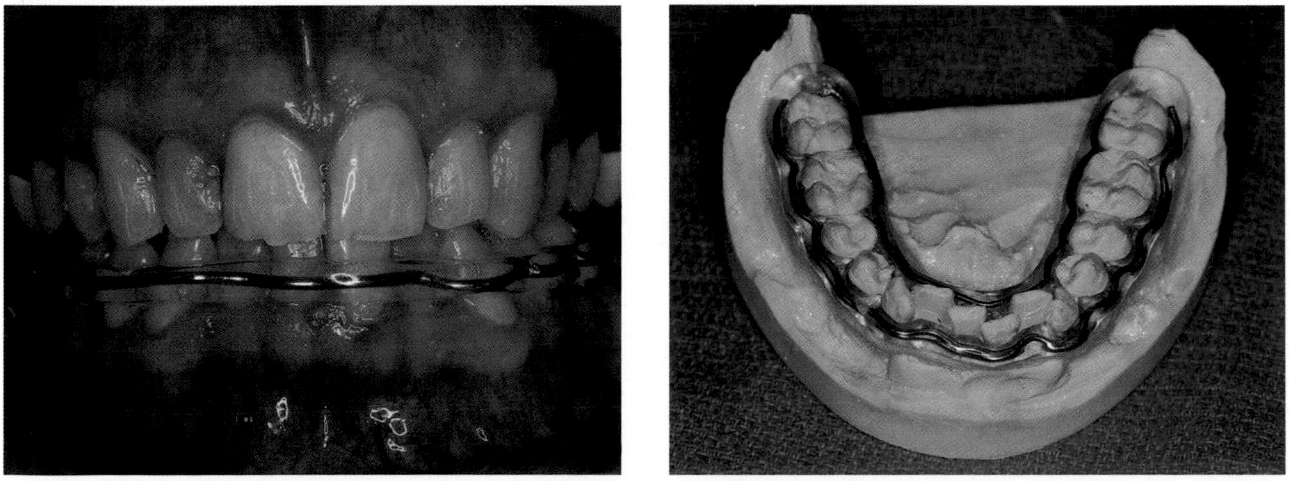

Figure 9.10 Mandibulotomy splint at the try-in appointment on the patient's teeth (a) and on a model (b).

in some cases for improving stability and retention. A large bulky graft also reduces the retention of the denture by obliterating the neutral zone in which teeth may be placed.

Patients with partial mandibulectomy and osseous/rigid fixation plate reconstruction may also be rehabilitated using variations of removable partial and full dentures if adequate support, stability and retention are present postoperatively. It is generally not acceptable to rest a denture on a fixation plate so some osseous support should be made available. In some instances a three-quarters or unilateral partial denture may be used if particular patient anatomy is conducive to it. Often providing a patient with a single side of contacting functional teeth is adequate to meet their needs. Once again communication between the practitioner and the patient is pivotal in reaching a satisfactory result.

The glossectomy patient presents different problems for the dentist in that, depending on the amount of tongue removed and the results of reconstruction there may be serious speech impairment. Following glossectomy the tongue may be physically smaller and deviated to one side. There are also usually clinically significant sensory and motor neural deficits that make speech even more difficult. Patients may be unable to make certain sounds such as 't', 'k', 'hard g' or 's'. In these patients alterations to upper and lower dentures or purposeful fabrication of a maxillary appliance with a lower palate may allow many of these sounds to be made (Figure 9.11). In these cases it is imperative that the dentist work in close contact with both the surgeon and the speech/language pathologist.

Implants

Osseointegrated implants will, in the future, play a greater role in the rehabilitation of the surgical oncology patients. Currently their use in irradiated jaws is at an early stage and their expense takes them out of the realm of possibility for most patients. Implants are placed following a thorough radiological examination and treatment planning session to ensure that there is adequate bone to allow their placement. No implant should be placed without consulting the radiation oncologist and gaining input as to the radiation dose at the proposed implant site. The lower the dose the safer it is to place implants. In addition implants should be placed only if they are prosthetically useful. For this reason it is wise for the surgeon to contact the prosthodontist prior to placing the implant to ensure that it can form an integral part of the final prosthesis.

Anaplastology/ocular prosthetics

A complete maxillofacial oncology service should ideally include as part of the restorative team an anaplastologist and an ocularist. The ocularist, among other services, fits the ocular prostheses in patients who have had surgical enucleation of the globe or surgical removal of the eye and surrounding structures. This is done using modified impressions of the residual eye contents. The ocularist may modify the socket or globe by adding and removing prosthetic material. They must select the correct pupil size, custom paint the iris to ensure that the eye is compatible with the remaining anatomy, is comfortable, is attractive, and allows the patient to maintain hygiene of the eye region (Figure 9.12) This is a gross oversim-

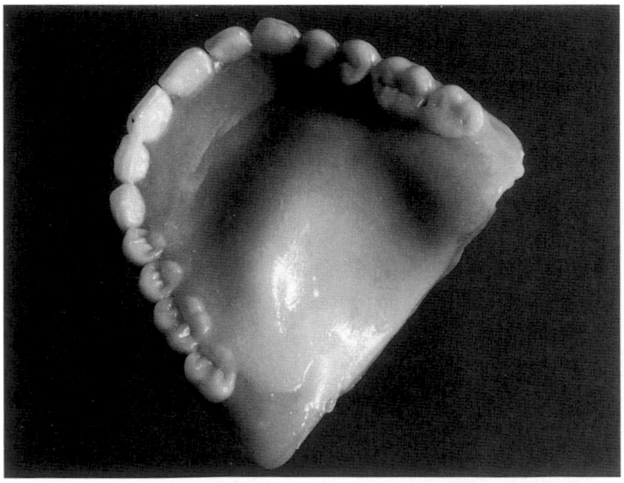

Figure 9.11 Addition of material to a maxillary appliance allows a deficient tongue to achieve contact with the palate so that a partial glossectomy patient can make speech sounds they normally would not be able to do.

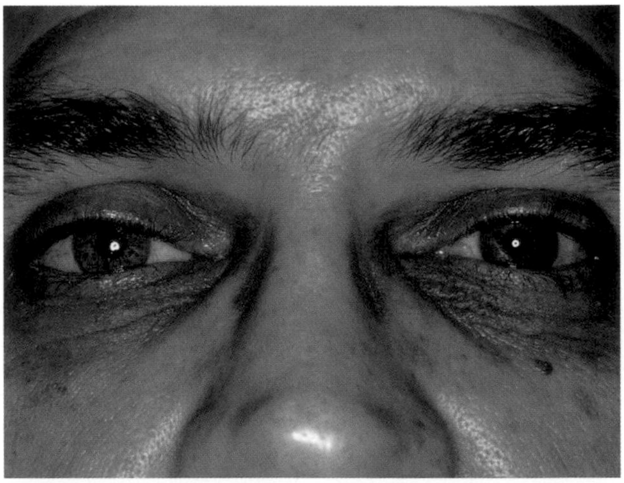

Figure 9.12 This patient has a well-fitting custom-made ocular prosthesis designed and made by a certified ocularist. It is difficult to tell which eye is the real one and which is the prosthetic one.

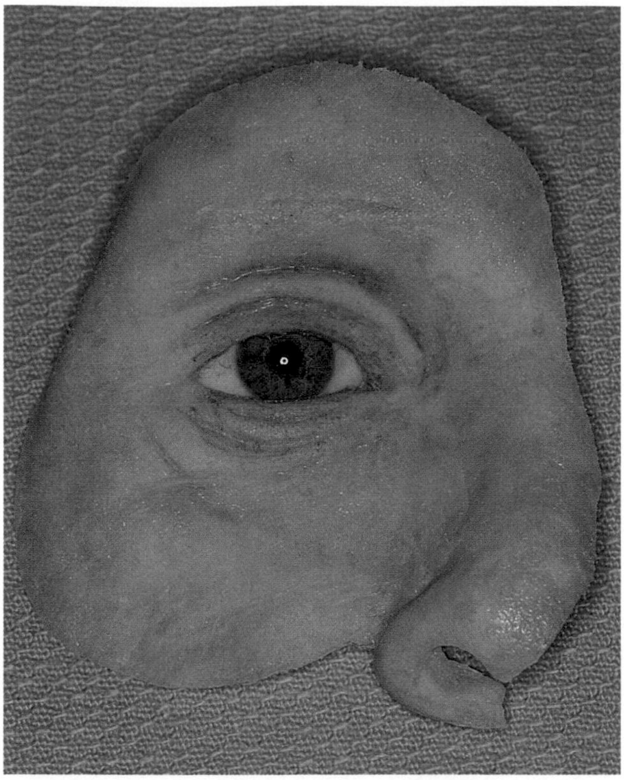

Figure 9.13 Integrated effort of anaplastologist, prosthodontist and ocularist results in an appliance which will reconstitute the missing portions of a patient's anatomy.

plification of the responsibilities of the ocularist. A more detailed description of the many functions of the ocularist may be found elsewhere.[17] In maxillofacial prosthetics the ocularist works with the prosthodontist and anaplastologist to ensure that any patients requiring prosthetic eyes receive a high-quality ocular prosthesis, which can function as an integral part of the prosthetic rehabilitation.

The anaplastologist performs a similar function as the ocularist and prosthodontist. He fabricates facial prostheses including nasal, peri-orbital, auricular and facial prostheses to replace facial components that are lost as a consequence of cancer surgery or radiation treatment. The anaplastologist like the ocularist must be part anatomist, part artist and part materials expert (Figure 9.13). The anaplastologist, prosthodontist, dentist, and ocularist work together with the surgeon to reconstitute the patient back to a level which allows them to function normally.

The long-term cancer survivor

The long-term head and neck cancer survivor can be integrated back into a general dental practice if the general practitioner is provided with either a resource person or obtains appropriate information for their care. Postradiation patients should be kept under close observation with a 3–6 monthly recall schedule and prompt management of any problem that may arise. These patients should be on life long topical neutral sodium fluoride gel application in custom fluoride trays as well as strict self-directed oral hygiene measures. Failure to do so will result in the development of post-radiation caries. If any invasive or extensive dental work is contemplated it is wise for the general practitioner to discuss the patient with the radiation oncologist or the dentist at the oncology centre. At the author's institution the patients are seen yearly to assess the general condition of the mouth. The patient must be cautioned to maintain their tobacco abstinence or if they still smoke be directed to their family physician or community resource person in an effort to get them to quit smoking.

Since oral cancer can recur, each follow-up examination should include an evaluation of the neck nodes and the oral and paraoral soft tissues. Visual examination by an experienced practitioner is likely the best method for spotting early cancers although toluidine-blue rinses have been postulated as a means of diagnosing very early cancers.[18] This author does not favour the use of these agents because of the high incidence of false positives and the likelihood that numerous unnecessary biopsies may be undertaken.[19]

There is a temptation to avoid doing radiographs on postradiation patients because of the misperception that these patients have had 'too much radiation already' or that the diagnostic radiation will 'cause' another cancer. Radiographs should be used when there is a probability that they will add to the diagnostic capability. The cancer patient, who is xerostomic, eating more highly refined carbohydrates, and may not be exercising superb oral hygiene is at greater risk of developing dental disease. For this reason more rather than fewer radiographs may need to be exposed.

In evaluating the postsurgical patient the prosthetic appliance should be examined for signs of deterioration, wear, and discoloration. The defect should be evaluated for cleanliness and recurrence and an assessment of fit and occlusion should be made. Appliances may wear out or require relining. If a patient is very content with their appliance it may be best to leave well enough alone. It is the patient who is the final arbiter of satisfaction with respect to fit and function. Whilst an appliance may not be 'prosthetically ideal', if a patient is content, and the appliance is not damaging adjacent hard or soft oral structures there is no need to fabricate a new appliance.

REFERENCES

1. Hughes CJ, Spiro RH. Carcinoma of the oropharynx. *A NZ J Surg* 1994; **64**: 302–306.
2. Bishay N, Petrikowski CG, Maxymiw WG, Lee L, Wood, RE. Optimum dental radiography in bone marrow transplant patients. *Oral Surg Oral Med Oral Pathol Oral Radiol Endod* 1999; **87**: 375–379.
3. Myers RE, Mitchell DL. Fluoride for the head and neck radiation patient. *Mil Med* 1988; **153**: 411–413.
4. Backstrom I, Funegard U, Andersson I, Franzen L, Johansson I. Dietary intake in head and neck irradiated patients with permanent dry mouths. *Eur J Cancer* 1995; **31B**: 253–257.
5. Tatum RC, Daniels R. The correlation of radiotherapy to salivary gland production and increased caries incidence: a caries control method. *Oral Med Oral Pathol Oral Radiol Endod* 1982; **52**: 9–11.
6. Niedermeier W, Matthaues C, Meyer C, Staar S, Muller RP, Schulze HJ. Radiation-induced hyposalivation and its treatment with oral pilocarpine. *Oral Med Oral Pathol Oral Radiol Endod* 1998; **86**: 541–549.
7. Wood RE, Maxymiw WG, McComb D. A clinical comparison of glass ionomer (polyalkenoate) and silver amalgam restorations in the treatment of class V caries in xerostomic head and neck cancer patients. *Oper Dent* 1993; **18**: 94–102.
8. Wood RE, McComb D, Hamilton M, Lee L, Maxymiw WG, Erickson R,. A clinical comparison of conventional glass ionomer cement restorations to bonded composite resin and hybrid glass-ionomer-resin restorations in the treatment of Class V caries in xerostomic head and neck radiation patients. *Oper Dent* (in press).
9. Maxymiw WG, Liu F-F, Wood RE. Post-radiation dental extractions without hyperbaric oxygen. *Oral Med Oral Pathol Oral Radiol Endod* 1991; **72**: 270–274.
10. Wong JK, Wood RE, McLean M. Conservative management of osteoradionecrosis. *Oral Med Oral Pathol Oral Radiol Endod* 1997; **84**: 16–21.
11. Merlano M, Benasso M, Cavallari M, Blengio F, Rosso M. Chemotherapy in head and neck cancer. *Eur J Cancer* 1994; **30B**: 283–289..
12. Greenberg MS, Cohen SG, McKitrick JC, Cassileth PA. The oral flora as a source of septicemia in patients with acute leukemia. *Oral Med Oral Pathol Oral Radiol Endod* 1982; **52**: 32–36.
13. Maxymiw WG, Wood RE, Anderson JD. The immediate role of the dentist in the maxillectomy patient. *J Otolaryngol* 1989; **18**: 303–305.
14. Adisman IK, Minsley GE. Maxillofacial prosthetics. In: Owall B, Kayser AF, Carlsson GE (eds). *Prosthodontics, Principles and Management Strategies.* London: Mosby-Wolfe, 1996; Chapter 5.
15. Laney WR. Restoration of acquired oral and perioral defects. In: Laney WR, Gibilisco JA (eds). *Diagnosis and Treatment in Prosthodontics.* Philadelphia: Lea and Febiger, 1983; Chapter 5.
16. Spiro RH, Gerold FP, Shah JP, Sessions RB, Strong EW. Mandibulotomy approach to oropharyngeal tumors. *Am J Surg* 1985; **150**: 466–469.
17. McFall JD. The role of the ocularist. *Adv Opthalmic Plast Reconstr Surg* 1990; **8**: 53–54.
18. Epstein J, Oakley C, Millner A et al. The utility of toluidine blue application as a diagnostic aid in patients previously treated for upper oropharyngeal carcinoma. *Oral Med Oral Pathol Oral Radiol Endod* 1997; **83**: 537–547.
19. Martin IC, Kerawal CJ, Reeds M. The application of toluidine blue as a diagnostic adjunct in the detection of epithelial dysplasia. *Oral Med Oral Pathol Oral Radiol Endod* 1998; **85**: 444–446.

10 Palliation of advanced head and neck cancer

John Williams and Karen Broadley

Introduction

Head and neck malignancies are rare and constitute less than 5% of all cancers in the western world with an average cure rate of about 50%. When the disease presents early, cure is possible in up to 90% but the patient may still be symptomatic as a result of treatment and they may benefit from many of the management strategies discussed in this chapter.

If the cancer is more advanced, either when it presents or when disease recurs or progresses, then emphasis may be less on cure but more on good symptom control. The need to palliate the distressing symptoms associated with advanced malignancy is of utmost importance.

Palliative care is best described as:

> '... the active total care of a person whose disease is no longer responsive to curative treatment. Control of pain, of other symptoms and of psychological, social and spiritual problems is paramount. The goal of palliative care is achievement of the best quality of life for patients and their families. Many aspects of palliative care are also applicable earlier in the course of the illness in conjunction with anti-cancer treatment.[1]

Although some of the common symptoms of head and neck malignancy may be due to treatment, they commonly occur as a result of disease progression. If further anti-cancer treatment is available this may be the most effective method of palliation. The potential benefits should be weighed up against the probable adverse effects and this information should be shared with the patient and their family before embarking upon treatment.

This chapter is primarily concerned with the practical management of physical problems arising from the cancer and/or its treatment. However, it cannot be overstated how important it is to also manage the psychological problems from which these patients suffer. This is evident when reflecting how socially important the structures of the face and neck are both from a functional (speech and swallow) and a psychosocial sense (aesthetic appearance). It is critical that the patient is treated holistically.

The main causes of symptoms in advanced head and neck cancer are:

1. Local disease causing infiltration, pressure or ulceration;
2. An incidental cause such as infection or coexisting illness;
3. Side effects from treatment with chemotherapy, radiotherapy, surgery or medication;
4. Distant spread with metastases for example in the lungs and bone.

Symptom control may be synonymous with the treatment of the neoplastic process either with surgery, radiotherapy or chemotherapy. Where these measures fail or are inappropriate, other symptom specific measures need to be employed. This chapter addresses some of the more common symptoms and their management.

In all situations medication should be kept simple and easy to swallow. Patients generally prefer liquids as mouth opening may be difficult. In addition, tablets may get stuck because of mechanical problems or lack of saliva. Liquids are essential with tube feeding and suppositories are useful where there is no upper gastrointestinal route of access. In other situations transdermal preparations or the subcutaneous route may be available and appropriate.

Pain

General considerations

Pain has been defined as 'an unpleasant sensory and emotional experience associated with actual or potential tissue damage'.[2] In patients with head and neck cancer, pain can occur following treatments such as surgery and radiotherapy (acute pain) or may be a longer-term problem associated with the disease process itself (chronic pain). Chronic pain patients may be debilitated with advanced disease or may have a stable condition with long life expectancy.

Effective pain control is essential for all patients with head and neck cancer because pain diminishes activity, appetite and sleep and may contribute to feelings of fear, anxiety and depression.[3] Head and neck cancer patients may also have the additional burden of difficulty in swallowing and talking and the presence of visible disease.

Recent developments in the understanding of pain physiology and pharmacology have indicated that pain transmission from the periphery to the brain is a complex process capable of modification and adaptation, known as *'plasticity'*.[4] Prolonged nociceptive input into the dorsal horn of the spinal cord can result in sensitization of receptors, which then facilitate further pain transmission. This process is also known as 'wind up'. The *N*-methyl *D*-aspartate receptor is involved in this process and is a potential target for analgesics that can block this receptor such as methadone or ketamine. A summary of recently identified pain pathways and neurotransmitters is illustrated in Figure 10.1 and recent advances in pain pharmacology and physiology and their clinical relevance are given in Table 10.1.

Because of the many different processes involved in pain transmission effective analgesia is more likely if many different classes of analgesic drug are used to treat pain. Additionally it is likely that involvement of a multidisciplinary team approach including

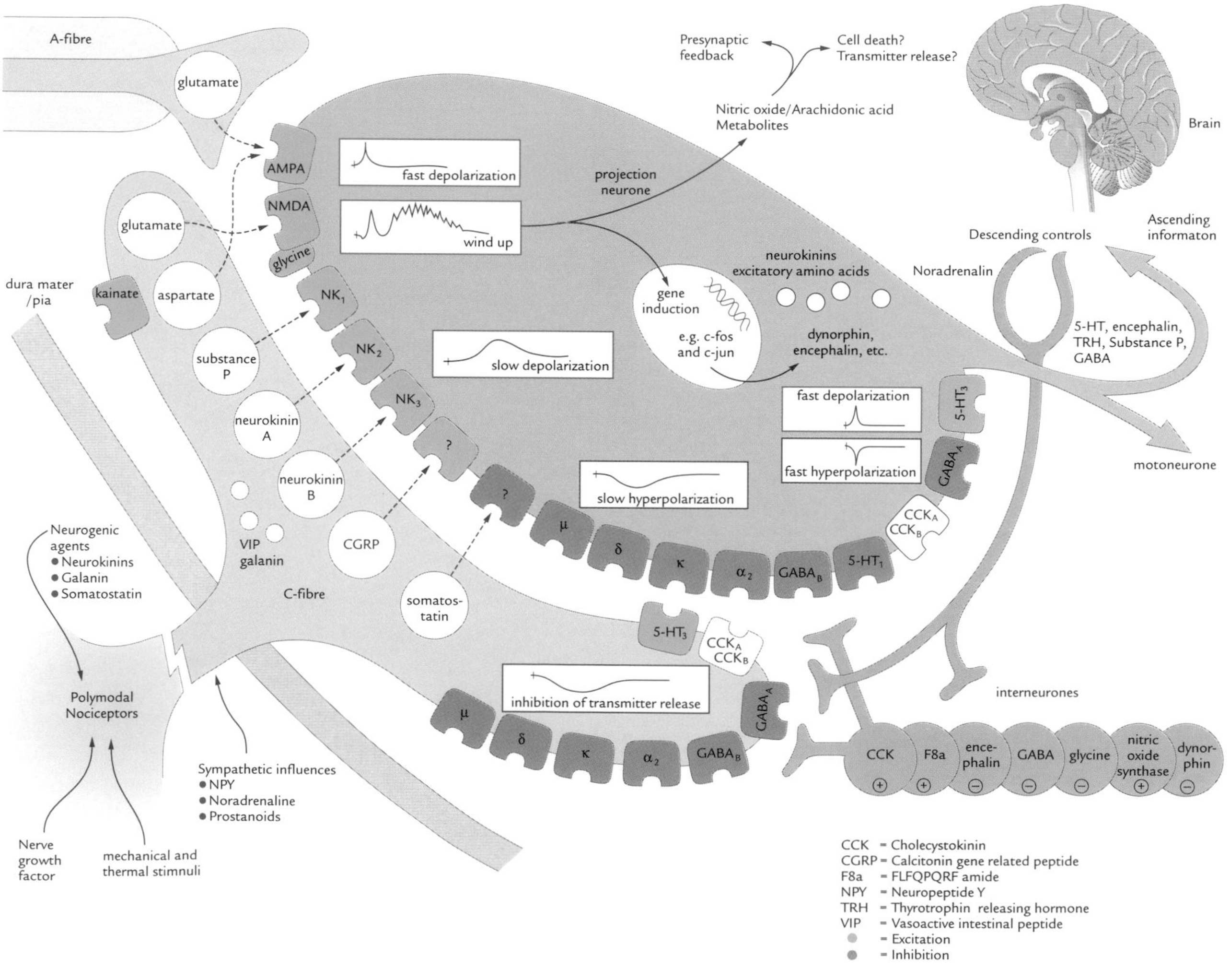

Figure 10.1 Cross-section through dorsal horn of spinal cord showing different stimulatory and inhibitory modulatory mechanisms.

Table 10.1 Recent advances in pain pharmacology and physiology and clinical relevance

Recent advance	Potential clinical relevance
Central nervous system plasticity and sensitization (wind up)	Treat pain early before long-term changes take place that may be difficult to reverse
NMDA receptor identified as being part of wind up process	NMDA-antagonist drugs such as methadone and ketamine may be effective
Evidence for the effectiveness of pre-emptive analgesia	Analgesic drugs given prior to a painful stimulus may be more effective
Evidence for the effectiveness of the multidisciplinary approach	Involve practitioners from other disciplines in treating chronic pain

specialists from different disciplines such as psychology, physiotherapy, surgery and palliative care would be beneficial.[5]

Pain assessment

Prior to commencement of analgesic therapy, patients with head and neck cancer pain should be investigated for the cause of the pain and the potential role of surgery, radiotherapy and chemotherapy in treating the cancer and relieving pain. This will involve a detailed history and examination and use of appropriate investigations such as MRI scan.

Pain syndromes in head and neck cancer

Acute pain

Acute pain can occur after surgery, radiotherapy or chemotherapy. Postsurgical pain is usually treated in either the postoperative recovery room or on the wards using opioids and other drugs such as NSAIDs. Occasionally postsurgical pain may become a more persistent problem due to damage or bruising to nerves at the time of surgery or due to the formation of painful neuromata. In particular this may occur following radical neck dissection or following other major head and neck procedures.

It is essential to treat acute postoperative pain aggressively as it is usually responsive to analgesic medication and there is some evidence that effective early treatment of acute pain may lead to a lower incidence of chronic pain problems.[6]

Pain following radiation therapy or chemotherapy usually presents as oral mucositis which develops during the second to fourth week after commencement of treatment. In patients who have difficulty in swallowing oral analgesics, this can be treated with either subcutaneous or intravenous opioids. Mucositis usually spontaneously resolves 3–4 weeks after cessation of therapy.[7]

Infection may play a role in exacerbating pain at any stage in the treatment of head and neck cancers. Infection may present as a worsening pain problem without any associated signs and symptoms such as fever, leukocytosis or signs of local infection.[8]

Chronic pain

Chronic pain in head and neck cancer patients may be classified into nociceptive or neuropathic pain syndromes. Figure 10.2 shows three different pain transmission states: (1) physiological pain transmission, where the pain impulses travel from the stimulus to the brain with minimal dorsal horn wind up; (2) nociceptive pain where there is some peripheral and central sensitization; and (3) neuropathic pain where there is abnormal wind up resulting in altered pain transmission and supersensitivity.

Nociceptive pain may be due to tumour pressure or infiltration into the mucosa or submucosa, which may lead to ulceration and infection. This may be exacerbated by local irritation with alcohol or acid, oedema and movement especially in dynamic structures such as the tongue and soft palate.

Bony infiltration can result in localized pain or, if there is direct pressure on a sensory nerve, pain in the distribution of the nerve. Cervical spine lesions may be a cause of both head and neck pain. Lesions may be as a result of cervical degeneration, metastases or surgical trauma.

Neuropathic pain can result after tumour pressure on a nerve or infiltration of a nerve. Typically this type of pain is characterized by lancinating or shooting pains in the distribution of the nerve, pain in a numb

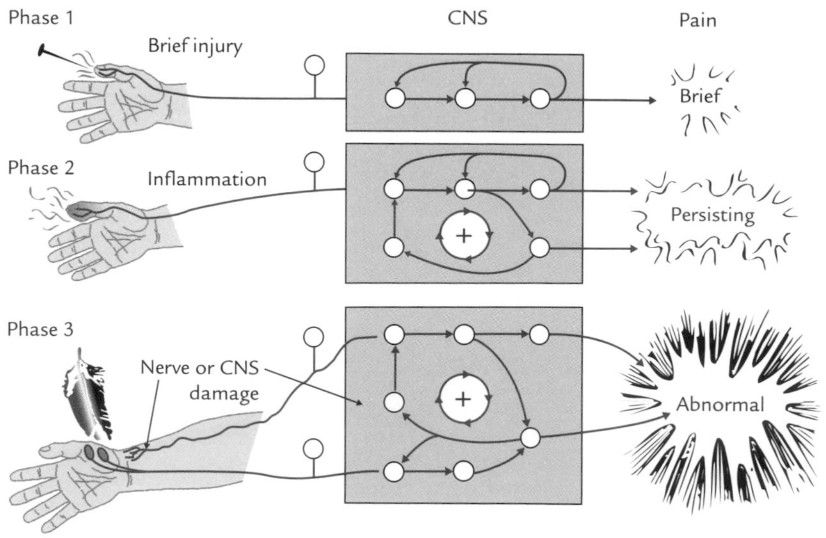

Figure 10.2 Three different pain transmission mechanisms; Phase 1, physiological pain; Phase 2, inflammatory pain; Phase 3, neuropathic pain.

Table 10.2 Neuropathic pain syndromes in head and neck cancer

Tumour	Neuropathic pain syndrome
Intraorbital	Sharp, lancinating pains in region of ophthalmic nerve
Maxillary antrum	Sharp, lancinating pains in distribution of maxillary nerve
Infratemporal fossa	Mandibular neuralgia, trismus, temporal pain
Nasopharynx, oropharynx, tonsillar region	Neuralgias in distribution of vagus and glossopharyngeal nerves
Postherpetic neuralgia	Commonly affects trigeminal nerve, stabbing pains, hyperaesthesia

area, burning pain and dysaesthesiae such as 'pins-and-needles.' Neuropathic pain syndromes are listed in Table 10.2.

Drug therapy

The majority of head and neck cancer pains can be managed using the WHO guidelines for the treatment of cancer pain.[9] This involves using non-invasive drug treatments according to a step-wise progression in drug dosages and by following the guidelines listed in Tables 10.3 and 10.4.

Head and neck cancer patients who are unable to swallow tablets can take these drugs enterally via gastrostomy or nasogastric tubes or rectal route. Patients unable to use any enteral route may require these drugs to be given either subcutaneously or intravenously.

Step 1. Non-opioid drugs
This group includes paracetamol, aspirin and other non-steroidal anti-inflammatory drugs (NSAIDS) such as ibuprofen, naproxen and diclofenac.

Table 10.3 WHO guidelines for relief of cancer pain

'The right drug at the right dose at the right time intervals'

- By the mouth
- By the clock
- By the ladder
- For the individual
- Use of adjuvant medication
- Attention to detail

Table 10.4 WHO analgesic ladder

Step 1 Non-opioid +/- adjuvant

Step 2 Opioid for mild to moderate pain +/- non-opioid +/- adjuvant

Step 3 Opioid for moderate to severe pain +/- non-opioid +/- adjuvant

NSAIDs work by inhibiting the cyclo-oxygenase enzyme responsible for producing prostaglandins, which contribute to the peripheral inflammatory response. NSAIDs are effective against nociceptive pain such as mucosal ulceration and bone pain. They are less effective for neuropathic pain.

All NSAIDs have the potential for adverse effects including haemorrhage, renal impairment and gastric erosion. They should be used with caution in patients with renal dysfunction or with a history of peptic ulcer.

Recent developments have included the development of NSAIDs such as meloxicam. As specific COX-2 antagonists, they do not antagonize the production of prostaglandins responsible for normal physiological functioning, and thus have the potential for fewer adverse effects.

Step 2. Opioids for mild to moderate pain

Opioids for mild to moderate pain (formerly known as weak opioids) include codeine, dihydrocodeine and dextropropoxyphene and combinations of these drugs with paracetamol such as co-proxamol and co-dydramol. Many of these combination preparations only have a small dose of weak opioid and some practitioners pass directly from step 1 to step 3 in patients with pain resistant to non-opioids.

Tramadol is a relatively new step 2 drug. It works as an opioid agonist and as an activator of CNS descending inhibitory systems, and is an alternative to codeine or dihydrocodeine.

Step 3. Opioids for moderate to severe pain

Immediate release preparations include morphine tablets such as Sevredol® or liquid morphine, Oramorph®.

Sustained-release preparations such as the twice daily MST® or the once daily MXL® are used in stable long-term pain conditions. MST® is available as a suspension that can pass down a feeding tube. In patients unable to take tablets, transdermal fentanyl may be an alternative. This preparation gives a sustained release of the strong opioid fentanyl, and may be associated with fewer adverse effects compared to MST®.

Alternative strong opioids in patients unable to take morphine, because of resistance or intolerance, include hydromorphone and oxycodone which are available in immediate and sustained-release preparations.

Opioid-induced side-effects

The main side-effects of opioid therapy include dry mouth, constipation, sedation and nausea. Dry mouth is difficult to treat as it may in part have been caused by the underlying disease process. All patients should be prescribed a laxative on commencement of opioids. A combined bowel stimulant and stool softener may be appropriate. About one-third of patients will need an anti-emetic.

Adjuvant drugs

This group of drugs can be used at all stages in the WHO ladder.[10] They include drugs that have another primary indication, such as the treatment of depression or epilepsy, but which also have analgesic properties or may contribute to pain relief (Table 10.5).

Neuropathic pain syndromes are often treated with this group of drugs in the first instance (Table 10.6).

Table 10.5 Adjuvant drugs used for neuropathic pain

Drug class	Examples
Antidepressant	Amitriptyline, dosulepin
Anticonvulsant	Carbamazepine, sodium valproate
Membrane stabilizer	Mexiletine, flecainide
Alpha-2-agonist	Clonazepam
Skeletal muscle relaxants	Diazepam, clonazepam

Table 10.6 Treatment of neuropathic pain

Nerve compression pain may respond to corticosteroids
Use adjuvant analgesics in first instance
Amitriptyline 25 mg at night, increase dose by 25 mg at weekly intervals according to response and side-effects
Consider use of gabapentin
Add sodium valproate or carbamazepine
There may be a gradation of response to opioids, in particular methadone may be useful
Mexiletine or flecainide
Consider subcutaneous ketamine

Other symptom problems

Nausea and vomiting

Nausea and vomiting occur in up to 50% of patients with advanced cancer, frequently together, although occasionally in isolation. Nausea and vomiting are generally multifactorial but there are commonly identifiable causes (Table 10.7). If a particular cause is thought to be reversible, it should be treated specifically. Frequently, however, this is not possible and anti-emetics are required.

There are many anti-emetics available, with different mechanisms of action and different uses (Table 10.8). Although in most cases the oral route is preferred, if intractable vomiting or mechanical problems prevent this, other routes must be considered. These include sublingual, rectal, subcutaneous and intravenous administration. A subcutaneous infusion or regular subcutaneous injections can be useful when rapid control is needed. Most of the commonly used anti-emetics can be combined in a syringe driver with morphine or diamorphine. Once symptoms improve, the patient may be converted back onto oral preparations.

Nutritional problems

Cachexia, a syndrome of anorexia and weight loss associated with cancer is often multifactorial in nature. The syndrome is characterized by a chronic abnormal metabolic state with abnormalities in carbohydrate, fat and protein metabolism. In patients

Table 10.7 Causes of nausea and vomiting

- Metabolic
  - Hypercalcaemia
  - Uraemia
- Raised intracranial pressure—cerebral metastases
- Drug induced
- Chemotherapy
- Radiotherapy
- Gastrointestinal cause
  - Constipation
  - Gastric distension and stasis
  - Bowel obstruction
- Pain
- Anxiety

Table 10.8 Commonly used anti-emetic drugs, their route of administration and uses

Drug	Usual dosages and route of administration	Typical dose in 24 hour subcutaneous infusion	Specific uses, apart from general anti-emetic
Cyclizine	50 mg PO/SC/IV tds	150 mg over 24 hours	Pharyngeal stimulation and vertigo
Haloperidol	1.5–3.0 mg PO/SC/IV od/bd	3–10 mg over 24 hours	Opioid-induced nausea and uraemia
Domperidone	10–20 mg PO; 30–60 mg PR tds/qds	Not available	Gastric stasis
Metoclopramide	10 mg PO/SC/IV tds	30 mg over 24 hours	Gastric stasis
Prochlorperazine	5–10 mg PO tds 3–6 mg buccal – bd 5 mg tds, 25 mg bd –PR	Not suitable	Vertigo
Levomepromazine	6.25–12.5 mg PO/SC od/bd	12.5– 25 mg over 24 hours	Where sedation is useful
Hyoscine	200–400 mg SC tds 1 mg transdermal, lasts 3 days	800–1200 μg over 24 hours	May improve sialorrhoea
Ondansetron	4–8 mg PO/IV bd	Has been used as a continuous infusion 8 mg over 24 hours	Chemotherapy or drug-induced nausea and nausea due to uraemia
Granisetron	1 mg PO bd 3 mg IV	Not known	Chemotherapy-induced nausea
Dexamethasone	4–16 mg PO/IV/SC od	4–16 mg (tends to precipitate when mixed with other drugs at high doses)	Raised intracranial pressure, liver metastases

od: once daily; bd: twice daily; tds: three times a day; qds; four times a day; stat: immediately; PO: by mouth; SC: subcutaneously; IV: intravenously; PR with head and neck cancer there is often a relative decline in food intake, hypophagia. Decreased appetite is a frequent complaint and is often more of a concern to the family than for the patient.

Hypophagia may result from chronic nausea either due to chemotherapy or radiotherapy. The disease itself or previous anti-cancer treatment may have caused changes in taste and smell (Table 10.9). Diminished saliva production will be an aggravating factor and there are often mechanical reasons due to tumour and treatment, which limit food intake (Table 10.10). The tumour may produce circulating products, which decrease the appetite. Cytokines, produced by the host in response to the tumour probably have a large role to play.

Nausea should be treated and practical advice given such as avoidance of meal preparation where possible. Small frequent meals are often best, together with dietary supplements. Appetite stimulants can be used but should be avoided when hypophagia is due to a mechanical reason. Studies in patients with non-endocrine responsive cancer show that progestogens such as megestrol acetate improve appetite and food intake and have in some cases been shown to stimulate weight gain. Corticosteroids have a beneficial effect on appetite and well-being, but rarely result in weight gain. Artificial cannabinoids also appear effective. All these drugs have side-effects which may not be tolerable for the patient.

Tube feeding is common in head and neck cancer patients. Patients are frequently malnourished when they present due to a multitude of factors and nasogastric feeding is used as a temporary measure whilst active treatment is being carried out. This allows for administration of medication in addition to nutritional intake. Generally nasogastric tubes are only used in the short term as the tube may cause chronic throat irritation, alar damage and aggravate oesophageal reflux. The appearance can be unacceptable to the patient and in addition they can be easily dislodged. If a more long-term solution is required then placement of a gastrostomy or jejunostomy tube can be performed using endoscopic- or radiological-guided placement.[11] Where there is significant obstruction due to disease then the latter method may be easier. If a fistula, previously used for speech, still exists between oesophagus and trachea and is no longer being used, then a long tube can be placed this way. Enteral feeding can take place overnight to minimize disruption during the day.

In all cases there can be problems such as tube blockage, dislodgment, leakage or skin infection. Patients may decide not to have a tube replaced if they have had many problems.

Table 10.9 Causes of taste changes in head and neck cancer

Surgical management of carcinoma of the oral cavity and tongue
Radiotherapy treatment for the same
Surgical or radiotherapeutic effect on the olfactory component of taste
Xerostomia
Stomatitis
Oral infections
Poor oral hygiene
Progressive local disease

Table 10.10 Causes of hypophagia

Difficulty in mastication: edentulous, pain, dry mouth
Functional dysphagia: treatment related, progression of cancer
Chronic nausea
Changes in taste
Aspiration

Mouth care

Patients who have been treated for head and neck cancer often have a dry mouth (xerostomia) and are more susceptible to local infections such as *Candida*. Medication used for either analgesia or anti-emesis can also aggravate an already dry mouth.

As disease progresses, ulceration may occur, which can be painful. It may be difficult for patients to keep a dental plate in position due to pain and cleansing may become impossible.

Many measures have been suggested to try and improve xerostomia. Water should be taken frequently and ice chips can be soothing. Pilocarpine capsules have been used in both xerostomia induced by radiation[12] and due to medication.[13] Some of the lubricating sprays such as Glandosane® are also helpful but need to be used frequently. Recent studies suggest that chewing sugar-free gum can improve the symptoms.

Fungal infections should be treated either with topical therapy such as nystatin suspension or systemic treatment such as fluconazole. Dentures, if worn, should also be treated.

Patients should be encouraged to maintain as good mouth care as possible, to use a soft toothbrush and an antibacterial mouthwash. In some situations when ulceration is a problem, then mouthwashes, which often contain alcohol, may be extremely painful. In such situations, bicarbonate of soda solution can be helpful.

Infection

Infection is common in head and neck patients, with cellulitis, localized tumour infections and orocutaneous fistulae contributing to more than 20% of febrile episodes in head and neck cancers.[14]

In some situations, improving local mouth care, cleansing and reducing secondary bacterial infections may reduce the risk of developing overwhelming sepsis. In many situations, however, antibiotics are required because of clinical signs of infection or because of increasing pain and discharge. In this situation, broad-spectrum antibiotics such as metronidazole and a penicillin are commonly used.

Fungating wounds

Fungating wounds occur as a result of local recurrence of disease, but may also be due to skin metastases or spread to the tracheostomy site or scar. A fungating tumour is distressing because of the appearance and the odour from necrotic tissue. Both of these can lead to social isolation and loss of intimacy between the patient and carers.

Pain can occur due to skin and muscle infiltration and may be aggravated as a result of inflammation due to treatment or supra-added infection. Pain can usually be managed effectively and treatment of infection may improve pain and also local swelling.

Where pain is a problem at the time of dressing changes, quick-acting opioid drugs given just prior to the procedure, either using immediate-release morphine or dextromoramide (Palfium), may help. These need to be given about 20–30 minutes before. Where the skin is generally sore, then topical local anaesthetic gels are useful as a short-term measure. These can be mixed with gel applied for wound debridement.

Odour

Necrotic tissue is susceptible to microbial colonization. Metronidazole gel has been shown to reduce odour and colonization, but does not treat overwhelming infection.[15] When odour is particularly offensive, then charcoal-containing dressings can be applied over the top of the wound dressing. Although it seems sensible to try and mask offensive smells with aromatherapy oils, this can make the unpleasant odour more noticeable, which may merely aggravate the problem.

Bleeding

Where there is capillary bleeding at the time of dressing changes, adrenaline soaks applied directly to the wound may reduce this. Many of the newer dressings such as the alginates are haemostatic. The dressings should be absorbent to prevent maceration of the surrounding skin, and fibre-free to reduce infection and allow for ease of removal. Gentle pressure should be applied to the bleeding points. If bleeding becomes more of a problem, it is essential to check there are no aggravating factors (discontinue aspirin or anti-coagulants, for example).

Tranexamic acid can be applied as a topical solution or given orally (0.5–1 g four times daily) to help with haemostasis. Where bleeding occurs from local lesions in the mouth, then tranexamic acid can be used as a mouth gargle and spat out. Where catastrophic bleeding is threatened and resuscitation is not appropriate, it may be appropriate to have medication to hand when the dressing is changed (crisis pack; see Table 10.11).

Table 10.11 Crisis pack

In the event of distress caused by sudden acute bleed or by upper respiratory obstruction:

1. 10–20 mg IV/IM midazolam
2. Diamorphine IV/IM equivalent to 4-hourly dose (if not on opioids, give 10–20 mg)

If distress continues, commence a subcutaneous pump

Where there is continued severe bleeding further management should be considered. Radiotherapy can be effective for superficial bleeding where there is still a possibility of its use. In some situations embolization has been used successfully.[16,17] However, it is not without significant risks, and should only be considered in patients who are relatively stable and are expected to have a fairly good quality of life for a while after the procedure.

Severe haemorrhage

This complication is feared by all health-care professionals and by those patients who are aware. A patient dying from exsanguination such as a 'carotid blowout' is a traumatic event for everyone. Severe bleeding though is not a common cause of death. In two series of head and neck patients referred for inpatient palliative care, two of 102 and one of 38 patients died in this manner.[18,19] It is a more likely occurrence after surgery where radiotherapy has been used in the past. In the series of 38 patients, 11 patients had repeated episodes of bleeding but these did not cause death. Most died as a result of pneumonia and general deterioration.[19]

Blood loss can occur from either the tumour bed or from erosion of a large vessel. Where major bleeding is likely to be a problem, it is often heralded by several minor bleeds. These can be extremely worrying for the patient and carers, as the timing cannot be predicted. If they occur at dressing changes at the time when health-care practitioners are within the house a crisis pack (Table 10.11) can be at the ready. It is always helpful for the patient to have a letter explaining their condition and how a bleed should be managed in Accident and Emergency, as it is likely that they will be taken to their nearest hospital rather than to a specialist centre. Should a bleed occur, then immediate pressure should be applied to the wound, and when the bleeding stops, a pressure dressing applied. When there is catastrophic bleeding such as a carotid blowout there is little time for medication to be drawn up and administered. In this situation it is important not to leave the patient alone but to remain at their side.

Fistulae and secretions/discharge

Where infection contributes to discharge, antibiotics may be appropriate. There may be excessive secretions, particularly where a fistula (or fistulae) has formed between the oral cavity and the skin. Liquid food and saliva can pour through and the most absorptive dressings are needed to reduce contact with the skin to prevent irritation. Where there is excessive saliva production (particularly where it cannot be swallowed), the role of an anticholinergic such as hyoscine or glycopyrronium can be considered. Hyoscine is available as a transmucosal preparation (Kwells®) or as a transdermal preparation that stays in place for 3 days (Scopaderm®).

Lymphoedema

Lymphoedematous swelling of the face can occur in small areas or more generally. The lymphatics may be damaged as a result of cancer, radiotherapy or surgery. In progressive disease there may be concomitant hypoalbuminaemia, and venous obstruction due to neck disease, which will exacerbate the condition. Infection can also be a causative factor as before. Lymphoedema is best managed when caught at an early stage. The skin should be protected by moisturizing it regularly and care should be given to avoid skin damage. If infection occurs, this should be treated rapidly with antibiotics. If cellulitis causes the patient to be systemically unwell then prophylactic antibiotics should be considered after a second episode.

In moderate or severe lymphoedema, the face can be uncomfortable as well as unsightly due to pressure and skin tightness. It can be a particular problem after lying down at night. During the day the lymphoedema will slowly decrease through the effect of gravity. It can be minimized by raising the head at night.

Discomfort and pain should be treated with appropriate analgesia. Occasionally diuretics can reduce the tightness of the face though they rarely help with swelling. High-dose steroids may benefit, reducing tumour bulk and perivascular oedema. If a trial of steroids fails to elicit any change, they should be stopped, as conversely they may also aggravate swelling and encourage candidal infection. Specialized massage of the face can improve lymphatic flow when there is no concomitant infection but should only be attempted by those experienced in its use. A compression dressing over absorbent dressings may be effective where skin is broken and weeping (lymphorrhoea) but comfort must not be compromised.

Dyspnoea

Dyspnoea may be due to concomitant disease such as bronchopneumonia or chronic obstructive airway disease, or may be due to cancer.

Many patients will have had a tracheostomy inserted during part of their cancer treatment. These can become blocked, with progression of local disease, secretions or blood. It requires skilled nursing to care for a difficult and sometimes distorted tracheostomy site. This is a common reason why such patients remain in hospital. When formation of a tracheostomy may give relief of symptoms in late-stage disease this should be considered. Whenever possible the patient and family should be involved in these discussions. It is always best to prevent a situation happening as an emergency but to plan it early as symptoms arise. Causes of dyspnoea and management are listed in Table 10.12.

Whatever the cause, breathlessness is a subjective symptom that is increasingly mentioned as a problem as a patient deteriorates. On occasions a specific cause cannot be found and it may be attributed to generalized weakness and debility. Anxiety is frequently present, which can make the feeling

Table 10.12 Common causes of dyspnoea with suggested managements

Due to disease	Specific treatment
Upper airway obstruction	Humidified air to reduce sticky secretions Consider tracheostomy if due to disease progression
Nasal obstruction	Surgery, stenting or laser treatment
SVCO	Radiotherapy or SVC stenting
Lung metastases	Symptomatic treatment
Lymphangitis carcinomatosis	Trial of high-dose steroids (12–16 mg dexamethasone a day)
Associated with the disease	
Pulmonary emboli	Anticoagulation as long as bleeding is not a problem
Bronchopneumonia	Antibiotics and bronchodilators
COAD	Bronchodilators

SVCO: superior vena cava obstruction; SVC: superior vena cava; COAD: chronic obstructive airways disease

worse. Fears of being suffocated and of breathing stopping during sleep are common and can make the night a worry. Reassurance is often needed and simple things such as company, a night-light and a fan can be helpful.

The general feeling of breathlessness can be improved by reducing anxiety and lowering the respiratory drive. Diazepam given in small doses (2–5 mg) morning and night together with regular oral morphine may help to achieve this. Respiratory depression tends not to be a problem when the drugs are introduced in low doses and titrated up.

Sudden attacks of breathlessness or panic attacks can be eased by sublingual lorazepam (0.5–1 mg), which acts rapidly.

If acute airway obstruction occurs such as blockage of the tracheostomy tube or an acute bleed compromises the airway, then sedation should be administered (Table 10.12). Helium-oxygen mixture has been used with tracheal obstruction, the rationale being that it is less viscous than air and may require less respiratory effort.

Hypercalcaemia

This is common in patients with head and neck cancers. Occasionally, the hypercalcaemia may be picked up as an incidental finding, but the symptoms, such as thirst, constipation and confusion are likely indicators. Management of mild hypercalcaemia may involve encouragement of oral fluid intake. At a higher level particularly with dehydration, then intravenous fluids may be indicated, together with the use of bisphosphonates given intravenously. On some occasions resistant hypercalcaemia can be a terminal event.

Communication problems

During early disease management, communication issues may have been a concern. In some situations, speech may just be understandable or the patient may use a mechanical device. As a patient becomes weaker or develops more extensive local disease, they may become harder to understand. In this situation, patients easily become frustrated and there is a need to spend more time with them to try and develop some form of communication. Where writing has been relied on, it becomes more difficult as weakness progresses. The niceties of speech and conversation become lost. Liaison with a speech therapist is essential.

The dying patient

When a patient is dying, all treatments, drugs and investigations that are not necessary should be discontinued. Analgesia and anti-emetics should be continued. Analgesic requirements can increase at this time and it is important that the patient is reviewed regularly. If terminal agitation or restlessness occurs it is important to exclude simple causes such as pain, urinary retention or faecal impaction. If there is renal impairment, accumulation of drugs may be an aggravating factor. Agitation is, however, often due to the dying process. Medications such as midazolam (initially 20–30 mg in 24 hours) or levomepromazine (12.5–50 mg initially in 24 hours) given subcutaneously by continuous infusion have been used to good effect.

Respiratory distress can be reduced with opioids and benzodiazepines given subcutaneously. If excess secretions are a problem, parenteral fluids should be stopped and hyoscine or glycopyrronium be added to the syringe driver. In some circumstances patients may require suction. On the whole, chestiness due to retained secretions tends to cause the family and staff more distress than the patient.

Other terminal events should be anticipated. Even if an anti-emetic is not required regularly, one should be prescribed in case it is needed. If haemorrhage is a possibility, then midazolam or another quick acting anxiolytic should be prescribed.

If the patient has expressed a wish about where they would like to die, efforts should be made to ensure the request is fulfilled. Most head and neck patients request to be on an inpatient unit where they are known. It may not be possible or appropriate however, to move a sick person in their last days. In any event the patient has a right to peaceful and, if possible, private surroundings with their family near. They should be allowed to die with dignity, with respect given their religious beliefs and customs.

REFERENCES

1. World Health Organization. *Cancer Pain and Palliative Care.* Technical Report Series 804. Geneva. 1990.
2. International Association for the Study of Pain, Subcommittee on Taxonomy. Part 2. Pain terms: a current list with definitions and notes on usage. *Pain* 1979; **6**: 249–52 (updated 1982, 1986).
3. Moinpour CM, Chapman CR. Pain management and quality of life in cancer patients. In: Lehmann RKA, Zech D (eds) *Transdermal Fentanyl: A New Approach to Prolonged Pain Control.* Berlin: Springer-Verlag, 1991; 42–63.
4. Dickenson AH. Recent advances in the physiology and pharmacology of pain: plasticity and its implications for clinical analgesia. *J Psychopharmacol* 1991; **5**: 342–351.
5. Flor H, Fydrich T, Turk DC. Efficacy of multidisciplinary pain treatment centers; a meta-analytic review. *Pain* 1992; **49**: 221–230.
6. McQuay HJ. Pre-emptive analgesia (Editorial). *Br J Anaesth* 1992; **69**: 1–3.
7. Weisseman DE. Cancer-associated pain syndromes. *Pain Digest* 1991; **1**: 92–99.
8. Bruera E, MacDonald N. Intractable pain in patients with advanced head and neck tumours: a possible role of local infection. *Cancer Treat Rep* 1986; **70**: 691–692.
9. World Health Organization 1986 Cancer Pain Relief and Palliative Care. Geneva, Switzerland.
10. World Health Organization 1990, Cancer Pain Relief and Palliative Care. Report of a WHO expert committee (WHO Technical Report Series, 804) Geneva, Switzerland.
11. Hunter JG, Lauretana L, Shellito PC. Percutaneous endoscopic gastrostomy in head and neck cancer patients. *Ann Surg* 1989; **210**: 42–46.
12. LeVeque FG, Montgomery M, Potter D et al. A multicenter, randomized, double-blind, placebo-controlled, dose-titration study of oral pilocarpine for treatment of radiation-induced xerostomia in head and neck cancer patients. *J Clin Oncol* 1993; **11**: 1124–1131.
13. Davies AN, Daniels C, Pugh R, Sharma K. A comparison of artificial saliva and pilocarpine in the management of xerostomia in patients with advanced cancer. *Palliat Med* 1998; **12**: 105–111.
14. Hussain M, Kish JA, Crane L et al. The role of infection in the morbidity and mortality of patients with head and neck cancer undergoing multimodality therapy. *Cancer* 1991; **67**: 716–721.
15. Newman V, Allwood M, Oakes RA. The use of metronidazole gel to control the smell of malodorous lesions. *Palliat Med* 1989; **3**: 303–305.
16. Wilner HI, Lazo A, Metes JJ et al. Embolization in cataclysmal hemorrhage caused by squamous cell carcinomas of the head and neck. *Radiol* 1987; **163**: 759–762.
17. Bhansali S, Wilner H, Jacobs JR. Arterial embolization for control of bleeding in advanced head and neck carcinoma. *J Laryngol Otol* 1986; **100**: 1289–1293.
18. Talmi YP, Bercovici M, Waller A et al. Home and inpatient hospice care of terminal head and neck cancer patients. *J Palliat Care* 1997; **13**:9–14.
19. Forbes K. Palliative care in patients with cancer of the head and neck. *Clin Otolaryngol* 1997; **22**: 117–122.

PART II

Mainly squamous neoplasms

11 Tumours of the oral cavity

Snehal G Patel, Daniel J Archer and J Michael Henk

Introduction

Tumours of the oral cavity are relatively uncommon compared to other head and neck sites such as the larynx, but the incidence and mortality rates for oral cancer, especially in younger men, have shown an increase in the UK and almost all the EC countries over the last few decades. The tumour and the consequences of its treatment can profoundly impact on one or more of the several important functions that the oral cavity normally serves. Alteration of functions such as mastication, speech, taste, swallowing, oral sensation and continence, and of body image can have a devastating impact on quality of life. Apart from the obvious goal of disease-free survival, these factors must be considered in treatment planning.

Surgical anatomy

The oral cavity extends from the vermilion border of the lips to an arbitrary plane bound by the circumvallate papillae of the tongue inferiorly and the junction of the hard and soft palate superiorly. It can be divided into two functional units; that which is bathed constantly in saliva and is subject to salivary flow and that which is relatively dry. The significance of this division is of practical importance in that surgery on the inferior saliva-bathed structures runs the risk of developing the potential complication of postoperative salivary fistula formation and that to the superior relatively dry area may be complicated by postoperative wound contracture and residual deformity. There may also be some significance in the relative exposure of the mucosa to potential salivary carcinogens and the relative incidence of local recurrence of disease in these two areas (Figure 11.1), an observation that is substantiated by a recent epidemiological study.[1] The oral cavity is divided into several anatomical subsites (Figure 11.2).

Lip

The lip includes only the vermilion surface or the portion that comes into contact with the opposing lip. This area is particularly vulnerable to cancer in the aged and those exposed to sun damage, the lower lip being more commonly affected. In European populations of spirit drinkers and cigarette smokers, squamous cancers at the commissures are more aggressive. At this site surgical excision involves difficult techniques for restoration of functional anatomy, and despite both surgery and radiotherapy in combination, local recurrence is more common.

The lips are supplied by the superior and inferior labial branches of the facial artery. The upper lip is supplied by the infraorbital branch of the maxillary nerve (V^2) while the lower lip is supplied by the mental branch of the inferior dental nerve (V^3). The muscles of the lower lip are supplied by the cervical branch of the facial nerve and the marginal mandibular branch which leaves the lower border of the parotid gland and crosses the inferior border of the mandible superficial to the facial vessels to reach the face beyond the anterior border of the masseter

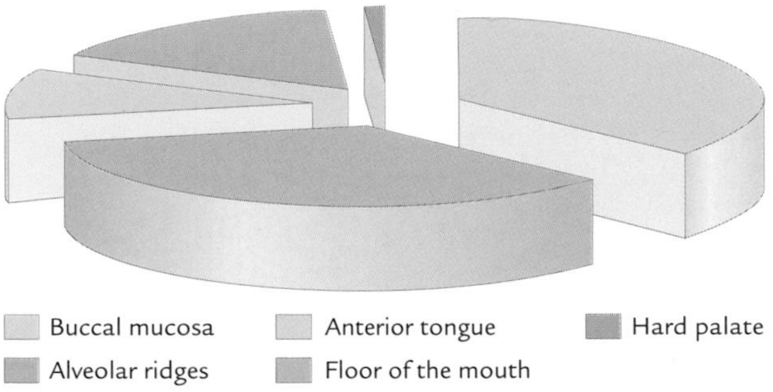

Figure 11.1 Distribution of sites of squamous carcinoma of the oral cavity.

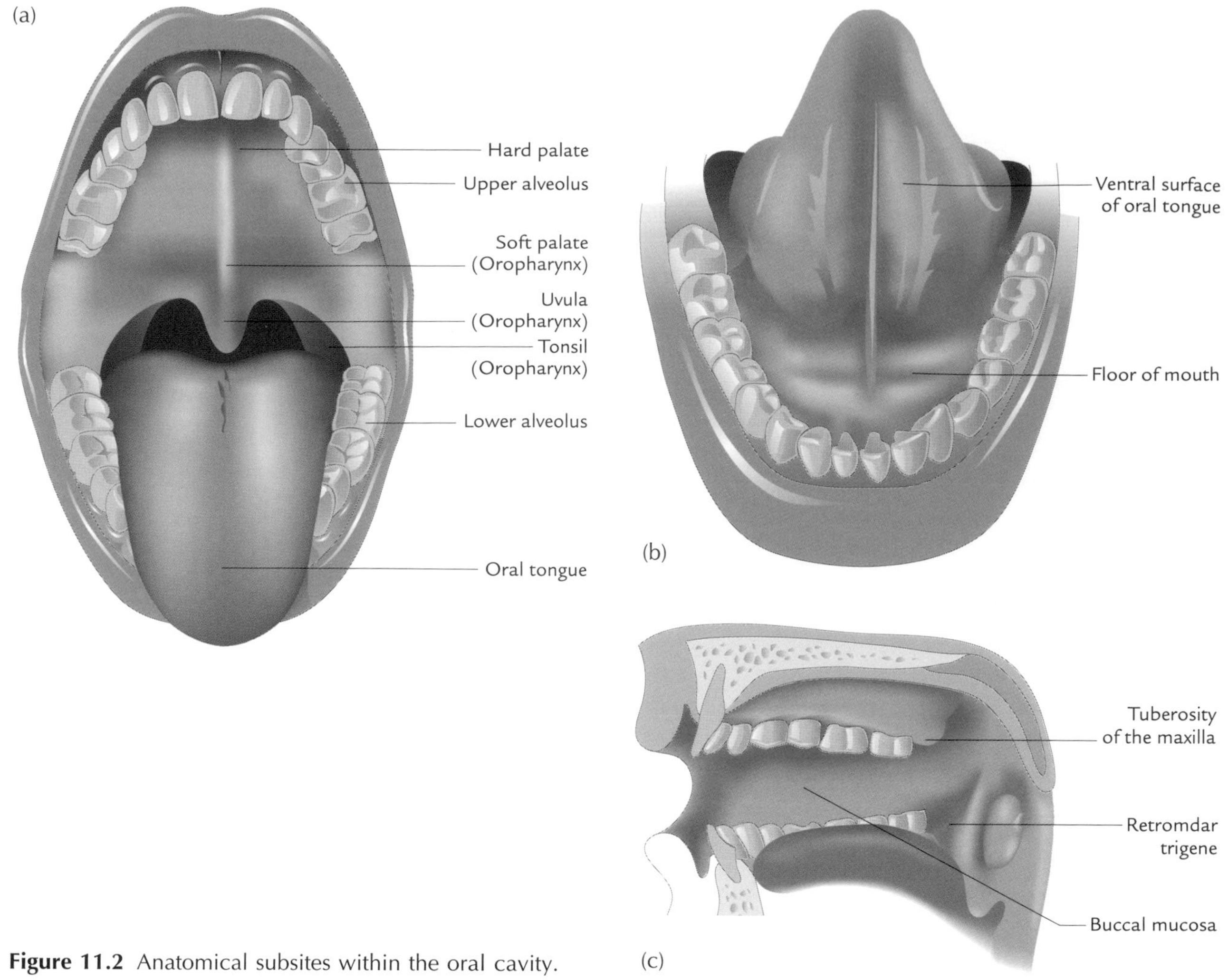

Figure 11.2 Anatomical subsites within the oral cavity.

muscle. The muscles of the upper lip and the orbicularis oris are supplied by the buccal branch of the facial nerve.

The upper lip drains lymph first into the buccal and parotid nodes, then into the prevascular facial node overlying the margin of the mandible and ultimately into the upper deep cervical nodes via the submandibular nodes. The lower lip drains into the submandibular nodes and then into the upper deep cervical nodes. The central portion of the lower lip drains first into the mental nodes and then to the submandibular and upper deep cervical nodes (level II) or directly to the omohyoid node (level III). Lesions of the central portions of the lips not uncommonly metastasize to nodes at level I on both sides.

Buccal mucosa

This site includes all the membrane lining of the inner surface of the cheeks and lips from the line of contact of opposing lips to the line of attachment of mucosa of the alveolar ridges and pterygomandibular raphe. The parotid (Stensen's) duct opens on a low papilla opposite the second upper molar tooth with the tiny openings of the ducts of the molar glands nearby.

The attached mucosa overlying the ascending ramus of the mandible from the level of the posterior surface of the last molar tooth to the apex superiorly, adjacent to the tuberosity of the maxilla constitutes the retromolar trigone. Tumours arising in this area are commonly not confined to it: indeed there is a quite common presentation of a tumour of the mandibular alveolus, often involving the posterior floor of mouth and passing superiorly to the maxillary tuberosity, thus in theory involving three primary sites.

The buccal mucosa derives its blood supply from branches of the transverse facial artery which runs along the parotid duct from its origin from the superficial temporal branch of the external carotid artery. Much of the buccal mucosa is supplied by the buccal branch of the mandibular branch of the trigeminal nerve. Lymph drains into the parotid, submental and, submandibular lymph nodes, and ultimately into the upper deep cervical nodes or to the facial node on the margin of the mandible and then to the submandibular lymph nodes.

Alveolar ridges

The alveolar ridges include only the alveolar processes of the mandible and the maxilla, and their covering mucosa. As the mucosa is intimately fused to the underlying periosteum tumours of both alveolar ridges may invade the alveolar bone of the jaws quite early in their natural history.

The lower alveolus receives its sensory innervation from the branches of the mandibular nerve (inferior alveolar, buccal and lingual nerves) while the upper alveolus is innervated by branches of the maxillary nerve (superior alveolar, greater palatine and nasopalatine nerves). The primary echelons of lymphatic drainage are the nodes in the submental and submandibular triangle. Tumours of the lower jaw are much more likely to metastasize to the neck than those of the upper jaw.

Floor of the mouth

The floor of the mouth is a horseshoe-shaped space overlying the mylohyoid and hyoglossus muscles, extending from the inner surface of the lower alveolar ridge to the undersurface of the tongue. Its posterior boundary is the base of the anterior pillar of the tonsil and the space is divided into two sides by the frenulum of the tongue. The mylohyoid muscles form the partition between the mouth above and neck below. The floor of the mouth contains the openings of the submandibular and sublingual salivary gland ducts. Surgery or radiotherapy to the anterior floor of the mouth may interfere with free salivary flow and can result in salivary gland obstruction, which may mimic lymphadenopathy. Lymphatic channels from the floor of the mouth drain to the submental and submandibular lymph nodes.

Hard palate

The hard palate is a semilunar area that extends from the inner surface of the superior alveolar ridge to the posterior edge of the palatine bone. Its mucosa is strongly united with the underlying periosteum, which in turn is secured to the bone by Sharpey's fibres. This mucoperiosteal fusion extends from the maxillary alveolus to the midline and ends posteriorly at the soft palate–hard palate junction. Over the horizontal plate of the palatine bone, however, the mucous membrane and periosteum are separated by a mass of mucous glands that may give rise to adenocarcinoma. The mucosa also contains numerous minor salivary glands from which minor salivary gland tumours may arise.

The hard palate is supplied by branches of the greater palatine artery, which emerges from the greater palatine foramen and passes laterally around the palate to enter the nose through the incisive foramen. The maxillary nerve supplies the greater part of the palate up to the incisive foramen by its greater palatine branch via the pterygopalatine ganglion while the premaxillary area between the incisors and incisive foramen is supplied by its nasopalatine branches. Lymphatic channels drain first to the retropharyngeal and then to the deep cervical nodes.

Anterior (oral) tongue

The freely mobile portion of the tongue extends anteriorly from the line of the circumvallate papillae to the undersurface of the tongue at the junction of the floor of mouth. It is composed of four areas: the tip, lateral borders, dorsum and the non-villous undersurface. The surface epithelium is keratinizing stratified squamous epithelium that is roughened by the presence of papillae. The dorsum of the anterior tongue bears no mucous or serous glands, these being concentrated mainly under the tip and the sides. Also under the tip, in a paramedian position on each side, open the tiny ducts of the anterior lingual glands.

The intrinsic muscles of the tongue (superior and inferior longitudinal, transverse and vertical) are not attached to bone and serve to alter the shape of the tongue during chewing, swallowing and articulation. The extrinsic muscles are attached to bone: genioglossus (mandible and hyoid), hyoglossus (hyoid), styloglossus (styloid process) and palatoglossus (hard palate). The genioglossus is the largest and makes up the bulk of the tongue. The extrinsic muscles stabilize the tongue and by their contraction alter its position as well as its shape.

The major arterial supply is from branches of the lingual artery, which is the third branch of the external carotid artery. Minor contributions come from the tonsillar branch of the facial artery and the ascending pharyngeal artery. The midline of the tongue is an avascular plane due to the tough fibrous septum which prevents anastomosis of blood vessels of the two muscular halves.

The lingual vein accompanies the lingual artery and usually joins the internal jugular vein near the greater cornu of the hyoid. The tip of the tongue is drained by the deep lingual vein that is visible ventrally on each side of the midline. It runs backwards superficially on the hyoglossus and is joined at its anterior border by the vein from the sublingual gland to form the vena comitans of the hypoglossal nerve, draining into either the lingual, facial or internal jugular veins. The hypoglossal nerve supplies all the muscles of the tongue except the palatoglossus, which is supplied by the pharyngeal plexus. The trigeminal component (cell bodies in the trigeminal ganglion) of the lingual nerve mediates common sensibility while the chorda tympani component (cell bodies in the geniculate ganglion of the facial nerve) mediates taste.

Although the lymphatic drainage of the tongue is extremely variable, as a general rule, the tip drains to the submental nodes while the rest of the anterior tongue drains to the submandibular nodes. A unique feature of these lymphatics is that lymph from one side may reach nodes of both sides of the neck, especially when ipsilateral channels are blocked. Patients may therefore require bilateral neck treatment to maximize locoregional control. Lymphatics from the tip of the tongue as from the anterior floor of the mouth may go directly from the submental nodes to the jugulo-omohyoid node at the junction of levels III and IV, thus missing out the submandibular and upper cervical nodes. This factor is extremely important in consideration of neck treatment for tumours at these sites.

Pathology

The vast majority of primary tumours of the oral cavity are squamous cell carcinomas but a variety of other pathological types can occur (Table 11.1). Squamous cancer typically presents as an obvious, exophytic, ulcerated lesion with a greyish necrotic base and an associated margin of induration (Figure 11.3). Other morphological types include the flat, superficial type, the endophytic type that infiltrates deeply, and the verrucous type which is covered with filiform projections. Histologically, the tumour consists of irregular nests, columns or strands of malignant epithelial cells infiltrating subepithelially.

Mucosal melanomas are particularly virulent tumours and are fortunately rare. Men are affected three times as commonly as women, and the palate (Figure 11.4) and gingiva are the commonest sites involved. Roughly a third of cases are preceded by melanosis and therefore, pigmented oral lesions should be carefully followed and biopsied if

Table 11.1 The histology of oral tumours

Mucosa	Squamous cell carcinoma Malignant melanoma
Minor salivary glands	Pleomorphic adenoma Mucoepidermoid tumours Adenoid cystic carcinoma Acinic cell tumours Other adenocarcinomas
Tumours of the bone	Giant cell lesions 'Reparative' granuloma 'Brown tumours' of hyperparathyroidism Giant cell tumour of bone Fibro-osseous lesions Fibrous dysplasia Ossifying fibroma Periapical cemental dysplasia ('cementoma') Chondrogenic neoplasms Chondroma Chondrosacroma Osteoid osteoma and osteoblastoma Cementoblastoma Ameloblastoma Osteogenic sarcoma Other tumours Histiocytosis X Primary lymphoma Multiple myeloma Ewing's sarcoma
Other neoplasms	Malignant lymphoma Burkitt's lymphoma Soft tissue sarcoma Kaposi's sarcoma Carcinosarcoma
Metastatic tumours	

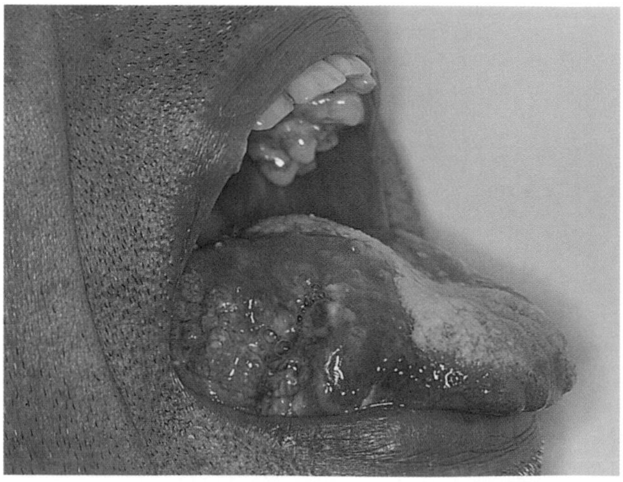

Figure 11.3 Squamous cell carcinoma of the tongue.

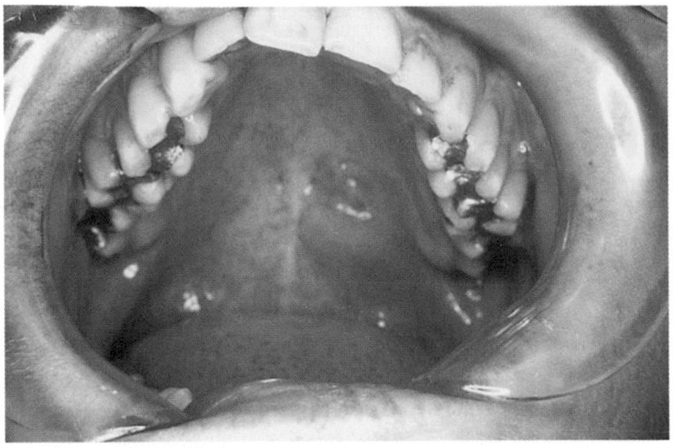

Figure 11.4 Malignant melanoma of the soft palate.

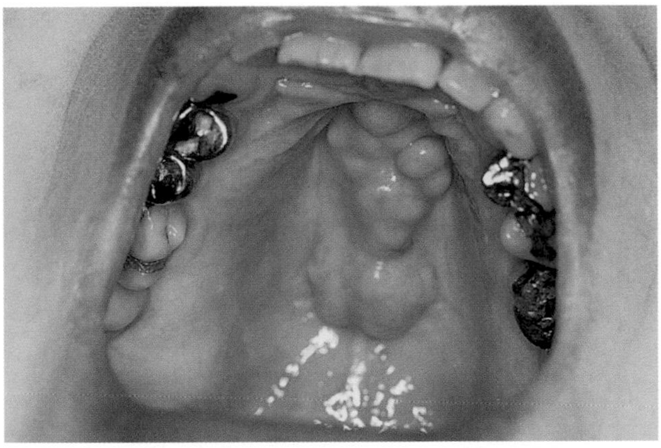

Figure 11.5 Pleomorphic adenoma arising from the minor salivary glands of the hard palate.

appropriate. Early diagnosis is often difficult, and the gross appearance can vary from a typically pigmented lesion to a non-pigmented, soft vascular tumour. Histological diagnosis of difficult cases may be aided by immunohistochemical demonstration of S100 protein.

Minor salivary gland tumours can arise anywhere in the mucosa of the upper aerodigestive tract. The majority of these are malignant but benign tumours do arise occasionally, especially on the hard palate. They appear as rounded masses with a smooth overlying mucosa (Figure 11.5) and may be confused with more benign swellings, for example torus palatinus on the palate (Figure 11.6).

An exceptional degree of interdisciplinary cooperation is required between clinician, radiologist and pathologist for diagnosis of bone tumours and tumour-like conditions. All of the tumours that affect bone elsewhere in the body can also occur in the facial skeleton. Imaging information should be made available to the pathologist as a given histological picture may be interpreted differently

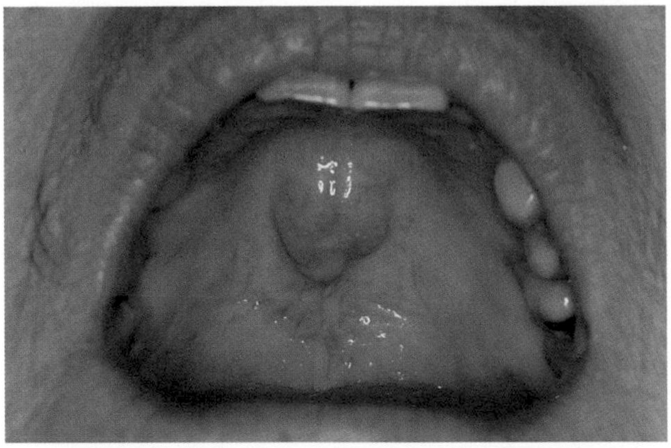

Figure 11.6 Torus palatinus of the hard palate.

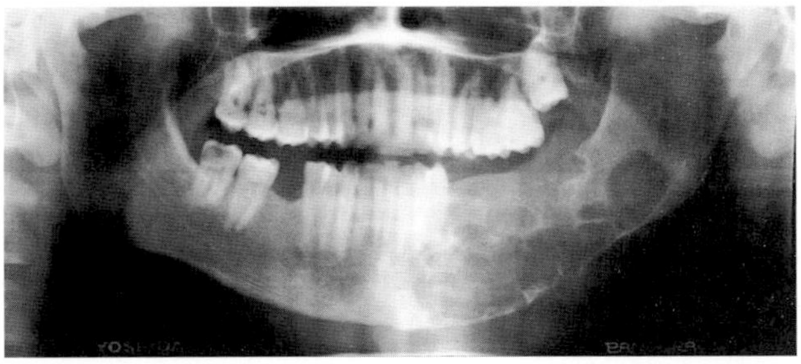

Figure 11.7 Orthopantomogram showing extensive bone destruction from an ameloblastoma of the right mandible.

depending upon its location in the skeleton. Odontogenic tumours of the jaw are derived from the dental soft and hard tissues, and may have a purely epithelial origin, a purely mesenchymal origin, or a mixture of both. The most important of these is the ameloblastoma (Figure 11.7), which is an epithelial neoplasm. The most frequent site of affliction is the molar region of the mandible and these tumours are locally aggressive, often producing extensive bone destruction.

Metastases to soft tissues of the oral cavity are extremely rare (0.1% of all oral malignancy) and arise most commonly from melanomas, breast, lung, or kidney. Metastases to the jaw are more common (1% of all oral malignancy), involve the mandible four times as commonly as the maxilla, and arise most frequently[2] from adenocarcinoma of the breast, prostate, gastrointestinal tract or hypernephroma of the kidney (Figures 11.8).

Epidemiology

The oral cavity ranks only twentieth on the list of cancers in the United Kingdom with approximately 1600 new cases and 850 deaths each year. The

(a)

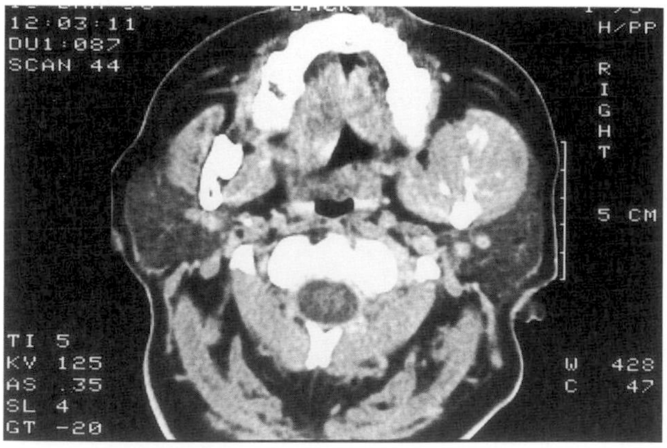

(b)

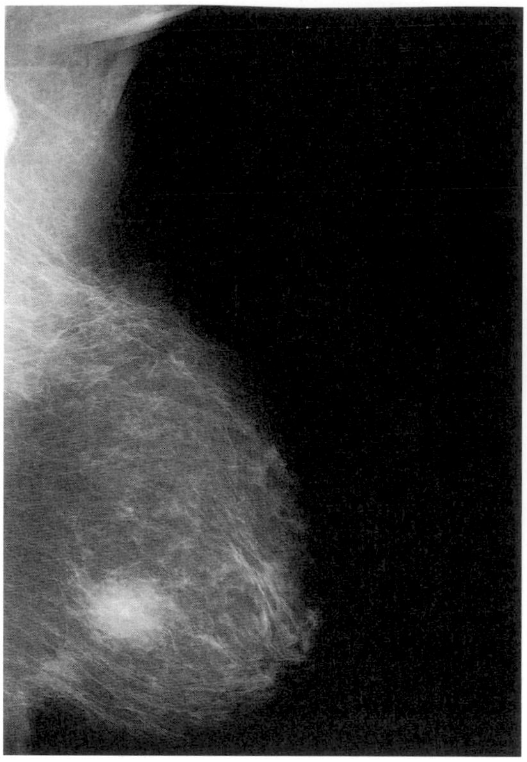

Figure 11.8 (a) CT scan demonstrates extensive osseous metastasis to the ascending ramus of the right mandible. (b) The primary tumour in the breast is clearly seen on mammography.

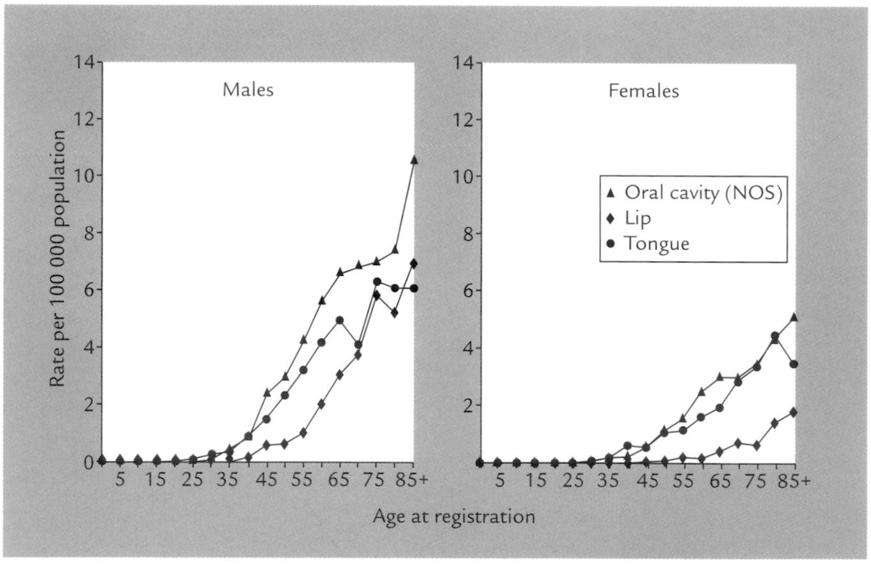

Figure 11.9 Age-specific incidence rates in England and Wales (1985–1987).

incidence and mortality rates have, however, shown an increasing trend in recent decades and oral cancer has the potential to become a more important health problem in the future.

The incidence and mortality rates from oral cancer are higher in Scotland than in England and Wales. While no clear pattern has been shown in Scotland,[3] there is a distinctly higher rate in the north with a north–south gradient in England and Wales.

Age and sex distribution

The incidence increases with age and about 85% of cases in Britain occur after the fifth decade (Figure 11.9) but in poorer countries the age range is much lower and oral cancer is seen in much younger people. The male:female ratio has decreased steadily over recent decades as the incidence rate in men has fallen more sharply relative to that in women. The male:female mortality ratio has similarly come down from 5:1 50 years ago to less than 2:1 at present.

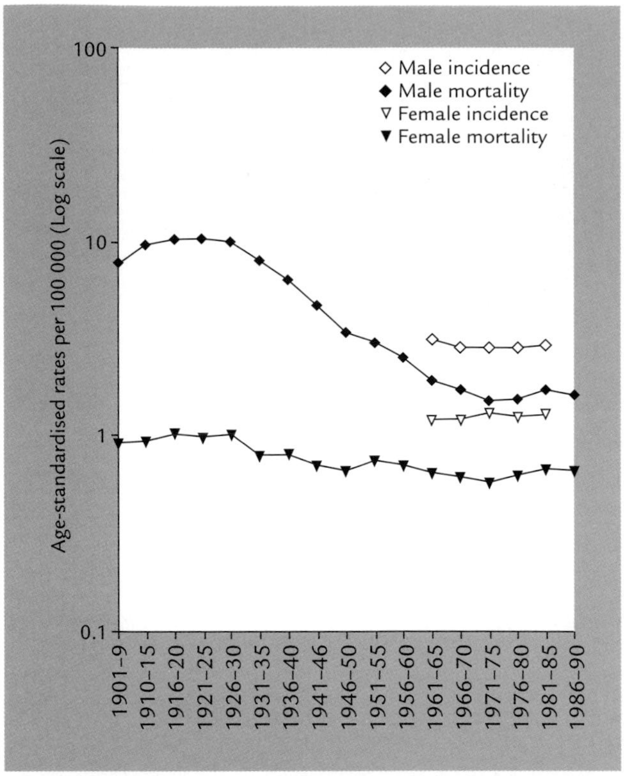

Figure 11.10 The incidence and mortality of oral cancer in England and Wales: 1901–1990.

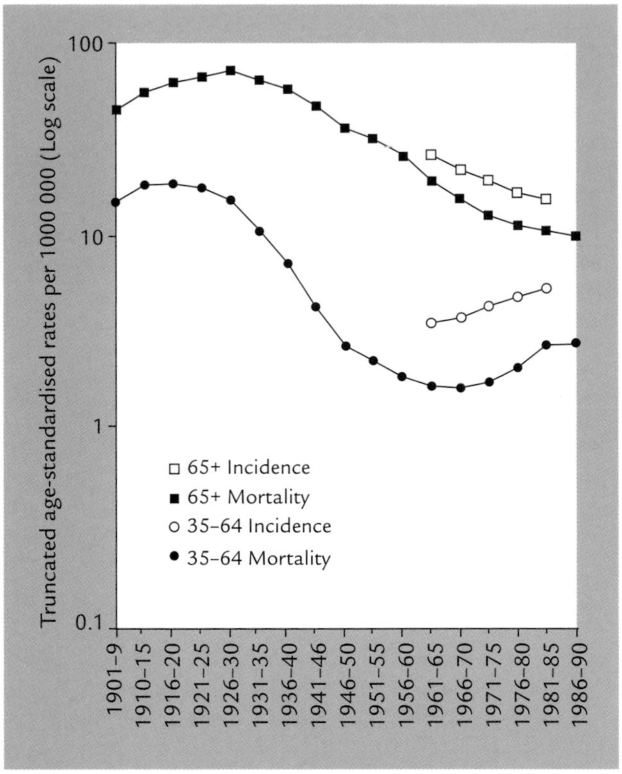

Figure 11.11 Increased incidence and mortality of oral cancer in younger males: England and Wales 1901–1990.

Trends

In England and Wales, although an overall reduction has been reported this century (Figure 11.10), a significant increase in incidence and mortality has been noted in younger males during the last 30 years[4] (Figure 11.11). Smilar trends have been noted in Scotland where the mortality from oral cancer declined until the 1970s. Following this period a substantial increase in both incidence and mortality has been reported in male cohorts born after 1910.[5] A similar increase has been reported from Northern Ireland from a study spanning 14 years.[6] Other European countries have also experienced an upward trend in younger birth cohorts of men,[7] and this has been attributed to increasing levels of alcohol consumption.[8] The role of smokeless tobacco has remained unresolved in the UK and there is no evidence that HIV disease has contributed to the rising incidence in young males.[9] Although the overall mortality from oral cancer in the United States has shown a decline of 19% over recent years, the incidence and survival rates during the same period have reportedly remained steady.[10]

Aetiological factors

The epidemiology of oral cancer reflects the importance of aetiological factors: smoking and alcohol drinking are the major risk factors in Caucasians while betel nut and tobacco consumption have been associated with oral cancer in the Asian section of the population.

Tobacco

A clear dose-response relationship has been demonstrated between tobacco exposure and oral cancer.[11] As many as 34 000 of the 56 000 estimated annual cases of oral cancer in India are thought to be tobacco induced and are therefore potentially avoidable.[12] Cigarette smoking, however, cannot be the sole aetiological factor as only a small percentage of smokers develop oral cancer, and genetic predisposition must be taken into account. Although the precise molecular targets of tobacco have eluded conclusive identification thus far, there is proof that significant tobacco and alcohol use is associated with a high frequency of p53 mutations.[13] Other genetic factors associated with increased risk include mutagen sensitivity,[14] which reflects a defect in DNA repair seen in conditions like xeroderma pigmentosum, Fanconi anaemia and ataxia telangiectasia.

Epidemiological studies from India have correlated the form and method of tobacco consumption to the site of involvement. 'Bidi' smoking (Figure 11.12) has been linked to cancer of the oral commissure and

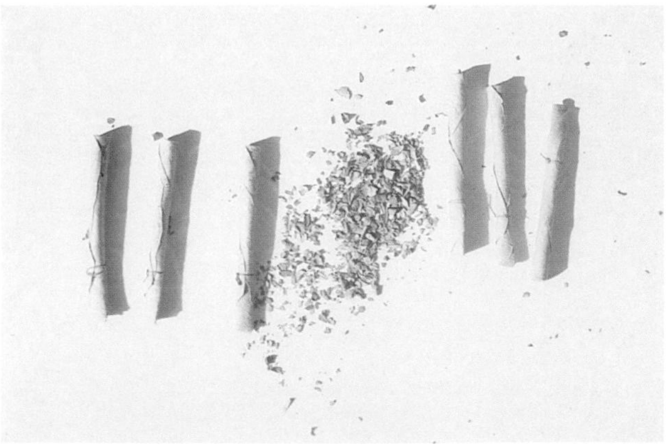

Figure 11.12 The 'bidi' is made of tobacco rolled up in a dried temburni leaf and is the most common form of tobacco use in India.

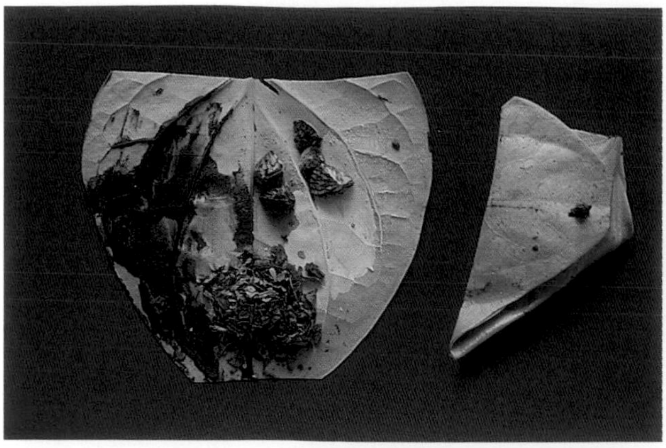

Figure 11.13 'Paan' is a quid of betel leaf (*Piper betel*) which contains areca nut, lime, other aromatic spices and may contain catechu and tobacco.

the tongue. 'Reverse smoking' ('Chutta')[15] is a practice peculiar to parts of India and has been linked with an increase in the incidence of cancer of the hard palate. The habit of chewing 'paan' has been linked to the increased risk of alveolobuccal cancer in the Indian subcontinent (Figure 11.13).[16] Khaini[17] is a mixture of tobacco and lime that is retained in the inferior gingivolabial sulcus and leads to cancer in this site.

Alcohol

There is strong evidence that alcohol acts synergistically with tobacco,[18] most probably because of a topical effect, and mucosal areas exposed to prolonged contact with alcohol are at increased risk. Others have proposed an independent effect,[19] and American[20] as well as French[21] studies have demonstrated a positive correlation of alcohol to oral cancer. This link has not been proved in the UK, probably because of the prohibition of unmatured, pot-stilled spirits containing toxic by-products.[22]

Premalignant lesions

Leukoplakia is a 'white patch or plaque that cannot be characterised clinically or pathologically as any other disease'.[23] It is important to realize that the term has no histological meaning and is often loosely used to imply a premalignant condition.

(i) Homogeneous leukoplakia (leukoplakia simplex)

This is the most common variety and lesions appear as homogeneous, sharply circumscribed, thickened whitish areas broken up by longitudinal fissures (Figure 11.14). They are generally hyperorthokeratotic but can less frequently be hyperparakeratotic on histological examination. Dysplastic changes are seen in only 2–5% of patients. Excision, at least in part may be necessary and after exclusion of risk factors such as smoking and tobacco use, these patients may be satisfactorily managed by follow-up at reasonable intervals along with maintenance of oral hygiene.

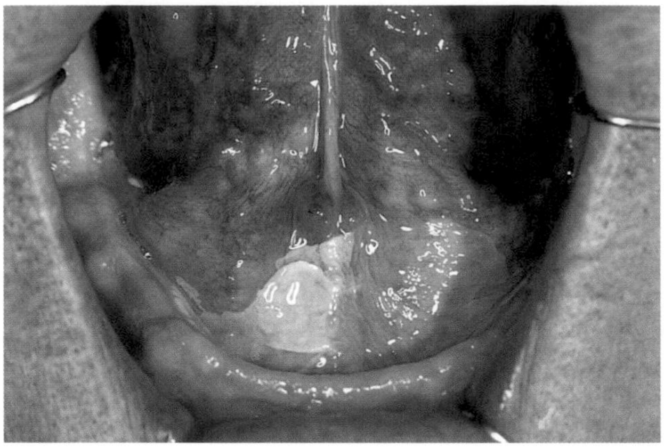

Figure 11.14 Homogenous leukoplakia of the anterior floor of mouth.

(ii) Non-homogeneous leukoplakia

Non-homogeneous leukoplakia can be nodular, speckled (erythroleukoplakia) or verrucous. Nodular and speckled lesions are usually associated with severe epithelial dysplasia and candida infection. Common light microscopic features of these lesions include hyperkeratosis, acanthosis, parakeratosis, widening of rete pegs, dyskeratosis, and carcinoma in situ, which is a term used to signify full thickness involvement of the mucosa by dysplasia. Verrucous leukoplakia has a warty surface and is often associated with dysplasia. This variety can develop into a squamous cell or verrucous carcinoma.

Malignant transformation in leukoplakic lesions
Malignant change in leukoplakia is often seen as thickening of the lesion, ulceration or development of indurated areas. Vital staining using toluidine blue[24] or Lugol's iodine[25] may be useful diagnostic adjuncts, especially in high-risk patients and as a method of ruling out false-negative clinical impressions. Suspicious lesions must be biopsied and in the absence of dysplasia less than 5% of lesions will develop malignant features. The presence of dysplasia, which is characterized by mitoses, pleomorphism, and prominent nucleoli, however, increases this risk to 15–30%.[26] Nodular lesions and lesions in the floor of mouth and the ventral surface of the tongue appear to be at increased risk,[27] as are lesions more than a centimetre in diameter.[28]

Management
Preventive measures include improvement of oral and dental hygiene, balanced diet, and avoidance of tobacco, spicy food and alcohol. Drug therapy may be instituted for treatment of oral candidiasis. The role of retinoids in the prevention of oral cancer remains controversial because of doubtful effectiveness and a low safety index.

Suspicious-looking lesions can be managed by either conventional excision biopsy with split skin grafting for resurfacing the defect or by laser excision.[29]

Regular follow-up of patients is crucial to detecting early carcinomatous change and may also serve to reinforce the implementation of preventative measures.

(iii) Erythroplakia
Erythroplakia is defined as a 'bright red velvety patch that cannot be characterised clinically or pathologically as being caused by any other condition' (Figure 11.15). These lesions are commonly associated with underlying epithelial dysplasia and in the presence of carcinoma in situ, 40% of patients will develop frank malignancy. On the whole malignancy is about 17 times commoner in erythroplakia as compared to leukoplakia.

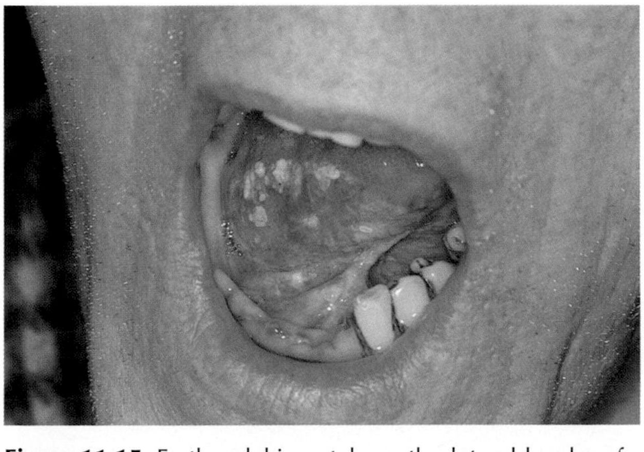

Figure 11.15 Erythroplakic patch on the lateral border of the tongue.

Other factors

A diet deficient in vitamin A is thought to predispose to oral cancer while fruits and vegetables have been found to have a protective effect.[30] Various epidemiological studies have implicated chronic irritation in carcinogenesis. Factors implicated include poor dental hygiene,[23] syphilis, chronic use of mouthwash[31] and marijuana smoking.[32] The herpes simplex virus (HSV-1) has long been suspected but has never been identified within oral cavity carcinoma.[33] Types 2, 11 and 16 of the human papilloma virus[34] have also been associated with oral cancer without conclusive proof. Immunosuppression associated with kidney transplantation and bone marrow transplant has been implicated in the development of oral cancer.[35] HIV-infected patients with AIDS are more prone to Kaposi's sarcoma and non-Hodgkin's lymphoma but squamous cancer can also occur.[36]

Site distribution

The importance of the 'cancer-prone crescent' has been known for several decades and its significance is related to the postulate that most oral cancers should occur in mucosa where saliva pools due to gravity exposing it to salivary carcinogens.[37] Moore and Catlin[38] reported a very interesting analysis of the site distribution of oral cancer in patients from two separate hospitals and showed that roughly 25% of lesions occurred in each of the two 'alveolar-lingual areas' (corresponding to the posterior floor of mouth and adjacent lateral border of tongue), 25% in the anterior floor of mouth, and 25% in the rest of the mouth. The distribution of oral cancer in developing countries is, however, very different and may be explained by certain habits peculiar to that population, for example betel quid chewing which contributes to the high incidence of buccal cancer in the Indian subcontinent (Table 11.2).[39]

Nodal metastases

Lymphatic spread of the tumour from the oral cavity into the neck generally follows a step-wise, orderly and predictable fashion. The lymph node basins of the neck have traditionally been described

Table 11.2 Site distribution in percentage of total cases of oral cancer

	Anterior tongue (%)	Floor of the mouth (%)	Buccal mucosa (%)	Alveolar ridges (%)	Hard palate (%)
United Kingdom	36	←	46	→	
USA[40]	36	35	10	16	3
France[41]	22	68	7	2	1
India[42]	22	4	43	18	3.5

as named groups of nodes but this had led to confusion in comparison of terminology. The Memorial Sloan-Kettering classification is a more precise system of describing the cervical nodes and is now well accepted.[43] The patient with a clinically negative neck is at highest risk of metastasis to levels I–III while about 15% patient with an N^+ neck are at risk of developing metastases at level IV in addition to the upper three levels.[44] Skip metastases to level IV do occur, missing out levels II and III, and are more commonly associated with cancer of the anterior tongue. Metastases to level V are however seen in only about 1% of patients with clinically palpable nodes at other levels and are almost never seen as skip metastases. This understanding of the patterns of nodal metastasis from lesions of the oral cavity has practical implications in the design of neck dissection for patients with oral cancer and these have been outlined elsewhere in this book.

The primary echelons of drainage from alveolar ridge cancers are levels I and II (Figure 11.16), but about 6% of tumours will metastasize to level V. The probability of lymph node metastases is directly related to T stage (70% for T4 with an average of 30%)[45,46] but mandibular ridge cancers have been shown to metastasize more frequently than those of the maxillary ridge.

Tumours of the floor of mouth drain initially to the submental and submandibular nodes (Figure 11.17) and 12–30% of early (T1–T2) lesions will have occult metastases depending upon the thickness of the lesion.[51] The incidence of lymph node metastases in larger lesions (T3–T4) is between 47 and 53%. The floor of the mouth therefore is a high-risk area for cervical nodal metastases and elective treatment of the neck should be considered in the initial management of selected patients.

Carcinoma of the oral tongue has the greatest propensity among all oral cancers for metastasis to the neck. The primary echelon of drainage is level II but other levels may be also involved (Figure 11.18). Depending upon the size of the primary tumour as many as 15–75% of patients will have neck metastases[47,48] and about 25% of patients will have occult nodal metastases at presentation.[51] The incidence of bilateral metastases is 25% while 3% of patients have only contralateral metastases, a pattern that is commoner in tumours that approach or cross the midline. The depth of invasion and tumour thickness seem to be significant predictors of lymph node metastasis.[51,52]

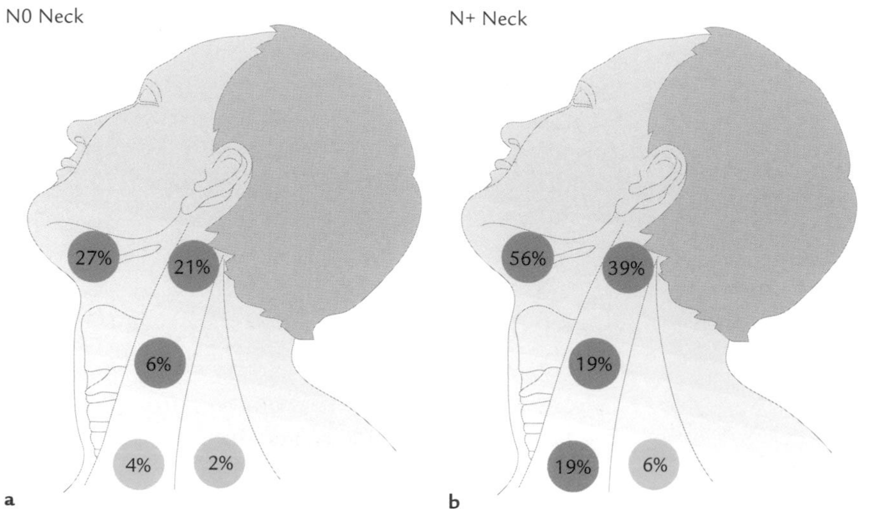

Figure 11.16 (a) Incidence of occult lymph node involvement in the clinically node negative patient with alveolar ridge cancer. (b) Incidence of lymph node metastasis in the clinically node-positive patient with alveolar ridge cancer.

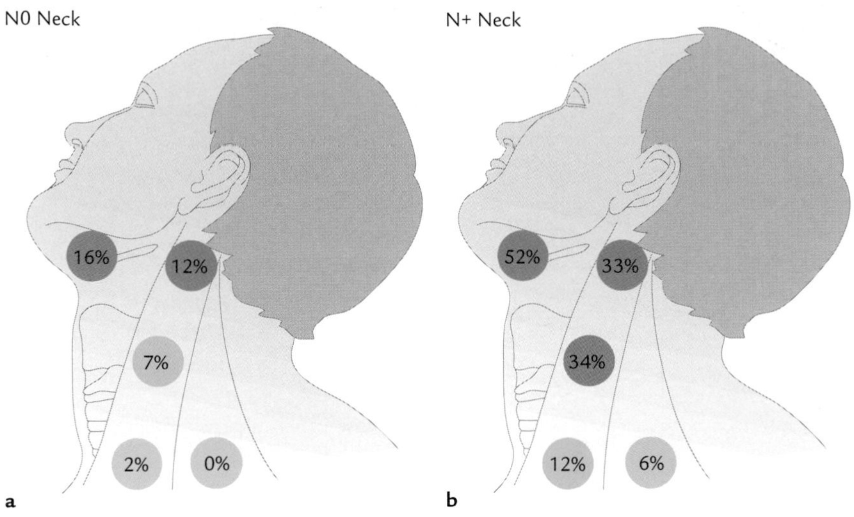

Figure 11.17 (a) Incidence of occult lymph node involvement in the clinically node-negative patient with cancer of the floor of mouth. (b) Incidence of lymph node metastasis in the clinically node-positive patient with cancer of the floor of mouth.

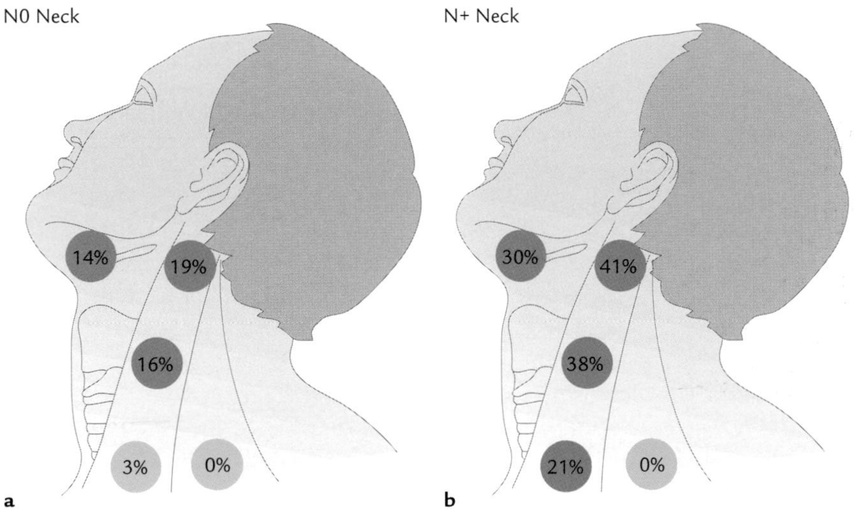

Figure 11.18 (a) Incidence of occult lymph node involvement in the clinically node negative patient with cancer of the oral tongue. (b) Incidence of lymph node metastasis in the clinically node-positive patient with cancer of the oral tongue.

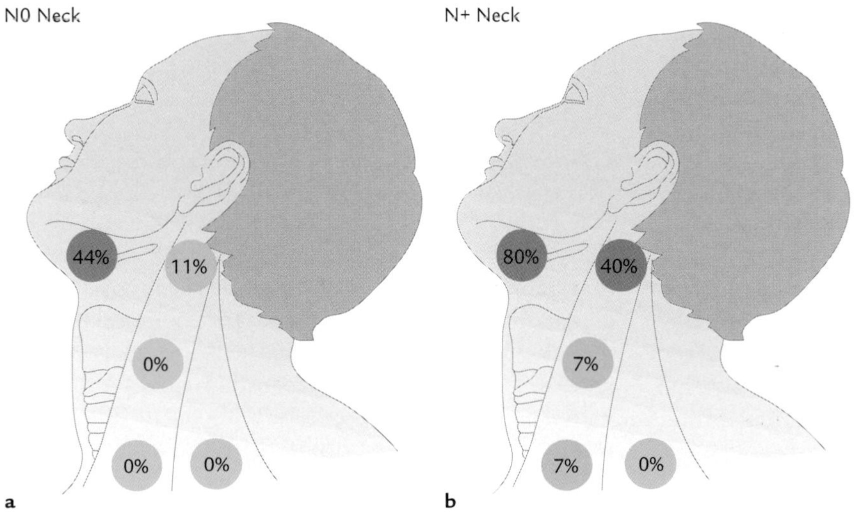

Figure 11.19 (a) Incidence of occult lymph node involvement in the clinically node-negative patient with cancer of the buccal mucosa. (b) Incidence of lymph node metastasis in the clinically node-positive patient with cancer of the buccal mucosa.

Only 10% of patients with buccal cancer have clinically significant neck nodes at presentation. The primary echelons are levels I and II (Figure 11.19). Tumour thickness is a significant prognostic factor: and the 5-year survival has been shown to be significantly better in tumours less than 6 mm thick as compared to deeper tumours.[49]

Table 11.3 Staging of primary tumour (T)

TX	Primary tumour cannot be assessed
T0	No evidence of primary tumour
Tis	Carcinoma in situ
T1	Tumour 2 cm or less in greatest dimension
T2	Tumour more than 2 cm but not more than 4 cm in greatest dimension
T3	Tumour more than 4 cm in greatest dimension
T4 (lip)	Tumour invades adjacent structures e.g., through cortical bone, inferior alveolar nerve, floor of mouth, skin of face
T4 (oral cavity)	Tumour invades adjacent structures e.g., through cortical bone, into deep (extrinsic) muscle of tongue, maxillary sinus, skin. (Superficial erosion alone of bone/tooth socket by gingival primary is not sufficient to classify a tumour as T4)

Table 11.4 Staging of regional lymph nodes (N)

NX	Regional lymph nodes cannot be assessed
N0	No regional lymph node metastasis
N1	Metastasis in a single ipsilateral lymph node, 3 cm or less in greatest dimension
N2a	Metastasis in a single ipsilateral lymph node more than 3 cm but not more than 6 cm in greatest dimension
N2b	Metastasis in multiple ipsilateral lymph nodes, none more than 6 cm in greatest dimension
N2c	Metastasis in bilateral or contralateral lymph nodes, none more than 6 cm in greatest dimension
N3	Metastasis in a lymph node more than 6 cm in greatest dimension

Note: Midline nodes are ipsilateral nodes

Table 11.5 Staging of distant metastases (M)

MX	Presence of distant metastases cannot be assessed
M0	No distant metastases
M1	Distant metastases

Table 11.6 Stage grouping of oral cancer

Stage I	T1N0M0
Stage II	T2N0M0
Stage III	T3N0M0
	T3N1M0
Stage IV	T1–3N2M0
	Any T, N3, M0
	Any T, Any N, M1

TNM staging

The clinical staging of a particular tumour consists of staging the primary tumour (Table 11.3), the neck (Table 11.4), and assessment for distant metastases (Table 11.5). This information can then be assimilated and a TNM stage grouping for the tumour is derived (Table 11.6).[50]

Although the TNM system is useful for comparing outcome after treatment with various modalities in tumours of similar severity, it is far from perfect as a prognostic indicator for individual patients. One of its major limitations is that it fails to take into consideration the prognostic implications of the third dimension or depth of invasion of the primary tumour. This aspect of tumour spread has been shown in various studies[51,52] to be a more reliable predictor of cervical nodal metastasis than the conventional T stage, especially for tumours of the tongue. However, until better prognosticators are available, the TNM system will continue to be the standard language of communication among clinicians treating oral and other cancers.

The biology and natural history of oral squamous cell carcinoma

Over four decades ago, Slaughter et al[53] hypothesized the role of 'field cancerization' in the aetiology of oral cancer. Their theory was based on the premise that an inherent instability of the mucosa of the entire upper aerodigestive tract combined with repeated carcinogenic insults leads to an increased risk of developing multiple independent premalignant and malignant foci. Until recently this theory was only indirectly supported by the observation of the high incidence of second primary tumours in patients with oral cancer. With advances in our understanding of tumour biology and molecular biology, there is now evidence to support this hypothesis.

Oral carcinogenesis appears to evolve through a complex, multistage process involving biomolecular changes that precede premalignant lesions which in turn precede invasive cancer. The exact sequence of events in human oral carcinogenesis has not yet been accurately mapped out and the following is only a synopsis of our current understanding of this complex process.

The genetic changes caused by exposure to carcinogens like tobacco and alcohol tend to accumulate over time in the entire mucosa exposed to this insult. Clonal malignant foci, however, develop only in specific sites where tumorigenesis is possible. The fundamental genetic events associated with carcinogenesis have not yet been established but several non-random chromosomal alterations such as those in chromosomes 1, 3, 5, 7, 8, 9, 10, 11, 13 and 17 have been identified.[54] The carcinogen-containing environment that initiated tumorigenesis also affects the adjacent tissue, and loss of heterozygosity and other chromosomal abnormalities have been demonstrated in this histologically normal tissue lending support to the field cancerization theory.[55]

The fundamental regulatory mechanism in carcinogenesis is thought to be the cellular balance between oncogenes and tumour suppressor genes. The proto-oncogenes stimulate cell growth and proliferation, and are under negative control of the tumour suppressor genes, which prevent overgrowth. A cancer may therefore arise either from activation of a proto-oncogene or due to loss of a tumour suppressor gene. Uncontrolled cell growth can be caused by only a single mutation of an oncogene, but deletion or mutation of both alleles of a tumour suppressor gene is necessary for the same effect. Numerous genetic events are required to cause a cancer, but the most frequently observed molecular abnormality is mutation of the p53 tumour suppressor gene which is seen in 40–70% of malignant lesions[56] and 20% of premalignant lesions.[57] Several other oncogenes and tumour suppressor genes have been studied but no clear relationship has been demonstrated with phenotypic behaviour or survival.

Once the cancer has developed, its phenotypic behaviour is dependent on complex microenvironmental and biologic systems. The capability of a tumour to invade and metastasize depends on its production of degradative enzymes, for example collagenase, plasminogen activators like urokinase, and cathepsin, as well as angiogenic factors, growth factors, cytokines, receptors, cell-surface properties and motility factors. The tumour milieu is also influenced by host factors such as stromal cells, nerve fibres and tumour-associated and tumour-infiltrating lymphocytes.

The tumour then increases in size both horizontally and vertically to invade adjacent and deep structures. It may present as a local mass, producing symptoms such as pain, airway obstruction, infection and haemorrhage, cranial nerve involvement secondary to invasion or fungation with fistula formation. Later on in the course of the disease there is invasion of the lymphatics leading to locoregional disease and usually late in the sequence there may be disseminated metastasis. Death is most commonly related to the effects of locoregional disease either due to direct invasion of vital structures or large nodal masses producing catastrophic haemorrhage.

Clinical presentation

Symptoms

Despite the fact that the oral cavity is an easily accessible site for both the patient and the physician, a surprisingly large number of oral tumours present late because of the painless and rather vague nature of the symptomatology. The relatively phlegmatic personality types associated with the major risk factors related to the disease may also contribute to the relatively advanced stage at presentation.

Tumours of the alveolar ridge commonly present with pain while chewing but patients may present with intermittent bleeding, loose teeth and edentulous patients may complain of ill-fitting dentures. The development of symptoms such as trismus and altered sensation or anaesthesia of the lower teeth and lip from involvement of the mandibular canal and the inferior alveolar nerve signify locally advanced disease.

Lesions in the floor of mouth are typically painful, infiltrative lesions that extend to invade bone anteriorly, muscles of the floor of mouth deeply or tongue posteriorly. Patients often complain of 'food getting trapped under the tongue.' Early spread to the alveolus and periosteum of the mandible is common; clinical fixation of the tumour to the mandible indicates periosteal involvement and direct bone invasion may be present in a high number of cases.

Tumours of the oral tongue usually start as a small ulcer that gradually infiltrates the musculature of the tongue until its normal motility is lost. An early lesion may appear as a small granular excrescence, which may arouse suspicion only because of a subtle difference from surrounding normal mucosa or because of the patient's anxiety about the nature of the lesion. More advanced tumours present either as exophytic or ulcerative lesions, which are usually quite evident.

Endophytic infiltrative lesions, however, may be more difficult to recognize and their extent may not be apparent until an adequate evaluation under a general anaesthetic is carried out. Patients may be aware of a difficulty swallowing or speaking, which becomes even more pronounced when the tumour spreads to the floor of the mouth. Cancer of the tongue is generally painful even in its early stage but lesions can be painless and this feature may contribute to a considerable delay in diagnosis. Any painful ulcer in the oral cavity that fails to heal within a week after a suspected irritant has been eliminated must be investigated by a biopsy. As the disease progresses the lesion may be the cause of an excruciating pain which may radiate to the neck or the ear. Cervical lymph node metastases occur early in the course of the disease and an occasional patient may present with a lump in the neck.

Buccal mucosal cancer, like that of the gums, is commoner in developing countries as a consequence of peculiar patterns of tobacco abuse amongst the population. Lesions may be papillary or erosive and are often located near the dental occlusal line where they are more likely to be traumatized. Leukoplakia of the surrounding mucosa may be a striking feature. Buccal cancers are more frequently exophytic than other oral cancers but they rarely present as T1 tumours because pain is not a prominent symptom. The presence of trismus indicates extension into pterygoid musculature and signifies locally advanced disease.

Physical examination

There should be a thorough examination of the lesion and the rest of the upper aerodigestive tract. Line drawings and photographic records of the tumour are extremely useful and provide a baseline for comparison on later occasions. A TNM-staged record at original examination is similarly essential and may incorporate information from further staging investigations.

Investigation

Radiological investigations including orthopantomogram, CT and MRI examination of the primary tumour and neck can provide valuable information, which must be used to stage the disease accurately. Imaging of bone may be necessary to detect involvement by the tumour or for planning surgical treatment, and is discussed later in this chapter.

Most accessible lesions may be adequately biopsied in the clinic, but thorough examination under general anaesthesia (EUA) offers the optimal conditions for assessment of the depth of invasion, tumour biopsy, and palpation of neck nodes. The value of routine panendoscopy of all upper aerodigestive tract mucosa for assessment of second primary tumours is doubtful and should probably be reserved for investigation of symptoms in high-risk individuals. Biopsy may be achieved with a knife, punch biopsy forceps, trucut needle or fine-needle aspiration. Each technique has its protagonists and each has its disadvantages extending from crush artefact to the potential risk of tumour seeding as a result of the biopsy technique. The clinician and the histologist are usually able to arrive at a protocol that suits their own and the patient's circumstances.

Occasionally a patient with an asymptomatic primary tumour may present with a neck node mass. Open neck node biopsy should only be used as an option of last resort when no primary can be found after examination of the entire upper aerodigestive tract under a general anaesthetic and when fine-needle aspiration cytology has proven unhelpful. Neck node sampling may compromise an adequate neck dissection in definitive management and should be reserved for the diagnosis of lymphoma when fine needle aspiration cytology suggests this as a diagnostic possibility.

Multidisciplinary clinic

The team approach to treatment planning cannot be overemphasized and a combined clinic with physicians, surgeons, radiotherapists, medical oncologists, nurses, dieticians, physiotherapy and rehabilitation staff is of great importance. In addition to allowing time to collate all clinical and investigational data the pretreatment phase allows discussion between doctor and patient and also with all those potentially involved in the future management of the patient including family, friends and other healthcare professionals. The emotional and spiritual needs of the patient must also be given due weight in this phase. The diagnosis and treatment plan are now explained carefully and clearly to the patient in terms that he or she can understand. It is also important that the patient realizes the potential for failure of treatment and that management of complications of treatment may require staged procedures over a long period of time, so that informed consent can be obtained.

Cessation of smoking in the period leading up to treatment, especially major surgery, is important in minimizing complications. In addition, a prospective study[58] has shown the adverse prognostic effect of continued tobacco consumption and advice to stop smoking is essential both from a prophylactic as well as from a therapeutic point of view.

For some patients, notably those with advanced disease or underlying medical conditions that militate against optimal treatment, non-standard treatment regimens must be entertained; options including clinical trials, supportive treatment, or even of no treatment at all other than supportive or palliative care may be discussed.

Treatment: general principles

Treatment of squamous carcinoma of the oral cavity is in general either by surgery or by radiation alone or in combination. Chemotherapy and new immunologically based treatment protocols are at the moment reserved for patients with what is considered to be incurable disease in normal terms or for those patients in whom conventional treatment has failed.

The choice of the best initial therapy for a particular patient must take into account a variety of interrelated factors (Figure 11.20). As with most other cancers, only a very general policy of treatment selection can be outlined, and the management of each patient must be tailored individually.

The chronological age by itself should not be a deterrent to aggressive treatment. Rather, the risk of treatment should be assessed based on intercurrent conditions, cardiopulmonary status and other factors. The patient's enthusiasm and acceptance of a particular plan of management also need to be taken into account. Treatment decisions may be influenced by the patient's lifestyle (i.e. unwillingness to give up smoking and alcohol) and by their occupation and socioeconomic status.

A multidisciplinary team approach is absolutely essential to ensure a favourable outcome and expertise in various medical specialties should be available to the head and neck unit. Physical and psychological support services play a vital role in posttreatment rehabilitation, which should be seamlessly integrated with overall management and with care in the community.

As single modality treatment using either radiation or surgery offers comparable control rates for early lesions (T1–2), other factors including functional results, compliance of the patient, cost of treatment and long-term sequelae must be considered. For more advanced lesions (stage III and IV), primary surgery followed by postoperative radiation therapy is generally accepted as standard treatment.

Treatment: surgical management

Surgical excision is one of the two mainstays of locoregional treatment of oral cancer. It allows histopathological assessment of the clearance margins of the tumour together with further information regarding tumour spread and dynamics. Considerable controversy has been generated in

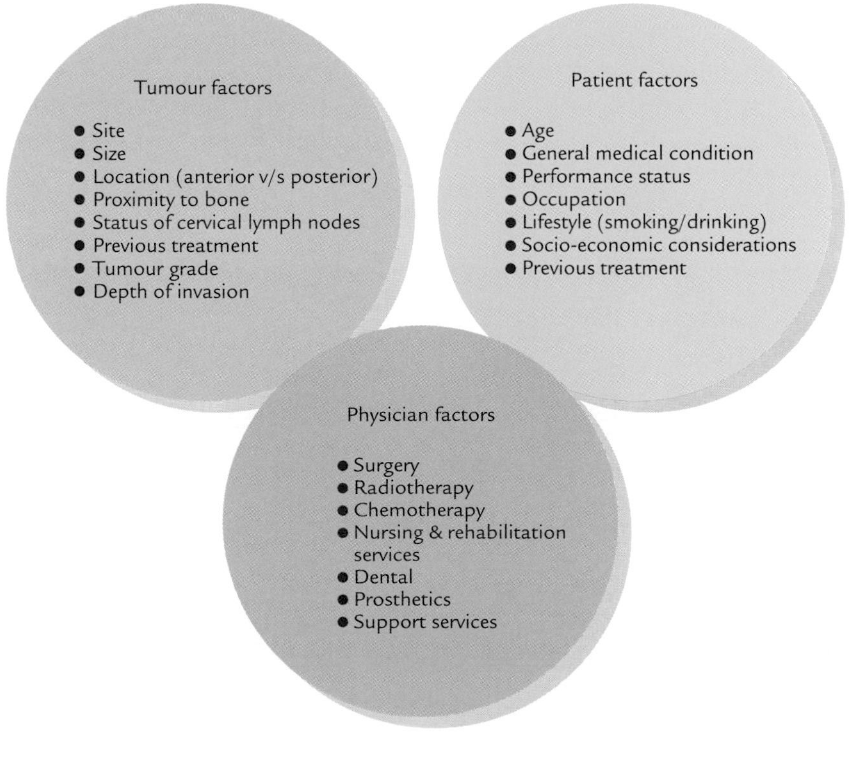

Figure 11.20 Factors determining the choice of initial treatment.

recent years over the comparison of results of surgery with radiation and it is important to choose the modality best suited to the individual patient.

A detailed description of operative procedures for cancer of the oral cavity is outside the scope of this chapter but some general principles are outlined below.

Access to the oral cavity

A detailed and meticulous examination, often under anaesthetic, must be undertaken before deciding the choice of surgical approach. Small, superficial, anteriorly located tumours can be easily resected per orally. Larger, infiltrative lesions, and those located more posteriorly will require more extensive surgical exposure using techniques such as cheek flaps or mandibulotomy. Some form of neck dissection is now regarded as mandatory except perhaps for the most superficial T1 lesion. This can be carried out either as an en bloc procedure or via a separate neck incision.

Transoral excision

Premalignant lesions and small, superficial tumours of the anterior floor of mouth, alveolus and tongue may be resected through the open mouth. (Figure 11.21). The ability to use this approach also depends on how wide the patient's mouth can be opened under anaesthetic as well as on other physical factors like the transverse diameter of the oral commissure and the size of the tongue. In general, one of the other more extensive approaches must be used if there is any doubt about the adequacy of surgical exposure. Laser vaporization may be used for superficial premalignant lesions but all other lesions must be excised using palpation to achieve adequate resection margins.

Cheek flaps

Tumours of the posterior oral cavity are not easily accessible transorally, and a cheek flap may give more adequate exposure in appropriate cases. An upper cheek flap is raised using a median upper lip split and carrying the incision around the nose with the corresponding mucosal incision in the upper gingivobuccal sulcus. The lower cheek flap requires a midline lip split that continues over the chin into the neck. The flap is raised subplatysmally but great care must be exercised not to strip the periosteum off the mandible. Accurate replacement of a cheek flap is facilitated by leaving a substantial mucosal cuff on the alveolar side. A midfacial degloving flap through bilateral gingivobuccal incisions is preferable in appropriate cases as this avoids midfacial scars. A visor flap can give access to both sides of the neck and avoids splitting the lip, but adequate mobilization results in division of both mental nerves with anaesthesia of the lip.

Mandibulotomy

Larger tumours of the lateral border of the tongue or those involving or extending onto the floor of the mouth may occasionally be resected transorally with a separate neck dissection approach but most require a lip-splitting mandibulotomy approach. Similarly, adequate surgical exposure of tumours located in the posterior oral cavity may be obtained using a mandibulotomy. The technical aspects of mandibulotomy have been discussed in Chapter 13.

Management of the mandible

Mechanism of invasion of the mandible

Tumours of the floor of the mouth, the ventral surface of the tongue and the gingivobuccal sulcus spread along the mucosa and submucosa to the adjacent gingiva. The mechanism of invasion of

(a)

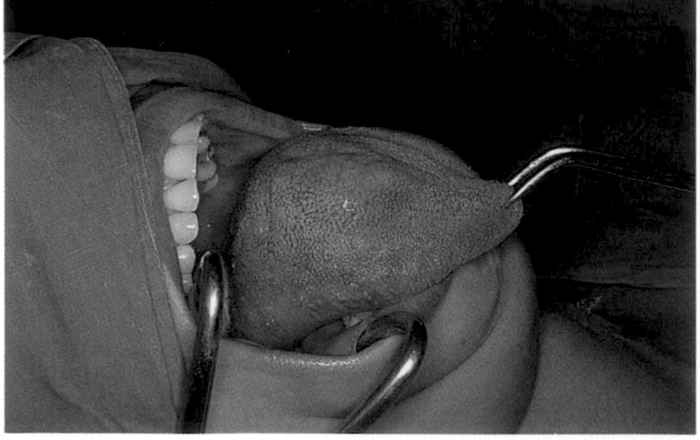

(b)

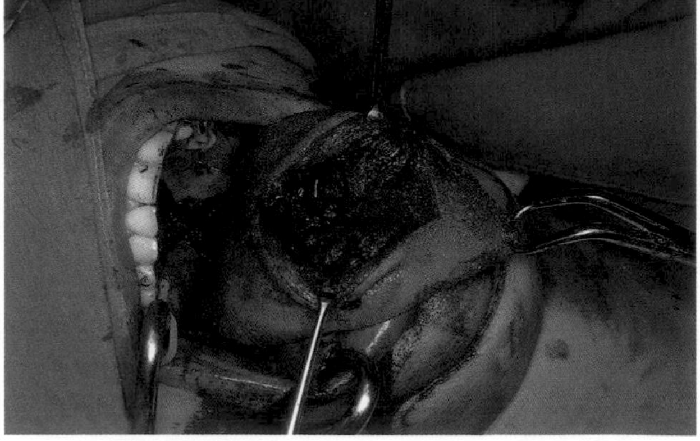

Figure 11.21 Transoral excision of a tongue tumour: (a) pre-excision; (b) postexcision.

these tumours into the mandible has been established[59,60] and we know that periosteum acts as a deterrent to mandibular invasion.[61] Apart from the obvious implication of upstaging of the tumour with bony invasion, involvement of the mandible increases the risk of invasion of the inferior alveolar nerve within the mandibular canal, and raises the possibility of perineural spread of the tumour towards the base of the skull. Figure 11.22 shows that in the dentate mandible, tumour creeps up from the gingiva, through the dental socket into the cancellous bone. In contrast, the edentulous mandible offers much less resistance and tumour invasion of cancellous bone occurs through the dental pores of the alveolar process (Figure 11.23).

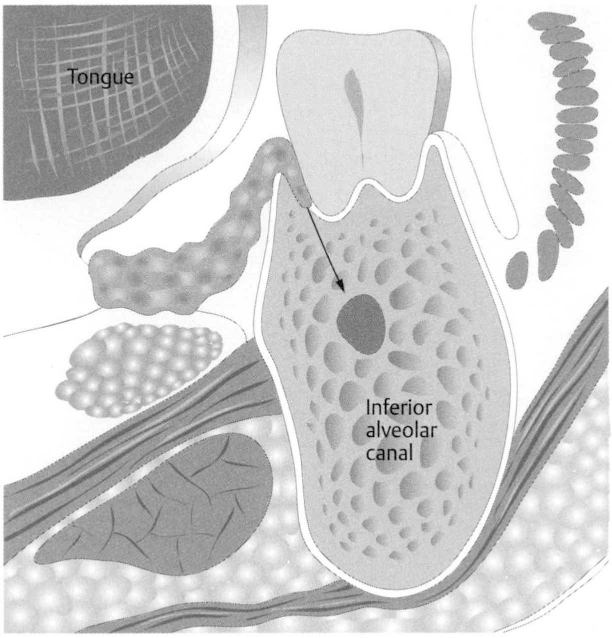

Figure 11.22 Route of mandibular invasion in the dentate mandible.

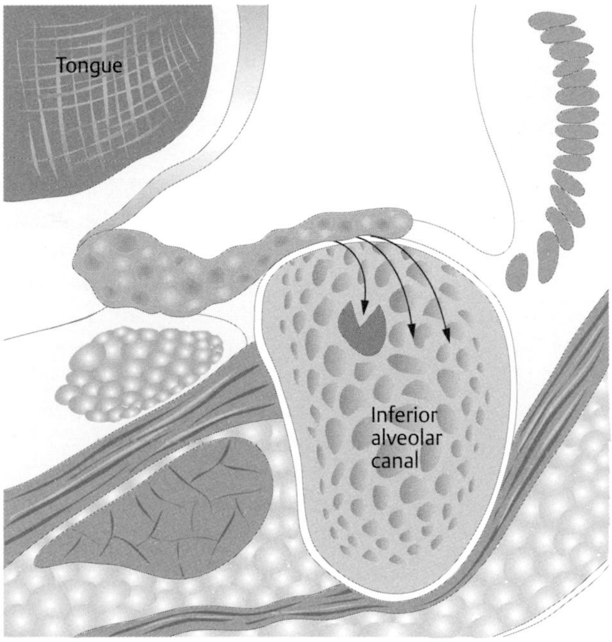

Figure 11.23 Route of mandibular invasion in the edentulous mandible.

Assessment of bony invasion

Early cortical invasion of the mandible is extremely difficult to image radiographically even with modern technology. A number of radiological investigations are available: plain radiography, cephalometric orthognathic films, orthopantomogram (OPG), dental occlusal films, radionuclide bone scans, CT scans, MR imaging and PET scans. The accuracy of conventional radiography in detecting early invasion is limited by the fact that 30–50% mineral loss must occur before the changes are radiologically apparent. The OPG (Figure 11.24) is currently the first line investigation but early invasion of the lingual cortex, especially in the region of the mental symphysis, may not be evident and intraoral dental films are indicated in patients with anterior floor of mouth lesions. Although its accuracy in demonstrating bone invasion in edentulous patients has been reported,[62] the accuracy of CT scanning in routine assessment of bony invasion is limited by artefacts produced by irregular dental sockets, other dental artefacts and by patient motion. However, 1:1 reconstruction of axial images may be useful in fabricating templates for planning accurate bony microvascular reconstruction. Computerized tomography multiplanar reformation (CT/MPR or Dentascan) is a computer software technique that uses information from CT scan slices to generate true cross-sectional images and panoramic views of the mandible and maxilla.[63] The oblique sagittal view on Dentascan reportedly allows accurate evaluation of both buccal and lingual cortical bone margins as well as clear visualization of the incisive and inferior alveolar canals.[64] The role of MR has also been investigated and reports indicate that while a negative study virtually excludes periosteal or cortical involvement, the overall usefulness of this investigation is hampered by the high rate of false-positive results in dental infections, previously irradiated mandibles and in osteoradionecrosis.[65] Bone scans, for example ^{99m}Tc-labelled diphosphonate are not specific and suffer from a high rate of false-positive results due to infections and inflammatory processes.[66] Overall,

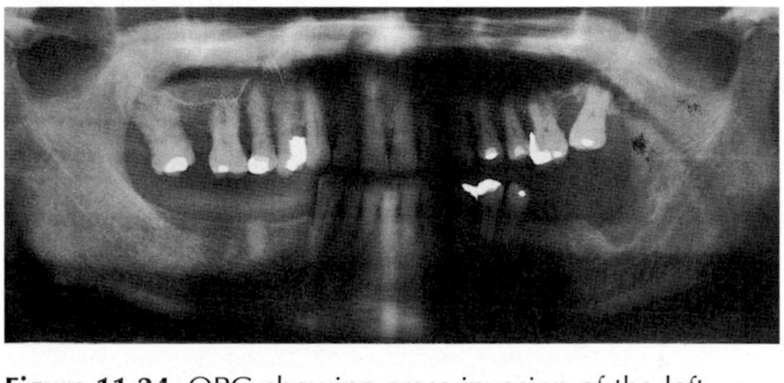

Figure 11.24 OPG showing gross invasion of the left mandible.

Table 11.7 Indications for marginal mandibulectomy

Primary tumour abutting against the mandible
Minimal involvement of the alveolar process
Minimal cortical erosion

clinical evaluation has been shown to be reliable in assessment of early bony invasion[67] but radiological investigation must be ordered if any form of bone resection and reconstruction are planned.

Marginal resection of the mandible

The understanding of tumour invasion into mandible enables the use of marginal resection of bone (Table 11.7) based on the observation that the cortical part of the bone containing the mandibular canal lies inferior to the dental roots and remains relatively uninvolved in early stage disease, and can be safely spared.

In practical terms, however, the ability to perform a marginal mandibulectomy in a given patient depends upon the vertical height of the body of the mandible (Figure 11.25). Resorption of the mandible with age results in recession of the alveolar process and the mandibular canal with the inferior alveolar nerve is at increased risk of involvement in these patients. Marginal resection in edentulous patients is fraught with danger as the residual bone is very liable to iatrogenic or spontaneous fracture. The risk of fracture after marginal resection can be minimized by using smooth, rounded cuts because sharp angles tend to concentrate the forces of stress and increase the chances of fracture (Figure 11.26).

Adequate tumour clearance in edentulous patients may necessitate a segmental mandibulectomy. Marginal mandibular resection is also best avoided in previously irradiated patients because of the more variable routes of tumour entry and multiple foci of tumour invasion coupled with the high risk of osteoradionecrosis. The indications of segmental resection are listed in Table 11.8, and resection of the normal

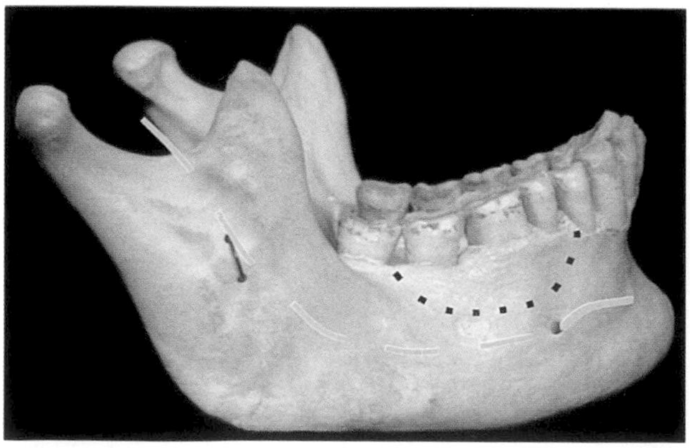

Figure 11.25 Significance of the vertical height of the mandible in relation to the mandibular canal.

Table 11.8 Indications for segmental mandibulectomy

Invasion of the mandibular canal and inferior alveolar nerve
Gross invasion of the mandible
Primary mandibular osseous tumour
Metastatic tumour to the mandible

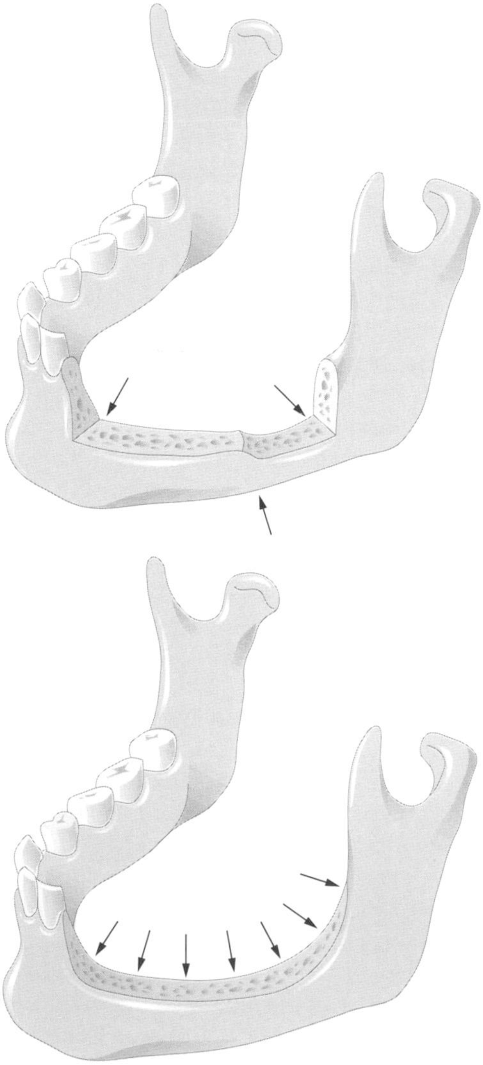

Figure 11.26 Sharp bony cuts in the mandible tend to concentrate the forces of stress and increase the chance of fracture after marginal resection. In contrast, a smooth, rounded resection distributes these forces more evenly and the residual mandible is therefore more resistant to fracture.

Table 11.9 Risk factors for nodal metastasis in patients with oral cancer

	High risk	Low risk
Subsite of the primary	Tongue and floor of mouth	Hard palate and lips
T stage	Advanced stage (T3–4)	Early stage (T1–2)
Depth of invasion	> 8 mm	< 2 mm
Histological grade	High grade	Low grade
Morphology of the primary tumour*	Infiltrative	Exophytic or verrucous Flat superficial
Other histopathological features*	Lymphatic permeation Vascular invasion Perineural invasion Invading front of tumour	Lymphocytic infiltration Pushing front of tumour

*These factors have not been shown to be statistically predictive of lymph node metastasis

uninvolved mandible to accomplish an en bloc resection can no longer be justified in view of the realization that there are no lymphatic channels passing through the mandible.

Management of the neck

The management of cervical lymph node metastases in the patient with head and neck cancer has been described in Chapter 16 but this section is a concise discussion of the problem with particular emphasis on oral cancer.

It is well known that although 60–70% of patients with early stage oral cancer will present with a clinically negative neck (N0), approximately 20–30% will have occult nodal metastasis if subjected to an elective neck dissection. Furthermore, about 30–50% of patients will eventually develop neck metastases during the course of their disease. It is also well recognized that metastasis to the cervical lymph nodes is the single most important prognostic factor in patients with head and neck cancer. The presence of a metastatic cervical node in a patient with oral cancer decreases the chance of cure by 50% when compared to those with similar primary tumours without nodal metastases.[68] It therefore follows that management of the neck is a crucial and integral part of overall management of the patient with oral cancer. Primaries at certain subsites such as the oral tongue and the floor of the mouth are more liable to metastasize to the neck, and prophylactic treatment of the neck should be considered in their initial management. Tumours at other sites such as the hard palate, the upper alveolus and the lips have a low rate of occult nodal metastasis and elective treatment of the neck may not be necessary in these patients.[69] The risk of nodal metastasis is related to several factors (Table 11.9) and these must be taken into consideration in planning of neck treatment.

If a decision is taken to treat the neck, a neck dissection is carried out when the treatment of the primary is surgical, especially when the neck has to be accessed for reconstruction of the primary defect. If the primary is being treated with irradiation, the neck can be included in the treatment plan. Only very rarely do the primary tumour and the neck need to be treated using different modalities.

Selection of the type of neck dissection

As described earlier, metastasis to the neck from an oral primary generally occurs in an orderly and predictable manner, most often involving levels I through III. In a patient with a clinically negative neck, the risk of metastasis to levels IV and V is very small and a supraomohyoid neck dissection (SOHND) would therefore adequately address the neck in these patients. For similar patients with tongue primaries, inclusion of level IV in the dissection is probably justified in view of the higher incidence of skip metastases. When a SOHND is carried out, suspicious nodes are sent for frozen section analysis and if positive, the modified radical neck dissection is completed (i.e. levels IV and V are removed) via a separate lower neck incision. A treatment policy combining SOHND with radiation therapy when indicated has resulted in failure rates of less than 10% in patients with clinically N0 necks.[70,71] While recognizing that each patient needs to be managed on an individual basis, our general policy of action if occult metastases are found on histopathological examination of the neck dissection specimen is outlined in Figure 11.27.

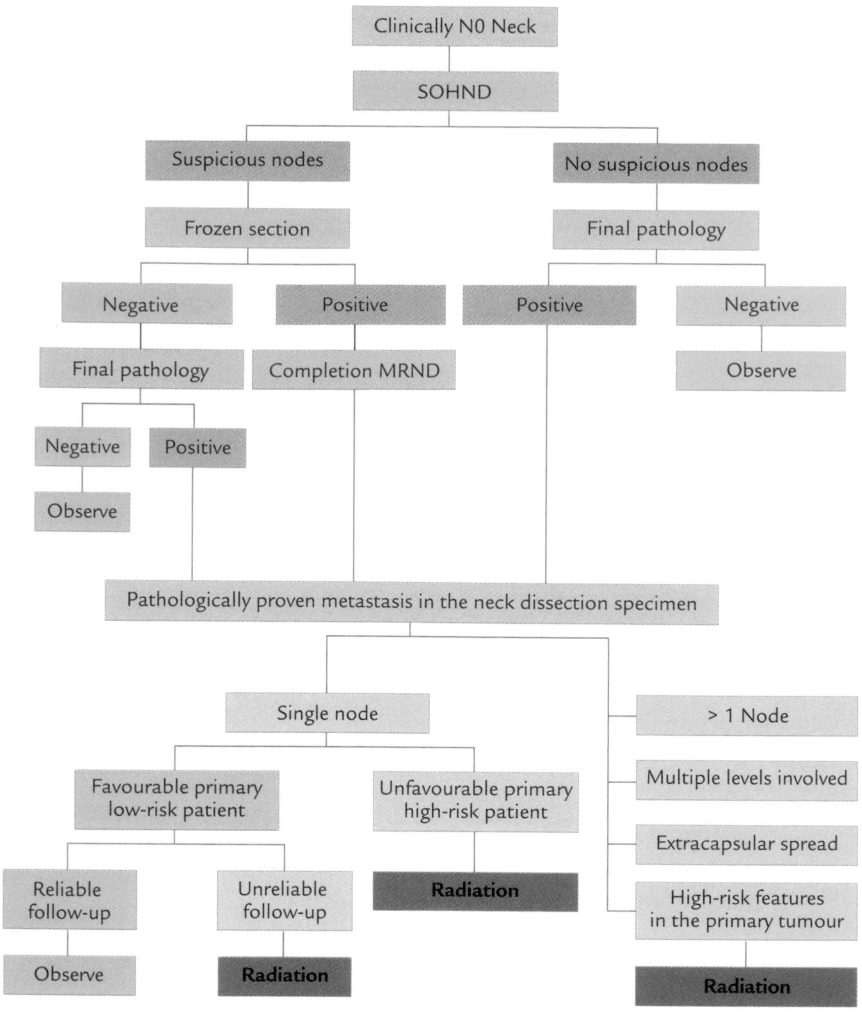

Figure 11.27 Algorithm for the surgical management of the clinically node negative neck in patients with oral cancer.

Favourable primary tumour
- Hard palate, lips
- Early T stage
- Verrucous primary
- Superficial flat lesions < 2 mm in depth

Low-risk patient
- No associated aetiological factors
- Can be relied upon to attend for follow-up

Unfavourable primary tumour
- Tongue, floor of mouth
- Advanced T stage
- Infiltrative lesion > 8 mm in depth
- Lymphatic and/or vascular invasion
- Perineural spread

High-risk patient
- Heavy smoker, especially if continues to smoke
- Alcohol abuser
- Poor oral hygiene
- Immunocompromised status
- Cannot be relied upon to attend for follow-up

In patients with palpable cervical nodes, levels I to IV are at highest risk. The choice of neck dissection in these patients depends largely on the individual patient but the general principle is that all five lymph node levels are dissected and the spinal accessory nerve is never sacrificed unless it is directly involved by tumour. The classical radical neck dissection is almost never indicated in the absence of direct infiltration of the relevant structures.

The classical radical neck dissection (RND) does, however, remain the gold standard against which the effectiveness of all other forms of neck dissection must be evaluated. When used alone, RND controls disease in the neck in more than 90% of N0 patients but as many as 60% of patients with bulky neck disease will recur. The control rate for patients with a clinically positive neck improves to more than 80% if postoperative radiation therapy is added.[72] For clinically N0 patients who are proven pathologically N0, failure rates of less than 10% have been reported.[73,74] The 30% of patients who have pathologically proven occult metastases following SOHND develop neck recurrence in 10–24%, depending upon the number of

Table 11.10 Indications for postoperative radiation therapy to the neck

Features of the primary tumour
- Advanced T stage:
  - Bulky tumour
  - Involvement of bone, nerves or skin
- High histological grade
- Positive surgical resection margins
- Lymphatic permeation
- Vascular invasion
- Perineural spread

Features of the cervical lymph nodes
- Single pathologically involved node in high risk patient and/or unfavourable primary tumour
- More than two pathologically involved nodes
- Involvement at more than one lymph node level in the neck
- Lymph node more than 3 cm in diameter (N2 or N3 stage)
- Presence of extracapsular spread
- Microscopic or gross residual disease in the neck

positive nodes and the presence of extracapsular extension. The addition of postoperative radiation reduces the failure rate in these patients to 0–15%. The appropriate use of postoperative radiation therapy (Table 11.10) in combination with modified radical neck dissection has resulted in comparable control rates to radical neck dissection for similar patients.[73] With lesions approaching or crossing the midline, bilateral neck dissections are carried out.

Reconstructive surgery

The ultimate functional outcome of surgical treatment depends a great deal upon choosing the appropriate reconstructive procedure. Reconstruction of the head and neck and mandibular reconstruction are discussed in detail in Chapters 27 and 28.

Radiotherapy

Radical radiotherapy is used in the following circumstances:

1. T2, and larger T1 tumours, where the chances of local control and survival are similar to those of radical surgery, but where the functional or cosmetic result is likely to be better;
2. For larger tumours where surgery is more appropriate, but the patient is medically unfit for, or refuses surgery;
3. Advanced, inoperable tumours.

Surgery is preferable to radical radiotherapy for larger and deeply infiltrating tumours. Radiotherapy should not be used in the presence of bone invasion, as the chance of success is low, and even if the malignant cells are eradicated, the bone usually fails to regenerate leading inevitably to troublesome osteoradionecrosis. Relative contraindications to radical radiotherapy include widespread field change and young age.

The success rate of radiotherapy is appreciably higher if some or all of the dose is administered by brachytherapy, rather than by external beam alone.[74,75] Wherever possible, unless the tumour is adjacent to bone, brachytherapy should be used. Our policy is to combine external beam and brachytherapy, giving 40 Gy to the primary and 50 Gy electively to the neck, followed by a further 35–40 Gy to the primary tumour by an interstitial implant. It has been claimed that the combination of the two modalities gives poorer results than brachytherapy alone,[76] but the probable reason was the time gap between the two of 3–4 weeks, allowing tumour cell repopulation. When the gap is no more than 1 week the results appear to be as good as those of brachytherapy alone.[77,78]

Long-term side-effects of radiotherapy include xerostomia with increased risk of dental caries; this is much less of a problem after brachytherapy than external beam, because of the smaller volume of normal mucosa irradiated. Necrotic ulcers of the soft tissues occasionally occur, more commonly after brachytherapy.

Osteoradionecrosis is a serious sequel to treatment with radiation and its management can be extremely challenging. The development of this complication can be largely prevented by a few simple precautions (Table 11.11). Diseased teeth within the treatment volume are the prime initiator of osteoradionecrosis and almost all bone necrosis occurs in patients who were dentulous prior to radiotherapy. Risk factors include the size and location of the lesion, the volume of the mandible within the radiation field, dosage more than 65 Gy and the health of the dentition. Three major pathological elements seem to be involved: periosteal and endosteal microangiopathy, primary or secondary osteomyelitis, and osteocyte damage.[79]

The onset of osteonecrosis is heralded by intractable local pain and a high index of suspicion is essential to early diagnosis. This is, however, not easy and the situation is often complicated by the need to exclude a local recurrence of tumour. It is important to avoid traumatizing the suspicious area with multiple biopsies, which only serve to worsen the problem. Currently used radiological investigations are not very specific and PET scanning may

Table 11.11 Prevention of osteoradionecrosis

Preradiotherapy
Avoid radiation therapy for tumours involving the mandible
Extract poor-prognosis teeth prior to starting treatment
Remove cysts and odontomes
Postradiotherapy
Stress on maintenance of oral and dental hygiene through and after radiation therapy
Avoid dental extraction, especially of multiple teeth after radiation therapy
Removal of caries and extirpation of pulps
Root canal therapy
Prevent tooth loss
Fluoride gel and mouthwashes
Chlorhexidine mouthwashes
Limit radiation caries with dental splint coverage

prove more useful in differentiating viable tumour tissue in a previously irradiated mandible from the necrosis and inflammation associated with osteoradionecrosis.[80]

Early and limited areas of osteoradionecrosis may be treated with conservative measures such as use of a water pik, debridement, long-term antibiotics and occasionally, hyperbaric oxygen. The use of systemic antibiotics remains controversial, but our policy is to use either a combination of metronidazole and a third generation cephalosporin or long-term tetracycline depending upon the extent and duration of bone exposure. We have tried topical therapy using gentamicin-impregnated methylmethacrylate beads with good results in selected cases. For more extensive necrosis, the conservative approach requires protracted treatment with an often disappointing outcome in terms of function and cosmesis. Selected patients with severe osteonecrosis may benefit from aggressive surgical excision of the necrotic mandible and immediate microvascular reconstruction.[81]

Follow-up and rehabilitation

Rehabilitation of the patient after treatment involves close cooperation with other health professionals including dieticians, speech therapists, dental surgeons, hygienists, and prosthodontists as discussed elsewhere.

Patients who have been treated for oral cancer require a regular periodic examination on a graduated time scale dependent upon assessment of the state of the primary site, locoregional disease and distant spread. The possibility of the occurrence of a second head and neck primary exists at a constant rate of about 4–7% of treated patients a year and thorough examination and a high suspicion are synergistic activities. While it is important for patients to stop abusing tobacco and alcohol, prevention strategies have not worked[82] and chemoprevention using agents such as retinoids has been under investigation.[83] Routine chemoprevention cannot, however, be recommended just yet because of the doubtful value and low index of safety of currently available agents.

Results of treatment

Alveolar ridge and retromolar trigone tumors

Surgery is the best option for patients with T1,2 lesions. Primary radiation is less feasible because the tendency of these tumours to invade through thin mucoperiosteum or tooth sockets placing the patient at increased risk for osteoradionecrosis. A brachytherapy technique using iridium wires looped over the gum is available for superficial lesions,[84] but is rarely used. Mucoperiosteal or minimal cortical invasion can be effectively managed by combining surgical excision of the lesion with a marginal mandibulectomy or partial maxillectomy, which can often be safely accomplished transorally (Figure 11.28). Posteriorly located lesions may be better accessed using an appropriately planned upper or lower cheek flap. Edentulous patients with 'pipestem' mandibles may however need segmental resection of their mandible for adequate tumour clearance. Elective neck dissection is carried out in most N0 cases en bloc with the primary or through a separate incision. More advanced tumours are best treated with combined modality treatment using surgery and radiation therapy. Surgery followed by postoperative radiation therapy is probably a better option compared to preoperative radiation which is associated with a higher risk of osteoradionecrosis. Resection of the mandible and/or maxilla may be required and functional outcome can be improved with osteomyocutaneous free tissue transfer[85] and osseointegrated implants as appropriate.

Surgery as the only modality of treatment has resulted in 5-year actuarial survival rates of 77% in early stage disease (stages I and II).[86] This figure drops sharply to 24% in patients with stage IV disease.[87] Radical radiotherapy is best avoided for tumours of the alveolar ridge because of the likelihood of bone invasion, unless surgery is not possible for any reason. Early tumours of the retromolar trigone, on the other hand, tend to respond better to radiotherapy, there being no difference in survival rates between surgery and radiotherapy.[88] Five-year survival rates of 88% for T1 and 69% for T2 tumours have been reported from a radical radiotherapy policy.[89] Some radiotherapy failures result from perineural spread in the direction of the infratemporal fossa and so it is important to irradiate an adequate superior margin.

Floor of the mouth

Equivalent control rates have been reported following surgery and radiation therapy for early tumours of the floor of mouth. Anterior and lateral floor of mouth lesions can be resected transorally (Figure 11.29) and the defect closed using mucosal advancement or a skin graft. Superficial lesions can be excised with little postoperative morbidity. The submandibular gland ducts need to be carefully dissected and transplanted laterally while excising lesions of the anterior floor of mouth. Interstitial

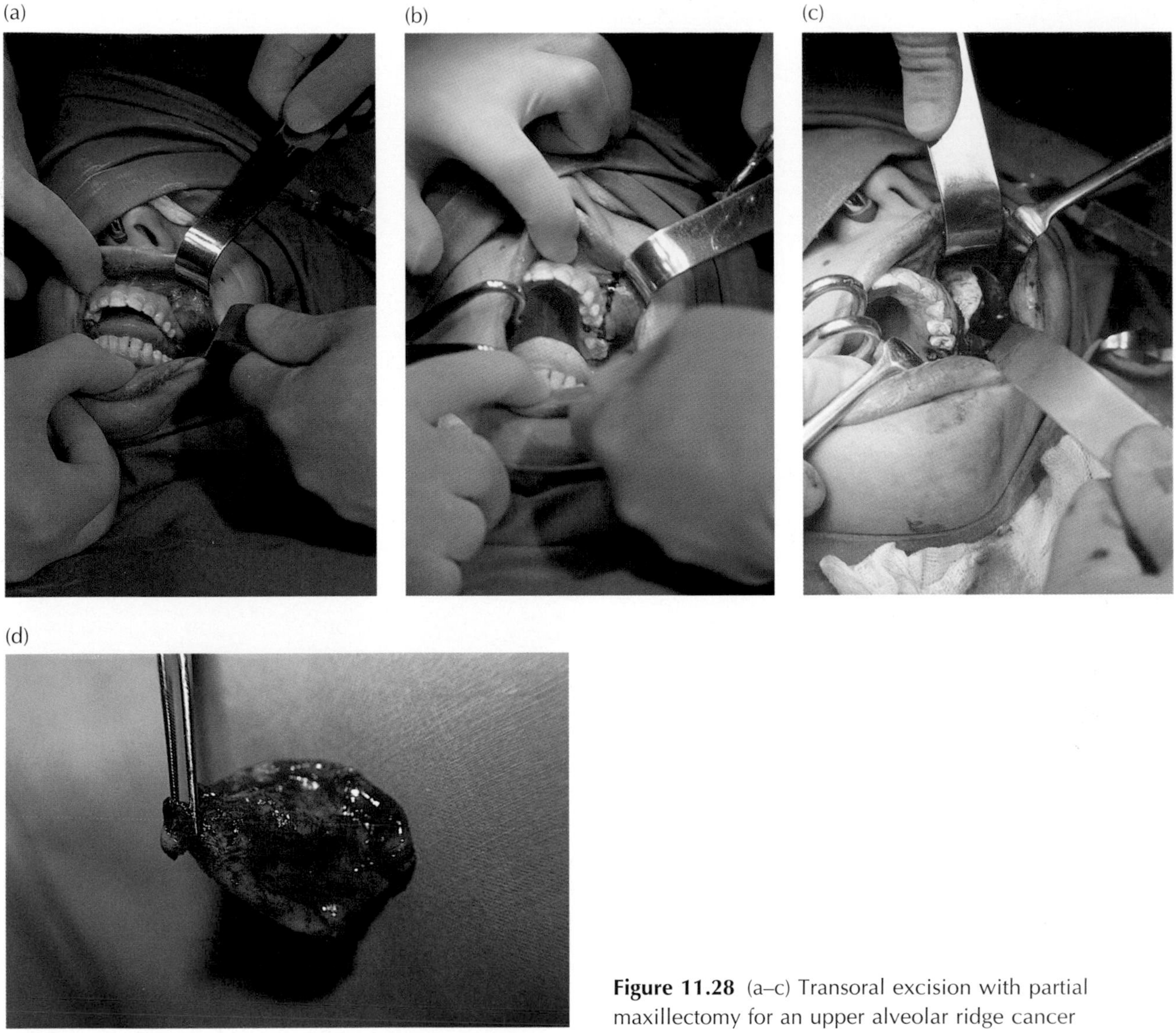

Figure 11.28 (a–c) Transoral excision with partial maxillectomy for an upper alveolar ridge cancer

implants have also been used[90] but radiation therapy is contraindicated as the primary modality of treatment in lesions that abut against or are tethered to the mandible. The management of the clinically N0 neck is controversial: most authors recommend elective neck dissection while some advocate neck dissection if the lesion is more than 4 mm thick.[52] Our practice is to carry out a supraomohyoid neck dissection and submit suspicious nodes for frozen section analysis with a view to a complete modified radical neck dissection if any node shows metastasis. Bilateral neck dissections are carried out for lesions approaching or crossing the midline. Locally advanced floor of mouth tumours are best treated using a combination of surgery and radiation therapy. Apart from the horizontal spread to involve mandibular bone, these lesions infiltrate the sublingual salivary gland and the space between the intrinsic tongue muscles and the genioglossus. Surgical excision of the floor of mouth cancers may therefore include partial glossectomy, marginal or segmental mandibulectomy, and reconstruction using skin grafts, pedicled flaps or microvascular tissue transfer. Patients are subjected to elective or therapeutic neck dissection and lesions that approach or cross the midline may need bilateral neck dissection. As discussed previously, postoperative radiation therapy is an integral part of the management when indicated.

The overall 5-year survival rates in patients with floor of mouth cancer reported in the literature are shown in Table 11.12. Early lesions (T1–T2) treated with surgery have a 10% local failure rate while failure in the neck (40%) is a bigger concern in patients with larger lesions (T3–T4). Radiation therapy for stage I tumours has a 6% local failure rate while 16% of stage II tumours will recur locally if treated with radiation alone.[96] Locoregionally advanced tumours (stage III) are treated with a combination of surgery and radiation therapy achieving a 79% 5-year actuarial local control.[99]

(a)

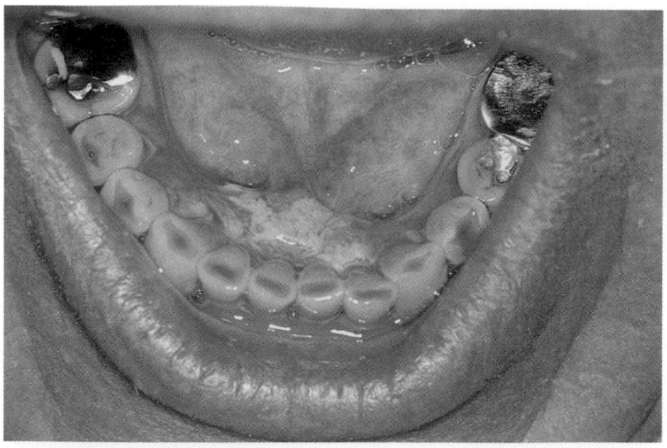

(b)

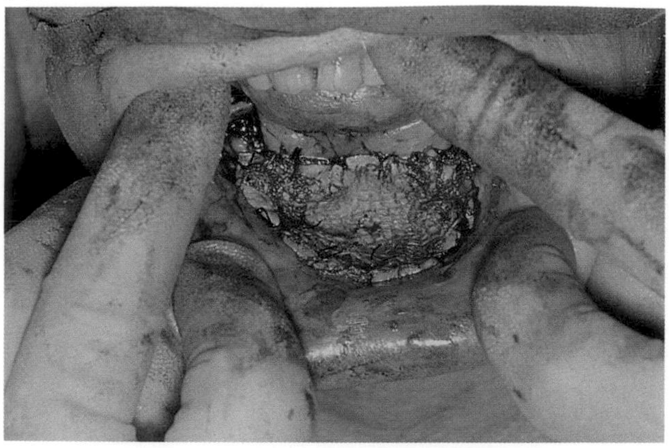

(c)

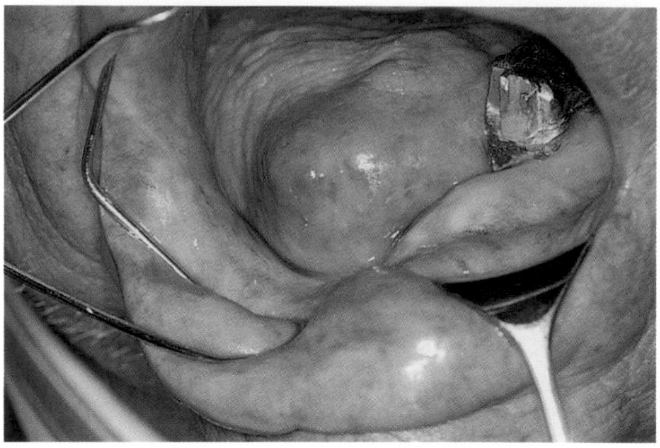

Figure 11.29 (a–c) Transoral excision and split skin graft for a cancer of the anterior floor of mouth.

Table 11.12 Overall 5-year survival (%) in patients with cancer of the floor of the mouth

Series	No. of patients	Stage I	Stage II	Stage III	Stage IV
Harrold[91]	634	69	49	25	7
Panje et al[92]	103	57	60	43	19
Nason et al[93]	198	69	64	46	26
Shaha et al[94]	320	88	80	66	32
Fu et al[95]	153	83	71	43	10

Table 11.13 Overall 5-year survival (%) in patients with cancer of the tongue

Series	No. of patients	Stage I	Stage II	Stage III	Stage IV
Callery et al[102]	252	75	60	40	20
Decroix and Ghossein[103]	602	59	45	25	13
Wallner et al[104]	424	68	50	33	20
Ildstad et al[105]	122	48	48	18	26
O'Brien et al[106]	97	73	62	–	–

Oral tongue

As with most other oral cancers, equivalent results have been reported with surgery and radiation therapy. ^{192}Ir implants have been used successfully in the treatment of these tumours and the functional results of radiation may be better than those after surgery, especially in the case of tumours on the dorsum and lateral border of the middle third. Lesions amenable to radiation include T1, and exophytic T2–T3 lesions with minimal infiltration. Transoral excision of smaller tumours can often be safely accomplished but surgical excision of larger T2 lesions with adequate margins most often results in a partial glossectomy. Reconstruction of the resultant defect using a free radial forearm flap gives good functional results and is our current treatment of choice.

The role of elective treatment of the clinically negative neck in the management of early tongue cancer continues to generate controversy and there have been reports in literature evaluating the predictive value of histological parameters such as the depth of tumour invasion.[53,54] Despite the lack of conclusive survival benefit in two prospective trials[54,96] in early oral cavity cancer, there seems to be unanimity in opinion regarding the importance of elective treatment of the neck in early tongue cancer.[97] Our practice of routine elective neck treatment for early tongue lesions is based on our observation[98] that patients whose necks had not been treated had a statistically significant increase in the rate of neck failure. Although the difference in actuarial 5-year survival rates between those whose necks were treated electively and those who had no elective treatment was not statistically significant (75 versus 65%; $P - 0.44$), there was a significant increase in risk for neck failure in the latter group (17% versus 43%; $P = 0.025$). Multivariate analysis of another group of our cases treated by brachytherapy showed that elective neck irradiation was a statistically significant favourable prognostic factor;[99] there was a similar finding in favour of elective neck dissection in a French study.[100] Additionally, as many as 67% of our patients who failed in the neck succumbed to their disease and it is our contention that the best chance for treatment of the neck is at initial presentation of the primary tumour.

Surgical excision of larger lesions may require a mandibulotomy or a lingual-releasing approach to gain access. Patients presenting with a clinically N0 neck should undergo a functional neck dissection while those with palpable nodes are treated with a modified or radical neck dissection. Discontinuous resection of the primary has been shown to be oncologically safe and we make no special effort to resect the neck nodes in continuity with the primary tumour.

The overall 5-year survival rates reported in major series in the literature are listed in Table 11.13. Local control of the tumour using primary radiation can be achieved in 80–85% of patients with early lesions (T1–T2) and in 68% of patients with T3 lesions.[111] Surgical excision gives local control in 85% of T1, 77% of T2 and only 50% of T3 lesions.[101] Despite combined treatment with surgery and radiation therapy only 35% of patients with advanced stage disease (stages III and IV) will survive 5 years, mainly as a result of recurrence in the neck.[110]

Buccal mucosa

As with other sites within the oral cavity, surgery and radiation therapy are equally effective in controlling T1 lesions. Smaller lesions can be excised transorally (Figure 11.30) with minimal functional sequelae while larger lesions that approach the commissure are probably best managed by radiation. Exophytic or superficial lesions can be managed by radiation therapy but infiltrative lesions are best managed by surgery. Patients with a clinically negative neck may be safely observed because, in contrast to other sites, fewer than 10% of patients fail in the neck.

Surgery combined with radiation therapy is the treatment of choice for more advanced tumour. Adequate exposure may be obtained by elevating a cheek flap. A full-thickness resection may be required if tumour invades into the buccal fat pad or the overlying skin. Other structures that need careful evaluation for invasion prior to surgery are the alveolar ridges and the mandible. Adequate clearance of tumour almost certainly necessitates resection of these structures and preoperative planning of bony cuts facilitates reconstruction and rehabilitation. The surgical defect is reconstructed using pedicled myocutaneous flaps or free tissue transfer. An ipsilateral neck dissection is carried out in all patients with locally advanced tumours irrespective of nodal status. In addition to the obvious advantage in terms of regional control, a modified neck dissection resecting the sternomastoid muscle may be essential if the pedicle of a myocutaneous flap has to be accommodated in that side of the neck.

Radiation therapy as a single modality offers limited control: 3-year disease-free survival is 85% for stage I, 63% for stage II, 41% for stage III and only 14% for stage IV patients.[107] Surgical excision as the only modality has slightly better results compared to radiation therapy: 5-year disease-free survival is 77% for stage I, 65% for stage II, 27% for stage III and 18% for stage IV patients.[108]

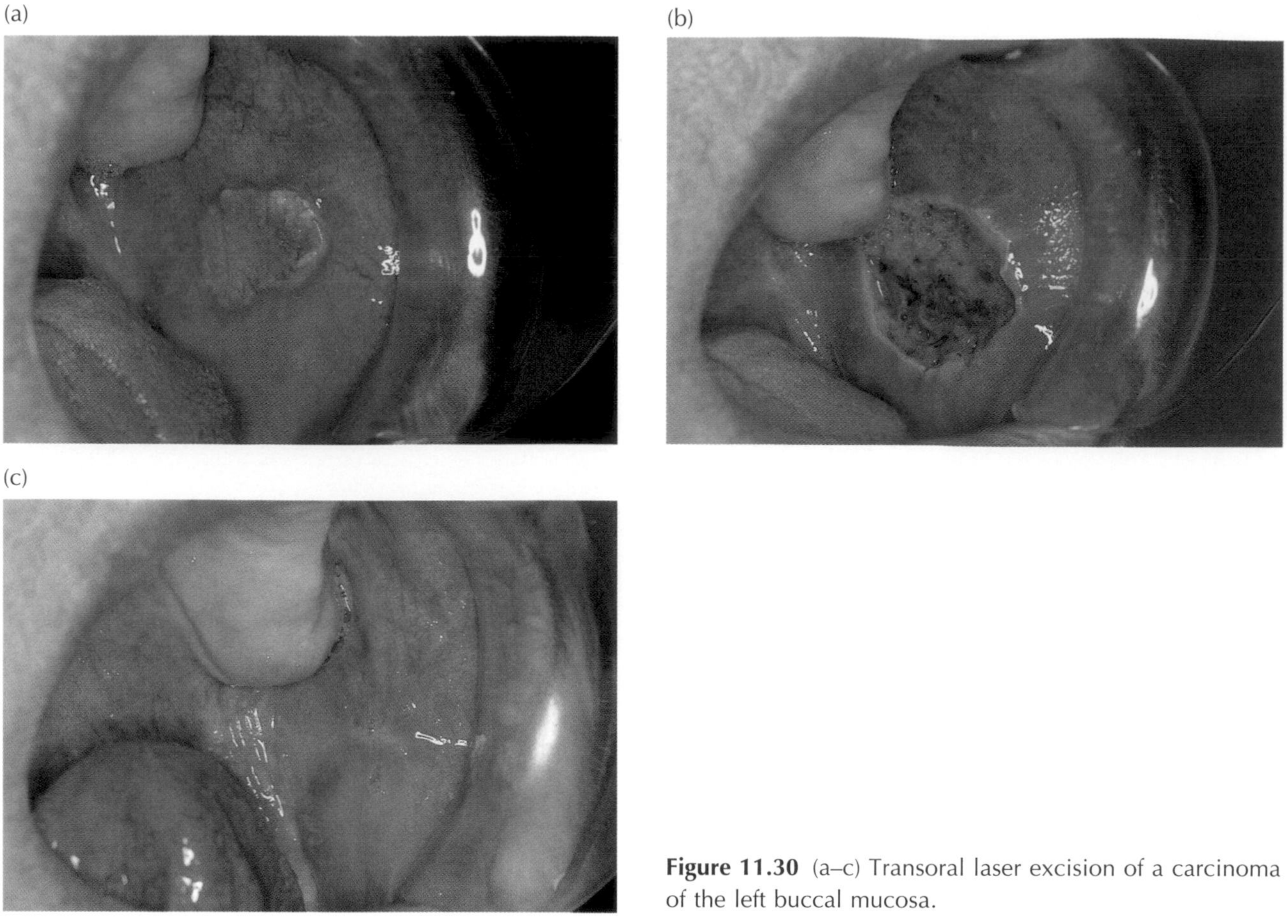

Figure 11.30 (a–c) Transoral laser excision of a carcinoma of the left buccal mucosa.

Oral cancer: the way ahead

Although treatment results for patients with oral cancer have improved considerably over the last several decades we have now reached a plateau in terms of survival because of the adverse effect of second and subsequent primary tumours in long-term survivors. Oral cancer provides a classic module where efforts towards fundamental research, preventive education, early diagnosis, effective treatment and rehabilitation can all pay handsome dividends. Future areas of research will concentrate on unravelling the molecular events predisposing to and causing cancer, and on identifying their timing during multistep carcinogenesis. If the mechanisms of invasion and metastasis can be identified, future therapeutic approaches could use targeted monoclonal antibodies or inhibitors to block key binding sites and prevent metastasis. Advances in molecular biology and biotechnology have already helped expand our capabilities for molecular and gene therapy. Gene intervention strategies may allow us to augment the body's immune response, deliver a toxic gene or metabolite, alter chemo- or radiation sensitivity or even induce death of specific cells. In addition to improving results in patients with established cancer, a detailed understanding of the molecular biology of the disease may make its prevention using genetic manipulation a real possibility.

REFERENCES

1. Jovanovic A, Schulten EA, Kostense PJ et al. Tobacco and alcohol related to the anatomical site of oral squamous cell carcinoma. *J Oral Pathol Med* 1993; **22**: 459–462.
2. Meyer I, Shklar G. Malignant tumors metastatic to the mouth and jaws. *Oral Surg* 1965; **20**: 350.
3. Kemp I et al. *Atlas of Cancer in Scotland* 1975–1980. IARC Scientific Publications No. 72. 1985.
4. Hindle I, Downer MC, Speight PM. The epidemiology of oral cancer. *Br J Oral Maxillofac Surg* 1996; **34**: 471–476.

5. Macfarlane GJ, Boyle P, Scully C. Oral cancer in Scotland: changing incidence and mortality. *Br Med J* 1992; **305**: 1121–1123.
6. Cowan CG, Gregg TA, Kee F. Trends in the incidence of histologically diagnosed intra-oral squamous cell carcinoma in Northern Ireland, 1975–1989. *Br Dent J* 1992; **173**: 231–233.
7. Boyle P, Macfarlane GJ, Scully C. Oral cancer: necessity for prevention strategies. *Lancet* 1993; **342**: 1129.
8. Moller H. Changing incidence of cancer of the tongue, oral cavity and pharynx in Denmark. *J Oral Pathol Med* 1989; **18**: 224–229.
9. Epstein JB, Scully C. Neoplastic disease in the head and neck of patients with AIDS. *Int J Oral Maxillofac Surg* 1992; **21**: 219–226.
10. Goldberg HI, Lockwood SA, Wyatt SW, Crossett LS. Trends and differentials in mortality from cancers of the oral cavity and pharynx in the United States: 1973–1987. *Cancer* 1994; **74**: 565–572.
11. Spitz MR, Fueger JJ, Goepfert H et al. Squamous cell carcinoma of the upper aerodigestive tract: a case comparison analysis. *Cancer* 1988; **61**: 203–208.
12. Jayant K, Notani PN. Epidemiology of oral cancer. In: Rao RS, Desai PB (eds). *Oral Cancer*. Tata Memorial Hospital, Bombay: Professional Education Division, 1991.
13. Brennan JA, Boyle JO, Koch WM et al. Association between cigarette smoking and mutation of the p53 gene in squamous cell carcinoma of the head and neck. *N Engl J Med* 1995; **332**: 712–717.
14. Schantz SP, Hsu TC. Head and neck cancer patients express increased clastogen-induced chromosome fragility. *Head Neck* 1989; **11**: 337–343.
15. Reddy CRRM. Carcinoma of hard palate in relation to reverse smoking of chuttas. *J Natl Cancer Inst* 1974; **53**: 615–619.
16. IARC Monographs on the evaluation of the carcinogenic risk of chemicals to the human. Tobacco habits other than smoking: betel-quid and areca nut chewing and some related nitrosamines. Lyon: International Agency for Research on Cancer, 1985: 37.
17. Mehta FS, Gupta PC, Daftary DK et al. An epidemiologic study of oral cancer and precancerous conditions among 101 761 villagers in Maharashtra, India. *Int J Cancer* 1972; **10**: 134–141.
18. McCoy DG, Wynder EL. Etiological and preventive implications in alcohol carcinogenesis. *Cancer Res* 1979; **39**: 2844–2850.
19. Mashberg A, Garfinkel L, Harris S. Alcohol as a primary risk factor in oral squamous carcinoma. *CA Cancer J Clin* 1981; **31**: 146–155.
20. Graham S, Dayal H, Rohrer T et al. Dentition, diet, tobacco, and alcohol in the epidemiology of oral cancer. *J Natl Cancer Inst* 1977; **59**: 1611–1618.
21. Szpirglas H. Alcohol et cancer buccaux. *Actual Odontostomatol* (Paris) 1976; **115**: 448–454.
22. Binnie WH. Epidemiology and aetiology of oral cancer in Britain. *Proc R Soc Med* 1976; **69**: 737–740.
23. Axell T, Holmstrup P, Kramer IRH et al. International seminar on oral leukoplakia and associated lesions to tobacco habits. *Community Dent Oral Epidemiol* 1984; **12**: 145.
24. Warnakulasuriya KA, Johnson NW. Sensitivity and specificity of OraScan toluidine blue mouthrinse in the detection of oral cancer and precancer. *J Oral Pathol Med* 1996; **25**: 97–103.
25. Epstein JB, Scully C, Spinelli J. Toluidine blue and Lugol's iodine application in the assessment of oral malignant disease and lesions at risk of malignancy. *J Oral Pathol Med* 1992; **21**: 160–163.
26. Silverman S Jr., Gorsky M, Lozada F. Oral leukoplakia and malignant transformation: a follow-up study of 257 patients. *Cancer* 1984; **53**: 563–568.
27. Kramer IR, El Labban N, Lee KW. The clinical features and risk of malignant transformation in sublingual keratosis. *Br Dent J* 1978; **144**: 171–180.
28. Inoue A, Uchida M, Kimura Y, Kazaoka N. Malignant progression of oral leukoplakia. *Gan To Kagaku Ryoho* 1989; **16**: 1650–1656.
29. Rhys Evans PH, Frame JW, Brandrick J. A review of carbon dioxide laser surgery in the oral cavity and pharynx. *J Laryngol Otol* 1986; **100**: 69–77.
30. McLaughlin JK, Gridley G, Block G, et al. Dietary factors in oral and pharyngeal cancer. *J Natl Cancer Inst* 1988; **80**: 1237–1243.
31. Wynder EL, Kabat G, Rosenberg S, Levenstein M. Oral cancer and mouthwash use. *J Natl Cancer Inst* 1983; **70**: 255–260.
32. Donald PJ. Marijuana smoking – possible cause of head and neck cancer in young patients. *Otolaryngol Head Neck Surg* 1986; **94**: 517–521.
33. Shillitoe EJ, Greenspan D, Greenspan JS, Silverman S Jr. Immunoglobulin class of antibody to herpes simplex virus in patients with oral cancer. *Cancer* 1983; **51**: 65–71.
34. Watts SL, Brewer EE, Fry TL. Human papillomavirus DNA types in squamous cell cancer of the head and neck. *Oral Surg Oral Med Oral Pathol* 1991; **7**: 701–707.
35. Fortner JG, Shiu MH. Organ transplantation and cancer. *Surg Clin North Am* 1974; **54**: 871–876.
36. Ficarra G, Eversole LE. HIV related tumors of the oral cavity. *Crit Rev Oral Biol Med* 1994; **5**: 159–185.
37. Lederman M. The anatomy of oral cancer. *J Laryngol Otol* 1964; **78**: 181.
38. Moore C, Catlin D. Anatomic origins and locations of oral cancer. *Am J Surg* 1967; **114**: 510–513.
39. Ahmed F, Islam KM. Site of predilection of oral cancer and its correlation with chewing and smokings habits—a study of 103 cases. *Bangladesh Med Res Counc Bull* 1990; **16**: 17–25.
40. O'Brien JC. Oropharyngeal tumours. *Selected Readings in Plastic Surgery Syllabus* 1984; **3**: 4.
41. Boffetta P, Mashberg A, Winkelmann R, Garfinkel L. Carcinogenic effect of tobacco smoking and alcohol drinking on anatomic sites of the oral cavity and oropharynx. *Int J Cancer* 1992; **52**: 530–533.
42. Desai PB, Rao RS, Dinshaw KA et al. *Hospital Cancer Registry: Annual Report 1993*. Bombay, India: Tata Memorial Hospital, 1993; 23.

43. Robbins KT, Medina JE, Wolfe GT et al. Standardizing neck dissection terminology. *Arch Otolaryngol Head Neck Surg* 1991; **117**: 601–605.
44. Shah JP, Candela FC, Poddar AK. The patterns of cervical lymph node metastases from squamous carcinoma of the oral cavity. *Cancer* 1990; **66**: 109–113.
45. Byers RM, Newman R, Russell N, Yue A. Results of treatment for squamous carcinoma of the lower gum. *Cancer* 1981; **47**: 2236–2238.
46. Willen R, Nathanson A. Squamous cell carcinoma of the gingiva. *Acta Otolaryngol* 1973; **75**: 299–300.
47. Lindberg R. Distribution of cervical lymph node metastases from squamous cell carcinoma of the upper respiratory and digestive tracts. *Cancer* 1972; **29**: 1446–1449.
48. Strong EW. Carcinoma of the tongue. *Otolaryngol Clin North Am* 1979; **12**: 107–113.
49. Urist MM, O'Brien CJ, Soong SJ et al. Squamous carcinoma of the buccal mucosa: analysis of prognostic factors. *Am J Surg* 1987; **154**: 411–414.
50. Beahrs OH, Henson DE, Hutter RVP, Kennedy BJ. *Manual for Staging of Cancer.* 4th edn. Philadelphia: JB Lippincott, 1992.
51. Spiro RH, Huvos AG, Wong GY et al. Predictive value of tumor thickness in squamous carcinoma confined to the tongue and floor of the mouth. *Am J Surg* 1986; **152**: 345–350.
52. Fakih AR, Rao RS, Borges AM, Patel AR. Elective versus therapeutic neck dissection in early carcinoma of the oral tongue. *Am J Surg* 1989; **158**: 309–313.
53. Slaughter DP, Southwick HW, Smejkal W. 'Field cancerization' in oral stratified squamous epithelium: clinical implications of multicentric origin. *Cancer* 1953; **6**: 963.
54. Lester EP, Tharapel SA. Chromosome abnormalities in squamous carcinoma cell lines of head and neck origin. Presented at the Third International Head and Neck Oncology Research Conference, Las Vegas, 1990.
55. van der Riet P, Nawroz H, Hruban RH et al. Frequent loss of chromosome 9 p21–22 early in head and neck cancer progression. *Cancer Res* 1994; **54**: 1156–1158.
56. Brachman DG, Graves D, Vokes E et al. Occurrence of p53 gene deletions and human papilloma virus infection in human head and neck cancer. *Cancer Res* 1992; **53**: 4832.
57. Boyle JO, Hakin J, Koch W et al. The incidence of p53 mutations increases with progression of head and neck cancer. *Cancer Res* 1993; **53**: 4477–4480.
58. Bundgaard T, Bentzen SM, Wildt J. The prognostic effect of tobacco and alcohol consumption in intraoral squamous cell carcinoma. *Eur J Cancer Oral Oncol* 1994; **30B**: 323–328.
59. McGregor AD, McDonald DG. Routes of entry of squamous cell carcinoma to the mandible. *Head Neck Surg* 1988; **10**: 294–301.
60. McGregor AD. Patterns of spread of squamous cell carcinoma in the mandible. *Head Neck* 1989; **11**: 457–461.
61. Marchetta FC, Sako K, Murphy JB. The periosteum of the mandible and intraoral carcinoma. *Am J Surg* 1971; **122**: 711–713.
62. Huntley TA, Busmanis I, Desmond P, Wiesenfeld D. Mandibular invasion by squamous cell carcinoma: a computed tomography and histological study. *Br J Oral Maxillofac Surg* 1996; **34**: 69–74.
63. King JM, Caldarelli DD, Petasnick JP. Dentascan—a new diagnostic method for evaluating mandibular and maxillary pathology. *Laryngoscope* 1992; **102**: 379–387.
64. Yanagisawa K, Friedman CD, Vining EM, Abrahams JJ. Dentascan imaging of the mandible and maxilla. *Head Neck* 1993; **15**: 1–7.
65. Chung TS, Yousem DM, Seigerman HM et al. MR of mandibular invasion in patients with oral and oropharyngeal malignant neoplasms. *Am J Neuroradiol* 1994; **15**: 1949–1955.
66. Ahuja RB, Soutar DS, Moule B et al. Comparative study of technetium-99m bone scans and orthopantomography in determining mandible invasion in intraoral squamous cell carcinoma. *Head Neck* 1990; **12**: 237–243.
67. Shaha AR. Preoperative evaluation of the mandible in patients with carcinoma of the floor of the mouth. *Head Neck* 1991; **13**: 398–402.
68. Shah JP, Andersen PE. Evolving role of modifications in neck dissection for oral squamous carcinoma. *Br J Oral Maxillofac Surg* 1995; **33**: 3–8.
69. Farr HW, Arthur K. Epidermoid carcinoma of the mouth and pharynx 1960–1964. *J Laryngol Otol* 1972; **86**: 243–253.
70. Spiro JD, Spiro RH, Shah JP, Sessions RB, Strong EW. Critical assessment of supraomohyoid neck dissection. *Am J Surg* 1988; **156**: 286–289.
71. Mannii JJ, van den Hoogen FJA. Supraomohyoid neck dissection with frozen section biopsy as a staging procedure in the clinically node-negative neck in carcinoma of the oral cavity. *Am J Surg* 1991; **162**: 373–376.
72. Tupchong L, Scott CB, Blitzer PH et al. Randomized study of preoperative versus postoperative radiation therapy in advanced head and neck carcinoma: long-term follow-up of RTOG study 73–03. *Int J Radiat Oncol Biol Phys* 1991; **20**: 21–28.
73. Andersen PE, Spiro RH, Cambronero E, Shah JP. The role of comprehensive neck dissection with preservation of the spinal accessory nerve in the clinically positive neck. *Am J Surg* 1994; **168**: 499–502.
74. Chu A, Fletcher GH. Incidence and cause of failure to control by irradiation the primary lesions in squamous cell carcinomas of the anterior two-thirds of the tongue and floor of mouth. *Am J Roentgenol* 1973; **117**: 502–508.
75. Wallner PE, Hanks GE, Kramer S, McLean CT. Patterns of care study: analysis of outcome survey data: anterior two-thirds of tongue and floor of mouth. *Am J Clin Oncol* 1986; **9**: 50–57.
76. Benk V, Mazeron JJ, Grimard L et al. Comparison of curietherapy versus external irradiation combined with

curietherapy in stage II squamous cell carcinoma of the mobile tongue. *Radiother Oncol* 1992; **18**: 339–347.
77. Pernot M, Malissard L, Hoffstetter S, et al. The study of tumoral, radiobiological, and general health factors that influence results and complications in a series of 448 oral tongue carcinomas treated exclusively by irradiation. *Int J Radiat Oncol Biol Phys* 1994; **29**: 673–679.
78. Henk JM. Treatment of oral cancer by interstitial irradiation using iridium-192. *Br J Oral Maxillofac Surg* 1992; **30**: 355–359.
79. Archer DJ. Osteoradionecrosis and the dental surgeon. In: Bloom HJ, Hanham IWF. *Head and Neck Oncology.* New York: Raven Press, 1986; 253–258.
80. Minn H, Aitasalo K, Happonen RP. Detection of cancer recurrence in irradiated mandible using positron emission tomography. *Eur Arch Otorhinolaryngol* 1993; **250**: 312–315.
81. Shaha AR, Cordeiro PG, Hidalgo DA et al. Resection and immediate microvascular reconstruction in the management of osteoradionecrosis of the mandible. *Head Neck* 1997; **19**: 406–411.
82. COMMIT Research Group Community intervention trial for smoking cessation (COMMIT): I. Cohort results from a four-year community intervention. *Am J Public Health* 1995; **85**: 183–192.
83. Lippman SM, Hong WK. Retinoid chemoprevention of upper aerodigestive tract carcinogenesis. In: DeVita VT, Hellman S, Rosenberg SA (eds) *Important Advances in Oncology.* Philadelphia: Lippincott, 1992, 93–109.
84. Alcock CJ, Paine CH, Weatherburn H. Interstitial radiotherapy in treatment of superficial tumours of the lower alveolar ridge. *Clin Radiol* 1984; **35**: 363–366.
85. Hidalgo DA. Aesthetic improvements in free-flap mandible reconstruction. *Am Soc Plast Reconst Surg* 1991; **88**: 574–585.
86. Cady B, Catlin D. Epidermoid carcinoma of the gum: a 20-year survey. *Cancer* 1969; **23**: 551–569.
87. Soo KC, Spiro RH, King W et al. Squamous carcinoma of the gingiva: an update. *Am J Surg* 1988; **156**: 281–285.
88. Byers RM, Fields RS, Anderson B et al. Treatment of squamous carcinoma of the retromolar trigone. *Am J Clin Oncol* 1984; **7**: 647–652.
89. Wang CC. *Radiation Therapy for Head and Neck Neoplasms* 2nd edn. Chicago: Year Book Medical Publishers, 1990.
90. Mazeron J, Grimard L, Raynal M et al. Iridium-192 curietherapy for T1 and T2 epidermoid carcinomas of the floor of mouth. *Int J Radiat Biol Phys* 1990; **18**: 1299–1306.
91. Harrold CC Jr. Management of cancer of the floor of mouth. *Am J Surg* 1971; **122**: 487–493.
92. Panje WR, Smith B, McCabe BF. Epidermoid carcinomas of the floor of mouth. Surgical therapy vs combined therapy vs radiation therapy. *Otolaryngol Head Neck Surg* 1980; **88**: 714.
93. Nason RW, Sako K, Beecroft WA et al. Surgical management of squamous cell carcinoma of the floor of mouth. *Am J Surg* 1989; **158**: 292–296.
94. Shaha AR, Spiro R, Shah JP. Squamous carcinoma of the floor of the mouth. *Am J Surg* 1984; **148**: 455–461.
95. Fu KK, Lichter A, Galante M. Carcinoma of the floor of mouth: an analysis of treatment results and the sites and causes and failures. *Int J Radiol Oncol Biol Phys* 1976; **1**: 829–837.
96. Vandenbrouck C, Sancho GH, Chassagne D, Cachiu SD. Elective vs Therapeutic neck dissection in epidermoid carcinoma of the oral cavity. Results of a randomized trial. *Cancer* 1980; **46**: 386–390.
97. DeSanto LW, Johnson JT, Million RR. Controversies: cost-effective management of T1N0 carcinoma of the tongue. *Head Neck* 1996; **18**: 573–576.
98. Yii NW, Patel SG, Rhys Evans PH, Breach NM. Management of the N0 neck in early cancer of the oral tongue. *Clin Otolaryngol* 1999; **24**: 75–79.
99. Dearnaley DP, Dardoufas C, A'Hern RP, Henk JM. Interstitial irradiation for carcinoma of the tongue and floor of mouth: Royal Marsden experience 1970–86. *Radiother Oncol* 1991; **21**: 1883–1892.
100. Piedbois P, Mazeron JJ, Haddad E et al. Stage I–II squamous carcinoma of the oral cavity treated by iridium-192: is elective neck dissection indicated? *Radiother Oncol* 1991; **21**: 100–106.
101. Spiro RH, Strong EW. Surgical treatment of carcinoma of the tongue. *Surg Clin North Am* 1974; **54**: 233–239.
102. Callery CD, Spiro RH, Strong EW. Changing trends in the management of squamous carcinoma of the tongue. *Am J Surg* 1984; **148**: 449–454.
103. Decroix Y, Ghossein NA. Experience of the Curie Institute in treatment of cancer of the mobile tongue: treatment policies and results. *Cancer* 1981; **47**: 503–508.
104. Wallner PE, Hanks GE, Kramer S, McLean CJ. Patterns of care study: analysis of outcome survey data–anterior two thirds of tongue and floor of mouth. *Am J Clin Oncol* 1986; **9**: 50–57.
105. Ildstad ST, Bigelow ME, Remensnyder JP. Squamous cell carcinoma of the mobile tongue: Clinical behavior and results of current therapeutic modalities. *Am J Surg* 1983; **145**: 443–449
106. O'Brien CJ, Lahr CJ, Soong SJ, Gandour MJ, Jones JM, Unst MM et al. Surgical treatment of early stage carcinoma of the oral tongue-would adjuvant treatment be beneficial? *Head Neck Surg* 1986; **8**: 401–408.
107. Nair M, Sankaranarayanan R, Padmanabhan TK. Evaluation of the role of radiation therapy in the management of carcinoma of the buccal mucosa. *Cancer* 1988; **61**: 1326–1331.
108. Bloom NO, Spiro RH. Carcinoma of the cheek mucosa: a retrospective analysis. *Am J Surg* 1980; **140**: 556–559.

12 Tumours of the nasopharynx

Christopher P Cottrill and Christopher M Nutting

Introduction

Nasopharyngeal tumours are biologically distinct from the more common head and neck tumours and are characterized by their propensity for early lymphatic and distant metastatic spread. Anatomical constraints, together with widespread lymphatic permeation effectively exclude curative surgery. Radical radiotherapy is the mainstay of treatment though increasingly this is being combined with chemotherapy.

Anatomy

The nasopharynx lies beneath the skull base, posterior to and continuous with the nasal cavities (Figure 12.1a, b). It is lined in part by pseudostratified columnar respiratory-type epithelium and also in part by non-keratinizing stratified squamous epithelium.

Anatomical relations

Roof and posterior wall

The sloping roof is continuous with the posterior wall. It is formed by the floor of the sphenoid sinus medially and the fibrocartilage of the foramina lacerum laterally (Figure 12.1a, b). The cavernous sinus with the internal carotid artery and cranial nerves III, IV, V and VI lies immediately above the foramen lacerum on each side (Figure 12.1c). The posterior wall overlies the basilar part of the occipital bone and the anterior arch of the atlas inferiorally. It is ridged, posteriorly, by the longus capitis muscles and beneath its fascial lining lie the medial retropharyngeal lymph nodes (Figure 12.1d).

Lateral walls

The Eustachian (auditory) tubes gain access to the nasopharynx through its lateral walls, which are themselves formed by the pharyngobasilar fascia reinforced inferiorally by the superior constrictor muscles. Viewed from the nasal cavities the upper and posterior aspects of the Eustachian tube orifices are marked by the cartilaginous tubal elevation behind which, on each side, lies the slit-like fossa of Rosenmüller. Immediately deep to the lateral wall lies the parapharyngeal space containing the internal carotid artery, cranial nerves IX, X, XI, XII, the internal jugular vein and lateral retropharyngeal lymph nodes (of Rouvière) (Figure 12.1d).

The pharyngeal fascia and fibrous foramen lacerum offer little resistance to direct invasion by malignant tumours of the nasopharynx. This and the frequent involvement of lateral retropharyngeal nodes explains the relatively common occurrence of cranial nerve palsies.

Floor

The floor is formed by the superior surface of the soft palate, which, in conjunction with the palatopharyngeal sphincter, serves to close the pharyngeal isthmus during swallowing, isolating the nasopharynx from the oropharynx below.

Lymphatic drainage and nerve supply

The mucosa is raised into several folds by the underlying musculature and contains variable aggregations of lymphoid tissue. The most prominent of these, especially in children, is the pharyngeal tonsil (or 'adenoids') lying in the midline and projecting forwards from the junction of the roof and posterior wall. The rich submucosal lymphatic plexus drains primarily to the retropharyngeal, upper deep posterior cervical (junctional) and jugulodigastric node groups.

The nerve supply to the nasopharyngeal mucosa is derived from the maxillary division of the trigeminal nerve via a small branch, the pharyngeal nerve, which arises in the pterygopalatine fossa, close to the pterygopalatine ganglion.

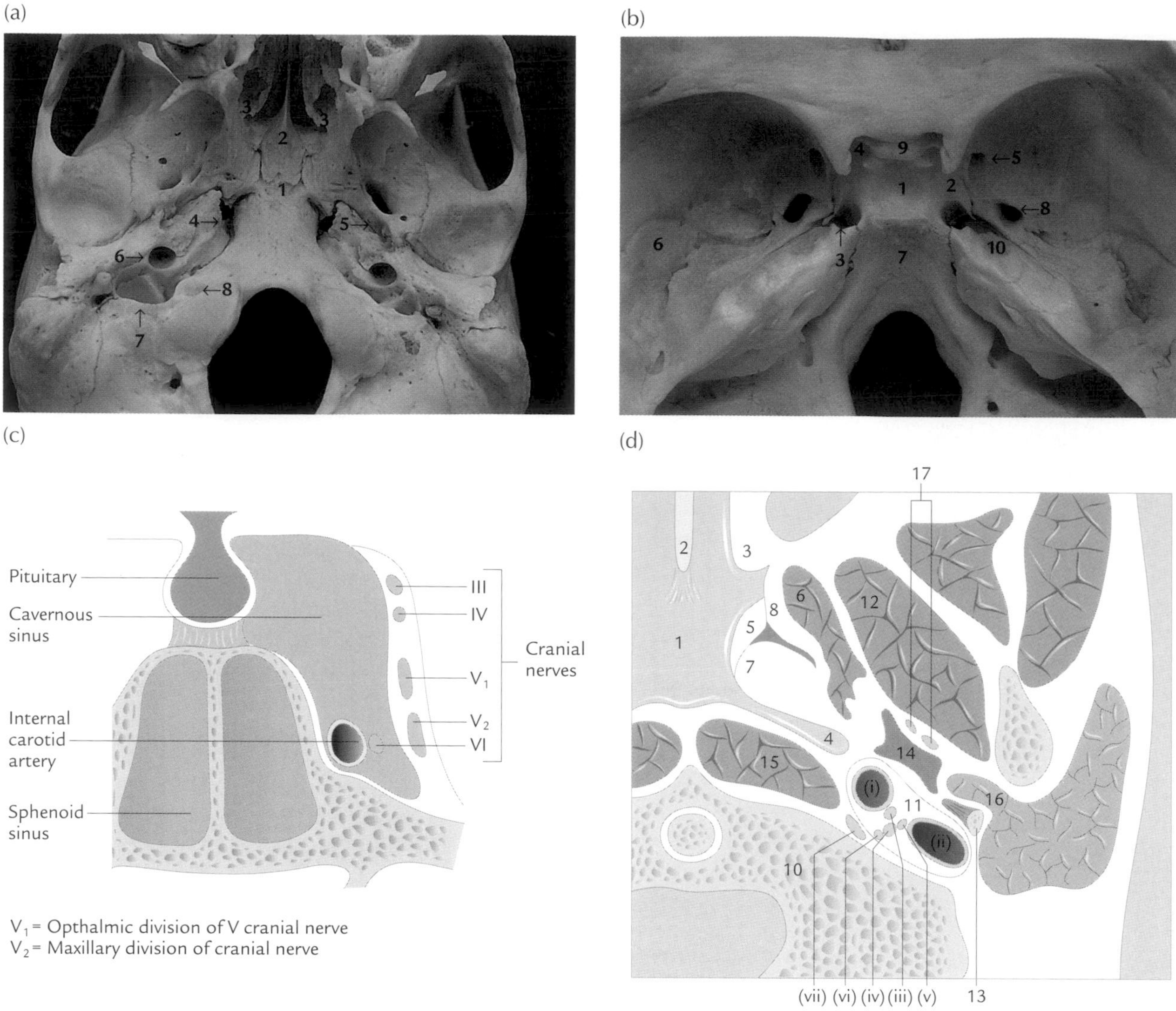

Figure 12.1

(a) Base of skull.
1: roof of nasopharynx;
2: posterior end of vomer;
3: posterior end of inferior turbinates;
4: foramen lacerum;
5: Eustachian tube orifice (bony portion);
6: carotid canal;
7: internal jugular canal;
8: hypoglossal canal;

(b) Middle cranial fossa.
1: Sella turcica;
2: carotid groove;
3: foramen lacerum;
4: optic canal;
5: foramen rotundum;
6: floor of middle cranial fossa;
7: clivus;
8: foramen ovale;
9: optic chiasm;
10: trigeminal ganglion impression.

(c) Cavernous sinus in coronal section

(d) Transverse section through the nasopharynx at the level of the atlas (C1).
1: roof of nasopharynx;
2: posterior end of vomer;
3: posterior end of inferior turbinates;
4: fossa of Rosenmuller;
5: Eustachian tube orifice;
6: Eustachian tube musculature;
7: posterior eustachian tube cushion;
8: anterior eustachian tube cushion;
9: posterior wall of nasopharynx;
10: C1;
11: carotid sheath and its contents;
- i) internal carotid artery (ICA);
- ii) internal jugular vein (IJV);
- iii) cranial nerve IX;
- iv) cranial nerve X;
- v) cranial nerve XI;
- vi) cranial nerve XII;
- vii) sympathetic trunk;

12: lateral pterygoid muscle;
13: styloid process and musculature;
14: parapharyngeal space;
15: longus capitus;
16: deep lobe of parotid;
17: cranial nerve V (branches of mandibular division).

(a) (b)

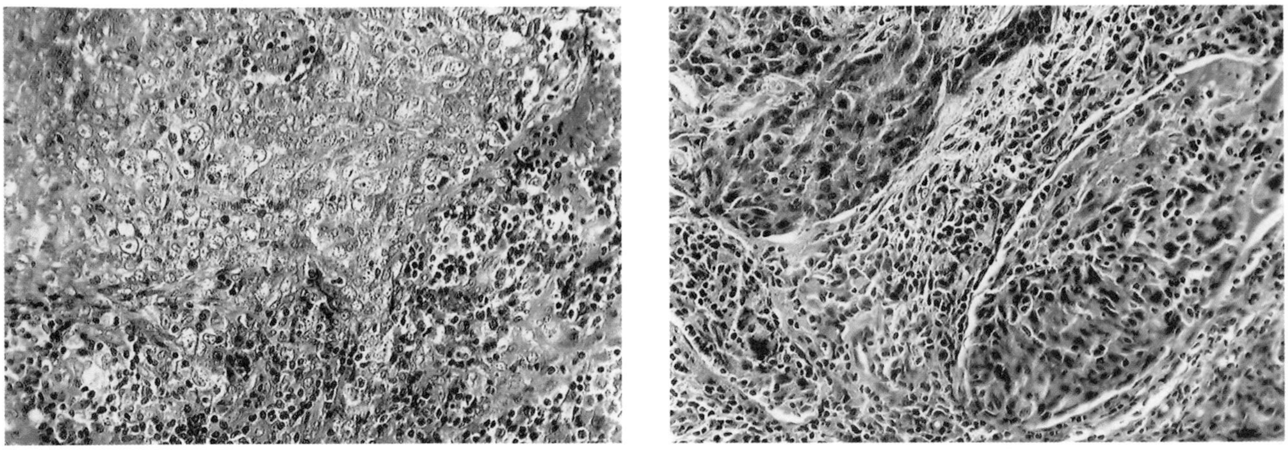

Figure 12.2 Photomicrographs of (a) undifferentiated carcinoma (UCNT) and (b) squamous cell carcinoma of the nasopharynx (haematoxylin and eosin). Both specimens show a background lymphocytic infiltrate illustrating that this is not a specific phenomenon.

Pathology

The pathological classification of nasopharyngeal tumours is described in Table 12.1. There have been many classifications proposed for nasopharyngeal carcinoma but in practical terms epidemiological and clinical features broadly define two groups, the squamous cell carcinomas (SCC) of varying degrees of differentiation and the undifferentiated carcinomas of nasopharyngeal type (UCNT) (Figure 12.2).[1,2] The WHO type 2 tumours are the most poorly defined with no clear morphological distinction between these and the undifferentiated carcinomas.[2]

The term lymphoepithelioma describes a carcinoma with a reactive lymphocytic infiltrate where the epithelial component may form well-defined aggregates (Regaud pattern) or be diffusely interspersed with inflammatory cells (Schmincke pattern). As the lymphocytic infiltrate has no clear prognostic significance these tumours are best categorized according to the features of the epithelial component which is invariably undifferentiated.

Table 12.1 Pathological classification of nasopharyngeal tumours

Benign tumours	
Juvenile angiofibroma	
Malignant tumours	
Nasopharyngeal carcinoma (NPC)	85%*
WHO type 1 – keratinizing squamous cell carcinoma	
WHO type 2 – non-keratinizing (differentiated) carcinoma	
WHO type 3 – undifferentiated carcinoma	
Non-Hodgkin's lymphoma (Hodgkin's lymphoma rare)	10%*
Adenoid cystic carcinoma	
Adenocarcinoma and minor salivary gland tumours	
Plasmacytoma	
Melanoma	
Sarcoma (especially rhabdomyosarcoma)	
Chordoma	

*Approximate proportion of all malignant tumours

Nasopharyngeal carcinoma

Epidemiology and pathogenesis

In the western hemisphere (the Americas and Europe) nasopharyngeal carcinoma (NPC) is rare with an annual incidence of around 0.5/100 000, accounting for 1–2% of all head and neck cancers. In contrast in southern China and Hong Kong the disease is endemic with annual incidence rates of up to 50/100 000.[3] This disparity is related to histopathological subtypes. In North American series keratinizing squamous cell carcinomas account for up to 68% of cases[4] whilst in the Far East over 95% are WHO type 2–3.[5] The incidence of UCNT is also high in Eskimo and native Alaskan populations[6] and moderately increased in Malaysia, north Africa and southern Europe.

Nasopharyngeal carcinoma is probably the result of complex interaction of genetic and environmental factors. Familial clusters of NPC are reported in endemic areas and emigrants from these areas carry with them an increased risk,[7] though this falls somewhat in successive generations.[8] In ethnic Chinese, NPC is associated with the concurrence of HLA types A2 and Bw46 (formerly B*sin*2).[9] The phenotype B17 carries a similar relative risk and, like Bw46, is associated with benign conditions characterized by immune dysfunction such as autoimmune thyrotoxicosis and systemic lupus erythematosis. B17 is said to be associated with younger-onset disease and possibly carries a poorer prognosis.[10] An HLA linkage study in affected sibling pairs suggests the presence of an NPC susceptibility gene closely linked to the HLA locus that may carry a relative risk of over 20.[11]

There is a strong association between UCNT and positive serology for Epstein–Barr virus (EBV) antigens.[12] Antibody titres (particularly IgA) to the viral capsid antigen (VCA) and early antigen complex (EA) have been correlated with the stage of the disease[13] and a fall reflects tumour response to therapy. Persistently elevated or rising antibody titres predict for progression or recurrence.[14,15] Clonal EBV DNA has been demonstrated in NPC as have the nuclear proteins necessary to ensure persistence of the viral genome with cell replication.[16] These observations imply that the virus is present from the start of the neoplastic process and could contribute to it. The EBV latent membrane protein LMP1, for example, has oncogenic and growth-stimulating properties.[16] It is conceivable that the genetic factors eluded to above influence the way in which an initial EBV infection is handled, allowing its persistence in a potentially oncogenic form. That reactivation of the latent virus occurs is suggested by the high incidence (96.6%) of antibodies to the EBV replication activator BZLF-1 (or 'ZEBRA') in NPC patients.[17]

Until recently it has been thought that squamous cell carcinoma of the nasopharynx is biologically distinct from UCNT, with no EBV association. However, in situ hybridization techniques have now demonstrated the presence of EBV-encoded RNA in all three histological types, though it is less abundant in well-differentiated tumours.[18] Whether SCC is associated with the same risk factors as for other head and neck sites is unclear, though there is certainly evidence to suggest that heavy smoking further increases the risk of UCNT in endemic areas.[19]

Environmental factors beyond EBV are likely to be important in UCNT. Ho[20] hypothesized that early childhood consumption of salted fish contributed to the high-risk of NPC in southern China and Hong Kong. This has been supported by a case-control study[21] and may also explain the high incidence of UCNT in Eskimos.[6] Fish preservation by salting leads to the accumulation of potentially carcinogenic nitrosamines.[20]

In general NPC affects a younger population than cancer at other head and neck sites. In endemic areas the incidence rises from age 20 to peak in the fourth and fifth decades.[19] In areas of lower risk the median age falls between the fifth and sixth decades but there is still a significant incidence in the under 30s, giving rise to a bimodal distribution, with an initial peak between 15 and 25 years. All NPC types show a male predominance of around 3:1.

Natural history

The majority of tumours arise in the region of the fossa of Rosenmüller or roof of the nasopharynx (Figure 12.3). By direct anterior extension the tumour may invade the posterior nasal cavity or extend inferiorly along the pharyngeal wall (Figure 12.4), on to the soft palate or down to the tonsil (Figure 12.5).

Involvement of the skull base at presentation has been reported in 35% of cases evaluated by CT scanning.[22] The tumour may invade the sphenoid sinus or gain access to the cavernous sinus through the fibrous tissue floor of the foramen lacerum (Figure 12.6). Here cranial nerves III–VI are vulnerable, with V and VI being most frequently involved clinically (Figure 12.7).

Parapharyngeal space involvement has been described in 35% to over 80%.[5,22–24] It may arise by direct tumour extension, particularly adjacent to the Eustachian tube where the lateral wall is relatively

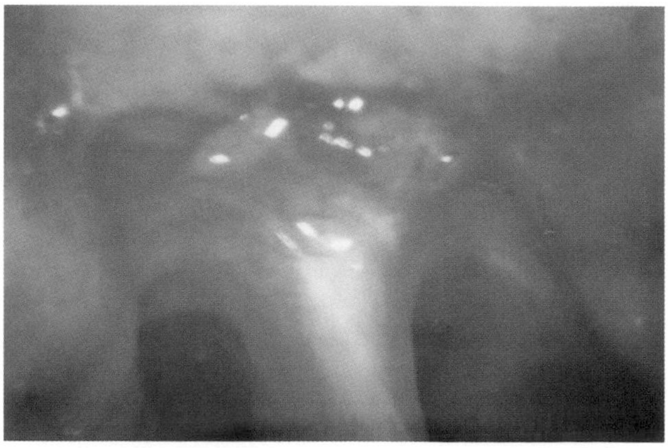

Figure 12.3 Endoscopic view of a small UCNT at the junction of the vomer with the clivus.

QMUL Library

Borrowed Items 24/09/2009 11:33

XXXXXX319X

Item Title	Due Date
An introduction to oral and m	29/09/2009
Oral and maxillofacial surger	29/09/2009
* Principles and practic[illegible]	22/10/2009

Amount Outs[illegible] : £4.00

* Indicates items borrowed today

Thank you for using this unit

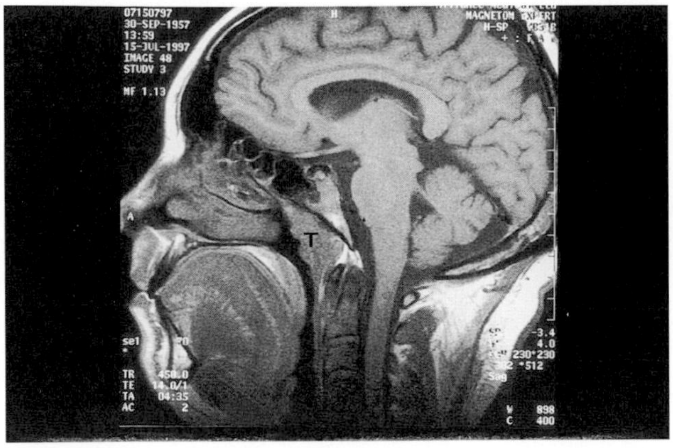

Figure 12.4 T1-weighted sagittal magnetic resonance image showing a UCNT (T) occupying the roof and posterior wall of the nasopharynx.

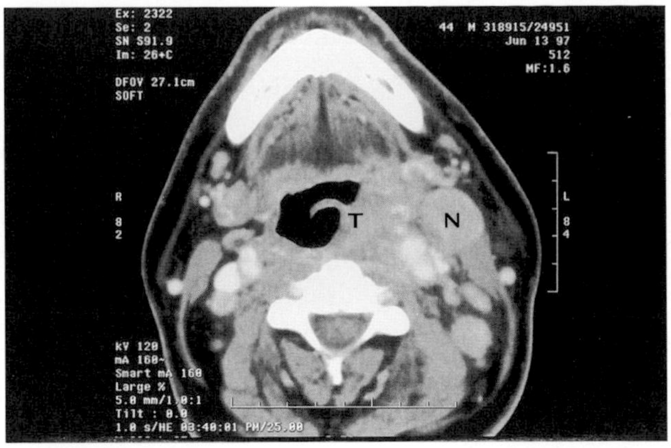

Figure 12.5 Contrast-enhanced CT scan showing invasion of the left lateral wall of the oropharynx by UCNT (T). Note the enlarged lymph nodes (N).

(a)

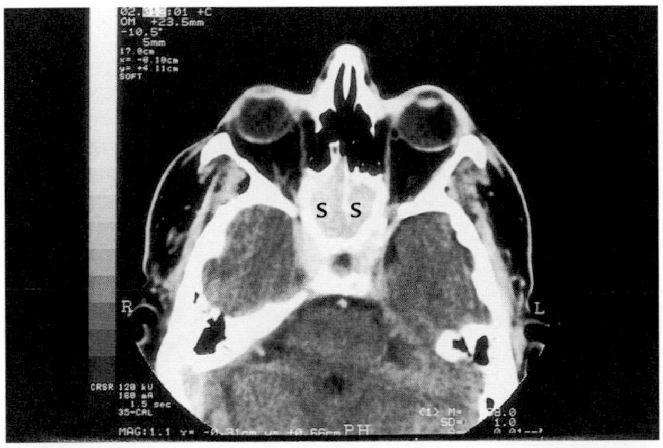

(b)

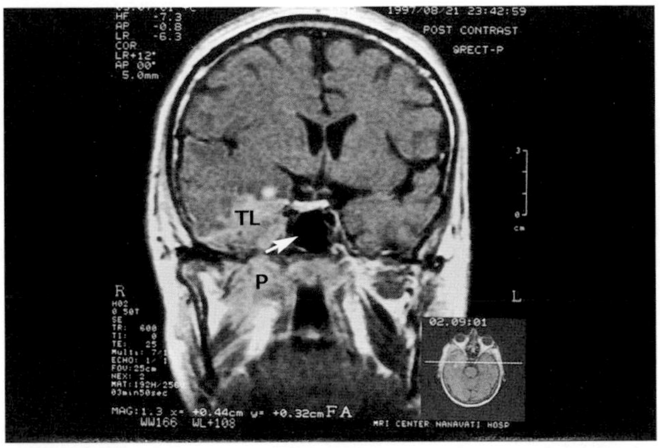

(c)

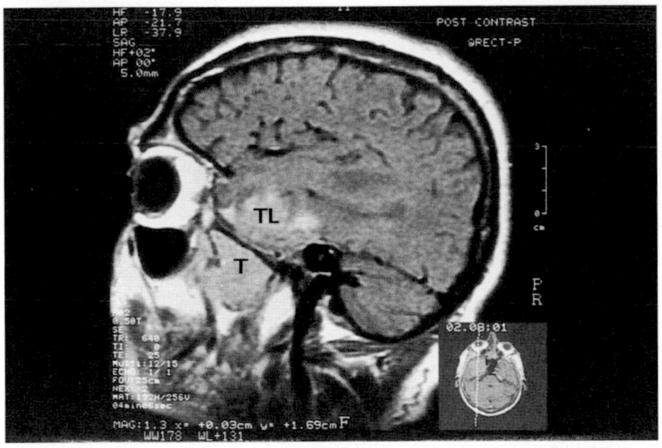

Figure 12.6 (a) Contrast-enhanced CT scan of the skull base showing tumour filling the sphenoid sinuses (S). (b) Gadolinium-enhanced coronal T1-weighted MR image showing UCNT in the right parapharyngeal space (P), extending through the foraminae of the skull base to involve the temporal lobe (TL) of the brain and cavernous sinus (arrow). (c) Sagittal image from the same series as (b). Primary UCNT (T) with extension into temporal lobe (TL).

deficient (Figure 12.8). Alternatively it can occur by expansion of involved parapharyngeal nodes (Figure 12.9). Either case may progress to involvement of lower cranial nerves (CN IX–XII) where they lie adjacent to the major vessels in the posterior part of the parapharyngeal space. From the parapharyngeal space the tumour can gain access to the middle cranial fossa (Figure 12.6) and cavernous sinus via the foramen ovale. Involvement of the pterygoid plates may lead to forward extension into the pterygopalatine fossa and beyond into the inferior orbital fissure. Alternatively tumour may invade the orbit via the ethmoid sinuses (Figure 12.10).

In a report of 628 patients, 7% had involvement of one or more of cranial nerves II–VIII, while 3.5% had involvement of the lower cranial nerves (IX–XII). Five patients had involvement of both groups.[22] In a

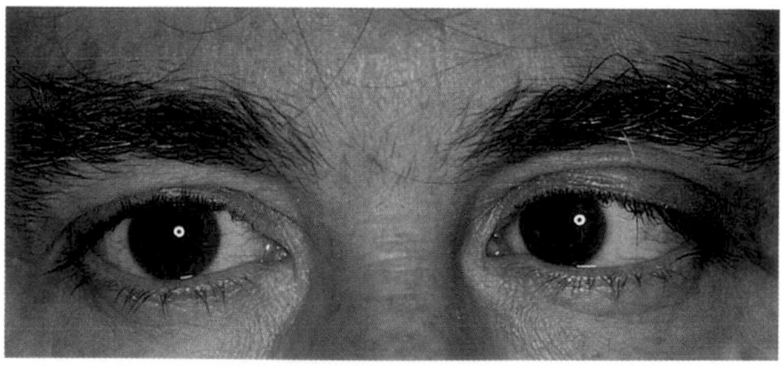

Figure 12.7 Right lateral rectus palsy.

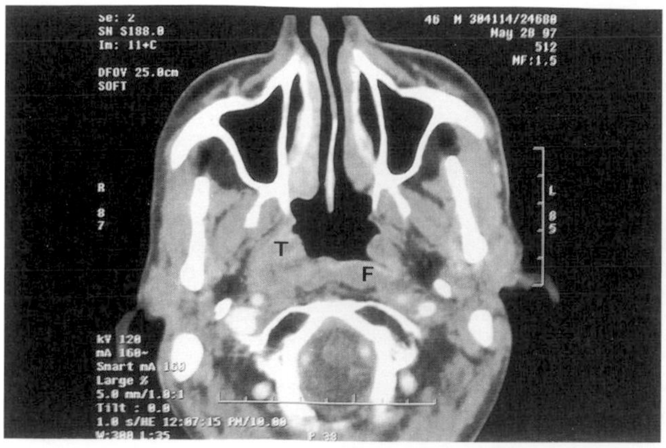

Figure 12.8 CT scan with intravenous contrast showing direct extension of a right-sided nasopharyngeal carcinoma (T) into the parapharyngeal space. Note how the tumour has obliterated the right fossa of Rosenmuller as compared to the normal fossa (F) on the left.

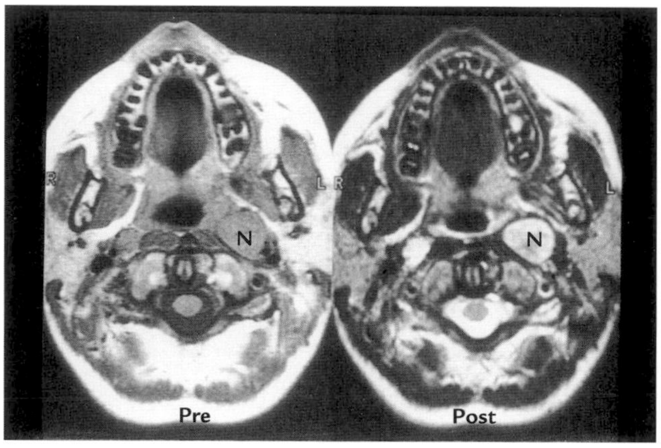

Figure 12.9 Paired T1-weighted MR images (pre- and postintravenous gadolinium) showing distortion of the left parapharyngeal space due to expansion of a retropharyngeal lymph node (N) by UCNT.

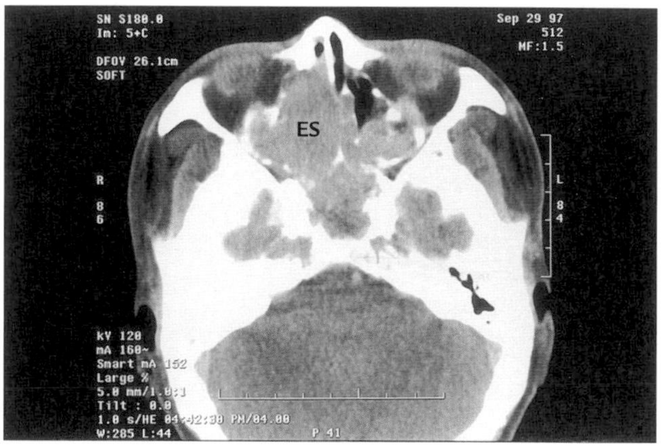

Figure 12.10 Contrast-enhanced CT scan showing expansion and destruction of the walls of the right ethmoid sinuses (ES) with extension of tumour into the right orbit.

(a) (b)

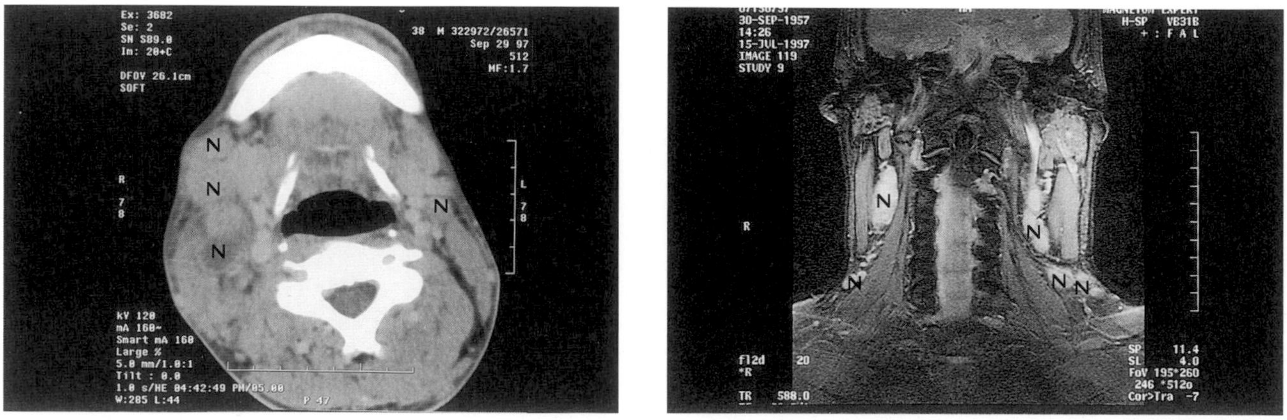

Figure 12.11 (a) Contrast-enhanced CT scan of the upper neck showing multiple involved nodes (N) in a patient with UCNT. (b) STIR sequence coronal MR image in a patient with bilateral lymphadenopathy (N) from UCNT.

series of 378 patients reported from the MD Anderson Cancer Center, 8% had one or more cranial nerve palsies, with CN VI being the most commonly involved.[25] In contrast, Lederman[26] described cranial nerve involvement in 26% of 218 patients at presentation and a similar figure (23.8%) was reported by Perez et al.[27]

Nasopharyngeal carcinoma is characterized by early and often bulky cervical lymph node involvement (Figure 12.11). Large series report between 63 and 79% lymph node involvement[22,24,25,27,28] with around 30% of patients having bilateral lymphadenopathy at diagnosis.[25,27] There has been no obvious increase in the reported incidence with the now routine use of CT scanning,[22,24] suggesting that nodal involvement is rarely subtle. The jugulodigastric (upper deep cervical) and posterior cervical (upper and middle) node groups are most frequently involved, followed by the middle deep cervical.[25,27,29] Submental, occipital or parotid nodal involvement is unusual. A lack of correlation between the stage of the primary tumour and the extent of nodal involvement has been consistently reported.[25,27,28] In keeping with this the nasopharynx is well recognized as the seat of an occult primary tumour in patients presenting with apparently isolated cervical lymphadenopathy. Cervical node relapse is reported to occur in 30% of untreated clinically node-negative necks.[30]

Distant metastases are found in 3–6% of patients at presentation[28,31] but ultimately develop in around 40%.[28,32] Bone is most commonly affected, followed by lung and liver. Bone marrow involvement is not uncommon in patients with metastatic disease and carries a poor prognosis.[33] Lymph node metastases beyond the neck, and not necessarily in contiguity, may occur at presentation or on relapse.[23]

Clinical features

The most common presenting complaint is of a lump in the neck, reflecting the frequency of nodal involvement. The primary itself may cause nasal blockage, discharge or bleeding and obstruction of the auditory tube can lead to otitis media with effusion (Figure 12.12) and otalgia. Bony destruction and expansion of the parapharyngeal space may result in a persistent deep-seated headache and direct invasion of CN V can give rise to trigeminal neuralgia.

Forward extension into the orbit can produce proptosis and diplopia as well as retro-orbital pain. With invasion of the cavernous sinus, palsies of CNs III, IV and VI can also lead to diplopia or even complete ophthalmoplegia.

Involvement of the soft palate and pharyngeal wall may be evidenced by a sore throat or odynophagia. Difficulty in swallowing can also occur through compromise of the lower cranial nerves in the parapharyngeal space when it may be associated with mucosal hypoaesthesia, disturbed taste, palatal incompetence, hemiglossal paralysis and weakness of the muscles innervated by the spinal accessory nerve.

Metastatic disease may present as extraregional lymphadenopathy, bone pain, respiratory symptoms or hepatomegaly. Several paraneoplastic syndromes have been described with NPC including hypertrophic osteoarthropathy, pyrexia of unknown origin and inappropriate ADH secretion. Metastatic disease may also be accompanied by a leukaemoid peripheral blood picture.[33]

Clinical assessment and investigation

A full history, particularly with respect to neurological symptoms and complaints implicating metastatic disease is essential. As radiotherapy is the primary treatment modality it is important to identify potentially complicating factors such as previous irradiation, smoking, alcohol abuse, poor nutrition and dental complaints.

Physical examination should be directed towards nasal cavities and nasopharynx with the aid of a rigid endoscopic optical rod or flexible nasoendoscope noting the extent of the primary tumour, which may be grossly exophytic, or simply loss of definition of the fossa of Rosenmüller. Extension to the soft palate, pharyngeal wall and oropharynx should be sought by both inspection and palpation. Evidence of lower cranial nerve deficits may be apparent from palatal or glossal paralysis and atrophy. A full evaluation of the remaining cranial nerves should include visual assessment and examination of the tympanic membranes.

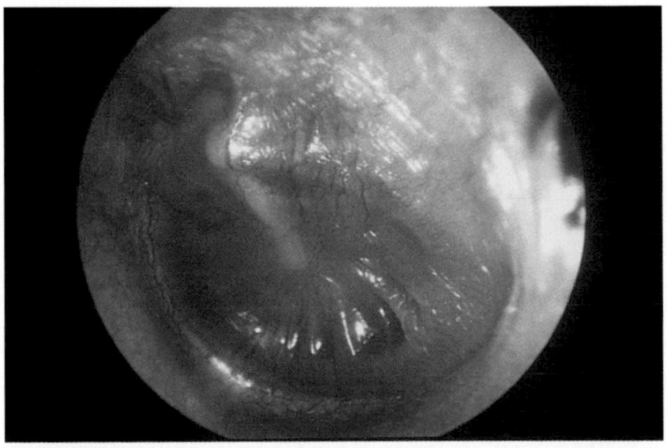

Figure 12.12 Chronic otitis media with effusion

The extent of nodal disease in the neck should be documented and further examination must include all other lymph node areas as these are potential sites of metastatic disease. Chest and abdominal examination should be directed towards the search for metastatic disease. Histological verification of a bulky tumour can be achieved through biopsy under local anaesthetic and endoscopic guidance in the clinic. Smaller and less accessible tumours should be biopsied at examination under general anaesthetic.

Appropriate imaging of the primary tumour is important not only for staging but for accurate radiotherapy planning. The choice between high resolution CT scanning and MRI is largely one of availability.[34] Since both techniques have their advantages and disadvantages in this setting they can be considered complementary. The superior spatial and contrast resolution of MRI make it the more sensitive investigation for the detection of subclinical tumours as well as for delineating soft tissue invasion in more extensive disease. Consequently some authors consider it the modality of choice.[35] However, bone involvement is more readily detected by CT and in a comparative study, more patients were up-staged by CT than MRI.[36] It is generally agreed that MRI is superior to CT for the detection of local recurrence and the imaging of treatment complications.[34–36]

As indicated earlier, serology for EBV, particularly IgA directed towards VCA and EA can be useful diagnostically and may have a role in screening for asymptomatic NPC in high-risk populations.[37] It can also be helpful in monitoring the response to therapy and in the diagnosis of relapse. The assay for IgG anti-ZEBRA antibodies is not yet in routine clinical use, though high titres appear to predict for the development of distant metastases.[17] While less specific, high serum lactate dehydrogenase (LDH) levels are also associated with metastatic disease.[38]

A summary of the recommended investigations is given in Table 12.2. Screening for metastatic disease is indicated in those patients with advanced nodal disease and any suspicious symptoms should be investigated. Finally, prior to embarking on radiotherapy a full dental assessment with completion of any restorative work is imperative.

Table 12.2 Recommended investigations in nasopharyngeal carcinoma

In all patients
Direct nasopharyngoscopy and biopsy of primary tumour
Full blood count
Biochemistry profile including liver function tests and lactate dehydrogenase (LDH)
Epstein–Barr virus serology (IgA anti-VCA, IgA anti-EA)
Chest X-ray
High resolution CT (with intravenous contrast) or MRI scan of the middle cranial fossa, skull base, nasopharynx, paranasal sinuses, neck and thoracic inlet
Orthopantomogram
In patients with advanced nodal disease (UICC N3) or when metastatic disease is suspected
Bone scan and plain radiographs of abnormal or symptomatic areas
Liver ultrasound scan
Supplementary tests
Baseline audiometry (if clinically indicated or prior to platinum chemotherapy)
Creatinine or EDTA clearance (prior to platinum chemotherapy)

Staging

A number of staging classifications have been proposed for NPC[20,39–42] but the two most commonly used have been those of Ho and the UICC (1989). As outlined in Table 12.3 these classifications are based on different criteria, particularly with respect to the N stage. An analysis of CT-staged patients treated at the Prince of Wales Hospital, Hong Kong suggests that the Ho classification is superior for the prediction of local failure, freedom from metastasis and overall survival.[43] A further refinement of the Ho classification, taking into account the prognostic significance of parapharyngeal involvement and intracranial extension, has been proposed by Teo (Table 12.3).[44] The major weakness of the 1989 UICC classification is the combination of a very heterogeneous group of patients in stage IV, while stages I and II are very similar in outcome and together account for only a small proportion of patients. These criticisms have been addressed in the 1997 system (Table 12.3),[41] which has also recognized the prognostic significance of supraclavicular node involvement as described by Ho.[20]

Prognostic factors

Age and sex

There is considerable disagreement in the literature as to whether these represent significant prognostic factors. Several studies report that the survival of patients under 40 is better.[45–47] Perez et al[27] report poorer local control and survival in patients over 50, whilst others find no age effect.[5,25] In a series of patients under 21, the prognosis was more favourable in those no more than 15 years old.[48] Ho[49]

Table 12.3 Staging classifications for nasopharyngeal carcinoma

Ho (1978)		Prince of Wales Hospital (1991)		UICC (1989)		UICC (1997)	
T1	Tumour limited to nasopharynx	T1	Tumour limited to nasopharynx	T1	Tumour limited to one wall of nasopharynx	T1	Tumour confined to nasopharynx
T2	Tumour beyond nasopharynx and into:	T2	Tumour beyond nasopharynx and into:	T2	Involvement of two or more walls of nasopharynx	T2	Tumour extends to soft tissue of oropharynx and/or nasal fossa
n	Nasal fossa	n	Nasal fossa	T3	Invasion of nasal cavity and/or oropharynx	T2a	Without parapharyngeal extension
o	Oropharynx	o	Oropharynx	T4	Invasion of skull base and/or cranial nerve(s)	T2b	With parapharyngeal extension
P	Parapharyngeal region	T3a	Involvement of skull base and/or parapharyngeal region			T3	Tumour invades bony structures and/or paranasal sinuses
T3a	Bone involvement below skull base including floor of sphenoid sinus	T3b	Cranial nerve palsy			T4	Tumour with intracranial extension and/or involvement of cranial nerves, infratemporal fossa, hypopharynx or orbit
T3b	Involvement of base of skull	T4	Intracranial extension				
T3c	Cranial nerve palsy						
T3d	Invasion of orbit, hypopharynx or infratemporal fossa						
N0	No palpable cervical nodes	N0	No palpable cervical nodes	N0	No palpable cervical nodes	N0	No regional lymph node metastasis
N1	Node(s) above skin crease extending laterally and backward from or just below thyroid notch	N1	Nodes above the supraclavicular fossa (N2f fixed nodes)	N1	Single unilateral node ≤ 3 cm	N1	Unilateral metastasis in lymph node(s), ≤ 6 cm, above the supraclavicular fossa
N2	Node(s) below skin crease but above supraclavicular fossa	N2	Supraclavicular fossa nodes (N3f fixed nodes)	N2a	Single ipsilateral node > 3 cm ≤ 6 cm	N2	Bilateral metastasis in lymph nodes, ≤ 6 cm, above the supraclavicular fossa
N3	Supraclavicular nodes			N2b	Multiple ipsilateral nodes ≤ 6 cm	N3	Metastasis in lymph node(s)
				N2c	Bilateral or contralateral nodes ≤ 6 cm	N3a	> 6 cm
				N3	Node(s) > 6 cm	N3b	In the supraclavicular fossa
M0	No distant metastases	M0	No distant metastases	M0	No distant metastases	M0	No distant metastases
M1	Distant metastases	M1	Distant metastases	M1	Distant metastases	M1	Distant metastases
Stage grouping		Stage grouping		Stage grouping		Stage grouping	
I	T1 N0	Ia	T1 N0	I	T1 N0	I	T1 N0
II	T2 and/or N1	Ib	T2 N0	II	T2 N0	IIA	T2a N0
III	T3 and/or N2	IIa	T1–2 N1–N1f	III	T3 N0, T1–3 N1	IIB	T1–2a N1, T2b N0–1
IV	N3 (any T)	IIb	T3 N0	IV	T4 N0–1	III	T1–2b N2, T2ab N2, T3 N0–2
V	M1	IIIa	T3 N1–N1f		N2–3 (any T)	IVA	T4 N0–2
		IIIb	T1–2 N2–N2f		M1 (any T, any N)	IVB	N3 (any T)
		IVa	T3 N2–N2f, T4 any N M0			IVB	M1 (any T any N)
		IVb	M1 (any T any N)				

did not find any influence of gender on prognosis but several later studies have suggested that males fare worse both in terms of local control and survival.[5,45–47]

Histological subtype

It is difficult to generalize on the influence of histological subtypes from the published evidence. Part of the problem lies in the widely variable classifications used but more importantly, the large series from endemic areas include few differentiated squamous cell carcinomas. Perhaps as a result, these series show no significant effect of histology on survival.[45–47] On the contrary, in a series from the Institut Gustave Roussy, in which half the patients had squamous cell carcinomas, the 5-year disease-free survival was significantly better in those patients with UCNT.[5] In support, two North American series suggest that histological subtype is a strong determinant of local control.[25,50] One of these[25] found that histological subtype also predicated for regional control and indeed, that within the squamous cell carcinomas, the poorly differentiated (grade III) cases showed better local and regional control when compared to lower grade SCCs. Santos et al[51] also report poorer local and regional control in SCC, reflected in worse 5-year survival figures.

In the Mallinckrodt Institute series[27] histological subtype had no influence on disease-free and overall survival but local control of T2–T3 SCCs was considerably poorer (33%) than with other histological types (83%). In the same series undifferentiated carcinomas and lymphoepitheliomas were more frequently associated with distant metastases (41%) than either non-keratinizing (21%) or keratinizing (6%) SCCs.

Taking all of these observations together, a reasonable overview would be that stage for stage, local–regional control is more likely to be a problem with differentiated SCC whilst UCNT has a greater chance of failing distantly. Either scenario carries an ominous prognosis.

Disease stage

The Ho classification is used in the large series reported from Hong Kong whilst western centres employ the UICC system. Centres in mainland China and Taiwan have used different systems again (for example the Shanghai[45] and Huang[40]). Whilst the details of these various Chinese systems can be criticized[44] their stage groupings do predict for survival.[28,40,45,46,49,52] There are no published series validating the 1989 UICC system but in a comparative study from Hong Kong its predictive value proved inferior to the Ho system.[43] In the absence of a unified system it is more instructive to consider the components of stage individually. Overall, the presence or absence of distant metastasis (M stage) is the dominant prognostic factor.

T stage

Despite the number and variation of staging systems used, there is general agreement that the extent of the primary tumour is a strong predictor for local control.[25,27,43,53] However, the value of subdividing disease confined to the nasopharynx (i.e. UICC 1989 T1 and T2) has been questioned[43,49] and systematic biopsy of all subsites has failed to demonstrate a correlation between the extent of involvement and local control.[54] Nevertheless, discrepant local failure rates for UICC (1989) stages T1 and T2 have been reported.[25,27] The 1997 revision of the UICC system no longer subdivides disease confined to the nasopharynx (Table 12.3).

The independent prognostic value of T stage for survival is unclear. Most series report outcomes for stage groupings from which it is impossible to determine the influence of primary stage, given the overriding effect of nodal involvement (see below). In multivariate analysis current T stage classifications offer a weak prognostic indicator.[24,27,46,53] Notwithstanding this uncertainty there are clearly factors related to the extent of primary tumour that influence both local control and survival.

Cranial nerve involvement clearly predicts for increased risk of local and distant failure and poorer survival.[47] Furthermore, it remains an independent predictor of poorer survival in multivariate analysis even when T stage does not.[22,27] Similarly, it predicts for local failure independently of T stage.[25] Involvement of the upper cranial nerves (II–VIII) is more ominous than the lower (IX–XII).[47] Invasion of the skull base in the absence of cranial nerve involvement is also associated with local and distant failure and a poorer outcome.[25,47] Intracranial extension of the primary tumour predicts a very poor prognosis and is frequently associated with distant failure.[22]

With the routine use of CT scanning it is clear that parapharyngeal extension (PPE) is common.[24,55] Chua et al[24] have defined three grades of involvement, with extensive parapharyngeal extension (grade 2–3) being associated with both local failure and distant metastases. The authors suggest that extensive PPE may lead to direct invasion of the vertebral (Batson's) venous plexus. Reporting the same association between PPE and metastatic disease, Teo et al assert that extensive parapharyngeal tumour is difficult to distinguish from retropharyngeal nodal metastasis and that the latter may explain the link with distant metastasis.[22]

N stage

In the absence of clinically apparent distant metastases, cervical lymph node involvement is the strongest prognostic factor in NPC. The huge Hong Kong series clearly demonstrate the ability of Ho's levels of nodal involvement[20] to predict for distant failure and consequently survival.[28,46,47] The 1989 UICC nodal classification also predicts for distant metastases[27] and both of these systems predict increasing regional failure with advanced nodal stage.[25,47] In contrast, there appears to be no correlation between failure at the primary site and nodal stage.[25,47]

In the 1970s Ho criticized the contemporary UICC system on its surgical basis, which, though appropriate for the majority of head and neck cancers, had little relevance to NPC and he was unable to demonstrate any prognostic significance for nodal laterality or fixity.[49] Although none of the current systems include fixity, recent Hong Kong series suggest that this is indeed a prognostic factor,[47,56,57] though of secondary importance to Ho's levels. The significance of maximum nodal size and laterality, on which the current UICC system is based, remains controversial.[47,56,58,59]

Treatment

Radiotherapy: general considerations

Radiotherapy remains the primary treatment modality for NPC. The use of neoadjuvant and concomitant chemotherapy, though increasingly applied, should still be considered investigational until the definitive results of randomized studies are available (see below).

The challenge in planning successful and safe radiotherapy to the nasopharynx and the surrounding pathways of local invasion becomes obvious from a simple consideration of the anatomy. A radiation dose exceeding the tolerance of most normal tissues must be delivered to a site intimately related to the brainstem, temporal lobes, pituitary gland and optic chiasm. Late radiation effects on other related structures such as the parotid glands, temporomandibular joints and oropharyngeal musculature can contribute significantly to late morbidity.

In view of the necessarily narrow field margins and the proximity of critical structures, head immobilization during treatment planning and delivery is essential. Our preference is to use a plastic immobilization shell covering the full face, neck and upper thorax in the supine position. The shell is drilled out or cut away over the treatment fields as far as practicable to retain the skin-sparing properties of the megavoltage treatment beams. A plastic mouth bite is used to depress the tongue and away from the palate and so out of the treatment volume.

Target volume

The treatment of the primary site offers an excellent example of the so-called 'shrinking field' technique. To facilitate this, accurate assessment of the extent of the gross tumour volume by a combination of clinical examination and CT or MRI scanning is essential. Whilst gross tumour will need to be treated to a minimum dose of 65 Gy, clinically uninvolved sites at risk of microscopic disease need not be treated beyond 50–55 Gy, allowing sparing of adjacent sensitive structures.

When the gross tumour volume (GTV) is limited to the nasopharynx the clinical target volume (CTV) should include (bilaterally) the posterior quarter of the orbit (i.e. behind the globe), the posterior half to one-third of the nasal fossa and maxillary sinus, the posterior ethmoid sinuses and the whole of the sphenoid sinus, the cavernous sinus with adjacent middle temporal fossa, the medial portion of the petrous temporal bone with the clivus and intervening fissure, the nasopharynx, the parapharyngeal tissues (including the medial pterygoid muscle, most of the adjacent lateral pterygoid muscle, the styloid process and jugular foramen) and the retropharyngeal space with the longus capitis muscle. Inferiorly the volume should include the whole of the soft palate and uvula with adjacent oropharynx. This volume will necessarily include the retro- and parapharyngeal nodes.

When there is extensive involvement of the nasal cavity the initial volume should include the whole of the nasal fossa, maxillary antrum and all ethmoid sinuses bilaterally. Similarly, tumour extension down the lateral or posterior pharyngeal wall will require the primary volume to be extended inferiorally (see Field arrangements below).

Once the areas of potential microscopic involvement have been treated to a dose of 50 Gy the primary volume can be further reduced, excluding critical structures such as the optic nerves, spinal cord and brainstem, to include the GTV with a 1–1.5 cm margin as the planning target volume (PTV).

Given the propensity of nodal involvement in NPC, the majority of patients will require therapy to all cervical node groups, with the exception of the rarely involved submental nodes.[29] In practice this means irradiation of both sides of the neck from the occiput to the sternal notch. Ho[49] questioned the need for elective nodal irradiation in clinically node-negative patients, quoting the results of a randomized study in which all cases of neck-only relapses in the unirradiated were successfully salvaged. The analysis, limited to T1N0 cases, showed no survival advantage for elective nodal irradiation. A further report from the same institute describing their subsequent experience with an observation policy in T1N0 (Ho) confirms successful salvage in the 30% of patients who relapsed in the neck.[30] However, the survival of this group was lower than those not relapsing, with an increased rate of distant metastases. Since it is impossible to determine whether the neck relapses contributed to the distant failure and given the psychological morbidity of any disease recurrence, the authors now recommend elective nodal irradiation.

Although there is little data on the relative rates of nodal involvement with histological type, it is the policy at the Royal Marsden Hospital to electively treat only the upper and middle (both deep and posterior) cervical nodes in the rare node-negative well-differentiated squamous carcinomas.

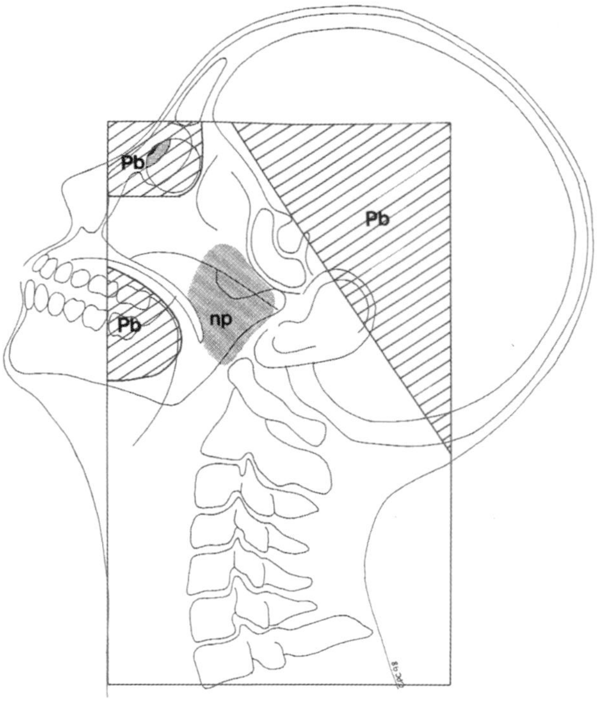

Figure 12.13 Diagram illustrating the borders and lead shielding (Pb) of the parallel-opposed lateral fields employed in the first phase of irradiation in NPC with bulky cervical lymphadenopathy. np: nasopharynx.

Field arrangements and radiation dose

The fields are simulated and treated with the patient immobilized in the supine position with the neck fully extended (chin elevated). At the Royal Marsden Hospital the field arrangement is essentially that described by Ho[60] with minor modifications. The primary site is treated in two or three phases and the neck in one or two depending on the bulk of disease. These phases run in succession with no planned gaps in treatment. Our accepted maximum doses to critical normal tissues over a 6–7 week course of treatment are: spinal cord and brainstem 45 Gy, optic nerve and retina 50 Gy and lens 10 Gy.

In patients with bulky cervical lymphadenopathy, particularly in the upper deep cervical or junctional region, or in those with extensive oropharyngeal involvement, the primary volume (as defined above) and both sides of the neck are treated in continuity with parallel opposed lateral fields extending inferiorally to the supraclavicular fossa (Figure 12.13). In those patients where the position of the shoulders prevents irradiation of the lowest neck nodes with lateral fields a single anterior field with midline shielding is matched to the inferior border of the lateral fields. This volume is treated isocentrically to a maximum intersection dose of 30 Gy in 15 fractions of 2 Gy treating all fields daily over 3 weeks. It is our practice to use 5 or 6 MV photons for this phase. If there is a rapid response of the nodal disease this phase may be curtailed at 20 Gy in favour of an earlier switch to the second phase.

In the second phase of treatment the same patient position is adopted, though a new shell may be required if there has been a significant change in the contour of the neck. The primary volume (as defined above) is treated with small parallel opposed fields with lead shielding to the anterior orbit, mouth, brainstem, spinal cord and posterior inferior corner of the field where it overlaps the neck fields (Figure 12.14). This volume is treated to a further 20–30 Gy (depending on the phase 1 dose) in 2-Gy daily fractions to bring the total dose to 50 Gy at the intersection point. Where possible high energy photons should be used to improve sparing of the temporomandibular joints. During this phase both sides of the neck are treated with parallel opposed anterior and posterior fields with midline shielding to the spinal cord and larynx plus infraclavicular shielding bilaterally. With the neck extended the upper border of these fields runs across the angle of the mandible and the occiput (Figure 12.14). Depending on the phase 1 dose the neck is treated to a further 30–40 Gy in daily 2-Gy fractions, specified at a point 3 cm lateral to the field centre, 2.5 cm deep to the anterior skin surface (neck reference point). This brings the total neck dose to 60 Gy. The sites of originally involved nodes are thereafter boosted with electron fields of appropriate energy for the treatment depth to a total dose of 65 Gy.

In the final phase of treatment to the primary site the volume is further reduced and localized to the site of the gross tumour at diagnosis with a 1–1.5 cm

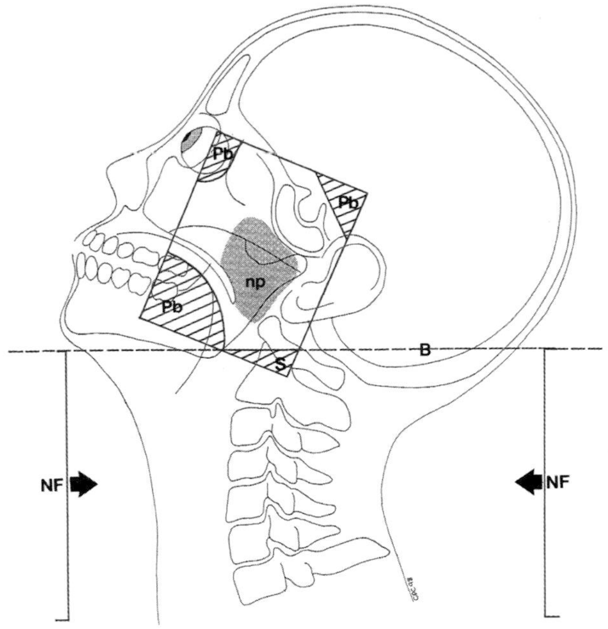

Figure 12.14 Diagram illustrating the extent of the lateral fields used to treat the nasopharynx and adjacent sites at risk of microscopic involvement. The upper border of the anterior and posterior parallel opposed neck fields (NF) is indicated (B) and the overlap is shielded (S). Pb: lead shielding, np: nasopharynx.

(a)

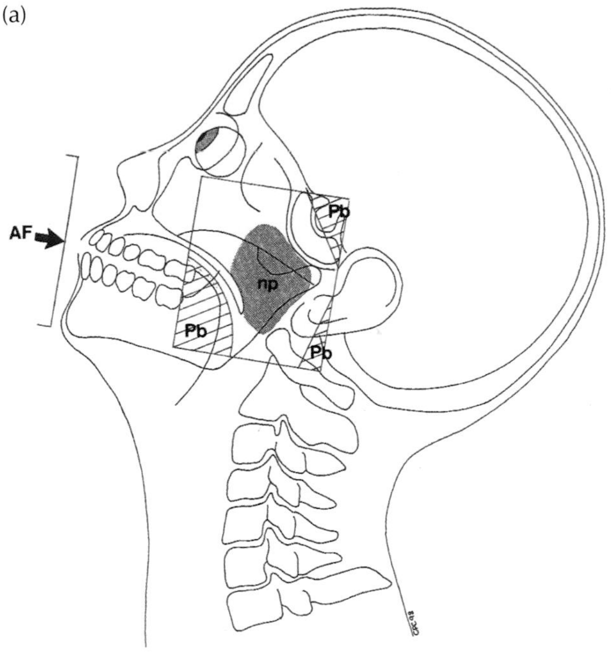

(b)

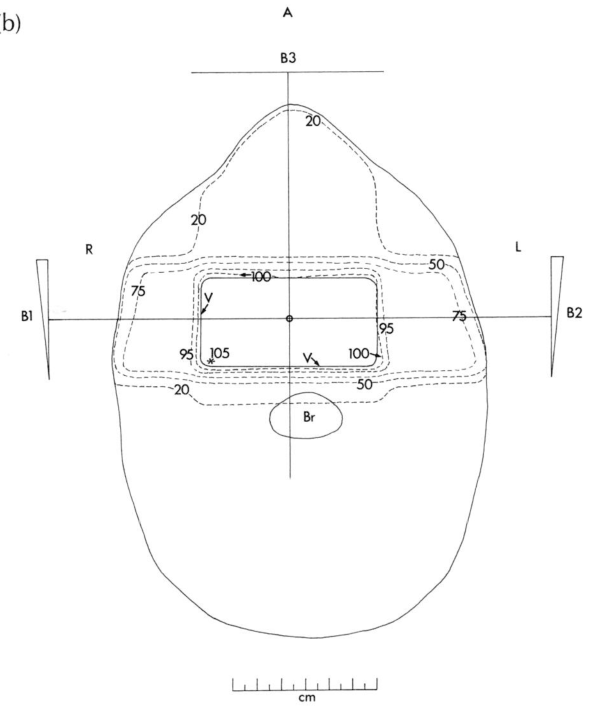

Figure 12.15 (a) Diagram indicating the field arrangement for the final phase of radiotherapy to the nasopharynx. AF: anterior field, Pb: lead shielding. (b) Dosimetry plan for the same field arrangement in a patient with bilateral parapharyngeal extension. The figures indicate percentage isodoses. V: target volume; Br: brainstem.

margin. This volume is treated with a three-field plan with an anterior field and two wedged opposed lateral fields (Figure 12.15). Undifferentiated carcinomas (UCNT) are treated to a further dose of 15 Gy in five daily fractions of 3 Gy (to a total dose of 65 Gy) whereas differentiated SCCs are treated to a further 20 Gy in daily fractions of 2 Gy (to a total dose of 70 Gy).

In patients without bulky nodal involvement we omit the initial large lateral fields, treating throughout with smaller lateral fields to the primary site (moving on to a three-field plan) with opposed anterior and posterior neck fields throughout. In the case of node-negative (on CT scan) well differentiated SCCs the lower border of the neck fields lies at the inferior border of the thyroid cartilage.

Although this protocol is generally applicable the precise volume treated to each dose level should be individually tailored according to the clinical and imaging information available. For example, disease extending into the nasal cavity may need to be treated with a three-field plan throughout and disease extending into the paranasal sinuses certainly will. The final phase of treatment must take into account any disease extension into the parapharyngeal region, which, when involved, should be included with an adequate margin.

It is our practice to use megavoltage photon beams throughout, except for boosting the sites of nodal involvement. We have no experience in the use of mixed photon and (anterior) electron fields for the treatment of disease extending into the nasal cavity as detailed by Ho.[60] Another technique outside of our experience but well described by the Hong Kong radiotherapists[47] is the use of a unilateral direct posterior oblique photon field to boost the parapharyngeal region. This is used at the end of a standard course of treatment and requires a new head cast with the patient's head turned to the contralateral side. The field lies behind the ipsilateral temporomandibular joint, anterior to the spinal cord and below both temporal lobes and the opposite eye. A further dose of up to 20 Gy in 2-Gy fractions is given by this field.[47] Examples of North American treatment techniques are described in detail by Fletcher and Million[61] and Perez.[4]

Three dimensional conformal radiotherapy

The introduction of CT planning and three-dimensional dose calculation have offered the opportunity for improvements in radiation treatment planning. CT scans of the head and neck region are used to localize the tumour and organs at risk in three-dimensional space. This requires the radiation oncologist to outline on each CT image the target volume and radiosensitive organs such as the spinal cord, brain stem, parotid glands and orbits. The outlined structures can be reconstructed in three dimensions and these images can be used to optimize beam direction and allows conformal beam shaping from the beams-eye-view.

Computer algorithms are used to calculate the dose distribution that can be examined in multiple planes. Dose-volume histograms can be generated to summarize the radiation dose received by the target volume and each radiosensitive normal tissue structure. These data can be used to predict complications of radiation therapy and allow further customization of the dose distribution for individual patients.

Three-dimensional conformal radiotherapy has been used to reduce the radiation dose to normal tissue structures with the aim of reducing radiation toxicity[62]. The therapeutic advantage of conformal radiotherapy can also be used to increase radiation dose to the target with the aim of increasing tumour control rates within currently acceptable toxicity levels.

Intensity-modulated radiotherapy

Intensity-modulated radiotherapy (IMRT) is a new and experimental method of radiation delivery. IMRT allows the delivery of radiation dose distributions with complex shapes, particularly where the required dose distribution is concave. This allows the delivery of high dose radiotherapy to tumours even when they are wrapped around a radiosensitive normal tissue structure such as the spinal cord or parotid gland. The question of which head and neck tumours have the most to gain from an IMRT approach remains unanswered at present, but theoretical advantages have been demonstrated for tumours of the nasopharynx, and others[63,64]. Current clinical trials are underway to prove the benefit of IMRT over current techniques[65].

Radiation dose, technique and local control

There is a considerable volume of literature discussing the question of a dose-response relationship in nasopharyngeal carcinoma (see Perez[4] for a detailed review). The evidence, such as it is, comes from retrospective reviews spanning the last five decades during which time there have been major changes in radiation oncology with the introduction of megavoltage treatment machines, the establishment of treatment simulation as standard practice and the use of computerized dosimetry. Furthermore, major advances in radiation biology have led to considerable changes in fractionation in line with our current understanding of the basis of late tissue morbidity. Not surprisingly many studies spanning several decades have shown improvements in local control in later cohorts, often accompanied by increasing radiation doses. The difficulty in establishing a dose-response relationship from such data is illustrated by the study of Marks and co-workers[66] who felt that improvement in local control owed more to technological advances than the increasing doses delivered. A later study from the same institute has suggested an improvement in local control for T1–T3 tumours treated to over 66 Gy, though very few patients received over 70 Gy.[27] There was no corresponding improvement for T4 tumours. A recent retrospective study from the MD Anderson Cancer Center found no evidence of a dose effect in multivariate analysis.[25]

The work of Yan and colleagues[67] has been cited as evidence of a dose-response effect. In a retrospective analysis they compared the outcome of patients with clinical evidence of residual disease at the primary site after standard treatment to 70 Gy who received no further therapy to those who were treated to a further 20–50 Gy with reduced fields. There was certainly improvement in the local control and 5-year survival in the 'boost' group but at the cost of increased severe radiation encephalomyelitis (17% versus. 5.5% in the 'observed group').

One should be cautious in ascribing the reduced rates of distant metastases and better survival to the improved local control as the two groups were not well matched for advanced T and N stage. Unfortunately, those patients with T3–T4 tumours at diagnosis seemed to benefit less from the boost treatment.

One should balance these arguments for dose escalation against the high rates of local control (73% at 5 years) achieved by Lee and associates in over 4000 patients, the vast majority of whom were treated to 64–66 Gy. Local control was significantly worse in those patients treated to 55–59 Gy compared to 64 Gy or above. Perhaps more importantly, for patients who were staged and planned with CT the 5-year local control rates were 88% for T1 (Ho), 83% for T2 (Ho) and 67% for T3 (Ho).

There have been no prospective studies on dose escalation reported and these would certainly be difficult to run outside endemic areas. The advent of three-dimensional conformal planning is likely to bring with it improved dose distributions with more uniform delivery of currently prescribed doses to the target volume, with perhaps lower risks of normal tissue complications.[68] In addition there is the potential for improved target definition with MRI. Improved dosimetry may therefore allow safe dose escalation but as yet it is difficult to identify those patients who will benefit.

Brown and colleagues have suggested that proton therapy can improve tumour dose distribution at depth whilst reducing the dose received by adjacent normal tissues.[69] Unfortunately such therapy is expensive and not yet widely available. On the other hand the nasopharynx is one of the sites most likely to benefit from intensity modulated radiation therapy (IMRT) for which the majority of modern linear accelerators can be adapted.[70]

The results of the recent CHART study (continuous hyperfractionated accelerated radiation therapy) in head and neck cancers indicate that tumour cell repopulation during the course of treatment is a very real phenomenon.[71] Accelerated radiotherapy thus offers an alternative approach to improving local control in NPC whilst hyperfractionation may improve the therapeutic ratio. Wang[72] has demonstrated that accelerated hyperfractionated treatment is feasible in NPC, with improved local control compared to historical controls treated once daily. There was no apparent increase in toxicity with the twice daily regimen. A prospective randomized study is needed to confirm these results.

In summary there may well be a modest dose-response effect between 55 and 70 Gy. However, in the absence of prospective data there is no clear indication to take the majority of patients beyond 70 Gy. Sadly, those patients who are at most risk of local relapse seem on present evidence to benefit least from dose escalation.[27,67] Technological advances and novel fractionation regimens may, however, permit more effective delivery of current doses and allow the safe escalation of dose in those patients most at risk of local failure with current standard therapy.

Intracavitary brachytherapy

Brachytherapy offers the potential for local delivery of high radiotherapy doses with rapid dose fall-off to spare neighbouring normal tissues. In addition the use of low-dose rate sources confers the added advantage of the sparing effect of low-dose rate on late morbidity. Some authors advocate the routine addition of a brachytherapy boost to the nasopharynx after completion of external beam therapy to 60–70 Gy and describe appropriate after-loading techniques.[52,73–75] Doses of 6–20 Gy in from one to three applications have been given using medium or high-dose rate systems. Wang[74] reported an improvement in local control with the addition of brachytherapy when compared to a non-randomized contemporary population but the local failure rate in the latter was rather higher than one might expect from recent megavoltage external beam series.[59]

From the published results it is not clear that the routine use of brachytherapy boosts confers any advantage over modern conformal external beam therapy. Tsao[76] advocates the selective use of brachytherapy in those patients with residual disease at the end of a standard course of external beam treatment and electively in all patients with well-differentiated SCCs where the risk of local failure is increased. At the Royal Marsden Hospital we do not use brachytherapy in the initial management of NPC, reserving its use for recurrent disease.

Radiotherapy: results of treatment

The multiplicity of staging systems and heterogeneity of patient populations make it impossible to compare results across series. In addition, many retrospective reports include patients staged before the advent of CT and treated without simulation on orthovoltage machines. Table 12.4 shows the results of Lee and colleagues[59] who treated over 4000 patients with megavoltage irradiation between 1976 and 1985. Only 12 patients in this series had WHO type 1 tumours. The improved result in more recently treated patients is typical of many retrospective NPC series and reflects a combination of factors such as stage migration after the introduction of CT scanning, improved target localization and a degree of dose escalation. Table 12.5 illustrates the results from three Western series, with all patients retrospectively staged using the UICC 1989 system.

Patterns of failure after radical radiotherapy

The time to failure is very consistent across the many series reported. Around 75% of recurrences, both locoregional and distant, occur within 2 years of treatment, 85–90% occurring within 3 years.

Table 12.4 Actuarial local control rates for NPC treated with megavoltage irradiation

Stage[99]	All patients (*N* = 4128) control at 10 years	Patients treated 1976–1980 (*N* = 2010) control at 5 years	Patients treated 1981–1985 (*N* = 2118) control at 5 years
T1	74	77	83
T2	72	69	79
T3 (all)	61	64	67
T3a	72		
T3b	66		
T3c	50		
T3d	35		

Data from Ho.[49]

Table 12.5 Actuarial local and regional control in western NPC series

Centre	SCC*	LC at (years)	T1	T2	T3	T4	N0	N1	N2a	N2b	N2c	N3
Mallinckrodt[23] 1956–1986 (*N* = 143)	54	10	85	75	67	40	82	86	72†			72
Gustave Roussy[4] 1960–1991 (*N* = 308)	46	5	63	62	68	54	66	57	58	56	54	57
MD Anderson[21] 1954–1992 (*N*= 378)	51	5	93	79	68	53	95	94	91	80	77	71
		10	87	75	63	45	95	94	91	77	74	71

LC: local control.
*Percentage squamous cell carcinoma in series.
†Figures for all N2 combined

Thereafter there are a small number of relapses occurring out to 5 and even 10 years.

Of 5037 patients treated at the Queen Elizabeth Hospital Hong Kong, half died of nasopharyngeal carcinoma.[28] Forty-six per cent of patients were known to be disease free at the time of last follow-up or death. Thirty per cent of patients had either persistent local disease or subsequently relapsed at the primary site and less than 15% of these were successfully salvaged by retreatment. Thirty-five per cent of patients either had or developed distant metastases, the actuarial 10-year metastasis-free rate being 59%. As indicated in Table 12.6, there was a strong correlation between the cumulative incidence of metastasis and nodal stage at diagnosis. Of those developing distant metastases, just over 40% had associated local or regional failure.

In a more recent series of 628 patients from Hong Kong treated in the CT era, 185 (29.5%) had failed after 2 years of follow-up.[77] Most of these[116] had developed distant metastases, three-quarters of whom had no evidence of local or regional recurrence. The 2-year actuarial local failure rate was just 12.7% from a series in which 76% had primary disease beyond the nasopharynx. Patients with bulky (> 4 cm) nodal disease were treated with

Table 12.6 Nasopharyngeal carcinoma: incidence of distant failure with node stage at diagnosis

	N0	N1	N2	N3
Lee et al[24] *N* = 5037 (Ho 1978 stage)	16	28	37	57
Petrovich et al[78] *N* = 107 (AJC 1977 stage)	17	18	33	46

neoadjuvant chemotherapy and all patients received bilateral neck radiotherapy. Of the 7% of patients who relapsed in the neck, the majority had associated local or distant failure.

In the Mallinckrodt Institute series of 143 patients, just over half died of NPC.[27] Two-thirds of patients had evidence of local recurrence at the time of death and one-third had relapsed in the neck. Nineteen per cent of patients developed distant metastases, two-thirds of whom had no evidence of locoregional recurrence at death. Of 256 patients treated at eight Veterans Administration Medical Centers between 1956–1978 only 10% were alive without evidence of recurrence at the time of reporting. Sixty-three per cent had failed at the primary site and only 4% died from distant metastases with locoregional control.[78] Once again distant failure correlated with nodal stage at diagnosis (Table 12.6). In a series from Memorial Sloan-Kettering Cancer Center, just over half of 107 NPC patients relapsed and of these the primary site was the first site of failure in 60%.[79] Hoppe and colleagues describe a 56% actuarial disease-free survival in 82 NPC patients. Of the 32 failures, 17 relapsed locally and 12 developed distant metastases with locoregional control.[80]

It is very difficult to generalize over such widely different series. However, it is clear that both locoregional and distant failure are major causes of death in nasopharyngeal carcinoma. In endemic areas despite the high rates of local control in recent series, significant numbers of patients still succumb from distant metastases. In the West, where squamous cell carcinomas are more prevalent it would appear that local relapse is a more significant cause of failure.

Complications of radiotherapy

The side-effects of radiotherapy are conventionally termed 'acute' or 'early' if they occur during or within 3 months of completion of a course of radiotherapy. Some of these are reversible, depending on the total dose delivered. 'Late' complications, developing at least 3 months and often years after a course of treatment are not reversible. The incidence increases with the total dose delivered and, unlike acute reactions, with increasing size of the individual daily fractions. It is likely that late reactions reflect the delayed expression of vascular damage with secondary ischaemia and fibrosis. The incidence, diagnosis and treatment of radiation complications in NPC have been reviewed in detail by Lee.[81] In general the severity of acute reactions and the incidence of late complications increase with the size of the volume irradiated to high dose. Consequently, both are more likely to increase with advanced stages of disease.

Acute complications

The majority of patients develop acute mucositis and in many this is likely to be confluent within the high-dose region.[25] Undernutrition and weight loss can easily occur as a result and close attention must be paid to the patient's diet. Salivary tissue responds rapidly to radiation and a transient early parotitis may occur that does not require specific therapy beyond reassurance.[81] Early loss of salivary function is not uncommon and the majority of patients will develop some degree of long-term xerostomia.[46,80] This, added to the common occurrence of reversible taste disturbance and anorexia will increase the potential for malnutrition. Nausea or vomiting, though rarely severe can occasionally occur.

Even with the skin-sparing effects of megavoltage irradiation, most patients will develop some degree of skin reaction that may extend to moist desquamation.[25] Where possible the immobilization cast should be drilled out or cut away to minimize build-up effects. Finally, most patients describe some degree of malaise.

Late complications

With its close relationship to the CNS the potential for serious neurological complications is considerable. Such sequelae can take over 2 years to be expressed[82] and since a large number of patients will have relapsed by that time it is difficult to get a realistic impression of the true complication rates. Sanguineti and associates[25] have estimated the actuarial incidence of RTOG grade 3–5 late complications to be 16, 19 and 29% at 5, 10 and 20 years respectively. In their study 12 of 378 (3%) patients died as a result of late complications, though 11 of these were treated between 1954 and 1971, before the routine use of treatment simulation and megavoltage irradiation. Indeed, as a result of improved technique the 10-year actuarial incidence of severe (grade 4 and 5) late complications has dropped to 5% in their most recent cohort of patients.

Neurological damage occurred in 451 of the 5037 patients reported by Lee and co-workers[28] and accounted for all but three of the 62 radiation-induced fatalities. In a series from Beijing of NPC patients treated to doses of up to 90 Gy or more, the incidence of neurological complications was 18.4%.[45] At conventional doses temporal lobe necrosis occurs in about 1% of patients[25,27] with a latent interval of 4 years.[83] It may present with temporal lobe epilepsy, the features of raised intracranial pressure or more vague symptoms such as personality changes.[83] Few patients have specific neurological signs and MRI scanning is the investigation of choice.[84] Early cases may respond to systemic steroids but these offer little benefit once extensive cystic change has occurred.[83]

Late radiation damage to the brainstem or spinal cord can be equally devastating. It has been variably reported in 0–3% of cases[25,27,46] and generally presents with progressive spastic paraparesis. Most patients will have long-tract motor signs and again MRI is the investigation of choice.[81] Sadly there is little treatment to offer beyond rehabilitation and supportive care. With modern CT imaging and planning, accurate patient immobilization and dosimetry this complication should be avoidable.

Other potential neurological complications include optic neuropathy and chiasmal damage, cranial nerve palsy and retinopathy. Again these should be avoidable with careful planning and attention to normal tissue dose limits. The lower cranial nerves appear to be most vulnerable,[46,80,82] presumably through late radiation changes in the parapharyngeal space.

Symptomatic hypopituitarism has been reported in 6%,[25] though much higher rates have been reported in patients investigated prospectively.[85] Radiation damage to the hypothalamus is thought to be the underlying cause with the growth hormone axis the most commonly affected followed by the gonadotrophins, corticotrophin and TSH.[85] Primary hypothyroidism may result from high-dose irradiation of the lower neck. Treating physicians should be aware of the possibility of long-term endocrine dysfunction in NPC survivors and periodic endocrine assessment is appropriate.

Serous otitis media has been reported in 7–18% of patients.[45,80,82] Myringotomy is required where this is persistent. Of more concern is the recent report from Queen Mary Hospital Hong Kong in which prospective audiological assessment of treated NPC patients detected persistent sensorineural hearing loss (SNHL) in 24% of ears tested.[86] High frequency was more affected than low frequencies. A similar number again developed transient SNHL. Fourteen per cent of ears developed serous otitis media, the majority within 2 years. A particularly high incidence of persistent SNHL (46.9%) was found in those ears with serous otitis media, compared to those without (19%, $P = 0.0013$). There was no evidence of enhanced radiation-induced SNHL in those patients given neoadjuvant cisplatin. The authors suggest that the presence of a middle ear effusion is a marker for increased risk of damage to the inner ear. Clearly it is important to limit the radiation dose to the audiological apparatus as far as possible.

Of the soft tissue and bone complications, trismus is reported in 3–12%,[25,45,66] moderate to severe neck fibrosis in 2–4%[25,27,82] and osteoradionecrosis (mandible, maxilla, skull base) in 2–3%.[25,27] As in all head and neck sites where significant volumes of salivary tissue are irradiated to high dose, long-term xerostomia predisposes to dental caries and close attention to oral hygiene is essential. Finally, radiation-induced second malignancies, particularly osteosarcoma have been described in long-term survivors but with an incidence of less than 1%.

Radiotherapy: treatment for local recurrence

Although chemotherapy may offer some palliative benefit in locally recurrent disease it does not offer the prospect of long-term control (see below). Some cases may be amenable to local surgery, perhaps combined with brachytherapy as discussed later. For the majority of local recurrences reirradiation offers the best hope for salvage. Obviously, given the risks of primary irradiation, retreatment to high dose carries a significant complication rate.

In the largest series of reirradiated patients Lee and colleagues[87] report an actuarial 5-year local salvage rate of 23% in 654 patients with local recurrence treated to a further 7.5–70 Gy (median 45.6 Gy) with external beam (82%), brachytherapy (6%) or a combination (12%). Despite close follow-up the majority of relapses were too bulky for brachytherapy alone. Fifty-one per cent of patients responded completely but over a third of these subsequently relapsed again after a median of 1.5 years. Not surprisingly salvage rates were better for more localized recurrences and were higher in those with less extensive primary tumours at first diagnosis. The estimated 5-year complication-free rate was 52%. One or more serious late complications was recorded in 168 patients (26%) including 20 cases of temporal lobe necrosis, 13 of whom died as a result. Most of the other complications were in the soft tissues, such as trismus (16%) but two patients died after massive haemorrhage from telangiectatic mucosa. Late complications were lower in those patients treated with more protracted fractionation (both courses) and in those treated by a combination of external beam and brachytherapy. There did not appear to be any association between the complication rate and the interval between courses of radiotherapy.

A report from the MD Anderson Cancer Center[88] describes a 35% actuarial 5-year local control rate after re-irradiation to a median total dose of 112 Gy. Eight of the 53 patients developed severe complications which proved fatal in five. The overall 5-year actuarial incidence of severe complications was 17%, reaching 39% in those patients receiving cumulative external beam doses of over 100 Gy. There was a suggestion of improved local control with fewer complications in those patients treated with a combination of external beam and intracavitary therapy. The authors found no dose-response relationship in this series but in 51 patients retreated with external beam radiotherapy with or without brachytherapy, Wang[89] reported improved survival in those treated to 60 Gy or more. However, those treated to lower doses tended to have more advanced recurrences.

There is clearly a role for repeat irradiation in those patients with recurrent NPC. From the published experience it seems that few patients have sufficiently localized disease to be treated by brachytherapy alone, though a combination of external beam and brachytherapy is to be preferred where practicable. Radical treatment is necessary to achieve salvage rates of around 35%, perhaps higher in more selected cases. It is clearly important to exclude metastasic disease before embarking on such retreatments. For localized disease a combination of surgery and perioperative brachytherapy is an option as discussed later. Isolated nodal relapses in the neck can be managed as described below.

Chemotherapy

There is a large body of evidence (reviewed by Altun[5]) demonstrating that nasopharyngeal carcinoma is highly sensitive to chemotherapy. The most active regimens contain cisplatin and two widely employed schedules are outlined in Table 12.7.[90,91]

Neoadjuvant chemotherapy

The rationale for combining primary (neoadjuvant or induction) chemotherapy with subsequent radiotherapy is two-fold. Firstly, cytotoxic reduction of bulky primary and nodal disease may enhance locoregional control and secondly, the eradication of systemic micrometastases at an early stage may reduce later distant relapses. Indeed, a number of studies have suggested that the addition of neoadjuvant chemotherapy can enhance local control and survival when compared to historical or non-randomized controls.[92–94] In contrast, Tannock and colleagues were unable to demonstrate a long-term benefit from neoadjuvant chemotherapy despite a 75% response rate.[95] Where side-effects have been reported, chemotherapy seems to be tolerated by most patients and has not resulted in reductions of radiotherapy dose subsequently delivered.

Table 12.7 Chemotherapy regimens used in nasopharyngeal carcinoma

BEC[80]	**3-weekly cycle**		
Bleomycin	15 IU	iv bolus	Day 1
Bleomycin	12 IU/m² per day	Continuous iv infusion	Days 1–5
Epirubicin	70 mg/m²	iv bolus	Day 1
Cisplatin	100 mg/m²	iv infusion	Day 1
PF[81]	**3-weekly cycle**		
Cisplatin	100 mg/m²	iv infusion	Day 1
5–Fluorouracil	1000 mg/m²	Continuous iv infusion	Days 1–5

See references for detailed schedules

Two randomized studies of neoadjuvant chemotherapy have been reported. In the first, Chan and coworkers[96] randomized 82 UCNT patients with Ho N3 or any N stage with nodal diameter of 4 cm or more, between their standard radiotherapy protocol and the same preceded and followed by chemotherapy. A modification of the PF schedule outlined in Table 12.7, in which the 5-fluorouracil was given for 3 rather than 5 days, was given for two cycles before the radiotherapy and for four cycles afterwards. Sixty-five per cent of patients responded to chemotherapy at the primary site and 81% in nodal disease. At the end of radiotherapy all of the combined arm patients were disease-free compared to 95% of the radiotherapy-only arm. The chemotherapy toxicity was much as one would anticipate for the regimen and there was no enhancement of the subsequent radiation toxicity. However, 46% of patients failed to complete the postradiation chemotherapy. After a median follow-up of 28.5 months there were no differences in 2-year survival, locoregional relapse rate, distant metastatic rate or relapse-free survival. While longer follow-up might reveal survival differences and the chemotherapy regimen could be criticized as suboptimal, the results suggest that a large survival benefit from induction chemotherapy is unlikely.

A second, larger, multicentre study has been reported by the International Nasopharynx Cancer Study Group.[90] Using the BEC protocol (Table 12.7) developed at the Institut Gustave Roussy, 339 patients were randomized between three cycles of induction chemotherapy followed by radiotherapy or radiotherapy alone. The same radiotherapy technique and dose was employed in both arms. Over 90% of patients had UCNT and the majority were T3–T4, N2c–N3. There were 14 treatment-related deaths (8%) in the chemotherapy arm compared to two (1%) in the radiotherapy-only arm, though there was no enhancement of radiotherapy toxicity. Ninety-one per cent of patients responded to the chemotherapy, with a complete response in 47%. After a median follow-up of 49 months tumour progression, recurrence or metastasis had occurred in 33% of the combined therapy patients compared to 55% of those receiving radiotherapy alone. The pattern of recurrence was the same in both groups suggesting that chemotherapy improved both locoregional control and distant failure rates. However, at the time of reporting there was no difference in overall survival. Only time will tell whether or not a true survival advantage has been masked by a short-term response of radiotherapy-only arm failures to salvage chemotherapy. The high chemotherapy-related death rate and relatively reduced compliance with radiotherapy in the combined arm may further hide a survival benefit from induction chemotherapy but the impression is that any advantage will be relatively small.

Concomitant chemotherapy

Chemotherapy given during the course of radical radiotherapy offers the potential for radiation sensitization in the tumour as well as the possibility of eradicating micrometastases. It also offers the risk of enhanced toxicity, with radiotherapy delays or even dose reductions as a result. Huang and colleagues reported that the introduction of a number of different low-dose concomitant regimens involving cyclophosphamide, methotrexate, cisplatin or bleomycin coincided with an improvement in local control and overall survival compared to historical series. However, many series report improved results over successive decades, for reasons discussed earlier, and without the use of chemotherapy. Turner and Tiver[97] report their experience with concomitant mitomycin C and 5-fluorouracil in 43 patients with advanced NPC. Over half of the radiotherapy courses were interrupted, for a median of 2 weeks, and there were two treatment-related deaths. With no obvious improvement over published results the authors could not support the continued use of this combined regimen. Souhami and Rabinowits[98] came to a similar conclusion after a trial of the same drugs with the addition of methotrexate. Again severe mucositis resulted in treatment interruptions and there was no clear improvement in survival.

The Radiation Therapy Oncology Group (RTOG) conducted a trial (RTOG 81-17) of cisplatin (100 mg/m^2 3-weekly × 3) given concomitantly with a standard course of irradiation for advanced SCC of the head and neck.[99] This study includes a group of 27 patients with advanced NPC which has been reported separately in comparison with historical controls treated by radiation alone.[100] All combined therapy patients reached a dose of at least 64.5 Gy while 19 of 27 completed three cycles of chemotherapy. A complete response at the end of therapy was seen in 24 (89%) and in all of those with poorly differentiated tumours. There was some degree of leukopenia in most patients, severe or life-threatening in four (15%). Moderate to severe mucositis occurred in 85% but there was no indication as to the frequency of treatment interruptions. However, in the main study the treatment time was over 70 days in 20% of those patients achieving over 64.5 Gy. There was a suggestion of improved local control and reduced distant failure in the stage IV NPC patients treated with combined therapy as compared to historical controls but the groups could not be considered directly comparable. The combined regimen formed the basis of the subsequent intergroup study (0099) discussed later.

Adjuvant chemotherapy

The aim of adjuvant chemotherapy, given after radical radiotherapy, is to reduce the high distant metastatic failure rate. It is unlikely to contribute significantly to locoregional control. Once again there is a suggestion from retrospective series that the introduction of adjuvant chemotherapy into NPC treatment protocols has improved disease-free and overall survival compared with historical controls treated with radiation alone.[101,102] In contrast, Teo and colleagues[103] found no reduction in distant metastases and indeed more rapid distant failure in a group of patients treated with both neoadjuvant and adjuvant platinum-based combination chemotherapy.

A large multicentre randomized trial co-ordinated by the Instituto Nazionale Tumori, Milan, failed to show any relapse-free or overall survival benefit for the addition of combination chemotherapy in patients in complete remission after radical radiotherapy for NPC.[104] In the chemotherapy arm patients received up to 12 cycles of vincristine, cyclophosphamide and doxorubicin. Although there were some problems with compliance in the chemotherapy arm and the schedule did not include cisplatin, the results do argue against the routine use of adjuvant chemotherapy in NPC.

Combined concomitant and adjuvant chemotherapy

The preliminary results of the Southwest Oncology Group co-ordinated Intergroup study 0099 (with the RTOG and ECOG) have been reported.[105] Patients with UICC (1989) stages III and IV NPC were randomized between standard radical radiotherapy (70 Gy in 35 fractions over 7 weeks) and the same with concomitant cisplatin (100 mg/m^2 day 1, 22, 43) followed by three cycles of adjuvant cisplatin plus 5-fluorouracil chemotherapy. The trial was closed prematurely on the advice of the Data Monitoring Committee when an interim analysis of 138 patients demonstrated a median progression-free survival of 13 months for the radiotherapy patients compared to 52 months for the combined arm. At a median follow-up of 40 months the median survival of the combined arm patients had not been reached, whilst that of the radiotherapy group was 30 months. There was an excess of deaths (39%) in the radiotherapy group compared to the combined arm (16%) with 2-year actuarial survivals 55% and 80% respectively. There was apparently no increase in radiotherapy toxicity with concomitant cisplatin.

Palliative chemotherapy

It was the encouraging responses of recurrent and metastatic NPC to systemic chemotherapy that led to its investigation in primary therapy as previously discussed. Choo and Tannock[106] have summarized the Princess Margaret Hospital experience of palliative chemotherapy in recurrent and metastatic NPC. With the application of lymphoma-type and cisplatin-based regimens response rates of 70% could be achieved with at least two of 30 patients surviving in complete remission for over 3 years. In this retrospective review they were unable to demonstrate a survival benefit for more aggressive chemotherapy and could not comment on its palliative benefits beyond objective tumour responses. Al-Kourainy and colleagues[107] report a 76% response rate to platinum-containing regimens in 12 patients treated with recurrent disease. Half of those treated with the PF regimen (as Table 12.7 but 4-weekly) responded completely, with one of three CRs maintained for over 5 years.

Altun et al[5] have described the evolution of palliative chemotherapy protocols at the Institut Gustave Roussy. Overall response rates of 50–75% have been achieved with platinum-based regimens including BEC (Table 12.7). Of 131 patients with metastatic disease treated between 1985 and 1991, 13 remained disease-free for more than 2 years and 11 of these were alive and in remission at up to 79 months. Long-term responses are described in both bony and visceral sites and it would seem that around 10% of patients will achieve durable remissions, perhaps cure with aggressive chemotherapy in metastatic disease. Obviously none of these regimens are without toxicity.

Surgery for recurrent disease

Nasopharyngeal relapse

The role of surgery in the event of local recurrence is one of definitive resection or to facilitate brachytherapy. Recurrent disease involving the skull base, cranial nerves or deep parapharyngeal space cannot be cured by aggressive surgery and in these circumstances high-dose reirradiation with its attendant risks remains the treatment of choice.

Primary surgery

Primary surgery has been advocated where recurrent disease remains relatively localized.[108] A number of approaches have been described (Table 12.8) and the results have been summarised by Morton and colleagues.[108] Wei and co-workers[109] reported a 42% local control at 3.5 years using a maxillary swing access technique. This was associated with a high palatal fistula rate, though the majority subsequently healed. Hsu et al[110] reported a 46% local cure rate after the selective use of surgery for recurrence. The results were described as excellent for recurrent stage T1 (rT1), good for rT2, fair for rT3 and palliative for rT4. These results reflect the extent of recurrence; from the least extensive, that is the roof of the nasopharynx, towards the ethmoid and oropharynx and thence to the most severe manifestations of deep parapharyngeal and skull base involvement. En bloc resection was only possible in some of the rT1 cases and recurrence into the skull base. Similarly, Fisch[111] was able to achieve local control in T1/2 recurrences but could only palliate T4 lesions where infiltration of the dura and cranial nerves prevented complete excision.

Surgery with interstitial brachytherapy

Surgery combined with interstitial brachytherapy has the potential advantage of reduced morbidity, as compared to external beam reirradiation, for moderately advanced local recurrence. In some approaches the surgical procedure has simply served to expose the nasopharynx, facilitating the implantation of radioactive iodine (^{125}I) seeds or gold (^{198}Au) grains into the tumour under direct vision.[115,116] Choy and co-workers[116] describe a 61–80% 5-year local control after gold grain implantation into persistent or recurrent disease via a transpalatal approach. Local control was poorer (44% at 5 years) in those patients with skull base erosion. The main complication was

Table 12.8 Surgical approaches to the nasopharynx

Type	Description	Reference
Anterior	Transnasal/transantral	Wilson [112]
	Le Fort 1 maxillotomy	Belmont[113]
Inferior	Palatal split	Fee et al[114]
	Transpalatal flap	Harrison et al[115]
	Transcervico-mandibulo-palatal	Morton et al[108]
Lateral	Infratemporal	Fisch[111]
Anterolateral	Maxillary swing	Wei et al[109]

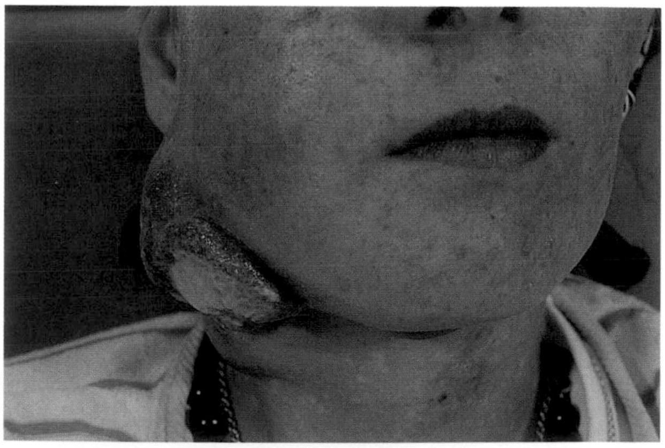

Figure 12.16 Fungating cervical lymphadenopathy.

Table 12.9 Surgical findings on neck dissection for cervical node relapse in NPC

Structures involved by tumour infiltration	Cases (%)
Sternomastoid muscle	26
Internal jugular vein	16
Floor of posterior triangle, carotid artery, vagus nerve	4
Disease adherent to but not infiltrating local structures (for example floor of posterior triangle, carotid artery)	28

Data from Wilson[108]

delayed onset headache which persisted for a median of 7 months and appeared to be related to the number of gold grains implanted. Seven of 43 patients developed palatal fistula that healed completely in six.

Another approach is to combine surgical resection with postoperative brachytherapy. Some of the cases described by Wei and colleagues[109] were treated in this manner. At the Royal Marsden Hospital we have developed a technique of combined surgical debulking, usually via the Le Fort 1 maxillotomy approach, with afterloading brachytherapy using either iridium (^{192}Ir) wires or the high-dose rate Microselectron (Nucleotron).[117] In either case between two and four catheters placed intraoperatively have been afterloaded delivering a dose of 60 Gy to the 85% reference isodose (low dose rate) or 36 Gy in 8–10 fractions (high-dose rate). Ten patients with recurrent disease were treated between 1989 and 1996 and at a median follow-up of 12 months (range 6–45 months) four patients remain alive and disease-free. There have been no major complications from the Le Fort 1 procedure but two patients developed asymptomatic osteoradionecrosis, which was managed conservatively.

Cervical relapse

Retreatment of the neck with high-dose external beam radiotherapy carries a high risk of soft tissue fibrosis and/or necrosis. Formal neck dissection is therefore the treatment of choice for cervical node relapse. Where extracapsular extension and fixity results in residual macroscopic disease, the procedure can be combined with afterloading brachytherapy as described elsewhere in this book. Where there is doubt about skin viability after neck dissection or if postoperative brachytherapy is planned, non-irradiated tissue cover (e.g. a pectoralis major flap) must be brought into the operative field.

Wei and colleagues[118] have described their experience of salvage surgery in 51 cases of nodal relapse after radical radiotherapy for NPC. Three-quarters of the patients presented with a single enlarged node with 86% presenting in cervical node regions II and upper V. In over half of the cases the node was fixed to underlying structures or skin (Figure 12.16 and Table 12.9) and 36% of clinically solitary nodal relapses were associated with multiple pathologically involved nodes at dissection. Fifteen per cent of single nodes were not malignant but all multiple nodal relapses were. Their policy of neck dissection, with or without brachytherapy was associated with a 38% 5-year actuarial survival and a 66% probability of neck control.[118] Lymph node mobility was the only significant independent prognostic factor for local control and survival.

REFERENCES

1. Micheau C, de The G, Orofiamma B et al. Practical value of classifying NPC into two major microscopical types. In: Grundman E, Krueger GRF, Ablashi DV (eds) *Cancer Campaign, Volume 5: Nasopharyngeal Carcinoma*. Stuttgart: Gustav Fisher, 1981; 51–57.
2. McGuire L, Suen M. Histopathology. In: van Hasselt A, Gibb A (eds) *Nasopharyngeal Carcinoma*. Hong Kong: The Chinese University Press, 1991.

3. Yu M. *Nasopharyngeal carcinoma: epidemiology and dietary factors.* IARC Scientific Publications, 1991; 104.
4. Perez CA. Nasopharynx. In: Perez CA, Brady LW (eds) *Principles and Practice of Radiation Oncology.* 2nd edn. Philadelphia: JB Lippincott, 1992; 617–643.
5. Altun M, Fandi A, Dupuis O et al. Undifferentiated nasopharyngeal cancer (UCNT): Current diagnostic and therapeutic aspects. *Int J Radiat Oncol Biol Phys* 1995; **32**: 857–887.
6. Lanier A, Bender T, Talbot M et al. Nasopharyngeal carcinoma in Alaskan Eskimos, Indians and Aleuts: a review of cases and study of Epstein–Barr virus, HLA, and environmental risk factors. *Cancer* 1980; **46**: 2100–2106.
7. Buell P. Nasopharynx cancer in Chinese of California. *Br J Cancer* 1965; **19**: 459–470.
8. King H, Haenzel W. Cancer mortality among foreign and native-born Chinese in the United States. *J Chron Dis* 1972; **26**: 623–646.
9. Chan S, Day N, Kunaratnam N, Simons M. HLA and nasopharyngeal carcinoma in Chinese—a further study. *Int J Cancer* 1983; **32**: 171–176.
10. Chan S, Day N, Khor T et al. HLA markers in the development and prognosis of NPC in Chinese. In: Grundman E, Krueger GRF, Ablashi DV (eds) *Cancer Campaign, Volume 5: Nasopharyngeal Carcinoma.* Stuttgart: Gustav Fischer, 1981: 205–211.
11. Lu S-J, Day N, Dagos L et al. Linkage of a nasopharyngeal carcinoma susceptibility locus to the HLA region. *Nature* 1990; **346**: 470–471.
12. Henle W, Henle G, Ho JHC et al. Antibodies to Epstein–Barr virus in nasopharyngeal carcinoma, other head and neck neoplasms and control groups. *J Nat Cancer Inst* 1970; **44**: 225–231.
13. Henle W, Ho JHC, Henle G et al. Antibodies to Epstein–Barr virus related antigens in nasopharyngeal carcinoma: comparison of active cases and long term survivors. *J Nat Cancer Inst* 1973; **51**: 361–369.
14. Henle W, Ho JHC, Henle G *et al.* Nasopharyngeal carcinoma: significance of changes in Epstein–Barr virus-related antibody patterns following therapy. *Int J Cancer* 1977; **20**: 663–672.
15. de-Vathaire F, Sancho-Garnier H, de The H et al. Prognostic value of EBV markers in the clinical management of nasopharyngeal carcinoma (NPC): a multicenter follow-up study. *Int J Cancer* 1988; **42**: 176–181.
16. Liebowitz D. Nasopharyngeal carcinoma: the Epstein–Barr virus association. *Semin Oncol* 1994; **21**: 376–381.
17. Yip T, Ngan R, Lau W et al. A possible prognostic role of immunoglobulin-G antibody against recombinant Epstein–Barr virus BZLF-1 transactivator protein ZEBRA in patients with nasopharyngeal carcinoma. *Cancer* 1994; **74**: 2414–2424.
18. Pathmanathan R, Prasad U, Chandrika G et al. Undifferentiated, nonkeratinizing and squamous cell carcinoma of the nasopharynx. Variants of Epstein–Barr virus-infected neoplasia. *Am J Pathol* 1995; **146**: 1355–1367.
19. Lin T, Chang H, Chen C et al. Risk factors for nasopharyngeal carcinoma. *Anticancer Res* 1986; **6**: 791–796.
20. Ho JHC. Stage classification of nasopharyngeal carcinoma: a review. In: de The G, Ito Y (eds) *Nasopharyngeal carcinoma: Etiology and Control.* Lyon: International Agency for Research on Cancer, 1978; **20**: 94–114.
21. Yu M, Ho J, Lai S, Henderson B. Cantonese-style salted fish as a cause of nasopharyngeal carcinoma: report of a case-control study in Hong Kong. *Cancer Res* 1986; **46**: 956–961.
22. Teo P, Shiu W, Leung S et al. Prognostic factors in nasopharyngeal carcinoma investigated by computer tomography. *Radiother Oncol* 1992; **23**: 79–93.
23. Cvitkovic E, Bachouchi M, Armand J. Nasopharyngeal carcinoma: biology, natural history, and therapeutic implications. *Haematol Oncol Clin North Am* 1991; **5**: 821–838.
24. Chua D, Sham J, Kwong D et al. Prognostic value of paranasopharyngeal extension of nasopharyngeal carcinoma. A significant factor in local control and distant metastasis. *Cancer* 1996; **78**: 202–210.
25. Sanguineti G, Geara F, Garden A et al. Carcinoma of the nasopharynx treated by radiotherapy alone: determinants of local and regional control. *Int J Radiat Oncol Biol Phys* 1997; **37**: 985–996.
26. Lederman M. *Cancer of the Nasopharynx: Its Natural History and Treatment.* Springfield, Illinois: Charles C Thomas, 1961.
27. Perez C, Devinini V, Marcial-Vega V et al. Carcinoma of the nasopharynx: factors affecting prognosis. *Int J Radiat Oncol Biol Phys* 1992; **23**: 271–280.
28. Lee A, Poon Y, Foo W et al. Retrospective analysis of 5037 patients with nasopharyngeal carcinoma treated during 1976–1985: overall survival and patterns of failure. *Int J Radiat Oncol Biol Phys* 1992; **23**: 261–270.
29. Fletcher G, Million R. Malignant tumors of the nasopharynx. *Am J Roentgenol Radium Ther Nucl Med* 1965; **93**: 44–55.
30. Lee A, Sham J, Poon Y et al. Treatment of stage I nasopharyngeal carcinoma: Analysis of the patterns of relapse and results of withholding elective neck irradiation. *Int J Radiat Oncol Biol Phys* 1989; **17**: 1183–1190.
31. Neel HI. Nasopharyngeal carcinoma: clinical presentation, diagnosis, treatment and prognosis. *Otolaryngol Clin North Am* 1985; **18**: 479–490.
32. Ahmad A, Stefani S. Distant metastases of nasopharyngeal carcinoma: a study of 256 male patients. *J Surg Oncol* 1986; **33**: 194–197.
33. Cvitkovic E, Bachouchi M, Boussen H et al. Leukemoid reaction, bone marrow invasion, fever of unknown origin, and metastatic pattern in the natural history of advanced undifferentiated carcinoma of nasopharyngeal type. *J Clin Oncol* 1993; **11**: 2434–2442.
34. Kreel L, Ma H, Metreweli C. Imaging. In: van Hasselt C, Gibb A (eds) *Nasopharyngeal Carcinoma.* Hong Kong: The Chinese University Press, 1991:

35. Mancuso A. Imaging in patients with head and neck cancer. In: Million R, Cassisi N (eds) *Management of Head and Neck Cancer: A Multidisciplinary Approach.* Philadelphia: JB Lippincott, 1994:
36. Olmi P, Fallai C, Colagrande S et al. Staging and follow-up of nasopharyngeal carcinoma: magnetic resonance imaging versus computerised tomography. *Int J Radiat Oncol Biol Phys* 1995; **32**: 795–800.
37. Yong-Sheng Z, Sham J, Ng M et al. Immunoglobulin A against viral capsid antigen of Epstein–Barr virus and indirect mirror examination of the nasopharynx in the detection of asymptomatic nasopharyngeal carcinoma. *Cancer* 1992; **69**: 3–7.
38. Liaw C-C, Wang C-H, Huang J-S et al. Serum lactate dehydrogenase level in patients with nasopharyngeal carcinoma. *Acta Oncol* 1997; **36**: 159–164.
39. Chang C, Liu T, Chang Y, Cao L. Radiation therapy of nasopharyngeal carcinoma. *Acta Radiolog Oncol* 1980; **19**: 433–438.
40. Huang S, Lui L, Lynn T-C. Nasopharyngeal cancer: study III. A review of 1206 patients treated with combined modalities. *Int J Radiat Oncol Biol Phys* 1985; **11**: 1789–1793.
41. UICC. *TNM Atlas.* 4th edn. Berlin: Springer-Verlag, 1997.
42. UICC. *TNM Atlas.* 3rd edn, 2nd Rev. Berlin: Springer-Verlag, 1992.
43. Teo P, Leung S, Yu P et al. Comparison of the Ho's, UICC and AJC stage classification for nasopharyngeal carcinoma (NPC). *Cancer* 1991; **67**: 434–439.
44. Teo P. Staging. In: van Hasselt C, Gibb A (eds) *Nasopharyngeal Carcinoma.* Hong Kong: The Chinese University Press, 1991.
45. Qin D, Hu Y, Yan J et al. Analysis of 1379 patients with nasopharyngeal carcinoma treated by radiation. *Cancer* 1988; **61**: 1117–1124.
46. Sham J, Choy D. Prognostic factors of nasopharyngeal carcinoma: a review of 759 patients. *Br J Radiol* 1990; **63**: 51–58.
47. Teo P, Yu P, Lee W et al. Significant prognosticators after primary radiotherapy in 903 nondisseminated nasopharyngeal carcinoma evaluated by computer tomography. *Int J Radiat Oncol Biol Phys* 1996; **36**: 291–304.
48. Ingersoll L, Shiao Y, Donaldson S et al. Nasopharyngeal carcinoma in the young: A combined MD Anderson and Stanford experience. *Int J Radiat Oncol Biol Phys* 1990; **19**: 881–887.
49. Ho JHC. An epidemiologic and clinical study of nasopharyngeal carcinoma. *Int J Radiat Oncol Biol Phys* 1978; **4**: 183–198.
50. Hoppe R, Williams J, Warnke R et al. Carcinoma of the nasopharynx: the significance of histology. *Int J Radiat Oncol Biol Phys* 1978; **4**: 199–205.
51. Santos J, Gonzalez C, Cuesta P et al. Impact of changes in the treatment of nasopharyngeal carcinoma: an experience of 30 years. *Radiother Oncol* 1995; **36**: 121–127.
52. Tang S, Lin F, Chen MS et al. Prognostic factors of nasopharyngeal carcinoma: a multivariate analysis. *Int J Radiat Oncol Biol Phys* 1990; **19**: 1143–1149.
53. Cellai E, Olmi P, Chiavacci A et al. Computed tomography in nasopharyngeal carcinoma: part II: impact on survival. *Int J Radiat Oncol Biol Phys* 1990; **19**: 1177–1182.
54. Sham J, Wei W, Nicholls J et al. Extent of nasopharyngeal carcinoma involvement inside the nasopharynx. Lack of prognostic value on local control. *Cancer* 1992; **69**: 854–859.
55. Yu Z, Xu G, Huang Y et al. Value of computed tomography in staging the primary lesion (T-staging) of nasopharyngeal carcinoma (NPC): an analysis of 54 patients with special reference to the parapharyngeal space. *Int J Radiat Oncol Biol Phys* 1985; **11**: 2143–2147.
56. Sham J, Choy D, Choi P. Nasopharyngeal carcinoma: the significance of neck node involvement in relation to the pattern of distant failure. *Br J Radiol* 1990; **63**: 108–113.
57. Lee A, Foo W, Chan D. Nasopharyngeal carcinoma: evaluation of N-staging by Ho and AJCC/UICC system. *Int J Radiat Oncol Biol Phys* 1994; **30** (Suppl. 1): 202.
58. Neel H, Taylor W, Pearson G. Prognostic determinants and a new view of staging for patients with nasopharyngeal carcinoma. *Ann Otolaryngol Rhinol Laryngol* 1985; **94**: 529–537.
59. Lee A, Law S, Foo W *et al.* Nasopharyngeal carcinoma: local control by megavoltage irradiation. *Br J Radiol* 1993; **66**: 528–536.
60. Ho JHC. Nasopharynx. In: Halnan K (ed.) *Treatment of Cancer.* London: Chapman and Hall, 1982: 249–267.
61. Fletcher G, Million R. Nasopharynx. In: Fletcher G (ed) *Textbook of Radiotherapy.* Philadelphia: Lea and Febiger, 1980: 364–383.
62. Leibel SA, Kutcher GJ, Harrison LB, Fass DE, Burman CM, Hunt MA et al. Improved dose distributions for 3D conformal boost treatments in carcinoma of the nasopharynx. *Int J Radiat Oncol Biol Phys.* 1991; **20**: 823–833
63. Hunt MA, Zelefsky MJ, Wolden S, Chui CS, LoSasso T, Rosenzweig K et al. Treatment planning and delivery of intensity-modulated radiation therapy for primary nasopharynx cancer. *Int J Radiat Oncol Biol Phys.* 2001; **49**: 623–632.
64. Xia P, Fu KK, Wong GW, Akazawa C, Verhey LJ. Comparison of treatment plans involving intensity-modulated radiotherapy for nasopharyngeal carcinoma. *Int J Radiat Oncol Biol Phys.* 2000; **48**: 329–337
65. Sultanem K, Shu HK, Xia P, Akazawa C, Quivey JM, Verhey LJ, Fu KK. Three-dimensional intensity-modulated radiotherapy in the treatment of nasopharyngeal carcinoma: the University of California-San Francisco experience. *Int J Radiat Oncol Biol Phys.* 2000; **48**: 711-722.
66. Marks J, Bedwinek J, Lee F et al. Dose-response analysis for nasopharyngeal carcinoma. An historical perspective. *Cancer* 1982; **50**: 1042–1050.
67. Yan J, Qin D, Hu Y et al. Management of local residual primary lesion of nasopharyngeal carcinoma (NPC): are higher doses beneficial? *Int J Radiat Oncol Biol Phys* 1989; **16**: 1465–1469.

68. Leibel S, Kutcher G, Harrison L et al. Improved dose distributions for 3D conformal boost treatments in carcinoma of the nasopharynx. *Int J Radiat Oncol Biol Phys* 1991; **20**: 823–833.
69. Brown A, Urie M, Chisin R et al. Proton therapy for carcinoma of the nasopharynx: a study in comparative treatment planning. *Int J Radiat Oncol Biol Phys* 1989; **16**: 1607–1614.
70. Webb S. *The Physics of Conformal Radiotherapy. Advances in Technology*. Bristol: Institute of Physics Publishing, 1997.
71. Saunders M, Dische S, Barrett A et al. Randomised multicentre trials of CHART vs. conventional radiotherapy in head and neck and non-small-cell lung cancer: an interim report. *Br J Cancer* 1996; **73**: 1455–1462.
72. Wang C. Accelerated hyperfractionation radiation therapy for carcinoma of the nasopharynx. *Cancer* 1989; **63**: 2461–2467.
73. Zhang Y, Liu T, Fi C. Intracavitary radiation treatment of nasopharyngeal carcinoma by the high dose rate afterloading technique. *Int J Radiat Oncol Biol Phys* 1989; **16**: 315–318.
74. Wang C. Improved local control of nasopharyngeal carcinoma after intracavitary brachytherapy boost. *Am J Clin Oncol* 1991; **14**: 5–8.
75. Kouvaris J, Plataniotis G, Sandilos C et al. Combined teletherapy and intracavitary brachytherapy boost for the treatment of nasopharyngeal carcinoma. *Radiother Oncol* 1996; **38**: 263–267.
76. Tsao S. Radiotherapy. In: van Hasselt C, Gibb A (eds) *Nasopharyngeal Carcinoma*. Hong Kong: The Chinese University Press, 1991.
77. Yu K, Teo P, Lee W et al. Patterns of early treatment failure in non-metastatic nasopharyngeal carcinoma: a study based on CT scanning. *Clin Oncol* 1994; **6**: 167–171.
78. Petrovich Z, Cox J, Middleton R et al. Advanced carcinoma of the nasopharynx. 2. Pattern of failure in 256 patients. *Radiother Oncol* 1985; **4**: 15–20.
79. Vikram B, Mishra U, Strong E et al. Patterns of failure in carcinoma of the nasopharynx: I. Failure at the primary site. *Int J Radiat Oncol Biol Phys* 1985; **11**: 1455–1459.
80. Hoppe R, Goffinet D, Bagshaw M. Carcinoma of the nasopharynx. Eighteen years' experience with megavoltage radiation therapy. *Cancer* 1976; **37**: 2605–2612.
81. Lee A. Complications of radiation therapy. In: van Hasselt C, Gibb A (eds) *Nasopharyngeal Carcinoma*. Hong Kong: The Chinese University Press, 1991.
82. Mesic J, Fletcher G, Goepfert H. Megavoltage irradiation of epithelial tumors of the nasopharynx. *Int J Radiat Oncol Biol Phys* 1981; **7**: 447–453.
83. Lee A, Ng S, Ho JHC et al. Clinical diagnosis of late temporal lobe necrosis following radiation therapy for nasopharyngeal carcinoma. *Cancer* 1988; **61**: 1535–1542.
84. Lee A, Cheng L, Ng S et al. Magnetic resonance imaging in the clinical diagnosis of late temporal lobe necrosis following radiotherapy for nasopharyngeal carcinoma. *Clin Radiol* 1990; **41**: 24–41.
85. Lam K, Tse V, Wang C et al. Effects of cranial irradiation on hypothalamic-pituitary function: a 5–year longitudinal study in patients with nasopharyngeal carcinoma. *Q J Med* 1991; **78**: 165–176.
86. Kwong D, Wei W, Sham J et al. Sensorineural hearing loss in patients treated for nasopharyngeal carcinoma: a prospective study of the effect of radiation and cisplatin treatment. *Int J Radiat Oncol Biol Phys* 1996; **36**: 281–289.
87. Lee A, Foo W, Law S et al. Reirradiation for recurrent nasopharyngeal carcinoma: factors affecting the therapeutic ratio and ways for improvement. *Int J Radiat Oncol Biol Phys* 1997; **38**: 43–52.
88. Pryzant R, Wendt C, Declos L et al. Re-treatment of nasopharyngeal carcinoma in 53 patients. *Int J Radiat Oncol Biol Phys* 1992; **22**: 941–947.
89. Wang C. Re-irradiation of recurrent nasopharyngeal carcinoma: treatment techniques and results. *Int J Radiat Oncol Biol Phys* 1987; **13**: 953–956.
90. International Nasopharynx Cancer Study Group. Preliminary results of a randomized trial comparing neoadjuvant chemotherapy (cisplatin, epirubicin, bleomycin) plus radiotherapy vs. radiotherapy alone in stage IV (≥ N2, M0) undifferentiated nasopharyngeal carcinoma: a positive effect on progression-free survival. *Int J Radiat Oncol Biol Phys* 1996; **35**: 463–469.
91. Dimery I, Peters L, Goepfert H et al. Effectiveness of combined induction chemotherapy and radiotherapy in advanced nasopharyngeal carcinoma. *J Clin Oncol* 1993; **11**: 1919–1928.
92. Khoury G, Paterson I. Nasopharyngeal carcinoma: a review of cases treated by radiotherapy and chemotherapy. *Clin Radiol* 1987; **38**: 17–20.
93. Atichartakarn V, Kraiphibul P, Clongsusuek P et al. Nasopharyngeal carcinoma: result of treatment with cis-diamminedichloroplatinum II, 5 fluorouracil and radiation therapy. *Int J Radiat Oncol Biol Phys* 1988; **14**: 461–469.
94. Garden A, Lippman S, Morrison W *et al.* Does induction chemotherapy have a role in the management of nasopharyngeal carcinoma? Results of treatment in the era of computerised tomography. *Int J Radiat Oncol Biol Phys* 1996; **36**: 1005–1012.
95. Tannock I, Payne D, Cummings B et al. Sequential chemotherapy and radiation for nasopharyngeal cancer: absence of long-term benefit despite a high rate of tumour response to chemotherapy. *J Clin Oncol* 1987; **5**: 629–634.
96. Chan A, Teo P, Leung T et al. A prospective randomized study of chemotherapy adjunctive to definitive radiotherapy in advanced nasopharyngeal carcinoma. *Int J Radiat Oncol Biol Phys* 1995; **33**: 569–577.
97. Turner S, Tiver K. Synchronous radiotherapy and chemotherapy in the treatment of nasopharyngeal carcinoma. *Int J Radiat Oncol Biol Phys* 1993; **27**: 371–377.

98. Souhami L, Rabinowits M. Combined treatment in carcinoma of the nasopharynx. *Laryngoscope* 1988; **98**: 881–883.
99. Marcial V, Pajak T, Mohuiddin M et al. Concomitant cisplatin chemotherapy and radiotherapy in advanced mucosal squamous cell carcinoma of the head and neck. *Cancer* 1990; **66**: 1861–1868.
100. Al-Sarraf M, Pajak T, Cooper J et al. Chemo-radiotherapy in patients with locally advanced nasopharyngeal carcinoma: a Radiation Therapy Oncology Group study. *J Clin Oncol* 1990; **8**: 1342–1351.
101. Rahima M, Rakowsky E, Barzilay J et al. Carcinoma of the nasopharynx. An analysis of 91 cases and a comparison of differing treatment approaches. *Cancer* 1986; **58**: 843–849.
102. Tsujii H, Kamada T, Tsuji H et al. Improved results in the treatment of nasopharyngeal carcinoma using combined radiotherapy and chemotherapy. *Cancer* 1989; **63**: 1668–1672.
103. Teo P, Ho J, Choy, D et al. Adjunctive chemotherapy to radical radiation therapy in the treatment of advanced nasopharyngeal carcinoma. *Int J Radiat Oncol Biol Phys* 1987; **13**: 679–685.
104. Rossi A, Molinari P, Boracchi P *et al.* Adjuvant chemotherapy with vincristine, cyclophosphamide and doxorubicin after radiotherapy in local-regional nasopharyngeal cancer: results of a 4-year multicenter randomized study. *J Clin Oncol* 1988; **6**: 1401–1410.
105. Al-Sarraf M, LeBlanc M, Giri P *et al.* Superiority of chemo-radiotherapy (CT-RT) vs. radiotherapy (RT) in patients (pts) with locally advanced nasopharyngeal cancer (NPC). Preliminary results of Intergroup 0099 (SWOG 8892, RTOG 8817, ECOG 2388) randomized study (meeting abstract). *Proc Ann Meeting of the American Society of Clinical Oncology* 1996; **15**: A882.
106. Choo R, Tannock I. Chemotherapy for recurrent or metastatic carcinoma of the nasopharynx. A review of the Princess Margaret Hospital experience. *Cancer* 1991; **68**: 2120–2124.
107. Al-Kourainy K, Crissman J, Ensley J et al. Excellent response to cis-platinum-based chemotherapy in patients with recurrent or previously untreated advanced nasopharyngeal carcinoma. *Am J Clin Oncol* 1988; **11**: 427–430.
108. Morton R, Liavaag P, McLean M et al. Transcervico-mandibulo-palatal approach for surgical salvage of recurrent nasopharyngeal cancer. *Head and Neck* 1996; **18**: 352–358.
109. Wei W, Ho C, Yuen P et al. Maxillary swing approach for resection of tumours in and around the nasopharynx. *Arch Otolaryngol Head Neck Surg* 1995; **121**: 638–642.
110. Hsu M, Ko J, Sheen T et al. Salvage surgery for recurrent nasopharyngeal carcinoma. *Arch Otolaryngol Head Neck Surg* 1997; **123**: 305–309.
111. Fisch U. The infratemporal fossa approach for nasopharyngeal tumours. *Laryngoscope* 1983; **93**: 36–43.
112. Wilson C. Observations on surgery of the nasopharynx. *Ann Otol Rhinol Laryngol* 1957; **66**: 5–40.
113. Belmont J. The Le Fort 1 osteotomy approach for nasopharyngeal and nasal fossa tumours. *Arch Otolaryngol Head Neck Surg* 1988; **114**: 751–754.
114. Fee W, Gilmer P, Goffinet D. Surgical management of recurrent nasopharyngeal carcinoma after radiation failure at the primary site. *Laryngoscope* 1988; **98**: 1220–1226.
115. Harrison L, Sessions R, Fass D et al. Nasopharyngeal brachytherapy with access via a transpalatal flap. *Am J Surg* 1992; **164**: 173–175.
116. Choy D, Sham J, Wei W et al. Transpalatal insertion of radioactive gold grain for the treatment of persistent and recurrent nasopharyngeal carcinoma. *Int J Radiat Oncol Biol Phys* 1993; **25**: 505–512.
117. Bliss P, Laing R, See A et al. Treatment of recurrent nasopharyngeal carcinoma by combined surgery and brachytherapy (in preparation).
118. Wei W, Lam K, Ho JHC et al. Efficacy of radical neck dissection for the control of cervical metastasis after radiotherapy for nasopharyngeal carcinoma. *Am J Surg* 1990; **160**: 439–442.

13 Tumours of the oropharynx

Peter H Rhys Evans, Snehal G Patel and J Michael Henk

Introduction

Tumours of the oropharynx are relatively infrequent with an incidence of 0.8 per 100 000 population per annum. For head and neck tumours, this is the commonest site for carcinomas of the pharynx. Functionally, the oropharynx is one the most critical sites in the upper aerodigestive tract since it is situated at the important bifurcation of the respiratory and digestive tract. Tumours at this site will affect swallowing, speech and ultimately the airway and, therefore, decisions about treatment are influenced, not only by the most optimal method of tumour ablation, but also by important functional considerations.

The oropharynx also includes important lymphatic structures in the base of tongue and tonsils which form part of Waldeyer's ring and, therefore, is a significant extranodal site for development of lymphomas, which have a quite different morphology and natural history to squamous carcinomas arising in this site.

Tumours may arise from any site within the oropharynx but there is considerable variation in the type and behaviour of tumours in these different sites even for squamous carcinoma. It is therefore of practical importance to divide the oropharynx into the palatine arch and the oropharynx proper (Table 13.1).[1] In general, squamous carcinomas of the palatine arch tend to be less aggressive and metastasize later than those elsewhere in the oropharynx.

Table 13.1 Divisions of the oropharynx

Palatine arch	
	Soft palate and uvula
	Anterior faucial pillar
Oropharynx proper	
	Lateral and posterior wall including the pharyngoepiglottic fold
	Base of tongue and vallecula
	Glossotonsillar sulcus
	Tonsillar fossa and posterior faucial pillar

Anatomical subsites

The oropharynx is the middle part of the pharynx and is functionally unique in that it forms the common conduit for the upper respiratory and digestive tracts. Superiorly it communicates through the velopalatine isthmus with the nasopharynx, anterosuperiorly through the palatoglossal arch with the oral cavity, and inferiorly it continues as the hypopharynx with an anteroinferior opening into the larynx. Each of these orifices is surrounded by a complex independent sphincter mechanism which controls the integrity of the opening during respiration and deglutition. Under normal circumstances these sphincters are functionally synchronized by cortical and local neuromuscular reflex pathways, but these can be easily disrupted under pathological conditions causing serious functional complications.

The oropharynx extends from the level of the hard palate above to the hyoid bone below (Figure 13.1). It is further subdivided into four main anatomical subsites for the purpose of tumour classification (Table 13.2).

Anterior wall

This comprises the base or posterior third of the tongue bounded anteriorly by the V-shaped line of circumvallate papillae. These commence laterally adjacent to the base of the palatoglossal fold and come to an apex in the midline at the vestigial foramen caecum (Figure 13.2). It extends caudally to include the valleculae at the junction of the base of the tongue with the lingual aspect of the epiglottis and both the lateral pharyngoepiglottic and the midline glosseoepiglottic folds. The epiglottis itself is classified as part of the supraglottic larynx. Laterally it extends to the margins of the tongue.

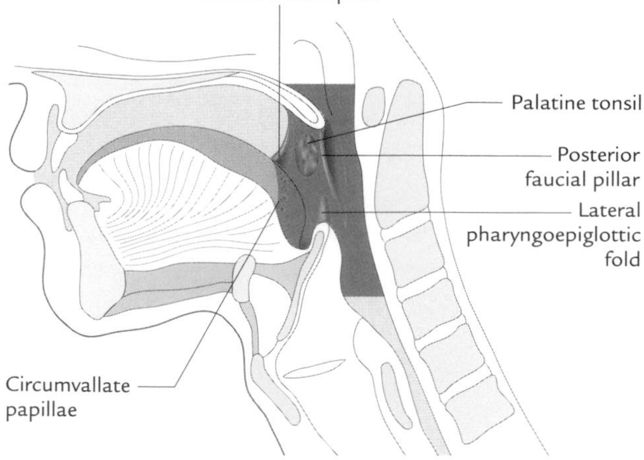

Figure 13.1 Divisions of the oropharynx.

Table 13.2 Anatomical subsites of the oropharynx
Anterior wall (glossoepiglottic area)
Tongue posterior to the circumvallate papillae (base of tongue)
Vallecula (but not the lingual surface of the epiglottis, which is now included in the larynx – suprahyoid epiglottis)
Lateral wall
Tonsil
Tonsillar fossa and faucial pillars
Glossotonsillar sulcus
Posterior wall
Superior wall
Inferior surface of the soft palate
Uvula

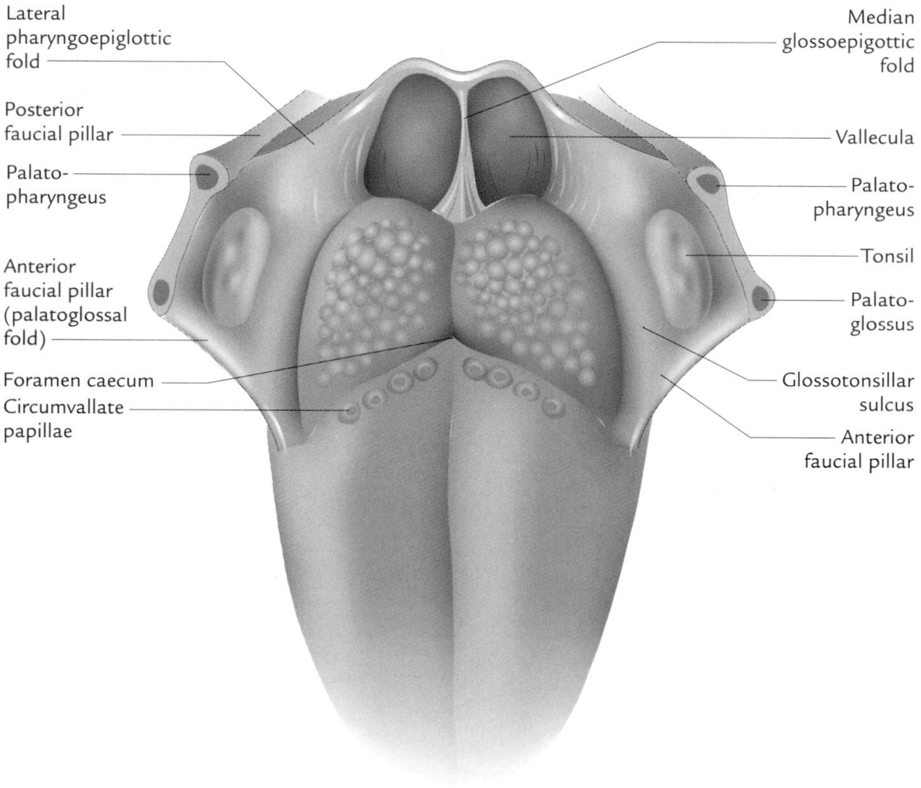

Figure 13.2 Dorsum of the tongue.

The base of the tongue is mostly covered with aggregates of lymphoid tissue forming the lingual tonsil. Mucous glands open onto the surface and also into the crypts of the lingual tonsil. The bulk of the tongue base is formed by the interlacing network of intrinsic (vertical and transverse) and extrinsic (styloglossus and hyoglossus) muscle bundles (Figure 13.3). The attached part or root of the tongue also contains the important vascular and nerve pedicles on each side. The septum linguae is a strong midline connective tissue septum. Small tumours at this site however may spread bilaterally via neurovascular bundles and thus compromise the function and viability of the whole tongue.

Vascular supply

The base of the tongue has a rich vascular supply from the lingual artery, which is the third branch of the external carotid artery. Normally there is a good collateral circulation from the facial artery so that

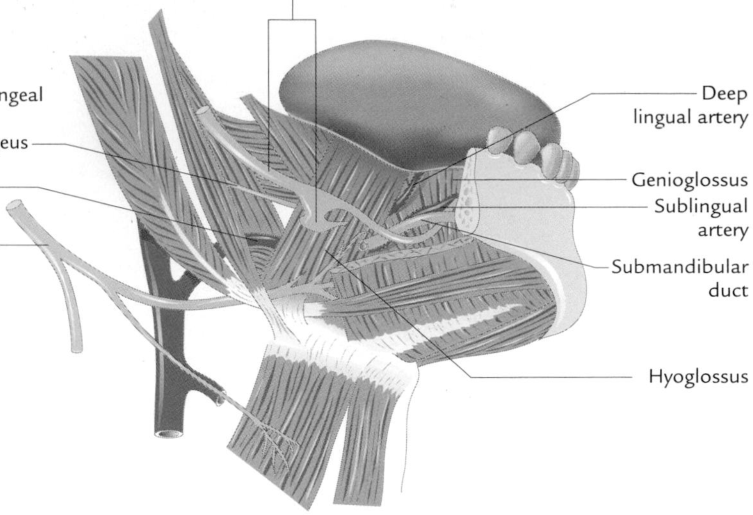

Figure 13.3 Innervation and musculature of the tongue.

ligation of the origin of the lingual artery does not significantly reduce bleeding. Venous drainage is via the deep lingual vein which accompanies the hypoglossal nerve, 'protecting' its superficial surface during dissection of the area.

Innervation

The afferent supply to the posterior part of the tongue is through the glossopharyngeal (IX) nerve except for a small area in the valleculae and adjacent part of the tongue mucosa, which is supplied by twigs from the superior laryngeal branch of the vagus (X). The glossopharyngeal nerve contains fibres both of general sensation and of taste, the latter especially distributed to the circumvallate papillae. The acute pain on swallowing, eating and talking associated with tumours of the tongue base, is an important clinical sign even in the absence of mucosal abnormality.

Motor innervation to the muscles of the tongue is via the hypoglossal (XII) nerve, which emerges between the internal jugular vein and internal carotid artery, descending to a point above the carotid bifurcation where it gives off the descendans hypoglossi branch of the ansa cervicalis. It curves forwards on the surface of the internal and external carotid arteries adjacent to the deep aspect of the jugulodigastric lymph node. Here it can be invaded by metastatic tumour or may need to be resected.

Lymphatic drainage

Lymphatics from the tongue posterior to the circumvallate papillae run downwards towards the hyoid bone where they pierce the pharyngeal wall to enter the nodes of the upper deep cervical chain (level II). Tumours typically drain into the largest of these nodes (jugulodigastric), which lies on the lateral aspect of the internal jugular vein, just below the inferior border of the posterior belly of digastric muscle (Figure 13.3). From here lymphatics normally drain sequentially to levels III, IV and V although under pathological conditions or following surgery to the neck there may be retrograde spread to level I, the retropharyngeal nodes or to the contralateral side of the neck. Tumours near the midline are more likely to exhibit bilateral spread.

Lateral wall

This includes the tonsil, the tonsillar fossae, the faucial pillars and more posteriorly the lateral pharyngeal wall, which merges into the posterior wall. The anterior boundary is the vertical fold of the palatoglossus muscle (anterior faucial pillar) which separates it from the oral cavity. The posterior faucial pillar is formed by the palatopharyngeus and deep to both muscles is the superior pharyngeal constrictor. Inferiorly the lateral wall includes the glossotonsillar sulcus, which separates it from the border of the tongue (Figure 13.2).

The tonsil is the largest aggregation of lymphoid tissue in Waldeyer's ring. It is characterized by deep crypts in which squamous carcinomas may arise without causing obvious surface ulceration. It has a distinct capsule which separates it from the superior constrictor and deep to that the contents of the parapharyngeal space (Figure 13.4).

Vascular supply

The tonsillar branch of the facial artery is the main supply with other branches from the lingual, the ascending palatine and superiorly from the lesser palatine arteries. The tonsillar and other pharyngeal veins drain into a plexus situated on the posterior wall of the pharynx, which communicates above with the pterygoid plexus and below with the superior thyroid and lingual veins or directly into the facial or internal jugular.[2] A separate ring-like

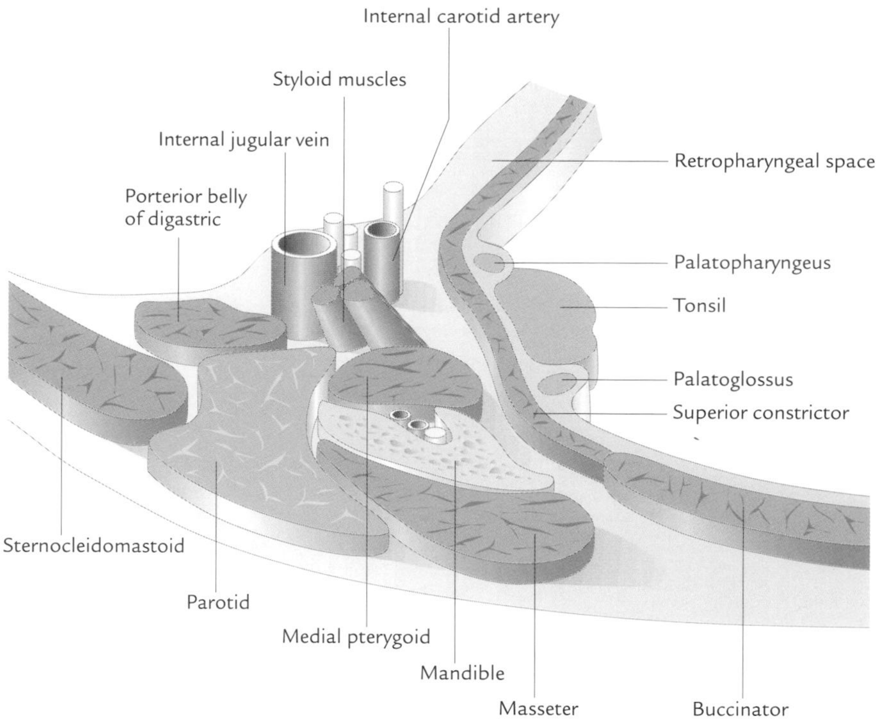

Figure 13.4 Deep relations of the tonsil.

submucosal pharyngeal plexus is situated around the entrance to the larynx and is particularly dense with veins 1–3 mm in diameter. It is arranged in two parts, one on the anterior and the other on the posterior wall of the pharynx, and is thought to be concerned with pressure adjustments accompanying swallowing.[3] It accounts for the increased vascularity noticed in this area during pharyngeal resections.

Innervation

The sensory innervation of the tonsillar region is via the glossopharyngeal nerve which passes forwards and lateral to the stylopharyngeus and deep to the lower pole of the tonsil. Tumours arising in the depths of the tonsillar crypts may invade branches of this exquisitely sensitive nerve causing pain and otalgia before surface ulceration becomes apparent. Sensation from the upper part of the tonsil is through descending branches of the lesser palatine nerves coursing through the sphenopalatine ganglion from the facial (VII) nerve.

The pharyngeal plexus provides the motor and most of the sensory innervation to the pharynx from branches of the glossopharyngeal and vagus nerves. The former contributes only sensation to the plexus, but the vagus supplies sensory fibres as well as all the motor fibres including those joining from the internal ramus of the accessory (XI) nerve. Loss of the glossopharyngeal nerve either from tumour invasion or from surgery will therefore impair sensation and the swallow reflex, but good function is maintained unless there is additional loss of the vagus or its pharyngeal branches at the skull base.

Lymphatic drainage

The oropharyngeal mucosa has a rich lymphatic network, especially the tonsils, which drain directly through the pharyngeal wall into the upper deep cervical (jugulodigastric) nodes. Large early metastatic deposits may present. This node has a tendency to undergo cystic degeneration in the presence of squamous carcinoma, it is often mistaken for a branchial cyst with serious consequences for the patient. In addition, fine-needle aspiration of the cystic fluid may often be acellular or non-diagnostic giving a false sense of security. It can never be said too often that in an adult, particularly where there is a history of smoking, an enlarged node that has been present for more than 1 month should be regarded as metastatic carcinoma until proved otherwise, irrespective of whether or not it has partly responded to antibiotics. Ultrasound-guided FNAC may help to take samples from the wall of the cyst rather than the fluid itself. From level II nodes drainage continues to levels III and IV.

Lymphatics from the upper lateral wall drain to the retropharyngeal nodes of which the only constant one is the node of Rouvier situated close to the skull base between the internal carotid artery and the lateral wall of the pharynx. Lymph from here drains into the deep cervical chain (levels II, III and IV)

Posterior wall

This extends superiorly from the level of the hard palate and Passavant's ridge down to the hyoid bone where the posterior pharyngeal wall is continuous with that of the hypopharynx. Laterally it curves forward to merge with the lateral wall. The mucosa is smooth and contains occasional small aggregates of lymphoid tissue. Deep to this are the overlapping posterior fibres of the superior and middle constrictor muscles that insert largely into each other in a midline pharyngeal raphe. The muscular wall with its thin covering of buccopharyngeal fascia is separated from the prevertebral fascia by an area of loose connective tissue forming the retropharyngeal space.

Vascular supply

The arterial supply of the posterior wall is from branches of the ascending pharyngeal and superior thyroid arteries. The venous drainage is through the pharyngeal plexus previously described.

Innervation

Details of the motor and sensory distribution of the vagus and glossopharyngeal nerves to the pharyngeal wall are described above.

Roof

The roof of the oropharynx is formed by the curved arch of the inferior surface of the soft palate and the uvula in the midline. There are numerous palatine glands opening onto the mucosa on the oral surface of the soft palate and they are especially abundant over the uvula. The palatine aponeurosis forms the skeletal framework of the soft palate and is firmly attached anteriorly to the posterior margin of the hard palate. The tensor and levator veli palatini muscles fuse with each other in the midline raphe and are responsible for closing off the nasopharynx during speech and swallowing. The palatoglossus and palatopharyngeus control the sphincteric action of the faucial pillars.

Vascular supply

The soft palate is supplied by the lesser palatine arteries, which are branches of the descending palatine from the maxillary artery. The venous drainage is mainly to the pharyngeal and pterygoid plexus.

Innervation

Sensory innervation from the soft palate is through fibres in the lesser palatine nerve via the pterygopalatine ganglion. All the muscles of the soft palate are supplied from the pharyngeal plexus from the vagus (X), with the exception of the tensor veli palatini, which is innervated by a branch from the mandibular nerve.

Lymphatic drainage

Lymphatic drainage is mainly to the upper deep cervical nodes (level II).

Histology

As with other sites in the upper aerodigestive tract, tumours may arise in the oropharynx from different epithelial elements and three main histological types are well recognized:

1. Squamous cell carcinoma from the squamous epithelium;
2. Lymphomas from the tonsils and lymphoid follicles in the base of the tongue;
3. Salivary gland tumours from minor salivary glands concentrated in the soft palate, uvula and the capsule of the tonsil.

Generally, in the upper aerodigestive tract squamous cell carcinoma accounts for about 90% of all malignant epithelial tumours. Because of the higher concentration of lymphoid tissue in the oropharynx and hence the greater proportion of non-Hodgkin's lymphoma (25%), the incidence of squamous carcinomas is less (70%) than in other sites in the upper aerodigestive tract. Salivary gland tumours and other rare tumours account for the remaining 5%.

1. Squamous cell carcinoma

Epidemiology

The incidence of oropharyngeal cancer varies considerably around the world but in most series it ranks second or third in order of frequency of head and neck cancers and in general it is not as common as laryngeal or oral cavity tumours. Approximately 500 new cases of squamous carcinoma of the oropharynx are registered annually in England and Wales with an incidence of 0.8 per 100 000 population per annum. This accounts for about 10.9% of all head and neck cancers compared with 36% occurring in the larynx and 18% in the oral cavity.[4]

In parts of Central Europe, South America and Asia the incidence is between 1.5–3% of all cancers and the relative frequency among head and neck carcinoma ranges from 18–25%.[5–7] Raised incidence rates (per 100 000 population per annum) are observed in the Netherlands Antilles (5.5) and Bombay (4.7) but these are overshadowed by the Bas-Rhin and Doubs regions of France where the incidence is 11.6 and 6.8 respectively. Other high values recorded are in Geneva (5.7), Slovenia (4.6) and Varese, Italy (4.1).[4]

The male to female ratio is about 2.5:1 and tumours are seen most frequently in the sixth decade in women and in the seventh decade in men.

Aetiological factors

Tobacco

As with other squamous carcinomas of the upper aerodigestive tract, tobacco is the most important factor and may be synergistic in its effect combined with alcohol consumption. There is a clear dose-response relationship between tobacco exposure and squamous carcinoma.[8] The nitrocarbon carcinogens in tobacco are relatively insoluble in normal saliva but are more soluble in alcohol and therefore are more readily absorbed into the surface epithelium. In normal cigarette smokers, the site of malignancy most commonly seen is within the capsule of the tonsil. Where additional alcohol consumption is an important factor, tumours also commonly arise in the glossotonsillar sulci and more posteriorly in the pharyngo-epiglottic fold. The reverse 'chutta' smoking habit seen in some areas of India, particularly in women, predisposes to carcinomas developing in the palatine arch.[9] 'Bidi' smoking in India also predisposes to development of tumours in the base of the tongue.

Cigarette smoking cannot be the sole aetiological factor as only a small percentage of smokers will develop carcinoma. Genetic factors associated with increased risk include: mutagen sensitivity,[10] which reflects a defect in DNA repair, including xeroderma pigmentosum, Fanconi anaemia and ataxia telangiectasia. Other genetic markers include induceability of cytochrome P450.[11]

Alcohol

A positive correlation between tobacco and alcohol consumption has been shown in Amercian[12] and French[13] studies. Interestingly this has not been shown to be the case in one study in the United Kingdom[14] probably because of prohibition of unmatured pot-stilled spirits containing toxic by-products. Mashberg et al[15] have also shown that mucosal areas exposed to prolonged contact with alcohol are at an increased risk.

Diet

McLaughlin et al[16] have shown the importance of dietary factors in predisposition of oral and pharyngeal cancer. Vitamin A deficiency predisposes to evolution of carcinoma and fruits and vegetables have been found to have protective effect. Ingestion of salted meat has also been shown to be a risk factor in oral cavity and pharyngeal carcinoma.[17] Chronic irritants, poor dental hygiene,[12] syphilis and marijuana smoking[18] have been identified as predisposing factors in upper aerodigestive tract carcinoma.

Viruses

Although an association has been identified between human papilloma virus (types 2,11,16) and the development of squamous carcinoma of the oropharynx[19] there is no molecular evidence to support a causal association.[20] Human immunodeficiency virus (HIV) also probably accelerates development of squamous cell carcinoma in high-risk patients.[21]

Immunosuppression

Kidney transplantation and the use of immunosuppressive drugs following marrow transplantation have also been shown to predispose to evolution of cancer.[22]

Genetic predisposition

Accumulation of p53 in tumour cell nuclei predicts a significantly increased risk of death, independent of tumour grade, stage and lymph node status.[23] The EGFR gene may be involved in pathogenesis[24] and chromosome 18 may be a possible site for a tumour suppressor gene deletion.[25]

Precancer

Precancerous lesions such as leukoplakia and erythroplakia do not have such significance in predisposition for oropharyngeal cancer as they do in squamous carcinoma of the oral cavity. There is an accepted predisposition for cancer development in certain conditions such as submucous fibrosis (Figure 13.5), which predisposes to tumours developing in the oropharynx particularly in the anterior palatoglossal fold.

Site distribution

The distribution of carcinomas at various sites in the oropharynx follows similar patterns to that seen in the oral cavity in that the sites most commonly affected are those in more prolonged contact with surface carcinogens.[26] The crypts of the tonsils, the

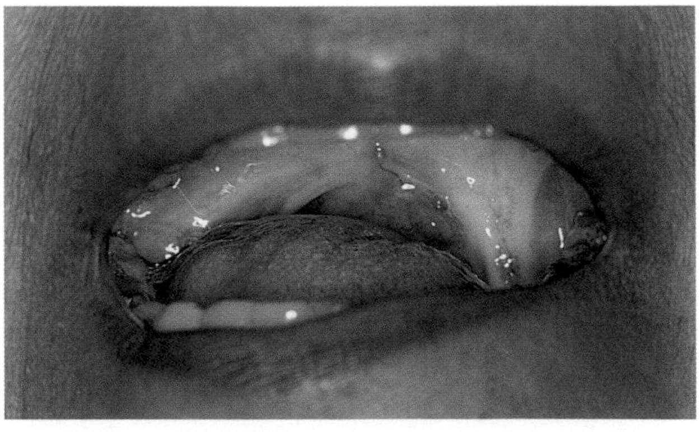

Figure 13.5 Oral submucous fibrosis, a condition that is associated with cancer developing in the anterior palatoglossal fold.

Table 13.3 Site distribution in the oropharynx

	Argentina 1970–1994[5]		UK 1983–1991[28]	
	Number	Percentage	Number	Percentage
Anterior wall	288	37.5	42	33
Lateral wall	333	43.5	73	57
Superior wall	119	15.5	8	6
Posterior wall	27	3.5	6	4
Total number	767	100	129	100

Table 13.4 Nodal metastases in oropharyngeal carcinoma

Site	Node positive (%)		Bilateral nodes (%)
	Henk[27]	Lindberg [29]	Lindberg[29]
Base of tongue	60	78	34
Tonsil	73	76	21
Soft palate	2	44	19
Anterior faucial pillar	—	45	7
Posterior wall	2	—	—

glossotonsillar sulci and the tongue base are bathed in saliva to a greater extent than the soft palate or posterior pharyngeal wall and are thus more common sites where smoking and alcohol are aetiological factors.

There is also considerable geographical variation in the incidence of squamous carcinoma at different sites due to environmental and other aetiological agents. The practice of 'reverse smoking' (Chutta) in women in certain parts of India is associated with a higher incidence of carcinoma of the soft and hard palate.[9] In France and other Mediterranean countries there is a higher incidence of oropharyngeal tumours than in the UK because of differences in tobacco and alcohol consumption. In these regions carcinoma is more common in the glossotonsillar sulcus and on the pharyngoepiglottic fold.

The commonest site for carcinoma in the oropharynx is the tonsil followed by the base of the tongue and these two sites account for between 80–90% of cases (Table 13.3). The soft palate and posterior wall are much less common and those tumours occurring on the posterior wall almost invariably are situated low down near the junction with the hypopharynx at the level of the hyoid.[5,27]

Nodal metastases

The incidence of nodal metastases is in the region of 65%[28] to 77%.[5]

Grade does not seem to be an influential factor since metastases are just as common with poorly differentiated lesions as with well-differentiated tumours. Site, however, does influence the occurrence of nodal disease because of the richer distribution of lymphatics in the tongue base and tonsillar fossae (Table 13.4). Tumours in these two sites have a high risk of metastatic nodal disease at presentation (76–78%) compared with 44–45% from lesions in the soft palate and anterior faucial pillar.[29]

The T stage of oropharyngeal carcinoma is based on size and as a group there does not appear to be any overall correlation between size and N stage since positive nodes are seen just as commonly with T1 as with T4 tumours (Table 13.5).[27] This is probably related to the dominant sites of the tonsil and to a lesser extent the tongue base because of their rich lymphatic drainage. For posterior wall and soft palate the numbers are too small for analysis but node metastases are generally not so commonly seen from smaller tumours at these sites.

For midline structures the risk of bilateral node involvement is much greater with base of tongue

Table 13.5 Clinical stage-wise distribution of tongue base and tonsil carcinoma[28]

	Base of tongue					Tonsil					Total
	N0	N1	N2	N3	N+ (%)	N0	N1	N2	N3	N+ (%)	
T1	1				0	7	7	7	2	69	24
T2	13	5	1	3	41	6	5	6	3	70	42
T3	1	5	2		87	5	4	4	5	72	26
T4	1	4	1	5	90	2	5	1	4	83	23
Total	16	14	4	8		20	21	18	14		115

tumours (34%) than soft palate (19%).[29] Tonsillar carcinoma is also more prone to bilateral disease (21%) than tumours on the adjacent anterior faucial pillar (7%).

Staging

The TNM classification of squamous cell carcinoma has undergone several changes but the accepted joint UICC/AJC classification for oropharyngeal tumours is shown in Tables 13.6 and 13.7 with the following provisions:

1. The classification only applies to squamous cell carcinoma;
2. There must be histological verification of the disease and the grade may range from well-differentiated to poorly differentiated or anaplastic carcinoma. Spindle cell or basal cell variants may be seen.
3. The extent and staging must include clinical, radiological and endoscopic findings.

Distant metastases at presentation are rarely seen but in large series the frequency may be in the region of 1–2%.[5] Long-term follow-up of patients with oropharyngeal carcinoma reveals a distant metastasis rate of 15% which is above the average (11%) for head and neck squamous carcinoma.[30] Synchronous (Figures 13.6 and 13.7) or metachronous primary tumours of the upper aerodigestive tract or lung are seen in about 10% of patients with squamous cell carcinoma of the oral cavity and oropharynx although in some countries where there is a high intake of tobacco and alcohol this incidence is as high as 20%.[1]

Table 13.6 Classification of primary tumour (UICC/AJC)

Tx	Tumour extent cannot be assessed
Tis	Carcinoma in situ
T0	No evidence of primary tumour
T1	Tumour 2 cm or less in its greatest dimension
T2	Tumour 2–4 cm in its greatest dimension
T3	Tumour more than 4 cm in its greatest dimension
T4	Tumour invading adjacent structures e.g. through cortical bone, soft tissue of neck, deep (extrinsic) muscles of the tongue

Table 13.7 Classification of cervical nodes

Nx	Regional lymph nodes cannot be assessed
N0	No evidence of cervical node involvement
N1	Single clinically positive homolateral node* up to 3 cm in greatest diameter
N2	Clinically positive nodes less than 6 cm in diameter:
N2a	Single clinically positive homolateral node 3–6 cm in diameter
N2b	Multiple clinically positive homolateral nodes, none greater than 6 cm in diameter
N2c	Clinically positive contralateral or bilateral nodes, none greater than 6 cm in diameter
N3	Massive homolateral, contralateral or bilateral node/s more than 6 cm in diameter

*Midline nodes are considered homolateral

Lymphoepithelioma

Otherwise known as undifferentiated carcinoma of nasopharyngeal type (UCNT) this variant of squamous carcinoma is found most commonly, as its name implies, in the nasopharynx. It is however also found in the tonsil and base of tongue. The squamous component may be extremely undifferentiated but the lymphoid element is composed of non-neoplastic lymphocytes that permeate widely throughout the tumour. Surface marker studies have shown these lymphoid cells to be reactive B cells, T helper and T suppressor cells. Metastases are characterized by the presence of only the squamous element similar to the primary tumour and do not contain lymphocytes.

The important clinical features of this tumour are its increased tendency to metastasize, similar to

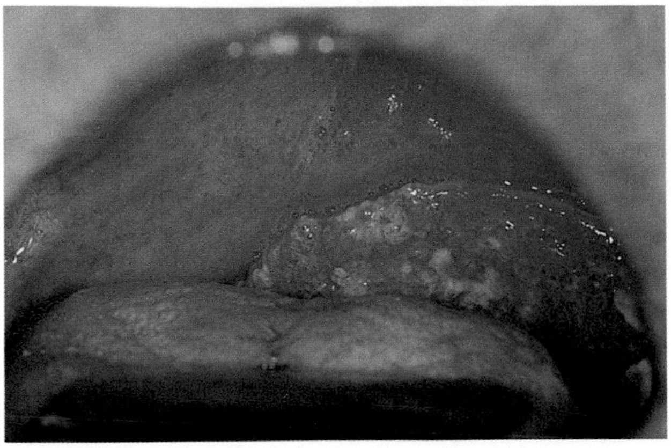

Figure 13.6 Patient presenting with a large ulcerating squamous carcinoma of the soft palate was also found on examination to have a synchronous asymptomatic squamous carcinoma of the floor of mouth (see Figure 13.7).

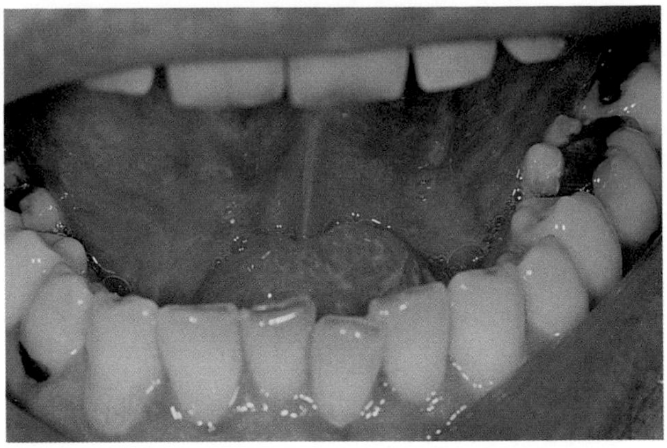

Figure 13.7 Patient with a synchronous asymptomatic squamous carcinoma of the floor of mouth (see Figure 13.6).

nasopharyngeal UCNT, and also its extreme radiosensitivity.

2. Lymphoma

Non-Hodgkin's lymphoma accounts for about 8% of oropharyngeal tumours,[31] the usual sites being the tonsil (5%) and base of tongue (3%), but more commonly presents in the head and neck as nodal metastases. The commonest type of lymphoma presenting in the oropharynx is the B cell lymphoma which is a large cell lymphoma of high-grade malignancy. T cell lymphomas are rare in the oropharynx but do show a well documented association with T lymphotrophic virus type 1 (HTLV-1) especially in Japan and the Caribbean countries.[32]

The classification of lymphomas has undergone major modifications over the past 20 years and a working formulation has been devised by the National Cancer Institute.[33] A comprehensive review of lymphomas of the oropharynx and head and neck is given elsewhere.[1]

3. Salivary gland tumours

Salivary gland tumours account for about 5% of all tumours of the oropharynx and the majority of such tumours arising from the minor salivary glands are malignant, in contrast to major salivary gland tumours, which are most commonly of a benign type.

Spiro has described a large series of minor salivary gland tumours, 3% of which affected the oropharynx and almost all of them arose in the tonsillar fossa.[34] The majority of these are adenoid cystic carcinomas and they behave in a similar way to those arising in other sites within the head and neck in that they do have a propensity to spread along nerve sheaths in the perineural lymphatics with late metastases to lymph nodes, lung and bone. Although the short-term prognosis for these tumours is very good with an 80% 5-year survival rate, eventually about 60–80% of patients die from or with metastatic disease.

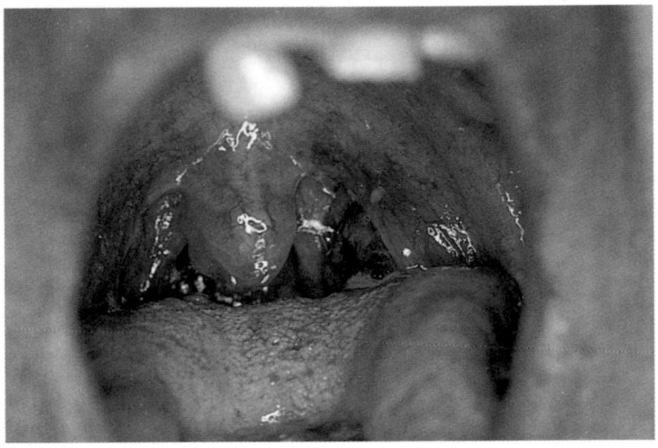

Figure 13.8 Metastatic malignant melanoma in the left tonsil from a primary located on skin of the back.

Metastatic disease

Metastases to the oropharynx from primaries outside the head and neck region are rare but are occasionally found (Figure 13.8).

Clinical presentation

Symptoms

Diagnosis of oropharyngeal carcinoma in its early stages is uncommon (Table 13.8) because of vague initial symptoms such as soreness or discomfort in the throat particularly on swallowing or otalgia are

Table 13.8 Tumour and node stage at presentation[27,35]

		T1	T2	T3	T4	Total
N0	Spiro et al[35]	11	24	16	3	54
	Henk[27]	8	19	6	3	36
N1	Spiro et al[35]	3	10	11	2	26
	Henk[27]	7	10	9	9	35
N2	Spiro et al[35]	8	7	14	2	31
	Henk[27]	7	7	6	2	22
N3	Spiro et al[35]	3	1	2	0	6
	Henk[27]	2	6	5	9	22
Total	Spiro et al[35]	25	42	43	7	117
	Henk[27]	24	42	26	23	115

Table 13.9 Overall staging at presentation[27,35]

	I (%)	II (%)	III (%)	IV (%)
Spiro et al[35]	9	20	34	35
Henk[27]	7	17	28	48

common. Only 7–10% of patients are Stage I at presentation,[27,35] roughly 20% are Stage II and about 70% are Stage III and IV (Table 13.9). Over two-thirds of patients will present with a neck lump which often can be misdiagnosed as a branchial cyst when it lies in the jugulodigastric region. Sometimes these nodes can rapidly enlarge due to haemorrhage or necrosis and they are often tender. Other symptoms include a foreign-body sensation in the throat or altered voice with a 'plum in the throat' quality. For more advanced tumours otalgia and throat pain become more pronounced and ulceration, necrosis and secondary infection may result in foul breath. There may also be progressive impairment of tongue movement affecting speech and swallowing.

Physical examination

A full clinical examination of the upper aerodigestive tract and the neck, including fibreoptic examination is essential. The extent of involvement is often misleading on inspection, and bimanual palpation of the tumour must be undertaken in all patients. The pharyngoglossoepiglottic folds and the posterior surface of the soft palate are blind spots that are not readily accessible to routine examination and the importance of a thorough examination cannot be overemphasized. Anterior faucial pillar, soft palate and tonsillar tumours may be visible with good lighting, but advanced lesions may be associated with trismus, which will make oral examination difficult. Surface appearance of squamous carcinomas is either ulcerative (Figure 13.9) or exophytic (Figure 13.10) although early lesions of the tonsil or tongue base arising in the lymphatic crypts may not be visible and may only be detectable on palpation under anaesthetic or following tonsillectomy. In general the exophytic tumour spreads superficially and may be associated with other areas of leukoplakia in the oral cavity; the ulcerative type invades deeply. Adenocarcinoma may present as a smooth lobulated swelling without surface ulceration (Figure 13.11). Malignant lymphoma typically causes nodular enlargements in the tonsil or tongue base (Figure 13.12).

Sensory and motor function should be assessed, particularly mobility of the tongue as well as fixation. A twelfth nerve paralysis causes wasting of the ipsilateral tongue with deviation to the affected side on protrusion, but in the early stages fasciculations may be apparent. Palatal movement may be impaired by the tumour mass but a palsy of the vagus nerve near the skull base will also cause weakness (and also a vocal cord palsy). Impaired sensation over the chin distribution of the mental nerve and the lateral part of the tongue is an ominous sign indicating invasion of the inferior alveolar nerve or the lingual nerve in the infratemporal fossa.

Fibreoptic examination either with a rigid or flexible scope under local anaesthetic has greatly enhanced the ease of examination of the pharynx and larynx, particularly in assessing the lower extent of the tumour and mobility of structures at or below the level of the hyoid. It is also valuable for estimating invasion of the nasopharynx. Indirect laryngoscopy with a mirror is no longer deemed sufficient for optimum assessment.

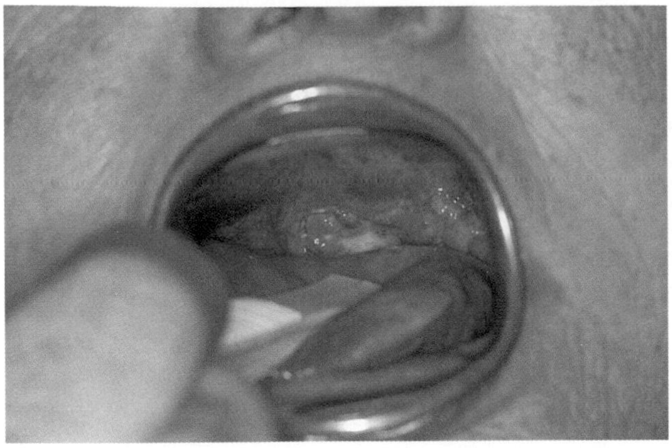

Figure 13.9 Squamous cell carcinoma of the soft palate (ulcerative type).

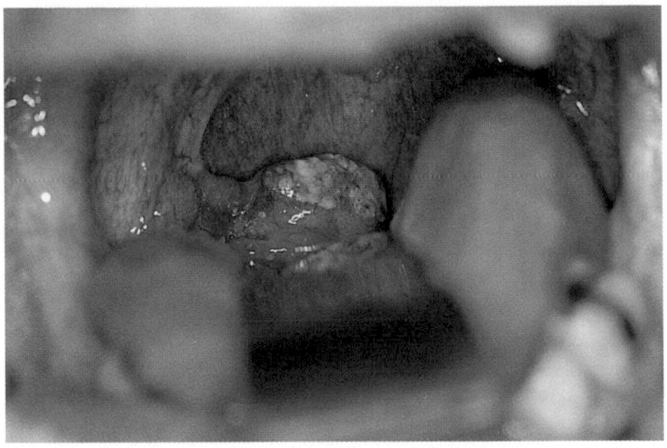

Figure 13.10 Squamous cell carcinoma of the right tonsil (exophytic type).

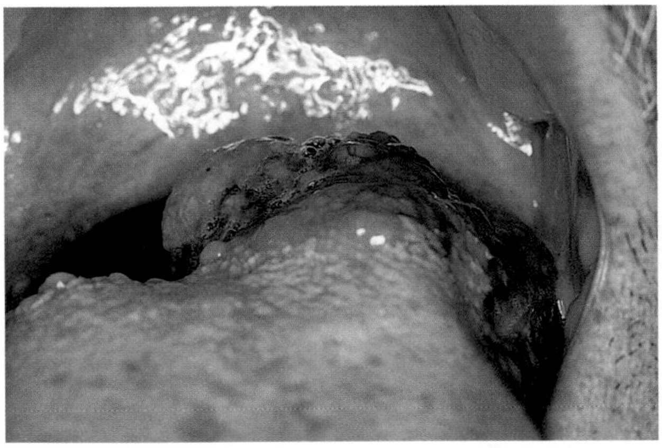

Figure 13.11 Adenocarcinoma of the base of the tongue.

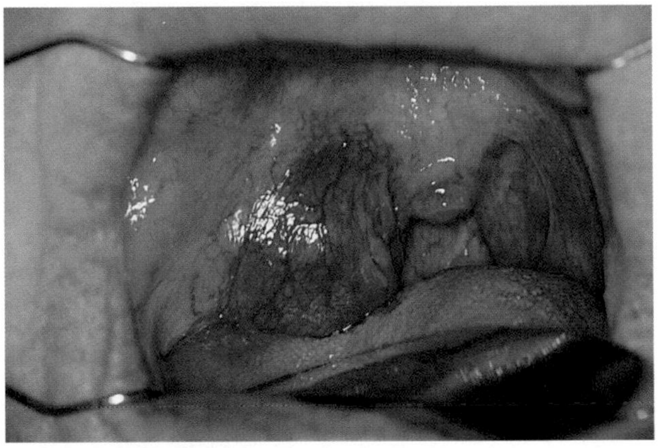

Figure 13.12 Lymphoma of the right tonsil.

Examination of the neck must be carried out systematically and each level must be carefully palpated to detect lymph node enlargement or deep invasion of the tumour. The deep cervical chain of nodes is particularly difficult to assess correctly especially if the patient has a thick neck or there is muscle spasm. At best, clinical examination of the neck has a 30% inaccuracy rate with 20% false negative and 10% false positive.

Nodal metastases from squamous cell carcinomas are typically hard and irregular and when small are generally mobile. As they enlarge, those in the deep cervical chain (levels II, III and IV) initially become attached to the structures in the carotid sheath and the overlying sternomastoid muscle with restriction of vertical mobility (Figure 13.13), but later become attached to the deeper structures in the prevertebral region with absolute fixation. Cystic degeneration or necrosis in a metastatic jugulodigastric node may cause rapid enlargement and may initially be confused for a branchial cyst, with potential delay in proper diagnosis. Lymphomatous nodes have a firm and rubbery consistency and are generally larger and multiple with matting together of adjacent nodes.

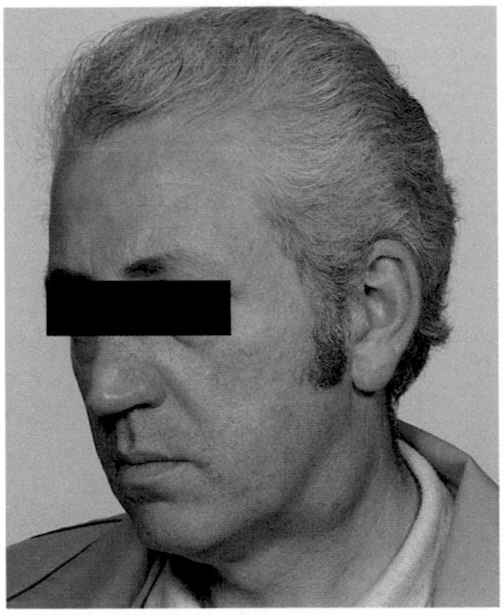

Figure 13.13 N3 metastasis from a T1 squamous cell carcinoma of the tonsil.

Investigations

Fine-needle aspiration cytology

Any suspicious swelling or node in the neck should have FNAC at initial consultation, which should allow rapid differentiation between a branchial cyst, lymphoma and squamous cell carcinoma. Aspiration of cystic fluid from a necrotic metastatic node may give a false negative result and should be repeated to sample the solid portion or wall of the cyst, if necessary under ultrasound guidance.

Radiological investigations

Orthopantomogram (OPG) may be necessary:

- To assess dentition prior to radiotherapy
- If a mandibulotomy is planned
- To show mandibular invasion.

Chest X-Ray (PA and lateral) is essential to rule out:

- Metastatic carcinoma
- Synchronous bronchial primary
- Coexisting acute or chronic pulmonary disease.

Suspicious lesions will need further investigation with chest CT scan, lung function studies or bronchoscopy.

CT and/or MRI of the head and neck are essential:

- For assessing the extent of the primary tumour and its relation to adjacent structures; an MRI is preferable to CT scan to show up small tongue-base tumours
- To assess any mandibular invasion, which is far better shown on CT scan
- For accurate evaluation of the neck to assess the presence, the site, the size and invasive potential of cervical lymphadenopathy and in particular their relation to the carotid artery. Following radiotherapy treatment to the neck these examinations are less dependable in accurately assessing disease in the carotid sheath because of postradiotherapy inflammation and fibrosis, which may be mistaken for tumour
- To assess clinically N0 necks, particularly in obese patients, those with a thick neck or where there is spasm, and help identify possible nodes in the deep cervical chain or parapharyngeal space
- To help distinguish between lymphoma and carcinomatous nodes.

Ultrasound examination

Ultrasound examination of the neck to detect metastatic nodal disease is more sensitive than palpation and has an specificity of about 75%. The specificity is improved to over 90% with the use of ultrasound-guided FNAC as compared with CT and MRI scans (approximately 80%).[36] This technique is very dependable in experienced hands but is not really practical in the routine head and neck clinic.

Examination under anaesthetic and biopsy

A biopsy may be taken under local anaesthetic in the clinic when appropriate and this may suffice in elderly or infirm patients where there may be unacceptable risks with a general anaesthetic. In all other patients a full examination of the upper aerodigestive tract under general anaesthesia is essential:

- For biopsy of the primary
- To look for a possible synchonous primary
- To assess fixation of the primary, for example to the mandible
- For bimanual palpation, particularly lesions of the tongue base
- To assess involvement of the pre-epiglottic space, larynx and hypopharynx
- To assess the neck and perform FNAC if necessary
- To assess the airway and carry out tracheostomy if necessary
- For PEG insertion if nutritional support is required
- For dental extraction prior to treatment
- For bone marrow aspirate in cases of lymphoma

Multidisciplinary clinic

Full evaluation of the patient with all investigations should be discussed in a joint assessment with:

- Head and neck surgeon
- Radiotherapist
- Medical oncologist
- Reconstructive surgeon
- Speech therapist
- Clinical nurse specialist
- Dietician

Treatment

General principles

Curative treatment of oropharyngeal carcinoma is either by surgery or radiotherapy or a combination of both. As with other head and neck cancers, chemotherapy and newer forms of biological therapy or immunotherapy do not give consistent results and at the moment are reserved for patients with advanced or recurrent disease following conventional therapy. Early disease (T1–2) is generally best treated by single modality, either radiotherapy or surgery, but for advanced lesions (stage III and IV) combined therapy with radical surgery followed by postoperative radiotherapy is generally accepted as giving the best chance of cure.

The most difficult dilemmas however in the treatment of oropharyngeal carcinoma concern the choice of optimal treatment for T3–4 tumours where radical surgery may well involve unacceptable loss of the larynx, tongue or both. In these instances, organ preservation using a combination of induction chemotherapy and radiation should be considered as an option.[37] In some situations curative treatment may not be applicable and palliative therapy may be the only option.

In a series of 127 patients with previously untreated squamous carcinoma of the oropharynx seen at the Royal Marsden Hospital between 1983 and 1991, the choice of treatment modality is given in Table 13.10.[28] The large majority (98) of patients received radiotherapy and 23 had primary surgery (21 with postoperative radiotherapy). In the early years neoadjuvant chemotherapy was given prior to irradiation (11) or surgery (4). Four patients had palliative treatment and two others died before therapy.

In general, the choice for the individual patient will depend on a number of factors. The site and size of the primary tumour is one of the most important factors in determining treatment. Where cure rates for surgery and radiotherapy are similar, the choice is usually that which causes least functional disability. Deeply ulcerative lesions of the oropharynx are best treated with initial surgery followed by postoperative radiation therapy as the results of salvage surgery in this setting are poor.[38]

The presence of nodal metastases in the neck at presentation will reduce the prognosis by about 50% and although radical radiotherapy may be effective in N0 and early N1 nodal disease, optimum treatment for N+ disease usually involves a combination of primary surgery with postoperative radiotherapy.

The influence of performance status on outcome was found to be the only significant treatment factor on multivariate analysis for the series of 127 oropharyngeal carcinoma patients seen at the Royal Marsden Hospital between 1983 and 1991 (Table 13.11).[28]

Table 13.10 Treatment of oropharyngeal carcinoma[28]

Radiotherapy	96	Salvage surgery in 13/96
Brachytherapy	2	
Surgery	23	Postoperative radiotherapy in 21/23
Palliative treatment	6	Two died before treatment
Total	127	

Table 13.11 The prognostic significance of performance status in outcome after treatment for oropharyngeal carcinoma[28]

		5-year survival (%)	3-year local recurrence free survival (%)
All patients		40	73
Performance status	0	54	80
	1	23	62
	2	0*	0*
Age		< 55 years	59
		55–64 years	50
		> 65 years	21

*$P < 0.01$.

Radiotherapy

Radiotherapy has been the major treatment modality for the past 80 years, as it is only quite recently that improved reconstructive techniques have made a surgical approach possible. Despite surgical advances there is evidence that primary treatment by radiotherapy gives equal survival rates and a better quality of life than primary surgical treatment, especially in the case of soft palate and base of tongue tumours.[39] Mostly radiotherapy is delivered solely by external beam techniques, but in some centres, especially in France, brachytherapy boosts are used. Because most cases of carcinoma of the oropharynx have in the past been treated by external beam, this disease has been the frequent subject of trials of new approaches in radiotherapy.

External beam radiotherapy

The results of external radiotherapy are best seen in large series from France and the USA, and show small but steady improvement in both local tumour control and survival since the advent of supervoltage therapy. Fletcher and Lindberg[40] reported a 5-year survival of 30% in patients treated at the MD Anderson hospital from 1954 to 1962, whereas Fein et al[41] reported a 5-year survival of 44% in patients treated at the University of Florida from 1964 to

1991, with an improvement in local control in recent years attributed to greater use of hyperfractionation (see below).

There are few reports of results from the UK, reflecting the relative rarity of the disease. A series of 144 patients was treated at the South Wales Radiotherapy Centre from the introduction of supervoltage radiotherapy in 1960 up to 1971.[27] They were treated according to the philosophy of the Christie Hospital in Manchester, namely irradiation of small, localized volumes over a 3-week period without elective nodal irradiation. A series of 127 patients treated at the Royal Marsden Hospital from 1983 to 1991[28] showed some improvement in survival (40% versus 28% at 5 years) and local control (71% versus 57% in radically irradiated patients), attributable to improvements in radiotherapy techniques and supportive care together with the use of elective nodal irradiation; the increase in survival was modest because of the influence of distant metastases and deaths from other causes.

Typical results from large recently reported series of tonsillar and base of tongue carcinomas treated by external beam in USA and France are shown in Tables 13.12 and 13.13. Results of treatment of carcinoma of the soft palate are generally similar to those of the tonsillar carcinoma but all series are relatively small. Carcinoma arising on the posterior wall of the oropharynx is so rare that there are no reliable treatment statistics.

Fractionation

The American College of Radiology 'patterns of fractionation' study reviewed the results of radiotherapy for tonsillar carcinoma in nine centres in UK, the USA and Canada that used different once-per-day fractionation schedules. No significant differences could be found between the widely used 2 Gy per day for 6½–7 weeks, and the 3 or 4 week schedules used at Manchester and Toronto.[44] There does however appear to be an advantage to using hyperfractionation. A regime using twice-daily fractions of 1.2 Gy to a total dose of 74–79 Gy was introduced at the University of Florida in 1978; retrospective comparison with daily fractionation revealed an improvement in local control for all sites and T stages especially the more advanced.[41] A multicentre controlled trial conducted by the EORTC compared 70 Gy given in daily fractions of 2 GY with 80.5 Gy in twice daily fractions of 1.15 Gy, both over the same time of 7 weeks; the hyperfractionated arm gave a significantly higher local control rate with no greater morbidity, but subgroup analysis showed that the advantage was confined to the T3 group.[45]

There is also some evidence of the benefits of accelerated radiotherapy. The CHART regime showed equal local control with reduced late morbidity,[46] while the EORTC trial of an accelerated hyperfractionated split-course regime led to a better local control rate but increased late morbidity.[47] The concomitant boost technique introduced at the MD Anderson Hospital shows promising early results, but which are yet to be confirmed in a randomized trial.[48] The DAHANCA-7 trial compared five against six 2 Gy fractions per week, to the same total dose; six fractions per week gave a higher local control rate, with increased early, but not late, morbidity.[49]

Hypoxia

There is evidence of the oxygen effect in radiotherapy of oropharyngeal carcinoma, as demonstrated by the early trials of irradiation in high pressure oxygen.[50] In the DAHANCA-5 trial of the hypoxic cell sensitizer nimorazole, 414 patients were randomized, of whom 187 had oropharyngeal carcinoma. The nimorazole group had a highly significantly better local control and disease-free rate, but the oropharynx cases were not reported separately.[51] The combination of nimorazole with six fractions per week in the DAHANCA-7 study appears to be the most effective regime yet studied.

Table 13.12 Local control rates for carcinoma of the tonsillar fossa

	No. of patients	T1 (%)	T2 (%)	T3 (%)	T4 (%)
Bataini et al[42] (France)	465	90	84	64	47
Fein et al [41] (USA)	200	87	79	71	44
Henk et al[28] (UK)	52	100	58	76	—

Table 13.13 Two–year actuarial local control rates for external beam radiotherapy of carcinoma of the base of tongue

	No. of patients	T1 (%)	T2 (%)	T3 (%)	T4 (%)
Jaulerry et al[43] (France)	166	96	57	45	23
Fein et al[41] (USA)	107	90	92	76	40
Henk et al[28] (UK)	33	—	78	72	—

Table 13.14 Comparison of local control rates of carcinoma of the base of tongue treated by external beam alone and combined external beam plus implant

Treatment technique	T1 (%)	T2 (%)	T3 (%)	T4 (%)
External beam	37/41 (90)	62/79 (78)	75/95 (79)	20/43 (47)
External beam plus implant	42/48 (88)	88/126 (70)	79/107 (74)	14/20 (70)

From Foote et al.[54]

Brachytherapy

Tumours at all sites in the oropharynx can be treated by interstitial implantation. Brachytherapists nowadays almost invariably use loops of plastic tubing, which are afterloaded with iridium-192 wire. The loops are inserted through either the lateral neck skin in the case of tonsillar and soft palate tumours[52] or the submental region in the case of base of tongue tumours.[53] Brachytherapy is used mainly as a 'boost' after external beam therapy; a course of external radiotherapy to a dose of 50–55 Gy is followed by an implant delivering a further 20–35 Gy.

Implantation of the oropharynx is technically difficult, and therefore applicable only in centres treating a large number of cases where the expertise can be acquired. Some brachytherapists use local anaesthesia, but usually general anaesthesia and often tracheostomy is needed. Severe haemorrhage is not uncommon. Although high local control rates have been reported using brachytherapy, Foote et al[54] comparing the results in six reports of combined external beam and brachytherapy with those of external beam alone at MD Anderson Hospital and the University of Florida (Table 13.14) concluded that both local control and morbidity were similar with the two methods, and that brachytherapy was not justified. For these reasons we rarely use brachytherapy, except occasionally for a second primary tumour in a patient who has already received radiotherapy.

Typical results of brachytherapy boosts are shown in Tables 13.15 and 13.16.

Nodal irradiation

In view of the high incidence of occult metastases in the clinically negative neck elective nodal irradiation is widely advocated. In any case the first echelon lymph nodes are in the path of the radiation beams with most radiotherapeutic techniques. Tumours of the base of tongue, soft palate and posterior wall are treated with lateral opposing beams, and the first echelon nodes (levels II and III) bilaterally are included. Well-lateralized T1–2N0 tonsillar carcinomas rarely give rise to contralateral nodal metastases, so irradiation can be limited to the primary tumour and homolateral nodes with consequent reduction of subsequent xerostomia.[57] Node-positive cases often have widespread subclinical nodal involvement, so elective irradiation of all node areas bilaterally is advisable.[58]

In node-positive cases in which the primary tumour is treated by radiotherapy alone, the management of the neck is controversial. Undifferentiated carcinoma, especially of the nasopharyngeal type,[59] is very radiosensitive and local control rates by radiotherapy are high so that

Table 13.15 Results of combined external beam and brachytherapy for carcinoma of the base of tongue

	No. of patients	2-year local control (%)	5-year survival (%)
Harrison et al[53]	36	87.5	87.5
Crook et al[55]	48	75	50
Puthawala et al[56]	70	83	33

Table 13.16 Local control rates of tonsillar fossa carcinoma by combined external beam and brachytherapy

No. of patients	T1 (%)	T2 (%)	T3 (%)
277	89	86	67

From Pernot et al.[52]

neck dissection is unnecessary. For other types of squamous carcinoma many authorities recommend neck dissection, either before or after radiotherapy to the primary. However, size for size primary tumours and nodal metastases in the same patient tend to be equally radiosensitive,[60] and radiotherapy failures at the primary site are as difficult to salvage surgically as nodal recurrences, in contrast to other head and neck sites such as the supraglottis. Therefore, in patients with small nodal metastases that become impalpable after radiotherapy there may be little or no gain from planned neck dissection. Peters et al reported only three isolated neck failures in a series of 62 node-positive patients managed by radiotherapy without planned neck dissection.[61]

Postoperative radiotherapy

The indications for postoperative radiotherapy are the same as for other head and neck sites, namely large or infiltrating primary tumours, close or positive resection margins, multiple nodal involvement or extracapsular spread from a nodal metastasis. We give 60 Gy to the primary site and involved nodal areas, or 66 Gy to areas where gross residual tumour is suspected. Where there is unilateral nodal involvement the opposite side of the neck is irradiated electively to a dose of 50 Gy.

Surgical management

Transoral excision

Early tumours of the tonsil, faucial arches and the soft palate may be adequately excised per orally. The resultant defect may be closed primarily, skin grafted or left to epithelialize. Larger tumours requiring bony resection, and more posteriorly located tumours require more extensive access and every effort must be made to carry out the surgical excision under direct vision. Selected, superficial early lesions, especially those involving the soft palate or posterior pharyngeal wall, may be resected using a transoral endoscopic laser[62] combined with discontinuous neck dissection as indicated.[63]

Transhyoid pharyngotomy

This is a useful approach to small tumours of the base of the tongue even in the presence of limited involvement of the supraglottic larynx. The hyoid bone is transected or excised and the vallecula is entered blindly (Figure 13.14). After resection of the tumour inferiorly from the neck, the resultant defect is closed primarily. Access is limited and the technique must be used only in very selected patients to excise small lesions. Great care must be exercised to avoid damaging the lingual artery and the hypoglossal nerve if any tongue remnant is preserved on the side of the lesion. The advantage of this technique is that it maintains the integrity of the mandible and preserves the mobility of the tongue by preventing scarring in the anterior oral cavity.[64] Larger tumours of the tonsil and base of the tongue may be excised using a combination of the transoral and transhyoid approaches.[65]

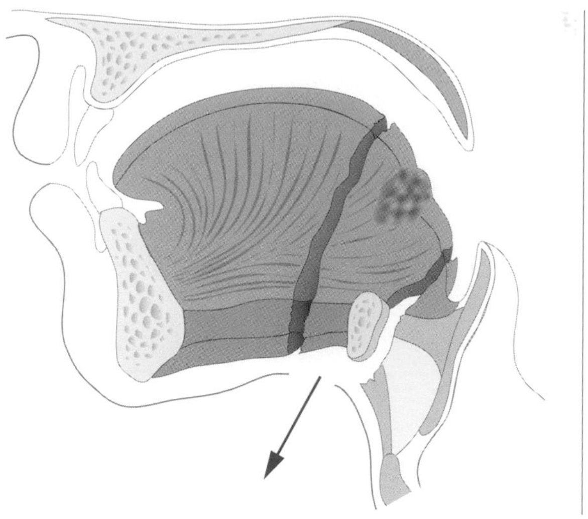

Figure 13.14 Transhyoid pharyngotomy.

Lateral pharyngotomy

Small lesions of the posterior and lateral pharyngeal walls may be excised through a lateral pharyngotomy. The mucosa of the pyriform sinus is stripped off the medial surface of the thyroid ala which is retracted anteriorly. The superior laryngeal nerve is carefully preserved and the pyriform sinus is entered in its superior aspect to gain access to the oropharynx. The superior extent of the mucosal incision is limited by the mandible, and this approach can be safely used in only selected instances.

Anterior midline glossotomy

The rare small, locally limited lesions of the base of the tongue may be resected via this approach. The tongue is bisected anteriorly in its relatively avascular midline to access the region of the base (Figure 13.15). After adequate resection of the tumour, the defect is closed primarily and the bisected halves of the anterior tongue are sutured back in layers. While the functional outcome of this operation is excellent, it must be stressed that only very small lesions in selected patients are suitable. Larger tumours cannot be adequately excised without creating a substantial soft tissue defect with a tongue remnant of doubtful viability, and one of the other more extensive approaches must be used in these patients.

Table 13.17 Features of the three types of mandibular osteotomy

	Lateral	Median	Paramedian
Site of osteotomy	Body or angle of mandible	Midline	Between lateral incisor and canine
Exposure	Limited	Good	Good
Dental extraction	May be required	One central incisor	Not required
Inferior alveolar nerve and vessels	Have to be transected	Spared	Spared
Division of genial muscles	Not required	Inevitable	Not required. Only the mylohyoid needs division
Mechanical stability	Poor because of unequal pull of muscles on the two mandibular segments	Good	Good
Fixation of osteotomy	May require intermaxillary fixation	Compression miniplates or stainless steel wire	Compression miniplates or stainless steel wire
Postoperative radiation therapy	Osteotomy lies within the lateral portal. Increased risk of complications	Lies outside the lateral portal. Safe	Lies outside the lateral portal. Safe

Mandibulotomy and mandibular swing

A mandibulotomy approach with paralingual extension, the so-called 'mandibular swing' has been used effectively for resection of advanced tumours of the oropharynx.[66] The extent of exposure and the functional consequences of the procedure depend a great deal on the site of the mandibular osteotomy. Three types of mandibulotomy have been described and the relative advantages and disadvantages of each have been outlined in Table 13.17.

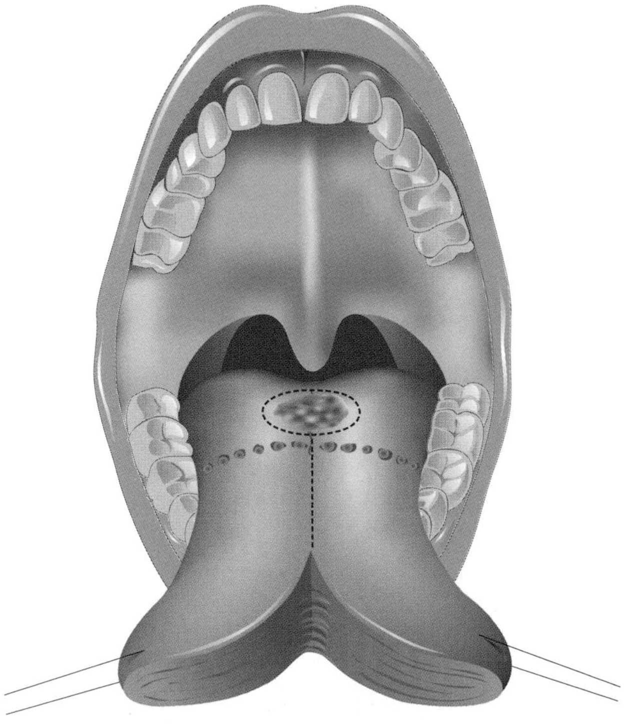

Figure 13.15 Anterior midline glossotomy may be used to approach selected, small lesions of the base of the tongue.

The paramedian mandibulotomy is designed to be anatomically less disruptive and results in lesser functional deficit postoperatively. It is also inherently more stable mechanically than a lateral osteotomy, and if radiation therapy becomes necessary, lies outside the limit of the lateral portal. These features along with the disadvantages of median (Figure 13.16) and lateral mandibulotomy make the paramedian mandibulotomy the procedure of choice in access to the oropharynx (Tables 13.18 and 13.19).

The lower lip is split, with a vermillion notch, in the midline. The gingivolabial sulcus is incised towards the side of the osteotomy leaving an adequate mucosal cuff to facilitate subsequent closure. The mandible is exposed by raising short cheek flaps bilaterally, dissecting in the plane above the periosteum and taking care to limit dissection to the point where the mental nerve exits the mental foramen. For a paramedian mandibulotomy, the osteotomy is sited between the lateral incisor and canine teeth. This is a natural area where the roots curve away from each other, and are at minimal risk of direct injury. There is considerable debate in the literature about the shape of the osteotomy; notched (Figure

Table 13.18 Disadvantages of lateral mandibulotomy

- Provides limited exposure
- Inferior alveolar nerve has to be transected leading to denervation of all teeth distal to the osteotomy and the skin in the mental area
- Causes interruption of endosteal supply to the mandibular segment and distal teeth
- Unequal muscular pull on the mandibular segments causes stress at the site of osteotomy and this may necessitate intermaxillary fixation, which may interfere with postoperative oral hygiene
- The mandibulotomy site lies directly within the lateral portal of radiation: may delay bony healing in radiated mandibles, and increase the risk of osteoradionecrosis if followed by postoperative radiation.

Table 13.19 Disadvantages of median mandibulotomy

- Requires extraction of one central incisor
- Division of the geniohyoid and genioglossus muscles, which arise from the genial tubercle interferes with normal mastication and swallowing

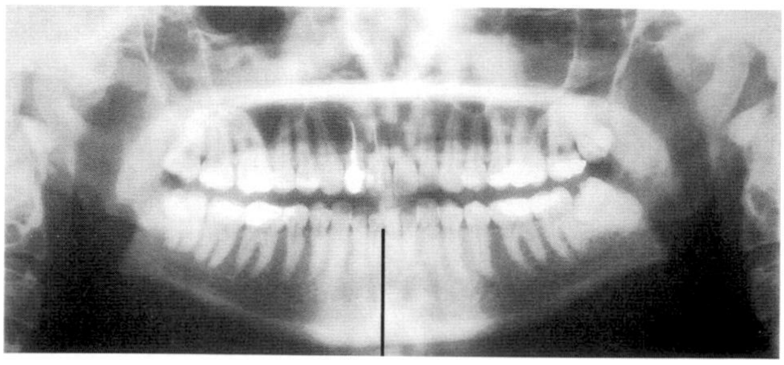

Figure 13.16 A median osteotomy.

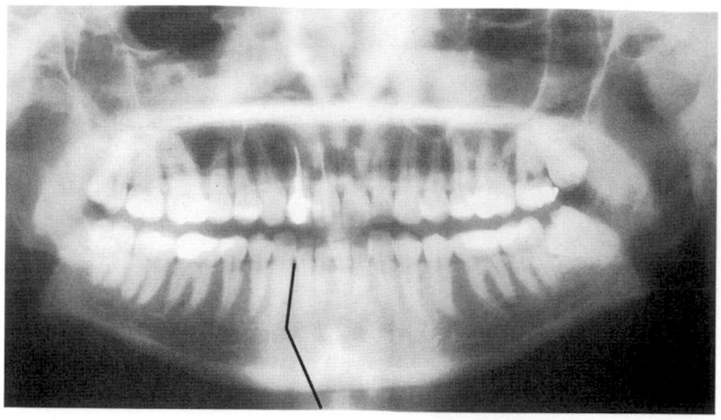

Figure 13.17 The notched paramedian osteotomy.

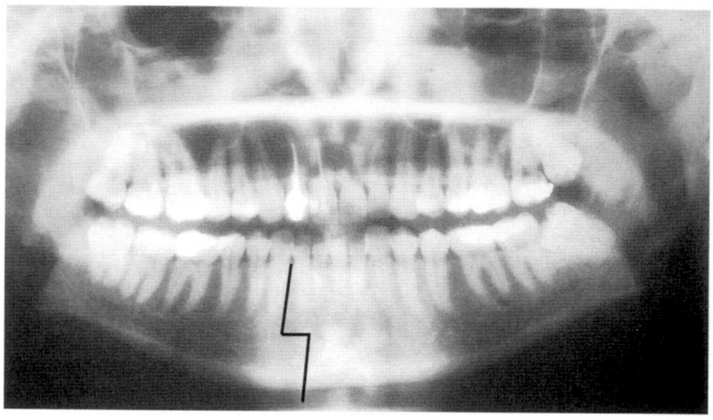

Figure 13.18 The horizontal cut of the step paramedian osteotomy must be carefully sited to avoid damaging the roots and at the same time must leave a reasonable thickness of bone on the inferior segment.

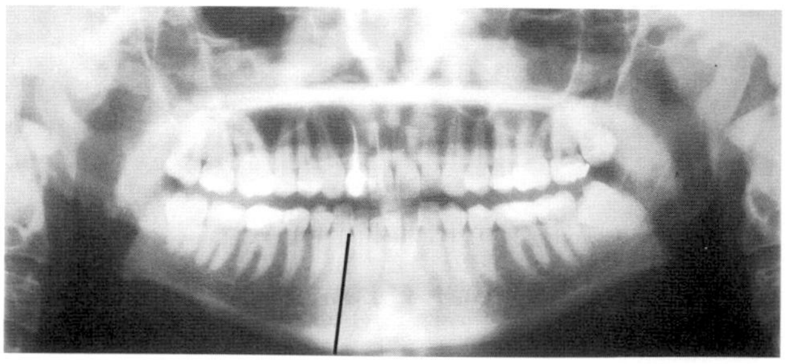

Figure 13.19 The straight paramedian osteotomy.

13.17) or step (Figure 13.18) osteotomies tend to be preferred over a straight one (Figure 13.19) because of their mechanical stability. Both these osteotomies are technically more demanding and the mandible is more liable to fracture if the horizontal cut of the stair-step is sited too close to the inferior border of the bone. An oscillating power saw with the appropriate attachments is essential for accurate bony cuts. The mucosa and muscles of the floor of the mouth are now incised posteriorly right up to the anterior pillar of the soft palate, and this requires transection of the lingual nerve and the styloglossus muscle which cross the field. The mandible can then be swung out laterally to expose the oropharynx (Figure 13.20).

Opinions regarding the type of fixation after mandibulotomy are divided, but no difference in stability and healing has been reported using either stainless steel wires or compression miniplates.[67] We prefer to use miniplates, and prelocalization of the plates across the osteotomy before the cuts are

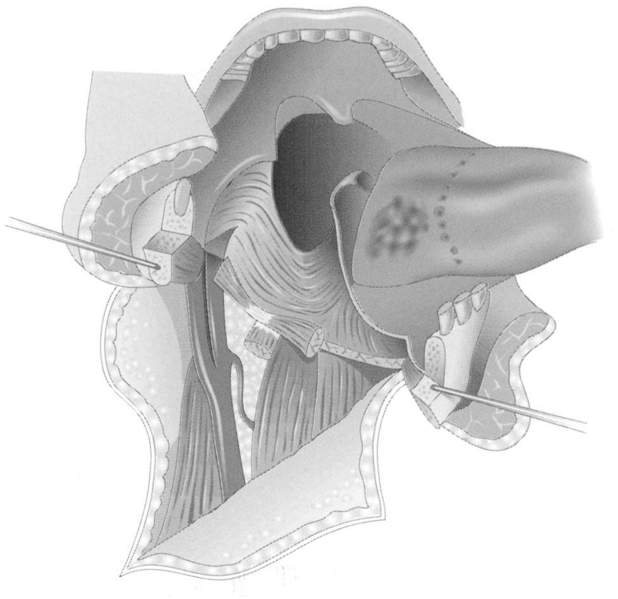

Figure 13.20 When the incision of the floor of the mouth is completed, the mandible can be swung out laterally to expose the tumour in the oropharynx.

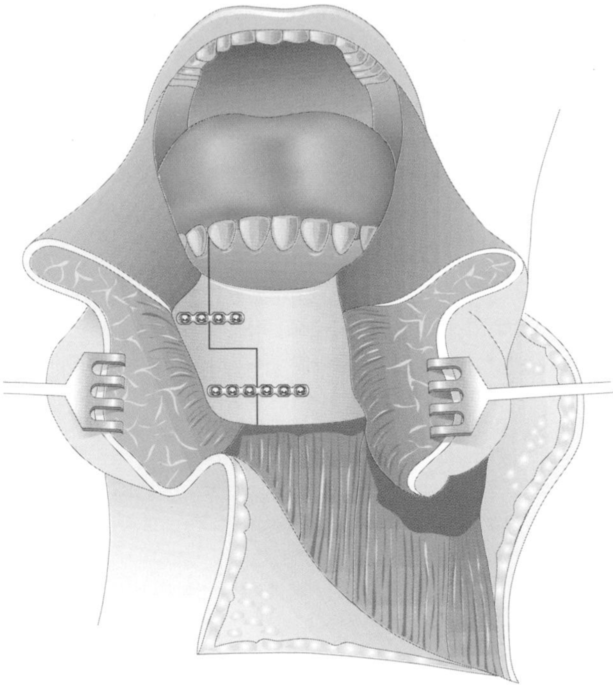

Figure 13.21 Miniplates are used to approximate the two halves of the mandible at the end of the procedure.

actually made allows accurate approximation at the end of the procedure. Two plates are used across the osteotomy on the anterior surface (Figure 13.21).

There are conflicting reports in the literature about the incidence of non-union and osteoradionecrosis after mandibulotomy in irradiated patients.[68,69] We prefer to avoid splitting the mandible in irradiated patients and rely on other approaches such as the floor of mouth, transhyoid or lateral pharyngotomy in these patients.

Floor of mouth (lingual-releasing) approach

This is an alternative to the more extensive mandibulotomy approach. It avoids splitting the mandible, especially in patients who have had previous irradiation and are at risk of non-union or osteoradionecrosis.

It is usually combined with neck dissection, and the superior laryngeal nerve is carefully dissected and preserved. The glossopharyngeal and lingual nerves are then dissected and preserved if a partial glossectomy is planned and part of the ipsilateral anterior tongue is to be preserved. Once the two nerves have been displaced downwards, the muscles of the floor of mouth are ready for incision. The hyoid bone may have to be resected depending upon the extent of the disease. The mucosa of the floor of the mouth is then incised, leaving an adequate cuff on the alveolus (Figure 13.22). The muscles of the floor of the mouth are divided and branches of the lingual artery need

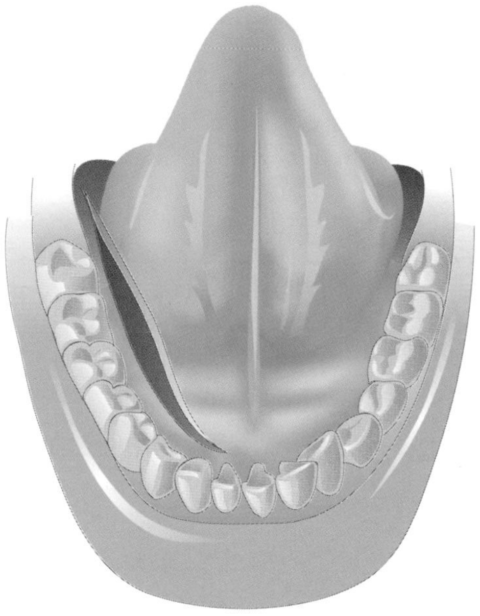

Figure 13.22 Incision of the mucosa of the floor of the mouth: leaving an adequate cuff on the alveolus facilitates subsequent closure.

ligation. The lingual nerve is divided posteriorly in the lateral floor of the mouth, and the tongue can then be drawn downwards into the neck. Lesions requiring partial excision of the tongue can often be excised by combining peroral excision with the floor of mouth approach. If a total glossectomy is planned, the opposite submandibular triangle is also dissected and the floor of the mouth is incised all around the tongue. When the incision of the floor of mouth is complete, the tongue can be pulled through into the neck and the tumour excised under direct vision. We have found this approach very useful, especially in patients who have had previous irradiation. The surgical defect after total glossectomy (Figure 13.23) is reconstructed using a free latissimus dorsi flap (Figure 13.24) as it results in excellent vertical movement and thus provides far better functional mobility and velopharyngeal closure for swallowing and speech than a tethered pedicled myocutaneous or cutaneous flap. Although the surgical access using this approach is good, suturing in a myocutaneous flap may not always be easy. A useful technique in closure is to place all the sutures approximating the inferior tip of the flap to the mucosa of the inferior edge of the defect, and then tying them transorally. The rest of the flap can be sutured in quite easily through the open mouth.

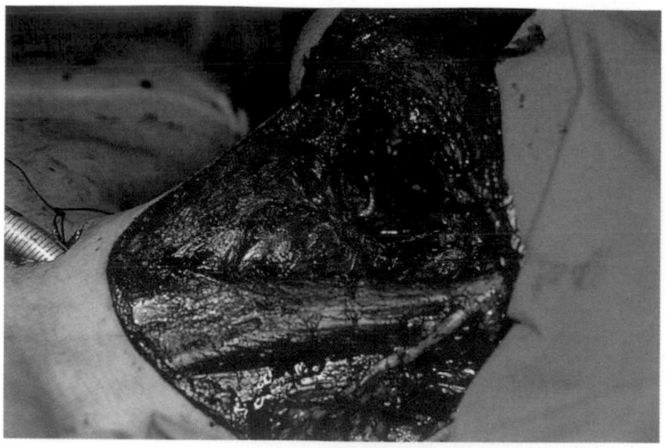

Figure 13.23 The surgical defect after total glossectomy using the floor of mouth lingual-releasing approach.

Resection of soft tissue

Resection of the tumour along with an adequate cuff of normal surrounding tissue forms the basis of good oncologic surgery. Nowhere is this principle more difficult to follow than in the base of the tongue, mainly because of the difficulty in judging the extent of the tumour through the nodular surface of the organ. The tumour must be carefully palpated to ensure adequate margins as excision proceeds but frozen section evaluation of the margins and the base of excision can minimize the chances of incomplete resection. Partial glossectomy may be oncologically adequate for limited tumours of the base of the tongue, but the anterior tongue can be salvaged only if the hypoglossal nerve and the blood supply via the lingual artery can be preserved on one side. Although a total glossectomy is a formidable procedure, it may be the only hope for survival in patients with locally advanced base of tongue tumours. Most patients requiring major glossectomy have conventionally been subjected to a total laryngectomy, either as a concomitant or subsequent procedure to prevent chronic aspiration.[70] The functional results after glossectomy are as greatly influenced by the volume of tongue lost as by the mobility, sensitivity and the shape of the tongue remnant. Significant advances in reconstructive surgery, prosthetics and speech therapy have, however, greatly contributed in reducing the incidence of prophylactic total laryngectomy in patients with good performance status.[71] Locally advanced tumours of the base of tongue involving adjacent sites require extended resections such as pharyngoglossectomy with complex reconstruction.

The salient technical aspects of excision of particular tumours within the oropharynx have been discussed under the relevant subsites.

(a)

(b)

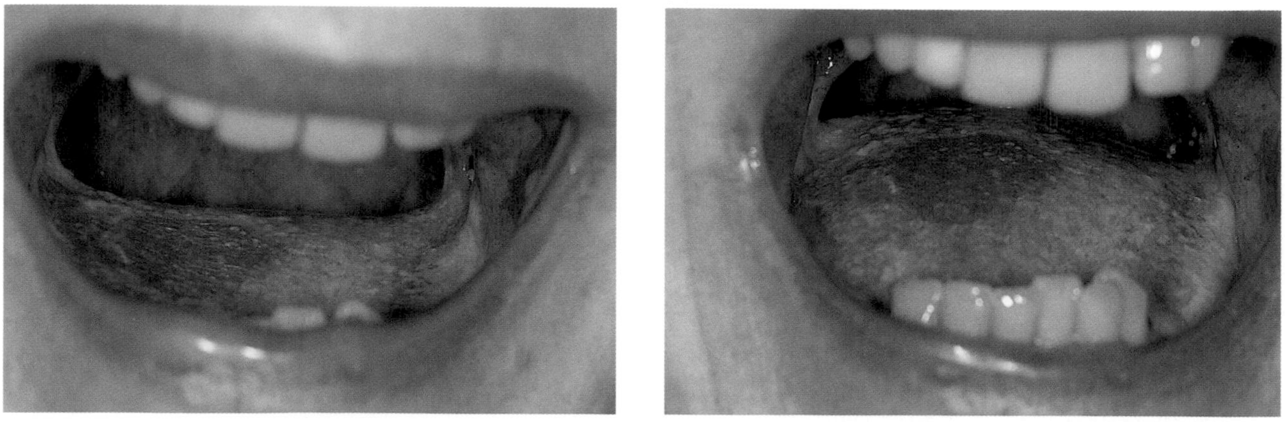

Figure 13.24 Free latissimus dorsi flap for reconstruction following total glossectomy showing excellent vertical movement that provides far better functional mobility and velopharyngeal closure for swallowing and speech than a tethered pedicled myocutaneous or cutaneous flap. (a) At rest; (b) on laryngeal elevation.

Management of the neck

As with other sites within the head and neck, the management of the clinically negative neck depends on the risk of occult metastases. Early lesions of the soft palate and the posterior pharyngeal wall are at low risk and the clinically negative neck in these patients may be safely observed. In all other patients, elective treatment of the N0 neck must be considered. The type of treatment of the N0 neck depends largely upon the mode of treatment of the primary; if the primary is treated with radiation therapy, the neck is included in the fields and if surgery is chosen for the primary, treatment of the neck is guided by the principles outlined in Figure 13.25. The uninvolved neck in well-lateralized lesions of the tonsil and tongue may be treated unilaterally but both sides need treatment in lesions approaching or involving the midline.

The histology of the primary tumour obviously plays an important role in deciding treatment of positive neck nodes; undifferentiated carcinoma of the nasopharyngeal type (UCNT) and lymphomas are radiosensitive and do not require primary surgery. For all other well-lateralized primary lesions with an N+ neck, surgical treatment must include a comprehensive neck dissection including all five levels. A modified radical neck dissection is the procedure of choice, preserving as many normal structures as possible to minimize the postoperative functional deficit. A radical neck dissection should be necessary only if the relevant structures are directly infiltrated by nodal disease. Bilaterally involved nodes can be treated with simultaneous bilateral neck dissection. The side with more advanced neck disease is dissected first aiming to preserve the internal jugular vein. At least one internal jugular vein must be preserved to minimize postoperative complications such as raised intracranial tension and oedema. Preservation of the external jugular veins may help venous drainage and reduce oedema of the skin flaps postoperatively. Postoperative radiation therapy is given for the usual indications, either due to adverse features of the primary or the neck nodes.

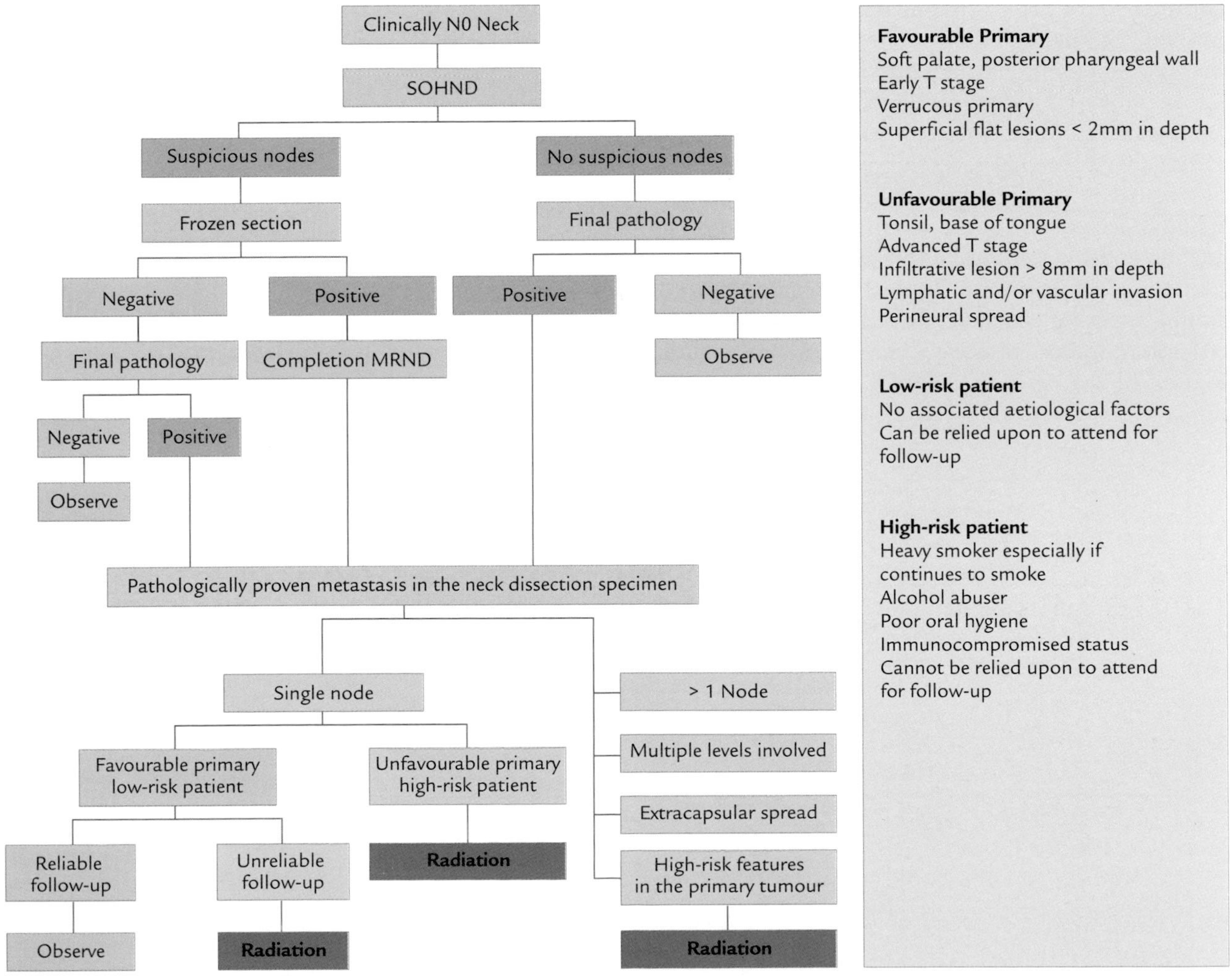

Figure 13.25 Algorithm for the surgical management of the clinically negative neck in patients with oropharyngeal carcinoma.

When the tumour is being treated with radical radiotherapy alone, a planned postradiotherapy neck dissection may be necessary for patients who have greater than N1 disease in the neck. Histopathological examination of the residual nodal tissue in such patients fails to demonstrate viable tumour in almost two-thirds of patients.[72] We have recently modified our approach to local excision and frozen section analysis of the residual node, followed by neck dissection only if viable tumour cells are demonstrated.

Around 50% of patients with stage III and IV oropharyngeal carcinoma have involvement of the retropharyngeal nodes.[73] Routine surgical procedures do not dissect these nodes but virtually all of these patients with locoregionally advanced disease require postoperative radiation therapy, and the retropharyngeal area can be easily included in the fields. One of the advantages in treating the clinically negative neck with primary radiation therapy is that this policy includes the retropharyngeal nodes which are not usually included in neck dissection.

Management of mandibular involvement

Invasion of the mandible is less common in oropharyngeal carcinoma as compared to oral cancer, but as with oral tumours, there is a high degree of correlation between clinical and histopathological findings.[74] Segmental resection of the mandible may be required in locally advanced oropharyngeal tumours, especially of the tonsil. Excellent access to all sites within the oropharynx can be obtained using a mandibulotomy, and the uninvolved mandible should never be resected solely to gain access to the tumour. Marginal resection of the ascending ramus (Figure 13.26) or inner table 'rim resection' of the mandible (Figure 13.27) may be carried out to obtain deep clearance in tumours of the tonsil or tongue base that abut against the periosteum of the body or ramus of the mandible.

Management of the airway and the larynx

Oropharyngeal tumours, by virtue of their location, can cause great difficulty in endotracheal intubation. This problem is compounded if the patient has trismus secondary to invasion of the pterygoid muscles. Fibreoptic endoscope-guided endotracheal intubation is an option, but in most instances it may be safer to perform a preliminary tracheostomy under local anaesthetic. The temporary tracheostomy may then be used to protect the airway in the postoperative period, especially in patients who have had a total glossectomy with flap reconstruction. Decannulation of the tracheostomy depends on a combination of factors including the efficacy of deglutition, the extent of aspiration and the performance status of the patient.

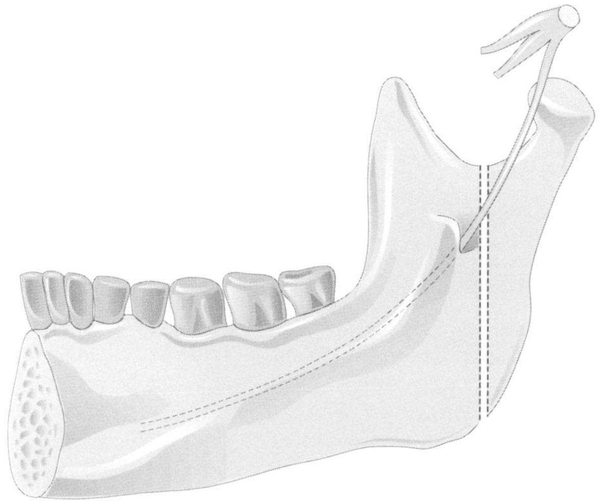

Figure 13.26 Marginal resection of the ascending ramus of the mandible for a posterior tonsullar tumour.

(a)

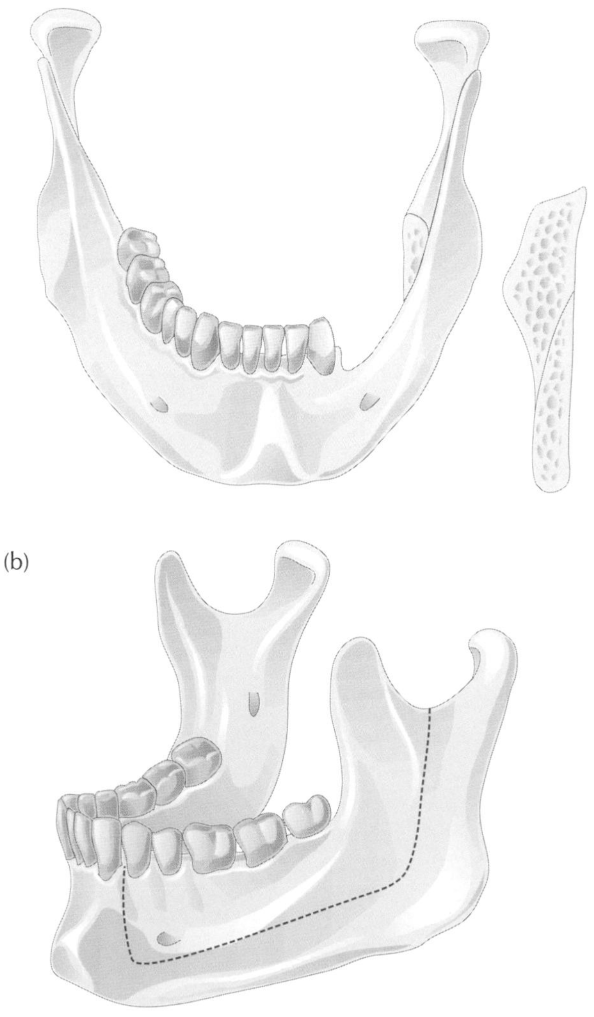

(b)

Figure 13.27 'Rim resection' of the mandible. (a) Inner cortical plate; (b) extended alveolar.

In selected patients who have had a limited excision of the base of the tongue with free radial forearm flap reconstruction, we have been able to avoid a tracheostomy by maintaining the patient on endotracheal tube ventilation overnight. The patient is extubated on the high dependency unit after endoscopic evaluation of the tongue and the flap by the surgeon and the anaesthetist. It is necessary to emphasize that this approach is used in very selected instances and requires a great deal of experience and judgement. It is always safer to perform a tracheostomy if there is any doubt whatsoever about the adequacy of the airway.

Tumours of the base of the tongue may break through the hyoepiglottic ligament and invade the pre-epiglottic space, or even the framework of the larynx. Depending upon the extent of involvement of the larynx, surgical excision of such lesions requires excision of the base of the tongue to be combined with either partial supraglottic or total laryngectomy. As a general rule, the performance status of the patient is a major factor when choosing between a partial and total laryngectomy; poor-risk patients will benefit from a total laryngectomy even when a supraglottic laryngectomy is technically feasible.

Reconstruction

Major soft tissue defects of the oropharynx can be broadly divided into those that require thin, pliable flaps for resurfacing and those that need bulkier myocutaneous flaps to provide volume. The posterior pharyngeal wall is an area that is best resurfaced using either a split skin graft or a free radial forearm flap. Substantial defects of the base of the tongue, tonsillar and lateral pharyngeal walls need reconstruction with myocutaneous flaps such as the pectoralis major or the latissimus dorsi pedicled flaps. While it is tempting to attempt primary closure of small defects of the base of the tongue, the best functional results are obtained by adequately replacing the volume of tongue lost and an appropriately planned myocutaneous flap should be used to provide adequate bulk and shape to the tongue remnant. Partial circumference defects of the pharynx are reconstructed using pedicled myocutaneous flaps while circumferential defects are best restored by a gastric pull-up or microvascular jejunal transfer. Mandibular continuity may be restored after segmental resection and these issues are discussed elsewhere in this book as are the individual reconstruction techniques.

Ancillary procedures such as laryngeal suspension and palatal augmentation may help improve functional results after major glossectomy.[71] Swallowing after a total glossectomy suffers from a lack of the 'oral phase' of swallowing. The 'oral hold' phase is lost and the bolus passes immediately to the oropharynx and then directly to the hypopharynx aided only by gravity. As a result, the material tends to pool in the pyriform sinuses and spills over into the larynx causing aspiration. A cricopharyngeal myotomy facilitates the passage of the bolus into the oesophagus and prevents the 'pharyngeal hold' phase of the swallowing sequence in glossectomized patients.

Role of tube feeding

Most patients with dysphagia and weight loss will have been on tube feeds preoperatively and this must be continued into the postoperative period. Percutaneous endoscopic gastrostomy must be considered at the time of the operation if tube feeding is anticipated for more than 10 days postoperatively, for example in patients who have had major glossectomy and reconstruction, and in those who have been planned for postoperative radiation therapy.

Salvage surgery and management of recurrences

Surgical salvage of recurrent tumours after radiation therapy is difficult because fibrosis makes palpation of the extent of the tumour inaccurate, and frozen section control of margins is extremely useful in this situation. Meticulous sharp dissection, avoidance of excessive diathermy charring and careful haemostasis contribute to minimizing postoperative complications with healing. Patients who have required partial or total pharyngeal reconstruction commence feeds on around the tenth postoperative day. Early detection of recurrence after surgery, especially in the presence of a flap is extremely difficult. A high index of suspicion based on symptoms such as localized pain is vital to timely diagnosis. The recurrence commonly involves the undersurface of the flap or the suture line, and although conventional imaging using CT or MR may aid detection,[75] a PET scan appears to be the most useful investigation in this setting available currently.[76]

Site-specific presentation, treatment and results

Carcinoma of the base of the tongue

Tumours of the base of the tongue are diagnosed late and as many as three-quarters of patients present with stage III or IV disease.[77] In addition, these tumours tend to infiltrate diffusely into the surrounding tissues and regional nodal metastases are more common. Consequently, treatment is difficult and the outcome, both in terms of function and survival, is poor.

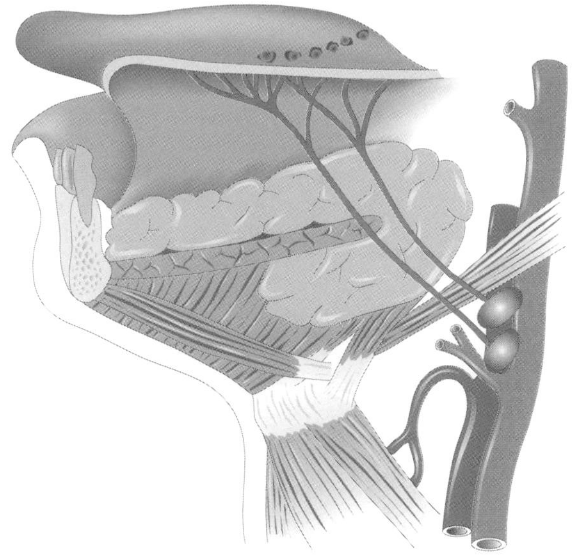

Figure 13.28 The base of the tongue drains lymph directly to level II nodes.

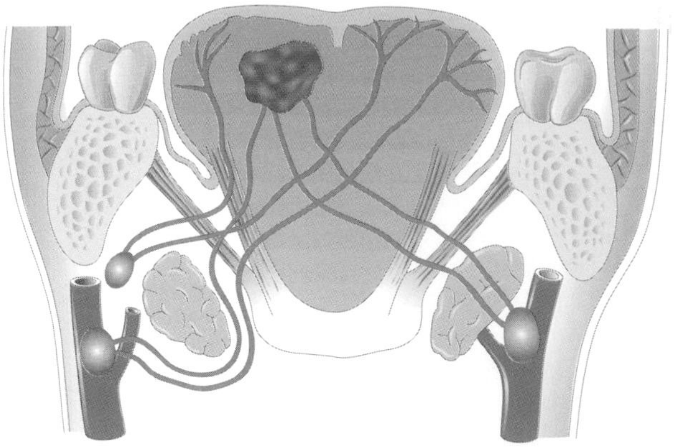

Figure 13.29 Cross-over lymphatics result in a high percentage of bilateral cervical nodal metastases.

Lymph node metastases

The most commonly involved nodes are those at levels II and III, but level IV is more commonly involved than oral cavity tumours (Figure 13.28). Bilateral lymphatic spread (Figure 13.29) occurs in approximately a third of patients and the risk of nodal metastasis progressively increases from 70% for T1 to 85% for T4 lesions.[29] As most tumours are treated with radiation therapy and do not undergo elective neck dissection, the actual risk of occult nodal metastases may be much higher than the reported figure of around 20%.

Treatment of early disease

Surgery and radiation therapy give equivalent results in the treatment of early lesions of the base of the tongue. Radiation therapy is generally favoured because it causes lesser functional deficit. In view of the high propensity of these lesions to metastasize to the lymph nodes, elective treatment of the clinically negative neck is an integral part of the treatment. Dissection of the neck is recommended in patients who present with clinically involved nodes.

Early lesions can be approached either transorally, by a lateral pharyngotomy or through a combination of transoral and transhyoid approaches. Adequate resection of small unilateral lesions usually results in a defect that can be reconstructed with good functional outcome using a free radial forearm flap.

Treatment of advanced disease

Radiation therapy may be used to treat most T3 lesions in combination with neck dissection for palpable nodes. In view of the diffuse infiltration associated with advanced lesions, surgical resection results in positive margins in about a quarter of the cases.[78] Radiation therapy is generally offered to patients with negative necks but salvage neck dissection can be performed in patients who have residual neck disease after a course of radical radiation. Alternatively, a neck dissection can be carried out at the same time as the implants when the primary tumour is treated with brachytherapy.

Some form of laryngeal resection may be required in locally advanced tumours of the base of the tongue as the hyoepiglottic ligament provides only a flimsy barrier to the pre-epiglottic space (Figure 13.30). Smaller lesions of the vallecula, which do not extend along the pharyngoepiglottic fold to involve the lateral pharyngeal wall, may be adequately encompassed by an extended supraglottic laryngectomy. The major problem of combining glossectomy with laryngeal resection is the impairment of normal

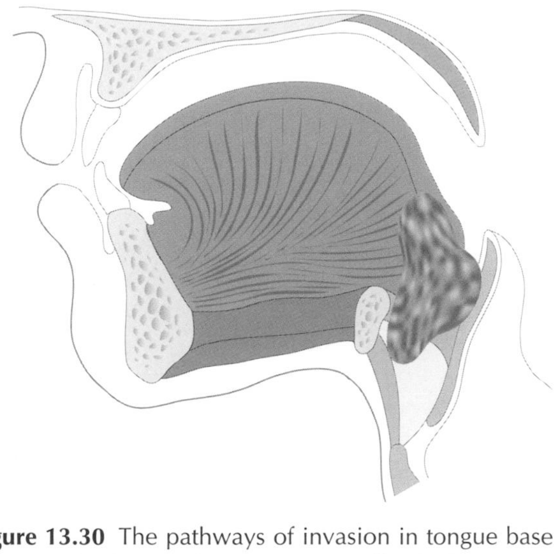

Figure 13.30 The pathways of invasion in tongue base tumours: the hyoepiglottic ligament offers little resistance to spread into the pre-epiglottic space.

Table 13.20 The functional results of surgical treatment of base of tongue tumours

Reference (No. of patients)	Survival	Total glossectomy	Mandibular resection (%)	Impaired swallowing (%)	'Useful' speech (%)	Severe aspiration (%)	Concomitant/interval laryngectomy (%)
Weber et al[78] (27)	51% at 2 years	27	?	56	92	11	0/8
Ruhl et al[80] (54)	41% at 5 years	54	?	?	?	?	?
Razack et al[81] (45)	20% at 5 years	45	49	69	84	37	40/13
Gehanno et al[82] (80)	65% at 1 year	80	?	49	39	?	?
Kraus et al[83] (100)	65% at 5 years	?	14	?	?	?	20

deglutition that results in chronic postoperative aspiration and pulmonary infection. The performance status of the patient must be taken into account when planning such a procedure and a total laryngectomy may often be the only surgical option available to protect the airway. Induction chemotherapy with radiation therapy may be tried in appropriate patients in an effort to preserve the larynx, keeping the option of surgery for salvage of failures.

Results of treatment

The results of treatment using radiation therapy have been discussed previously. Early lesions of the base of the tongue can be controlled using surgery in approximately 85% of cases. As in many other upper aerodigestive tract tumours, the morphology of the tumour is a major determinant of outcome: exophytic tumours do much better than infiltrative, endophytic tumour. A retrospective functional evaluation has confirmed that radiation therapy provides a better posttreatment performance status than surgery for both early as well as advanced tumours.[79] There are, however, no prospective randomized trials in literature comparing the oncologic and functional results of surgery alone with either radiation alone or combined treatment. The functional results of surgical treatment of base of tongue tumours as reported in the literature are listed in Table 13.20. Any attempt at comparison of these results is meaningless, as most reports are based on subjective evaluations, and the ones that have used objective parameters cannot be compared because of a lack of standardization.

Although most centres use a combined modality treatment policy when indicated, the results of surgery alone in the treatment of base of tongue tumours have been reported from the Mayo Clinic.[84] A total of 55 patients, almost 75% with stage III or IV tumours, underwent complete surgical excision without pre- or postoperative chemotherapy or irradiation. Failure in the neck (44%) was the main cause of treatment failure with local recurrence in 22% and distant metastases in 13%. Surgical mortality was 4% and the cause-specific survival at 5 years was 65%. The stage-wise survival has been listed in Table 13.21. Not surprisingly, the authors have concluded that patients with advanced neck disease should be considered for adjuvant radiotherapy.

Table 13.21 Survival rates in patients treated for carcinoma of the base of the tongue

Reference	Follow-up (years)	Stage I (%)	Stage II (%)	Stage III (%)	Stage IV (%)
Thawley et al[85]	5	50	44	45	28
Weber et al[78]	5	100	72	50	30
Barrs et al[86]	3	68	55	55	11
Kraus et al[83]	5	77	77	64	59
Foote et al[84]	5	60	48	76	20–35*

*Tumours were staged based on the American Joint Committee on Cancer, 1988 recommendations.

The survival rates for cancer of the base of tongue do not vary much between stages I and III but stage IV patients have a generally poor outcome (Table 13.21).

Carcinoma of the tonsil

Tumours of the tonsillar pillar tend to be more superficial than those of the tonsillar fossa which tend to present as bulky tumours. As they progress, these tumours spread to involve the adjacent structures. Tonsillar tumours present in stage III or IV in as many as 75% cases, mainly because symptoms like pain and dysphagia occur relatively late. Other symptoms include mass in the neck, weight loss, and if the pterygoid muscles are involved, trismus (Figure 13.31). Lesions originating at the inferior pole of the tonsil may be visible only on endoscopic examination, and thorough bimanual palpation is necessary to establish their extent.

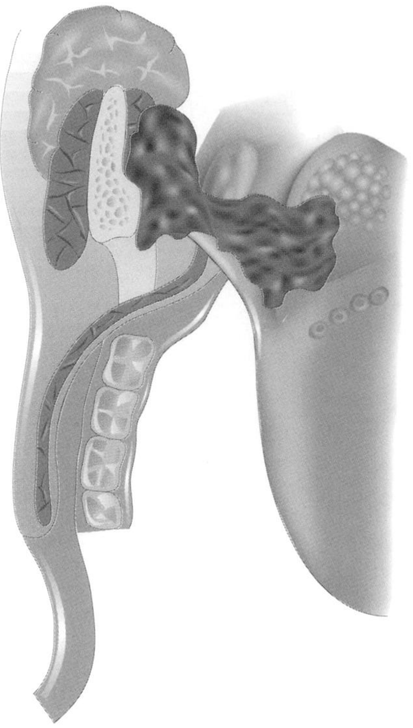

Figure 13.31 Trismus is an ominous clinical sign caused by invasion of tonsillar tumours into the pterygoid muscles.

Lymph node metastases

Lymphatics from the tonsillar region drain into the jugulodigastric nodes and also into the nodes of the submandibular and upper posterior triangles. Tumours involving the tonsillar pillars present with lymph node involvement less frequently (38% of T2 lesions) as compared to tonsillar fossa tumours (68% of T2 lesions). Likewise, contralateral metastases are commoner with tonsillar fossa tumours and about 55% of patients present with advanced stage (N2–3) neck disease.[29] Lesions of the posterior tonsillar pillar are more prone to metastasize to the spinal accessory and upper posterior triangle nodes.

Treatment of early lesions

Early lesions of the tonsillar region can be treated using a single-modality approach. If surgery is chosen as an option, transoral resection is generally possible and every effort must be undertaken to ensure adequate margins. In patients with limited mouth opening one of the other approaches described previously, such as lateral pharyngotomy or mandibulotomy, is to be preferred. Tumours abutting against the periosteum of the mandible may need marginal resection including the coronoid process (Figure 13.26). A neck dissection is an integral part of treatment, even for patients with a clinically negative neck in view of the high risk of lymph node metastasis.

An early, asymptomatic lesion arising deep within a tonsillar crypt may present with a metastatic neck node, the so-called 'unknown primary'. Optimal management of these patients must include a meticulous endoscopic evaluation of the entire upper aerodigestive tract, and if no lesion is obvious, an ipsilateral tonsillectomy is the only reliable method to detect a small, tonsillar crypt primary.

Equivalent results can be obtained using radiation therapy alone for the treatment of early tonsillar tumours.[87] It offers excellent cure rates with a potentially better functional outcome. As with surgical management, elective treatment of the negative neck must be undertaken and it is usually possible to avoid irradiating the contralateral neck for well-lateralized lesions.

Treatment of advanced lesions

Surgery combined with postoperative radiation therapy has been conventionally used in the treatment of advanced lesions but radiation alone for the primary combined with neck dissection for involved nodes has been reported.[88] A policy of radiation alone needs to be very selective as it has been shown that endophytic T3–4 lesions do not respond well to radiation and are best managed by surgery and postoperative radiation. Exophytic T3 lesions, on the other hand, can be managed by external beam radiation with or without interstitial implants and a neck dissection for involved lymph nodes. Adequate surgical resection of advanced tonsillar tumours has conventionally required a mandibulectomy, the so-called 'tonsil commando' operation (Figure 13.32).

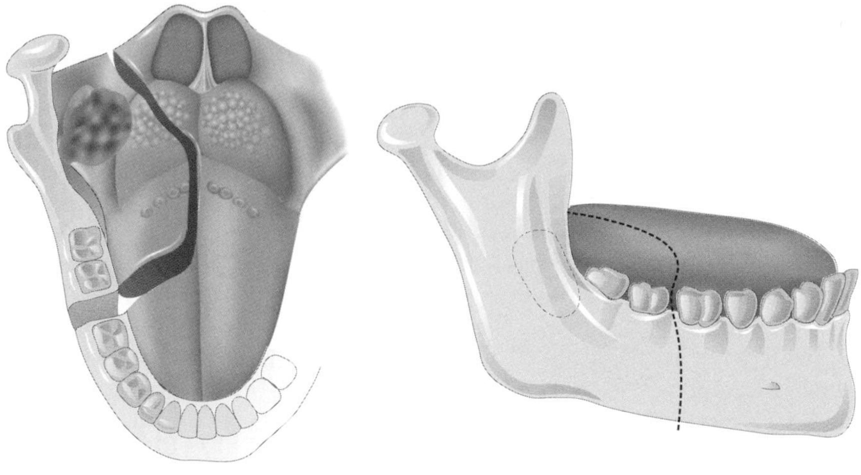

Figure 13.32 Composite resection of an advanced tonsillar tumour including the mandible: the 'tonsil commando' operation.

Involvement of the inferior alveolar nerve is an ominous sign, and is commoner in elderly patients with edentulous mandibles. Conservation mandibular surgery is hazardous in patients with resorbed, edentulous mandibles but for most other patients whose tumours do not directly invade the mandible, optimal functional results may be obtained using segmental resection combined with reconstruction and osseointegrated implants.

Results of treatment

Although surgical resection alone is not commonly used for early tonsillar cancer, excellent control rates have been reported for such a policy.[89] When the disease has spread to extend to the base of the tongue or lateral pharyngeal wall, the local recurrence rates for surgery alone tend to be unacceptable (47 and 33%, respectively).[90]

The results of treatment for more advanced lesions are uniformly poor (Table 13.22). Most authors recommend surgery combined with postoperative radiation, although there are advocates of radiation therapy alone, reserving surgery for salvage.[91] Some authors[87,92] have shown a survival benefit for combination therapy in the treatment of advanced tonsillar carcinoma while others[93] could not demonstrate any advantage in treating stage III and IV disease using a combined modality approach. While these studies were based on retrospective data, the RTOG 73–03 study[94] compared preoperative radiation therapy (50 Gy) plus surgery, surgery plus postoperative radiation therapy (60 Gy), and radiation therapy alone (65–70 Gy) with surgery reserved for salvage in a prospective randomized setting. No benefit could be demonstrated, either in terms of locoregional control or in survival, on comparison of results of the three methods of treatment. The study, however, did not stratify the patient population into subsites and the conclusions cannot be reliably applied to any one site such as the tonsil.

We currently prefer postoperative, rather than preoperative radiation therapy for advanced lesions because it allows more reliable assessment of locoregional extent of the disease and surgical margins, and is also associated with a lower rate of surgical complications. The choice of treatment and the sequence of therapy must however be tailored to the individual patient with the aim to cure the disease with the least functional deficit.

Carcinoma of the pharyngeal wall

Tumours of the posterior pharyngeal wall tend to present late. Common symptoms at presentation

Table 13.22 Results of treatment of tonsillar carcinoma

Reference	No. of patients	Follow-up (years)	Stage I (%)	Stage II (%)	Stage III (%)	Stage IV (%)
Perez et al[87]	218	3	76	40	42	25
Spiro and Spiro[93]	117	3	89	83	58	49
Dasmahapatra et al[92]	174	5	83	72	23	15
Amornmarn et al[95]	185	5	100	73	52	21
Mizono et al[96]	171	5	92	77	56	29
Givens et al[97]	104	5	93	57	27	17

include dysphagia, odynophagia, mass in the neck, weight loss, and bleeding. Tumours in this location tend to be more superficial and less bulky than those at other sites within the oropharynx, but they can be associated with extensive submucosal spread and 'skip' areas. Most tumours originate at the junction between the oropharynx and the hypopharynx. The tumour may spread superiorly to the nasopharynx, inferiorly to the pyriform sinuses and hypopharynx, and posteriorly to infiltrate the prevertebral fascia.

Tumours of the posterior pharyngeal wall have a higher than usual rate of second primary tumours (37% in one series[98]), and the importance of a meticulous examination of the entire upper aerodigestive tract cannot be overemphasized in these patients.

Lymph node metastases

The primary echelons of drainage are the retropharyngeal nodes and the nodes at levels II and III. The incidence of lymph node metastasis corresponds to the T stage and rises from 25% for T1 lesions to over 75% for T4 tumours.[99]

Treatment of early lesions

Transoral excision may be possible for small lesions in patients with good mouth opening when the lower limit of the tumour is well visible. For most other tumours, a transhyoid or lateral pharyngotomy approach can be used to resect the lesion. The avascular retropharyngeal space acts as a good plane of cleavage and the tumour can usually be easily separated from the underlying prevertebral fascia, which is very rarely involved in early lesions. Alternative approaches like the median labiomandibular glossotomy and mandibular swing are more extensive and are usually reserved for more advanced lesions. Reconstruction of the defect commonly entails a split thickness skin graft or a free radial forearm flap. The functional results of surgery, even for small lesions, are far from optimal because of impairment of swallowing that results from denervation and resection of the pharyngeal musculature. Surgery is generally not extensive enough to encompass the retropharyngeal nodes and postoperative radiation therapy to the neck may be indicated in high-risk patients.

Treatment of advanced lesions

Advanced tumours of the posterior pharyngeal wall are treated using surgery combined with postoperative radiation therapy. An important issue in deciding resectability is involvement of the prevertebral fascia and underlying structures. CT and MR reliably detect advanced infiltration, but early involvement of the fascia is most often apparent only at operation. Resection of locally advanced pharyngeal wall tumours usually entails a total laryngopharyngectomy. The resultant defect may be reconstructed using one of the various available options like tubed fasciocutaneous or myocutaneous flaps, gastric transposition, or microvascular free jejunal transfer. These operations have been discussed in detail elsewhere in this book but currently, the free jejunal transfer is the procedure of choice for reconstructing circumferential pharyngeal defects as it allows early return to swallowing with the minimum of physiological disturbance. Postoperative radiation therapy is recommended in view of the high incidence of retropharyngeal node involvement and locoregional failure.

Results of treatment

Tumour classification is often difficult because by the time they are detected, most lesions involve two separate anatomical regions, each having its own distinct classification; tumours of the oropharynx are also classified by size while those of the hypopharynx are classified by site of involvement. This, combined with the fact that these are rare tumours, makes comparison of treatment modalities difficult.

Radiation therapy alone has limited effectiveness in treatment mainly because of the technical difficulty in delivering adequate doses to tissue in such close proximity to the spinal cord, but also because these tumours are not very radiosensitive.

The predominant feature of surgical treatment of these tumours is the high incidence of local failure that ranges between 30[99] and 40%.[98] The probability of local recurrence is directly related to stage (16% for stage I and 63% for stage IV) and salvage rates are only about 40%. Table 13.23 lists the results of treatment of posterior pharyngeal wall tumours reported in the literature.

Carcinoma of the soft palate

The anterior surface of the palate tends to be the most commonly involved and the posterior surface is spared until the tumour is well advanced. Most lesions tend to be superficial and start as leukoplakia or as raised lesions. Clinical diagnosis may be difficult in heavy smokers as leukoplakic areas on the palate are very common in this population. Also, delineation of the extent of a biopsy-proven lesion may be difficult because of the keratinization of the mucosa associated with heavy smoking. Common presenting symptoms include bleeding and a sore throat, but patients may complain of altered speech or swallowing. As the tumour advances, it may spread to involve the tonsillar pillars, the base of the

Table 13.23 Results of treatment of posterior pharyngeal wall carcinoma

Reference	No. of patients	Treatment*	Follow-up (years)	Survival (%)
Wang[100]	36	R	3	25
Pene et al[101]	131	S, R	5	3
Marks et al[102]	51	R±C	3	14
Schwaab et al[103]	24	C±R	3	60
			5	25
Jaulerry et al[104]	98	R	3	30
			5	14
Spiro et al[98]	78	S±R	2	49
			5	32

*R: radiation; S: surgery; C: chemotherapy.

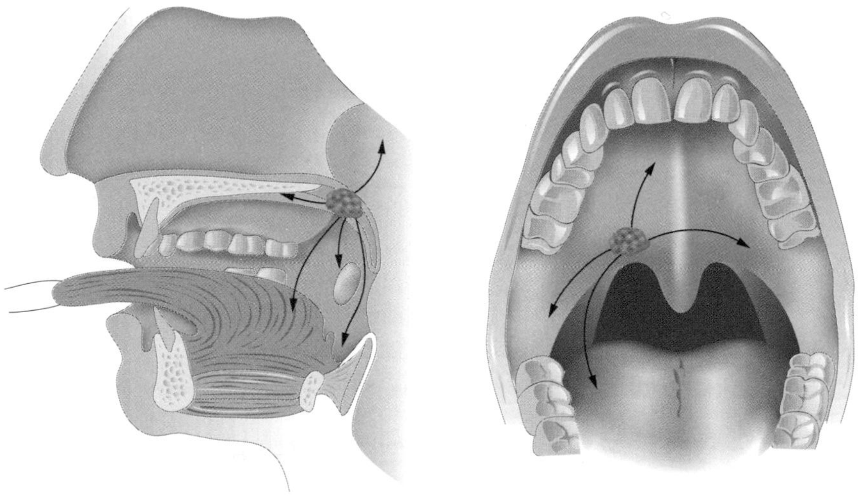

Figure 13.33 Pathways of local spread of tumours of the soft palate.

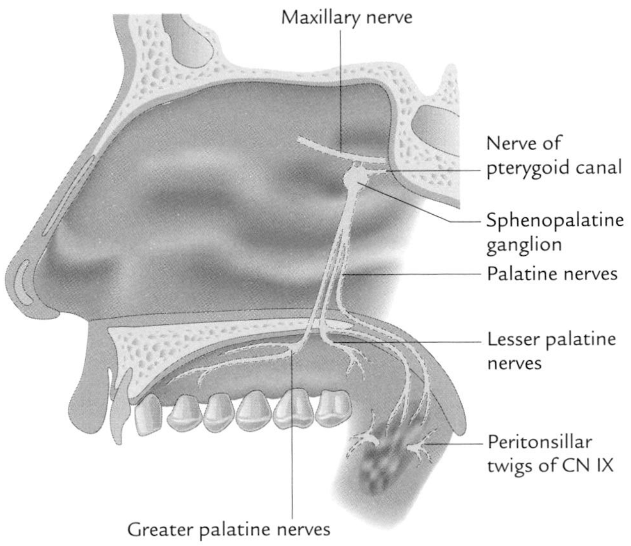

Figure 13.34 Involvement of the nerves of the palate results in pain, and the tumour may extend cranially along this path.

tongue or the nasopharynx (Figure 13.33). Involvement of the pharyngeal muscles results in pain as may extension along the palatine nerves (Figure 13.34).

Lymph node metastases

Primary drainage is to the upper jugulodigastric and the retropharyngeal nodes (Figure 13.35). About 30% of patients present with clinically positive neck nodes but extension of the tumour to involve the tonsillar fossa increases this risk. Occult nodal metastases occur in 16% of patients and about 15% of patients who have a midline primary lesion will have bilateral or contralateral neck metastases.[105]

Treatment of early disease

The treatment of carcinoma of the soft palate is essentially by radiation therapy because surgical excision of all but the very small lesions results in

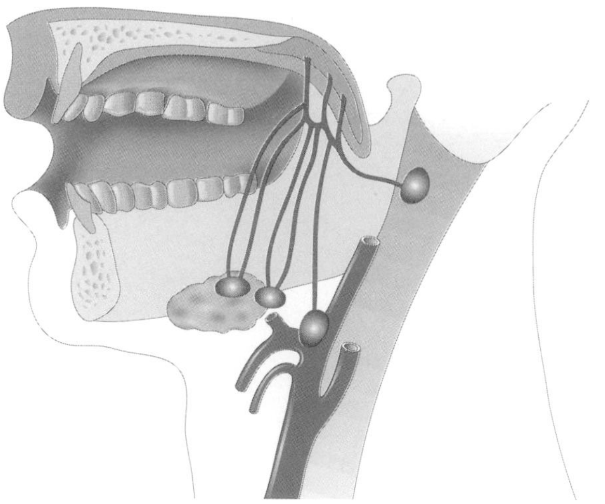

Figure 13.35 Lymphatic drainage of the soft palate.

unacceptable functional deficit such as nasal speech, regurgitation and difficulty swallowing. Small primary tumours with clinically positive nodes can be treated with radical radiation to the primary and the neck, surgery being reserved for salvage of failures. Brachytherapy has been used in treatment of small lesions[106] and has the advantage of sparing the major salivary glands from significant radiation, with a decreased risk of xerostomia.

Treatment of advanced disease

As with other sites, advanced tumours of the soft palate are also best managed using surgery combined with postoperative radiation therapy. Local control rates for T3 and T4 tumours with continuous-course radiation are 45% and 25%, respectively, and the results of salvage surgery in these patients are poor.[107]

Results of treatment

Overall 5-year survival rates range from 80–90% for stage I and II to 30–60% for stage III and IV lesions.[108] The results of treatment reported in the literature are listed in Table 13.24.

Follow-up and rehabilitation

Rehabilitation of patients who have had surgery for oropharyngeal tumours is often a prolonged and painstaking process. Apart from a great deal of patience, successful rehabilitation requires close co-operation between the surgeon, the speech therapist, the dietitian, the nursing staff and the physiotherapist. Palatal augmentation prostheses and videofluoroscopy are useful adjuncts to rehabilitation.

The time scale of posttreatment follow-up for these patients is identical to that for other head and neck patients but it is vitally important to examine them thoroughly using palpation, fibreoptic endoscopy and imaging as appropriate. Recurrences under a flap reconstruction are notoriously difficult to detect and judicious use of imaging must be combined with examination and biopsy under anaesthetic in suspicious cases.

Table 13.24 Results of treatment for carcinoma of the soft palate

Reference	No. of patients	Treatment*	Follow-up (years)	Survival (%)
Esche et al[109]	43	I±R	3	81
			5	64
Keus et al[110]	146	R	3	59
			5	53
Leemans et al[111]	52	S, R, C, L	5	77
Medini et al[112]	24	R	3	81

*I: Interstitial implant; R: external radiation; S: surgery; C: chemotherapy; L: laser resection.

REFERENCES

1. Rhys Evans PH. Tumours of the oropharynx and lymphomas of the head and neck. In Kerr AG (ed.) *Scott-Brown's Otolaryngology*, Vol. 5, 6th edn, London: Butterworth, 1997.
2. Hollinshead WH. In: *Anatomy for Surgeons: Volume 1 The Head and Neck*. 3rd edn. Philadelphia: Harper and Row, 1982.
3. Batson OV. Veins of the pharynx. *Arch Otolaryngol* 1942; **36**: 212.
4. Powell J, Robin PE. Cancer of the head and neck: the present state. In: Rhys Evans PH, Robin PE, Fielding JWL (eds). *Head and Neck Cancer*. London: Castle House Publications, 1983.
5. Pradier RN, Califano L. Cancer of the oropharynx. In: Shah J, Johnson J (eds) *Proceedings of the 4th International Conference on Head and Neck Cancer*. 1996.
6. Marandas P, Marandas N. Tumeurs malignes de l'oropharynx: epidemiologie, diagnostic, traitment. *La Reveu du Practicien* (Paris) 1995; **45**: 623–628.
7. Biorklund A, Wennesberg J. Epidemiology of cancer of the oral cavity and oropharynx. Recent results. *Cancer Res* (Germany) 1994; **134**: 1–8.
8. Spitz MR, Fueger JJ, Goepfert H et al. Squamous cell carcinoma of the upper aerodigestive tract: a case comparison analysis. *Cancer* 1988; **61**: 203–208.
9. Reddy CRRM. Carcinoma of hard palate in relation to reverse smoking of chuttas. *JNCI* 1974; **53**: 615–619.
10. Schantz SP, Hsu TC. Mutagen-induced chromosome fragility within peripheral blood lymphocytes of head and neck cancer patients. *Head Neck*. 1989; **11**: 337–342.
11. Guengerich FP. Roles of cytochrome p-450 enzymes in chemical carcinogenesis and cancer chemotherapy. *Cancer Res* 1988; **48**: 2946–2954.
12. Graham S, Dayal H, Rohrer T et al. Dentition, diet, tobacco, and alcohol in the epidemiology of oral cancer. *J Natl Cancer Inst* 1977; **59**: 1611–1618.
13. Szpirglas H. Alcohol et cancer buccaux. Actualites Odontostomatol Paris. No. 1976; **115**: 448–454.
14. Binnie WH. Epidemiology and aetiology of oral cancer in Britain. *Proc R Soc Med* 1976; **69**: 737–740.
15. Mashberg A, Garfinkel L, Harris S. Alcohol as a preliminary risk factor in oral squamous carcinoma. *CA Cancer J Clin* 1981; **31**: 146–155.
16. McLaughlin JK, Gridley G, Block G et al. Dietary factors in oral and pharyngeal cancer. *JNCI* 1988; **80**: 1237–1243.
17. DeStefani E, Orregia F, Ronco A et al. Salted meat consumption as a risk factor for cancer of the oral cavity and pharynx: a case control study from Uruguay. *Cancer Epidemiol Biomarkers Prev* 1994; **3**: 381–385.
18. Donald PJ. Marijuana smoking: possible cause of head and neck cancer in young patients. Otolaryngol Head Neck Surg 1986; **94**: 517–521.
19. Watts SL et al. Human papillomavirus DNA types in squamous cell cancer of the head and neck. *Oral Surg Oral Med Oral Pathol* 1991; **7**: 701–707.
20. Frazer IH, Leonard JH, Schonrock J et al. HPV DNA in oropharyngeal squamous cell cancers: comparison of results from four DNA detection methods. *Pathology* 1993; **25**: 138–143.
21. Singh B, Balwally AN, Shaha AR et al. Upper aerodigestive tract SCC. The human immunodeficiency virus connection. *Arch Otolaryngol Head Neck Surg* 1996; **122**: 639–643.
22. Fortner JC, Shiu MH. *Organ transplantation and cancer. Surg Clin North Am* 1974; **54**: 871.
23. Caminero MJ, Nunez F, Suarez C et al. Detection of p53 protein in oropharyngeal carcinoma. Prognostic implications. *Arch Otolaryngol Head Neck Surg* 1996; **122**: 769–772.
24. Saranath D, Panchal RG, Nair R et al. Amplification and overexpression of epidermal growth factor receptor gene in human oropharyngeal cancer. *Eur J Cancer B Oral Oncol* 1992; **28B**: 139–143.
25. Rowley H, Jones AS, Field JK. Chromosome 18: a possible site for a tumor suppressor gene deletion in squamous cell carcinoma of the head and neck. *Clin Otolaryngol* 1995; **20**: 266–271.
26. Moore C, Catlin D. Anatomic origins and locations of oral cancer. *Am J Surg* 1967; **114**: 510–513.
27. Henk JM. Results of radiotherapy for carcinoma of the oropharynx. *Clin Otolaryngol* 1978; **3**; 137–143.
28. Henk JM, A'Hern RP, Taylor K. Carcinoma of the oropharynx in the United Kingdom. In: Johnson JT, Didolkar MS (eds) *Head and Neck Cancer*. Vol 3. Amsterdam: Excerpta Medica, 1992; 779–784.
29. Lindberg RD. Distribution of cervical lymph node metastases from squamous cell carcinoma of the upper respiratory and digestive tracts. *Cancer* 1972; **29**: 1446–1450.
30. Million RR, Cassisi NJ. Oropharynx. In: Million RR, Cassisi NJ (eds) *Management of Head and Neck Cancer: A Multidisciplinary Approach*. Philadelphia: Lippincott, 1984.
31. Stell PM, Nash JRG. Tumours of the oropharynx. In: Kerr AG (ed.) *Scott-Brown's Otolaryngology*, Vol. 5, 6th edn, London: Butterworth, 1997.
32. Million RR. The lymphomatous diseases. In: Fletcher GH (ed.) *Textbook of Radiotherapy*, Philadelphia: Lea and Febiger, 1980.
33. National Cancer Institute sponsored study of classifications of Non-Hodgkins Lymphoma. *Cancer* 1982; **49**: 2112–2135.
34. Spiro RH, Koss LG, Hajdu SI, Strong EW. Tumours of minor salivary gland origin: a clinicopathologic study of 492 cases. *Cancer* 1973; **31**: 117–129.
35. Spiro RH, Alfonso AE, Farr HW, Strong EW. Cervical node metastasis from epidermoid carcinoma of the oral cavity and oropharynx. A critical assessment of current staging. *Am J Surg* 1974; **128**: 562–567.
36. Castelijns JA, van den Brekel MW. Imaging of lymphadenopathy in the neck. *Eur Radiol*. 2002; **12**: 727–738.

37. Pfister DG, Harrison LB, Strong EW et al. Organ-function preservation in advanced oropharynx cancer: results with induction chemotherapy and radiation. *J Clin Oncol* 1995; **13**: 671–80.
38. Rodriguez J, Point D, Brunin F et al. Surgery of the oropharynx after radiotherapy. *Bull Cancer Radiother* 1996; **83**: 24–30.
39. Harrison LB, Zelefsky MJ, Armstrong JG et al. Performance status after treatment for squamous cell cancer of the base of tongue: a comparison of primary radiation therapy versus primary surgery. *Int J Radiat Oncol Biol Phys* 1994; **30**: 953–957.
40. Fletcher GH, Lindberg RD. Squamous cell carcinoma of the tonsillar area and palatine arch. *Am J Roentgenol Radium Ther Nucl Med* 1966; **96**: 574–587.
41. Fein DA, Lee RW, Amos WR et al. Oropharyngeal carcinoma treated with radiotherapy: a 30-year experience. *Int J Radiat Oncol Biol Phys* 1996; **34**: 289–296.
42. Bataini JP, Asselain B, Jaulerry CH et al. A multivariate primary tumour control analysis in 465 patients treated by radical radiotherapy for cancer of the tonsillar region: clinical and treatment parameters as prognostic factors. *Radiother Oncol* 1989; **14**: 265–277.
43. Jaulerry C, Rodriguez J, Brunin F et al. Results of radiation therapy in carcinoma of the base of tongue: the Curie Institute experience with about 166 cases. *Cancer* 1991; **67**: 1532–1538.
44. Withers HR, Peters LJ, Taylor JMG et al. Local control of carcinoma of the tonsil by radiation therapy: an analysis of patterns of fractionation in nine institutions. *Int J Radiat Oncol Biol Phys* 1995; **33**: 549–562.
45. Horiot JC, le Fur T, N'Guyen C et al. Hyperfractionation compared with conventional radiotherapy in oropharyngeal carcinoma. *Eur J Cancer* **26**: 1990; 779–780.
46. Dische S, Saunders M, Barrett A et al. A randomised multicentre trial of CHART versus conventional radiotherapy in head and neck cancer. *Radiother Oncol* 1997; **44**: 123–137.
47. Horiot JC, Bontemps P, le Fur R et al. An overview of the EORTC accelerated and hyperfractionated radiotherapy trials in head and neck cancer. *Radiother Oncol* 1996; **40**: S30.
48. Mak AC, Morrison WH, Garden AS et al. Base-of-tongue carcinoma: treatment results using concomitant boost radiotherapy. *Int J Radiat Oncol Biol Phys* 1995; **33**: 289–296.
49. Overgaard J, Saad Hansen H, Sapra W et al. Conventional radiotherapy as the primary treatment of squamous-cell carcinoma of the head and neck. A randomized multicentre study of 5 versus 6 fractions per week: preliminary report from the DAHANCA 6 and 7 trial. *Radiother Oncol* 1996; **40**: S31.
50. Henk JM. Late results of a trial of hyperbaric oxygen and radiotherapy in head and neck cancer: a rationale of hypoxic sensitizers? *Int J Radiat Oncol Biol Phys* 1986; **12**: 1339–1341.
51. Overgaard J, Hansen HS, Overgaard M et al. A randomized double-blind phase III study of nimorazole as a hypoxic radiosensitizer of primary radiotherapy in supraglottic larynx and pharynx carcinoma. Results of the Danish Head and Neck Cancer Study (DAHANCA) protocol 5–85. *Radiother Oncol* 1998; **46**: 135–146.
52. Pernot M, Malissard MD, Taghlan A et al. Velotonsillar squamous cell carcinoma: 277 cases treated by combined external irradiation and brachytherapy: results according to extension, localization and dose rate. *Int J Radiat Oncol Biol Phys* 1992; **21**: 715–723.
53. Harrison LB, Zelefsky MJ, Sessions RB et al. Base-of-tongue cancer treated with external beam irradiation plus brachytherapy: oncologic and functional outcome. *Radiology* 1992; **184**: 267–270.
54. Foote RL, Parsons JT, Mendenhall WM et al. Is interstitial implantation essential for successful radiotherapeutic treatment of base of tongue carcinoma? *Int J Radiat Oncol Biol Phys* 1990; **18**: 1293–1298.
55. Crook J, Mazeron JJ, Marinello G et al. Combined external irradiation and interstitial implantation for T1 and T2 epidermoid carcinomas of the base of tongue: the Creteil experience (1971–1981). *Int J Radiat Oncol Biol Phys* 1988; **14**: 105–114.
56. Puthawala AA, Nisar Syed AM, Eads DL et al. Limited external beam and interstitial 192iridium irradiation in the treatment of carcinoma of the base of tongue: a ten-year experience. *Int J Radiat Oncol Biol Phys* 1988; **14**: 839–848.
57. Murthy AK, Hendrickson FR. Is contralateral neck treatment necessary in early carcinoma of the tonsil? *Int J Radiat Oncol Biol Phys* 1980; **6**: 91–94.
58. Fletcher GH. Elective irradiation of subclinical disease in cancer of the head and neck. *Cancer* 1972; **29**: 1450–1454.
59. Klijanienko J, Micheau C, Azli N et al. Undifferentiated carcinoma of nasopharyngeal type of tonsil. *Arch Otolaryngol Head Neck Surg* 1989; **115**: 731–736.
60. Henk JM. Radiosensitivity of lymph node metastases. *Proc R Soc Med* 1975; **68**: 85–86.
61. Peters LJ, Weber RS, Morrison WH. Neck surgery in patients with primary oropharyngeal cancer treated by radiotherapy. *Head Neck* 1996; **18**: 552–559.
62. Rhys Evans PH, Frame JW, Brandrick J. A review of carbon dioxide laser surgery in the oral cavity and pharynx. *J Laryngol Otol* 1986; **100**: 69–77.
63. Eckel HE, Volling P, Pototschnig C et al. Transoral laser resection with staged discontinuous neck dissection for oral cavity and oropharynx squamous cell carcinoma. *Laryngoscope* 1995; **105**: 53–60.
64. Zeitels SM, Vaughan CW. Suprahyoid pharyngotomy for oropharynx cancer including the tongue base. *Arch Otolaryngol Head Neck Surg* 1991; **117**: 757–760.
65. Civantos F, Wenig BL. Transhyoid resection of tongue base and tonsil tumours. *Otolaryngol Head Neck Surg* 1994; **111**: 59–62.
66. Spiro RH, Gerold FP, Shah JP et al. Mandibulotomy approach to oropharyngeal tumours. *Am J Surg* 1985; **150**: 466–469.

67. Shah JP, Kumarawamy SV, Kulkarni V. Comparative evaluation of fixation methods after mandibulotomy for oropharyngeal tumours. *Am J Surg* 1993; **166**: 431–434.
68. Dubner S, Spiro RH. Median mandibulotomy: a critical assessment. *Head Neck* 1991; **13**: 389–393.
69. Altman K, Bailey BM. Non-union of mandibulotomy sites following irradiation for squamous cell carcinoma of the oral cavity. *Br J Oral Maxillofac Surg* 1996; **34**: 62–65.
70. Krespi YP, Sissons GA. Reconstruction after total or subtotal glossectomy. *Am J Surg* 1983; **146**: 488–492.
71. Weber RS, Ohlms L, Bowman J, Jacob R, Goepfert H. Functional results after total or near total glossectomy with laryngeal preservation. *Arch Otolaryngol Head Neck Surg* 1991; **117**: 512–515.
72. Boyd TS, Harari PM, Tannehill SP et al. Planned postradiotherapy neck dissection in patients with advanced head and neck cancer. *Head Neck* 1998; **20**: 132–137.
73. Hasegawa Y, Matsuura H. Retropharyngeal node dissection in cancer of the oropharynx and hypopharynx. *Head Neck* 1994; **16**: 173–180.
74. Jones AS, England J, Hamilton J et al. Mandibular invasion in patients with oral and oropharyngeal squamous carcinoma. *Clin Otolaryngol* 1997; **22**: 239–245.
75. Hudgins PA, Burson JG, Gussack GS, Grist WJ. CT and MR appearance of recurrent malignant head and neck neoplasms after resection and flap reconstruction. *Am J Neuroradiol* 1994; **15**: 1689–1694.
76. McGuirt WF, Greven K, Williams D III et al. PET scanning in head and neck oncology: a review. *Head Neck* 1998; **20**: 208–215.
77. Riley RW, Fee WE Jr, Goffinet D et al. Squamous cell carcinoma of the base of the tongue. *Otolaryngol Head Neck Surg* 1983; **91**: 143–150.
78. Weber R, Gidley P, Morrison W et al. Treatment selection for carcinoma of the base of tongue. *Am J Surg* 1990; **160**: 415–419.
79. Harrison LB, Zelefsky MJ, Armstrong JG et al. Performance status after treatment for squamous cell cancer of the base of tongue: a comparison of primary surgery versus primary surgery. *Int J Radiat Oncol Biol Phys* 1994; **30**: 953–957.
80. Ruhl CM, Gleich LL, Gluckman JL. Survival, function and quality of life after total glossectomy. *Laryngoscope* 1997; **107**: 1316–1321.
81. Razack MS, Sako K, Bakamjian VY, Shedd DP. Total glossectomy. *Am J Surg* 1983; **146**: 509–511.
82. Gehanno P, Guedon C, Barry B et al. Advanced carcinoma of the tongue: total glossectomy without total laryngectomy. Review of 80 cases. *Laryngoscope* 1992; **102**: 1369–1371.
83. Kraus DH, Vastola AP, Huvos AG, Spiro RH. Surgical management of squamous cell carcinoma of the base of the tongue. *Am J Surg* 1993; **166**: 384–388.
84. Foote RL, Olsen KD, Davis DL et al. Base of tongue carcinoma: patterns of failure and predictors of recurrence after surgery alone. *Head Neck* 1993; **15**: 300–307.
85. Thawley SE, Simpson JR, Marks JE et al. Preoperative irradiation and surgery for carcinoma of the base of the tongue. *Ann Otol Rhinol Laryngol* 1983; **92**: 485–490.
86. Barrs DM, DeSanto LW, O'Fallo WM. Squamous cell carcinoma at the tonsil and tongue-base regions. *Arch Otolaryngol* 1979; **105**: 479–485.
87. Perez CA, Purdy JA, Breaux SR et al. Carcinoma of the tonsillar fossa: a non-randomized comparison of preoperative radiation and surgery and irradiation alone: long-term results. *Cancer* 1982; **50**: 2314–2322.
88. Pernot M, Malissard L, Hoffstetter S et al. Influence of tumoral, radiobiological and general factors on local control and survival of a series of 361 tumors of the velotonsillar area treated by exclusive irradiation (external beam irradiation and brachytherapy or brachytherapy alone). *Int J Radiat Oncol Biol Phys* 1994; **30**: 1051–1057.
89. Remmler D, Medina JE, Byers RM et al. Treatment of choice for squamous cell carcinoma of the tonsillar fossa. *Head Neck Surg* 1985; **7**: 206–211.
90. Tong D, Laramore GE, Griffen TW et al. Carcinoma of the tonsil region: results of external irradiation. *Cancer* 1982; **49**: 2009–2014.
91. Mendenhall W, Parsons J, Cassisi N et al. Squamous cell carcinoma of the tonsillar area treated with radical irradiation. *Radiother Oncol* 1987; **10**: 23–30.
92. Dasmahapatra K, Mohit-Tabatabai M, Rush B et al. Cancer of the tonsil: improved survival with combination therapy. *Cancer* 1986; **57**: 451–455.
93. Spiro J, Spiro R. Carcinoma of the tonsillar fossa: an update. *Arch Otol Head Neck Surg* 1989; **115**: 1186–1189.
94. Kramer S, Gelber R, Snow J et al. Combination radiation therapy and surgery in the management of advanced head and neck cancer: the final report of study 73–03 of the Radiation Therapy Oncology Group. *Head Neck Surg* 1987; **10**: 19–30.
95. Amornmarn R, Prempree T, Jaiwatana J, Wizenberg MJ. Radiation management of carcinoma of the tonsillar region. *Cancer* 1984; **54**: 1293–1299.
96. Mizono GS, Diaz RF, Fu KK, Boles R. Carcinoma of the tonsillar region. *Laryngoscope* 1986; **96**: 240–244.
97. Givens CD, Johns ME, Cantrell RW. Carcinoma of the tonsil: analysis of 162 cases. *Arch Otolaryngol* 1981; **107**: 730–734.
98. Spiro RH, Kelly J, Vega AL et al. Squamous carcinoma of the posterior pharyngeal wall. *Am J Surg* 1990; **160**: 420–423.
99. Guillamondegui OM, Meoz R, Jesse RH. Surgical treatment of squamous cell carcinoma of the pharyngeal walls. *Am J Surg* 1978; **136**: 474–476.
100. Wang CC. Radiotherapeutic management of carcinoma of the posterior pharyngeal wall. *Cancer* 1971; **27**: 894–896.
101. Pene F, Avedian V, Eschwege F et al. A retrospective study of 131 cases of carcinoma of the posterior pharyngeal wall. *Cancer* 1978; **42**: 2490–2493.

102. Marks JE, Freeman RB, Lee F, Ogura JH. Pharyngeal wall cancer: an analysis of treatment results, complications and patterns of failure. *Int J Radiat Oncol Biol Phys* 1978; **4**: 587–593.
103. Schwaab G, Vandenbrouck C, Luboinski B, Rhys Evans P. Les carcinomes de la paroi posteriure du pharynx traites par chirurgie premiere. *J Eur Radiother* 1983; **4**: 175–179.
104. Jaulerry C, Brunin F, Rodriguez J et al. Carcinomas of the posterior pharyngeal wall. Experience of the Institut Curie. Analysis of the results of radiotherapy. *Ann Otolaryngol Chir Cervicofac* 1986; **103**: 559–563.
105. Lindberg RD, Barkley HT, Jesse RH, Fletcher GH. Evolution of the clinically negative neck in patients with squamous cell carcinoma of the faucial arch. *Am J Roentgenol Radium Ther Nucl Med* 1971; **111**: 60–65.
106. Mazeron JJ, Marinello G, Crook J et al. Definitive radiation treatment for early stage carcinomas of the soft palate and uvula: the indications for iridium-192 implantation. *Int J Radiat Oncol Biol Phys* 1987; **13**: 1829–1837.
107. Amdur RJ, Mendenhall WM, Parsons JT et al. Carcinoma of the soft palate treated with irradiation: analysis of results and complications. *Radiother Oncol* 1987; **9**: 185–194.
108. Weber RS, Peters LJ, Wolf PS, Guillamondegui O. Squamous cell carcinoma of the soft palate, uvula and anterior faucial pillar. *Otolaryngol Head Neck Surg* 1988; **99**: 16–23.
109. Esche BA, Haie CM, Gerbaulet AP et al. Interstitial and external radiotherapy in carcinoma of the soft palate and uvula. *Int J Radiat Oncol Biol Phys* 1988; **15**: 619–625.
110. Keus RB, Pontvert D, Brunin F et al. Results of irradiation in squamous cell carcinoma of the soft palate and uvula. *Radiother Oncol* 1988; **11**: 311–317.
111. Leemans CR, Engelbrecht WJ, Tiwari R, Deville WL, Karim AB, van der Waal I, Snow GB. Carcinoma of the soft palate and anterior tonsillar pillar. *Laryngoscope* 1994; **104**: 1477–1481.
112. Medini E, Medini A, Gapany M, Levitt SH. External beam radiation therapy for squamous cell carcinoma of the soft palate. *Int J Radiat Oncol Biol Phys* 1997; **38**: 507–511.

14 Tumours of the hypopharynx

Paul Q Montgomery, Peter H Rhys Evans and J Michael Henk

Introduction

Hypopharyngeal tumours have one of the worst survival rates for any head and neck site and are associated with significant morbidity. This is due to several factors. Early symptoms are often vague and many patients are diagnosed at a late stage in the disease when the local tumour is advanced and nodal metastases are frequently present. Progressive dysphagia over several months prior to diagnosis may reduce the patient to a poor physical state with a correspondingly increased risk of morbidity and mortality following treatment. The larynx is frequently involved, although in the early stages of the disease hoarseness is not a common symptom. If radiotherapy is given for anything other than a small lesion, particularly near the lower part of the hypopharynx, there is a significant risk of continued dysphagia because of postradiation circumferential cicatrization. For those patients who recur after primary radiotherapy, salvage surgery is associated with an increased risk of complications and may not be feasible. Primary total laryngectomy with partial or total pharyngectomy may offer the best chance of cure but with a very severe reduction in quality of life. The optimum curative treatment for more advanced disease at this site involves one of the most complex operations in head and neck surgery which is associated with significant morbidity and mortality.

The concept of 'organ preservation' with neoadjuvant chemotherapy as a predictor of radiosensitivity has offered a rational basis to avoid less mutilating treatment although its long-term value in terms of cure has yet to be proven. Finally, the complex management of these tumours exemplifies the essential need for a multidisciplinary team approach.

Surgical anatomy

The hypopharynx is that part of the pharynx that extends from the level of the hyoid cartilage superiorly to the lower border of the cricoid cartilage. It is divided into three subsites: the piriform fossae; the postcricoid region; and the posterior pharyngeal wall (Figure 14.1).[1,2]

Piriform fossa

Relations

Each piriform fossa is analogous to an inverted pyramid with a (superior) base, medial and lateral walls and an (inferior) apex.[1–4] The base is formed by the hypopharyngeal aspect of the lateral pharyngoepiglottic and adjacent aryepiglottic folds. The apex is at the confluence of the medial and lateral walls at the entrance of the cervical oesophagus at or just below the inferior border of the cricopharyngeus muscle. The medial wall of the hypopharynx includes the lateral surface of the aryepiglottic fold, the arytenoid and cricoid cartilages, and is related to the paraglottic space, the laryngeal ventricle, saccule and the intrinsic muscles of the larynx. A distinction is made by some authors[5,6] between the superior aspect of the medial wall (aryepiglottic fold: part of the epilarynx) and the inferior aspect (the piriform fossa proper) as the prognosis of squamous cell carcinomas in the former site is better. The lateral wall of the piriform fossa is formed by the inferior constrictor (thyropharyngeus and cricopharyngeus muscles), and deep to this the internal branches of the superior laryngeal neurovascular bundle, the hyoid, thyrohyoid membrane and thyroid ala. A descriptive distinction is also made between the upper 'membranous' and lower 'cartilaginous' piriform fossa, that part of the lateral wall mucosa which is, respectively, adjacent to the thyrohyoid membrane and the cartilaginous thyroid ala.[7]

Innervation

Sensation is via the glossopharyngeal and vagal cranial nerves through the pharyngeal plexus. Lesions within the piriform fossa may cause a sensation medial to the sternomastoid muscle and lateral to the thyroid ala. The common origin of Arnold's nerve to the external auditory canal and the internal branch of the superior laryngeal nerve from the vagus results in the phenomenon of referred otalgia associated with invasive piriform lesions.[8] Motor

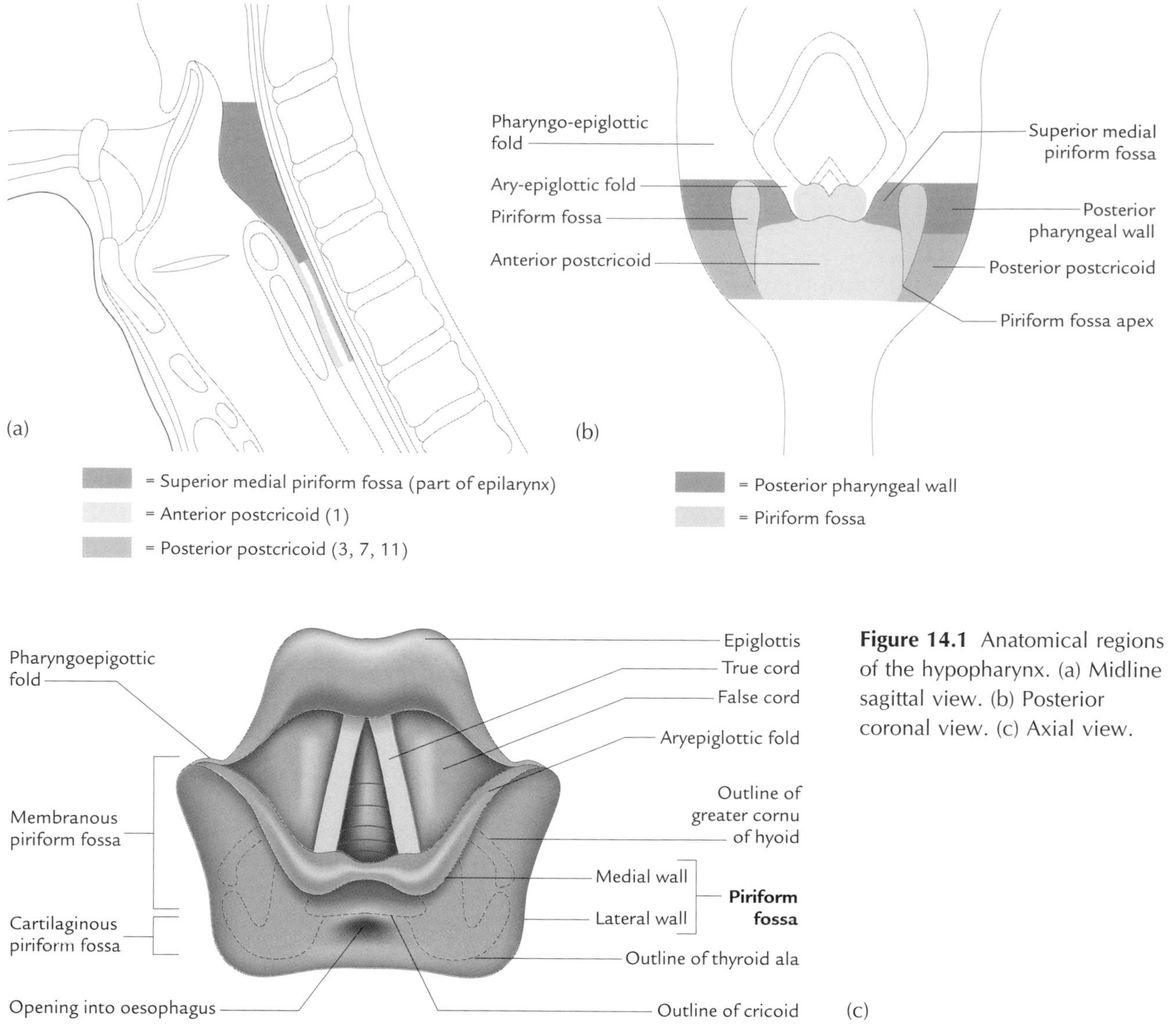

Figure 14.1 Anatomical regions of the hypopharynx. (a) Midline sagittal view. (b) Posterior coronal view. (c) Axial view.

innervation is via the pharyngeal plexus and the recurrent laryngeal nerve from the vagus.

Lymphatic drainage

Lymphatic channels draining the piriform fossa pierce the thyrohyoid membrane (with associated nodes at the lateral margin of the thyrohyoid muscle) to follow the superior laryngeal artery where they drain into three main lymph node groups: the subdigastric nodes, the lateral jugular nodes and the jugular nodes below the common facial vein. Pathological studies suggest that midjugular nodes (level III) drain twice the lymphatic flow as the upper (level II) or lower jugular nodes (level IV).[9] Hasegawa and Matsuura[10] noted the significance of retropharyngeal nodes in the lymphatic drainage of the piriform fossa in advanced carcinoma (Figure 14.2).

Postcricoid

The postcricoid area is the anterior (laryngeal) surface extending from the superior aspect of the arytenoid cartilages to the inferior border of the cricoid cartilage. Silver,[3] Ogura et al[11] and Million and Cassisi[7] also included the opposing posterior pharyngeal mucosal surface enclosed by cricopharyngeus, thus regarding this subsite as a circumferential surface.

Relations

Deep to the mucosa are the arytenoids, the cricoarytenoid joints, the cricoid and the interarytenoid and posterior cricoarytenoid muscles. Inferiorly, any tumour growth on the anterior (laryngeal) surface below the cricoid, towards the oesophagus, brings the tumour into direct relationship with the trachealis muscle and recurrent laryngeal nerves.

Innervation

Sensation is through the glossopharyngeal and vagus nerves via the pharyngeal plexus.[8] Lesions produce a globus sensation, prior to true dysphagia, at the level of the suprasternal notch.

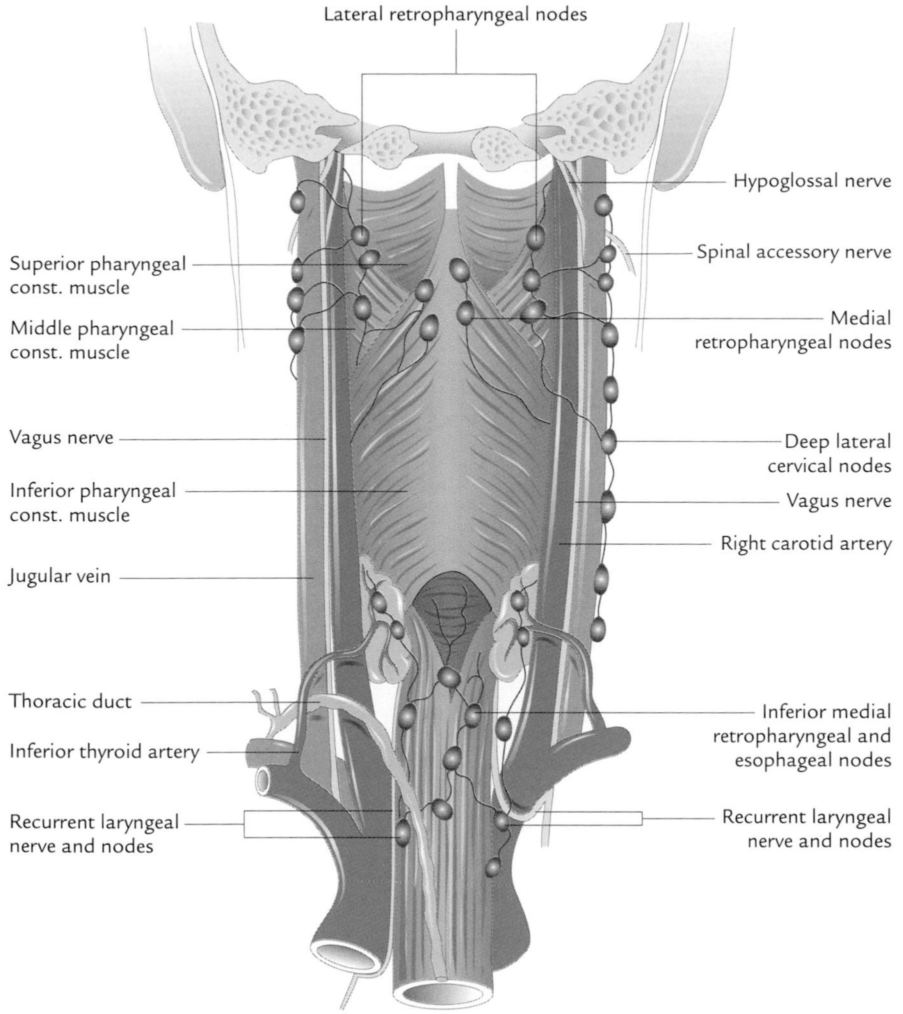

Figure 14.2 Lymphatic drainage of the hypopharynx viewed posteriorly.

Lymphatic drainage

The postcricoid mucosa may drain directly through the muscular layer to local lymph nodes or pass submucosally then pierce the muscular layer. Thus midline flow is not only bilateral,[12] it is submucosal and this has surgical implications as to the extent of resection. The lymphatics drain to the nodes associated with the recurrent laryngeal nerve in the paratracheal and oesophageal grooves (Figure 14.2) and then: to level IV; or to ascend with the lymphatic drainage of the piriform fossa (levels II and III); or to drain down into the superior mediastinum.[8]

Posterior pharyngeal wall

The posterior wall of the hypopharynx extends from the horizontal level of the floor of the vallecula to the inferior border of the cricoid[1] and laterally it merges into the piriform fossa (Figure 14.1). In the UICC definition[1] it is implicit that the term 'posterior pharyngeal wall' includes the lateral walls of the hypopharynx. It is difficult to define precisely and has a maximum anteroposterior extent of 2 cm.[7] Pure lateral pharyngeal wall lesions are correspondingly very rare (7% of oro- and hypopharyngeal tumours.[13]) The deep relations of the lateral wall are significantly different to those of the posterior wall. Local control, recurrence and survival between the two areas is similar for T1/2/3 growths[14] but T4 lesions of the posterior pharyngeal wall have a much poorer local control than those of the lateral pharyngeal wall (29% versus 68%).[15]

Relations

The deep relation of the lateral aspect of the posterior pharyngeal wall is the lateral pharyngeal space containing the carotid sheath whereas that of the posterior aspect of the posterior pharyngeal wall is the prevertebral fascia and muscles.

Innervation

This is from the glossopharyngeal and vagus nerves via the pharyngeal plexus, the superior and recurrent laryngeal nerves.[8]

Lymphatic drainage

The posterior pharyngeal wall lymphatics may drain bilaterally, passing to the lateral retropharyngeal nodes or the internal jugular nodes (levels II and

III).[9,16] Hasegawa and Matsuura[10] and Ballantyne[18] highlighted the significance of the retropharyngeal nodes in the lymphatic drainage of the posterior pharyngeal wall in advanced carcinoma.

Histology

The vast majority of lesions are squamous cell carcinomas but occasional other tumour types such as sarcomas, chondrosarcomas, adenocarcinomas, lymphomas and melanomas have been reported. Lederman[19] reported squamous cell carcinoma in 99.5% of cases with 0.1% sarcomas. However, sarcomas may be overreported as some may in fact be pseudosarcoma variants of squamous cell carcinoma (pleomorphic carcinoma; spindle cell carcinoma).

Epidemiology

The hypopharynx is a rare site for tumours, accounting for approximately 10% of all squamous cell carcinomas of the upper aerodigestive tract.[3] The overall incidence in the Western world is 1 per 100 000 per year. There is a very high incidence in northern France[20] of 14.8 per 100 000 per annum accounting for 18% of all UADT lesions (Table 14.1).

The distribution by subsite indicates that piriform fossa lesions are the commonest subsite in North America and France whereas postcricoid lesions appear more commonly in Northern Europe (Table 14.2).

The mean age at presentation of hypopharyngeal tumours is approximately 60 years. Piriform fossa and posterior pharyngeal wall lesions demonstrate the typical male predominance: for piriform fossa lesions this sex difference is marked in North America (approximately 5–20 males to 1 female[29–31]) and extreme in France with ratios of nearly 50:1.[6,32] Postcricoid lesions, unlike all other sites, show a consistent moderate female preponderance (approximately 1.5:1 female to male ratio).[12,21,28,33,34]

Table 14.1 Incidence of hypopharyngeal carcinoma per 100 000 per year

Sweden[21]	0.84
USA[8]	1
Canada[22]	0.75
UK[23]	0.7
France[20]	14.8

Aetiology

As with all head and neck squamous cell carcinomas there is a significant association with alcohol and smoking which also act synergistically. Postcricoid carcinoma is associated with previous radiation exposure; variously reported in 4–7% of cases[12,21,35] and sideropenic dysphagia[12,28,33] (4–6% have a history of Patterson Brown-Kelly (Plummer-Vinson) syndrome with the prevalence being 1%[21]). Radiation exposure has also been implicated in posterior pharyngeal wall carcinomas.[36]

Staging systems

The UICC/AJC[1] have agreed a common staging system for hypopharyngeal tumours (Table 14.3).

Piriform fossa

The UICC/AJC[1] system, as applied to the piriform fossa, is generally accepted by most centres as the reporting system of choice in its ability to reflect the natural history and prognoses of lesions at this subsite. Bataini[6] excludes the superior part of the piriform aspect of the aryepiglottic fold, which he regards as part of the epilarynx, where tumours have a better prognosis. Other systems have been used[6,11] in an attempt to reflect the natural history/prognosis of the disease. It is worth noting that a tumour may progress from a 'T1' to 'T4' without intermediate 'T' stages depending on its position and direction of spread (see below).

Postcricoid

Prior to 1997 the UICC/AJC system attracted criticism as tumour length was not included. This was a

Table 14.2 Distribution by site of hypopharyngeal carcinoma

Site	France[6]	Canada[22]	USA[24]	Brazil[25]	Belgium[26]	UK[27]	Finland[28]
Piriform fossa (%)	90	85	59	97	89	60	52
Posterior pharyngeal wall (%)	7	8	35	3	9	5	18
Postcricoid (%)	3	7	6	—	2	35	30

significant omission as tumour length relates to the degree of invasion through the muscle coat to the adventitia, circumferential spread and into the thyroid gland.[37] Other staging systems therefore evolved to address this issue[11,33] and in 1997 the UICC/AJC system was amended to include length.

Posterior pharyngeal wall

As with postcricoid lesions the pre 1997 UICC/AJC system was criticized as the size of the lesions was not taken into account. T1 lesions would not only include the smallest invasive lesion but also a massive lesion completely occupying the posterior pharyngeal wall and thus many clinicians used the size-based UICC[1] oropharyngeal system. Another consideration was that posterior pharyngeal wall carcinomas often arise at the junction of the oro- and hypopharynx creating a dilemma as to which UICC[1] system should be used. Pene et al[38] and Schwaab et al[39] suggested a compromise classification for all posterior pharyngeal wall carcinomas. The 1997 UICC/AJC classification includes both site and size criteria to answer these issues.

Table 14.3 Staging system for hypopharyngeal tumours[1]

T1	One subsite of the hypopharynx and 2 cm or less in greatest dimension
T2	More than one subsite of the hypopharynx or an adjacent site, or measures more than 2 cm but not more than 4 cm in greatest dimension, without fixation of hemilarynx
T3	Tumour measures more than 4 cm in greatest dimension, or with fixation of hemilarynx
T4	Tumour invades adjacent structures (e.g. thyroid/cricoid cartilage, carotid artery, soft tissues of the neck, prevertebral fascia/muscles, thyroid, and/or cervical oesophagus)
NX	Regional lymph nodes cannot be assessed
N0	No regional lymph node metastasis
N1	Metastasis in a single ipsilateral lymph node, 3 cm or less in greatest dimension
N2a	Metastasis in a single ipsilateral lymph node more than 3 cm but not more than 6 cm in greatest dimension
N2b	Metastasis in multiple ipsilateral lymph nodes, none more than 6 cm in greatest dimension
N2c	Metastasis in bilateral or contralateral lymph nodes, none more than 6 cm in greatest dimension
N3	Metastasis in a lymph node more than 6 cm in greatest dimension

Stage grouping

Stage 0	Tis	N0	M0
Stage I	T1	N0	M0
Stage II	T2	N0	M0
Stage III	T3	N0	M0
	T1	N1	M0
	T2	N1	M0
	T3	N1	M0
Stage IVA	T4	N0,1	M0
	Any T	N2	M0
Stage IVB	Any T	N3	M0
Stage IVC	Any T	Any N	M1

Note: midline nodes are considered ipsilateral nodes.

Natural history: symptoms

Piriform fossa

Unilateral sore throat and dysphagia are common symptoms of intraluminal growth although their onset may be late. As these symptoms become more severe they are associated with weight loss. Otalgia is associated with invasion through the pharyngeal wall and hoarseness from involvement of laryngeal musculature (Table 14.4).[26] The profuse lymphatic drainage from the piriform fossa results in early nodal metastases and up to 75% of patients have pathologically involved nodes on presentation of which at least 10% are bilateral.[40,41]

Postcricoid

Rapid onset of dysphagia is common with 50% of patients having symptoms for less than 3 months.[33] Other symptoms such as voice change are common because of the proximity of the larynx. Large retropharyngeal nodes may produce occipital and nape of the neck pain radiating to the retrorbital area (Table 14.4).[8]

Table 14.4 Symptoms of hypopharyngeal carcinoma

Symptoms	Piriform fossa[26] (%)	Postcricoid[12,33] (%)		Posterior wall[42] (%)
Dysphagia	41	99	90	46
Odynophagia	18	—	18	60
Otalgia	9	—	9	14
Hoarseness	31	20	15	11
Neck lump	—	—	7	14
Weight loss	—	54	—	—
Dyspnoea	1	—	—	—

Posterior pharyngeal wall

Dysphagia and sore throat are common symptoms but the primary complaint of a neck mass has been reported in 18% of cases; 10% are asymptomatic and found incidentally.[43] As with postcricoid lesions large retropharyngeal nodes may produce occipital and nape of the neck pain radiating to the retrorbital area (Table 14.4).[8]

Natural history: clinicopathological features

Piriform fossa

Primary tumour

Piriform fossa lesions behave in a similar manner to transglottic rather than supraglottic laryngeal tumours.[21] The appearance is usually classified as either exophytic or endophytic with the former having generally a better prognosis. Tani et al[44] reported 20% of tumours predominantly medial, 35% lateral and 45% involving both walls (Figure 14.3). The majority of lesions present late (Table 14.5) with vocal cord immobility and/or cartilage invasion present in over 80%.

Lateral and apical extension is associated with invasion of cartilage[29] and submucosal spread may be beyond 10 mm.[46] Superiorly, the base of the tongue is at risk if extension is beyond the lateral pharyngoepiglottic fold into the vallecula.[29]

Cervical oesophageal involvement is seen less commonly than with primary postcricoid tumours but apical spread is an ominous sign as it is associated with a high probability of invasion of the thyroid and cricoid cartilages.[29] Involvement of the tracheo-oesophageal groove and cricopharyngeus occurs by deep extension after postcricoid involvement.[3]

Medial invasion is via the paraglottic space into the larynx (Figure 14.4) and thence through the cricothyroid membrane to involve the lower border of the

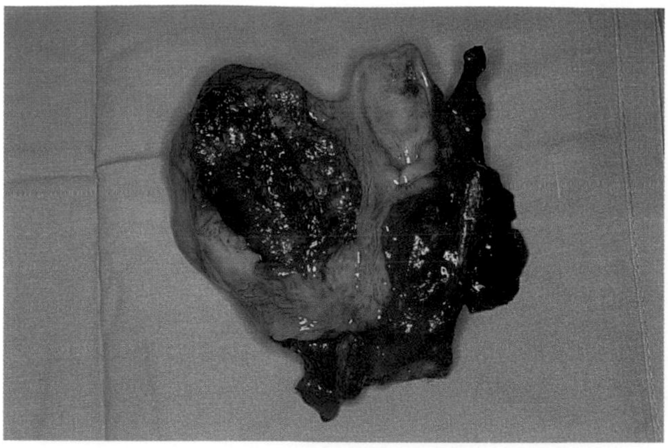

Figure 14.3 Piriform fossa tumour involving medial and lateral walls.

Table 14.5 Percentage T stage distribution at presentation

T stage	Kirchner (AJC 1973)[29]	El Badawi et al (AJC 1977)[45]
T1	5	5
T2	4	12
T3	91	38
T4	—	45

(a)

(b)

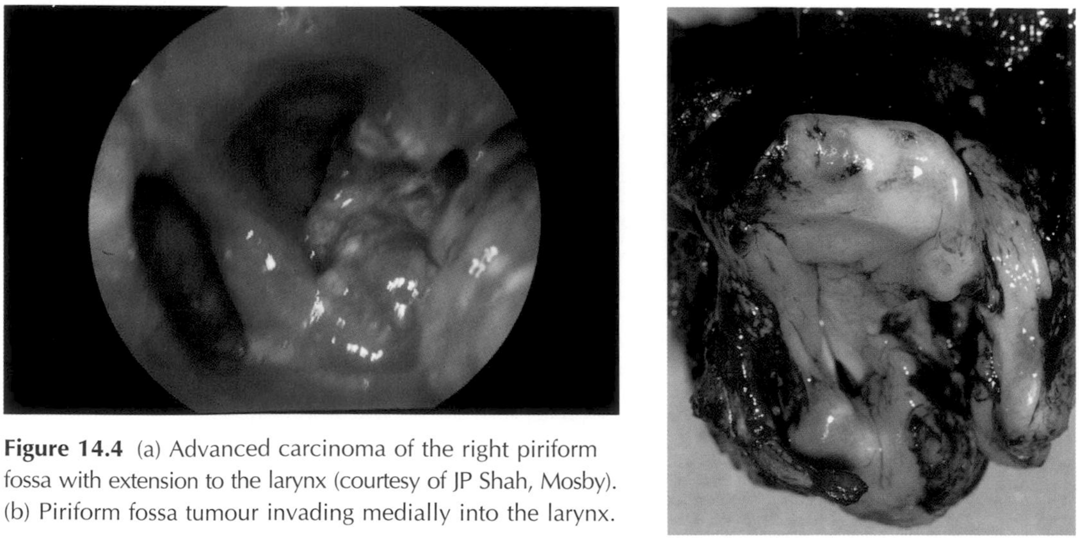

Figure 14.4 (a) Advanced carcinoma of the right piriform fossa with extension to the larynx (courtesy of JP Shah, Mosby). (b) Piriform fossa tumour invading medially into the larynx.

thyroid and upper border of the cricoid cartilage.[29] Olofssen and Van Nostrand[21] noted invasion of the laryngeal muscles in 42% of cases with spread to the false cord in 16%, pre-epiglottic invasion in 5% and tracheal invasion in 5%. Tani et al[44] found that tumours originating on the medial wall, which had extended to the posterior pharyngeal wall or postcricoid region, had all extended into the laryngeal structures.

Tumours of the lateral wall are associated with cartilaginous involvement in 55%, predominantly the posterior border of the thyroid cartilage,[29] and invasion of the thyroid gland in 11%.[21] Superficially tumours may spread onto the posterior pharyngeal wall. Tumours on the lateral wall may penetrate through the pharyngeal wall into the neck without necessarily causing vocal cord fixation, so T1/2 lesions may progress directly to a T4 lesion without a T3 stage.[44]

Tani et al[44] reported normal vocal cord mobility in 20% of cases, partial mobility in 10% and fixed cord in 70% of cases and found that fixation of the cords was strongly associated with intrinsic laryngeal muscle invasion. Involvement of the arytenoid cartilage or cricoarytenoid joint occurred in only 30% of cases and all of these had significant invasion of the intrinsic laryngeal muscles. Tani suggested that in medially based tumours a T1 lesion may progress to a T3 lesion due to involvement of the intrinsic laryngeal muscles without passing through the T2 stage.[44]

Kirchner also found that limitation of vocal cord mobility or fixation was due to invasion of the posterior cricoarytenoid or interarytenoid muscles.[47] Olofsson and Van Nostrand[21] noted that in cases of vocal cord fixation, 42% showed invasion of the intrinsic laryngeal muscles and invasion of the cricoarytenoid joint in 16%. Perineural invasion of the recurrent laryngeal nerve is quite common but is unlikely to be the primary cause of vocal cord fixation.[21]

Kirchner highlighted the problem of understaging with 47% of clinical T3 lesions having cartilage invasion (Figure 14.5)[29] mainly associated with apical and lateral surface extension. None of the T1 or T2 tumours had histological involvement of cartilage. Tani et al[44] pointed out that cartilage involvement was more likely to be contact rather than invasion (Table 14.6) and concluded that the arytenoid cartilage diverts spread either anteromedially to the thyroarytenoid muscle or posteromedially towards the cricoarytenoid joint (seldom invading it) and thence to the postcricoid laryngeal muscles.

Olofssen and Van Nostrand[21] found 42% of pharyngolaryngectomy specimens had thyroid lamina invasion with half of these extending beyond the larynx, 58% involving one or more laryngeal cartilages and epiglottic invasion occurring in 5%.

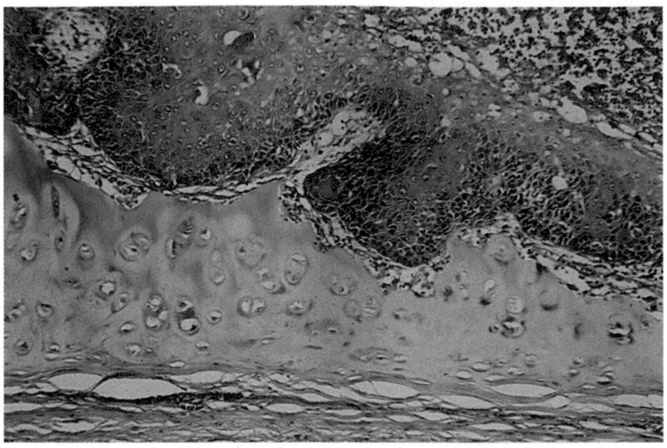

Figure 14.5 Laryngeal cartilage invasion by tumour.

Table 14.6 Analysis of cartilage involvement in piriform fossa lesions[44]

Cartilage	'Involvement' (%)	Contact (%)	Invasion (%)
Thyroid	90	60	30
Cricoid	45	40	5
Arytenoid	50	All	None

Table 14.7 Stage groupings (1988 AJC) at presentation for piriform fossa lesions

Stage	Bataini et al[6] (%)	El Badawi et al[45] (%)
I	3	6
II	4	22
III	50	38
IV	43	34

Regional metastasis

Neck metastasis at presentation is common and the majority of piriform fossa lesions are stage III/IV reflecting a large primary tumour and a high propensity for nodal metastasis (Table 14.7).

Kirchner[29] reported an incidence of 57%, Harrison[46] 65%, Million and Cassisi[40] 75% and Olofssen 63%.[21] In those who had no palpable disease and who had an elective neck dissection, 60% had

Table 14.8 Correlation of clinical with pathological nodal state[29]

	pN+ve (%)	pN–ve (%)
cN+ve	72	28
cN–ve	60	40

Table 14.9 Patterns of histologically proven cervical node metastases related to clinical nodal status[16]

Lymph node region	cN–ve (%)	cN+ve (%)
I	0	6
II	15	72
III	8	72
IV	0	47
V	0	8

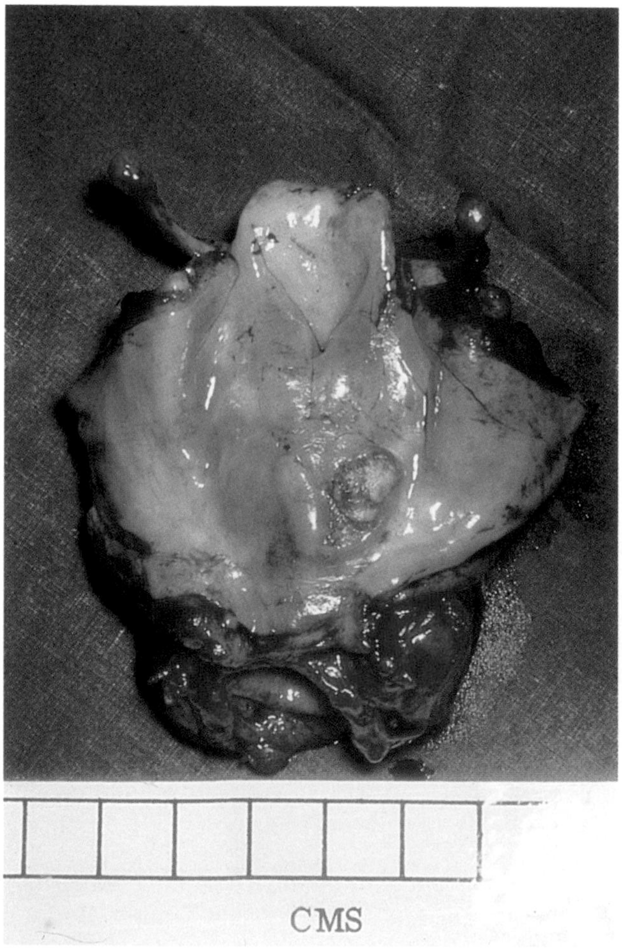

Figure 14.6 Small postcricoid carcinoma.

micrometastases.[29,41] In patients who had palpable neck disease (cN+ve) there was a significant false positive rate of 28% (Table 14.8).[29]

Levels II and III are mainly at risk of micrometastases in cN negative necks[16] but in cN positive patients the pattern of nodal spread suggests that all levels were at significant risk of metastasis (Table 14.9). Involvement of levels I or V is unlikely without simultaneous nodes in levels II, III and IV being present. Patients classified as cN1 were in fact pN2b in 75% of cases (i.e. more than one node involved).

Retropharyngeal node involvement has been found in 56% of patients with T2/3 lesions[10] and bilateral and contralateral nodal disease has been reported in 3–30%[10,27,48] associated with advancing T stage but not with tumour differentiation.[29] Involvement of paratracheal nodes is much lower in hypopharyngeal tumours (8.3%) than with cervical oesophageal carcinoma (71%).[49]

Second primaries

Approximately 6% of patients develop second primaries.[50]

Postcricoid

Primary tumour

Small tumours are unusual (Figure 14.6) and macroscopic mucosal spread at presentation is often extensive (Tables 14.10 and 14.13) with involvement of the piriform fossa and/or the posterior pharyngeal wall in 20–50% of cases. Willatt et al[37] found 35% had a longitudinal macroscopic extension of over 5 cm. Tumours greater than 5 cm in length were associated with circumferential involvement of the hypopharynx and invasion of the thyroid.

The extent of submucosal spread beyond the macroscopic tumour edge is of critical importance as it influences both the radiotherapy fields and the extent of resection and the mode of reconstruction. Davidge-Pitts and Mannel[51] found submucosal spread 5–10 mm above the superior macroscopic extent of the tumour. Inferiorly the average macroscopic extension into the cervical oesophagus was 10 mm with a further 6–30 mm (average 15 mm) of submucosal spread. In Harrison's series[52] submucosal spread was found 5 mm inferiorly and 10 mm superior to the macroscopic margin.

Vocal cord immobility or hemilaryngeal fixation in postcricoid carcinoma is due to direct spread into the paraglottic space or to involvement of the recurrent

Table 14.10 T stage presentation for postcricoid carcinoma

T stage	Stell et al[12] (%)	Farrington et al[33] (%)	Tandon et al[34] (%)	Olofsson and Van Nostrand[21] (%)
T1	32	8	0	27
T2	62	26	17	49
T3	6	24	39	19
T4	—	43	43	5

Table 14.11 Nodal status in postcricoid carcinoma

Nodel status	Stell et al[12] (%)	Pingree et al[53] (%)	Tandon et al[34] (%)	Harrison[46] (%)
N0	67	65	74	48
N+	33	35	26	52

laryngeal nerve. It is a late feature and may be associated with laryngeal cartilage invasion in 26%.[37]

Olofsson and Van Nostrand[21] found that 43% of postcricoid tumours at laryngectomy had invasion of the cricoid cartilage and 14% had involvement of the trachea and thyroid gland.

Regional metastasis

The incidence of cervical node involvement in postcricoid tumours is in the region of 33–52%[12,46] of which a quarter may be bilateral or fixed (Tables 14.11 and 14.12).

Unrecognized spread to paratracheal and lower deep cervical nodes may result in stomal and tracheal ulceration.[46] Hasegawa and Matsuura[10] noted that retropharyngeal nodes were involved in 75% of patients with advanced (stage III/IV) postcricoid primaries.

Table 14.12 Incidence of nodal involvement as related to T stage

T stage	Stell et al[12] (%)	Farrington et al[33] (%)	Tandon et al[34] (%)
T1	34	6	0
T2	38	17	25
T3	50	38	11
T4	—	50	40

Node involvement is associated with a 50% incidence of vocal cord paralysis and 40% of patients will have tumours longer than 5 cm.[30] Like piriform fossa tumours the majority of postcricoid lesions are stage III/IV at presentation (Table 14.13).

Table 14.13 Stage grouping presentation of postcricoid lesions

Stage	Stell et al[12] (%)	Farrington et al[33] (%)	Pingree et al[53] (%)	Tandon et al[34] (%)	Olofsson and Van Nostrand[21] (%)
I	21	7	{15.5} (I–II)	0	21
II	37	21		13	36
III	22	23	{77.6} (III–IV)	39	25
IV	20	49		48	18

Distant metastases and second primaries
Distant metastases from postcricoid carcinomas are rare at presentation with an incidence of between 0 and 2%.[12,21,33,37] The 2% incidence of second primaries[12,50] is less than for piriform fossa tumours (6%).

Patient status
Patients with postcricoid cancer may be unsuitable for radical therapy not only due to very advanced disease but also due to severe weight loss secondary to dysphagia and/or concomitant disease which precludes radical treatment. Jones et al[54] found 25% unsuitable for any treatment and Stell et al[12] noted that in the 30% who had no treatment, half were unsuitable because of poor general health.

Posterior pharyngeal wall

Primary tumour
The commonest site of origin is at the orohypopharyngeal junction:[38,39] 80% are ulcerative/infiltrative[38,39] and 20% are nodular (with a better prognosis). The majority (64%) of tumours (Figure 14.7) are larger than 4 cm at presentation while 8% are under 2 cm, 14% are 2–3 cm and 14% are 3–4 cm.[38]

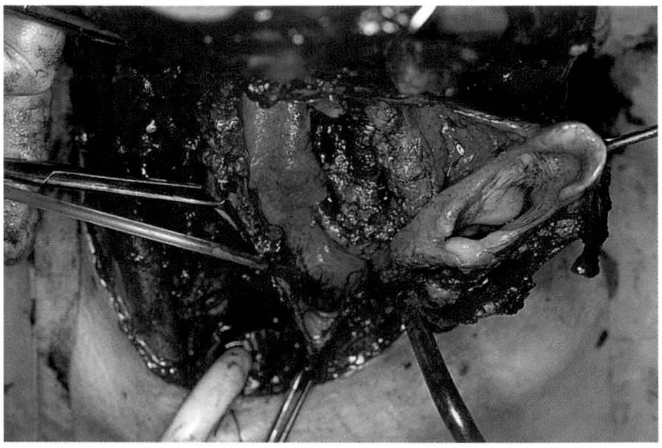

Figure 14.7 Posterior hypopharyngeal wall tumour.

Table 14.14 T stage presentation of posterior hypopharyngeal wall tumours (site-based (%))

T stage	Spiro et al[43]	Pene et al[38]	Teichgraeber and McConnel[55]
T1	14	7	10
T2	48	15	26
T3	23	78	30
T4	15	—	33

Over 85% of tumours (using the site-dependent T system) are T2–4 lesions (Table 14.14) and, in addition, 38–78% are associated with cord fixation.[38,43,55]

Once through the pharyngeal wall these tumours may involve the prevertebral fascia, which acts as a barrier to spread, and laterally through the parapharyngeal space to involve structures of the carotid sheath.[7] These extensions are rare at presentation but are not uncommon with recurrent disease following primary radiotherapy.

Regional metastasis
The first echelon of nodes to be involved in posterior hypopharyngeal wall tumours are levels II, III and retropharyngeal.[36] Candela's study of elective and therapeutic neck dissections also showed that once the neck was clinically positive all nodal levels were pathologically involved at a significant rate with 20%, 84%, 72%, 40% and 21% in levels I, II, III, IV and V, respectively.[16] It was also noted that involvement of the submandibular (I) or posterior triangles (V) did not occur without cN positive nodes in II, III and IV. Three-quarters of clinically N1 necks had multiple histologically involved nodes involved (pN2) and thus levels I and V were at significant risk. Retropharyngeal node involvement is in the region of 42%,[18] rising to 67% with stage III/IV disease.[10]

Overall, the incidence of nodal disease is between 35 and 45% and is associated with increasing T stage with the incidence of nodal disease being 33%, 10–12%, 40–77% and 50–80% at T1, T2, T3 and T4, respectively.[36,43,55]

Stage grouping
As with other hypopharyngeal carcinomas, very few cases present as stage I and two-thirds of patients have stages III or IV disease (Table 14.15).[36,43,55]

Distant metastasis and second primaries
Distant metastases are seen more frequently on presentation (3–10%) than with postcricoid lesions.[38,55] There is often a history (37%) of previous malignancy of the upper aerodigestive tract (50% laryngeal, 33% oral) and 10% may be found incidently as part of a diagnostic work-up for another primary.[43] Teichgraeber et al[55] reported 20% with metachronous and 3% synchronous second carcinomas with two-thirds of metachronous carcinomas occuring in the upper aerodigestive tract.

Table 14.15 Posterior hypopharyngeal wall staging at presentation (%)

Stage	Spiro et al[43]	Jones and Stell[36]	Teichgraeber and McConnel[55]*
I	9	26	6
II	37	16	23
III	29	26	16
IV	25	32	55

*Orohypopharyngeal (using an unspecified TNM system in 1985).

Investigations

A barium swallow, to determine the upper and lower extent of the tumour as well as any distortion or displacement of the pharyngeal/oesophageal lumen, should be carried out before endoscopy to reduce the risk of perforation. Endoscopic examination under general anaesthetic is essential to determine the mucosal extent and the presence of deep fixation. It should also include oesophagoscopy, laryngoscopy and bronchoscopy to further assess the involvement of adjacent structures and to investigate the possibility of second primaries. Imaging should include CT, and ideally MRI, of the neck and superior mediastinum to assess local extension and cervical, paratracheal, retropharyngeal and mediastinal nodal disease. Fine needle aspiration of any suspicious nodes sould be performed. The search for distant metastasis (chest X-ray, CT chest and liver ultrasound) is important for accurate clinical staging.

Treatment

General comments

The treatment of hypopharyngeal carcinoma has been one of the most challenging and controversial areas in the head and neck surgery. There is potential conflict between organ (larynx) preservation, optimum quality of life and survival. Management is therefore a complex assessment of: tumour factors (i.e. the response of the tumour to treatment modalities); patient factors (i.e. the wishes of the patient, their ability to attend follow-up, and physical and psychological health); physician factors (i.e. the ability of the physician to deliver effectively the treatment modality of choice); evidence factors (i.e the quality of the scientific base underpinning treatment).

Tumour factors

Tumour size

Larger and deeply infiltrating tumours are less likely to be controlled with radiotherapy because of high 'tumour load' and an associated higher proportion of hypoxic radioresistant cells. Tumours with true invasion of cartilage, rather than just 'contact' are also less likely to be cured with radiotherapy.

Nodal stage

The presence of neck metastases is usually a strong indication for primary surgical treatment of the neck disease, particularly for N2–3 disease where capsular rupture is frequently present. Persistent or recurrent tumour in the neck after radiotherapy is difficult to diagnose and salvage surgery rarely succeeds. It is generally accepted that the high incidence of micrometastases in cN negative necks requires elective treatment of the neck.

Patient factors

Patient preferences

It is of paramount importance that the patient is given balanced information concerning the benefits and disadvantages of the range of treatment options available. This helps them to choose what is appropriate to the perception of their needs.

Performance status

This group of patients are often debilitated by a period of progressive dysphagia and weight loss and are thus often poor candidates for either surgery or radiotherapy. It is important to consider, at a very early stage, some form of hyperalimentation irrespective of the choice of treatment to avoid the debilitating effects of weight loss alone.

Follow-up

In a proportion of patients whose tumour persists or recurs after radical radiotherapy, long-term survival can still be achieved by salvage surgery. Successful salvage surgery can only be achieved with meticulous follow-up and early diagnosis. Where regular visits are not feasable or the patient's attendance unpredictable, radiotherapy alone may not be the optimum primary treatment choice.

Physician factors

The multidisciplinary team dealing with the patient must not only have an appreciation of the best treatment choice but also must know their ability to deliver the treatment modality of choice with acceptable levels of morbidity, peri-operative mortality and survival. Referral to another centre may be appropriate.

Evidence factors

There are few randomized controlled trials on management of hypopharyngeal tumours with most of the literature on this subject being anecdotal and poorly controlled. There is also a lack of data on the 'quality of life' consequences of each treatment modality.

Treatment of the piriform fossa

Primary tumour

Radiotherapy

For T1 and early T2 lesions without nodal metastases, treatment to the primary site may be given from lateral fields to a dose of 50 Gy in 25 fractions to the entire volume, then reducing fields to cover the primary site only with a further 15 Gy in five fractions. In patients with more advanced local disease where surgery is unsuitable for any reason, consideration should be given to radical irradiation of primary and neck using one of the protocols aiming to improve the effectiveness of radiotherapy.

Surgery

As most tumours are advanced at presentation the mainstay of surgical treatment is total laryngectomy with partial or total pharyngectomy with reconstruction of the pharyngeal defect and voice restoration. For the rare early lesions in young healthy individual with good respiratory function, partial pharyngectomy or partial pharyngolaryngectomy should be considered. The surgical indications are set out in Table 14.16.

Table 14.16 Indications for partial/conservation surgery[56,57]

The true cords and arytenoids must be freely mobile and free of gross tumour involvement
No involvement of the apex of the piriform sinus
No thyroid cartilage invasion
No postcricoid involvement

These criteria are highly selective for early tumours of the upper lateral wall of the piriform fossa provided that the patient's cardiorespiratory function is good. There is general agreement with Kirchner[29] that salvage conservation surgery is contraindicated for radiotherapy recurrence because of unpredictable invasion patterns and poor healing.

Partial hypopharyngeal surgery is an evolving field and work by Steiner et al[58–61] using transoral CO_2 laser microsurgery on hypopharyngeal lesions (92% piriform fossa in origin) has shown promising results. It has the advantage of not precluding further endoscopic resection, conventional partial or radical resections or radiotherapy. Nodal disease is treated using selective or radical unilateral or bilateral neck dissection for both cN negative and cN positive disease. Adjuvant chemoradiotherapy is based on pT and pN data.

Reconstruction surgery

Resections of the medial wall of the piriform fossa combined with total laryngectomy may be closed primarily provided that there is a residual pharyngeal circumference of at least 6–7 cm. Anything less than this will require a skin 'patch', either a pectoralis major or latissimus dorsi myocutaneous flap (Figure 14.8), which are straightforward and highly dependable in this situation, or a more complex free radial forearm flap.[62] Steiner et al[58] have been resecting both these and lower piriform fossa lesions and allowing the defect to heal by secondary intention with little associated morbidity.

In lower piriform fossa lesions the resultant defect is typically a circumferential pharyngeal defect requiring a 'tubed' reconstruction of some kind either a free jejunal graft or a tubed pectoralis major flap or latissimus dorsi flap (Figure 14.9).[62]

With postcricoid involvement the resultant defect is of a circumferential pharyngo-oesophageal type. (See treatment of postcricoid carcinoma for further discussion.)

Regional disease

Radiotherapy

In a clinically node-negative neck, elective irradiation of levels II, III and IV is advisable because of the high incidence of micrometastases. In node-positive patients the entire lymphatic drainage of the neck must be treated including the contralateral deep cervical chain, which is involved in about 15% of cases.[48] Up to 44 Gy can safely be given to the whole neck. For the second phase of treatment alternatives are oblique fields, or lateral fields anterior to the cord plus electron fields to the posterior part of the neck.

(a)

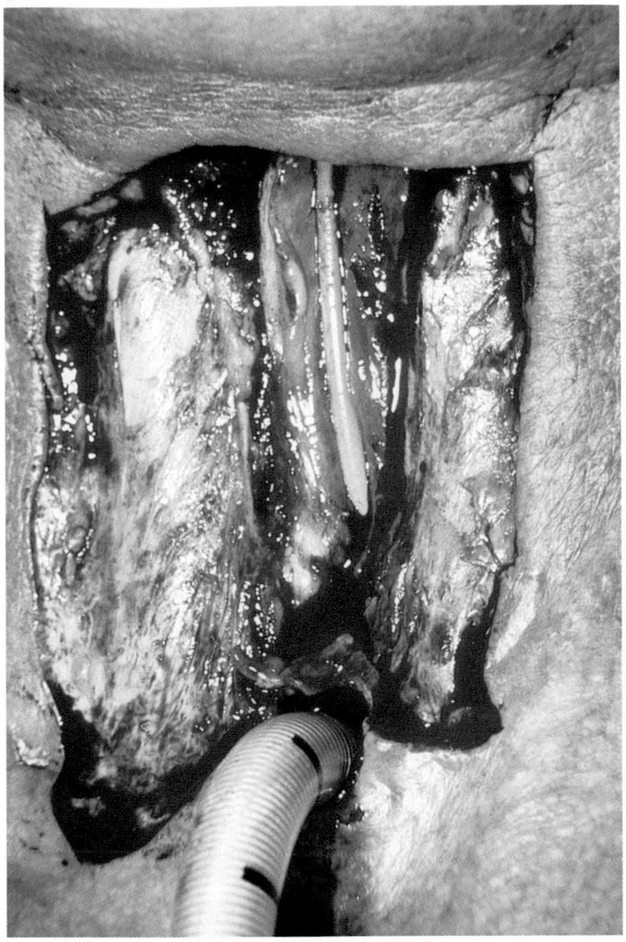

(b)

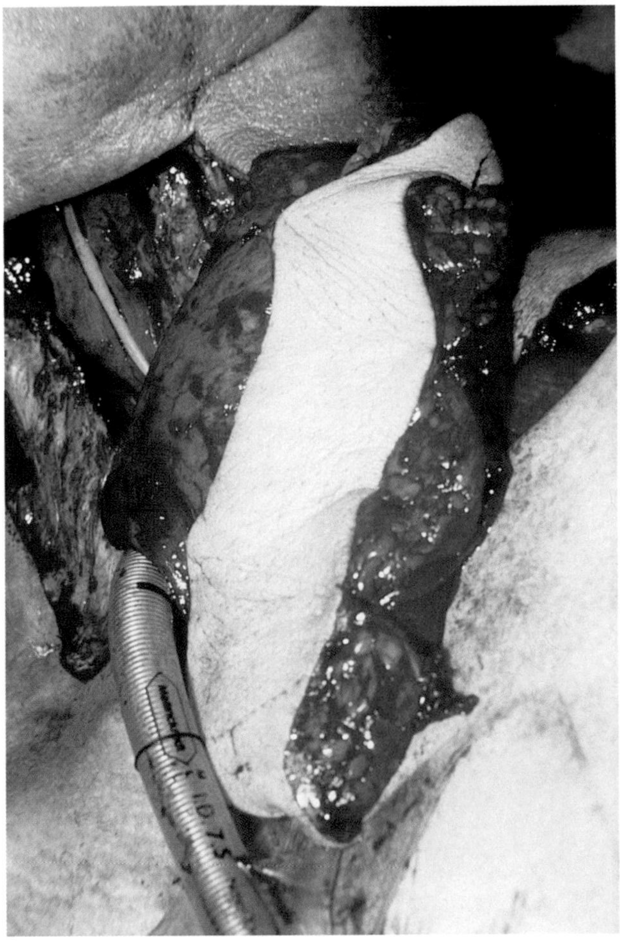

(c)

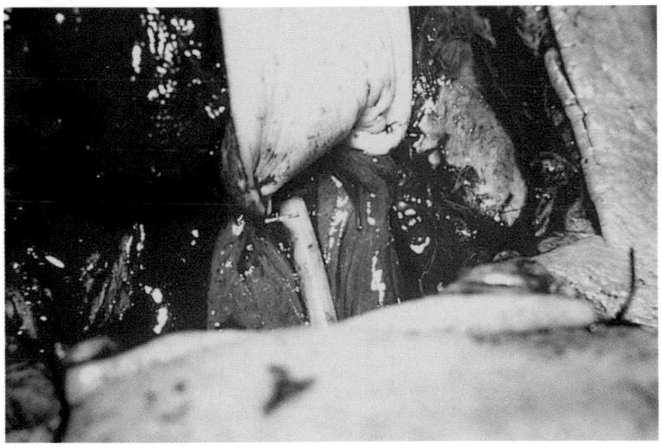

Figure 14.8 (a) Hypopharyngeal defect following subtotal pharyngolaryngectomy, leaving posterior strip of mucosa. (b) Latissimus dorsi flap raised. (c) Flap being sutured into position.

Surgery

Surgical staging (i.e. the removal of level II, III and IV nodes) of the cN negative neck gives a clearer understanding of disease progression, allows the selective use of adjuvant chemoradiotherapy and has therapeutic value in pN+ disease as well as low morbidity. In the cN positive neck surgery is more likely to achieve regional control for large or multiple nodes. In N1 disease radiotherapy is a good alternative for nodes under 2 cm in diameter, but for larger nodes there is an increased risk of extracapsular spread and central necrosis with a corresponding reduction in control if radiotherapy alone is used.

Combined radiotherapy/surgery

If radical radiotherapy has been given, particularly when the primary tumour is small and there is a reasonable chance of sparing the larynx, any residual

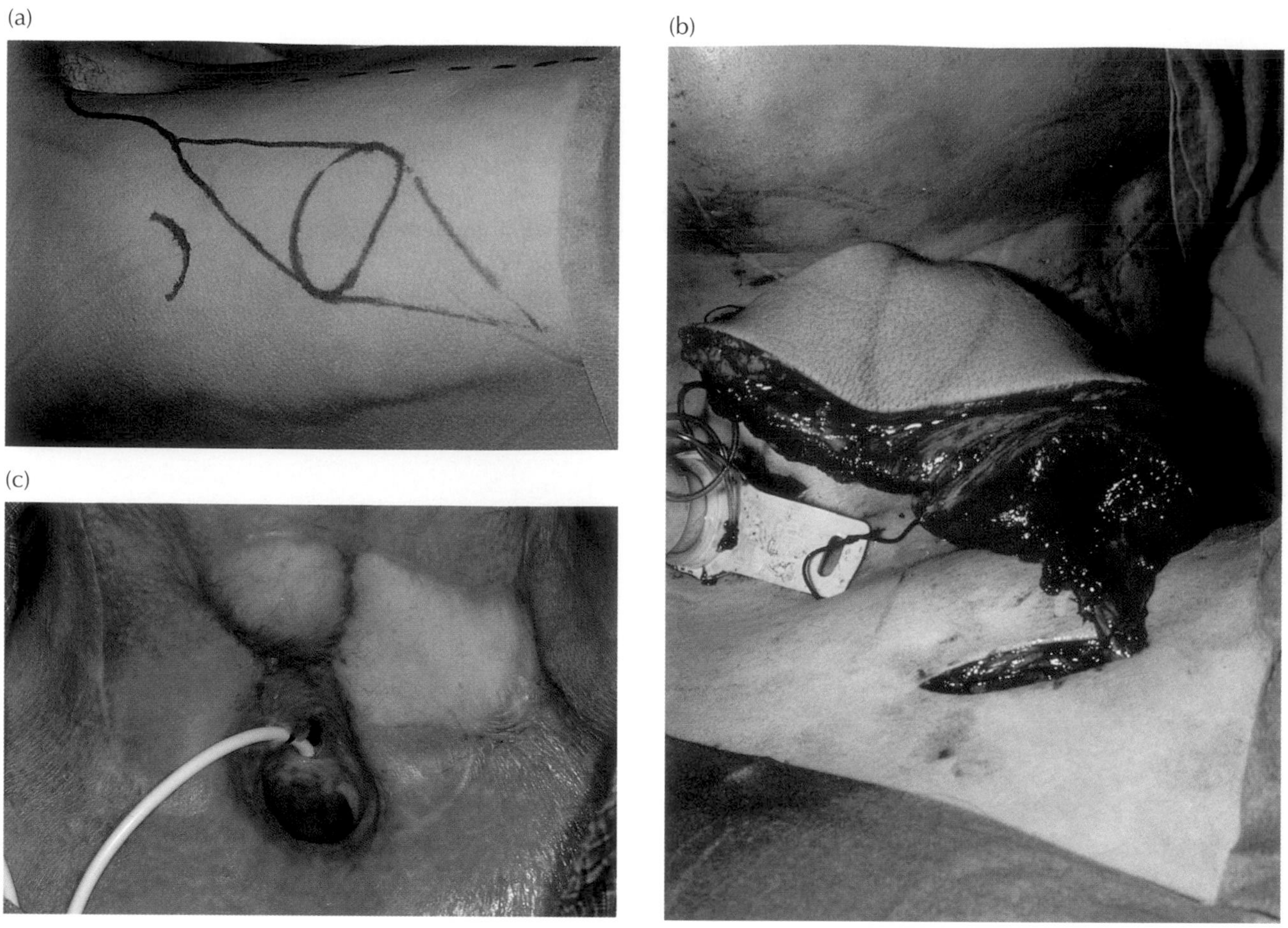

Figure 14.9 (a) Latissimus dorsi flap used for circumferential reconstruction of the hypopharynx and anterior neck skin defect. (b) Flap raised. (c) Six months postoperation (note large tracheo-oesophageal fistula tract requiring subsequent closure with a sternomastoid flap).

node(s) or even significant thickening at the node site should be excised at about 6–8 weeks after completion of treatment.

Shrinkage of the metastatic nodes as a result of treatment is not sufficient to guarantee radiotherapeutic cure, even in the absence of positive cytology. CT scanning is unreliable after radiotherapy; therefore, two strategies may be employed; either a relatively low threshold for elective neck dissections if there is clinical or CT evidence of abnormality or the combined use of a PET scan and subsequent ultrasound-guided fine-needle aspiration which may help to differentiate between residual fibrosis and persistent disease. For N2–3 disease, cure with radiotherapy alone is unlikely and an interval neck dissection at 6–8 weeks is almost always necessary unless there is total disappearance of all lymphadenopathy.

Retropharyngeal nodes should be cleared if involvement is suspected on a CT scan or by palpation at operation.

Treatment of the postcricoid

General comments

As with all patients with a resectable head and neck cancer a fundamental management decision has to be made between primary surgery and postoperative radiotherapy versus primary radiotherapy (with salvage surgery). The advantage of primary surgery in postcricoid carcinoma is immediate restitution of swallow and reasonable cure rates, but the disadvantages are loss of the larynx and the morbidity and mortality associated with resection and reconstruction.

The option of no treatment results in a rapid and unpleasant demise of the patient with 50% dead at 6 weeks, 90% at 4 months and 100% at 9 months.[33] The results of palliative radiotherapy, however, are only marginally better with 50% dead at 5 months, 90% dead at 12 months and none surviving 4 years.[33]

Primary tumour

Radiotherapy
Postcricoid tumours are often large and infiltrate down the cervical oesophagus. This large volume is difficult to irradiate to an adequate but safe dose. In some cases the disease may be encompassed by lateral angled-down fields, but often this technique gives an inadequate dose to the lower part of the target volume at the thoracic inlet. An alternative is to treat the primary tumour and cervical region with anterior oblique fields.

Surgery
The aim of surgeryis to eradicate the cancer with the minimum morbidity and mortality. This will result in a circumferential defect with the loss of the larynx. Minimal oncological clearance of the inferior margin requires resection at least 3 cm beyond the macroscopic extent thus resulting in a total laryngo-pharygectomy. For maximal oncological clearance, eradicating possible submucosal oesophageal skip lesions, the entire oesophagus is removed in continuity thus resulting in a total laryngo-pharyngoesophagectomy.

The choice between the two approaches is determed by the inferior extent of the tumour into the thoracic inlet, the presence and estimated probability of skip lesions, the ability of the patient to tolerate a trans-thoracic resection and reconstruction and the technical feasibility of performing a jejuno-oesophageal anastamosis.

Involvement of the tracheo-oesophageal groove/ posterior tracheal wall is also an important consideration. It is often difficult to dissect low in the neck and care must be taken to avoid tearing the trachealis muscle as this can rapidly dissect towards the carina with associated ventilatory difficulties.[3] Extensive tracheal resection may require a low suprasternal tracheostomy or even a manubrial resection.

Reconstruction surgery
Oncological clearance is of paramount importance and dictates the extent of resection and thus determines the method of reconstruction.

If it is possible to perform a jejunoesophageal anastamosis with oncological safety then a jejunal interposition may be preferable, in some patients, to the morbidity and mortality of gastric transposition. It should be noted that jejunal interposition is not without hazard as it involves two bowel anastomoses and two microvascular anastomoses.

Limited involvement of the upper trachea may necessitate a small deltopectoral flap for reconstruction.

Whichever technique of resection and reconstruction is chosen it should only be performed by experienced teams.

Regional disease

Radiotherapy
Both the superior mediastinum and the upper cervical nodes may be involved (level II) and radiotherapy should cover levels II, III, IV, paratracheal and retropharyngeal areas as well as level V if there is palpable disease. The neck nodes may be treated separately with an anterior split field.

Surgery
In N0 necks levels II, III, IV, paratracheal and retropharyngeal are cleared on both sides because of bilateral lymphatic drainage. If there is palpable disease at levels II, III or IV, level V should also be dissected as well as the superior mediastinum if there is radiological or palpable disease in this area using, if necessary, an upper sternotomy approach.[63]

Treatment of the posterior pharyngeal wall

Primary tumour

Radiotherapy
Radiotherapy requires accurate planning with lateral fields because of the close proximity of the spinal cord. Full thickness tumour infiltration of the posterior wall may often result in a large necrotic ulcer on the prevertebral fascia and anterior spinal ligament. This is frequently painful and due to the poor vascularity in this area may take a long time to heal.

Surgery
The size of the lesion dictates the extent of the resection and reconstruction (Table 14.17) but the most important functional consideration is whether the larynx is removed or retained. The age and health status of the patient must also be taken into consideration.

Larynx preservation
For small tumours confined to the posterior wall excision can be achieved through a lateral pharyngotomy. To minimize the risk of postoperative complications several points of surgical technique are important:

Table 14.17 Methods of resection and reconstruction[43]

Resection		Percentage
Transoral local resection		12
Transhyoid/anterior pharyngotomy		12
Lateral pharyngotomy		11
Median labiomandibular glossotomy		11
Mandibular swing, paralingual extension		11
Pharyngo-oesophagectomy		2
Pharyngolaryngectomy		16
Pharyngolaryngo-oesophagectomy		21
Circumferential pharyngectomy		5
Reconstruction (by site staging)		
T1	Split skin graft	100
T2	Split skin graft	29
	Deltopectoral flap	29
	Pectoralis major flap	21
	Gastric transfer	7
	Radial forearm free flap	14
T3	Deltopectoral flap	20
	Pectoralis major flap	20
	Gastric transfer	60
T4	Gastric transfer	100

1. The posterior margin of the thyroid cartilage may be removed to improve access.
2. The main postoperative risk is from aspiration because of loss of sensation and muscular activity on the posterior pharyngeal wall. Identification and preservation of the internal and external branches of the superior laryngeal nerve is therefore essential.
3. A small defect may be left to granulate and epithelialize or may be covered with a split skin graft (Figure 14.10a). Larger resections extending onto the lateral pharyngeal wall in very selected cases may be suitable for reconstruction with a free radial forearm flap (Figure 14.10b) or jejunum. In our experience more bulky flaps do not give a satisfactory functional result.
4. Temporary tracheostomy and insertion of a PEG are required to minimize the risk of aspiration but even so, rehabilitation may be prolonged.
5. Postoperative problems of healing and aspiration are much more likely in salvage surgery following previous irradiation.

Many tumours of the posterior pharyngeal wall and selected patients with recurrence following irradiation require total laryngectomy in addition to pharyngeal resection. It may be possible to safely retain mucosa of the postcricoid region and some of the piriform fossa in which case a myocutaneous skin paddle may be the most effective method of reconstruction.

Regional disease

Radiotherapy

In node negative patients a radical dose is given to the primary (and retropharyngeal nodes) and elective irradiation of node levels II, III and IV bilaterally. The technique used involves lateral fields of 50 Gy in 25 fractions to the entire volume, reducing the fields to cover the primary only with a further 15 Gy in five fractions. In node-positive disease level V nodes should also be included and planned interval neck dissection for any persistent nodal abnormality.

Nodal metastases are often bilateral and primarily involve levels II, III and retropharyngeal nodes. If surgery for the primary is the treatment of choice with a cN negative neck a bilateral selective dissection of levels II, III, IV and retropharyngeal nodes is

(a)

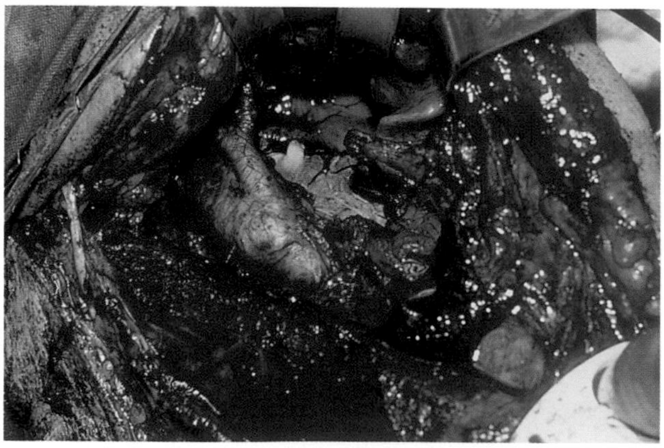

(b)

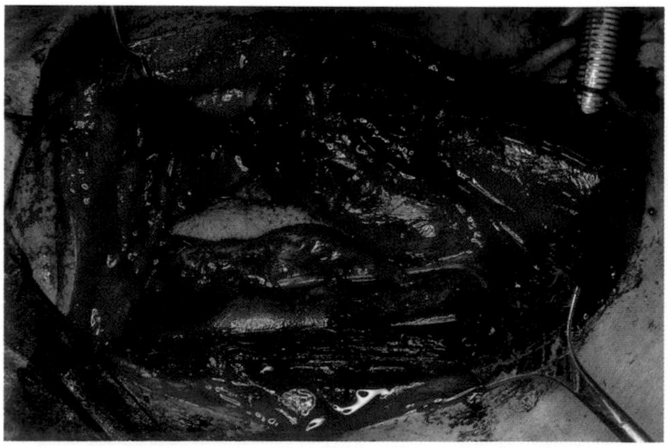

Figure 14.10 (a) Skin graft for defect on posterior pharyngeal wall. (b) Radial forearm free flap for defect on posterior pharyngeal wall extending on to the lateral pharyngeal wall.

advisable with a full (modified) radical neck dissection where the neck is clinically involved.

Results of treatment comparing radiation and surgery

The literature consists of three fundamental groups of papers. The first group comprises studies of primary radiotherapy with or without chemotherapy and salvage surgery. The results tend to be stratified by stage groupings rather than by the T system and are thus less able to deliver the 'answers' that surgeons want. Regimes have changed radically over time making comparisons difficult between different institutions.

The second group is composed of studies of primary surgery with or without postoperative radiation. These results tend to be stratified by the T system. The results of surgery depend mainly on the skill of the surgical team with wide variations (6–50%) in mortality rate. Patients who survive the operation have a high chance of cure and recent advances in voice rehabilitation have greatly improved quality of life considerations. Direct comparisons between individual techniques and different institutions are again difficult as these have changed over time.

The third group comprises studies of primary radiotherapy with or without chemotherapy and salvage surgery compared with primary surgery with or without postoperative radiation. Unless these studies are prospective randomized controlled trials in which the comparison groups are matched, the results make valid conclusions very difficult

Treatment results: piriform fossa

General comments

The goal of treatment is to ablate disease and preserve a functional laryngopharynx. The piriform fossa is the only hypopharyngeal subsite that has had treatment outcomes, comparing primary surgery with primary radiotherapy investigated using a randomized controlled trial. The rest of the literature consists of non-randomized studies.

Randomized controlled trial data comparing surgery with radiation: The EORTC Organ Preservation Study[64]

This is one of the few prospective controlled randomized trials in head and neck oncology and is the only one that compares the results of chemoradiation and surgery in hypopharyngeal carcinoma. In this study the EORTC Head and Neck Cancer Cooperative Group investigated the effect of chemoselection followed by radiation in T2-4, N0-2ab (and operable N3) piriform fossa lesions, in which the control was radical surgery and postoperative radiation.

The trial was designed to have a chemoselection arm in which patients received cis-platinum and 5-fluorouracil as chemoselectors for irradiation.[65] Chemoresponders were treated with radical radiotherapy and salvage surgery if necessary or possible. Non-responders were assumed to be relatively radioinsensitive and had immediate surgery followed by postoperative irradiation. These were compared with the control arm where all patients were treated with primary radical surgery and post-operative radiation. Patients were prospectively randomized into each arm and subsequently matched for tumour staging, age and sex. The outcome was evaluated in terms of overall survival, local/regional/distant control and preservation of a functional larynx.

The results showed that survival in the chemoselection arm was better at 3 years (57% versus 43%) than in those undergoing surgery but the 5-year survival remained similar (30% versus 35%). This may be due to later appearance of distant metastases in the chemotherapy group leading to a better 3-year survival but this effect does not last long enough to impact on the 5-survival.[66] Survivors in the chemoselection arm had a 50% chance of retaining a functioning larynx at 3 years and at 5 years. All the survivors in the primary surgical arm had undergone total laryngectomy. Those patients who had a complete response to chemotherapy had a 64% and 58% chance of retaining a functioning larynx at 3 and 5 years, respectively. None of the T4 lesions in the chemoselection had a complete response and therefore all had primary surgery. The relapse pattern was equal in both arms with respect to local and locoregional failures. This latter aspect is unusual as most other reports indicate poorer locoregional control with radiation alone and may be attributable to the chemotherapy. Thirty-six percent of patients in the surgery arm developed distant metastases as compared with 25% in the chemoselection arm.

Forastiere[67] and Stockwell[68] comment that this trial should be viewed as an alternative therapy for the informed patient desiring voice preservation and mandates enrolment in investigational protocols, if feasible. Forastiere states that it is too soon to adopt this as a new standard and also advises caution because the functional and productive quality of life of patients treated by chemotherapy and radiotherapy treatment programs is not established.[67]

In 1999 Lefebvre[66,69] commented that preservation regimes have not jeopardized survival and have allowed preservation of the larynx. In addition meta-analysis of this study, the GETTEC study (a study similar to the Veterans Affairs (VA) study but including T3 larynx disease) and the VA study showed no significant difference in survival but a laryngeal preservation rate of 53%. The analysis by subgroups of patients may vary both positively and negatively according to anatomical subsite, biological profiles and tumour extension. This method of selection may be only one of many strategies used to detect those patients who are suitable for either laryngeal preservation or ablation as the best treatment for them. He concludes that surgery remains, in some cases, the best solution and suggests that a larynx-preserving approach cannot be considered as a standard, and remains in the field of clinical research.

The power of the EORTC study is not only in the results that it gives but also in its design i.e. a randomized controlled trial. It is imperative clinicians investigating the use of these and other modalities investigate their efficacy with an equally robust methodology.

Non-randomized controlled trial data: Primary Radiotherapy

Million and Cassisi[70] reviewed the policy of radical irradiation for carcinoma of the piriform fossa between 1964 and 1978 and reported that irradiation gave high levels of local control for early (Tl and T2) lesions, but more advanced lesions were associated with significantly lower survival (Tables 14.18 and 14.19).

Failure of T1 lesions was mainly due to apical involvement in laterally originating lesions with 100% control with irradiation for anteriorly and medially originating lesions and 63% control for laterally originating lesions. Apical involvement is a poor prognostic sign due to the high probability of early cartilagenous involvement and understaging.

Million and Cassisi[70] recommended that T1 and favourable T2/3 lesions (i.e. no apical involvement) should be treated with primary irradiation and salvage surgery. Unfavourable T2/3 lesions (with apical involvement) may be managed with a policy of either: (a) primary surgery with postoperative radiation; or (b) primary irradiation to a level of 50 Gy provided that if the response is poor (e.g. failure of return of vocal cord mobility) early salvage surgery should be advised.

They also recommended T4 lesions require primary surgery with postoperative irrradiation.

From the same institution Mendenhall et al[71] in 1987 reviewed all stages of piriform fossa lesions treated with irradiation and salvage surgery from 1964 to 1984. It was again noted that local control for T1–3 lesions was good but there was no success with T4 lesions (ultimate local control was 89%, 90%, 60% and 0% at T1, T2, T3 and T4, respectively[71]). The determinate survival was also proportionately reduced in stage III/IV disease with 5-year determinate survival at 100% for stages I and II and 62% and 45% for stages III and IV, respectively.

Bataini et al[6] reported a series of 434 piriform fossa carcinomas (excluding the epilarynx as these had a 15% better overall survival) treated with primary radiotherapy and salvage surgery at the Institut Curie using the 1972 UICC staging system in which T3

Table 14.18 Ultimate local control with primary irradiation[58]

T stage	Local control (%)
T1	79
T2	90
T3	50
T4	14

Table 14.19 Survival with radiation in relation to stage[70]

	Determinate survival	
Stage	2 years (%)	5 years (%)
I/II	83	66
III	73	43
IV	55	11
Overall	64	32

Table 14.20 Survival as related to T stage[6]

	Determinate survival	
T stage	2 years (%)	5 years (%)
T1	56	49
T2	62	48
T3	52	39
Overall	54	41

lesions in 1972 are equivalent to T3/4 lesions using the 1997 system (Table 14.20). The cause-specific survival was twice the absolute survival indicating the high level of intercurrent disease and second primaries. In T1/2 lesions local control was significantly better if the dose level was greater than or equal to 65 Gy (65%) as compared with less than 65 Gy (36%). T3 lesions showed no dose-related improvement between 50 Gy and 75 Gy.

Mendenhall et al[72] also compared radiotherapy alone or followed by neck dissection for T1/2 lesions. The 5-year rates of local control and ultimate local control were 88% and 94% for stage I and 79% and 91% for stage II disease. When grouped for stage the cause-specific survival was 100% for I and II , 83% for III, and 51% for IV. He concluded that comparison with available data from series using conservation surgery showed similar rates of local control and survival but less risk of fatal and non-fatal complications.

Primary Surgery

Conventional conservation surgery

Conservation of the larynx with primary surgery is achievable in a proportion of carefully selected early lesions. In 1980, Ogura et al[73] found that partial laryngopharyngectomy and low-dose preoperative radiation in selected cases resulted in a 59% 3-year actuarial survival with 52% of patients treated by conservation surgery. Barton[74] found the 5-year determinate survival was 55% when treating 22 selected cases of early piriform fossa carcinoma with partial laryngopharyngectomy. Czaja and Gluckman, however, noted that the rare hypopharyngeal lesions, which were amenable to partial pharyngectomy had a local recurrence rate of 44%. This high recurrence rate was thought to be due to submucosal disease and 'skip lesions' and they suggested that limited resection for early hypopharyngeal lesions was ill-advised.[75]

Conservation transoral laser microsurgery of hypopharyngeal (predominantly piriform) cancer

Steiner[58–61] has used transoral laser microsurgery, neck dissection and early radiotherapy for hypopharyngeal cancer (92% piriform fossa lesions) aiming at complete locoregional tumour resection with laryngopharyngeal function preservation. The group consisted of 70% of patients with stage III/IV disease (previously untreated). With a median follow-up of 104 months the reported results were that four patients required a temporary tracheostomy and none had a laryngectomy. The 5-year crude survival was 64% (83% adjusted survival rate) with 17% dying of the hypopharyngeal cancer, 10% of second primaries and 10% of intercurrent diseases. These very promising results need further evaluation.

Radical surgery

El Badawi et al[45] at MD Anderson found that primary surgery and postoperative irradiation for predominantly T3/4 lesions gave an actuarial survival at 2 and 5 years of 55% and 40%. Locoregional recurrence rates were halved by primary surgery and radiotherapy as compared to radiotherapy alone.

Surgery compared with radiotherapy

In the 1987 series from the Institut Gustave-Roussy, Van den Brouck et al[32] reports two groups treated with primary surgery or radiotherapy. The radiotherapy group had a greater proportion of T2 tumours with the primary surgery group having more T3 lesions (Table 14.21). The overall survival was higher with surgery compared with radiation even though the lesions treated with radiation were generally earlier. Locoregional recurrence was also much higher in the radiotherapy group (Table 14.22). This paper[32] suggests that survival is higher with surgery alone compared to irradiation for advanced disease and that locoregional recurrence is much higher with radiation alone. They conclude that the strategy of primary surgery followed by postoperative radiation appeared to be the better course.

Table 14.21 T stage distribution of two treatment modalities[32]

T stage	Radiotherapy (%)	Surgery (%)
T1	13	14
T2	26	3
T3	54	78
T4	8	5

Table 14.22 Survival and locoregional recurrence rates related to treatment modality[32]

	Overall survival (%)		Locoregional recurrence (%)
	3 years	5 years	
Radiotherapy	25	14	44
Surgery	48	33	17.5

Table 14.23 Determinate survival as related to nodal status[6]

Nodel status	Determinate survival (%) 2 years	5 years
N0	60	48
N1	62	50
N2	30	28
N3	40	30

Management of regional disease

Primary radiotherapy

Bataini et al[6] found survival was significant affected by nodal status (Table 14.23). Metastases of less than or equal to 3 cm showed a significantly improved control if the dose was greater than or equal to 65 Gy compared with less than 65 Gy (93% versus 40%). For nodes greater than 3 cm a significantly improved control was obtained if the dose was greater than or equal to 70 Gy compared with less than or equal to 65 Gy (79% versus 23%).

Radiotherapy and surgery compared

Million and Cassisi[70] found irradiation with or without neck dissection very successful in controlling N0 and N1 neck disease but combination therapy was required for more advanced disease and this became progressively less effective (Table 14.24).

Salvage surgery

Million and Cassisi[70] noted the policy of salvage surgery resulted in an increase in local control from 57% to 65%. In local failures after primary irradiation only one-third had attempted salvage surgery, of which 60% were successful.

At the Princess Margaret Hospital, Toronto, 54% of patients developed locoregional failure alone for hypopharyngeal lesions (85% piriform) after irradiation.[22] Of these only 45% underwent salvage surgery, which was successful in only one in four cases. The overall locoregional control was 41% composed of 35% from radiation alone and 6% from salvage surgery. Bataini et al[6] found that locoregional failure occurred in approximately half of irradiated cases (local failure: 52%; regional failure: 18%; and locoregional failure: 30%). Salvage surgery was employed in only 4% of recurrent cases of which none was successful if the recurrence was local and only 20% if regional. Salvage surgery therefore only increased the overall survival by 0.5%, highlighting the difficulties and limitations of salvage surgery following high-dose irradiation.

It would appear that the role of salvage surgery for piriform fossa lesions contributes a modest component in the overall survival of between 0.5%[6] and 8%.[70]

Treatment results: postcricoid

General comments

There are no randomized controlled trials and therefore one can draw only very limited conclusions.

Primary radiotherapy

In a large series from the UK, treated with radiotherapy (96% of cases) and salvage surgery Farrington et al[33] reported a cause-specific 5-year survival in the radically treated group of 22% (Table 14.25). Survival decreased significantly with lesions more than 2 cm in length and for tumours over 4 cm the survival at 5 years was less than 5% (Table 14.26). In addition vocal cord palsy was a very poor prognostic feature (Table 14.27) irrespective of the treatment modality.

Table 14.24 Neck disease control related to treatment modality[70]

Nodal status	Irradiation alone (%)	Irradiation and surgery (%)
N0	100	—
N1	65	100
N2	65	83
N3	0	40

Table 14.25 Primary radiotherapy: cause-specific survival[33]

T stage	Cause-specific survival by year (%) 1	2	3	4	5
T1 (< 2 cm)	80	70	55	50	50
T2 (2–4 cm)	55	40	25	20	20
T3 (> 4 cm)	30	20	10	5	3
T4	25	10	5	5	3

Table 14.26 Tumour length correlated to actuarial survival[33]

Tumour length (cm)	Actuarial survival by year (%)		
	1	2	5
< 5	60	40	30
> 5	30	23	20

Table 14.27 Vocal palsy correlated to actuarial survival[33]

	Actuarial survival by year (%)		
	1	2	5
Vocal cord palsy	15	10	0
No vocal cord palsy	45	45	35

Primary irradiation compared with primary surgery

Axon et al[69] compared the effect of surgery or radiotherapy in treating postcricoid carcinoma and recommended that surgery was a better method of improving survival especially in patients with no nodal disease. In this series, however, the surgical group consisted of 69% stage III/IV whereas the radiotherapy arm had 71% stage I/II. In addition, 28% of patients in the surgical arm had had previous radiotherapy. There was a 14% peri-operative mortality, an average stay of 22 days, 17% incidence of gastric reflux and 5% requiring repeated dilation. The radiotherapy group had minimal complications with 20% undergoing salvage surgery. The 5-year survival figures for surgery verses radiotherapy were: 45% and 23% irrespective of nodal status; 63% and 25% without nodes; and 10% and 0% with nodes.

Stell et al[12] reported a series of postcricoid carcinomas where early lesions (stage I/II) were treated with radiotherapy, but more advanced tumours and patients with nodal involvement were treated with primary surgery using either flap or viscus repair. The 5-year survival for the surgical group repaired with a flap was 32% with radiotherapy being approximately 22%. The additional 10% overall survival advantage for those patients treated with primary surgery and a flap repair occurred despite the fact that the lesions in this group were more advanced (Table 14.28).

In a subsequent paper Stell et al[76] reported a 38% 5-year survival in patients treated with primary

Table 14.28 Crude survival[12]

	Crude survival by year (%)				
	1	2	3	4	5
Early (T1/2 N0): R/T	50	40	32	25	22
Advanced: surgery + flap	63	46	40	35	32
Advanced: surgery + viscus	10	5	5	5	5

irradiation and also in a group treated surgically and reconstructed with a flap. (Those with a visceral repair had only a 10% 5-year survival.) The radiotherapy group included T1 and small T2 lesions with a vertical length not greater than 5 cm and with no cervical nodes. Those in the surgery group included tumours greater than 5 cm in length and/or had cervical nodes or had radiorecurrent disease. It was concluded that early lesions should be treated with primary radiotherapy and surgery used for larger or recurrent tumours, but again the problem with this report is that the groups are non-comparable.

Harrison and Thompson[35] reported a series of 101 gastric transpositions (including 45% salvage operation after failed radiotherapy). The lesions were predominantly postcricoid (66%) in origin (19% piriform fossa, 9% cervical oesophagus, 4% larynx, 1% posterior pharynx and 1% thyroid). The survival rates (68%, 65%, 63% and 58% at 1, 2, 3 and 5 years, respectively) were high despite the fact that almost half of the patients were treated for recurrent disease following previous irradiation. This report clearly demonstrates that one of the fundamental issues about complex radical head and neck surgery is that it should only be carried out by an experienced surgical team and not on an occasional basis. The excellent results in this series, even for recurrent cases, reflect the low hospital mortality rate of 11%, which in the latter part of the study fell to 6%. Overall results showed that two-thirds of patients survived the first year, with 58% having a 5-year survival.

Salvage surgery

Following irradiation Farrington et al[33] found a recurrence rate of 75% of whom only 10% were thought to be suitable for salvage surgery with 25% success (i.e. one-twelfth of recurrences are successfully salvaged).[54] The cause-specific survival at 5 years was 22% (20% as a result of successful radiotherapy and an additional 2% with salvage). This compares with a 58% 5-year actuarial survival where surgery is advocated.[35]

Table 14.29 Nodal disease and survival (%)[12]

Nodal disease	Survival by year (%) 1	2	3	4	5
N0	35	28	27	27	24
N1	30	20	12	5	3
N2	15	0	0	0	0
N3	22	12	0	0	0

Table 14.30 Survival related to T stage[77]

	Crude 5-year survival (%)		Determinate 5-year survival (%)	
T stage	N–ve	N+ve	N–ve	N+ve
T1	43	20	50	n/c
T2	50	0	50	n/c
T3/4	0	0	n/c	n/c
Overall	36	10	39	14

n/c = no comment.

Management of regional disease

As at other sites nodal disease correlates with poor survival (Table 14.29) and advanced cases respond better to a combination of surgery and radiotherapy.

Treatment results: posterior pharyngeal wall

General comments

There are again no randomized controlled trials and the literature is sparse with all published series being very small. Most report the combined results of treatment of carcinomas of the posterior walls of the hypopharynx and the oropharynx and consequently it is impossible to compare the outcomes of different methods of treatment with any certainty.

Primary radiotherapy

In one of the very few reports of a series of posterior hypopharyngeal wall carcinomas treated by radical radiotherapy Talton et al[77] reported overall crude and cause-specific survival of 36–39% (Table 14.30) with nodal disease diminishing survival. Recurrence was seen in 79% of cases but radiotherapy was recommended as the treatment of choice. Meoz-Mendez et al[78] reported the results of radical radiotherapy at the MD Anderson Hospital for the posterior pharyngeal wall including hypopharynx and oropharynx with recurrence at the primary site associated with increasing T stage. Local failure was 9%, 27%, 39% and 63% for stages T1, T2, T3 and T4, respectively.

Pene et al[38] reported a group of oro- and hypopharyngeal malignancies predominantly treated with radiotherapy. Lesions over 4 cm had a worse prognosis than smaller tumours. The degree of lymph node involvement did not appear to affect survival. Seventy-five percent of patients died of local disease. The overall 5-(crude) year survival was 3% and local control was achieved in 69% of lesions under 4 cm and 10% in larger tumours.

Fein et al[15] from the University of Florida found the results of radiotherapy were no worse than surgery. At 2 years, local control was 100%, 76%, 51% and 25% for stages T1, T2, T3 and T4, respectively. However 11% developed radiotherapy complications with one patient dying after developing quadriplegia secondary to a peridural abscess and 2% developed severe soft tissue necrosis of the posterior pharyngeal wall.

Son and Kacinski[17] reported the use of combination brachytherapy and external beam radiotherapy in sequence for 14 pharyngeal wall cancers. For hypopharyngeal cancers local control was obtained in 80% of cases with an average follow-up of 3 years and the actuarial survival rate for oro- and hypopharyngeal wall tumours was 82% at 2 and 5 years.

Primary surgery

In a series of 78 patients with oro- and hypopharyngeal lesions, with surgery as the main treatment modality (76%) to both the primary site and neck, Spiro et al[43] found that the overall 2- and 5-year actuarial survival was 49% and 32%. For lesions confined to the posterior pharyngeal wall the overall 2- and 5-year actuarial survival was 58% and 34%. For stage I/II disease the overall 2- and 5-year actuarial survival was four times better than stage IV disease. In the N0 neck the overall 2- and 5-year actuarial survival was 61% and 41%. Local recurrence occurred in 41% of patients, regional failure in 21% and distant metastasis in 9%.

In Pene et al's series[38] primary surgery with postoperative radiotherapy was employed in only 7% of cases, in earlier lesions (mainly T1/2) with minimal nodal disease and fitter/younger patients giving a crude 5-year survival of 30%. Their recommendation of surgical treatment for the rare early lesions to reduce the risk of local recurrence was borne out by a subsequent publication.[39] Pene concluded that primary surgery with postoperative radiotherapy is indicated in tumours confined to the mucosa of the posterior pharyngeal wall without invasion of the lateral wall or adjacent structures. They also comment that at first presentation the extent of the disease frequently indicates the use of radiotherapy only.

Primary surgery compared to primary radiotherapy

In the Liverpool series, Jones and Stell.[36] found no difference in survival between primary surgery and primary irradiation when treatment was adjusted for stage with a 5-year stage I survival of 45–50%. There were no 5-year survivors for stage II, III and IV disease. Marks et al[13] reported preoperative radiotherapy and surgery for oro- and hypopharyngeal lesions verses radiotherapy and salvage surgery. The two groups were age, sex and tumour stage comparable. In the primary surgery group there was a 20% survival advantage at 5 years (Table 14.31) but a higher complication rate (11% major and 89% lesser versus 5% major and 48% lesser). They recommended surgical intervention with pre- or postoperative radiotherapy as the primary modality of treatment.

Table 14.31 Survival with primary surgery or radiotherapy[13]

	Actuarial survival by year (%)			
	1	2	3	5
Preoperative radiotherapy and surgery	70	40	30	25
Radiotherapy	50	30	15	5

Treatment results: conclusion

Hypopharyngeal cancer provides one of the clearest examples in the management of head and neck tumours where referral to an experienced multidisciplinary team is essential for optimum survival and quality of life for the patient. It is a rare disease and should not be treated on an occasional basis. A careful balanced view should be given between the obvious potential benefits of larynx-preserving radiotherapy and conservation surgery, which may be appropriate in early selected lesions, and the survival advantage of radical surgery for more advanced tumours. The management of these cases should be undertaken by an experienced multidisciplinary team.

From the above review it is evident that there is a need for high-quality trials to justify not only the introduction of new therapies but also to support present practice. It would be ideal, where possible, for most patients to be entered into trials.

Whatever choice is thought by the multidisciplinary team to be the 'best' for the patient, it is essential that the patient is given a balanced view of all options and their wishes being of paramount importance.

Piriform fossa

In early stage disease radical radiotherapy is recommended although surgery is justified in those institutions with very significant expertise in partial laryngopharyngeal surgery (conventional and laser endoscopic techniques). A prospective RCT would be appropriate for patients receiving laser endoscopic resection or radiotherapy.

More advanced stage disease (unfavourable T2, T3/4) is probably better treated by total laryngectomy, partial pharyngectomy and reconstruction with postoperative radiotherapy, provided the tumour is resectable and the patient fit for operation. However, the work of Steiner and the EORTC organ preservation study suggests that alternative strategies may, if verified, result in the retention of functional larynges without impairing survival.

Postcricoid

For non-circumferential disease radiotherapy is probably the treatment of choice as it allows organ preservation and a reasonable probability of cure and restoration of swallow. Circumferential lesions and advanced lesions present a greater dilemma; the literature would suggest that cure and restoration of swallow are best achieved by surgery and post-operative radiotherapy performed in those institutions with very significant expertise.

Posterior pharyngeal wall

Using a size-based T classification, early lesions (T1/2) are probably best treated with surgery and postoperative radiotherapy provided that the surgery causes minimal functional impairment and the patient is not at risk of significant aspiration. Larger tumours are best treated by radical combined therapy or palliated with radiotherapy.

Management of the neck in hypopharyngeal lesions

N0/1 disease is equally well controlled with surgery or radiotherapy alone, whereas N2/3 requires combined surgical clearance and postoperative radiotherapy for optimal results.

REFERENCES

1. Sobin LH, Wittekind Ch (eds). *TNM Classification of malignant tumours.* 5th edn. UICC/AJC. New York: John Wiley, 1997.
2. Beahrs OH, Henson DE, Hutter RVP, Myers ME (eds) *Manual for Staging of Cancer; American Joint Committee on Cancer.* 3rd edn. New York: JB Lippincott, 1988.
3. Silver CE *Surgery for Cancer of the Larynx and Related Structures.* 2nd edn. Philadelphia: WB Saunders 1996.
4. Warwick R, Williams PL (eds) *Gray's Anatomy.* 35th edn. London: Longman, 1978.
5. Lefebvre JL, Castelain B, De La Torre JC et al. Lymph node invasion in hypopharyngeal and lateral epilarynx carcinoma: a prognostic factor *Head Neck Surg* 1987; **10**: 14–18.
6. Bataini P, Brugere J, Bemier J et al. Results of radiotherapeutic treatment of carcinoma of the pyriform sinus: experience of the Institut Curie. *Int J Radiat Oncol Biol Phys* 1982; **8**: 1277–1286.
7. Million RR, Cassisi NJ (eds). *Management of Head and Neck Cancer: A Multidisciplinary Approach.* Philadelphia: JB Lippincott, 1994.
8. Myers EN, Suen JY. Cancer of the hypopharynx and cervical esophagus. In: *Cancer of the Head and Neck* 3rd edn. Philadelphia: WB Saunders, 1996; 423–438.
9. Haagensen CD, Feind CR, Herter FP et al. In: *The Lymphatics in Cancer* Philadelphia: WB Saunders, 1972; 171.
10. Hasegawa Y, Matsuura H. Retropharyngeal node dissection in cancer of the oropharynx and hypopharynx. *Head Neck* 1994; **16**: 173–180.
11. Ogura JH, Sessions DG, Spector G et al. Long term therapeutic results: cancer of the larynx and hypopharynx. Preliminary report, *Laryngoscope* 1974; **85**: 1746–1761.
12. Stell PM, Carden EA, Hibbert J, Dalby JE. Post cricoid carcinoma. *Clin Oncol* 1978; **4**: 215–226.
13. Marks JE, Smith PG, Sessions DG. Pharyngeal wall cancer: a reappraisal after comparison of treatment methods. *Arch Otolarygol* 1985; **111**: 79–85.
14. Barzan L, Barra S, Franchin G et al. Squamous cell carcinoma of the posterior pharyngeal wall: characteristics compared with the lateral wall. *J Laryngol Otol* 1995; **109**: 120–125.
15. Fein DA, Mendenhall WM, Parsons JT et al. Pharyngeal wall carcinoma treated with radiotherapy: impact of treatment technique and fractionation. *Int J Radiat Oncol Biol Phys* 1993; **26**: 751–757.
16. Candela FC, Kothari K, Shah JP. Patterns of cervical node metastases from squamous carcinoma of the oropharynx and hypopharynx. *Head Neck* 1990; **12**: 197–203.
17. Son YH, Kacinski BM. Therapeutic concepts of brachytherapy/megavoltage in sequence for pharyngeal wall cancers. Results of integrated dose therapy. *Cancer* 1987; **59**: 1268–1273.
18. Ballantyne AJ. Principles of surgical management of cancer of the pharyngeal walls. *Cancer* 1967; **20**: 663–667.
19. Lederman M. Cancer of the pharynx. *J Laryngol Otol* 1967; **81**: 151–172.
20. Adenis L, Lefebvre JL, Cambier L. Registre des cancers des voies aerodigestives superieures des departements du Nord et du Pas-de-Calais 1984–1986. *Bull Cancer Paris* 1988; **75**: 745–750.
21. Olofsson J, Van Nostrand AWP. Growth and spread of laryngeal and hypopharyngeal carcinoma with reflections on the effect of preoperative irradiation: 139 cases studied by whole organ serial sectioning. *Acta Otolaryngol Suppl* 1973; **308**: 1–84.
22. Keane TJ, Hawkins NV, Beale FA et al. Carcinoma of the hypopharynx: results of primary radical radiation therapy. *Int J Radiat Oncol Biol Phys* 1983; **9**: 659–664.
23. Raine CH, Stell PM, Dalby J. Squamous cell carcinomas of the posterior wall of the hypopharynx. *J Laryngol Otol* 1982; **96**: 997–1004.
24. Shah JP, Shaha AR, Spiro RH, Strong EW. Carcinoma of the hypopharynx. *Am J Surg* 1976; **132**: 439–443.
25. Rapoport A, Franco EL. Prognostic factors and relative risk in hypopharyngeal cancer – related parameters concerning stage, therapeutics and evolution. *Rev Paul Med* 1993; **111**: 337–343.
26. Van den Bogaert W, Ostyn F, Van der Schueren E. Hypopharyngeal cancer: results of treatment with radiotherapy alone and combinations of surgery and radiotherapy. *Radiother Oncol* 1985; **3**: 311–318.
27. Stell PM. Cancer of the hypopharynx. *J R Coll Surg Edinb* 1973; **18**: 20–30.
28. Kajanti M, Mantyla M. Carcinoma of the hypopharynx. *Acta Oncol* 1990; **29**: 903–907.
29. Kirchner JA. Pyriform sinus cancer: a clinical and laboratory study. *Ann Otolaryngol* 1975; **84**: 793–803.
30. Eisbach KJ, Krause CJ. Carcinoma of the pyriform sinus. A comparison of treatment modalities. *Laryngoscope* 1977; **87**: 1904–1910.

31. Driscoll WG, Nagorsky MJ, Cantrell RW, Johns ME. Carcinoma of the piriform sinus: analysis of 102 cases. *Laryngoscope* 1983; **93**: 556–560.
32. Van den Brouck C, Eschwege F, De La Rochefordiere A et al. Squamous cell carcinoma of the pyriform sinius: a retrospective study of 351 cases treated at the Institut Gustave-Roussy. *Head Neck Surg* 1987; **10**: 4–13.
33. Farrington WT, Weighill JS, Jones PH. Post-cricoid carcinoma (ten-year retrospective study). *J Laryngol Otol* 1986; **100**: 79–84.
34. Tandon DA, Bahadur S, Chatterji TK, Rath GK. Carcinoma of the hypopharynx: results of combined therapy. *Indian J Cancer* 1991; **28**: 131–138.
35. Harrison DFN, Thompson AE. Pharyngolaryngoesophagectomy with pharyngogastric anastamosis for cancer of the hypopharynx: review of 101 operations. *Head Neck Surg* 1986; **8**: 418–428.
36. Jones AS, Stell PM. Squamous cell carcinoma of the posterior pharyngeal wall. *Clin Otolaryngol* 1991; **16**: 462–465.
37. Willatt DJ, Jackson SR, McCormick MS et al. Vocal cord paralysis and tumour length in staging postcricoid cancer. *Eur J Surg Oncol* 1987; **13**: 131–137.
38. Pene F, Avedian V, Eschwege F et al. A retrospective study of 131 cases of carcinoma of the posterior pharyngeal wall. *Cancer* 1978; **42**: 2490–2493.
39. Schwaab G, Vandenbrouck C, Luboinski B, Rhys Evans P. Les carcinomas de la paroi posterieure du pharynx traites par chirurgie premiere. *J Eur Radiother* 1983; **4**: 175–179.
40. Million RR, Cassisi NJ (eds). In: *Management of Head and Neck Cancer: A Multidisciplinary Approach.* Philadelphia: JB Lippincott, 1984.
41. Ogura JH, Biller BF, Wette R. Elective neck dissection for pharyngeal and laryngeal cancers: an evaluation. *Ann Otol Rhinol Laryngol* 1971; **80**: 646–653.
42. Lederman M. The role of irradiation in the treatment of the hypopharynx, postcricoid and cervical oesophagus. In: Conley J (ed.) *Proceedings of the International Workshop on Cancer of the Head and Neck.* London: Butterworth, 1967; 347.
43. Spiro RH, Kelly J, Vega AL et al. Squamous carcinoma of the posterior pharyngeal wall. *Am J Surg* 1990; **160**: 420–423.
44. Tani M, Amatsu M. Discrepancies between clinical and histopathologic diagnosis in T3 pyriform sinus cancer *Laryngoscope* 1987; **97**: 93–96.
45. El Badawi SA, Goepfert H, Fletcher GH, et al. Squamous cell carcinoma of the pyriform sinus. *Laryngoscope* 1982; **92**: 357–364.
46. Harrison DFN. Pathology of hypopharyngeal cancer in relation to surgical management. *J Laryngol Otol* 1970; **84**: 349–366.
47. Kirchner JA. One hundred laryngeal cancers studied by serial section. *Ann Otol Rhinol Laryngol* 1969; **78**: 689–709.
48. Lindberg R. Distribution of cervical lymph node metastases from squamous cell carcinoma of the upper respiratory and digestive tracts. *Cancer* 1972; **29**: 1446–1449.
49. Weber RS, Marvel J, Smith P et al. Paratracheal lymph node dissection for carcinoma of the larynx, hypopharynx and cervical oesophagus *Otolaryngol Head Neck Surg* 1993; **108**: 11–17.
50. Dalley VM. Cancer of the laryngopharynx. *J Laryngol Otol* 1968; **82**: 407–420.
51. Davidge-Pitts KJ, Mannel A. Pharyngolaryngectomy with extrathoracic esophagectomy. *Head Neck Surg* 1983; **6**: 571–574.
52. Harrison DFN. Malignant disease of the hypopharynx: surgical pathology of hypopharyngeal neoplasms. *J Laryngol Otol* 1971; **85**: 1215–1218.
53. Pingree TF, Davis RK, Reichman O, Derrick L. Treatment of hypopharyngeal carcinoma: a 10-year review of 1362 cases. *Laryngoscope* 1987; **97**: 901–904.
54. Jones PH, Farrington WT, Weighill JS. Surgical salvage in postcricoid cancer. *J Laryngol Otol* 1986; **100**: 85–95.
55. Teichgraeber JF, McConnel FMS. Treatment of posterior pharyngeal wall carcinoma. *Otolaryngol Head Neck Surg* 1979; **94**: 287–290.
56. Freeman RB, Marks JE, Ogura JH. Voice preservation in treatment of carcinoma of the pyriform sinus. *Laryngoscope* 1979; **89**: 1855–1863.
57. Marks JE, Kurnik B, Powers WE, Ogura JH. Carcinoma of the pyriform sinus: an analysis of treatment results and patters of failure. *Cancer* 1978; **41**: 1008–1015.
58. Steiner W, Stenglein C, Fietkau R, Sauerbrei W. Therapy of hypopharyngeal cancer. Part IV: Long-term results of transoral laser microsurgery of hypopharyngeal cancer. *HNO* 1994; **42**: 147–156.
59. Steiner W. Therapy of hypopharyngeal cancer. Part III: the concept of minimally invasive therapy of cancers of the upper aerodigestive tract with special reference to hypopharyngeal cancer and trans-oral laser microsurgery. *HNO* 1994; **42**: 104–112.
60. Steiner W. Therapy of hypopharyngeal cancer. Part V: Discussion of long-term results of transoral laser microsurgery of hypopharyngeal cancer. *HNO* 1994; **42**: 157–165.
61. Ambrosch P, Brinck U, Fischer G, Steiner W. Special aspects of histopathological diagnosis in laser microsurgery of cancers of the upper aerodigestive tract. *Laryngorhinootologie* 1994; **73**: 78–83.
62. Lam KH, Ho CM, Lau WF et al. Immediate reconstruction of pharyngoesophageal defects. *Arch Otolaryngol Head Neck Surg* **115**: 608–612.
63. Ladas G, Rhys Evans PH, Goldstraw P. Anterior cervical transsternal approach for the resection of benign tumours at the thoracic inlet. *Ann Thorac Surg* 1999; **67**: 785–789.
64. Lefebvre JL, Chevalier D, Luboinski B et al. Larynx preservation in pyriform sinus cancer: preliminary results of a European Organization for Research and Treatment of Cancer phase III trial. *J Natl Cancer Inst* 1996; **88**: 890–899.
65. Lefebvre JL. Organ preservation... where do we stand? *Acta Otorhinolaryngol Belg* 1999; **53**: 223–225.
66. Lefebvre JL. What is the role of primary surgery in the treatment of laryngeal and hypopharyngeal cancer: Hayes Martin Lecture. *Arch Otolaryngol Head Neck Surg* 2000; **126**: 285–288.

67. Forastiere A. Another look at induction chemotherapy for organ preservation in patients with head and neck cancer. *J Natl Cancer Institute* 1996; **88**: 855–856.
68. Stockwell S. EORTC Trial: larynx preservation does not jeopardize survival in hypopharyngeal cancer. *Oncol Times* 1996; **8**: 11–12.
69. Axon PR, Woolford TJ, Hargreaves P et al. A comparison of surgery and radiotherapy in the management of post-carcinoma. *Clin Otolaryngol* 1997; **22**: 370–374.
70. Million RR, Cassisi NJ. Radical irradiation for carcinoma of the pyriform sinus. *Laryngoscope* 1981; **91**: 439–450.
71. Mendenhall WM, Parsons JT, Cassisi NJ, Million RR. Squamous cell carcinoma of the pyriform sinus treated with radical radiation therapy. *Radiother Oncol* 1987; **9**: 201–208.
72. Mendenhall WM, Parsons JT, Stringer SP et al. Radiotherapy alone or combined with neck dissection for T1–T2 carcinoma of the pyriform sinus: an alternative to conservation surgery. *Int J Radiat Oncol Biol Phys* 1993; **27**: 1017–1027.
73. Ogura JH, Marks JE, Freeman RB. Results of conservation surgery for cancers of the supraglottis and pyriform sinus. *Laryngoscope* 1980; **90**: 591–600.
74. Barton RT. Surgical treatment of carcinoma of the pyriform sinus. *Arch Otolaryngol* 1973; **97**: 337–339.
75. Czaja J, Gluckman JL. Surgical management of early-stage hypopharyngeal carcinoma. *Ann Otol Rhinol Laryngol* 1997; **106**: 909–913.
76. Stell PM, Rarnadan MF, Dalby JE et al. Management of postcricoid carcinoma. *Clin Otolaryngol* 1982; **7**: 145–152.
77. Talton BM, Elkon D, Kim JA. Cancer of the posterior hypopharyngeal wall. *Int J Radiat Oncol Biol Phys* 1981; **7**: 597–599.
78. Meoz-Mendez RT, Fletcher GH, Guillamondegui OM, Peters LJ. Analysis of the results of irradiation in the treatment of squamous cell carcinomas of the pharyngeal walls. *Int J Radiat Oncol Biol Phys* 1978; **4**: 579–585.

15 Tumours of the larynx

Snehal G Patel, Peter Rhys-Evans and Paul Q Montgomery

Introduction

Impairment of laryngeal function from disease and/or its treatment results in gross disturbances in breathing, speech, and swallowing with profound impact on the patient's lifestyle and self esteem. The successful management of laryngeal cancer is dependent as much upon individualizing the plan of management to suit the particular patient and their expectations, as on close co-operation among members of a Head and Neck multidisciplinary team.

Surgical anatomy

The larynx is divided into three distinct regions based on topographical landmarks (Figure 15.1). The supraglottis comprises the laryngeal epiglottis, false cords, ventricles, aryepiglottic folds and arytenoids. The glottis includes the true vocal cords, and the anterior and posterior commissures. The subglottis begins 10 mm below the level of the free margin of the vocal cords and extends to the inferior edge of the cricoid cartilage. In Europe, especially France, the larynx is also described as being divisible into an 'epilarynx' (or the 'marginal zone') and an 'endolarynx'. This distinction is based on the similar natural history of tumours of the epilaryngeal region and those arising in the adjacent hypopharynx. The epilarynx consists of the free border and posterior surface of the suprahyoid epiglottis (anterior epilarynx), the aryepiglottic fold (lateral epilarynx), arytenoids and interarytenoid incisure (posterior epilarynx) and the 'endolarynx' consists of the infrahyoid supraglottis (infrahyoid epiglottis, false cords and ventricles), glottis and subglottis.

Laryngeal spaces

The concept of laryngeal spaces is vital to understanding the growth and spread of laryngeal cancer

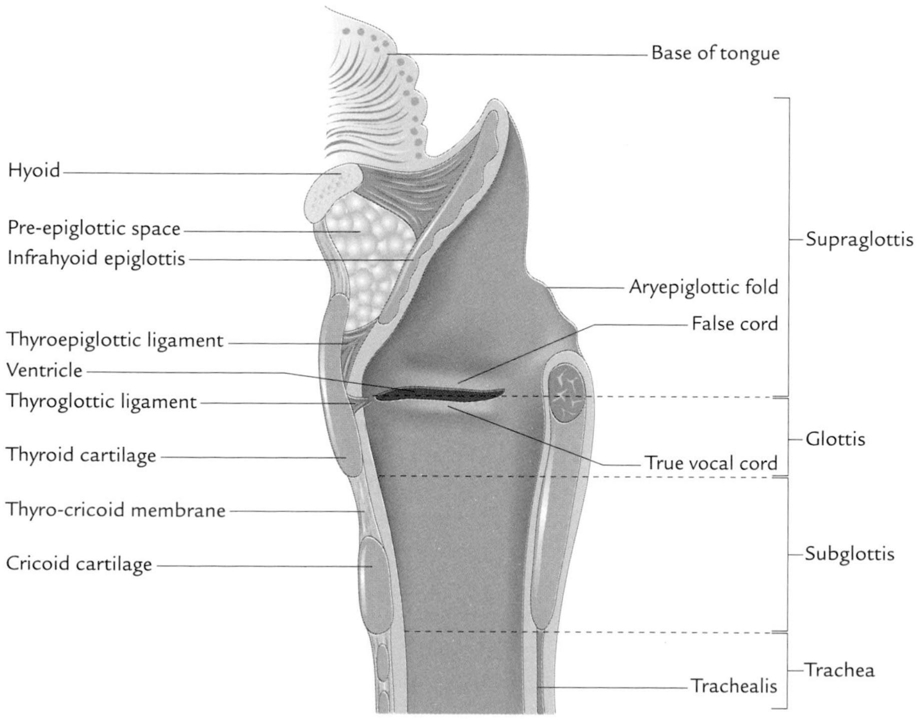

Figure 15.1 Anatomical divisions of the larynx.

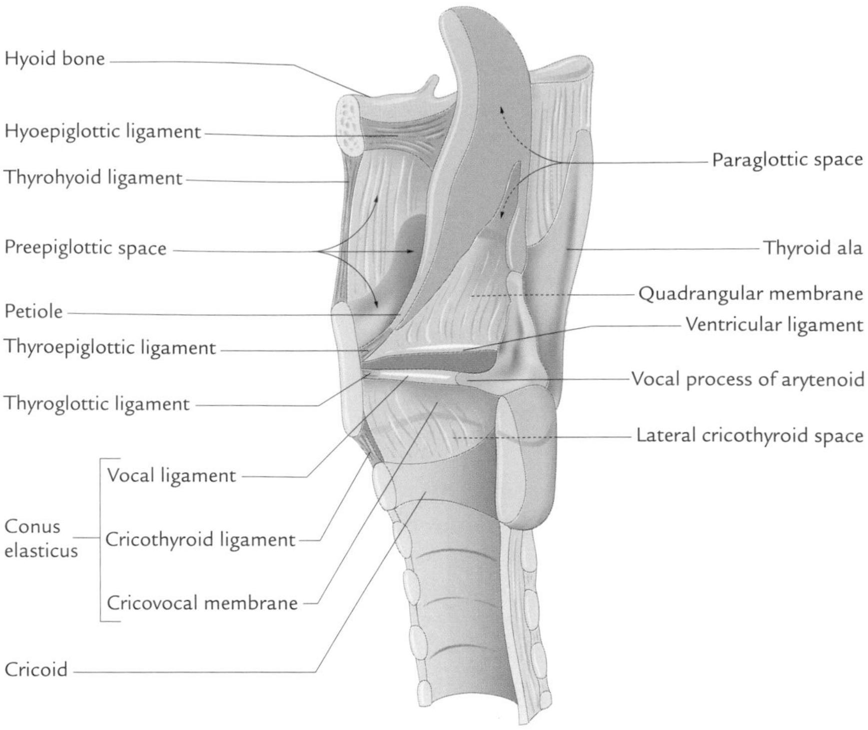

Figure 15.2 Laryngeal spaces and structures.

and therefore, to the understanding of the principles of conservation laryngeal surgery.

The pre-epiglottic space (of Boyer) is a funnel-shaped space bounded anteriorly by the upper part of the thyroid cartilage and thyrohyoid membrane down to the insertion of the thyroepiglottic ligament, superiorly by the hyoepiglottic ligament, and posteriorly by the epiglottis and the quadrangular membrane (Figure 15.2). It is continuous laterally with the paraglottic space and contains adipose and areolar tissue along with lymphatic channels. Tumours in an infrahyoid location at the base of the epiglottis tend to spread into the pre-epiglottic space and have a poorer prognosis than those located in the suprahyoid epiglottis.

The paraglottic space is bound anterolaterally by the thyroid cartilage, inferomedially by the cricovocal membrane, superomedially by the ventricle and quadrangular membrane, and posteriorly by the pyriform sinus mucosa. It contains the thyroarytenoid and vocalis muscles surrounded by the paramycium that separates these muscles from the adipose tissue of the posterior projection of the pre-epiglottic space. This space is therefore in continuity with the pre-epiglottic space and also the paralaryngeal tissues of the neck through the lateral cricothyroid space. The latter is an important route for the extralaryngeal spread of cancer.

The lamina propria of the mucosa over the true vocal cords is composed of three layers. The superficial layer immediately underneath the epithelium consists of loose fibrous tissue and is named Reinke's space. This space is almost devoid of blood vessels and lymphatics and thus affords resistance to the spread of early glottic cancers. The intermediate and deep layers of the lamina propria consist of elastic and collagenous fibres that form the vocal ligament.

Lymphatic drainage

As with the vascular supply, the glottis constitutes a watershed that divides the larynx into two units that have a distinct embryological derivation.[1,2] The supraglottic larynx is drained by lymphatics that run along the superior thyroid artery and drain into the nodes at level II. The vocal cords and their subepithelial spaces are largely devoid of lymphatics, which explains the relative rarity of cervical nodal metastases in glottic cancer. The subepithelial lymphatic vessels, which are densely concentrated in the region of the arytenoids, thin out progressively anteriorly and are sparsest in the anterior third of the cords.[3] The subglottis has a superficial lymphatic plexus that drains into three main pedicles: one anterior and two posterior. The anterior pedicle pierces the cricothyroid membrane and drains into the prelaryngeal or Delphian node, which in turn drains into the pretracheal and supraclavicular nodes. The paired posterolateral pedicles pierce the cricotracheal membrane to drain into the paratracheal and other superior mediastinal nodes.

Surgical applications of laryngeal anatomy

The structure of the larynx and the arrangement of its membranes and cartilages (Figure 15.3) plays an important role in the way laryngeal tumours spread.

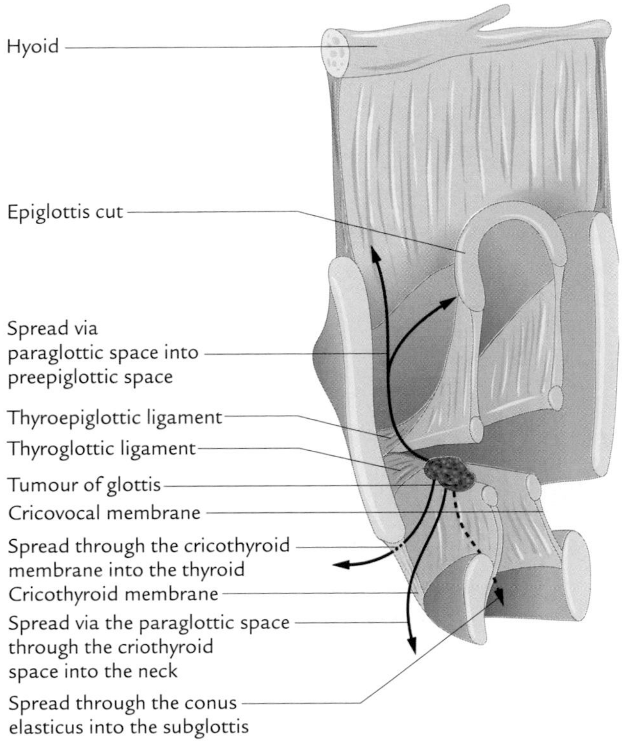

Figure 15.3 Laryngeal spaces and tumour spread.

1. The conus elasticus resists the inferior spread of glottic tumours and therefore subglottic extension is a relatively late and ominous manifestation of glottic carcinoma;
2. Tumours involving the anterior commissure frequently invade the adjacent thyroid cartilage as the internal perichondrium is deficient at this site. Similarly, the external perichondrium is thinner near the midline and thickens laterally. In addition the tumour may escape the larynx via the cricothyroid membrane;
3. The paraglottic space containing the vocalis muscle is deficient laterally at the lateral cricothyroid space through which glottic tumours can spread into the neck. Some glottic cancers may be understaged as clinical evaluation of this extension is difficult. The paraglottic space also communicates with the pre-epiglottic space, and glottic cancer may extend into the supraglottic larynx through this route;
4. Epiglottic carcinoma can spread directly into the pre-epiglottic space through dehiscences in the epiglottic cartilage, and this space must be resected completely during a supraglottic laryngectomy (Figure 15.4).

Histological variants

The histology of the tumour has an impact on the management of the patient and the eventual outcome (Table 15.1).[4] Although the vast majority of primary tumours of the larynx are squamous cell carcinomas, a variety of other pathological types can occur.

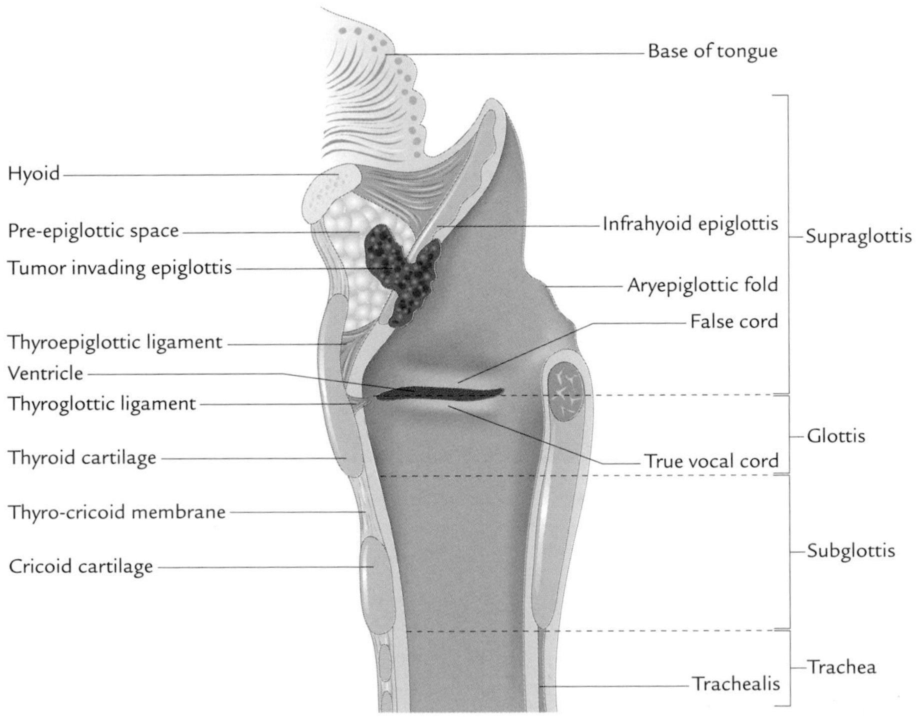

Figure 15.4 Infrahyoid epiglottic tumours gain direct access to the pre-epiglottic space through epiglottic dehiscences.

Table 15.1 Histological type and survival

Histological type	5-year survival rate (%)	10-year survival rate (%)
Verrucous squamous cell carcinoma	95	
Chondrosarcoma	90	
Mucoepidermoid carcinoma	80	
Squamous cell carcinoma	68	
Spindle cell carcinoma	68	
Atypical carcinoid	48	30
Melanoma	20	
Basaloid squamous cell carcinoma	17.5	
Small cell neuroendocrine carcinoma	5	

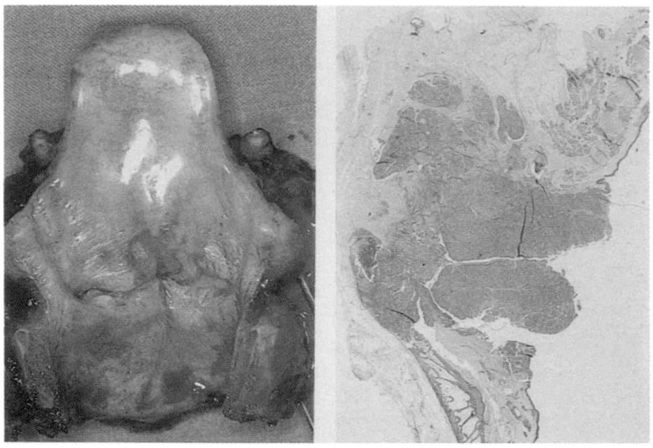

Figure 15.5 Squamous cell carcinoma of vocal cord.

Squamous cell cancers (Figure 15.5) comprise 85–90% of all laryngeal neoplasms. The majority of vocal cord carcinomas are well to moderately differentiated, and almost always arise in the anterior half from the epithelium of the membranous part of the glottis. The inferior arcuate line, which is the boundary separating the squamous and columnar epithelium, is a common site of origin.

Verrucous carcinomas (Figure 15.6) are a highly differentiated variant of squamous cell carcinoma that constitute about 1–4% of laryngeal neoplasms and about 1–2% of vocal cord tumours. Their importance lies in the fact that they present diagnostic difficulties to both the clinician and the pathologist, as the lesion that appears clinically malignant may only show histologically benign features. Human papillomavirus DNA sequences have been found in the tumour and in the adjacent normal tissue, pointing to a possible aetiological link.[5] The tumour is locally invasive but has very little tendency to metastasize. The surface of the tumour shows characteristic papillary fronds with prominent hyperkeratosis.

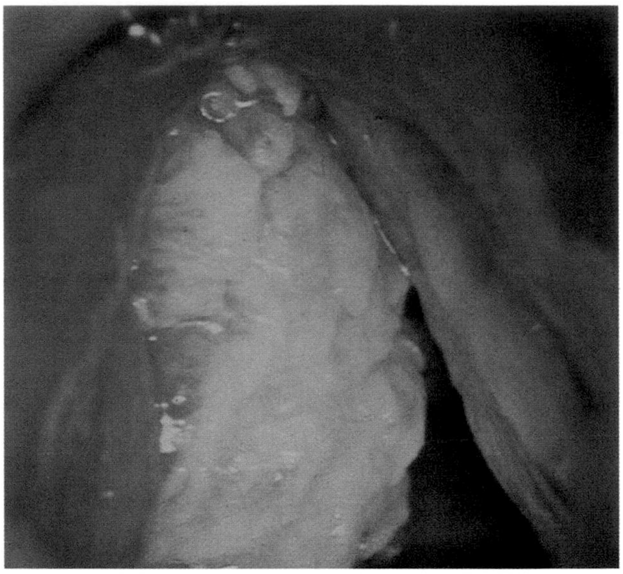

Figure 15.6 Verrucous carcinomas of the glottis.

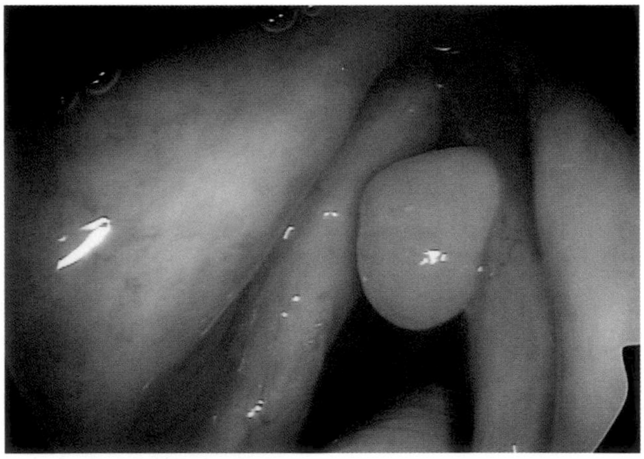

Figure 15.7 Spindle cell carcinoma of the vocal cord.

Spindle cell carcinoma

Most laryngeal tumours that have been previously classified as laryngeal sarcomas are now thought to be a biphasic variant of squamous cell carcinoma (Figure 15.7) with a predominant pseudosarcomatous component. The incidence of these spindle cell carcinomas is difficult to assess reliably because of differences in histological interpretation. These tumours most commonly arise in the vocal cords especially in the region of the anterior commissure.

Basaloid squamous cell carcinoma

This is a biologically aggressive biphasic variant of squamous cell carcinoma with a high propensity to regional and distant metastases (the latter may be seen even in the absence of cervical nodes).[6]

Neuroendocrine tumours

Atypical carcinoid tumour is the most frequent neuroendocrine tumour of the larynx and can be mistaken for a laryngeal paraganglioma. The vast majority (90%) occur in the supraglottis and some are associated with the carcinoid syndrome.[7] Cervical nodal metastasis is seen in 43% of cases, distant metastases in 45%, and painful skin or subcutaneous metastases in 22% of patients. Surgical excision must be preceded by detailed metastatic work-up. Elevated calcitonin levels are considered specific markers and may be used to monitor therapy.[8]

Small cell neuroendocrine tumours ('oat cell' carcinoma) are rare but extremely aggressive. They account for only 0.5% of all laryngeal neoplasms but almost 75% of patients die of widespread metastases. They are most commonly seen in males who are in their fifth or sixth decades of life and who have been heavy smokers. Cervical nodal metastasis is seen in half of all patients, and distant spread most commonly involves the liver, lungs, bone, and bone marrow. A detailed metastatic work-up, including CT scans of the lung and brain, bone and brain scintigraphy, and bone marrow aspiration biopsy, is mandatory at diagnosis. The tumour is associated with various paraneoplastic syndromes and the work-up must encompass this possibility.

Mucosal melanomas

Primary melanoma of the larynx is extremely rare with only about 50 reported cases so far.[9] It is commonly a tumour of elderly male caucasians and the majority are found in the supraglottis. Histological diagnosis of difficult cases may be aided by immunohistochemical demonstration of S100 protein and by electron microscopy. The differential diagnosis includes metastasis to the larynx from a cutaneous primary, which must be ruled out before treatment commences. The incidence of lymphatic metastasis is low, and elective neck dissection is not routinely indicated.

Other tumour types

Adenoid cystic carcinoma is an uncommon tumour that is unusual in many ways. It affects males and females almost equally and approximately two-thirds of tumours occur in the subglottis, often as a smooth submucosal mass.[10] The tumour has a high tendency to recur locally and to metastasize to the lungs in the absence of cervical nodal metastases.

Mucoepidermoid carcinomas are rare tumours that may metastasize to the neck and the lungs. The histological grade of the tumour determines survival: 5-year survival in low-grade tumours is 90–100% while that for high-grade tumours is 50%.[11]

Sarcomas of the larynx are uncommon, and chondrosarcoma (Figure 15.8) is the most common mesenchymal malignancy. It most commonly involves the cricoid cartilage with the thyroid cartilage, the arytenoids and the epiglottis being more rarely affected. Chondrosarcomas are slow growing tumours with a high potential for local recurrence. Lymphatic and distant metastases are rare.

Lymphomas of the larynx are predominantly of the B cell variety.

Epidemiology of laryngeal cancer

Tumours of the larynx constitute about 3.5% of all new malignancies diagnosed annually world-wide. They cause about 200 000 deaths, which is about 1% of all deaths from cancer.[12] Squamous cell carcinoma of the larynx has, over the years, been the most frequent malignant tumour of the upper aerodigestive tract in Europe, but recent increases in the incidence of oral and oropharyngeal cancer have narrowed the gap.

World-wide distribution

The incidence of laryngeal cancer generally ranges from 2.5 to 17.2 per 100 000 per year. The highest incidence of laryngeal carcinoma has been reported from the Basque Country, Spain (20.4) and the lowest incidence for men from Qidong, China (0.1).[13] Other areas of high incidence include Brazil (15.1) and North Thailand (18.4). European countries with a high incidence in males include France (15.6), Poland (11.9), and Italy (10.1) but on the whole, laryngeal cancer constitutes only 3% of the total number of new cases of cancer recorded in the EC in 1990.[14]

(a)

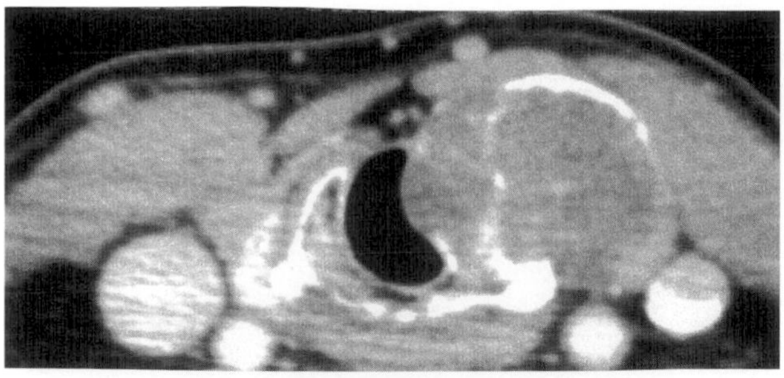

Figure 15.8 Chondrosarcoma of the larynx. (a) CT; (b) resected larynx; (c) histological section

(b)

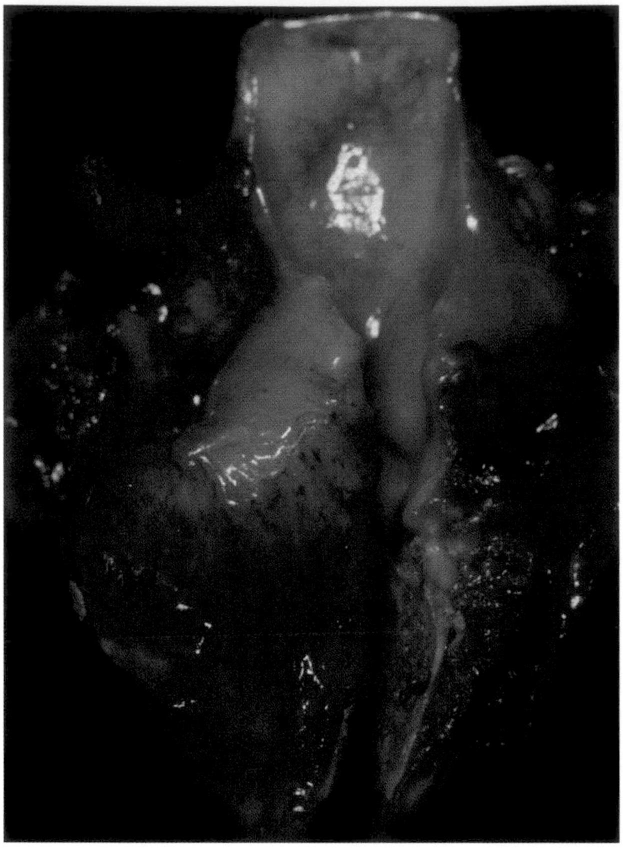

(c

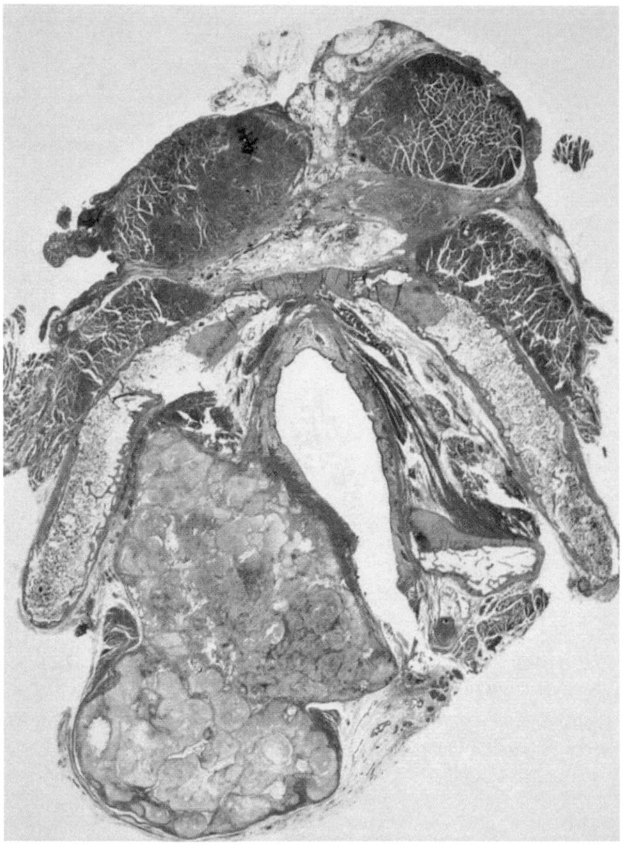

Cancer of the larynx is not a common disease in the United Kingdom, as indeed in the rest of the European Community. It ranks fifteenth on the list of common cancers in males in the UK and the age-standardized (world population) incidence rate for men was 4.4 and that for women was 0.8 per 100 000 in 1990. Within the UK, Scotland and Ireland have higher incidence rates as compared to England and Wales (Table 15.2).

Age and sex distribution

The age group most commonly affected is 50–70 years, women being affected at a younger age than males.[15] The male to female ratio, which used to be heavily biased towards males at 9:1, has come down to approximately 5:1 due to the increasing trend of smoking among females. In the United States, incidence rates continue to rise at 1.6% per year for white females while the corresponding rate in white males has decreased at 0.6% each year; the rates for both black men and women have been on the increase and the male:female ratio in this population has therefore not changed significantly. In patients younger than 35 years, however, the incidence in males and females is equal.[16] Another difference among the sexes is that supraglottic carcinoma is more frequent in women; according to one study 64% of laryngeal carcinomas were supraglottic in women against 46% in men.[17]

Trends

The trends in incidence rates in males have been variable, with decreases in France and Italy, increases in Denmark and Germany, but little change in the

Table 15.2 Comparison of age-standardized incidence rates for laryngeal cancer within the UK for 1990

	Males		Females	
	Cases	ASR (W)*	Cases	ASR (W)*
England and Wales	1665	4.5	368	0.8
Scotland	215	6.2	56	1.3
Ireland	121	6.2	30	1.3

*Age-standardized incidence (world population) rates.

other EC countries. There has been a slightly increasing trend in both males and females within the UK. Cohort analyses in the United States have revealed a decline in the rate for laryngeal cancer among white women born during the latter half of the 1800s, increasing among those born between 1895 and 1920, and decreasing thereafter. Cohort-specific patterns are much less remarkable for white men while the increases for laryngeal cancers among non-white males born after 1900 have been steep and have not yet reversed direction as they have for whites.[18]

Aetiological factors

Squamous cell carcinoma of the larynx is a preventable disease resulting from an interplay of numerous aetiological factors such as chronic consumption of tobacco and/or alcohol, environmental carcinogens, socioeconomic status, occupational hazards, dietary factors and genetic susceptibility.

Tobacco

Smoking is, without doubt, the major risk factor for laryngeal cancer. Tobacco smoke contains more than 30 different carcinogenic agents such as polycyclic aromatic hydrocarbons and nitrosamines. Nicotine from tobacco is not carcinogenic by itself, but burning tobacco releases the tar, that contains numerous carcinogens, notably methylcholanthrene, benzopyrene and benzanthracene. These carcinogens reach the epithelial cellular surface in the tobacco smoke or dissolved in saliva. These substances are then broken down by cellular enzymes like arylhydrocarbon hydroxylase into epoxides that bind to DNA and RNA, and cause genetic damage that can result in cancer. A dose-dependent increase in risk of laryngeal cancer has been demonstrated in case-control studies; patients smoking more than 40 cigarettes a day are 13 times more likely to die of laryngeal cancer than non-smokers.[19] Smoking non-filter cigarettes[20] and/or black (air-cured) tobacco[21] has been linked to higher risk due to the higher exposure to carcinogens. The Heidelberg case-control study estimated a nine-fold increase in the tobacco-associated relative risk in heavy smokers independent of alcohol consumption.[22] The role of passive or 'second-hand' smoking in cancer of the larynx is not clear. Apart from the aetiological role of tobacco smoking, its importance in prognosis of patients who develop laryngeal cancer is also relevant. It has been shown that patients who survive 3 years or more after treatment of laryngeal cancer and who continue to smoke, are seven times more likely to develop a second primary cancer.

Alcohol

Recent epidemiological studies have proved the long-suspected association between chronic alcohol consumption and the risk of laryngeal cancer. While chronic alcohol consumption is an independent dose-dependent risk factor by itself, in conjunction with chronic tobacco use, the risk multiplies several fold.[23] Alcohol is presumed to act as a cocarcinogen and acts both locally as well as systemically through various mechanisms at different stages during initiation and promotion. Carcinogenesis is also influenced by the malnutrition and depletion of protective vitamins and minerals that accompany chronic alcoholism.[24] Within the larynx, the epilarynx (laryngeal inlet), which overlaps the digestive tract on its exterior, is at greater risk from chronic alcohol consumption as compared to the endolarynx (glottis and subglottis) presumably because the latter site does not come into direct contact with alcohol.

Diet

A multicentre case-control study from Europe showed that high intake of fruit, vegetables, vegetable oil, fish, and low intake of butter and preserved meats were associated with reduced risk of both epilaryngeal and endolaryngeal cancers after adjustment for alcohol, tobacco, socioeconomic status and nutrition.[25] High intake of vitamins C and E, riboflavine, iron, zinc and selenium, and a high polyunsaturated/saturated fatty acid ratio in diet were also found to have a protective effect. The micronutrients act as antioxidants and/or inducers of differentiation, and are thought to inhibit carcinogenesis at different stages. Therefore, foods like fruit, salad, vegetables and dairy products may have a protective effect against the risk of laryngeal cancer.

Socioeconomic status

Laryngeal cancer has been associated with lower social class due to poor health care, smoking, drinking, dietary habits, and exposure to environmental and occupational carcinogens. This association has also been demonstrated in south-west England where the incidence of laryngeal carcinoma has shown a gradual increase with increasing deprivation.[26] The Heidelberg case-contol study[22] showed an increased independent relative risk for people of low educational standard and unskilled workers.

The impact of air pollution has resulted in a two-to-three-fold increase in the risk for laryngeal cancer in heavily industrialized cities as compared to rural populations.[27] In Third World countries, indoor air pollution by emission products of fossil fuel single stoves is a major risk factor.[28] Burning lignite, hard coal, oil or wood in these stoves causes an emission of high concentrations of carcinogenic combustion products such as polycyclic hydrocarbons into the indoor air, and their use in confined spaces increases the risk many fold.

Viruses

The role of the human papillomaviruses (HPV) in the production of laryngeal papillomas and malignant tumours remains controversial.[29] While a study from Denmark[30] could detect HPV infection in only one out of 30 (3.3%) dysplastic lesions, HPV DNA sequences from strains 16 and 33 of the virus were isolated from 40% of laryngeal tumours.[31] This finding must be interpreted in view of the fact that another study isolated HPV type 11 from 25% of normal human larynges.[32] A recent report on 179 patients treated for recurrent laryngeal papillomatosis found carcinoma in 1.7% of histologically verified papillomas.[33] The risk of developing carcinoma increases 16-fold for patients whose laryngeal papillomas have been treated with irradiation.[34]

At the present level of our understanding, perhaps more significant than the aetiological link between HPV infection and laryngeal cancer is the prognostic importance of finding HPV sequences in patients with laryngeal cancer. A study from the MD Anderson Cancer Center has reported that detection of HPV DNA in laryngeal tumours was significantly related to decreased survival independent of the stage of the tumour.[35]

Occupation

Blue collar workers exposed to asbestos, metal dusts, diesel exhaust, sulphuric acid mists, tar products and other inorganic and organic agents may have an increased risk of laryngeal cancer.[36] Although the carcinogenic effect of these agents may be important independently, the high incidence of tobacco and alcohol consumption in this social group must be taken into consideration. A high risk for wood-related occupations such as furniture making and woodworking has been reported in a case-control study from Spain.[37]

Genetic susceptibility

Enzymes such as glutathione S-transferase (GST) are involved in the detoxification of several tobacco smoke-derived carcinogens. It is therefore possible that deficiency of isoenzymes of GST due to homozygous deletion of the GSTM1 and GSTT1 genes (the null genotypes) may modulate susceptibility to smoking-induced cancers. A recent study from France has shown an increased risk in the GSTM1 null genotype among smokers of 20 g/day or less but not among heavier smokers.[38] Indirect evidence of a genetic predisposition to laryngeal cancer is provided by studies on familial laryngeal cancer and in patients with the Lynch syndrome[39] and Bloom's syndrome.[40]

Hormones

Epidemiological studies have shown that laryngeal cancer is predominantly a disease affecting men. It is, therefore, conceivable that hormonal changes might play an important role in the development and prognosis of laryngeal cancer. The role of hormonal receptors and hormonal manipulation has been investigated.[41,42] One report has identified the estradiol receptor content of the tumour as a good indicator of prognosis, with the estradiol-positive group enjoying a better disease-free survival.[43]

Ionizing radiation

The use of ionizing radiation in the treatment of benign conditions such as thyrotoxicosis, tuberculosis, and skin conditions has been associated with development of laryngeal carcinoma and sarcoma.[44] Radiation-induced sarcoma may also follow treatment of laryngeal cancer with radiation therapy.[45,46]

Precancer

Leukoplakia is a descriptive clinical term for a white patch on the mucosa and has no histologic or prognostic significance. Examination of most laryngeal leukoplakic patches reveals keratosis, a histological term used to describe complete replacement of superficial epithelial cells by keratin filaments with dissolution of the nuclei. Laryngeal keratosis is only a superficially visible manifestation of an underlying pathological process that can range from simple hyperplasia to invasive squamous carcinoma. The rate of malignant transformation of these lesions varies from 1 to 40% depending on the grade of dysplasia present. These lesions are almost always found on the true vocal cords and are usually bilateral (67%).[47] Clinical signs of high risk include: erythroplakia, surface granularity, increased keratin thickness, increased size, recurrence after conservative excision, and long duration.

The abundance and variety of histological terms used in the literature has led to confusion in attempts to describe the pathogenesis of malignant transformation of precancerous laryngeal lesions. Regardless of the other histological descriptives used, the most important practical indicator of potential to malignant change is the presence and the degree of dysplasia in the lesion. A 5-year follow-up of 147 patients who had hyperplastic laryngeal lesions with varying keratosis and/or dysplasia found carcinoma in 7.8% of patients whose initial specimens showed mild dysplasia. By contrast, as many as 55% of those who had moderate dysplasia in their original lesions progressed to severe dysplasia or carcinoma.[48] More than 20 schemes of classification of laryngeal dysplasia have been proposed but none is in common use. Five histological parameters have been described as reliable indicators of malignant potential: abnormal mitotic figures, mitotic activity, stromal inflammation, maturation level, and nuclear pleomorphism.[49] Factors such as surface morphology and the amount of keratinization, nucleolar prominence and poikilocytosis were not found significant.

Other factors

Chronic oesophagogastric reflux disease has been linked to an increase in cancers of the anterior two-thirds of the vocal cords.[50] Similarly, a correlation between laryngeal cancer and chronic hypertrophic laryngitis, which was seen in 6% of all vocal cord cancers, has been suggested without any epidemiological proof.[51]

Site distribution

The pattern of distribution of squamous cancer within the larynx appears to be related to the type of carcinogenic insult. In the UK and the US, the vast majority of laryngeal cancers may be related to smoking tobacco and therefore, the vocal cords are the most commonly affected. In contrast, the supraglottis, which is more exposed to other carcinogenic influences such as alcohol, is more frequently involved in countries like France which have a relatively higher per capita consumption (Table 15.3).

Table 15.3 Site distribution in percentage of total cases of laryngeal cancer

	Supraglottis (%)	Glottis (%)	Subglottis (%)
United Kingdom[52]	27	69	4
USA[53]	31	56	1
India[54]	71	28.6	0.2
France[55]	60	30	

Natural history of laryngeal cancer

The Primary

Supraglottic carcinoma

Although there are no doubts about the distinct embryological origin of the supraglottis, no actual anatomical barrier has been found in the body of the ventricle to support the traditional division of the larynx into the supraglottic, glottic and subglottic areas.[56,57] Tumours of the supraglottis generally tend to spread in an upward direction, an observation that has been verified by isotope injection studies.[58] When the isotope is injected into the false vocal fold, it fills up the paraglottic space laterally and then spreads into the pre-epiglottic space and the aryepiglottic folds superiorly. Inferior spread into the deep aspect of the vocal fold via the paraglottic space is seen only after a large volume of isotope has been injected. Tumours of the infrahyoid epiglottis spread anteriorly into the pre-epiglottic space. The perichondrium of the epiglottis and the thyroepiglottic ligament act as the first barriers to anterior spread. Once this barrier is breached, the tumour enters the pre-epiglottic space through fenestrations in the epiglottic cartilage. Within the space, the tumour grows with a 'pushing' margin and therefore, invasion of the hyoid bone is rare. Preservation of the hyoid bone during supraglottic laryngectomy is therefore safe in most patients, and may decrease postoperative problems with swallowing. Tumours that are restricted to above the ventricle almost never

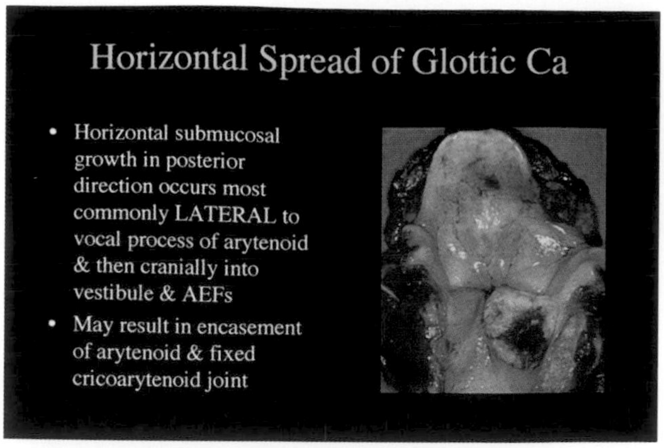

Figure 15.9 Glottic cancer.

invade the thyroid cartilage and its outer perichondrium can be safely preserved during supraglottic laryngectomy. Inferior spread in the region of the anterior commissure is limited by the anterior commissure tendon and the 'x-space,' which is a completely avascular triangular zone at the upper anterior end of the vocal cords separating the supraglottis from the glottis.

Tumours of the 'marginal zone', which is the suprahyoid epiglottis and the aryepiglottic folds, behave much more aggressively and are significantly more prone to lymphatic metastases. Once the tumour breaks through the quadrangular membrane to invade the adjacent medial wall of the pyriform sinus, it has ready access to the rich lymphatic supply of the vallecula or tongue base.

Glottic carcinoma

Cancers of the glottis are contained locally in the early stage by four major barriers: the vocal ligament, the anterior commissure, the thyroglottic ligament, and the conus elasticus. The thyroglottic ligament is that part of the conus elasticus which fans out from the anterior free border (the anterior vocal ligament) in an anterior and lateral direction thus covering the superior surface of the vocalis muscle to attach to the medial aspect of the thyroid lamina with the vocalis muscle. Its importance is that it acts as a barrier to tumour spread of anteriorly sited vocal cord cancers (Figures 15.9).

Tumours of the free margin of the true vocal cords are initially confined to the underlying Reinke's space by the vocal ligament. The tumour often spreads on the mucosal surface to involve the entire length of the cord, but once it breaches the vocal ligament and infiltrates the underlying thyroarytenoid (vocalis) muscle, vocal cord mobility is affected.

Tumours of the anterior commissure lie in close anatomical proximity to the thyroid cartilage and an important clinical decision in their management is assessment of cartilage invasion. Tumour cells have been shown growing along collagen bundles of the anterior commissure tendon, which provides them with access to the thyroid cartilage.[59] As this area is deficient in perichondrium at the site of attachment of the anterior commissure tendon, subclinical invasion by the tumour is likely. On laryngeal serial sections, however, thyroid cartilage invasion has been shown only in tumours that extend upward at the anterior commissure to involve the base of the epiglottis. Clinical evaluation of cancers involving this site should, therefore, be supplemented by imaging in an effort to determine early cartilage invasion.

Cancer of the middle and posterior true cords tends to spread laterally. After the barrier of the Reinke's space is overcome, superior spread into the ventricle is hampered by the thyroglottic ligament, which is an extension of the vocal ligament along the floor of the ventricle. Lateral spread into the thyroarytenoid muscle produces vocal cord fixation. The conus elasticus resists inferior spread, but once through it, the tumour can spread laterally into the paraglottic space or it may be deflected medially into the submucosa of the subglottis. Invasion of the paraglottic space may also occur by tumour spread along the superior surface of the vocal cord upwards and laterally into the ventricle, above the thyroglottic ligament. From the paraglottic space, the tumour spreads inferiorly and may breach the cricothyroid membrane to invade the thyroid gland and soft tissues of the neck. The inner perichondrium of the cartilage and the thyroid cartilage itself are effective barriers to tumour spread. Transglottic tumours and glottic cancers with more than 1 cm of subglottic extension are most likely to invade into the thyroid cartilage. Areas of ossification are at highest risk of invasion due to the better vascularity and biochemical changes associated with bone formation. The inferior rim of the thyroid cartilage and the superior rim of the cricoid cartilage are areas of early ossification that border the cricothyroid space. These ossified rims of the cricothyroid space are at increased risk of involvement as tumour spreads from the paraglottic space into the neck through the cricothyroid membrane and space.

Subglottic carcinoma

Primary tumours of the subglottis are rare and not much is known about the pathology and pathways of their spread. These tumours can extend submucosally in a superior direction through the conus elasticus to produce vocal cord fixation. The hypopharynx and oesophagus may be involved by posterior spread beneath the cricoid cartilage, and subepithelial spread along the mucous glands may allow spread to the cricothyroid membrane and cricoid cartilage.[60]

Lymphatic nodal metastases

As with other sites within the head and neck, cervical lymphatic metastasis in cancer of the larynx is the single most important determinant of prognosis. While there are no doubts about the importance of treating palpable cervical nodes, considerable controversy exists in the literature regarding management of the clinically negative neck.

Supraglottic carcinoma

Cancers of the supraglottic larynx are significantly more likely to present with cervical nodal metastasis compared to other laryngeal subsites. The incidence of occult metastasis in supraglottic carcinoma ranges from 20% to 50% depending on the T stage of the primary. The overall rate of nodal metastasis is also related to the T stage (Table 15.4).

The primary echelons of nodal drainage are levels II, III and IV (Table 15.5). In the clinically negative neck, micrometastases were found in 37% of patients with levels II and III being the most frequently involved. Occult metastases at levels I and V were found on pathological examination in only 6% and 1% respectively.[61] The patients who had occult metastases at levels I and V respectively had metastases at other levels. Surgical treatment of the clinically N0 or N1 neck may, therefore, safely include levels II, III and IV while levels I and V need to be dissected only for higher neck stages and for T4 primaries. For patients presenting with clinically obvious nodes, the incidence of involvement of levels I and V is up to 11% and 6% respectively. Level V is almost never involved in the absence of nodal disease at other more proximal levels while level I involvement is generally associated with adverse features of the primary tumour such as extralaryngeal spread, either into the soft tissues of the neck or the base of the tongue, or high grade.

Within the supraglottis, tumours of the marginal zone, which includes the suprahyoid epiglottis and the aryepiglottic folds have a greater propensity to neck metastases compared to those of the infrahyoid epiglottis (Table 15.6).

Glottic carcinoma

The risk of lymphatic metastases from carcinoma of the true vocal cords is relatively lower than that for supraglottic carcinoma. Since most early glottic cancers are treated using radiation therapy, the incidence of occult cervical metastasis has been reported only for surgically treated higher stage primaries, and ranges from 10% for T3 to 29% for T4 tumours.[63] The overall rate of metastasis is less than

Table 15.4 The overall (occult and clinical) incidence of lymphatic metastasis in supraglottic carcinoma

Stage of the primary tumour	Incidence (%)
T1	5–25
T2	30–70
T3–T4	65–80

Table 15.6 The incidence of lymphatic metastasis in supraglottic carcinoma according to subsite[62]

	Marginal zone (%)	Infrahyoid epiglottis (%)
Clinically N+ at presentation	48–57	32–41
Occult metastases	20–38	14–16

Table 15.5 The levels of nodal involvement in supraglottic cancer[61]

Level of nodal involvement	Clinically N0 neck (%)	Clinically N+ neck (%)	
		Immediate RND*	Subsequent RND*
I	6	5	11
II	18	62	63
III	18	53	68
IV	9	31	37
V	1	0	6

•Radical neck dissection

Table 15.7 The levels of nodal involvement in glottic cancer[61]

Level of nodal involvement	Clinically N0 neck (%)	Clinically N+ neck (%)	
		Immediate RND*	Subsequent RND*
I	0	15	6
II	21	54	38
III	29	61	75
IV	7	15	28
V	7	8	0

•Radical neck dissection

5% for T1, 5–10% for T2, 10–20% for T3, and 25–40% for T4 tumours.[64,65] The primary echelons of drainage are levels II, III and IV (Table 15.7). As with other laryngeal tumours, isolated involvement of levels I and V is uncommon. Tumours of the vocal cords rarely metastasize bilaterally or into the contralateral neck except in the presence of extensive supra- or subglottic involvement or invasion of the thyroid cartilage.

In a study of 92 whole organ laryngeal sections, about 9% revealed involvement of the Delphian or cricothyroid lymph node, and involvement seemed to be dependent more on the anatomic location of the primary tumour rather than its size.[66] Most tumours that metastasize to the Delphian node lie in an anterior location. Tumours that involve the conus elasticus, subglottis or cricoid cartilage anteriorly are at high risk of involving the Delphian node which, in turn, is associated with an increased risk of paratracheal node involvement and stomal recurrence. While a positive Delphian node may be not be relevant to the technique of total laryngectomy, it is an important consideration in the planning and performance of partial laryngeal surgery. The probability of total laryngectomy is much greater in these patients compared to other similar sized tumours. It is generally agreed that involvement of the Delphian node is associated with a poor outcome.[67]

Subglottic carcinoma

The overall incidence of cervical lymphatic metastasis from primary subglottic carcinoma is less than 20%. The incidence of paratracheal node involvement is, however, much higher at 50–65%.[68,69] Mediastinal nodes may be involved in a high percentage of cases, with one series reporting an incidence of 46%.[70] These statistics underscore the importance of treating the paratracheal nodes in management of subglottic cancers.

Distant metastases

The lung is the most commonly affected systemic site followed by the mediastinum, bone, and liver. About 15% of patients with supraglottic cancers and 3% with glottic cancers will develop distant metastases within 2 years of diagnosis.[71] The development of distant metastases is generally preceded by locoregional failure, but one study has reported that 11% of supraglottic and 7% of glottic carcinomas developed distant metastases in the absence of local failure or neck recurrence.[72]

Squamous cell carcinoma of the larynx is characterized by the relatively high incidence of second primary tumours. Most of these develop in the lungs and are more likely after supraglottic rather than glottic primaries. The incidence of second primary tumours increases linearly with time; 11–19% of patients develop second primary tumours within 5 years of treatment which increases to 30% at 10 years.[73] The value of routine chest radiography during follow-up is debatable. In a study of 556 patients with laryngeal carcinoma, yearly chest radiographs detected lung cancer in 12.4% patients. At diagnosis 68% of patients were asymptomatic but their survival averaged only 10 months against 4 months for the symptomatic patients.[74]

Staging

The use of the most recent version of the UICC/AJC rules for staging is mandatory (Tables 15.8–15.11). However, the TNM system (and associated stage grouping) is far from perfect as a prognostic indicator for individual patients. For instance, stage III includes patients with T3N0 as well as those with T1–3N1 tumours. The prognostic impact of positive lymph nodes is well recognized and must be considered in planning treatment. The staging system gives

Table 15.8 T staging of supraglottic tumours

Tx	Primary tumour cannot be assessed
T0	No evidence of primary tumour
T1	Tumour limited to one subsite of supraglottis with normal vocal cord mobility
T2	Tumour invades mucosa of more than one adjacent subsite of supraglottis or glottis or region outside supraglottis (e.g. base of tongue, vallecula, medial wall of pyriform sinus) without fixation of the larynx
T3	Tumour limited to larynx with vocal cord fixation and/or invades postcricoid area and/or pre-epiglottic tissues
T4	Tumour invades through thyroid cartilage and/or extends into soft tissues of the neck, thyroid and/or oesophagus

Table 15.9 T staging of glottic tumours

Tx	Primary tumour cannot be assessed
T0	No evidence of primary tumour
Tis	Carcinoma in situ
T1	Tumour limited to vocal cord(s) with normal mobility (may involve anterior or posterior commissures)
T1a	Tumour limited to one vocal cord
T1b	Tumour involves both vocal cords
T2	Tumour extends to supraglottis and/or subglottis and/or with impaired vocal cord mobility
T3	Tumour limited to larynx with vocal cord fixation
T4	Tumour invades through thyroid cartilage and/or extends beyond larynx (e.g. to trachea, soft tissues of the neck, thyroid, pharynx, etc)

no consideration to the biological behaviour of the primary tumour; an exophytic T1 tumour of the free edge of the vocal cord behaves very differently from a similarly staged superficial tumour that extends across the anterior commissure to involve both the cords. The TNM system is, however, the most widely accepted staging system and does provide a means of comparison of treatment methods and results.

Clinical presentation

Symptoms

The common symptoms of laryngeal cancer are hoarseness, sore throat, dysphagia and odynophagia. Hoarseness is an early symptom of glottic cancer but may be seen later in advanced supraglottic or

Table 15.10 T staging of subglottic tumours

Tx	Primary tumour cannot be assessed
T0	No evidence of primary tumour
Tis	Carcinoma in situ
T1	Tumour limited to subglottis
T2	Tumour extends to vocal cord(s) with normal or impaired mobility
T3	Tumour limited to larynx with vocal cord fixation
T4	Tumour invades through cricoid or thyroid cartilage and/or extends into soft tissues of the neck, thyroid and/or oesophagus

Table 15.11 TNM stage grouping for laryngeal tumours

	Tis	T1	T2	T3	T4
N0	0	I	II	III	IV
N1	n/a	III	III	III	IV
N2	n/a	IV	IV	IV	IV
N3	n/a	IV	IV	IV	IV

subglottic tumours signifying spread to the vocal cord, arytenoid or cricoarytenoid joint. Paraglottic spread can occur submucosally from these sites to produce hoarseness without any mucosal irregularity. Sore throat and dysphagia are more commonly associated with supraglottic tumours and odynophagia signifies involvement of the hypopharynx or base of tongue. Referred otalgia generally indicates base of tongue involvement, but may also be seen in tumours that have extended into the neck through cartilage. Ulceration and bleeding from exophytic tumours may present as haemoptysis. Dyspnoea and stridor occur with bulky supraglottic tumours or in the presence of vocal cord fixation. A neck mass almost always indicates lymphatic metastasis but may result from direct extension of the tumour into the soft tissues of the neck.

Physical examination and investigation

Clinical examination is limited by the fact that certain areas of the larynx are inaccessible to both visualization and palpation, and involvement of these structures has an important bearing on staging as well as management. Information from radiological imaging and operative endoscopy must be utilized in conjunction with physical findings to document an accurate pretreatment TNM staged record.

Supraglottic tumours are frequently understaged because the pre-epiglottic and paraglottic spaces cannot be assessed clinically. Infrahyoid tumours of the epiglottis are especially prone to invade the pre-epiglottic space. A study found invasion of the pre-epiglottic space in 89% of infrahyoid tumours as against none in suprahyoid tumours.[75] Both CT and MRI can detect invasion of the pre-epiglottic space, but MRI has the advantage of being able to provide sagittal images. Signs of pre-epiglottic space invasion include loss of normal fat density, and absent visualization of the superior extent of the lateral cricoarytenoid muscle.[76] Radiographic assessment is also useful to assess subglottic extension and the status of the laryngeal ventricle in glottic primaries. Although both CT and MRI are excellent for assessing subglottic extension, coronal MR reconstruction may be better at delineating ventricular and paraglottic submucosal spread. MRI may also be superior at differentiating thyroarytenoid muscle invasion from involvement of the cricoarytenoid joint as the cause of vocal cord fixation.[76] The value of CT in detecting cartilage invasion is doubtful because of the inconsistent mineralization patterns. If the sclerotic appearance of the cartilage is taken as a radiologic marker, only 46% of patients actually show histologic features of cartilage invasion.[77] Another study found microscopic invasion of the thyroid cartilage in as many as 50% of clinically and radiologically staged T3 tumours of the glottis.[78] Table 15.12 shows the radiological and clinical criteria that may be used to predict an increased risk of cartilage invasion in glottic cancers.

Positron emission tomography using fluorine-labelled deoxyglucose (FDG-PET) is as yet under investigation, and produces cross-sectional images depending upon the location and concentration of radionuclide-labeled radiotracers. Apart from the technical difficulty of having a cyclotron in close proximity to the imaging facility to produce the radioactive isotopes, its major disadvantage is the lack of anatomical detail on the image. Four months onwards after completion of treatment, it has been reported to be superior to any imaging modality currently available in differentiating recurrent tumour from postradiation soft tissue changes. Based on preliminary evidence, its major role appears to be in the evaluation of the postradiotherapy patient.[79]

Table 15.12 Radiological and clinical predictors of cartilage invasion in glottic cancer

	Risk (%)
Paraglottic spread	74
Extensive cartilage ossification	73
Extensive involvement of anterior commissure	67
Tumour > 2 cm	66
Vocal cord fixation	54

After Nakayama and Brandenburg.[78]

The role of routine oesophagoscopy in asymptomatic patients is controversial. The incidence of synchronous oesophageal primaries in patients with head and neck cancer is about 1–2%, and retrospective studies have not demonstrated any survival advantage for patients whose tumours were discovered using routine oesophagoscopy.[80] Oesophagoscopy is therefore recommended only to investigate symptoms such as difficulty swallowing.

Treatment

General principles

Treatment of the patient with laryngeal cancer, as for patients suffering from other cancers, must provide the best chance for cure while minimizing potential adverse effects on the normal laryngeal functions of phonation, protection of the airway and respiration. The psychosocial effects of loss of normal laryngeal function can be crippling and optimal treatment planning must be individually tailored based on a variety of interrelated factors. The patient's age, their occupation, ability to read and write, general health and co-morbid conditions, lifestyle issues such as refusal to stop smoking, distance from the hospital and family status need to be taken into account while planning treatment. The patient's opinion and preference for a particular treatment should be factored into the process of decision making.

While the chronological age by itself is not a deterrent to aggressive treatment, the risk of treatment associated with intercurrent conditions and the cardiopulmonary status generally prevalent in this population may modify treatment approaches considerably. Patients who are technically amenable to conservation laryngeal surgery may be unsuitable due to medical conditions such as chronic obstructive pulmonary disease or congestive heart failure. The pretreatment phase must be utilized to reinforce lifestyle issues such as cessation of smoking and alcohol abuse. In addition to joint treatment planning by the surgical, radiation and medical oncology teams, multidisciplinary input from speech therapists, physiotherapists, nutritionists, and psychological and social support services is invaluable to achieving a favourable outcome. Patients planned for total laryngectomy may benefit from meeting others who have tolerated the procedure well, and where available, the services of laryngectomee clubs must be utilized routinely.

Early laryngeal cancer (stages I and II) responds equally well to either radiation or surgery. Treatment decisions, therefore, must be based on the other factors mentioned previously and generally include functional results, compliance of the patient and long-term sequelae. Lesions that are more advanced (stages III and IV) have been traditionally treated with primary surgery followed by postoperative radiation therapy. This approach invariably translates into loss of the larynx with all its attendant physical and psychosocial effects. The effects of the loss of voice following total laryngectomy have been offset to a large extent by improved techniques for voice rehabilitation. The psychological effects of laryngectomy, however, are related as much to loss of voice as they are to other factors such as the need for a permanent tracheostoma.[81] This realization has led to the investigation and acceptance of larynx-preserving approaches using induction chemotherapy and radiation therapy, which may be offered to patients with advanced tumours.

Follow-up and rehabilitation

Rehabilitation of the patient after treatment involves close co-operation with other health professionals including the speech therapist, dietician, and nursing staff. The follow-up schedule must incorporate appropriate evaluation of the patient by these members of the treating team at regular intervals. In addition to a thorough examination of the head and neck region, a yearly chest radiograph may be useful, although its value in improving outcome of second primary lung cancer remains unproven.

Results of treatment

Carcinoma in situ

Carcinoma in situ is characterized by complete replacement of normal squamous epithelium by malignant cells that do not extend beyond the basement membrane. Clinically, these lesions may be seen as leukoplakia, erythroplasia, or hyperkeratosis, and management is based on the histological diagnosis. The pathological distinction between severe dysplasia and carcinoma in situ (CIS) is largely subjective but this may not be of practical importance as both carry a significant risk for development of invasive carcinoma. The incidence of CIS ranges from 1 to 15% of laryngeal tumours.[82] Most patients are males in their sixth decade of life and the anterior half of the true cords is the most common location. A review of 468 patients with laryngeal CIS found that 33–90% of untreated cases and 30% of treated patients eventually developed invasive carcinoma.[82]

Microinvasive carcinoma has the same cellular features as CIS but with discrete foci of invasion of the basement membrane. Most microinvasive lesions eventually progress to frankly invasive carcinoma.

The management of CIS and microinvasive carcinoma is controversial. Proponents of radiation therapy cite the better posttreatment voice quality as its major advantage. Table 15.13 shows the results of radiation therapy in the treatment of CIS.

Although radiation therapy may cure individual lesions, it provides no assurance that another lesion will not develop in an already diseased and unstable mucosa. Surgical treatment, on the other hand, has equivalent control rates (Table 15.14) with the advantage of repeatability. Excellent cure rates and functional results have been reported after endoscopic laser procedures.[87] Laser ablation may be used either primarily, or preferably, if biopsy of the

Table 15.13 Results of radiation therapy in the treatment of CIS

Reference	No. of patients	Local recurrence (%)	Total laryngectomy (%)	Survival
Pene and Fletcher[83]	79	11–26	11	—
Doyle et al[84]	22	4.5	—	95% at 5 years
Elman et al[85]	69	17–25	14	
Small et al[86]	415	20	—	96% after salvage surgery

Table 15.14 Results of surgical treatment for CIS and microinvasive carcinoma

Reference	No. of patients	Type of procedure	Local failure (%)	Total laryngectomy (%)	Survival
Lillie and DeSanto[88]	8	Endoscopic cordectomy	—	0	100% at 6 years
	33	Endoscopic biopsy + diathermy	15	3	100% at 5 years
Miller and Fisher[89]	100	Stripping	25		
	60	Laryngofissure + cordectomy	6.6		
Small et al[86]	248	Stripping	40		96%
	50	Endoscopic laser resection	8		100% after salvage surgery or RT

deep epithelial margin of the specimen after vocal cord stripping shows microinvasion. Radiation therapy is recommended for:

- Recurrence after one or more vocal cord strippings;
- Lesions that recur relatively soon after vocal cord stripping;
- Patients whose voice quality is critical to their livelihood (e.g. professional singers, etc.);
- Poor operative risk;
- Patients who are unlikely to attend for regular follow-up;
- Lesions that are not easily accessible to endoscopic ablation (e.g. anterior commissure lesions).

Patients must be encouraged to stop smoking and there must be regular follow-up after treatment.

Supraglottic cancer

Treatment options in supraglottic carcinoma include primary radiation therapy, endoscopic surgery, partial or total laryngectomy, combined therapy, and larynx-preserving chemoradiation therapy. Curative radiation therapy has been used effectively for small tumours and selected advanced lesions, reserving surgery to salvage failures. Alternatively, primary partial laryngectomy has been used for small lesions and total laryngectomy for advanced tumours. As discussed previously, the stage of the tumour is not the only factor that influences choice of treatment. The treatment decision is individualized to each patient based on a combination of factors such as the performance status, cardiopulmonary function, and the choice of the patient, in addition to the philosophy of the treating team.

Early disease

Stage I and II disease may be controlled with equal results using surgery or radiation therapy. Surgery controls T1 cancer in 90–95% patients and T2 lesions in 80–90%[90,91] while the corresponding rates for primary radiation therapy are slightly lower at 80–90% for T1 and 70–80% for T2 tumours.[92,93] The difference in control rates between surgery and radiation therapy become comparable when the effect of surgical salvage is added to the results of primary radiation (Table 15.15).

Primary radiation therapy with surgical salvage of failures is an attractive option because it provides an opportunity to preserve laryngeal function without compromising ultimate control rates. However, evaluation of the irradiated larynx for recurrent cancer is difficult on both physical as well as radiological examination. As a result, by the time they are detected, many recurrent cancers may not be amenable to conservation surgery. Although supraglottic laryngectomy can be performed safely in selected patients who fail radiation therapy, eligibility criteria are very stringent.

Endoscopic resection of early supraglottic tumours has been reported with good results. En bloc resection of 22 patients with T1 or T2 lesions without any further treatment resulted in 100% local control at 2 years.[97] This form of therapy has been especially popular in Germany, and its use in management of more advanced lesions has been successfully reported as part of a combined modality approach.[98] These authors reported a 72.6% 5-year overall survival in 43 patients with stage I–II (laser excision ± neck dissection) and 48% in stage III–IV disease (laser excision ± neck dissection ± radiation therapy). They report a laryngeal preservation rate of 70% in pT3–4 tumours, with a technique of blockwise, piecemeal resection of advanced laryngeal tumours which challenges traditional oncologic surgery.

Table 15.15 Results of primary radiation therapy in early stage supraglottic cancer

Reference	No. of patients	Local control (%)	Regional control (%)	Larynx preserved (%)	Ultimate control (postsalvage)	Survival
Goepfert et al[94]	147	T1 88 T2 81	≅ 90	T1 88.5 T2 77	T1 96 T2 97	T1 100% T2 80%
Weems et al[95]	39	T1 92 T2 81	T1 90 T2 76	T1 94 T2 84	T1 100 T2 76	Determinate 5-year survival T1 100% T2 100%
Nakfoor et al[96]	18	T1 96 T2 86	T1 85 T2 93	T1 96 T2 80	T1 96 T2 93	5-year disease-free survival T1 78% T2 82%

Advanced disease

Treatment results in stage III and IV supraglottic cancer depend mainly upon the presence of cervical lymph node metastases and their control. Control rates for patients treated with combined modalities have improved considerably from the traditionally quoted figures of 20–40%,[103] but overall survival has remained static. As in other head and neck sites, this is due to attrition of survival rates by deaths from distant metastases and second primary tumours. Primary radiation therapy by itself has been reported to control about 60% of T3 and 40–50% of T4 tumours.[104,105] Surgery is no longer used as a single modality in these patients, but a 50–70% cure rate has been reported (Table 15.16).

Combining surgery with postoperative radiation therapy has resulted in improved local-regional control but as described above, has not improved overall survival (Table 15.17).

The alternative approach of radical radiation therapy reserving surgery for salvage of failures, has been shown to produce equivalent local control to primary surgery or surgery combined with postoperative radiation, and with the advantage of larynx preservation in successfully treated patients (Table 15.18).

The arguments against using primary radical radiation for advanced tumours have been difficulty in monitoring these patients for local recurrence because of laryngeal oedema, and the reported dangers of postoperative complications if laryngectomy is required for salvage. The advent of larynx-preservation therapy has resulted in a change of attitude, and the indications of primary total laryngectomy have diminished (see later).

Overall, local failures after treatment occur in about 10%, regional failures in about 15–20%, and distant metastases in about 10–30% of patients with supraglottic cancer. Most patients die of second primary tumours (20–25%) or other intercurrent illness (20%), and Table 15.19 is a compilation of survival results according to stage of the disease.

Management of the neck

The supraglottis is a high-risk site for lymphatic metastases to the neck: 30–70% of patients with primaries larger than T2 have clinical or occult cervical nodes and about half of those with neck involvement have bilateral metastases.[99] Management of the patient who presents with clinically palpable nodes is well established, and may involve surgery and/or radiation as appropriate. A general principle is that if both the primary and the neck can be effectively treated using the same modality, combination therapy is avoided, but obviously, treatment needs to be individualized. The approach to the clinically negative neck, however, continues to be debated. Bocca[90] was one of the first to show that bilateral elective neck dissection can result in improved regional control. In a recent report of over 1000 cases, he demonstrated a 30–50% reduction in neck failure and a 78% 5-year overall survival using this approach.[99] It has also been shown that as many as two-thirds of patients who have occult neck metastasis in a unilateral radical neck dissection specimen died of the cancer, and almost 80% failed in the opposite neck.[100] Some authors have reported the relative ineffectiveness of radiation therapy in preventing neck failure.[101,102] We believe that the elective treatment of both sides of the neck needs to be incorporated into the treatment plan. The mode of treatment of the primary generally dictates the method used to treat the neck. If surgery is chosen

Table 15.16 The results of surgery in advanced supraglottic cancer

Reference	Treatment	T3/stage III (%)	T4/stage IV (%)
Ogura et al[106]	Partial/total laryngectomy	71*	63*
		63†	43†
Alajmo et al[107]	Total laryngectomy	53†	52†
DeSanto[108]	Partial/total laryngectomy	97‡	90‡
		75§	52§
Goepfert et al[109]	Partial/total laryngectomy	70§	32§

*3-year control; †5-year survival; ‡local control; §5-year cause-specific survival.

Table 15.17 The results of surgery combined with postoperative radiation therapy in advanced supraglottic cancer

Reference	Surgery	T3/stage III (%)	T4/stage IV (%)
Flynn et al[110]	Total laryngectomy	54*	
Goepfert et al[109]	Total laryngectomy	60†	35†
Burstein and Calcaterra[111]	Partial laryngectomy	90†	
Weems et al[112]	Partial/total laryngectomy	94‡	83‡
		100§	50§
Lee et al[113]**	Partial laryngectomy	91¶	

*5-year disease-free survival; †5-year cause-specific survival; ‡local control; §5-year determinate survival; ¶5-year disease-specific survival.
**36 of 60 patients were stage III or IV.

Table 15.18 The results of primary radical radiation therapy for advanced supraglottic carcinoma

Reference	No. of patients	Local control		Neck control		Larynx preservation		Survival	
		Stage	(%)	Stage	(%)	Stage	(%)	Stage	(%)
Harwood et al[114]*	136	T3N0	56	N1	56			T3N0	69
		T4N0	52	N3	39		64	T4N0	63
Karim et al[115]	81	T3-4N0	72†	T3-4N0	100†		67	T3-4N0	51‡
		T3-4N+	66†	T3-4N+	89†			T3-4N+	29‡
Mendenhall et al[116]§	—	T3	61	Stage III	59	T3	69	Stage III	45
		T4	33	Stage IVA	57	T4	57	Stage IVA	44
				Stage IVB	43			Stage IVB	24
Vermund et al[117]	216	Stage III	86	Stage III	90.5		74	Stage III	74¶
		Stage IV	72	Stage IV	78			Stage IV	45¶

*5-year figures; †3-year control rates; ‡5-year actuarial disease-free survival; §5-year statistics, AJCC 1983 staging; ¶5-year disease-free survival.

Table 15.19 5-year survival rates in squamous cell carcinoma of the supraglottic larynx

Reference	No. of patients	Stage I (%)	Stage II (%)	Stage III (%)	Stage IV (%)
Flynn et al[118]	234	93	49	50	33
Fu et al[119]	173	64	80	35	10
Shah and Tollefson[120]	290	83	72	42	0
Coates et al[121]	212	69	73	51	—
DeSanto[122]	236	80	65	62	52
Goepfert et al[109]	251	100	68	59	32
Weems et al[112]	195	100	93	58	54

for the primary tumour, neck dissection can be safely restricted to include bilateral levels II, III and IV only, as isolated involvement of levels I or V is rare.

Glottic cancer

Tumours of the true vocal cords present earlier than other laryngeal tumours because they produce hoarseness. In addition, because of sparse lymphatics, nodal metastasis is not a significant problem in these patients. These factors are generally combined with predicted impact of a particular regime on quality of voice to select treatment. Although radiation often impairs voice, the quality is generally better than that following surgery. Small cancers with mobile cords are effectively treated using radiation therapy. Advanced tumours have traditionally been treated using surgery with or without radiation therapy, but an additional option now available, albeit in the protocol setting, is chemoradiation therapy.

Early disease

The management and results of treatment of carcinoma in situ have been discussed previously. Invasive stage I and II cancers can be controlled equally effectively by radiation or surgery. Patients treated successfully with either modality retain lung-powered laryngeal speech. Surgery is slightly better at controlling these tumours than radiotherapy, but the advantage is lost when results of surgical salvage of radiation failures are considered. The main advantage of radiation therapy is that it generally results in a superior quality of voice but should the treatment fail, the rate of total laryngectomy has been reported to range between 50 and 70%.[123] The quality of voice after surgical treatment is an inverse function of the vocal cord mass resected, and primary conservation surgery suffers from the major drawback of leaving the patient with a voice that may be classified 'good' in only about a third of patients. Recent approaches have sought to combine the advantages of both modalities by using conservation surgery to salvage radiation failures, and this is probably the optimal therapeutic option for most patients with early glottic cancer.

Table 15.20 is a summary of local control rates and results of radiation therapy for T1–2 glottic cancer.

The treatment of choice in T1 and most T2 cancers is radiation therapy. Consequently, there are few series that report the results of primary conservation surgery in early glottic cancer (Table 15.21).

There is, however, a subset of patients whose tumours are thought by some to be less responsive to radiation therapy: lesions with impaired cord mobility, some larger T2 lesions, involvement of the anterior commissure, and subglottic extension. The impact of impaired cord mobility on local control prompted the proposal to subclassify T2 tumours into T2a (with normal mobility) and T2b (with impaired mobility). Involvement of the subglottis has been shown to worsen results of radiation therapy,[118,135] but the impact of anterior commissure involvement in T1 tumours is controversial. Several studies have reported equivalent local control rates in the region of 85–95% irrespective of involvement of the commissure.[126,128,136] For T2 cancers, there may be a negative impact of commissure involvement: local recurrence rates of 40 versus 13% if the commissure was free.[126]

Surgical salvage of limited stage failures after primary radiation therapy can be safely and effectively undertaken using conservation laryngectomy in properly selected patients. Table 15.22 shows the oncologic results of salvage partial laryngectomy. Laryngeal function does not necessarily have to be

Table 15.20 Results of radical radiation therapy in early glottic cancer

Reference	T1				T2			
	Local control			Voice preserved	Local control			Voice preserved
	No. of patients	Initial (%)	Ultimate (%)		No. of patients	Initial (%)	Ultimate (%)	
Mendenhall et al[124]	171	93	97	95	108	75	93	80
Kelly et al[125]	95	94	100	99	53	76	90	78
Pellitteri et al[126]	113	93	98	95	48	73	92	79
Small et al[127]	103	89	97	89	—	—	—	—
Fein et al[128]	132	95	98	96	—	—	—	—
Howell-Burke et al[129]	—	—	—	—	114	68	94	74
Guiney et al[130]	—	—	—	—	26	69	77	69

Table 15.21 Local control rates after primary conservation surgery in early glottic cancer

Reference	T1			T2		
	No. of patients	Initial (%)	Ultimate (%)	No. of patients	Initial (%)	Ultimate (%)
Ogura et al[131]	205	87	?	55	82	?
Laccourreye et al[132]	308	86.8	?	107	77.7	?
Johnson et al[133]	54	98	100	38	82	89
Thomas et al[134]	159	93	95	—	—	—

Table 15.22 The results of salvage vertical partial laryngectomy

Reference	No. of patients	Initial control (*N* (%))	Salvaged (*N* (%))	Ultimate local control (*N* (%))
Lavey and Calcaterra[138]*	251	206 (82)	34	240 (96)
DelGaudio et al[139]	22	18 (82)	2	20 (93)
Schwaab et al[140]	6	4 (66)	2	6 (100)
Lydiatt et al[141]	21	15 (71)	3	18 (85.7)
McLaughlin et al[142]	6	4 (66)	1	5 (83)
Watters et al[137]	25	18 (72)	6	24 (96)
Total	331	265 (80)	48/66 (72)	313 (94.5)

*Reported a review of 251 patients in 14 previously published series along with their own experience.

sacrificed in order to achieve local control of disease, and reserving total laryngectomy as the ultimate option for salvage provides more patients the chance for conservation of laryngeal function with no compromise in ultimate survival.[137]

In choosing a treatment strategy for an individual patient, the clinician must balance the expected control rate against the quality of voice. This is difficult because no objective measures of speech evaluation are available to define 'good' voice.

Investigations such as videostroboscopy and aerodynamic studies have been reported without much consistency in results,[143] and some studies have found that patients' perception of their own voice tends to be more forgiving than any objective assessment. Therefore, factors other than quality of voice must also be considered when recommending one treatment over another.

Advanced disease

It is generally accepted that more advanced glottic lesions causing invasion of cartilage, cord fixation or demonstrating direct extralaryngeal spread, are better treated with a combination of surgery and radiation. Surgical treatment of advanced glottic lesions generally consists of a total laryngectomy. The controversy over choice between primary laryngectomy and radiation with salvage laryngectomy has been stirred up again with the results of 'larynx-preservation' protocols demonstrating that almost two-thirds of patients can retain a functional larynx without any compromise in survival with the use of chemoradiation.

Radical radiation therapy with salvage laryngectomy of failures has been used at some centres, local control ranging from 40 to 60% and ultimate survival around 50–70%.[144,145] Some patients clearly respond better than others, and this has led some authors to subclassify locally advanced glottic cancers into 'favourable' (restricted to one hemilarynx, without airway obstruction) and 'unfavourable' cancers.[146] Other factors that may make the lesion more resistant to treatment with radical radiation and surgical salvage include tumour volume greater than 3.5 cm^3, involvement of the paraglottic space or the face of the arytenoid. It has also been reported that stage for stage, response rates are greater in females than in males[147] but no satisfactory explanation for this effect is available. Surgical salvage rates of about 50–65% after failure of radical radiation therapy have been reported and about 55–70% of all survivors of this approach will retain a functional larynx. Success with this form of therapy requires very careful and rigorous follow-up, especially since early detection of recurrence in radiated larynges is difficult. The other disadvantage can be the increased likelihood of postoperative complications after salvage laryngectomy.

Surgical treatment of advanced glottic lesions generally involves total laryngectomy and the results of primary total laryngectomy are listed in Table 15.23.

As discussed previously, conservation surgery using vertical partial laryngectomy can be safely carried out in a very select group of T3 patients. The oncologic effectiveness of this operation is demonstrated by Table 15.24. Despite these acceptable control rates, it is important to realize that only a very small number of patients with cord fixation are

Table 15.23 Primary laryngectomy in treatment of advanced glottic carcinoma

Reference	No. of patients and stage	Treatment*	Results† Percentage	Results† Description
Ogura et al[131]	88 T3N0–1	TL alone	68	Cure rate
	13 T4N0–1		54	Cure rate
Leroux-Robert[148]	40 T3	TL alone	57	Cure rate
	7 T4		14	Cure rate
Skolnik et al[149]	135 T3	TL alone	45	Cure rate
DeSanto[150]	63 T3N0	TL alone	98	Local control
			80	5-year survival
Johnson et al[151]	144 T3	TL±ND±PORT	T3 94	Local control
	34 T4		79	2-year DFS
			T4 86	Local control
			58	2-year DFS
Razack et al[152]	128 T3-4	TL±ND	95	Local control
			53	5-year survival (63% After salvage RT)

*TL: total laryngectomy; ND: neck dissection; PORT: postoperative radiation therapy.
†DFS: disease-free survival; RT: radiation therapy

Table 15.24 The results of conservation surgery in T3 glottic cancer

Reference	No. of patients	Treatment*	Results: Percentage	Results: Description
Som[153]	26	VPL	58	Cure rate
Lesinski et al[154]	18	VPL	83	Local control
Biller and Lawson[155]	26	VPL	73	Disease-free survival
Kessler et al[156]	27	VPL	85	Local control

*VPL: vertical partial laryngectomy.

suitable for conservation surgery. Hemilaryngectomy and its various modifications may be successfully used by surgeons experienced in the use of such procedures, but even in the best of hands, there is considerable morbidity associated with these extended resections.

The impact of adding routine postoperative radiation in advanced glottic cancer is controversial because local disease is controlled well with surgery, and lymphatic metastases are not as common as for other laryngeal tumours. Postoperative radiotherapy is beneficial in the presence of high-risk features of the primary tumour (invasion of the cartilage or extralaryngeal spread, involvement of the subglottis, adjacent hypopharynx or base of tongue) or high-volume neck disease. Another indication may be for prevention of stomal recurrence in patients who have had to undergo emergency tracheostomy or have pathologically involved paratracheal nodes, and in these patients, the lower edge of the radiation field must be modified to include the permanent tracheostome and the upper mediastinum.

Management of the neck

The overall incidence of lymphatic nodal metastases in glottic cancer is considerably lower than that for other laryngeal subsites. The risk for occult nodal metastases is directly dependent on the volume of the primary tumour, and ranges from 10% for T3 to about 30% for T4 tumours. Therefore, elective treatment of the neck in early lesions is not recommended. For more advanced tumours, however, the ipsilateral neck needs to be addressed during surgery, and dissection can be confined to levels II, III, and IV ('jugular node dissection'). This procedure has an accuracy of about 80% in identifying occult nodal metastases.[157] Postoperative radiation therapy is added according to the usual indications, and it may be elected to irradiate both sides of the neck depending upon the perceived risk of failure. If the primary treatment is radical radiation therapy, both sides of the neck are electively radiated in the hope of preventing subsequent neck metastases, which are difficult to control in this setting.

The overall survival for patients with early stage glottic cancer is in the range of 85–90% while the corresponding rates drop to around 65–70% for stage III and as low as 20% for stage IV tumours (Table 15.25).

Subglottic cancer

Primary

Primary cancers of the subglottic larynx are extremely rare (about 1% of laryngeal cancer) and generally present in an advanced stage. Apart from squamous cancers, other histological types like minor salivary gland tumours, cartilaginous tumours and soft tissue sarcomas may arise in this region. The subglottis is much more frequently invaded by glottic carcinoma, and these should be distinguished from primary subglottic carcinoma. As these are rare tumours, no large series exist and no meaningful comparison of treatment plans is possible. A comprehensive review of 185 patients with subglottic cancer reported in 20 series showed a 5-year survival of only 36% in 127 radiated patients and 42% in 58 who were treated with primary surgery.[165] Individual series have, however, reported better results (Tables 15.26 and 15.27).

Management of the neck

As described previously, the incidence of cervical nodal metastases in primary subglottic cancers is less than 20%, but the involvement of paratracheal nodal metastasis is estimated to be 50% or higher. Only clinically or radiologically positive nodes are treated, and elective cervical node dissection is not recommended based on the relatively low rate of neck failure (8%) in patients who are treated with laryngectomy alone.[69] The high rate of paratracheal

Table 15.25 Results of treatment in patients with squamous cell carcinoma of the true vocal cords

Reference	No. of patients	Stage I (%)	Stage II (%)	Stage III (%)	Stage IV (%)	Description
Skolnick et al[158]	264	82	70	53	20	5-year overall survival
Yuen et al[159]	192	—	—	80	63	5-year overall survival
Kaplan et al[160]	283	96	88	65	57*	5-year overall survival
Hendrickson et al[161]	525	82	68	61	37	4-year disease-free survival
Kelly et al[162]	148	82	79	—	—	3-year overall survival
Mainpang et al[163]	143	93	83	—	—	5-year overall survival
Fujii et al[164]	687	98	91	74	52	5-year relative survival

Table 15.26 The results of radical radiation therapy in subglottic cancer

Reference	No. of patients	Treatment	Results	
			Percentage	Description
Haylock and Deutsch[166]	23	Radiation ± surgical salvage	78	2-year disease-free survival
Warde et al[167]	23	Radiation	70	Local control for T1-3
			36	Local control for T4
Guedea et al[168]	6	Radiation	50	Local control for T2
			66	Local control for T4
Dahm et al[169]	6 (Stage I–II)	Radiation	33	5-year disease-free survival

Table 15.27 The results of primary surgery in subglottic cancer

Reference	No. of patients	Treatment	Results	
			Percentage	Description
Stell and Tobin[170]	45	Wide-field laryngectomy	53	Local control
Sessions et al[171]	3	Total laryngectomy ± neck dissection	66	5-year disease-free survival
Shaha and Shah[69]	16	Partial laryngectomy for stage I–II	100	Local control in stage I–II
		Wide-field laryngectomy for stage III–IV	77	Local control in stage III–IV
		Neck dissection for cN+ only		
Dahm et al[172]	12	Partial/total laryngectomy ± neck dissection for stage I–II	44	5-year disease-free survival in stage I–II
		Total laryngectomy + neck dissection ± radiation for III–IV	33	5-year disease-free survival in stage III–IV

nodal involvement, on the other hand, mandates elective treatment of these nodes in all patients.

Early stage disease is rare, and these patients should be given the chance of larynx preservation using primary radiation therapy. More advanced disease is best treated by laryngectomy with bilateral paratracheal node dissection, and ipsilateral or total thyroidectomy followed up by postoperative radiation therapy if indicated.

'Larynx preservation' therapy

Until the 1980s, the standard treatment for advanced stage laryngeal cancer consisted of total laryngectomy and/or radiation therapy in one of two settings: radical radiation with surgical salvage, or total laryngectomy with postoperative radiation. Although the first approach resulted in some patients retaining a functional larynx, recurrences were associated with significant reduction in survival. In the early 1980s, several clinical trials demonstrated high response rates of head and neck squamous cancers to induction chemotherapy,[173,174] and this observation was used to incorporate induction chemotherapy followed by radiotherapy in the treatment of laryngeal cancer. The goal of this strategy was to preserve laryngeal function without significantly reducing survival. Around this time, the issue of quality of life after treatment of cancer was being pushed into the limelight, and the debate was that some patients may be willing to sacrifice higher probability of cure in the hope of preserving function. The classic 'fireman study' of 1981[81] has often been quoted in this regard: healthy firemen and businessmen were given questionnaires addressing death from laryngeal cancer and the impact of total laryngectomy on their decision regarding their choice of treatment. Not surprisingly, some of these individuals were willing to accept alternative therapy even if it reduced their chance of survival. While the shortcomings of drawing conclusions from hypothetical questions posed to normal, healthy people are obvious, the study helped focus attention on the importance of providing patients with both laryngeal function and reasonable survival. In 1991, the Department of Veterans Affairs Laryngeal Cancer Study Group published the results of its landmark trial[175] comparing conventional treatment (surgery with postoperative radiation) and induction chemotherapy followed by radiation therapy in patients with advanced laryngeal cancer. Survival in each arm was equal at 68%, but as many as 64% of patients in the chemoradiation arm retained a functional larynx. The EORTC has also been active in this respect and the results of a phase III randomized trial of larynx-preserving therapy in advanced hypopharyngeal cancer showed results similar to the VALCSG trial.[176] They are now evaluating chemotherapy versus combined chemoradiation in larynx and hypopharyngeal carcinoma (EORTC 24954) in parallel to another randomized trial comparing definitive radiation therapy versus combined chemoradiotherapy (EORTC 22954).

The VALCSG trial has been the only large larynx-specific randomized trial but the results of this study paved the way for several other trials (Table 15.28) that evaluated this approach for other advanced head and neck cancers. The rationale for the use of induction chemotherapy has been the observation that it 'downstages' tumours, which then may permit cure with radiation. The mechanism of action of this effect has been debated extensively, and chemotherapy is believed to act either by sensitizing cancer cells or by selecting patients whose tumours are more likely to respond to radiation therapy.

As of now, there are many unanswered questions regarding the role of chemotherapy and its combination with radiation in the management of advanced stage laryngeal cancer. An ongoing co-operative intergroup phase III trial (RTOG 91-11) will hopefully provide some answers. This study has three treatment arms: irradiation only, irradiation with concurrent cisplatinum and induction chemotherapy using cisplatinum and 5-fluorouracil followed by surgery in non-responders and additional chemoradiation in responders. The primary endpoint is survival with preservation of laryngeal function, and the study has recruited a third of the targeted 546 patients. It is hoped that the results of this study will settle the debate whether chemotherapy does more than merely sensitize cancer cells to radiation therapy, and will help define the role of concurrent chemoradiation as compared to radiation therapy alone in advanced stage laryngeal cancer.

Most chemotherapy regimens employ a combination of cisplatinum and 5-fluorouracil but equivalent locoregional control and survival results have been achieved combining cisplatin with other drugs such as bleomycin or vinblastine.[184] Other studies have tried to improve the results of chemotherapy by adding leucovorin to the standard regimen of cisplatin-5-fluorouracil with mixed results; there was no improvement in toxicity or overall response in one study,[185] while two others have reported overall response rates of about 80%.[186,187] Newer approaches include the use of paclitaxel in combination with cisplatin and ifosfamide[188] and intra-arterial high-dose cisplatin concurrently with radiation therapy.[189] A major disadvantage of using chemotherapy before radiation therapy is the likelihood of significantly delaying the definitive treatment due to side-effects of chemotherapy.

As of now, standard therapy for advanced laryngeal cancer remains total laryngectomy combined with postoperative radiation as appropriate. A policy of primary radiation therapy and salvage laryngectomy may be a reasonable alternative, and has been used by some centres with comparable control rates. The role of chemotherapy remains investigational, and although there is general agreement of the importance of larynx-preserving treatment approaches, at the present time, such regimens are recommended only as part of a research protocol.

Table 15.28 Results of studies evaluating multimodality treatment for advanced laryngeal cancer[177]

Reference	No. of patients	Sites*	Treatment†	Stage III (%)	Stage IV (%)	Supraglottic (%)	N1–3 (%)	CR+PR‡ (%)	2-year survival (%)§	Larynx preservation (%)	Locoregional failure (%)	Distant failure (%)
Jacobs et al[178]	30	L, OC, OP, HP	C/RT	37	67	—	83	90	52	—	33	20
Demard et al[179]	50	L, HP¶	C/RT	54	10	—	28	74	—	—	—	—
VALCSG[75]	166	—	C/RT	56	44	63	48	85	68	64	20	11**
	166		S/RT	57	43	62	43	—	68	—	7	17
Pfister et al[180]	13	L, OP¶, HP	C/RT	43	55	77	63	85	77	68	31	8
Karp et al[181]	14	L, HP¶	C/RT	21	71	—	50	71	50	79	21	21
Urba et al[182]	8	L, OC, OP, HP, Sinus¶	C/RT	36	57	—	74	84	75	75	—	—
Clayman et al[183]	26	L, HP¶	C/RT	68	28	65	—	75	68	65	—	—
	52		S/RT	—	—	65	—	—	81	—	—	—

*OC: oral cavity; OP: oropharynx; HP: hypopharynx; L: larynx.
†C/RT: induction chemotherapy + radiation and surgery for salvage; S/RT: Surgery followed by postoperative radiation therapy.
‡CR, PR: usual definitions of complete and partial response apply.
§Data are for disease-specific survival when this information was available, otherwise data are for overall survival.
¶ Study included both larynx and other site, but statistics refer to patients with laryngeal primaries.
**Statistically significant improvement ($P < 0.05$) over other arm of study.

Voice rehabilitation and speech therapy

This is discussed in detail elsewhere.

Laryngeal cancer: the way ahead

As the aetiological factors and the basic molecular mechanism of carcinogenesis become clearer, greater emphasis will be placed on the prevention and early treatment of laryngeal cancer. Progress in the surgery of laryngeal cancer seems to have plateaued, but there is tremendous scope for improvement of reconstructive techniques after partial resections of the larynx in order to achieve good function in the remnant organ. Improved techniques in planning and delivering radiation therapy have considerably decreased the morbidity associated with such treatment. Chemoradiation using newer agents may result in an improvement in survival in addition to the already proven benefit of laryngeal organ preservation. Biological markers that reliably predict resistance to chemoradiation need to be identified, so that this subgroup could be treated more aggressively or offered surgery without a trial of larynx preservation. There seems to be some promise in markers such as p53 overexpression, p105 labelling, S-phase fraction labelling and potential doubling time.[190–192] An in vitro histoculture drug sensitivity has demonstrated the ability to predict which patients may respond favourably to chemotherapy,[193] but much study will be required before these tests come into routine clinical practice. Viral vectors have been used to transfer the p53 tumour suppressor gene into squamous cell carcinoma of the human lung[194] and several centres are investigating the application of gene therapy in head and neck cancer. The role of laryngeal transplantation has been explored for quite some time now, and interest in the subject has been renewed mainly because microvascular reconstruction is now an everyday routine in head and neck surgery. Parallel to the advances in microsurgical technique, improvements in immunosuppressive agents have now made laryngeal transplantation look more feasible. However, the major technical problem in achieving successful functional outcome remains reinnervation of the transplanted organ. Various techniques have been tried and the use of growth factors has not improved success. The possibility of using gene therapy to aid, and possibly guide, nerve regeneration needs to be explored. Apart from the difficulty in reinnervating the transplanted larynx, there are numerous other technical issues that are unresolved. The central question is the wisdom of immunosuppressing patients who are already at risk of developing subsequent malignant tumours. Although laryngeal transplant after laryngectomy for cancer may not become routine clinical practice for a while, there already is cause for optimism on the technical front. The first true human laryngeal transplant was carried out on 4 January 1998 at the Cleveland Clinic in Philadelphia, USA.[195]

In summary, future research and developments need to focus not only on understanding the basic mechanisms of the disease and how to prevent it, but efforts must also be made to help those who have been unfortunate to develop the disease and suffer its consequences.

REFERENCES

1. Pressman JJ et al. Further studies upon the submucosal compartments and lymphatics by the injection of dyes and radioisotopes. *Ann Otol Rhinol Laryngol* 1956; **65**: 963.
2. Welsh LW, Welsh JJ, Rizzo TA Jr. Laryngeal spaces and lymphatics: current anatomic concepts. *Ann Otol Rhinol Laryngol* 1983; **105**: 19–31.
3. Werner JA, Schunke M, Rudert H et al. Description and clinical importance of the lymphatics of the vocal fold. *Otolaryngol Head Neck Surg* 1990; **102**: 13–19.
4. Ferlito A, Rinaldo A, Devaney KO et al. Impact of phenotype on treatment and prognosis of laryngeal malignancies. *J Laryngol Otol* 1998; **112**: 710–714.
5. Fliss DM, Noble Topham SE, McLachlin M et al. Laryngeal verrucous carcinoma: a clinicopathologic study and detection of human papillomavirus using polymerase chain reaction. *Laryngoscope* 1994; **104**: 146–152.
6. Ferlito A, Altavilla G, Rinaldo A, Doglioni C. Basaloid squamous cell carcinoma of the larynx and hypopharynx. A clinicopathological study of 15 new cases with review of the literature. *Ann Otol Rhinol Laryngol* 1997; **106**: 1024–1035.
7. Overholt SM, Donovan DT, Schwartz MR et al. Neuroendocrine neoplasms of the larynx. *Laryngoscope* 1995; **105**: 789–794.
8. Batsakis JG, El-Naggar AK, Luna MA. Neuroendocrine tumours of the larynx. *Ann Otol Rhinol Laryngol* 1992; **101**: 710–714.
9. Wenig BM. Laryngeal mucosal malignant melanoma. A clinicopathologic, immunohistochemical, and ultrastructural study of four patients and a review of the literature. *Cancer* 1995; **75**: 1568–1577.

10. Batsakis JG, Luna MA, El-Naggar AK. Nonsquamous carcinomas of the larynx. *Ann Otol Rhinol Laryngol* 1992; **101**: 1024–1026.
11. Hyams VJ, Heffner DK. Laryngeal pathology. In: Tucker HM (ed.) *The Larynx*. 2nd edn. New York: Thieme, 1993; 35–80.
12. Cantrell RW. The current status of laryngeal cancer. In: Inouye T, Fukuda H, Sato T, Hinohara T (eds) *Recent Advances in Bronchesophagology*. Amsterdam: Excerpta Medica, 1990; 3–12.
13. Parkin DM, Muir CS, Whelan S et al (eds). *Cancer Incidence in Five Continents*. Vol. VI. IARC Scientific Publication No. 120. Lyon: World Health Organization, International Agency for Research on Cancer, 1992.
14. Esteve J, Kricker A, Ferlay J, Parkin DM (eds). In: *Facts and Figures of Cancer in the European Community*. International Agency for Research on Cancer Commission of the European Communities. Lyon: World Health Organization, 1993.
15. Maier H, Tisch M. Epidemiology of laryngeal cancer. In: Kleinsasser O, Glanz H, Olofsson J (eds). *Advances in Laryngology in Europe*. Elsevier: Amsterdam, 1997; 129–133.
16. Schottenfield S. Alcohol as a co-factor in the etiology of cancer. *Cancer* 1979; **43**: 1962–1966.
17. Wynder EL, Covey LS, Mabuchi K, Mushinski M. Environmental factors in cancer of the larynx: a second look. *Cancer* 1976; **38**: 1591–1601.
18. Devessa SS, Blot WJ, Fraumeni JF Jr. Cohort trends in mortality from oral, esophageal and laryngeal cancers in the United States. *Epidemiology* 1990; **1**: 116–121.
19. Hoffman D, Melkian A, Adams JD et al. New aspects of tobacco carcinogenesis. *Carcinogenesis* 1985; **8**: 239–256.
20. Maier H, Dietz A, Gewelke U et al. Tobacco and alcohol and the risk of head and neck cancer. *Clin Invest* 1992; **70**: 320–327.
21. Sancho-Garnier J, Theobald S. Black (air-cured) and blond (flue-cured) tobacco and cancer risk: pharynx and larynx cancer. *Eur J Cancer* 1993; **29A**: 273–276.
22. Maier H, Tisch M. Epidemiology of laryngeal cancer: results of the Heidelberg case-control study. *Acta Otolaryngol Suppl (Stockh)* 1997; **527**: 160–164.
23. Tuyns AJ, Esteve J, Raymond R et al. Cancer of the larynx/hypopharynx, tobacco and alcohol: IARC international case-control study in Turin and Varese (Italy), Zaragossa and Navarro (Spain), Geneva (Switzerland) and Calvados (France). *Int J Cancer* 1988; **41**: 483–491.
24. Brugere J, Guenel P, Leclerc A, Rodriguez J. Differential effects of tobacco and alcohol in cancer of the larynx, pharynx and mouth. *Cancer* 1986; **57**: 391–395.
25. Esteve J, Riboli E, Pequignot G et al. Diet and cancers of the larynx and hypopharynx: the IARC multi-center study in southwestern Europe. *Cancer Causes Control* 1996; **7**: 240–252.
26. Thorne P, Etherington D, Birchall MA. Head and neck cancer in the south west of England: influence of socio-economic status on incidence and second primary tumours. *Eur J Surg Oncol* 1997; **23**: 503–508.
27. Doll R. The epidemiology of cancer. *Cancer* 1980; **45**: 2475–2485.
28. World Health Statistics Annual 1983, Geneva: World Health Organization, 1983.
29. Clayman GL, Stewart MG, Weber RS et al. Human papillomavirus in laryngeal and hypopharyngeal carcinomas. *Arch Otolaryngol Head Neck Surg* 1993; **120**: 743–748.
30. Lindeberg H, Krogdahl A. Laryngeal dysplasia and the human papillomavirus. *Clin Otolaryngol* 1997; **22**: 382–386.
31. Morgan DW, Abdullah V, Quiney R, Myint S. Human papilloma virus and carcinoma of the laryngopharynx. *J Laryngol Otol* 1991; **105**: 288–290.
32. Nunez DA, Astley SM, Lewis FA, Wells M. Human papilloma viruses: a study of their prevalence in the normal larynx. *J Laryngol Otol* 1994; **108**: 319–320.
33. Klozar J, Taudy M, Betka J, Kana R. Laryngeal papilloma: precancerous condition? *Acta Otolaryngol Suppl (Stockh)* 1997; **527**: 100–102.
34. Lindeberg H, Elbrond O. Malignant tumours in patients with a history of multiple laryngeal papillomas: the significance of irradiation. *Clin Otolaryngol* 1991; **16**: 149–151.
35. Clayman GL, Stewart MG, Weber RS et al. Human papillomavirus in laryngeal and hypopharyngeal carcinomas. Relationship to survival. *Arch Otolaryngol Head Neck Surg* 1994; **120**: 743–748.
36. Elwood JM, Pearson JCG, Skippen DH, Jackson SM. Alcohol, smoking, social and occupational factors in the etiology of cancer of the oral cavity, pharynx and larynx. *Int J Cancer* 1984; **34**: 603–612.
37. Pollan M, Lopez Abente G. Wood-related occupations and laryngeal cancer. *Cancer Detect Prev* 1995; **19**: 250–257.
38. Jourenkova N, Reinikainen M, Bouchardy C et al. Larynx cancer risk in relation to glutathione S-transferase M1 and T1 genotypes and tobacco smoking. *Cancer Epidemiol Biomarkers Prev* 1998; **7**: 19–23.
39. Lynch HT, Kriegler M, Christiansen TA et al. Laryngeal carcinoma in a Lynch syndrome II kindred. *Cancer* 1988; **62**: 1007–1013.
40. Berkower AS, Biller JF. Head and neck cancer associated with Bloom's syndrome. *Laryngoscope* 1988; **98**: 746–749.
41. Mattox DE, Von Hoff DD, McGuire WL. Androgen receptors and antiandrogen therapy for laryngeal carcinoma. *Arch Otolaryngol* 1984; **110**: 721–724.
42. Urba SG, Carey THE, Kudla-Hatch V et al. Tamoxifen therapy in patients with recurrent laryngeal carcinoma. *Laryngoscope* 1990; **100**: 76–78.
43. Remenar E, Szamel I, Buda B et al. 'Why men?' Hormones and hormone receptors in male head and neck cancer patients. In: Kleinsasser O, Glanz O, Olofsson J (eds) *Advances in Laryngology in Europe*. Elsevier: Amsterdam, 1997.
44. Baker DC, Weismann B. Postirradiation carcinoma of the larynx. *Ann Otol* 1971; **80**: 634–637.

45. van der Laan BFAM, Baris G, Gregor RTh et al. Radiation-induced tumors of the head and neck. *J Otol Laryngol* 1995; **109**: 346–349.
46. Glaubiger DL, Casler JD, Garrett WL et al. Chondrosarcoma of the larynx after radiation treatment for vocal cord cancer. *Cancer* 1991; **68**: 1828–1831.
47. Bouquot JE, Gnepp DR. Laryngeal precancer: a review of the literature, commentary, and comparison with oral leukoplakia. *Head Neck* 1991; **13**: 488–497.
48. Hojslet PE, Nielsen VM, Palvio D. Premalignant lesions of the larynx. A follow-up study. *Acta Otolaryngol (Stockh)* 1989; **107**: 150–155.
49. Blackwell KE, Fu YS, Calcaterra TC. Laryngeal dysplasia. A clinicopathologic study. *Cancer* 1995; **15**: 457–463.
50. Morrison MD. Is chronic gastroesophageal reflux a causative factor in glottic carcinoma? *Otolaryngol Head Neck Surg* 1988; **99**: 370–373.
51. Glanz H, Kleinsasser O. Chronic laryngitis and carcinoma. *Arch Otorhinolaryngol* 1976; **212**: 57–75.
52. Data from the Royal Marsden Hospital Head and Neck Cancer Database. Personal communication with Roger A'hern, Department of Computing and Statistics, Royal Marsden Hospital, London, September 1998.
53. Shah JP, Karnell LH, Hoffman HT et al. Patterns of care for cancer of the larynx in the United States. *Arch Otolaryngol Head Neck Surg* 1997; **123**: 475–483.
54. Desai PB, Rao RS, Dinshaw KA et al. *Hospital Cancer Registry Annual Report 1993*. Bombay: Tata Memorial Hospital.
55. Robin PE, Powell J, Holme GM et al. Incidence. In: *Cancer of the Larynx (Clinical Cancer Monographs*. Vol. 2). New York, NY: Stockton Press, 1989; 64–65.
56. Kirchner JA, Carter D. Intralaryngeal barriers to the spread of cancer. *Acta Otolaryngol (Stockh)* 1987; **103**: 503–513.
57. Kirchner JA. Glottic-supraglottic barrier: fact or fantasy? *Ann Otol Rhinol Laryngol* 1997; **106**: 700–704.
58. Welsh LW, Welsh JJ, Rizzo TA. Internal anatomy of the larynx and the spread of cancer. *Ann Otol Rhinol Laryngol* 1989; **98**: 228–234.
59. Yeager VL, Archer CR. Anatomical routes for cancer invasion of laryngeal cartilages. *Laryngoscope* 1982; **92**: 449–452.
60. Bridger GP, Nassar VH. Carcinoma in situ involving the laryngeal mucous glands. *Arch Otolaryngol* 1971; **94**: 389–400.
61. Candela FC, Shah J, Jacques DP et al. Patterns of cervical node metastases from squamous carcinoma of the larynx. *Arch Otolaryngol Head Neck Surg* 1990; **116**: 432–435.
62. Marks JE, Breaux S, Smith PG et al. The need for elective irradiation of occult lymphatic metastases from cancers of the larynx and pyriform sinus. *Head Neck* 1985; **8**: 3–8.
63. Johnson JT, Myers EN, Hao SP et al. Outcome of open surgical therapy for glottic carcinoma. *Ann Otol Rhinol Laryngol* 1993; **102**: 752–755.
64. Daly CJ, Strong EW. Carcinoma of the glottic larynx. *Am J Surg* 1975; **130**: 489–492.
65. Jesse RH. The evaluation and treatment of patients with extensive squamous cancer of the vocal cords. *Laryngoscope* 1975; **85**: 1424–1429.
66. Thaler ER, Montone K, Tucker J, Weinstein GS. Delphian lymph node in laryngeal carcinoma: a whole organ study. *Laryngoscope* 1997; **107**: 332–334.
67. Olsen K, DeSanto LW, Pearson BW. Positive Delphian lymph node: clinical significance in laryngeal cancer. *Laryngoscope* 1987; **97**: 1033–1037.
68. Harrison DF. The pathology and management of subglottic cancer. *Ann Otol Rhinol Laryngol* 1971; **80**: 6–12.
69. Shaha AR, Shah JP. Carcinoma of the subglottic larynx. *Am J Surg* 1982; **144**: 456–458.
70. Lamprecht J, Lamprecht A, Kurten-Rothes R. Mediastinal involvement in cancers of the subglottis. *Laryngol Rhinol Otol (Stuttg)* 1987; **66**: 88–90.
71. Merino OR, Lindberg RD, Fletcher GH. An analysis of distant metastases from squamous cell carcinoma of the upper respiratory and digestive tracts. *Cancer* 1977; **40**: 145–151.
72. Johnson JT. Carcinoma of the larynx: Selective approach to the management of cervical lymphatics. *Ear Nose Throat J* 1994; **73**: 303–305.
73. Rovirosa A, Beullmunt J, Lopez A et al. The incidence of second neoplasms in advanced laryngeal cancer. Impact on survival. *Med Clin (Barc)* 1994; **102**: 121–124.
74. Engelen AM, Stalpers LJ, Manni JJ et al. Yearly chest radiography in the early detection of lung cancer following laryngeal cancer. *Eur Arch Otorhinolaryngol* 1992; **249**: 364–369.
75. Zeitels SM ,Vaughan CW. Preepiglottic space invasion in 'early' epiglottic cancer. *Ann Otol Rhinol Laryngol* 1991; **100**: 789–792.
76. Mancuso AA. Evaluation and staging of laryngeal and hypopharyngeal cancer by computed tomography and magnetic resonance imaging. In: Silver CE (ed.) *Laryngeal Cancer*. New York: Thieme, 1991.
77. Munoz A, Ramos A, Ferrando J et al. Laryngeal carcinoma: sclerotic appearance of the cricoid and arytenoid cartilage. CT-pathologic correlation. *Radiology* 1993; **189**: 433–437.
78. Nakayama M, Brandenburg JH. Clinical underestimation of laryngeal cancer. Predictive indicators. *Arch Otolaryngol Head Neck Surg* 1993; **119**: 950–957.
79. McGuirt WF, Greven K, Williams D et al. PET scanning in head and neck oncology: a review. *Head Neck* 1998; **20**: 208–215.
80. Atabek U, Mohit-Tabatabai MA, Rush BF et al. Impact of esophageal screening in patients with head and neck cancer. *Am Surg* 1990; **56**: 289–292.
81. McNeil BJ, Weichselbaum R, Pauker SG. Speech and survival: tradeoffs between quality and quantity of life in laryngeal cancer. *N Engl J Med* 1981; **305**: 982–987.
82. Ferlito A, Polidoro F, Rossi M. Pathological basis and clinical aspects of treatment policy in carcinoma-in-situ of the larynx. *J Laryngol Otol* 1981; **95**: 141–154.
83. Pene F, Fletcher GH. Results in irradiation of in situ carcinoma of the vocal cords. *Cancer* 1976; **37**: 2586–2590.

84. Doyle PJ, Flores A, Douglas GS. Carcinoma in situ of the larynx. *Laryngoscope* 1977; **87**: 310–316.
85. Elman AJ, Goodman M, Wang CC et al. In situ carcinoma of the vocal cords. *Cancer* 1979; **43**: 2422–2428.
86. Small W Jr, Mittal BB, Brand WN et al. Role of radiation therapy in the management of carcinoma in situ of the larynx. *Laryngoscope* 1993; **103**: 663–667.
87. Mahieu HF, Patel P, Annyas AA et al. Carbon dioxide laser vaporization in early glottic carcinoma. *Arch Otolaryngol Head Neck Surg* 1994; **120**: 383–387.
88. Lillie JC, DeSanto LW. Transoral surgery of early cordal carcinoma. *Ann Otol Rhinol Laryngol* 1973; **77**: 92–96.
89. Miller AH, Fisher HR. Symposium of carcinoma of the larynx: clues to the life history of carcinoma in situ of the larynx. *Laryngoscope* 1971; **81**: 1475–1480.
90. Bocca E. Supraglottic cancer. *Laryngoscope* 1975; **85**: 1318–1326.
91. Soo KC, Shah JP, Gopinath KS et al. Analysis of prognostic variables and results after supraglottic partial laryngectomy. *Am J Surg* 1988; **156**: 301–305.
92. Harwood AR, Beale FA, Cummings BJ et al. Management of early supraglottic laryngeal carcinoma by irradiation with surgery in reserve. *Arch Otolaryngol* 1983; **109**: 583–585.
93. Mendenhall WM, Parsons JT, Stringer SP et al. Carcinoma of the supraglottic larynx: a basis for comparing the results of radiotherapy and surgery. *Head Neck* 1990; **12**: 204–209.
94. Goepfert H, Jesse RH, Fletcher GH, Hamberger A. Optimal treatment for technically resectable squamous cell carcinoma of the supraglottic larynx. *Laryngoscope* 1975; **85**: 14–32.
95. Weems DH, Mendenhall WM, Parsons JT et al. Squamous cell carcinoma of the supraglottic larynx treated with surgery and/or radiation therapy. *Int J Radiat Oncol Biol Phys* 1987; **13**: 1483–1487.
96. Nakfoor BM, Spiro IJ, Wang CC et al. Results of accelerated radiotherapy for supraglottic carcinoma: a Massachusetts General Hospital and Massachusetts Eye and Ear Infirmary experience. *Head Neck* 1998; **20**: 379–384.
97. Zeitels SM, Koufman JA, Davis RK et al. Endoscopic treatment of supraglottic and hypopharynx cancer. *Laryngoscope* 1994; **104**: 71–78.
98. Ambrosch P, Martin A, Kron M, Steiner W. Results of transoral laser microsurgery for supraglottic carcinomas. In Kleinsasser O, Glanz H, Olofsson J (eds) *Advances in Laryngology in Europe.* Amsterdam: Elsevier, 1997; 286–290.
99. Bocca E, Pignataro O, Oldini C. Supraglottic laryngectomy: 30 years of experience. *Ann Otol Rhinol Laryngol* 1983; **92**: 14–18.
100. Levendag P, Sessions R, Vikram B et al. The problem of neck relapse in early stage supraglottic larynx cancer. *Cancer* 1989; **63**: 345–348.
101. Goffinet DR, Gilbert EH, Weller SA. Irradiation of clinically uninvolved cervical lymph nodes. *Can J Otolaryngol* 1975; **4**: 927–932.
102. Suarez C, Llorente JL, Nunez F et al. Neck dissection with or without postoperative radiation therapy in supraglottic carcinomas. *Otolaryngol Head Neck Surg* 1993; **109**: 3–9.
103. Siirala U, Paavolainen M. The problem of advanced supraglottic carcinoma. *Laryngoscope* 1975; **85**: 1633–1642.
104. Harwood AR, Beale FA, Cummings BJ et al. Supraglottic laryngeal carcinoma: an analysis of dose-time-volume factors in 410 patients. *Int J Radiat Oncol Biol Phys* 1983; **9**: 311–319.
105. Mendenhall WM, Million RR, Cassisi NJ. Squamous cell carcinoma of the supraglottic larynx treated with radical irradiation: analysis of the treatment parameters and results. *Int J Radiat Oncol Biol Phys* 1984; **10**: 2223–2230.
106. Ogura JH, Marks JE, Freeman RB. Results of conservation surgery for cancers of the supraglottis and pyriform sinus. *Laryngoscope* 1980; **90**: 591–600.
107. Alajmo E, Fini-Storchi O, Polli G. Five-year results of 1000 patients operated on for cancer of the larynx. *Acta Otolaryngol (Stockh)* 1976; **82**: 437–439.
108. DeSanto LW. Cancer of the supraglottic larynx: a review of 260 patients. *Otolaryngol Head Neck Surg* 1985; **93**: 705–711.
109. Goepfert JH, Jesse RH, Fletcher GH, Hamberger A. Optimal treatment for technically resectable squamous cell carcinoma of the supraglottic larynx. *Laryngoscope* 1975; **85**: 14–32.
110. Flynn MB, Jesse RH, Lindberg RD. Surgery and irradiation in the treatment of squamous cell cancer of the supraglottic larynx. *Am J Surg* 1972; **124**: 477–481.
111. Burstein FD, Calcaterra TC. Supraglottic laryngectomy: series report and analysis of results. *Laryngoscope* 1985; **95**: 833–836.
112. Weems DH, Mendenhall WM, Parsons JT et al. Squamous cell carcinoma of the supraglottic larynx treated with surgery and/or radiation therapy. *Int J Radiat Oncol Biol Phys* 1987; **13**: 1483–1487.
113. Lee NK, Goepfert H, Wendt CD. Supraglottic laryngectomy for intermediate-stage cancer: UTMD Anderson Cancer Center Experience with combined therapy. *Laryngoscope* 1990; **100**: 831–836.
114. Harwood AR, Beale FA, Cummings BJ et al. Supraglottic laryngeal carcinoma: an analysis of dose-time-volume factors in 410 patients. *Int J Radiat Oncol Biol Phys* 1983; **9**: 311–319.
115. Karim AB, Kralendonk JH, Njo KH et al. Radiation therapy for advanced (T3-T4N0-N3M0) laryngeal carcinoma: the need for a change of strategy: a radiotherapeutic view-point. *Int J Radiat Oncol Biol Phys* 1987; **13**: 1625–1633.
116. Mendenhall WM, Million RR, Cassisi NJ. Squamous cell carcinoma of the supraglottic larynx treated with radical irradiation: analysis of the treatment parameters and results. *Int J Radiat Oncol Biol Phys* 1984; **10**: 2223–2230.
117. Vermund H, Boysen M, Evensen JF et al. Recurrence after different primary treatment for cancer of the supraglottic larynx. *Acta Oncol* 1998; **37**: 167–173.

118. Flynn MB, Jesse RH, Lindberg RD. Surgery and irradiation in the treatment of squamous cell cancer of the supraglottic larynx. *Am J Surg* 1972; **124**: 477–481.
119. Fu KK, Eisenberg L, Dedo HH, Philips TL. Results of integrated management of supraglottic carcinoma. *Cancer* 1977; **40**: 2874–2881.
120. Shah JP, Tollefsen HR. Epidermoid carcinoma of the supraglottic larynx. Role of neck dissection in initial surgical treatment. *Am J Surg* 1974; **128**: 494–499.
121. Coates HL, DeSanto LW, Devine KD, Elveback LR. Carcinoma of the supraglottic larynx. *Arch Otolaryngol* 1976; **102**: 686–689.
122. DeSanto LW. Early supraglottic cancer. *Ann Otorhinolaryngol* 1990; **99**: 593–597.
123. Morris MR, Canonico D, Blank C. A critical review of radiotherapy in the management of T1 glottic carcinoma. *Am J Otolaryngol* 1994; **15**: 276–280.
124. Mendenhall WM, Parson JT, Stringer SP et al. T1–T2 vocal cord carcinoma: a basis for comparing the results of radiotherapy and surgery. *Head Neck Surg* 1988; **10**: 373–377.
125. Kelly MD, Spaulding CA, Constable WC et al. Definitive radiotherapy in the management of stage I and II carcinomas of the glottis. *Ann Otol Rhinol Laryngol* 1989; **98**: 235–239.
126. Pellitteri PK, Kennedy TL, Vrabec DP et al. Radiotherapy: the mainstay in the treatment of early glottic carcinoma. *Arch Otolaryngol Head Neck Surg* 1991; **117**: 297–301.
127. Small W Jr, Mittal BB, Brand WN et al. Results of radiation therapy in early glottic carcinoma: multivariate analysis of prognostic and radiation therapy variables. *Radiology* 1992; **183**: 789–794.
128. Fein DA, Mendenhall WM, Parson JT et al. T1–T2 squamous cell carcinoma of the glottic larynx treated with radiotherapy: a multivariate analysis of variable potentially influencing local control. *Int J Radiat Oncol Biol Phys* 1993; **25**: 605–611.
129. Howell-Burke D, Peters LJ, Goepfert H et al. T2 glottic cancer: recurrence, salvage, and survival after definitive radiotherapy. *Arch Otolaryngol Head Neck Surg* 1990; **116**: 830–835.
130. Guiney M, Smith J, Hughes P. Radiation therapy of glottic carcinomas: Peter MacCallum Cancer Institute experience. *Aust NZ J Surg* 1992; **62**: 622–627.
131. Ogura JH, Sessions DG, Spector GJ. Analysis of surgical therapy for epidermoid carcinoma of the laryngeal glottis. *Laryngoscope* 1975; **85**: 1522–1530.
132. Laccourreye O, Weinstein G, Trotoux J et al. Vertical partial laryngectomy: a critical analysis of local recurrence. *Ann Otol Rhinol Laryngol* 1991; **100**: 68–71.
133. Johnson JT, Myers EN, Hao SP et al. Outcome of open surgical therapy for glottic carcinoma. *Ann Otol Laryngol Rhinol* 1993; **102**: 752–755.
134. Thomas JV, Olsen KD, Neel HB et al. Early glottic carcinoma treated with open laryngeal procedures. *Arch Otolaryngol Head Neck Surg* 1994; **120**: 264–268.
135. Kersh CR, Kelly SM, Parkin JL et al. Early glottic carcinoma: patterns and predictors of relapse after definitive radiotherapy. *South Med J* 1990; **83**: 374–378.
136. Rudoltz MS, Benammar A, Mohiuddin M. Prognostic factors for local control and survival in T1 squamous cell carcinoma of the glottis. *Int J Radiat Oncol Biol Phys* 1993; **26**: 767–772.
137. Watters GW, Patel SG, Rhys Evans PH. Partial laryngectomy for recurrent laryngeal carcinoma. *Clin Otolaryngol* 2000; **25**: 146–152.
138. Lavey RS, Calcaterra TC. Partial laryngectomy for glottic cancer after high-dose radiotherapy. *Am J Surg* 1991; **172**: 662–664.
139. DelGaudio JM, Fleming DJ, Esclamado RM et al. Hemilaryngectomy for glottic carcinoma after radiation therapy failure. *Arch Otolaryngol Head Neck Surg* 1994; **120**: 959–963.
140. Schwaab G, Mamelle G, Lartigau E et al. Surgical salvage treatment of T1/T2 glottic carcinoma after failure of radiotherapy. *Am J Surg* 1994; **168**: 474–475.
141. Lydiatt WM, Shah JP, Lydiatt KM. Conservation surgery for recurrent carcinoma of the glottic larynx. *Am J Surg* 1996; **172**: 662–664.
142. McLaughlin MP, Parsons JT, Fein DA et al. Salvage surgery after radiotherapy failure in T1–T2 squamous cell carcinoma of the glottic larynx. *Head Neck* 1996; **18**: 229–235.
143. McGuirt WF, Koufman JA, Blalock D et al. Voice analysis of patients with endoscopically treated early laryngeal carcinoma. *Ann Otol Rhinol Laryngol* 1992; **101**: 142–146.
144. Robson NL, Oswal VH, Flood LM. Radiation therapy of laryngeal cancer: a twenty year experience. *J Laryngol Otol* 1990; **104**: 699–703.
145. Mendenhall WM, Parson JT, Stringer SP et al. Stage T3 squamous cell carcinoma of the glottic larynx: a comparison of laryngectomy and irradiation. *Int J Radiat Oncol Biol Phys* 1992; **23**: 725–732.
146. Million RR. The larynx ... so to speak: everything I wanted to know about laryngeal cancer I learned in the last 32 years. *Int J Radiat Oncol Biol Phys* 1992; **23**: 691–704.
147. Wang CC. Factors influencing the success of radiation therapy for T2 and T3 glottic carcinomas. Importance of cord mobility and sex. *Am J Clin Oncol* 1986; **9**: 517–520.
148. Leroux-Robert JL. A statistical study of 620 laryngeal carcinomas of the glottic region personally operated upon more than five years ago. *Laryngoscope* 1975; **85**: 1440–1466.
149. Skolnik EM, Yee KF, Wheatley MA, Martin LO. Carcinoma of the laryngeal glottis: therapy and end results. *Laryngoscope* 1975; **85**: 1453–1466.
150. DeSanto LW. T3 glottic cancer. Options and consequences of the options. *Laryngoscope* 1984; **94**: 1311–1315.
151. Johnson JT, Myers EN, Hao SP et al. Outcome of open surgical therapy for glottic carcinoma. *Ann Otol Rhinol Laryngol* 1993; **102**: 752–755.

152. Razack MS, Maipang T, Sako K et al. Management of advanced glottic carcinomas. *Am J Surg* 1989; **158**: 318–320.
153. Som ML. Cordal cancer with extension to vocal process. *Laryngoscope* 1975; **85**: 1298–1307.
154. Lesinski SG, Bauer WC, Ogura JH. Hemilaryngectomy for T3 (fixed cord) epidermoid carcinoma of larynx. *Laryngoscope* 1976; **86**: 1563–1571.
155. Biller HF, Lawson W. Partial laryngectomy for vocal cord cancer with marked limitation or fixation of the vocal cord. *Laryngoscope* 1986; **96**: 61–64.
156. Kessler DJ, Trapp TK, Calcaterra TC. The treatment of T3 glottic carcinoma with vertical partial laryngectomy. *Arch Otolaryngol Head Neck Surg* 1987; **113**: 1196–1199.
157. Spiro RH, Gallo O, Shah JP. Selective jugular node dissection in patients with squamous carcinoma of the larynx or pharynx. *Am J Surg* 1993; **166**: 399–402.
158. Skolnik EM, Yee KF, Wheatley MA, Martin LO. Carcinoma of the laryngeal glottis: therapy and end results. *Laryngoscope* 1975; **85**: 1453–1466.
159. Yuen A, Medina JE, Goepfert H et al. Management of stage T3 and T4 glottic carcinomas. *Am J Surg* 1984; **148**: 467–472.
160. Kaplan MJ, Johns ME, Clark DA, Cantrell RW. Glottic carcinoma. The roles of surgery and irradiation. *Cancer* 1984; **15**: 2641–2648.
161. Hendrickson FR. Radiation therapy treatment of larynx cancers. *Cancer* 1985; **55**: 2058–2061.
162. Kelly MD, Hahn SS, Spaulding CA et al. Definitive radiotherapy in the management of stage I and II carcinomas of the glottis. *Ann Otol Rhinol Laryngol* 1989; **98**: 235–239.
163. Mainpang T, Razack MS, Sako K, Chen TY. Surgical salvage for recurrent 'early' glottic cancers. *J Surg Oncol* 1989; **40**: 32–33.
164. Fujii R, Sato T, Yoshino K et al. A clinical study of 1079 patients with laryngeal cancer. Article in Japanese – Medline Abstract. *Nippon Jibiinkoka Gakkai Kaiho* 1997; **100**: 856–863.
165. Vermund H. Role of radiotherapy in cancer of the larynx as related to the TNM system of staging. A review. *Cancer* 1970; **25**: 485–504.
166. Haylock BJ, Deutsch GP. Primary radiotherapy for subglottic carcinoma. *Clin Oncol (R Coll Radiol)* 1993; **5**: 143–146.
167. Warde P, Harwood A, Keane T. Carcinoma of the subglottis. Results of initial radical radiation. *Arch Otolaryngol Head Neck Surg* 1987; **113**: 1228–1229.
168. Guedea F, Parsons JT, Mendenhall WM et al. Primary subglottic cancer: results of radical radiation therapy. *Int J Radiat Oncol Biol Phys* 1991; **21**: 1607–1611.
169. Dahm JD, Sessions DG, Paniello RC, Harvey J. Primary subglottic cancer. *Laryngoscope* 1998; **108**: 741–746.
170. Stell PM, Tobin KE. The behavior of cancer affecting the subglottic space. *Can J Otolaryngol* 1975; **4**: 612–617.
171. Sessions DG, Ogura JH, Fried MP. Carcinoma of the subglottic area. *Laryngoscope* 1975; **85**: 1417–1423.
172. Dahm JD, Sessions DG, Paniello RC, Harvey J. Primary subglottic cancer. *Laryngoscope* 1998; **108**: 741–746.
173. Hong WK, Shapshay SM, Bhutani R et al. Induction chemotherapy in advanced squamous head and neck carcinoma with high-dose cis-platinum and bleomycin infusion. *Cancer* 1979; **44**: 19–25.
174. Weaver A, Flemming S, Kish J et al. Cis-platinum and 5-fluorouracil as induction therapy for advanced head and neck cancer. *Am J Surg* 1982; **144**: 445–448.
175. The Department of Veterans Affairs Laryngeal Cancer Study Group. Induction chemotherapy plus radiation compared with surgery plus radiation in patients with advanced laryngeal cancer. *N Engl J Med* 1991; **324**: 1685–1690.
176. Lefebvre J, Chevalier D, Luboinski B et al. Larynx preservation in pyriform sinus cancer: preliminary results of a European Organization for Research and Treatment of Cancer Phase III trial. *J Natl Cancer Inst* 1996; **88**: 890–899.
177. Carew JF, Shah JP. Advances in multimodality therapy for laryngeal cancer. *CA Cancer J Clin* 1998; **48**: 211–228.
178. Jacobs C, Goffinet DR, Goffinet L et al. Chemotherapy as a substitute for surgery in the treatment of advanced resectable head and neck cancer: a report from the Northern California Oncology Group. *Cancer* 1987; **60**: 1178–1183.
179. Demard F, Chauvel P, Santini J et al. Response to chemotherapy as justification for modification of the therapeutic strategy for pharyngolaryngeal carcinomas. *Head Neck* 1990; **12**: 225–231.
180. Pfister DG, Strong E, Harrison L et al. Larynx preservation with combined chemotherapy and radiation therapy in advanced but resectable head and neck cancer. *J Clin Oncol* 1991; **9**: 850–859.
181. Karp DD, Vaughan CW, Carter R, et al. Larynx preservation using induction chemotherapy plus radiation therapy as an alternative to laryngectomy in advanced head and neck cancer: a long-term follow-up report. *Am J Clin Oncol* 1991; **14**: 273–279.
182. Urba SG, Forastiere AA, Wolf GT et al. Intensive induction chemotherapy and radiation for organ preservation in patients with advanced resectable head and neck carcinoma. *J Clin Oncol* 1994; **12**: 946–953.
183. Clayman GL, Weber RS, Guillamondegui O et al. Laryngeal preservation for advanced laryngeal and hypopharyngeal cancers. *Arch Otolaryngol Head Neck Surg* 1995; **121**: 219–223.
184. Pfister DG, Armstrong J, Strong E et al. A matched-pair analysis of cisplatin/5-fluorouracil versus other cisplatin-based regimens as induction chemotherapy for larynx preservation treatment. *Proc Am Soc Clin Oncol* 1993; **12**: 280.
185. Pfister DG, Bajorin D, Motzer R et al. Cisplatin, fluorouracil and leucovorin: increased toxicity without improved response in squamous cell head and neck cancer. *Arch Otolaryngol Head Neck Surg* 1994; **120**: 89–95.
186. Vokes EE, Weichselbaum RR, Mick R et al. Favorable long-term survival following induction chemotherapy with cisplatin, fluorouracil, and leucovorin and

concomitant chemoradiotherapy for locally advanced head and neck cancer. *J Natl Cancer Inst* 1992; **84**: 877–882.

187. Clark JR, Busse PM, Norris CM Jr et al. Induction chemotherapy with cisplatin, fluorouracil, and high-dose leucovorin for squamous cell carcinoma of the head and neck: long-term results. *J Clin Oncol* 1997; **15**: 3100–3110.
188. Shin DM, Glisson BS, Khuri FR et al. Phase II trial of paclitaxel, ifosfamide, and cisplatin in patients with recurrent head and neck squamous cell carcinoma. *J Clin Oncol* 1998; **16**: 1325–1330.
189. Robbins KT, Fontanesi J, Wong FS et al. A novel organ preservation protocol for advanced carcinoma of the larynx and pharynx. *Arch Otolaryngol Head Neck Surg* 1996; **122**: 853–837.
190. Truelson JM, Fisher SG, Beals TE et al. DNA content and histologic growth pattern correlate with prognosis in patients with advanced squamous carcinoma of the larynx. Department of Veterans Affairs Cooperative Laryngeal Cancer Study Group. *Cancer* 1992; **70**: 56–62.
191. Corvo R, Giaretti W, Sanguineti G et al. In vivo cell kinetics in head and neck squamous cell carcinomas predicts local control and helps guide radiotherapy regimen. *J Clin Oncol* 1995; **13**: 1843–1850.
192. Fu KK, Hammond E, Pajak TF et al. Flow cytometric quantification of the proliferation-associated nuclear antigen p105 and DNA content in advanced head and neck cancer: results of RTOG 91–08. *Int J Radiat Oncol Biol Phys* 1994; **29**: 661–671.
193. Robbins KT, Connors KM, Storniolo AM. Sponge-gel-supported histoculture drug-response assay for head and neck cancer: correlations with clinical response to cisplatin. *Arch Otolaryngol Head Neck Surg* 1994; **120**: 288–292.
194. Roth JA, Nguyen D, Lawrence DD et al. Retrovirus-mediated wild-type p53 gene transfer to tumors of patients with lung cancer. *Nature Med* 1996; **2**: 985–991.
195. Affleck J. A sound operation? Docs debate benefits, risks of first larynx transplant. *Philadelphia Daily News*, Jan 10, 1998.

16 Management of the neck

John K Joe, Snehal G Patel and Ashok R Shaha

Introduction

The prognostic significance of cervical lymph node status in squamous cell carcinoma of the upper aerodigestive tract is well recognized. Metastases to regional lymph nodes reduce 5-year survival rates to nearly one-half that of patients with disease confined to the primary site.[1] Appropriate management of the neck is therefore critical in planning treatment for patients with squamous cell carcinoma of the upper aerodigestive tract.

The management of metastases to regional cervical lymph nodes outlined in this chapter includes an overview of the relevant anatomy of the neck, a brief discussion of the biological mechanisms of lymphatic metastases, diagnostic evaluation, disease staging, and treatment principles. The major focus of this discussion will be on lymphatic metastases from squamous cell carcinoma, but a brief mention will be made regarding other malignancies of the head and neck, such as those of the salivary glands or thyroid, and cutaneous melanoma.

The anatomy and biology of cervical lymphatic metastases

It has been estimated that about 300 of the 800 lymph nodes in the human body are located in the head and neck region. To standardize reporting and facilitate communication, lymph node groups of the neck are classified into different levels. Cervical lymph nodes are categorized into five nodal levels, as illustrated in Figure 16.1. It has been suggested that these five nodal levels be further subdivided into a and b components to differentiate regions in close proximity anatomically but with potentially distinct patterns of lymphatic drainage.[2] Such subclassification of these nodal levels however has not become standard nomenclature. Regional lymph node levels of the anterior neck and superior mediastinum are illustrated in Figure 16.2. Table 16.1 lists the clinical and surgical landmarks used to describe these levels.

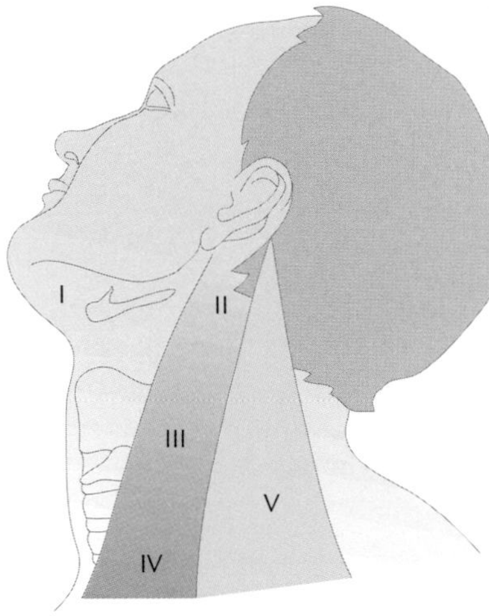

Figure 16.1 Lateral view of the neck to demonstrate the boundaries of lymph node levels I–V.

Other cervical lymph node groups relevant to patterns of nodal metastasis but lacking a standardized nodal level classification include lymph nodes of the retropharyngeal, facial, intraparotid, preauricular, postauricular, and suboccipital regions.

The biology of lymphatic metastasis

Despite the continuing advances in our knowledge regarding the molecular mechanisms involved in primary carcinogenesis, many questions persist as to how malignant cells metastasize to regional

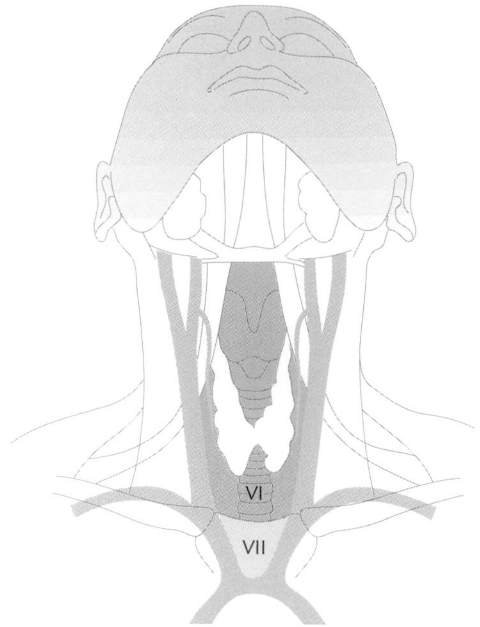

Figure 16.2 Regional lymph node levels of the anterior neck and superior mediastinum.

lymphatics. The frustration in our inability to delineate fully these molecular events is further compounded when considering the prognostic significance of nodal metastases in head and neck squamous cell carcinoma (HNSCC).

Molecular events in carcinogenesis and nodal metastasis

The development of malignant tumors at the primary site appears to be the result of multiple accumulated genetic alterations.[3] These genetic mutations must occur in the correct number and sequence for cancer to develop, a progression of genetic events first described by Fearon and Vogelstein for colorectal tumorigenesis.[4] A genetic progression model for head and neck cancer has been established demonstrating the multiple steps involved in the expansion and migration of clonally related preneoplastic cells.[5]

Once a primary malignancy progresses from carcinoma in situ to a microinvasive carcinoma to an invasive carcinoma extending into the surrounding stroma, the probability increases for metastasis to regional lymphatics. The primary processes involved in the complex cascade of invasion include changes in adhesion between cells, proteolytic degradation of the extracellular matrix, cellular migration, and angiogenesis.[6–8] This cascade has yet to be completely characterized, but our present understanding is summarized by the following molecular events: cell–cell adhesion between tumor cells decreases as adhesion between tumor cells and the extracellular matrix increases (Figure 16.3). Matrix metalloproteases (MMPs) provide enzymatic degradation of the basement membrane, giving way to

Table 16.1 Clinical and surgical landmarks for description of node levels

Node level	Clinical landmarks	Surgical landmarks
Level I	Submental and submandibular triangles	Lower border of the body of the mandible superiorly, posterior belly of the diagastric muscle posteriorly, and hyoid bone inferiorly
Level II	Upper jugular lymph nodes	Base of skull superiorly, posterior belly of diagastric muscle anteriorly, posterior border of the sternocleidomastoid muscle posteriorly, and hyoid bone inferiorly
Level III	Middle jugular lymph nodes	Hyoid bone superiorly, lateral limit of the sternohyoid muscle anteriorly, the posterior border of sternocleidomastoid muscle posteriorly, and cricothyroid membrane inferiorly
Level IV	Lower jugular lymph nodes	Cricothyroid membrane superiorly, lateral limit of the sternohyoid muscle anteriorly, posterior border of the sternocleidomastoid muscle posteriorly, and clavicle inferiorly
Level V	Posterior triangle lymph nodes	Posterior border of sternocleidomastoid muscle anteriorly, anterior border of the trapezius muscle posteriorly, and clavicle inferiorly
Level VI	Anterior compartment of the neck	Hyoid bone superiorly, suprasternal notch inferiorly, and medial border of the carotid sheath on either side of the neck laterally
Level VII	Superior mediastinal lymph nodes	Suprasternal notch superiorly

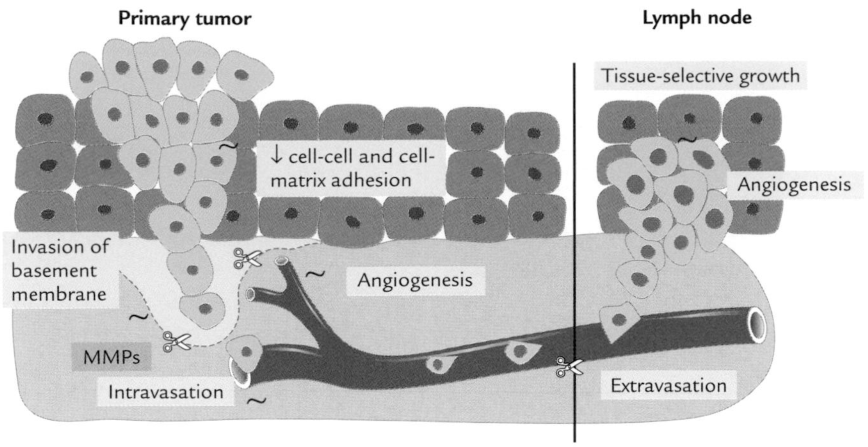

Figure 16.3 Cascade of events leading up to lymphatic metastases.

cellular motility and migration, further assisted by neovascularization. Endothelial cell ligands continue this cascade, facilitating the passage of tumor cells to and from the circulation. This cascade highlights the complex interaction between the lymphatic and hematogenous patterns of circulation, underscoring the importance of considering the two systems as interrelated, and not distinct entities, in the mechanism of metastasis.

Patterns of cervical lymphatic flow

Prior to the development of these molecular techniques, Ugo Fisch used contrast cervical lymphography to characterize the pathways of circulation through the lymphatics in the neck.[9] It was noted that following retroauricular injection of contrast, the cervical lymphatic network filled in an orderly sequence. Lymph nodes in the region of the upper lateral neck termed the 'junctional area' by Fisch filled with contrast first. Direct connections from the 'junctional area' then filled separately to the jugular nodes, to the supraclavicular nodes, and to the nodes along the spinal accessory nerve in the lower posterior triangle. Radiation therapy with conventional X-rays and with cobalt-60 was found to markedly decrease the caliber and number of lymph vessels, as well as the size and the number of cervical lymph nodes. These postradiation changes resulted in disturbance in the normal filling of the cervical lymphatic system, with the main route of lymph flow directed towards the jugular chain. Following radical neck dissection, Fisch noted that collateral lymphatic circulation developed through one of two mechanisms. Collateral circulation developed either by submental diversion through preexisting lymphatic channels (following unilateral neck dissection), or by retrograde flow to the subcutaneous and dermal lymphatic network of the neck (following bilateral neck dissection or unilateral neck dissection with postoperative radiation therapy).

Immunological aspects of nodal metastasis and lymphadenectomy

A subject not often broached in the literature of managing cervical nodal metastases concerns the immunological implications involved in nodal metastasis and in lymph node removal. Previous studies have shown a hierarchical immunomodulatory relationship between the primary tumor and its draining lymphatics in HNSCC.[10,11] These studies demonstrate that natural killer (NK) cell activity of lymph nodes positive for metastatic HNSCC was significantly diminished compared to uninvolved lymph nodes, and that interleukin-2 (IL-2)- activated cytotoxicity of lymph nodes closer to the primary tumor was depressed compared to lymph nodes further away from the primary site. These studies suggest an immunosuppressive effect of the primary tumor and lymph nodes in close proximity to the primary tumor, possibly by soluble suppressive factors. Inhibition of host immune responses in this manner has been proposed to play a role in perpetuating the spread of metastatic foci throughout cervical lymphatics.

The clinical significance of the immunity of regional lymphatics in HNSCC has been debated. In a double-blinded retrospective study, Berlinger et al determined that an absence of histological signs of lymph node immunologic activity on light microscopy negatively impacted on 5-year survival rates in patients with squamous cell carcinoma (SCC) of the larynx, pharynx, and oral cavity.[12] Gilmore and his colleagues however concluded in a double-blinded retrospective analysis of radical neck dissection specimens that immunologic activity in lymph nodes by light microscopy did not correlate with survival outcome in patients with SCC of the larynx.[13] A criticism applicable to both these reports is that neither study controlled for preoperative radiotherapy, which is known to affect cervical lymphatic drainage. Studying patients with oral cavity SCC undergoing elective neck dissection,

Cernea et al found that certain lymph node reactivity patterns on light microscopy (e.g. sinus histiocytosis) were more likely to predict local, regional, or distant recurrence than others (e.g. presence of germinal centers) in patients with N0 necks.[14]

In light of the immunosuppressive mechanisms involved in HNSCC metastatic to cervical lymph nodes, attempts have been made to stimulate lymphokine-activated killer cells using regional injection of recombinant IL-2.[15] Although augmented cytotoxic effects of NK cells have been observed in vivo, immunotherapy remains an experimental modality requiring further study in the treatment of HNSCC.

Another immunological question relevant to nodal metastases from HNSCC concerns the effect of neck dissection on host immunity. Using skin homografts in immunocompetent cancer patients, Griffiths found that removal of regional lymph nodes in the head and neck, axilla, and groin did not significantly alter host immunity.[16] Collateral lymphatic circulation was re-established, and the remaining immune cells were observed to compensate for those lymph nodes that had been removed. Thus, regional lymphadenectomy did not inhibit local host response against homografts in this study. It has been suggested that the histologic pattern of lymph node reactivity by light microscopy may not correlate with immunomodulatory activity in patients with HNSCC.[17]

Patterns of cervical lymphatic metastasis

Characteristics of the primary tumor influencing nodal metastasis

Various characteristics of the primary tumor may influence the frequency of cervical nodal metastases. Such characteristics include site of origin, size, T stage, location, and histomorphologic presentation. As illustrated in Table 16.2, certain primary sites have an increased predilection to metastasize to cervical lymph nodes. For example, in the oral cavity, cancers of the floor of mouth and tongue are more likely to present with regional lymph node metastases than those arising from the hard palate. Increasing size or advanced T stage of the primary tumor also increases the risk for nodal metastases. The anatomic location of the primary tumor is also important. As a general rule, the risk for lymph node metastasis increases for tumors located more posteriorly, for example oropharyngeal cancers are at higher risk than most oral cavity tumors. Similarly, within the laryngopharynx, the risk for nodal metastases increases centrifugally: glottic primaries are at lowest risk, while pyriform fossa and other hypopharyngeal

Table 16.2 The incidence of cervical lymph node metastasis by site of the primary tumor in previously untreated patients. (Percentages are approximate and are based on a review of the literature)

Site	Clinically abnormal nodes at presentation (%)	Incidence of occult nodal metastases (%)	Regional failure with observation of the neck (%)
Oral cavity			
Oral tongue	35–55	25–30	25–35
Floor of mouth	25–35	15–25	20–30
Gum and hard palate	15–25	5–15	10–15
Buccal mucosa	15–25	10–20	10–15
Oropharynx			
Tonsillar fossa	40–50	45–55	?*
Base of the tongue	40–50	40–50	?*
Soft palate	25–30	30–35	35–40*
Pharyngeal wall	35–45	35–45	?*
Nasopharynx	60–70	?†	?*
Hypopharynx	60–70	65–70	?*
Larynx			
Supraglottic	35–45	25–35	25–30
Glottic	< 5	< 5	< 5
Major salivary glands	15–20	5–10	10–15
Differentiated thyroid carcinoma	35–40	60–65	20–25

*Percentages not known or unreliable as most patients receive radiation therapy to the neck during initial treatment
†Percentages not known as initial treatment is largely non-surgical.

Table 16.3 Distribution of cervical lymph node metastases from squamous cell carcinoma of the upper aerodigestive tract in N0 patients[21]

Lymph node level	Oral cavity (%)	Oropharynx (%)	Hypopharynx (%)	Larynx (%)
I	58	7	0	14
II	51	80	75	52
III	26	60	75	55
IV	9	27	0	24
V	2	7	0	7

tumors metastasize quite frequently. Histomorphologic characteristics of the primary tumor that increase the risk of nodal metastasis include an endophytic, rather than exophytic, appearance, poorer degree of differentiation, and increased depth of invasion. Spiro and colleagues found that the risk of cervical metastasis approached 40% in patients with primary tumors of the floor of mouth and oral tongue which were greater than 2 mm in thickness.[18] Other histologic factors predisposing to a higher rate of lymphatic metastases include lymphatic and vascular invasion by tumor, and perineural infiltration.[19]

Predictable patterns of nodal metastasis

Appropriate management of cervical lymph nodes is based on the orderly and predictable spread of regional metastases based on the primary site.[20,21] Lymph nodes at highest risk for metastasis from carcinoma of the oral cavity are located at levels I, II, and III. Carcinoma of the nasopharynx often presents initially with lymph node metastases situated in the posterior triangle at level V or the superior deep jugular nodes at level II. Cancers of the oropharynx, hypopharynx, and larynx tend to spread first to lymph nodes at levels II, III, and IV. Nodal metastases from thyroid carcinoma typically present in the central compartment, at levels VI and VII, before extending to either or both lateral necks.

These patterns of cervical lymph node metastasis described above are not exclusive of other nodal levels, but rather predict those first echelon nodes at highest risk for initial involvement, based on the location of the primary tumor in the head and neck. As illustrated in Table 16.3, tumors arising in the oral cavity are more likely to present with nodal metastases at levels I, II, and III. Initial involvement of level IV is much less common, and metastases at level V on presentation are even more infrequent. A topic of ongoing debate in the literature however concerns the concept of 'skip metastases,' or metastases to inferior cervical nodes at levels III or IV in the absence of demonstrable involvement at levels I and II.[22] However, the likelihood of failure at level IV following supraomohyoid neck dissection (encompassing levels I through III) for oral cavity cancer is low.[23] The reported failure rate at level IV in the absence of nodal involvement of levels I through III following supraomohyoid neck dissection is approximately 5%.[24,25]

The orderly and predictable pattern of metastases no longer remains reliable once lymphatic drainage is altered following surgery or radiation. As described above, alterations in normal lymphatic architecture may result in nodal metastases presenting at unexpected sites so that selective neck dissections in these settings are inadequate for both staging and treatment.

Clinical evaluation of nodal metastases

History and physical examination

When evaluating a patient with a neck mass suspicious for cervical nodal metastases, one cannot overemphasize the need for a systematic, comprehensive medical history and physical examination of the head and neck. Salient features of the history and physical examination are summarized in Table 16.4.

Should the primary tumor prove elusive during the physical exam, particular attention must be directed to sites of the head and the neck where a primary lesion may remain occult, for example the tonsil and the base of tongue. The fiberoptic laryngoscope has proven invaluable in examining and photographically documenting the nasopharynx, laryngopharynx, and pyriform sinuses in the office setting.

Table 16.4 Salient features in the history and physical examination of a patient presenting with a cervical nodal mass

Clinical history
Otalgia (possibly referred)
Epistaxis
Trismus
Dysphagia
Odynophagia
Dysarthria
Globus sensation
Hoarseness
Dyspnea
Hemoptysis
Weight loss or other constitutional symptoms
Past medical history
Previous history of malignancy
Previous history of radiation exposure
Social history
Tobacco use
Alcohol use
Occupational exposures, including sun exposure
Family history
Family history of malignancy
Physical examination
Overview of functional status and nourishment
Comprehensive examination of the skin of the scalp, face and neck
Otoscopy
Anterior rhinoscopy
Test symmetry of the somatosensory function of the lower divisions of the trigeminal nerve (V2 and V3)
Test maximal interincisal (or interalveolar, if edentulous) distance
Assess dentition
Assess voluntary movement of the tongue
Bimanual palpation of oral cavity and oropharynx
Indirect mirror laryngoscopy or fiberoptic nasopharyngolaryngoscopy
Bimanual palpation of thyroid gland
Bimanual palpation of all cervical lymph node levels

Diagnostic imaging

Errors may occur in the clinical assessment of regional lymph nodes by palpation alone,[26] especially in patients with a short, stout neck, in patients with fibrotic changes secondary to previous radiotherapy, and in patients with metastatic lymph nodes at sites typically inaccessible by routine physical examination, such as the parapharyngeal space.[27] In the presence of adequate clinical suspicion, imaging is also helpful in excluding other histologies, such as carotid body tumors or schwannomas, and can guide the clinician to the appropriate path along the diagnostic algorithm. Imaging modalities currently available in routine clinical practice include ultrasonography, computed tomography (CT), and magnetic resonance imaging (MRI) scans, and positron emission tomography (PET) scans. Other modalities, such as single positron emission computer tomography (SPECT) scans are currently under evaluation and presently have little application in clinical practice.

Relevant imaging should be undertaken prior to manipulation of the primary tumor or neck nodes, in order to maximize the information obtained from these studies. Inflammation and obliteration of tissue planes from a recent biopsy may not only create difficulty in interpreting anatomic relations, but also cause artefacts on functional imaging studies, such as PET scans.

Computed tomography and magnetic resonance imaging

There is no substitute for a systematic, comprehensive examination of the neck; however, imaging studies provide valuable supplemental information of regional lymph node status. The sensitivity of CT and MRI for accurately detecting nodal metastases has been reported as 84% and 92%, respectively.[28] Although the presence of metastatic involvement of a lymph node is a histologic, not a radiologic diagnosis, there are characteristic changes apparent on CT and MRI suggestive of metastatic squamous cell carcinoma, including rim enhancement, central necrosis, and nodal size in excess of 1 cm in diameter. Lymphoma of the head and neck typically presents radiographically as solid, homogeneous lymph nodes that are isointense with muscle.

Despite the advantages afforded by these imaging modalities, limitations of both CT and MRI include difficulty differentiating reactive soft tissue inflammation or postradiotherapy fibrosis from residual or recurrent carcinoma. Furthermore, cervical lymph node size does not always correlate with the presence of tumor involvement. Although larger metastatic lymph nodes indicate greater tumor volume, a small lymph node less than 1 cm in diameter may still harbor foci of tumor cells. Conversely, lymph node size greater than 1 cm in diameter does not automatically herald metastatic cancer, since reactive lymphadenopathy following infection, inflammation, or surgical intervention may result in lymph nodes of such size. Another disadvantage of CT is that scatter artefact from dental fillings may result in poor image resolution.

Ultrasonography

Ultrasonography is a useful diagnostic imaging modality, which has been reported to be extremely sensitive in accurately characterizing cervical lymph nodes metastatic for SCC.[29] Advantages of ultrasonography include its relative low cost, easy on-screen nodal measurement, low patient burden, and facility for guided fine-needle aspiration.[30]

In spite of its high sensitivity (97%), a potential confounding factor in ultrasound examination of cervical lymph nodes is a low rate of specificity (32%) for the evaluation of metastatic HNSCC.[29] Another disadvantage of ultrasonography is that the results are dependent on the experience of the investigator.[31]

Positron emission tomography

PET scanning is a functional imaging modality that measures the metabolic rate of tissue using radioisotopes and is based on the principle that malignant tumors have higher metabolic rates compared to normal tissues. Glucose metabolism can be characterized following the administration of radiolabeled ^{18}-F-2-fluoro-2-deoxy-D-glucose (FDG). Although ^{18}FDG-PET imaging lacks the anatomic detail afforded by CT or MRI scans, it relies on metabolic activity from glucose transport, rather than gross lymph node size, to indicate metastatic foci. Sites of increased metabolic activity are reflected on PET scans by higher body weight-based standardized uptake values (SUV_{BW}). Such a physiologic study aims to reduce the false-negative rate of CT and MRI by identifying metastatic lymph nodes smaller than 1 cm. However, like these conventional imaging techniques, ^{18}FDG-PET is prone to the false–positive tendency of suggesting erroneously that reactive lymphadenopathy may be metastatic cancer.

Evaluation of ^{18}FDG-PET for accurately identifying nodal metastases demonstrates results comparable to those of CT or MRI. Kau et al found the sensitivity and specificity of ^{18}FDG-PET to be 87% and 94% respectively, compared to 65% and 47% respectively for CT, and 88% and 41% respectively for MRI in patients with HNSCC metastatic to cervical lymph nodes.[32] Prospective comparison of ^{18}FDG-PET with CT, MRI, and ultrasound demonstrated superior sensitivity and specificity of ^{18}FDG-PET for detecting cervical lymph node metastases from HNSCC.[31] Other reports have suggested that ^{18}FDG-PET is particularly useful when the findings on conventional CT imaging are equivocal for nodal metastases.[33] The lower limit in terms of resolution of ^{18}FDG-PET for detection of abnormal lymph nodes has not been clearly delineated, but accurate identification of metastatic SCC in cervical lymph nodes less than 5 mm in diameter has been reported.[34]

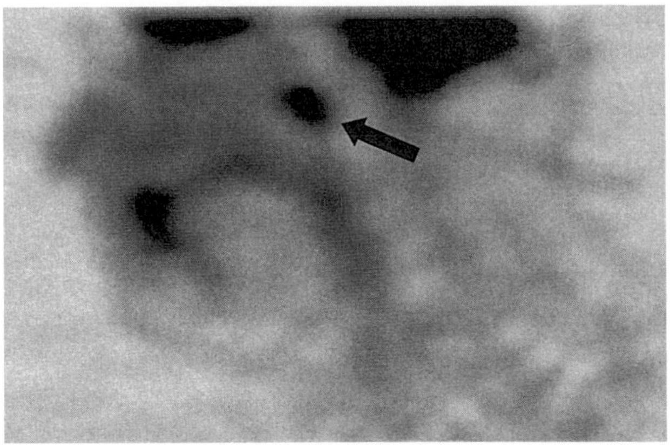

Figure 16.4 ^{18}FDG-PET scan of a patient with an 'unknown' primary showing intense activity in the nasopharynx. Nasopharyngoscopy had failed to reveal any mucosal abnormality and the patient was returned to the operating room for repeat examination and biopsy based on the PET findings. Histopathologic examination of the nasopharyngeal biopsy specimen confirmed the presence of squamous carcinoma.

Newer technologies are aimed at improving accuracy by combining functional information from ^{18}FDG-PET with the anatomic resolution of MRI or CT scans.[35]

^{18}FDG-PET may be of benefit in patients with cervical nodal metastases from an unknown primary (Figure 16.4). Some studies have suggested a beneficial contribution of ^{18}FDG-PET in elucidating the primary tumor,[36] while other reports have concluded that it did not significantly improve detection of the primary tumor and was hindered by false-positive results.[37] It is not surprising to have controversy over the utility of an imaging modality still relatively novel. However, an area where ^{18}FDG-PET seems particularly beneficial is the detection of recurrent HNSCC following radiation therapy.[38] To the extent that PET imaging is predicated on tissue metabolism, tumor cells should theoretically possess greater metabolic activity and express increased levels of glucose transporters, compared to edematous, scarred, or most normal tissues.[39] Furthermore, clinical response to concurrent radiation therapy and chemotherapy for HNSCC is mirrored by a decrease in tumor hypermetabolism on serial ^{18}FDG-PET scans before, during, and after therapy.[40]

Some authors have suggested that the indications for ^{18}FDG-PET may extend beyond the N+ neck, and may also include patients without clinically apparent nodal metastases on presentation (N0 neck). Patients whose primary tumor is in a high-risk location for occult regional metastatic disease may be appropriate candidates for evaluation by ^{18}FDG-PET.[41] However the current limited availability and greater expense of ^{18}FDG-PET may prohibit its routine use in patients with head and neck cancer.[42] The low yield associated with ^{18}FDG-PET in identifying intrathoracic second primaries or metastases from HNSCC not otherwise apparent on routine work-up has resulted in some authors suggesting that routine inclusion of the thorax in imaging a patient otherwise without pulmonary symptoms is unnecessary.[43]

However, for differentiated thyroid carcinoma, whole-body ^{18}FDG-PET imaging has been shown to be a useful tool for detecting recurrent and/or metastatic disease in patients who present with serially rising thyroglobulin levels but negative ^{131}I and thallium-201 (^{201}T1) scans following total thyroidectomy.[44] Certain thyroid tumors such as Hürthle cell carcinoma or poorly differentiated variants exhibit higher ^{18}FDG uptake so that tumors that are less radioactive iodine-avid are generally better imaged on ^{18}FDG-PET scan.

As our understanding of the uses and limitations of ^{18}FDG-PET scanning increases, the potential for delineating appropriate indications for patients with head and neck cancer becomes more likely. Several questions however persist in the interim. For the N+ neck, what minimum time should elapse following treatment intervention (e.g. neck dissection or radiotherapy) before attempting ^{18}FDG-PET scanning for residual or recurrent disease, in order to minimize false-positive imaging results due to inflammation or reactive changes? What is the prognostic significance of the absolute SUV_{BW} value? Previous studies have found no correlation between SUV_{BW} and histologic grade of tumor in nodal metastases from HNSCC, possibly due to the heterogeneity of tumor cell clones or differential expression of glucose metabolism induced by oncogenic alteration.[31]

Newer technologies

In light of the high cost associated with ^{18}FDG-PET, single photon emission computer tomography (SPECT) scans using ^{18}FDG and thallium-201 have been evaluated as less expensive modalities. Unfortunately, the resolution of SPECT scanners is currently inferior to PET scanners.[42]

Endoscopy

Endoscopic examination of the upper aerodigestive tract under anesthesia allows thorough inspection of the primary tumor as well as evaluation for second primary tumors, with the ability to biopsy suspicious sites. The oropharynx, hypopharynx, larynx, and esophagus should be examined in a systematic fashion through direct laryngoscopy and esophagoscopy.

Histologic diagnosis

The diagnosis of metastatic cancer is made histologically, and so pathologic confirmation should be obtained for clinically and radiologically suspicious nodes.

Fine-needle aspiration

Fine-needle aspiration (FNA) is an accurate, reliable procedure with minimal morbidity and may be performed in an outpatient setting, allowing for quick cytologic interpretation of suspicious neck masses. A diagnosis of metastatic epidermoid carcinoma may be distinguished from other malignant conditions, such as lymphoma, adenocarcinoma, or thyroid carcinoma. In addition, benign conditions, such as tuberculosis, chronic lymphadenitis, and hyperplastic lymph nodes, may be ruled out.[45] Sensitivity and specificity of FNA of masses of the head and neck have been reported as 97% and 96% respectively.[46] Immunohistochemical staining for markers such as thyroglobulin, calcitonin, cytokeratin and mucin may be performed on the cellular aspirate to classify the histology if necessary.

Masses at sites in the head and neck inaccessible on routine examination (e.g. retropharyngeal lymph nodes) may be sampled under image guidance using CT, MRI, or ultrasonography.[47–49]

An important caveat to remember regarding FNA concerns misinterpretation of cytologic results. A finding of epithelial cells in the presence of clear or straw-colored fluid on aspiration is occasionally misinterpreted as branchial cleft carcinoma, rather than cystic degeneration of a metastatic lymph node which is the more likely diagnosis in an adult. Metastases from squamous carcinoma of certain sites, such as the tonsil or base of tongue, and from well-differentiated thyroid carcinomas are often cystic and therefore more likely to such misinterpretation. True branchial cleft cyst carcinoma is an extremely rare condition, with few cases in the literature that satisfy all criteria originally proposed by Martin et al.[50,51] Repeat fine-needle aspiration, using image guidance if appropriate, should be considered following an initial non-diagnostic FNA. A metastatic lymph node with a necrotic center may occasionally yield a non-diagnostic specimen because of cellular debris in the hypoxic core, with viable tumor cells undetected at the periphery of the lymph node.

Core-needle biopsy

Should a repeat fine-needle biopsy performed for an initial non-diagnostic specimen fail to yield a diagnosis, one may consider a core-needle biopsy of the neck mass. The larger caliber of the needle generally provides an adequate specimen for cytologic and histologic evaluation. Core biopsy is typically not necessary for metastatic HNSCC, since a properly executed FNA should easily elucidate this diagnosis. It may, however, be useful in selected instances such as when malignant lymphoma is suspected. Extreme caution should be exercised when performing a core biopsy on a mass in the vicinity of the great vessels of the neck. Preprocedure imaging or radiographic-guided biopsy technique may reduce the risk of inadvertent injury to the major vasculature of the neck.

Open biopsy

The prognostic impact of open biopsy of a metastatic neck node during the work-up of a patient with squamous cell carcinoma of the head and neck remains controversial. Unfortunately, data from retrospective reviews[52–55] that have shown 'no adverse impact on overall outcome' are quoted to justify the practice. Ill-planned biopsy incisions create unwarranted difficulties with surgical planning during the definitive surgical operation. If the patient needs a subsequent neck dissection it may need resection of structures that would ordinarily be spared, in order to fully excise contaminated tissue planes and scar from the previous open biopsy. In addition, therapy may be delayed if the patient develops wound complications from the biopsy, and there have been anecdotal reports of fungation of the tumor through the biopsy site. An open biopsy of a suspicious neck node should therefore be discouraged in most instances.

Open neck node biopsy does have a role in selected instances, particularly when the FNA suggests lymphoma. In such circumstances, the open neck node biopsy should be planned in such a manner that the incision scar be excised with the surgical specimen should biopsy results demonstrate squamous cell carcinoma, necessitating subsequent neck dissection. At the time of open biopsy, communication with the pathologist is critical to facilitate the correct diagnosis. If lymphoma is the suspected diagnosis, the cervical nodal specimen should be transported to the pathology lab fresh (not fixed in formalin) to allow proper tissue typing. If mycobacterial infection is the suspected diagnosis, the microbiology lab should be contacted ahead of time to determine whether special handling or media is necessary.

Histopathologic diagnosis

An important consideration in the accurate detection of nodal metastases concerns the sensitivity of routine histopathologic examination of nodal specimens. Intraoperative labeling of cervical nodal levels with tags may facilitate orientation for accurate pathologic reporting, but this practice is not widely utilized. Surgical pathology departments at different institutions may have different policies regarding the routine sampling of neck dissection specimens to evaluate for metastatic lymph nodes. Standard sectioning techniques result in microscopic examination of only a small portion of the nodal contents excised. Serial microscopic sectioning of all lymph nodes would improve the sensitivity of detection over traditional hematoxylin and eosin (H&E) staining, but at significant expense of time and manpower. Furthermore, the prognostic significance of such micrometastases from HNSCC detected by serial sectioning is not known.[56] To improve on detection for occult nodal metastases, different immunohistochemical markers, such as proliferating cell nuclear antigen, MIB-1, E-cadherin, and c-myc, have been investigated for HNSCC.[57,58] Likewise, immunohistochemistry for S-100 has been studied as a predictive marker of occult nodal metastases from malignant melanoma.[59] Further study however is necessary to determine the prognostic significance of these immunohistochemical markers.

For cutaneous melanoma, the reverse transcriptase-polymerase chain reaction (RT-PCR) assay has been utilized as a sensitive technique to detect submicroscopic lymph node metastases.[60] Shivers et al have reported a significant difference in disease-free survival and overall survival between pathologically negative, RT-PCR positive and pathologically negative, RT-PCR negative patient groups undergoing lymphatic mapping and sentinel lymph node biopsy for malignant melanoma.[61] Although the ability to detect metastasis at the cellular, and even molecular level exists, the prognostic significance of these findings remains to be determined. A multicenter national trial in the US called the Sunbelt Melanoma Trial is currently ongoing to determine the optimal treatment for submicroscopic disease histologically negative, but positive by RT-PCR.[62] Such data is critical before considering including molecular staging in the evaluation of patients.

Diagnosis of the unknown primary

The work-up of squamous cell carcinoma metastatic to a cervical lymph node with an unknown primary represents a diagnostic challenge. Careful evaluation of the head and neck for an undetected primary

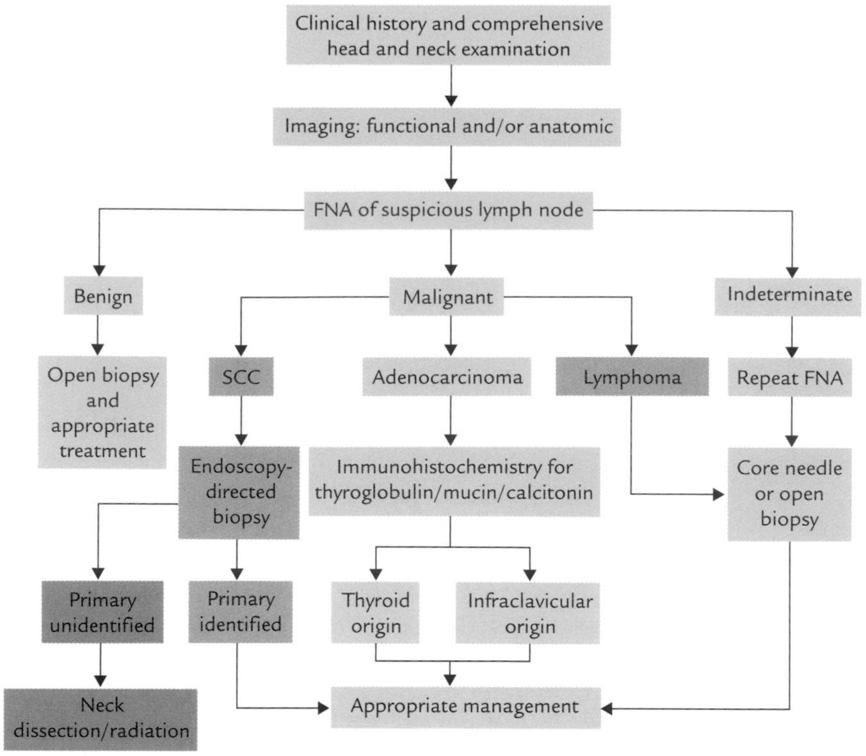

Figure 16.5 Algorithm for the work-up for a metastatic cervical lymph node with a suspected unknown primary.

tumor is critical.[63] Location of the metastatic lymph node may suggest the primary site.[64] Although primary malignancies for cervical metastases in the lateral neck often arise from the oral cavity or oropharynx, squamous cell carcinoma more inferiorly in the neck at the supraclavicular region may herald primary lesions at the hypopharynx, cervical esophagus, or thyroid gland.

Supraclavicular metastases may also arise from an infraclavicular primary, such as carcinoma of the lung, breast, or stomach. The skin of the head and neck should be thoroughly examined to rule out cutaneous malignancy, which may not have been brought to light during the history taking, particularly if treated in the distant past. Sites of potential occult primaries should be carefully evaluated, including the nasopharynx, base of tongue, and pyriform sinuses. The benefit of fiberoptic nasopharyngolaryngoscopy in the office setting may be illustrated by a series of three reports from Memorial Sloan-Kettering Cancer Center.[65–67] The most recent study found that the proportion of patients in whom occult primary tumors were subsequently identified dropped with each subsequent report from 31% to 15% to 12%. This decrease was largely attributed to improvements in technology which facilitated the identification of small primary tumors on initial evaluation.

With histologic diagnosis of squamous cell carcinoma, attempts to identify the primary tumor should include direct laryngoscopy and esophagoscopy in the operating room. Bronchoscopy with bronchial washings has been advocated in the work-up of an unknown primary. Although controversial, the yield from routine bronchoscopy in the absence of clinical symptoms or signs and without abnormalities on chest X-ray may be low. Also controversial is the manner in which biopsies to determine the primary site should be performed. Rather than 'blind' biopsies sampling tissues from various sites in the upper aerodigestive tract, biopsies directed by areas of suspicion based on preoperative clinical evaluation may be a more suitable approach. Some authors have advocated routine tonsillectomy to rule out microscopic tumor, especially within the tonsillar crypts.[68,69]

Should the primary tumor continue to be elusive despite thorough endoscopic examination, the pathologist may be requested to perform additional stains on the cytologic aspirate. Thyroglobulin or calcitonin stain may be requested if the diagnosis of thyroid malignancy is entertained. Epstein–Barr virus (EBV) titer may be requested if nasopharyngeal carcinoma is suspected. An algorithm for the approach to a metastatic cervical lymph node with an unknown primary is depicted in Figure 16.5.

Staging and prognosis

The staging system of regional metastases to cervical lymph nodes established by the American Joint

Table 16.5 Staging system of regional lymph nodes (N stage) for squamous cell carcinoma of the upper aerodigestive tract excluding nasopharynx

Nx	Regional lymph nodes cannot be assessed
N0	No regional lymph node metastasis
N1	Metastasis in a single ipsilateral lymph node, 3 cm or less in greatest dimension
N2a	Metastasis in a single ipsilateral lymph node more than 3 cm but not more than 6 cm in greatest dimension
N2b	Metastasis in multiple ipsilateral lymph nodes, none more than 6 cm in greatest dimension
N2c	Metastasis in bilateral or contralateral lymph nodes, none more than 6 cm in greatest dimension
N3	Metastasis in a lymph node more than 6 cm in greatest dimension

Table 16.6 Staging system of regional lymph nodes (N stage) for squamous cell carcinoma of the nasopharynx

Nx	Regional lymph nodes cannot be assessed
N0	No regional lymph node metastasis
N1	Unilateral metastasis in lymph node(s) 6 cm or less in greatest dimension, above the supraclavicular fossa
N2	Bilateral metastasis in lymph node(s) 6 cm or less in greatest dimension, above the supraclavicular fossa
N3a	Metastasis in a lymph node greater
N3b	Metastatic lymph node extension to the supraclavicular fossa

Table 16.7 Staging system of regional lymph nodes (N stage) for thyroid carcinoma. Regional lymph nodes are the cervical and upper mediastinal lymph nodes

Nx	Regional lymph nodes cannot be assessed
N0	No regional lymph node metastasis
N1	Regional lymph node metastasis
N1a	Metastasis in ipsilateral cervical lymph node(s)
N1b	Metastasis in bilateral, midline, or contralateral cervical or mediastinal lymph node(s)

Committee on Cancer (AJCC) is outlined in Tables 16.5–16.7.[70]

Characteristics of nodal metastases influencing outcome

The presence of cervical lymph node metastases results in decreased survival rates compared to those free of nodal metastases. However, various characteristics of the involved cervical lymph nodes can themselves impact on outcome. The current TNM staging system takes some of these into account, such as size, laterality, and number of involved lymph nodes. However, extracapsular spread (ECS) of carcinoma in cervical lymph nodes, which is probably the single-most important predictor of poor prognosis has not been included. ECS has been associated with increased rates of regional nodal recurrence,[71] as well as significantly decreased survival rates.[72] Multivariate analysis has demonstrated that extracapsular spread is an independent predictor of survival.[73] The location of metastatic disease within the neck is also of prognostic value; as a general rule, the incidence of distant metastasis increases with, and prognosis worsens with, more inferiorly located cervical metastases.[74,75]

Principles of treatment

Despite the shortcomings of the current AJCC staging system, N staging of cervical metastases from HNSCC is useful in guiding treatment planning. Early stage (N1) regional lymph node metastases may be treated equally well with surgery or radiation therapy, with the treatment modality usually in keeping with that of the primary tumor. For more advanced cervical metastases (N2 or N3), combined therapy with surgery and postoperative radiation therapy is usually necessary. Management of the N0 neck is a subject fraught with considerable controversy. Details of the treatment strategies applicable to the clinically N+ neck and the N0 neck follow later in this chapter.

Surgery

Traditional surgical management of cervical nodal metastases entails comprehensive neck dissection with or without preservation of certain anatomic structures, such as the spinal accessory nerve (XI), internal jugular vein (IJV), and the sternocleidomastoid muscle (SCM) when technically and oncologically feasible. There has been a continuing trend towards more selective procedures, sparing not only the XI, IJV, and SCM, but also lymph node groups thought to be at low risk for metastases.

History of neck dissection

Early attempts to resect cervical lymph nodes were met with pessimism. In the mid-nineteenth century, Chelius wrote 'Once the growth in the mouth has spread to the submaxillary gland complete removal of the disease is impossible.'[76] Towards the end of the nineteenth century however innovative surgical approaches incorporated regional lymph nodes during resection of tumors of the oral cavity. In 1880, Kocher described excising upper cervical lymph nodes at the time of resection of a cancer of the tongue.[77] In 1906, Crile was the first to describe a systematic, comprehensive approach to dissect cervical lymph nodes, including removal of the sternocleidomastoid muscle, internal jugular vein, and spinal accessory nerve.[78] This procedure was popularized by Martin and colleagues, who described in 1951 the indications and technique of the so-called 'radical neck dissection.'[79]

Classification of neck dissections

The classical radical neck dissection is the gold standard of lymphadenectomy for clinically apparent lymphatic metastases and consists of surgical clearing of nodal lymphatics from all five levels of the neck. Included in the specimen with the cervical lymphatics are the sternocleidomastoid and omohyoid muscles, spinal accessory nerve, internal jugular vein, submandibular gland and tail of the parotid.

Functional morbidity associated with radical neck dissection arises primarily from sacrifice of one or more of the following structures: the spinal accessory nerve, the sternocleidomastoid muscle, and the internal jugular vein. Sacrifice of the spinal accessory nerve results in loss of innervation to the trapezius muscle. The patient is unable to abduct the arm fully and suffers from chronic pain and stiffness of the shoulder. Destabilization of the shoulder results in a 'winged scapula' deformity and increases the risk for sternoclavicular subluxation.[80] Resection of the sternocleidomastoid muscle gives the appearance of platysmal banding and removes a layer of cover for the carotid artery, potentially important in the irradiated neck. Sacrifice of the internal jugular vein may result in significant facial edema and possibly neurovascular compromise, particularly following bilateral radical neck dissection and laryngopharyngectomy that disrupts collateral drainage into Batson's prevertebral venous plexus.

In light of the functional morbidity and cosmetic deformity associated with radical neck dissection, modifications to the procedure have been described. A classification scheme previously described to standardize nomenclature of the different types of neck dissection is listed in Table 16.8.[81]

Table 16.8 Classification of neck dissections

Comprehensive neck dissection
Classical radical neck dissection (RND)
Type I modified radical neck dissection (MRND I)
Type II modified radical neck dissection (MRND II)
Type III modified radical neck dissection (MRND III)
Extended radical neck dissection (ERND)
Selective neck dissection
Supraomohyoid neck dissection (SOHND)
Lateral neck dissection (LND)
Posterolateral neck dissection (PLND)

Comprehensive neck dissection

Comprehensive neck dissection refers to those procedures that remove cervical lymph nodes from levels I through V. This category includes the aforementioned radical neck dissection, as well as the following modifications to this technique. Type I modified radical neck dissection selectively preserves the spinal accessory nerve. Type II modified radical neck dissection preserves the spinal accessory nerve and sternocleidomastoid muscle but sacrifices the internal jugular vein. Type III modified neck dissection (functional neck dissection) preserves the spinal accessory nerve, sternocleidomastoid muscle, and internal jugular vein. Extended radical neck dissection is also included in the category of comprehensive neck dissection. In addition to those structures removed in the standard radical neck dissection, extended radical neck dissection includes nodal groups not typically removed during the dissection, such as retropharyngeal or parapharyngeal lymph nodes. Alternatively, extended radical neck dissection includes non-lymphatic structures not typically removed during the dissection, such as the carotid artery or hypoglossal nerve. The routine reporting of structures preserved or resected in comparison to the standard radical neck dissection is paramount for all procedures included in the category of comprehensive neck dissection.

Selective neck dissection

In contrast to comprehensive neck dissections, procedures in this category selectively remove cervical lymph node groups at certain levels, while preserving the spinal accessory nerve, sternocleidomastoid muscle, and internal jugular vein. Supraomohyoid neck dissection removes lymph nodes at levels I, II, and III. Lateral neck dissection (jugular neck dissection) removes lymph nodes at levels II, III, and IV. Posterolateral neck dissection removes lymph nodes at levels II through V, as well as suboccipital nodes and postauricular nodes.

Nodal yields in neck dissection

An area for which there is no easy answer concerns the impact of nodal count following neck dissection. Retrospective analyses that have quantified nodal counts exenterated in neck dissection illustrate the variation of nodal yields among different surgeons.[82–86] These studies demonstrate that the mean number of lymph nodes harvested during radical neck dissection has ranged from 22 to 39 nodes. Certainly, both the technical expertise of the surgeon performing the neck dissection and the meticulousness of the pathologist examining the specimen affect the absolute number of the nodal yield. As described above, more sensitive detection techniques, such as serial sectioning or PCR, may further increase the number of pathologically positive lymph nodes over conventional H&E evaluation. There are no good data correlating the number of lymph nodes harvested during neck dissection and outcome regarding regional recurrence or survival. The absence of such data to suggest what constitutes an adequate neck dissection is particularly important in light of the increasing acceptance of more selective procedures. The absence of standardized nomenclature characterizing the minimum number of cervical lymph nodes resected to qualify a procedure as a neck dissection is evident in the fifth edition of the AJCC Cancer Staging Manual, indicating that 'a selective neck dissection will ordinarily include six or more lymph nodes and a radical or modified radical neck dissection will ordinarily include 10 or more lymph nodes'.[70] These small numbers suggested could result in a wide variety of surgical procedures yielding markedly different numbers of nodes harvested, and yet these procedures would all be grouped under the general heading of 'neck dissection.'

Radiation therapy

General principles of radiotherapy summarized by Wang include; the generally favorable radioresponsiveness of most early stage head and neck squamous cell carcinomas; a well-oxygenated environment provides an ideal setting for therapeutic radiation; invasion of bone or deep muscle portends a poorer response to radiotherapy; and neck dissection, with or without adjuvant irradiation, is the preferred treatment for large cervical metastases.[87] Heterogeneity among radiosensitivity may be due to several factors, including tumor volume, intrinsic cellular radiosensitivity, clonogen density, and hypoxia.[88] In light of this heterogeneity, molecular markers to predict radiosensitivity have been investigated, including Ki-67 immunohistochemistry,[89] as well as assays for p53 mutation, or *bcl*-2 expression.[90] The prognostic significance of such molecular markers has yet to be determined.

Definitive radiation therapy

Definitive radiotherapy shares comparable results with surgical treatment for N0 and N1 neck disease. SCC arising from certain subsites in the head and neck is particularly radiosensitive, such as the nasopharynx and lymphoepithelial carcinoma of the tonsil. Even advanced cervical metastases from these primary tumors respond well to definitive radiotherapy, reserving planned neck dissection for residual disease. Although a variety of different fractionation schemes may be employed, definitive radiotherapy generally delivers 60–70 Gy through a shrinking field technique over 6–7.5 weeks.

Adjuvant radiation therapy

Advanced cervical lymphatic metastases (N2 or N3) from most sites of the head and neck usually require a combination of neck dissection and radiation therapy. Early reports combining neck dissection and preoperative radiation therapy demonstrated reduction in regional recurrence, particularly for advanced nodal disease.[91] The final report of study 73-03 of the Radiation Therapy Oncology Group did not demonstrate a statistically significant difference in survival between preoperative versus postoperative radiation therapy for advanced HNSCC, although locoregional control was improved in the patients receiving postoperative radiation therapy.[92] The standard timing of radiation therapy when combined with neck dissection is currently in an adjuvant setting. The advantages of delivering radiation therapy after surgery include the ability to deliver a greater dose of radiation in the postoperative setting (usually 60–70 Gy over 6–7 weeks), than preoperatively (typically 45 Gy over 4–5 weeks); and the additional information gleaned during neck dissection to plan for appropriate portals of radiation therapy, based on the surgical extent of tumor. Potential disadvantages associated with postoperative radiation therapy include possible contamination of tissue planes with tumor during surgical manipulation, or delayed wound healing from complications following neck dissection may delay the administration of radiation therapy. The ideal time to initiate postoperative radiotherapy has been recommended as between 4 and 6 weeks following surgery, in light of the risk for increased locoregional failure.[93]

Indications for adjuvant radiotherapy include metastatic lymph node size greater than 3 cm, multiple positive nodes, extracapsular lymph node extension, microscopic or gross residual disease and adverse features of the primary tumor such as positive surgical margins, vascular and lymphatic invasion or perineural infiltration. Adjuvant radiation therapy has been shown to improve locoregional control and survival in the presence of extracapsular spread or positive resection margins following surgery.[94] Postoperative radiotherapy however should not be construed as a panacea for an inadequate operation. Silver clips placed intraoperatively are useful to mark the extent of gross residual disease if adjuvant radiation therapy is planned, in order to facilitate planning for electron boost.

The decision to employ postoperative radiation therapy for HNSCC metastatic to cervical lymph nodes with an unknown primary mirrors that for nodal metastases from a known primary source. N1 disease without extracapsular extension can be managed by neck dissection alone,[95] whereas more advanced nodal disease requires postoperative radiation therapy to both sides of the neck, as well as to putative mucosal sites in the pharyngeal axis, particularly in the presence of extracapsular extension.[96]

Neck dissection is the preferred modality for salvage. Irradiation for surgical failure in the neck is associated with worse survival rates compared to salvage neck dissection following failed radiotherapy.[97]

Brachytherapy

Treatment options for patients with nodal recurrence or gross persistent disease following previous irradiation to the neck include neck dissection with intraoperative radiation therapy, where a single dose of high intensity external beam radiotherapy is employed, or neck dissection with brachytherapy. As illustrated in Figure 16.6, ^{121}I-Dexon mesh or afterloading catheters with ^{191}Ir wires may be used for brachytherapy. Care must be taken to protect the carotid artery when brachytherapy is employed. Either pedicled muscle flaps, or vascularized free flaps are suitable tissue coverage to minimize carotid exposure, when employing brachytherapy for gross residual or recurrent nodal disease.

Concurrent chemoradiation therapy

Concurrent chemotherapy and radiation therapy has been demonstrated to provide improved disease control and survival rates over sequential chemo-

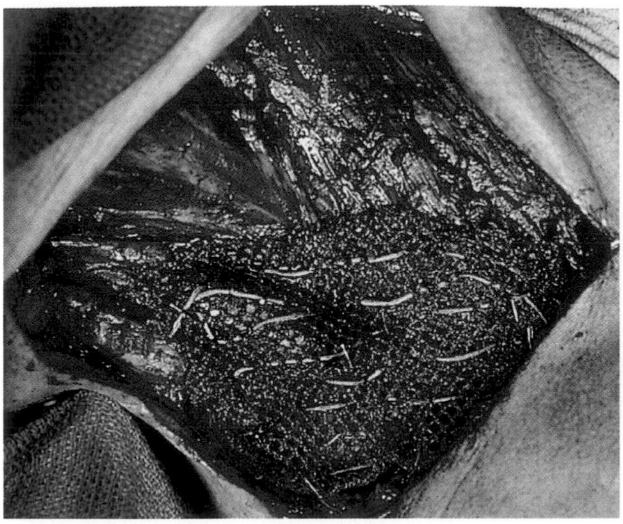

Figure 16.6 This patient had a regional recurrence following previous neck dissection and postoperative radiation therapy for a squamous carcinoma of the tonsil. The recurrent tumor was excised leaving gross residual disease in the region of the carotid bifurcation. A ^{121}I-Dexon mesh was sutured in place to deliver brachytherapy to the residual tumor.

radiation or radiation therapy alone, when utilized in an organ preservation approach for advanced SCC of the head and neck.[98–101] However, despite the improved benefit of concurrent chemoradiation, an area for which very little data exists is the optimal management of nodal metastases in a concurrent approach. Because of the paucity of data, a number of controversies persist regarding the optimal treatment of the neck in concurrent chemoradiation.

Assessing response to chemoradiation

One such controversy involves the optimal method to assess response in the neck following concurrent chemoradiation. There is no diagnostic technique that universally detects persistent nodal disease after concurrent chemoradiation. Clinical evaluation of the response to non-surgical therapy is difficult. Induration and erythema, combined with fibrosis and edema, obscure accurate assessment. Anatomic-based diagnostic imaging, such as CT, MRI, and ultrasonography, all fall short of consistently demonstrating persistent or recurrent tumor following chemotherapy or radiation therapy. As discussed previously, ^{18}FDG-PET scanning has been shown to correlate with clinical response to concurrent chemoradiation before, during, and after therapy.[40] Further study however is necessary prior to the adoption of PET scanning as the standard of care in evaluating the neck following chemoradiation.

Histological evaluation of posttreatment neck dissection specimens may be prone to error. Viable tumor cells may exist deep within muscle, fibrous, and lymphatic tissue particularly with advanced nodal metastases with a propensity for extracapsular extension into surrounding structures.

Biopsy specimens in a previously treated area may be falsely negative as a result of sampling artefacts that miss focally dispersed residual tumor. The utility of less invasive biopsy techniques such as fine-needle aspiration may be difficult to quantify, as a specimen interpreted as negative for malignancy does not rule out the possibility of viable tumor. Previous studies have demonstrated the controversy as to the predictive value of tumor response by clinical evaluation, and histologic evidence of residual disease.[102] The discrepancy between observed clinical response and histologic assessment of tumor persistence may in part be due to our present inability to distinguish viable tumor cells reliably on routine sectioning and H&E staining. Ghosting of dead cells with residual squamous architecture may not be evident for weeks following radiation therapy.

Necessity for neck dissection

Our present inability to reliably detect the histologic presence of residual viable tumor in nodal metastases following concurrent chemoradiation underscores the controversies in neck management that follow. Should a neck dissection be a planned component in the concurrent radiotherapy strategy?

There is little controversy surrounding the N0 neck, or the N1 neck for primary tumors known to be particularly radioresponsive, such as nasopharyngeal carcinoma or lymphoepithelial carcinoma of the tonsil. For other sites in the head and neck however considerable controversy persists as to the ideal management of nodal metastases in concurrent chemoradiation.

Data investigating the optimal management of the neck in concurrent chemoradiation regimens are sparse. Koch and colleagues studied a sample of 22 patients with cancer of the oral cavity, oropharynx, and hypopharynx treated with concurrent chemoradiation.[103] This study utilized planned neck dissection for nodal disease greater than 3 cm in size 8 weeks following chemoradiation. These authors questioned the value of planned postchemoradiation neck dissection, stating that three of five planned dissections yielded no viable cancer in the specimen. However, no further evidence regarding the impact of neck dissection on nodal recurrence is provided to further support this conclusion. The small patient sample size in this study, as well as the omission as to how tumor cells were evaluated for viability, makes interpreting these data difficult.

Lavertu and colleagues reported different conclusions based on 53 patients with stage III and IV head and neck cancer with N2 or N3 disease.[104] All patients with N2 or N3 disease were planned to undergo neck dissection 4–6 weeks following concurrent chemoradiation. For patients demonstrating less than a complete response in the neck after concurrent chemoradiation, 47% of nodal specimens were found to have tumor. However, in patients with a complete response in the neck after concurrent therapy, 22% of these complete responders were found to have the presence of tumor in the nodal specimens. This pathologic positivity was demonstrated to negatively impact on disease-specific survival. In light of this degree of pathological positivity in complete responders (greater than 20%), these authors concluded that all patients presenting with N2 or N3 disease should undergo planned neck dissection. Furthermore, they demonstrated a lower rate of nodal recurrence following neck dissection, and the inability to salvage nodal failure in patients who had not undergone neck dissection.

Timing of neck dissection

Despite the paucity of comparative data for concurrent chemoradiation, it appears from the preceding discussion that planned neck dissection may be considered for all N1 patients exhibiting less than a complete response, and for all N2 and N3 disease. If neck dissection is to be included in concurrent chemoradiation regimens, when should it occur? Again, there is no data to suggest an optimal time. Nevertheless, surgery should not be undertaken so early as to make dissection difficult due to hyperemia and excessive intraoperative bleeding. On the other hand, neck dissection should not be performed so late as to have fibrotic changes in the soft tissues of the neck complicate the operative procedure.

Type of neck dissection

Consequent to the realization that in previously treated patients where aberrant lymphatic pathways may result in unpredictable lymphatic spread, selective neck dissection is less ideal after concurrent chemoradiation.

Most authors who advocate posttreatment neck dissection have been performing radical or modified radical neck dissection preserving the spinal accessory nerve. Robbins and colleagues however have advocated the use of selective neck dissection after targeted intra-arterial chemoradiation, citing a regional control rate of 91% after a median follow-up of 36 months.[105]

In summary, there are no randomized trials investigating the management of the neck following concurrent chemoradiation. For the N1 neck exhibiting complete response, there appears to be little controversy that this neck may be safely observed. For the N+ neck exhibiting less than a complete response, it would be appropriate to proceed with neck dissection. In the absence of convincing data to the contrary, the patient with an N2 or N3 neck that exhibits a complete response to treatment should be managed with a planned neck dissection.

Adjuvant combined therapy

In light of the poor prognosis associated with advanced nodal metastases, the utility of adjuvant radiation therapy combined with chemotherapy following surgical treatment has been investigated. A randomized trial from France demonstrated reduced locoregional failure rates following concomitant cisplatin and radiation compared to radiation therapy alone (23% versus 41%), for patients with stage III or IV HNSCC with extracapsular spread of tumor in lymph node metastases.[106] Overall survival, and disease-free survival were also improved in the concurrent chemoradiation arm compared to the arm treated with radiation therapy alone. The addition of chemotherapy however was not found to improve the rate of distant metastases.

Management of cervical metastases from squamous cell carcinoma of the head and neck

Management of the clinically positive neck

As previously mentioned, early stage (N1) regional lymph node metastases may be treated equally well with surgery or radiation therapy, with the treatment modality usually in keeping with that of the primary tumor. For more advanced cervical metastases (N2 or N3), combined therapy with surgery and postoperative radiation therapy is indicated. Certain tumors, such as nasopharyngeal carcinoma or lymphoepithelial carcinoma of the tonsil, however typically respond well to radiation with/without chemotherapy without the need for routine neck dissection.

Special mention should be made with regard to advanced nodal metastases encasing the carotid. Although carotid artery resection has been reported by some authors, the risk of locoregional failure is substantial because of the high likelihood of leaving residual disease at other sites such as the skull base, pharynx or prevertebral region. In addition, the risk of neurological sequelae from carotid manipulation may preclude the practice of carotid resection for advanced HNSCC. Balloon test occlusion demonstrating adequate collateral circulation has been suggested to avoid neurovascular complications from carotid resection. However, neurological injury is still possible from embolization of a clot in the carotid. Furthermore, reconstruction of the carotid from saphenous vein or synthetic materials risks catastrophic hemorrhage from carotid rupture in the event of regional recurrence.

Management of the clinically negative neck

An issue of ongoing controversy concerns the management of the neck in patients without clinical evidence of regional nodal metastases (the N0 neck). Lymphatic metastases occur in a predictable fashion through sequential spread. Although previous surgery or irradiation may result in aberrant lymphatic drainage, there are well-established first echelon lymph nodes at highest risk for metastases depending on the primary site of cancer. Pathologic evidence of micrometastases has been observed on gross section in up to 33% of elective neck dissection specimens. More sensitive detection methods such as serial sectioning or polymerase chain reaction (PCR) may result in an even higher prevalence. In light of the propensity for various sites of the oral cavity and oropharynx to spread to regional lymphatics and the high risk of nodal recurrence, what constitutes the ideal approach to the N0 neck? Is the best approach observation or treatment? If treatment is chosen, is elective neck dissection or elective neck irradiation the optimal modality?

In light of the tumor characteristics influencing the propensity for nodal metastases, it has been suggested that if the probability of metastases to cervical lymph nodes exceeds 20%, then treatment of the neck is warranted.[107] The need for appropriate management of the clinically negative neck has been demonstrated by the fact that patients whose clinically negative necks are observed tend to fail with regionally advanced disease, that is difficult to salvage.[108]

Elective neck dissection

It has been reported that there is no survival advantage offered by elective neck dissection when compared to observation.[109] However, as previously mentioned, when observation is used for the neck at risk for metastasis, patients tend to fail with advanced nodal disease, even with close follow-up.[108] Elective neck dissection has been shown to be improve locoregional control, and may therefore positively impact on the quality of the patient's survival.[110]

One criticism of elective neck dissection has focused on potential complications from the procedure. In light of the morbidity associated with the radical neck dissection, there has been the trend towards selective, rather than comprehensive neck dissection, based on the predictable pattern of cervical lymph node metastases. Suarez described in 1963 that the sternocleidomastoid muscle, internal jugular vein, and spinal accessory nerve may be preserved during neck dissection without compromising sound oncologic principles.[111] Bocca popularized this technique as the 'functional' neck dissection.[112] Selective neck dissection has been demonstrated to be an oncologically sound procedure, providing effective treatment for the N0 neck.[86] Supraomohyoid neck dissection (SOHND), selective lymphadenectomy clearing cervical nodal levels I, II, and III, has been recommended for N0 patients with primary squamous cell carcinomas of the oral cavity.[21,113] Other reports have extended the indication for SOHND for primary tumors in the oral cavity to include not only N0 necks, but also N1 necks without evidence of extracapsular spread.[25,114] A proposed limitation of the SOHND for primary tumors of the oral tongue concerns the potential for 'skip metastases,' or metastases to inferior cervical nodes at levels III or IV in the absence of demonstrable involvement at levels I and II.[22] The risk of isolated level IV involvement in the absence of other cervical metastases is sufficiently low as to obviate the need for routine addition of level IV to the SOHND for the N0 neck with most oral cavity primary tumors with the exception of the oral tongue.[23] Meticulous care should be exercised in the region of level IV to prevent inadvertent injury either to the thoracic duct on the left side of the neck or to the main lymphatic duct on the right side of the neck.

Based on the predictable spread of cervical nodal metastases, SOHND may not be sufficient for the N0 neck with a primary arising in the oropharynx. The risk for level IV spread is higher from primary tumors of the oropharynx compared to those arising from the oral cavity. Thus, an anterolateral neck dissection encompassing levels II, III, and IV of the deep jugular chain has been advocated for N0 necks with an oropharyngeal primary.[21]

For primary tumors of the oral cavity or oropharynx, the risk of level V involvement has been shown to be minimal when only one level is involved, unless level IV is the involved level, or unless multiple levels are involved.[115] Level V therefore is not routinely included in the selective lymphadenectomy of N0 necks for primaries of the oral cavity or oropharynx.

Sentinel node mapping for mucosal squamous cell carcinoma of the head and neck

In this era of more selective neck dissections, the utility of sentinel node biopsy, which is clinically useful for treatment of cutaneous melanoma, has been investigated for primaries of the oral cavity.[116] The applicability of this technique may, however, be limited because not only is the incidence and implication of metastases from squamous carcinoma distinct from melanoma, but the morbidity and functional outcome after a staging procedure such as SOHND are minimal.

Elective neck irradiation

The theoretical advantages of treating the N0 neck with surgical lymphadenectomy include pathologic staging information, preparation of donor and recipient vessels for microvascular reconstruction, and avoidance of the morbidity associated with radiotherapy. However, elective neck irradiation has been shown to provide lymph node failure rates of less than 5% when the primary lesion has been adequately controlled.[117,118] In fact, no significant differences in regional recurrence have been demonstrated following treatment with elective neck irradiation, compared to elective neck dissection.[119]

The modality chosen to address the clinically negative neck may be largely influenced by philosophy of the treating physician and by the treatment planned for the primary tumor. Nevertheless, as a general rule, the treatment modality for the primary tumor is used concurrently to address occult metastases in the clinically negative neck if the risk is appreciable.

Management of neck metastases from an unknown primary

The detailed evaluation of the patient with cervical metastases from an unknown primary has been discussed above. The management of the neck in these patients follows similar principles as those in patients with a clinically positive neck and an identified primary. As a general rule, even patients with N1 disease from an unknown primary benefit from neck dissection because the additional pathologic information that becomes available may help plan further treatment. However, metastatic lymph nodes at level IV are not recommended for neck dissection if the primary site is believed to lie below the level of the clavicles, unless the patient complains of compressive symptoms. Data from Memorial Sloan-Kettering have compared institutional outcome data from patients treated for cervical metastases with an unknown primary from the years of 1977 and 1990 to those treated from 1965 to 1976.

In the cohort of patients treated from 1977 to 1990, control of the treated neck had improved from 50% to 74%, presumably from the addition of adjuvant radiation therapy following neck dissection. Five-year survival (45%) however had not significantly improved.

The standard type of neck dissection employed for cervical metastases with an occult primary involves comprehensive neck dissection, with or without preservation of the spinal accessory nerve.

Management of cervical metastases from salivary neoplasms

Routine elective neck dissection for salivary gland malignancies is not advocated as occult cervical metastases are uncommon.[120] Significant risk factors for occult nodal metastases from cancers of the major salivary glands include primary tumor size greater than 4 cm in size (20% versus 4%), and high tumor grade (49% versus 7%).[121] For clinically apparent nodal metastases, the benefit of adjuvant radiotherapy has been demonstrated in a matched-pair analysis of patients receiving combined surgery and postoperative radiotherapy compared to patients treated with surgery only.[122] Five-year determinate survival for the combined therapy group was improved compared to the group undergoing surgery only (48.9% versus 18.7%), and locoregional control was improved as well (69.1% versus 40.2%). The benefit of postoperative radiation therapy was especially pronounced in patients with high-stage and high-grade primary tumors.

Fast neutron radiotherapy is available at select institutions and has been suggested as effective treatment for locally advanced adenoid cystic carcinoma of the head and neck.[123] However, its role in the management of nodal disease remains undefined.

Management of cervical metastases from thyroid carcinoma

Clinically apparent nodal metastases from differentiated thyroid cancer are approached with dissection of the central compartment, as well as type III modified radical neck dissection. The presence of nodal metastases has not been shown in a matched-pair analysis to result in a decrease in survival if appropriately managed, although it was associated with an increase in local recurrence.[124] In this study, patients older than 45 years of age with N1 disease had 20-year survival rates lower than that of patients with N0 disease, although this difference did not reach statistical significance.

Patients with bulky nodal disease are at increased risk for distant metastases, especially to the lung. Radioactive iodine therapy after total thyroidectomy and appropriate neck dissection is recommended in this situation. Radioactive iodine dosimetry 4–6 weeks after surgery is used to identify any residual thyroid tissue, followed by RAI ablative treatment. RAI treatment requires a hypothyroid state to elevate the patient's serum thyroid stimulating hormone (TSH) for optimal concentration of iodine. Traditionally, this hypothyroid state has been effected by cessation of supplemental thyroxine for 4–6 weeks prior to RAI dosimetry and treatment. Patients often complain of debilitating symptoms of hypothyroidism, including fatigue and difficulty with concentration. In light of these unpleasant side-effects associated with several weeks of symptomatic hypothyroidism, a relatively recent advance has been the use of recombinant human TSH to elevate the patient's serum TSH in order to increase RAI uptake. Recombinant human TSH allows for elevated serum TSH without the debilitating symptoms of clinical hypothyroidism. Further studies are necessary however before recombinant human TSH supplants the traditional hypothyroid approach as standard therapy for RAI.

As previously mentioned, poorly differentiated tumors and thyroid cancer in older patients do not concentrate RAI effectively, and these patients may have to be treated either with external beam radiation or high dose RAI on an empiric basis. External beam radiotherapy is not typically utilized for differentiated thyroid cancer and is usually reserved for bulky gross residual or recurrent disease and for anaplastic thyroid cancer.

Management of cervical metastases from melanoma

Regional nodal metastases are relatively rare in thin cutaneous melanomas (less than 1 mm in thickness) of the head and neck region and elective neck dissection (END) is therefore not recommended. Thicker lesions (greater than 4 mm) are associated with a high incidence of distant metastases and therefore END is unlikely to impact on survival in this population. The role of END in patients with intermediate thickness (1.0–4 mm thick) melanomas continues to be debated, as only about 15% of patients will have histologically demonstrable metastatic nodes so that the remaining 85% may be considered to have undergone an unnecessary procedure. Four randomized trials[125–128] and a large, retrospective study[129] in patients with intermediate thickness melanomas have failed to demonstrate any improvement in survival following END. Sentinel lymph node biopsy (SLNB) for cutaneous head and neck melanoma has the potential to avoid the morbidity of routine elective nodal dissections while at the same time accurately and pathologically staging the regional nodes at risk for micrometastases. The usefulness and reliability of the technique has been well described in numerous publications since it was first reported in 1990.[130] In our experience, a negative SLNB correctly predicted regional nodal control in 47/48 (98%) patients but missed one of the five (20%) patients who had regional lymphatic disease. The 2-year disease-specific survival for SLN-negative patients was 93% compared to 50% for SLN-positive patients ($P = \mathrm{NS}$).[131] SLN mapping is a reliable indicator of the status of the draining lymphatic basins but patients with negative SLN(s) will need to be observed for longer periods to understand the true implications of the procedure.

Clinically apparent regional lymphatic spread to the parotid gland or to cervical lymph nodes should be managed with superficial parotidectomy and neck dissection, with likely adjuvant radiation therapy. Originally believed to be a radioresistant tumor, cutaneous melanoma has a radiation response different from that of squamous cell carcinoma, demonstrating effective tumor cell death at a higher dose per fraction than that of SCC. As a result, hypofractionation schemes utilizing large-dose fractions have been employed. Adjuvant hypofractionated radiotherapy has been shown to improve 5-year actuarial locoregional control rates for patients with stage II and III disease.[132]

Complications of treatment

Surgery

Sacrifice of the spinal accessory nerve, sternocleidomastoid muscle, and internal jugular vein during radical neck dissection results in functional morbidity and cosmetic deformity described earlier in the chapter.

Air embolism refers to inadvertent entry of air into the cervical venous system and may occur following laceration of the internal jugular vein. Clinical signs include a precipitous drop in systolic blood pressure, cardiac output, and oxygen saturation, and an audible 'to-and-fro' murmur. Further operating should cease immediately, and the following steps instituted: nitrous inhalation anesthesia should be terminated and the patient ventilated with 100% oxygen; the patient should be positioned in the left lateral decubitus position to trap the air embolus in the right atrium; aspiration of the air embolus may then be performed through cardiac puncture or central venous catheterization.

Chylous fistulae may be prevented by meticulous identification and ligation of the thoracic duct prior to division. The terminal branches of the thoracic duct on the left neck are at risk for inadvertent injury during dissection of lymph nodes at level IV. Intraoperative chylous leaks may be recognized by the extravasation of milky fluid at the lower neck, particularly with increased intrathoracic pressure by the Valsalva maneuver. Recognition of chylous fistulae intraoperatively should be treated immediately with suture ligatures or hemoclips. Postoperative chylous fistulae manifest with marked increase in output of milky fluid in suction drains. Conservative management of postoperative chylous fistulae includes cessation of wall suction, with drains on self-suction only; pressure dressings; and low-fat nutritional support. Failure of conservative measures warrants return to the operating room for surgical intervention.

Non-surgical treatment

In addition to side-effects of mucositis and xerostomia, major complications of external beam radiotherapy for SCC of the oral cavity and oropharynx include osteoradionecrosis, pathologic fracture, or ulceration of mucous membranes.[133] The risk of osteoradionecrosis necessitates comprehensive dental care prior to the initiation of radiotherapy.[134]

Complications associated with radioactive iodine therapy following total thyroidectomy for differentiated thyroid cancer include self-limited parotitis. High cumulative doses of RAI have been associated with bone-marrow depression and pulmonary fibrosis.

Conclusion

The prognostic significance of cervical metastases from head and neck squamous cell carcinoma necessitates sound management of clinically apparent nodal metastases, as well as thorough screening for detection of occult regional spread. Adequate treatment planning requires recognition of the relevant anatomy as well as ongoing study into our understanding of the biological mechanisms involved. Further study is necessary to complement our armamentarium particularly in managing advanced cervical metastases, where locoregional control rates remain suboptimal.

REFERENCES

1. Shah JP. Cancer of the upper aerodigestive tract. In: Alfonso AE, Gardner B (eds) *The Practice of Cancer Surgery*. New York: Appleton-Century-Crofts, 1982.
2. Robbins KT. Classification of neck dissection: current concepts and future considerations. *Otolaryngol Clin North Am* 1998; **31**: 639–655.
3. Knudson AG, Jr. Hereditary cancer, oncogenes, and antioncogenes. *Cancer Res* 1985; **45**: 1437–1443.
4. Fearon ER, Vogelstein B. A genetic model for colorectal tumorigenesis. Cell 1990; **61**: 759–767.
5. Califano J, van der RP, Westra W et al. Genetic progression model for head and neck cancer: implications for field cancerization. *Cancer Res* 1996; **56**: 2488–2492.
6. Liotta LA. Tumor invasion and metastases: role of the extracellular matrix: Rhoads Memorial Award lecture. *Cancer Res* 1986; **46**: 1–7.
7. Petruzzelli GJ, Benefield J, Yong S. Mechanism of lymph node metastases: current concepts. *Otolaryngol Clin North Am* 1998; **31**: 585–599.
8. Charoenrat P, Modjtahedi H, Rhys-Evans P et al. Epidermal growth factor-like ligands differentially up-regulate matrix metalloproteinase 9 in head and neck squamous carcinoma cells. *Cancer Res* 2000; **60**: 1121–1128.
9. Fisch UP. Cervical lymph flow in man following radiation and surgery. *Trans Am Acad Ophthalmol Otolaryngol* 1965; **69**: 846–868.
10. Mickel RA, Kessler DJ, Taylor JM, Lichtenstein A. Natural killer cell cytotoxicity in the peripheral blood, cervical lymph nodes, and tumor of head and neck cancer patients. *Cancer Res* 1988; **48**: 5017–5022.
11. Wang MB, Lichtenstein A, Mickel RA. Hierarchical immunosuppression of regional lymph nodes in patients with head and neck squamous cell carcinoma. *Otolaryngol Head Neck Surg* 1991; **105**: 517–527.
12. Berlinger NT, Tsakraklides V, Pollak K et al. Prognostic significance of lymph node histology in patients with squamous cell carcinoma of the larynx, pharynx, or oral cavity. *Laryngoscope* 1976; **86**: 792–803.
13. Gilmore BB, Repola DA, Batsakis JG. Carcinoma of the larynx: lymph node reaction patterns. *Laryngoscope* 1978; **88**: 1333–1338.
14. Cernea C, Montenegro F, Castro I et al. Prognostic significance of lymph node reactivity in the control of pathologic negative node squamous cell carcinomas of the oral cavity. *Am J Surg* 1997; **174**: 548–551.
15. Rivoltini L, Gambacorti-Passerini C, Squadrelli-Saraceno M et al. In vivo interleukin 2–induced activation of lymphokine-activated killer cells and tumor cytotoxic T-cells in cervical lymph nodes of patients with head and neck tumors. *Cancer Res* 1990; **50**: 5551–5557.
16. Griffiths CO Jr. Radical neck dissection. Should it be performed with excision of the primary tumor in the presence of clinically uninvolved regional lymph nodes? Effects of regional lymphadenectomy on immunity to simulated new growths in man. *Am J Surg* 1968; **116**: 559–570.
17. Houck JR, Jr., Panje WR, McCormick KJ, Merrick RH. Immunomodulatory activity in regional lymph nodes. *Arch Otolaryngol* 1983; **109**: 785–788.
18. Spiro RH, Huvos AG, Wong GY et al. Predictive value of tumor thickness in squamous carcinoma confined to the tongue and floor of the mouth. *Am J Surg* 1986; **152**: 345–350.
19. Kowalski LP, Medina JE. Nodal metastases: predictive factors. *Otolaryngol Clin North Am* 1998; **31**: 621–637.
20. Lindberg R. Distribution of cervical lymph node metastases from squamous cell carcinoma of the upper respiratory and digestive tracts. *Cancer* 1972; **29**: 1446–1449.
21. Shah JP. Patterns of cervical lymph node metastasis from squamous carcinomas of the upper aerodigestive tract. *Am J Surg* 1990; **160**: 405–409.
22. Byers RM, Weber RS, Andrews T et al. Frequency and therapeutic implications of 'skip metastases' in the neck from squamous carcinoma of the oral tongue [see comments]. *Head Neck* 1997; **19**: 14–19.
23. O'Brien CJ, Traynor SJ, McNeil E et al. The use of clinical criteria alone in the management of the clinically negative neck among patients with squamous cell carcinoma of the oral cavity and oropharynx. *Arch Otolaryngol Head Neck Surg* 2000; **126**: 360–365.
24. Spiro RH, Morgan GJ, Strong EW, Shah JP. Supraomohyoid neck dissection. *Am J Surg* 1996; **172**: 650–653.
25. Medina JE, Byers RM. Supraomohyoid neck dissection: rationale, indications, and surgical technique. *Head Neck* 1989; **11**: 111–122.
26. Woolgar JA. Pathology of the N0 neck. *Br J Oral Maxillofac Surg* 1999; **37**: 205–209.
27. Shah JP. Cervical lymph node metastases: diagnostic, therapeutic, and prognostic implications. *Oncology (Huntingt)* 1990; **4**: 61–69.
28. Hillsamer PJ, Schuller DE, McGhee RB Jr et al. Improving diagnostic accuracy of cervical metastases with computed tomography and magnetic resonance imaging [see comments]. *Arch Otolaryngol Head Neck Surg* 1990; **116**: 1297–1301.
29. Baatenburg De Jong RJ, Rongen RJ, Lameris JS et al. Metastatic neck disease. Palpation vs ultrasound examination. *Arch Otolaryngol Head Neck Surg* 1989; **115**: 689–690.
30. van den Brekel MW, Castelijns JA, Snow GB. Diagnostic evaluation of the neck. *Otolaryngol Clin North Am* 1998; **31**: 601–620.
31. Adams S, Baum RP, Stuckensen T et al. Prospective comparison of 18F-FDG PET with conventional imaging modalities (CT, MRI, US) in lymph node staging of head and neck cancer. *Eur J Nucl Med* 1998; **25**: 1255–1260.
32. Kau RJ, Alexiou C, Laubenbacher C et al. Lymph node detection of head and neck squamous cell carcinomas

by positron emission tomography with fluorodeoxyglucose F 18 in a routine clinical setting. *Arch Otolaryngol Head Neck Surg* 1999; **125**: 1322–1328.
33. McGuirt WF, Williams DW, III, Keyes JW, Jr et al. A comparative diagnostic study of head and neck nodal metastases using positron emission tomography. *Laryngoscope* 1995; **105**:373–375.
34. Bailet JW, Abemayor E, Jabour BA et al. Positron emission tomography: a new, precise imaging modality for detection of primary head and neck tumors and assessment of cervical adenopathy. *Laryngoscope* 1992; **102**: 281–288.
35. Fusion of positron emission tomography (PET) and magnetic resonance imaging (MRI) in head and neck cancer. Paper presentation. 5th International Conference on Head and Neck Cancer. San Francisco. July 2000.
36. Jungehulsing M, Scheidhauer K, Damm M et al. 2[F]-fluoro-2-deoxy-D-glucose positron emission tomography is a sensitive tool for the detection of occult primary cancer (carcinoma of unknown primary syndrome) with head and neck lymph node manifestation. *Otolaryngol Head Neck Surg* 2000; **123**: 294–301.
37. Greven KM, Keyes JW Jr, Williams DW III et al. Occult primary tumors of the head and neck: lack of benefit from positron emission tomography imaging with 2-[F-^{18}]fluoro-2-deoxy-D-glucose. *Cancer* 1999; **86**: 114–118.
38. Bailet JW, Sercarz JA, Abemayor E et al. The use of positron emission tomography for early detection of recurrent head and neck squamous cell carcinoma in postradiotherapy patients. *Laryngoscope* 1995; **105**: 135–139.
39. Farber LA, Benard F, Machtay M et al. Detection of recurrent head and neck squamous cell carcinomas after radiation therapy with 2-18F-fluoro-2-deoxy-D-glucose positron emission tomography. *Laryngoscope* 1999; **109**: 970–975.
40. Berlangieri SU, Brizel DM, Scher RL et al. Pilot study of positron emission tomography in patients with advanced head and neck cancer receiving radiotherapy and chemotherapy. *Head Neck* 1994; **16**: 340–346.
41. Myers LL, Wax MK, Nabi H et al. Positron emission tomography in the evaluation of the N0 neck. *Laryngoscope* 1998; **108**: 232–236.
42. McGuirt WF, Greven K, Williams D III et al. PET scanning in head and neck oncology: a review. *Head Neck* 1998; **20**: 208–215.
43. Keyes JW Jr, Chen MY, Watson NE Jr et al. FDG PET evaluation of head and neck cancer: value of imaging the thorax. *Head Neck* 2000; **22**: 105–110.
44. Muros MA, Llamas-Elvira JM, Ramirez-Navarro A T et al. Utility of fluorine-18–fluorodeoxyglucose positron emission tomography in differentiated thyroid carcinoma with negative radioiodine scans and elevated serum thyroglobulin levels. *Am J Surg* 2000; **179**: 457–461.
45. Shaha A, Webber C, Marti J. Fine-needle aspiration in the diagnosis of cervical lymphadenopathy. *Am J Surg* 1986; **152**: 420–423.
46. Peters BR, Schnadig VJ, Quinn FB Jr et al. Interobserver variability in the interpretation of fine-needle aspiration biopsy of head and neck masses. *Arch Otolaryngol Head Neck Surg* 1989; **115**: 1438–1442.
47. Robbins KT, vanSonnenberg E, Casola G, Varney RR. Image-guided needle biopsy of inaccessible head and neck lesions. *Arch Otolaryngol Head Neck Surg* 1990; **116**: 957–961.
48. Davis SP, Anand VK, Dhillon G. Magnetic resonance navigation for head and neck lesions. *Laryngoscope* 1999; **109**: 862–867.
49. Baatenburg De Jong RJ, Knegt P, Verwoerd CD. Reduction of the number of neck treatments in patients with head and neck cancer. *Cancer* 1993; **71**: 2312–2318.
50. Martin H, Morfit HM, Ehrlich H. The case of branchiogenic cancer (malignant branchioma). *Ann Surg* 1950; **132**: 867–887.
51. Singh B, Balwally AN, Sundaram K et al. Branchial cleft cyst carcinoma: myth or reality? *Ann Otol Rhinol Laryngol* 1998; **107**: 519–524.
52. Mack Y, Parsons JT, Mendenhall WM et al. Squamous cell carcinoma of the head and neck: management after excisional biopsy of a solitary metastatic neck node. *Int J Radiat Oncol Biol Phys* 1993; **25**: 619–622.
53. Ellis ER, Mendenhall WM, Rao PV et al. Incisional or excisional neck-node biopsy before definitive radiotherapy, alone or followed by neck dissection. *Head Neck* 1991; **13**: 177–183.
54. Parsons JT, Million RR, Cassisi NJ. The influence of excisional or incisional biopsy of metastatic neck nodes on the management of head and neck cancer. *Int J Radiat Oncol Biol Phys* 1985; **11**: 1447–1454.
55. Robbins KT, Cole R, Marvel J et al. The violated neck: cervical node biopsy prior to definitive treatment. *Otolaryngol Head Neck Surg* 1986; **94**: 605–610.
56. Ambrosch P, Brinck U. Detection of nodal micrometastases in head and neck cancer by serial sectioning and immunostaining. *Oncology (Huntingt)* 1996; **10**: 1221–1226.
57. Franchi A, Gallo O, Boddi V, Santucci M. Prediction of occult neck metastases in laryngeal carcinoma: role of proliferating cell nuclear antigen, MIB-1, and E-cadherin immunohistochemical determination. *Clin Cancer Res* 1996; **2**: 1801–1808.
58. Gapany M, Pavelic ZP, Kelley DJ et al. Immunohistochemical detection of c-myc protein in head and neck tumors. *Arch Otolaryngol Head Neck Surg* 1994; **120**: 255–259.
59. Cochran AJ, Wen DR, Morton DL. Occult tumor cells in the lymph nodes of patients with pathological stage I malignant melanoma. An immunohistological study. *Am J Surg Pathol* 1988; **12**: 612–618.
60. Wang X, Heller R, VanVoorhis N et al. Detection of submicroscopic lymph node metastases with polymerase chain reaction in patients with malignant melanoma. *Ann Surg* 1994; **220**: 768–774.
61. Shivers SC, Wang X, Li W et al. Molecular staging of malignant melanoma: correlation with clinical outcome. *JAMA* 1998; **280**: 1410–1415.

62. McMasters KM, Reintgen D, Edwards MJ et al. Sunbelt Melanoma Trial (SMT): A multicenter trial of adjuvant interferon alpha-2b for melanoma patients with early lymph node metastasis detected by lymphatic mapping and sentinel lymph node biopsy. Sunbelt Melanoma Trial Operations Manual. 1996. www.sunbeltmelanoma.com.
63. Shaha AR. The unknown primary. In: Lucente FE (ed.) *AAO-HNS Instruction Courses*. St Louis: Mosby-Year Book, 1995; 199–204.
64. Johnson JT, Newman RK. The anatomic location of neck metastasis from occult squamous cell carcinoma. *Otolaryngol Head Neck Surg* 1981; **89**: 54–58.
65. Barrie JR, Knapper WH, Strong EW. Cervical nodal metastases of unknown origin. *Am J Surg* 1970; **120**: 466–470.
66. Spiro RH, DeRose G, Strong EW. Cervical node metastasis of occult origin. *Am J Surg* 1983; **146**: 441–446.
67. Davidson BJ, Spiro RH, Patel S et al. Cervical metastases of occult origin: the impact of combined modality therapy. *Am J Surg* 1994; **168**: 395–399.
68. Randall DA, Johnstone PA, Foss RD, Martin PJ. Tonsillectomy in diagnosis of the unknown primary tumor of the head and neck. *Otolaryngol Head Neck Surg* 2000; **122**: 52–55.
69. Koch WM, Bhatti N, Williams MF, Eisele DW. Oncologic rationale for bilateral tonsillectomy in head and neck squamous cell carcinoma of unknown primary source. *Otolaryngol Head Neck Surg* 2001; **124**: 331–333.
70. American Joint Committee on Cancer. *AJCC Cancer Staging Manual*. 5th edn. New York: Lippincott-Raven, 1997.
71. Snow GB, Annyas AA, van Slooten EA et al. Prognostic factors of neck node metastasis. *Clin Otolaryngol* 1982; **7**: 185–192.
72. Johnson JT, Barnes EL, Myers EN et al. The extracapsular spread of tumors in cervical node metastasis. *Arch Otolaryngol* 1981; **107**: 725–729.
73. Noguchi M, Kido Y, Kubota H et al. Prognostic factors and relative risk for survival in N1–3 oral squamous cell carcinoma: a multivariate analysis using Cox's hazard model. *Br J Oral Maxillofac Surg* 1999; **37**: 433–437.
74. Glanz H, Popella C. Intrinsic weakness of the N/pN classification and proposal of a new pN classification. Presented at the 5th International Conference on Head and Neck Cancer, San Francisco, July 2000.
75. Kowalski LP, Bagietto R, Lara JR et al. Prognostic significance of the distribution of neck node metastasis from oral carcinoma. *Head Neck* 2000; **22**: 207–214.
76. Chelius JM. *A System of Surgery*. Philadelphia: Lea and Blanchard, 1847.
77. Kocher ET. Uber radicalheilung des Krebses. *Deutsche Chir* 1880; **13**: 134–166.
78. Crile GW. Excision of cancer of the head and neck with special reference to the plan of dissection based on one hundred and thirty-two operations. *JAMA* 1906; **47**: 1780–1786.
79. Martin H, DelValle B, Ehrlich H, Cahan WG. Neck dissection. *Cancer* 1951; **4**: 441–499.
80. Schuller DE, Reiches NA, Hamaker RC et al. Analysis of disability resulting from treatment including radical neck dissection or modified neck dissection. *Head Neck Surg* 1983; **6**: 551–558.
81. Robbins KT, Medina JE, Wolfe GT et al. Standardizing neck dissection terminology. Official report of the Academy's Committee for Head and Neck Surgery and Oncology [see comments]. *Arch Otolaryngol Head Neck Surg* 1991; **117**: 601–605.
82. Agrama MT, Reiter D, Topham AK, Keane WM. Node counts in neck dissection: are they useful in outcomes research? *Otolaryngol Head Neck Surg* 2001; **124**: 433–435.
83. Bhattacharyya N. The effects of more conservative neck dissections and radiotherapy on nodal yields from the neck. *Arch Otolaryngol Head Neck Surg* 1998; **124**: 412–416.
84. Busaba NY, Fabian RL. Extent of lymphadenectomy achieved by various modifications of neck dissection: a pathologic analysis. *Laryngoscope* 1999; **109**:212–215.
85. Friedman M, Lim JW, Dickey W et al. Quantification of lymph nodes in selective neck dissection. *Laryngoscope* 1999; **109**: 368–370.
86. Shah JP, Candela FC, Poddar AK. The patterns of cervical lymph node metastases from squamous carcinoma of the oral cavity. *Cancer* 1990; **66**: 109–113.
87. Wang CC. Radiation therapy in the management of oral malignant disease. *Otolaryngol Clin North Am* 1979; **12**: 73–80.
88. Bentzen SM, Thames HD. Tumor volume and local control probability: clinical data and radiobiological interpretations. *Int J Radiat Oncol Biol Phys* 1996; **36**: 247–251.
89. Mothersill C, Seymour CB, O'Brien A, Hennessy T. Proliferation of normal and malignant human epithelial cells post irradiation. *Acta Oncol* 1991; **30**: 851–858.
90. Ravi D, Ramadas K, Mathew BS et al. Apoptosis, angiogenesis and proliferation: trifunctional measure of tumour response to radiotherapy for oral cancer. *Oral Oncol* 2001; **37**: 164–171.
91. Strong EW. Preoperative radiation and radical neck dissection. *Surg Clin North Am* 1969; **49**: 271–276.
92. Kramer S, Gelber RD, Snow JB et al. Combined radiation therapy and surgery in the management of advanced head and neck cancer: final report of study 73-03 of the Radiation Therapy Oncology Group. *Head Neck Surg* 1987; **10**: 19–30.
93. Vikram B, Strong EW, Shah JP, Spiro R. Failure in the neck following multimodality treatment for advanced head and neck cancer. *Head Neck Surg* 1984; **6**: 724–729.
94. Huang DT, Johnson CR, Schmidt-Ullrich R, Grimes M. Postoperative radiotherapy in head and neck carcinoma with extracapsular lymph node extension and/or positive resection margins: a comparative study. *Int J Radiat Oncol Biol Phys* 1992; **23**: 737–742.
95. Coster JR, Foote RL, Olsen KD et al. Cervical nodal metastasis of squamous cell carcinoma of unknown

origin: indications for withholding radiation therapy. *Int J Radiat Oncol Biol Phys* 1992; **23**: 743–749.
96. Colletier PJ, Garden AS, Morrison WH et al. Postoperative radiation for squamous cell carcinoma metastatic to cervical lymph nodes from an unknown primary site: outcomes and patterns of failure. *Head Neck* 1998; **20**: 674–681.
97. Khafif RA, Rafla S, Tepper P et al. Effectiveness of radiotherapy with radical neck dissection in cancers of the head and neck. *Arch Otolaryngol Head Neck Surg* 1991; **117**: 196–199.
98. Adelstein DJ, Saxton JP, Lavertu P et al. A phase III randomized trial comparing concurrent chemotherapy and radiotherapy with radiotherapy alone in resectable stage III and IV squamous cell head and neck cancer: preliminary results. *Head Neck* 1997; **19**: 567–575.
99. Calais G, Alfonsi M, Bardet E et al. Randomized trial of radiation therapy versus concomitant chemotherapy and radiation therapy for advanced-stage oropharynx carcinoma. *J Natl Cancer Inst* 1999; **91**: 2081–2086.
100. Al Sarraf M, LeBlanc M, Giri PG et al. Chemoradiotherapy versus radiotherapy in patients with advanced nasopharyngeal cancer: phase III randomized Intergroup study 0099. *J Clin Oncol* 1998; **16**: 1310–1317.
101. Taylor SG, Murthy AK, Vannetzel JM et al. Randomized comparison of neoadjuvant cisplatin and fluorouracil infusion followed by radiation versus concomitant treatment in advanced head and neck cancer. *J Clin Oncol* 1994; **12**: 385–395.
102. Wang SJ, Wang MB, Calcaterra TC. Radiotherapy followed by neck dissection for small head and neck cancers with advanced cervical metastases. *Ann Otol Rhinol Laryngol* 1999; **108**: 128–131.
103. Koch WM, Lee DJ, Eisele DW et al. Chemoradiotherapy for organ preservation in oral and pharyngeal carcinoma. *Arch Otolaryngol Head Neck Surg* 1995; **121**: 974–980.
104. Lavertu P, Adelstein DJ, Saxton JP et al. Management of the neck in a randomized trial comparing concurrent chemotherapy and radiotherapy with radiotherapy alone in resectable stage III and IV squamous cell head and neck cancer. *Head Neck* 1997; **19**: 559–566.
105. Robbins KT, Wong FS, Kumar P et al. Efficacy of targeted chemoradiation and planned selective neck dissection to control bulky nodal disease in advanced head and neck cancer. *Arch Otolaryngol Head Neck Surg* 1999; **125**: 670–675.
106. Bachaud JM, Cohen-Jonathan E, Alzieu C et al. Combined postoperative radiotherapy and weekly cisplatin infusion for locally advanced head and neck carcinoma: final report of a randomized trial. *Int J Radiat Oncol Biol Phys* 1996; **36**: 999–1004.
107. Weiss MH, Harrison LB, Isaacs RS. Use of decision analysis in planning a management strategy for the stage N0 neck. *Arch Otolaryngol Head Neck Surg* 1994; **120**: 699–702.
108. Andersen PE, Cambronero E, Shaha AR, Shah JP. The extent of neck disease after regional failure during observation of the N0 neck. *Am J Surg* 1996; **172**: 689–691.
109. Vandenbrouck C, Sancho-Garnier H, Chassagne D et al. Elective versus therapeutic radical neck dissection in epidermoid carcinoma of the oral cavity: results of a randomized clinical trial. *Cancer* 1980; **46**: 386–390.
110. Hughes CJ, Gallo O, Spiro RH, Shah JP. Management of occult neck metastases in oral cavity squamous carcinoma. *Am J Surg* 1993; **166**: 380–383.
111. Suarez O. El problema se las metastasis linfticas y alejadas del cancer de laringe e hipofaringe. *Rev Otorhinolaryngol* 1963; **23**: 83–89.
112. Bocca E, Pignataro O. A conservation technique in radical neck dissection. *Ann Otol Rhinol Laryngol* 1967; **76**: 975–987.
113. Spiro JD, Spiro RH, Shah JP et al. Critical assessment of supraomohyoid neck dissection. *Am J Surg* 1988; **156**: 286–289.
114. Byers RM. Modified neck dissection. A study of 967 cases from 1970 to 1980. *Am J Surg* 1985; **150**: 414–421.
115. Davidson BJ, Kulkarny V, Delacure MD, Shah JP. Posterior triangle metastases of squamous cell carcinoma of the upper aerodigestive tract. *Am J Surg* 1993; **166**: 395–398.
116. Koch WM, Choti MA, Civelek AC et al. Gamma probe-directed biopsy of the sentinel node in oral squamous cell carcinoma. *Arch Otolaryngol Head Neck Surg* 1998; **124**: 455–459.
117. Rabuzzi DD, Chung CT, Sagerman RH. Prophylactic neck irradiation. *Arch Otolaryngol* 1980; **106**: 454–455.
118. Mendenhall WM, Million RR, Cassisi NJ. Elective neck irradiation in squamous-cell carcinoma of the head and neck. *Head Neck Surg* 1980; **3**: 15–20.
119. Weissler MC, Weigel MT, Rosenman JG, Silver JR. Treatment of the clinically negative neck in advanced cancer of the head and neck. *Arch Otolaryngol Head Neck Surg* 1989; **115**: 691–694.
120. McGuirt WF. Management of occult metastatic disease from salivary gland neoplasms. *Arch Otolaryngol Head Neck Surg* 1989; **115**: 322–325.
121. Armstrong JG, Harrison LB, Thaler HT et al. The indications for elective treatment of the neck in cancer of the major salivary glands. *Cancer* 1992; **69**: 615–619.
122. Armstrong JG, Harrison LB, Spiro RH et al. Malignant tumors of major salivary gland origin. A matched-pair analysis of the role of combined surgery and postoperative radiotherapy. *Arch Otolaryngol Head Neck Surg* 1990; **116**: 290–293.
123. Douglas JG, Laramore GE, Austin-Seymour M et al. Treatment of locally advanced adenoid cystic carcinoma of the head and neck with neutron radiotherapy. *Int J Radiat Oncol Biol Phys* 2000; **46**: 551–557.
124. Hughes CJ, Shaha AR, Shah JP, Loree TR. Impact of lymph node metastasis in differentiated carcinoma of the thyroid: a matched-pair analysis. *Head Neck* 1996; **18**: 127–132.
125. Balch CM, Soong SJ, Bartolucci AA et al. Efficacy of an elective regional lymph node dissection of 1 to 4 mm

thick melanomas for patients 60 years of age and younger. *Ann Surg* 1996; **224**: 255–263.

126. Balch CM, Cascinelli N, Sim FH et al. Elective lymph node dissection: results of prospective randomized surgical trials. In: Balch CM (ed.) *Cutaneous Oncology.* St. Louis: Quality Medical Publishing, 1998; 209–226.
127. Sim FH, Taylor WF, Ivins JC et al. A prospective randomized study of the efficacy of routine elective lymphadenectomy in management of malignant melanoma. Preliminary results. *Cancer* 1978; **41**: 948–956.
128. Veronesi U, Adamus J, Bandiera DC et al. Inefficacy of immediate node dissection in stage 1 melanoma of the limbs. *N Engl J Med* 1977; **297**: 627–630.
129. Coates AS, Ingvar CI, Petersen-Schaefer K et al. Elective lymph node dissection in patients with primary melanoma of the trunk and limbs treated at the Sydney Melanoma unit from 1960 to 1991. *J Am Coll Surg* 1995; **180**: 402–409.
130. Morton DL, Cagle LA, Wong JH et al. Intraoperative lymphatic mapping and selective lymphadenectomy: technical details of a new procedure for clinical stage I melanoma. Presented at the Annual Meeting of the Society of Surgical Oncology. Washington DC, 1990.
131. Patel SG, Coit DG, Shaha AR et al. Sentinel lymph node biopsy for cutaneous head and neck melanomas. *Arch Otolaryngol Head Neck Surg.* 2002; **128**: 285–291.
132. Ang KK, Peters LJ, Weber RS et al. Postoperative radiotherapy for cutaneous melanoma of the head and neck region. *Int J Radiat Oncol Biol Phys* 1994; **30**: 795–798.
133. Larson DL, Lindberg RD, Lane E, Goepfert H. Major complications of radiotherapy in cancer of the oral cavity and oropharynx. A 10 year retrospective study. *Am J Surg* 1983; **146**: 531–536.
134. Marx RE, Johnson RP. Studies in the radiobiology of osteoradionecrosis and their clinical significance. *Oral Surg Oral Med Oral Pathol* 1987; **64**: 379–390.

PART III

Mainly non-squamous neoplasms

17 Tumours of the upper jaw and anterior skull base

Valerie J Lund

Selected anatomy

The maxillary and anterior ethmoidal sinuses arise as out-pouchings from the lateral nasal wall at an early stage of fetal development. At birth small maxillary, ethmoid and sphenoid sinuses are present. The sphenoid may be regarded as embryologically arising from a posterior ethmoidal cell whilst the frontal sinuses do not begin to develop until some months after birth and should be regarded developmentally as deriving from the anterior ethmoidal system.

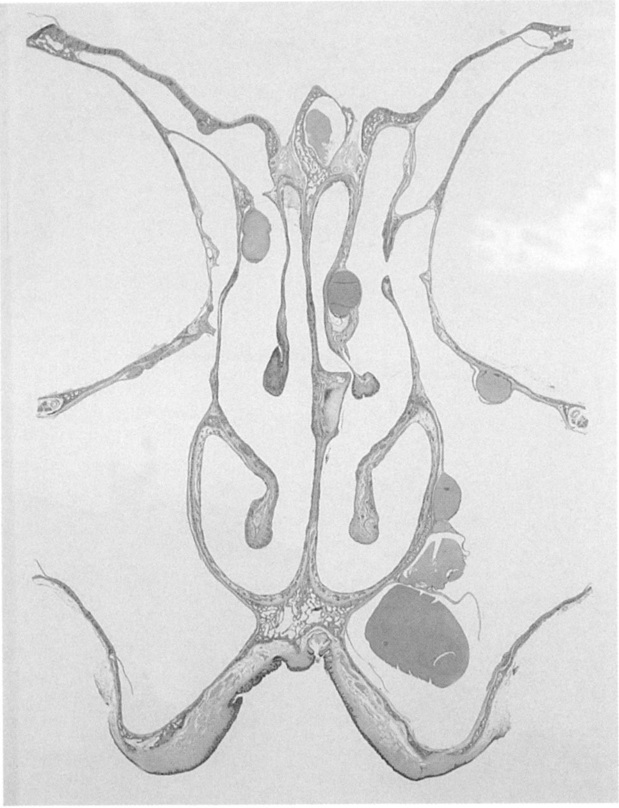

Figure 17.1 A coronal section from midfacial block (haematoxylin and eosin) showing proximity of orbit and anterior cranial fossa to nasal cavity and paranasal sinuses.

The maxillary, frontal and anterior ethmoidal cells drain into the middle meatus. This area together with the middle turbinate, which overlies it, is a frequent site for deposition of carcinogenic particulate matter. The posterior ethmoids drain into the superior meatus whilst the sphenoid sinus drains most posterosuperiorly into the sphenoethmoidal recess.

All the paranasal sinuses have an intimate relationship with the orbit from which they are divided by relatively thin and sometimes dehiscent bone, for example the lamina papyracea, the infraorbital canal, whilst the frontal and ethmoidal sinuses together with the superior nasal cavity are directly related to the anterior cranial fossa (Figure 17.1). Similarly diseases of the sphenoid may spread into the cavernous sinus and middle cranial fossa (and involve the internal carotid artery). Thus, although the lymphatic drainage of the sinuses and nasal cavity is poor, disease may spread directly into adjacent structures with catastrophic results.

Classification

Site

The late presentation of patients often makes it difficult to distinguish the exact origin of sinonasal malignancy. The maxillary sinus is regarded as the commonest site but lesions often arise within the middle meatus, involving the ethmoids, nasal cavity and maxillary antrum from an early stage of the disease. The ICD code 160, which also includes the

Table 17.1 Range of sinonasal neoplasia

	Benign	Malignant
Epithelial		
Epidermoid/Squamous	Papilloma	Carcinoma (spindle cell, verrucous, transitional)
Non-epidermoid	Adenoma	Adenoid cystic carcinoma
	Monomorphic	Adenocarcinoma
	Pleomorphic	Mucoepidermoid carcinoma
	Oncocytoma	Acinic cell carcinoma
		Metastases
Neuroectodermal	Meningioma	Malignant melanoma
		Olfactory neuroblastoma
	Neurofibroma	Neurofibroma
	Glioma	Neuroendocrine carcinoma
		Melanotic neuroectodermal tumour of infancy
Odontogenic tumours	Ameloblastoma	
	Calcifying epithelial odontogenic tumour	
Mesenchymal		
Vascular	Haemangioma	Angiosarcoma
	Capillary	Kaposi's sarcoma
	Cavernous	Haemangiopericytoma
	Angiofibroma	
	Angiomyolipoma	
	Paraganglioma	
	Glomus tumours	
Muscular	Leiomyoma	Leiomyosarcoma
	Rhabdomyoma	Rhabdomyosarcoma
Cartilaginous	Chondroma	Chondrosarcoma (mesenchymal)
	Chondroblastoma	
Osseous	Fibro-osseous lesions	Osteogenic sarcoma
	Fibrous dysplasia	
	Ossifying fibroma	
	Giant cell tumour	
	'Brown' tumour of hyperparathyroidism	
	Osteoma	
	Osteoblastoma	
Lymphoreticular		Burkitt's lymphoma
		Non-Hodgkin's lymphoma
		Extramedullary plasmacytoma
		Midline destructive lesions (T cell lymphoma)
	Chordoma	
	Eosinophilic granuloma	
	Fibroma	Fibrosarcoma
	Lipoma	Liposarcoma
	Myxoma	Malignant fibrous histiocytoma
		Ewing's sarcoma
		Alveolar soft part sarcoma

middle ear, does not separate individual paranasal sinuses though primary malignancy of the frontal and sphenoid sinuses is extremely rare.

Histology

The sinonasal region suffers from the greatest histological diversity in the body and every tumour type, both benign and malignant can be encountered (Table 17.1). Nonetheless, squamous cell carcinoma is the commonest malignancy, as in the rest of the aerodigestive tract and epithelial tumours predominate overall.

Accurate histological diagnosis can prove difficult because of the rarity and diversity of these tumours. The term 'anaplastic' should be treated with caution as when immunohistochemistry is performed these tumours may prove to be poorly differentiated squamous cell carcinoma, an olfactory neuroblastoma, malignant melanoma or lymphoma.

Metastatic spread, the sine qua non of malignancy, is infrequently encountered as patients more often die of local disease before secondary spread is manifest. By contrast the concept of a benign tumour must be re-evaluated in this area due to the proximity of vital structures.

Natural history

General considerations

Presentation

From the maxilla the tumour may spread into the nasal cavity producing nasal obstruction, and discharge that may be blood-stained. Involvement of the infraorbital canal may produce pain and paraesthesia in the distribution of the infraorbital nerve, extension into the soft tissues of the cheek or spread into the orbit (Figure 17.2). This may produce displacement of the globe with proptosis, diplopia, epiphora and chemosis; infiltration of the orbital structures leads to fixation of the globe and visual loss. Extension through the maxillary floor may occur through the dental roots to produce loosening of the teeth and/or a malignant oroantral fistula or erosion of the hard palate producing a mass or ulceration. Posterior extension into the pterygoid and infratemporal fossa may produce pain and trismus (Figure 17.3).

Spread from the ethmoid sinuses will involve the nasal cavity on one or both sides and the orbit with symptoms as before. Superior extension into the anterior cranial fossa is generally silent and not associated with headache, CSF leaks or meningitis (Figure 17.4).

(a)

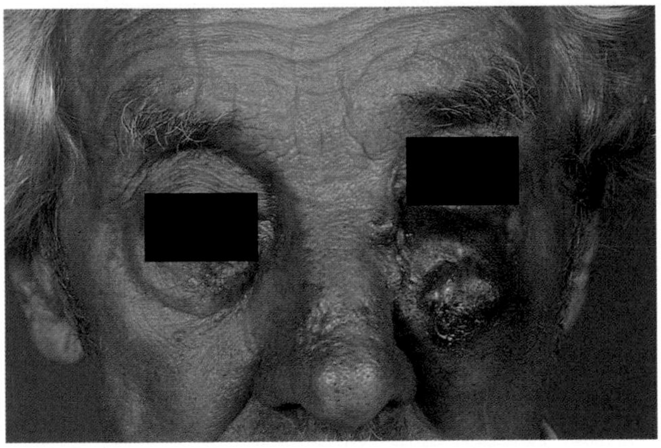

(b)

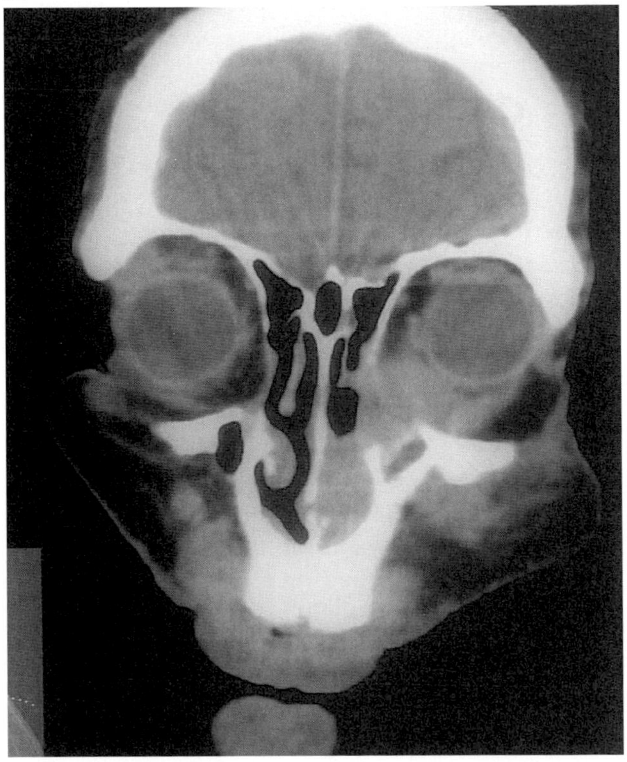

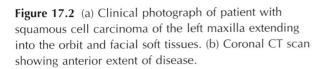

Figure 17.2 (a) Clinical photograph of patient with squamous cell carcinoma of the left maxilla extending into the orbit and facial soft tissues. (b) Coronal CT scan showing anterior extent of disease.

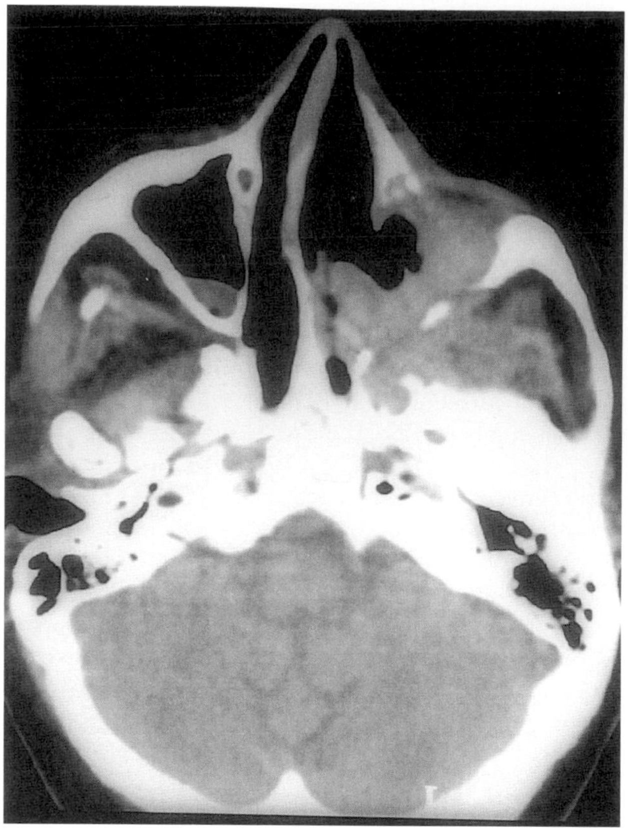

Figure 17.3 Axial CT scan in patient with recurrent squamous cell carcinoma showing infiltration of pterygoid and infratemporal regions.

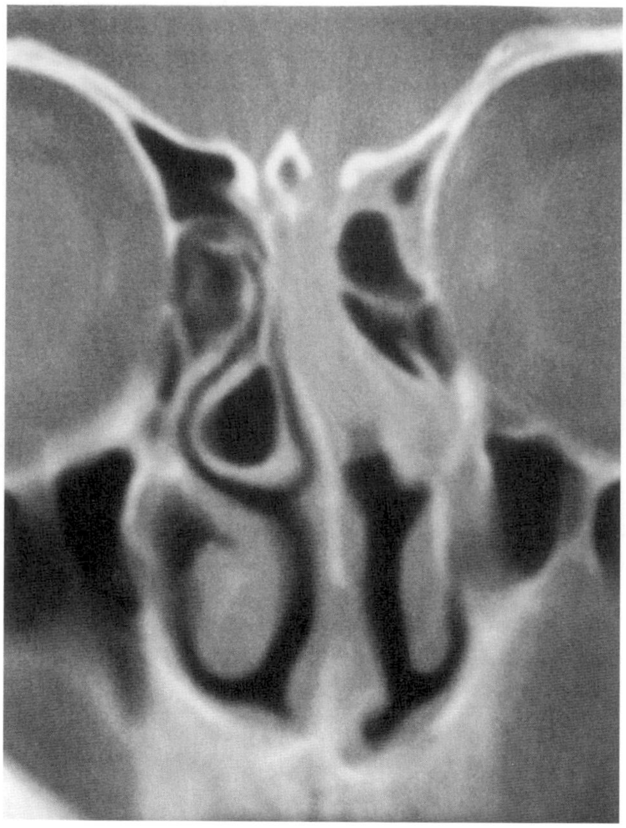

Figure 17.4 Coronal CT scan showing extension of olfactory neuroblastoma into anterior cranial fossa with early erosion of the cribriform niche. By kind permission of Dr GAS Lloyd.

The middle cranial fossa may also be extensively involved at presentation either from the anterior cranial fossa or via the orbital apex (Figure 17.5). Specific cranial nerve palsies may also result from involvement of the cavernous sinus (either via the orbital apex or sphenoid sinus) or from tumour spread through the foramen ovale.

Tumours of the nasal cavity in addition to symptoms of blockage, discharge and occasionally bleeding may obstruct the Eustachian tube producing a serous otitis media, spread around the maxillary spine to affect the hard palate and anteriorly infiltrate, erode and/or splay the nasal bones to produce a mass in the region of the glabella (Figure 17.6).

Epidemiology

A number of occupations have been linked with the development of sinonasal malignancy. In 1968 Acheson et al[1] observed a high frequency of adenocarcinoma of the ethmoids in the woodworkers of the High Wycombe area, which has been subsequently confirmed from many other parts of the world. The association is with hard wood dust exposure, for example mahogany where fine dust of no more than 5 μm diameter is deposited in the middle meatus.[2,3] The relative risk for a woodworker developing adenocarcinoma is 70 times normal. Adenocarcinoma has also been associated with the manufacture of chrome pigment, isopropyl alcohol, textiles, clothing, leather and shoes though many patients with adenocarcinoma have no predisposing factors.[4]

Squamous cell carcinoma has been linked with nickel refining, exposure to soft wood dust and historically with radium dial painting and mustard gas manufacture.[5] Cigarette smoking and alcohol have less impact in this area than elsewhere in the head and neck.

Incidence

Sinonasal malignancy is rare, constituting approximately 3% of head and neck cancer (excluding tumours of the external nose). Global figures suggest an incidence of less than 1 per 100 000 people per year in most countries though occupational factors may produce regional differences.

Sex ratio

The male to female ratio for sinonasal malignancy is approximately 2:1 except where occupational factors impact.

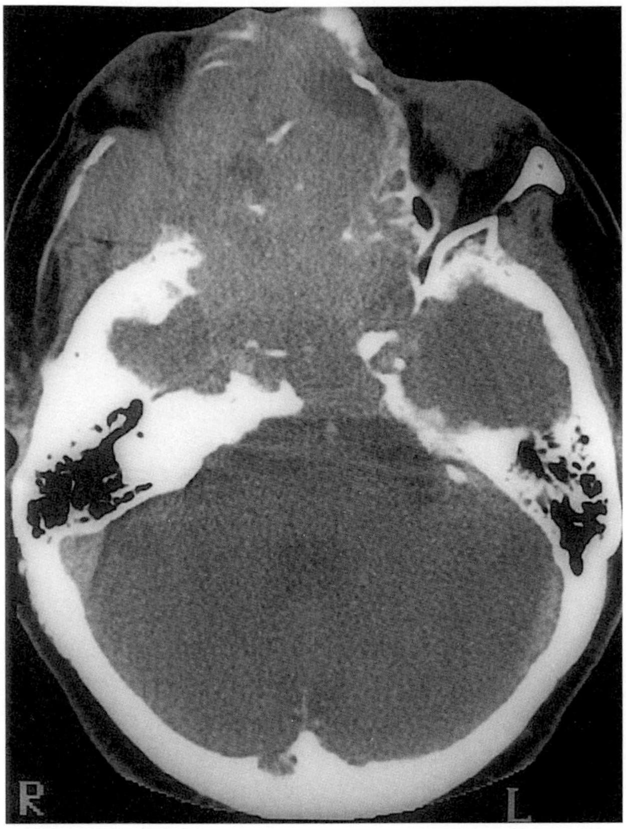

Figure 17.5 Axial CT scan showing extensive poorly differentiated squamous cell carcinoma affecting the anterior and middle cranial fossae.

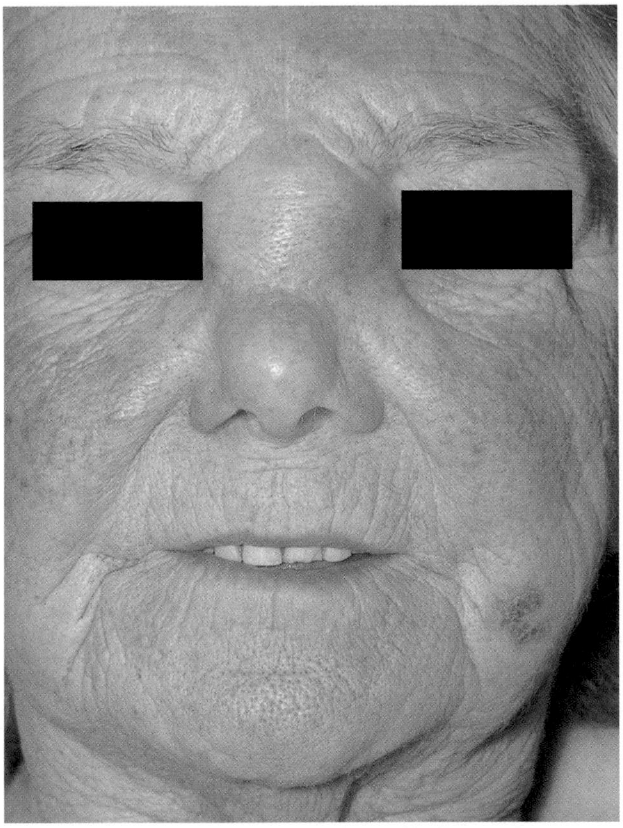

Figure 17.6 Clinical photograph showing infiltration of glabellar region by adenocarcinoma.

Age range

In our own cohort of nearly 600 cases the age range is 5–88 years with the majority presenting between 50 and 69.

Pathophysiology/modes of spread

Sinonasal malignancy impacts most dramatically by local spread into the adjacent structures such as the orbit, skull base, cheek, oral cavity, nasopharynx, pterygoid and infratemporal fossae.

Lymphatic spread

The relatively poor lymphatic drainage of the nose and paranasal sinuses means that cervical lymphadenopathy is relatively uncommon at presentation and is generally less than 10% during the course of the disease depending on the histology. The submandibular and jugulodigastric nodes are most frequently affected, particularly from squamous cell carcinoma of the vestibule and columella where the cervical lymphadenopathy may be bilateral.

Haematological spread

Haematological spread to bone, brain, lung, liver and skin is also uncommon, generally occurring in the later stages of malignancies. (Figures 17.7–17.9). Adenoid cystic carcinoma is well-known for its ability to spread along perineural lymphatics, but may also embolize along adjacent cranial nerves and not infrequently metastases to the lungs.

Prognostic factors

These relate to the extent of disease and histology. A multivariant analysis of 209 patients undergoing craniofacial resection for malignant tumours primarily of the ethmoid and nasal cavity demonstrated infiltration of the brain (as opposed to tumour onto dura) followed by infiltration of the orbit as the worst prognostic factors.[6] From the maxilla, extensions into the pterygoid and infratemporal fossae offer the worst outcome. Tumours of the columella and nasal vestibule also have a poor survival largely due to bilateral lymphatic spread to the submandibular and jugulodigastric nodes at an early stage of disease.

Similarly, although rare, secondary deposits in the bone, brain, lung and liver invariably herald a rapid demise with the exception of adenoid cystic carcinoma where patients may survive up to 7 or 8 years with widespread pulmonary metastases.

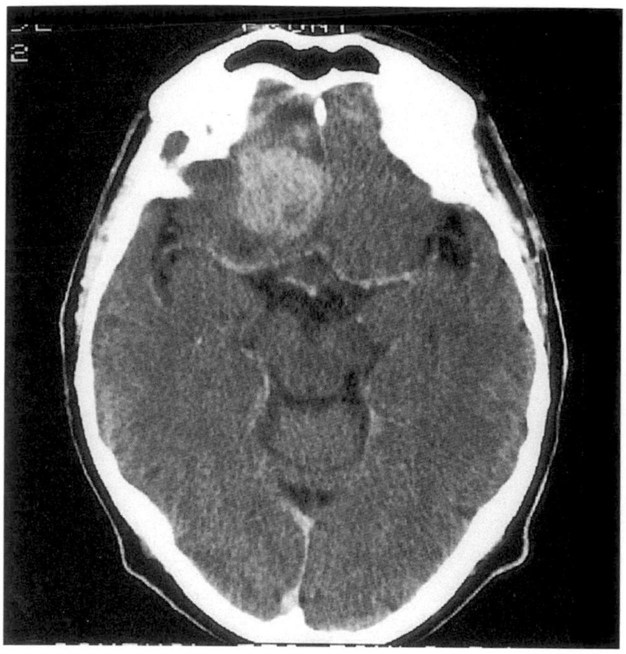

Figure 17.7 Axial CT scan of brain showing secondary deposit in frontal lobe of squamous cell carcinoma.

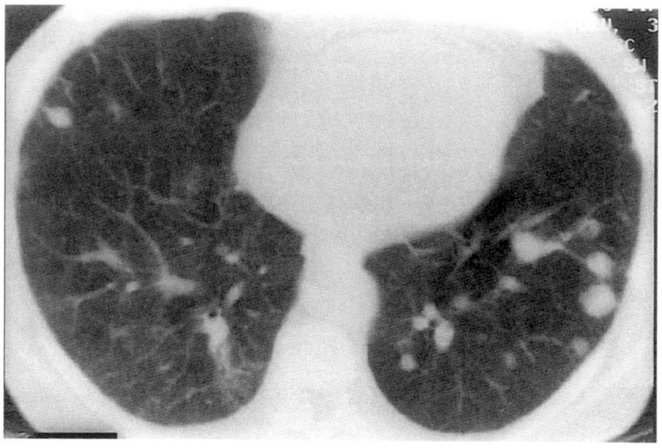

Figure 17.8 Axial CT scan of lung showing multiple deposits from squamous cell carcinoma of the antroethmoid.

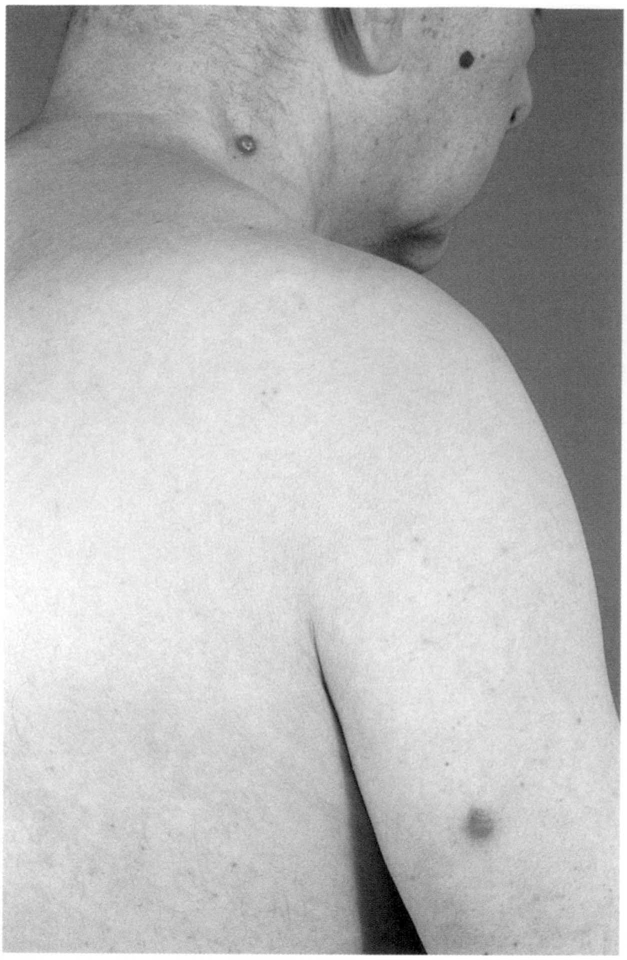

Figure 17.9 Clinical photograph showing skin metastases on neck and upper arm from poorly differentiated squamous cell carcinoma.

Results of treatment/survival

Sinonasal malignancy is rare and the different pathologies behave in very different ways. Consequently it is rather difficult to give an overall view of survival as this will depend upon the composition and size of the cohort and its length of follow-up. Indeed the concept of 'benign' is arguably irrelevant in an area where any progressive disease, for example an extracranial meningioma may result in bilateral blindness and the death of a patient even without the capability of metastatic spread.

In the cohort of 209 patients undergoing craniofacial resection is considered, the overall actuarial survival for the whole group was 51% at 5 years and 41% at 10 years.[6] The actuarial disease-free survival for malignant tumours was 44% at 5 years and 32% at 10 years. This group consisted of 167 individuals, comprising 20 different pathologies. Adenocarcinoma constituted the largest group (42) followed by olfactory neuroblastoma (26), squamous cell carcinoma (25) and chondrosarcoma (19). For benign tumours, actuarial disease-free survival was 75% at both 5 and 10 years (Figure 17.10). This group included 17 different pathologies, of which seven cases were meningioma.[6] Local recurrence usually occurred within the first 2 years, which should be considered to be residual disease though in some individuals disease reappeared many years later, up to 14 years after surgery in one case of olfactory neuroblastoma. Twenty-four patients are known to have died with metastatic disease with or without evidence of local recurrence. The commonest sites were bone (nine cases; brain: eight cases; and cervical lymph nodes: seven cases).

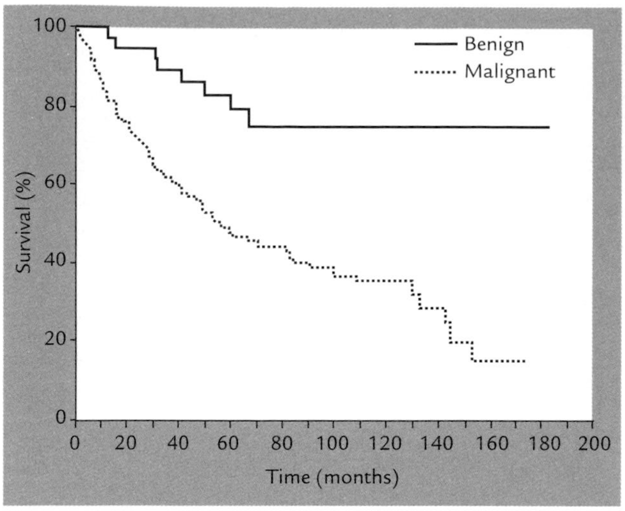

Figure 17.10 Actuarial survival Kaplan-Meier curve in 209 craniofacial patients.[6]

Consideration by histology/subsite

Squamous cell carcinoma of the maxillary sinus

Presentation

The tumour must break out of the maxillary sinus to present with symptoms related to the adjacent nasal cavity, orbit, cheek or pterygopalatine fossa. The most frequent symptoms at first onset are cheek swelling (29%), nasal obstruction (28%) and epistaxis (20%) and there is a reported average delay of 3–6 months before final diagnosis.[7]

Epidemiology

An association has been described with soft wood exposure but it is interesting that in Japan where maxillary sinus carcinoma has an unusually high incidence, there appears to be little relationship with their traditional woodworking industry.[8] Radium dial painting and mustard gas production manifested a high risk with exposure as short as 6 months, but are now happily obsolete. Workers in the sintering and roasting processes in the nickel industry have a risk that increases with age and duration of exposure.[9] Nickel and chromium are found as traces in home-made snuff, which is used in South Africa by the indigenous black population who have a high incidence of advantage antroethmoidal cancer.[10] Exposure to irradiation and the radiological contrast agent, thorium dioxide are also carcinogenic[11] though the relationship with smoking and chronic infection is small if any. The incidence of malignant transformation of inverted papilloma has been greatly overestimated in the literature, largely due to incorrect diagnosis of the initial material. The true incidence of squamous cell carcinoma arising de novo in inverted papilloma is probably of the order of 1–2%.[12]

Incidence

Squamous cell carcinoma is the commonest of sinonasal histologies, comprising over 60% of most series though this will vary depending upon the interests of the unit concerned. An incidence of 1/100 000 population per year is quoted for the United Kingdom, but 2.6/100 000 for men in Japan, Nigeria and Jamaica.

Sex ratio and age range

The sex ratio for squamous cell carcinoma is 1.7:1 male to female, while the age range is 19–90 years, with an average of 60 years.

Pathophysiology/modes of spread

The tumour makes use of areas of natural weakness such as the inferior orbital fissure or ethmoid labyrinth and early diagnosis with the tumour still confined within the maxilla is rare. Dura and orbital periosteum will resist disease for some time but once breached, there is rapid infiltration of the brain and orbit. Extension into the nasopharynx is occasionally associated with spread up the Eustachian tubes, with tumour presenting in the middle ear cavity. Cervical lymphadenopathy is present in approximately 10% of patients at initial presentation. Distant metastases are uncommon at presentation though may be found at autopsy in the lungs, liver and bone.

Prognostic factors

Some authors have tried to link prognosis to the degree of differentiation.[13,14] However, local spread into the orbital structures, frontal lobes and pterygopalatine fossa and the presence of systemic metastases are of much greater prognostic significance.

Several sub-groups of squamous cell carcinoma have been described. Verrucous carcinoma is a slow growing squamous cell carcinoma that is locally aggressive but rarely metastasizes. Anaplastic carcinoma may be a poorly differentiated squamous cell carcinoma but must be differentiated from other small cell tumours such as olfactory neuroblastoma and lymphoma. Spindle cell carcinoma or carcinosarcoma should be regarded as an aggressive squamous cell carcinoma. Transitional or cylindric cell carcinoma should be regarded as a poorly differentiated non-keratinizing squamous cell carcinoma.

Results of treatment/survival

Combined radiotherapy and surgery have remained the gold standard with 5-year survival rates of between 35% and 48%.[15–17] Most recurrences occur within 2 years and local recurrence is the prime cause of death. Radiotherapy may be given before or after surgery and the surgery varies from partial maxillectomy to total or radical maxillectomy with orbital clearance or craniofacial resection.

Results in excess of 50% have been claimed for topical 5-fluorouracil applied via a palatal fenestration and combined with repeated debulking in Japan and Holland[18,19] though results have not been reported from other departments.

Adenocarcinoma

Presentation

Nasal obstruction, discharge, unilateral epistaxis, pain, epiphora and other orbital symptoms are common (Figure 17.11) and occasionally it presents as a midline glabellar mass with involvement of the frontal bone (Figure 17.6).

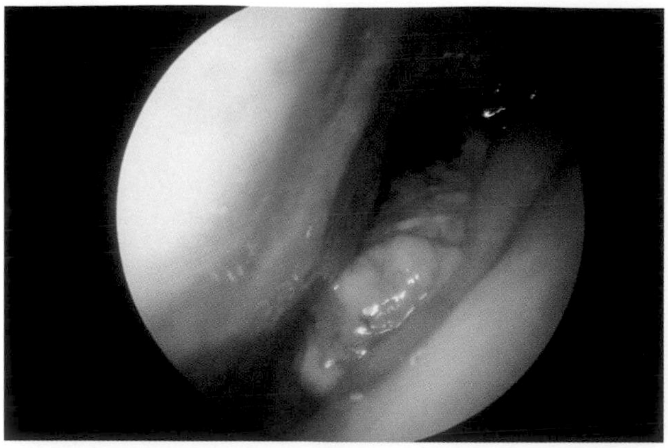

Figure 17.11 Endoscopic photograph of adenocarcinoma in left middle meatus.

Epidemiology

Incidence, sex ratio and age range

There is an incidence of 4–12% of sinonasal malignancies.[20] The sex ratio is 4:1 male to female, and increasing to 11:1 in the older age group, which reflects longer previous carcinogenic exposure. There is an age range of 9–90 years, with an average of 50–60 years with higher grade tumours presenting in slightly older patients.[21]

Pathophysiology/modes of spread

The tumour generally arises within the middle meatus spreading into the orbit, to the contralateral ethmoid and through the anterior skull base at an early stage. The nasopharynx may be involved by spread from the sphenoethmoidal recess. Cervical metastases are clinically palpable in 2–3% of cases at presentation.

Prognostic factors

Improved prognosis is said to occur with low-grade adenocarcinomas[21] though disputed by others.[22] Sex, age, site, size, histological type and the presence of cervical metastases have also been cited as prognostic factors. The worst prognostic factor in our own group of 60 patients is frontal lobe infiltration with no survivors beyond 12 months.

Results of treatment/survival

Craniofacial resection (ususally combined with radiotherapy) offers optimum long-term survival. In the past the majority of cases were managed by a radical maxillectomy or extended lateral rhinotomy frequently with sacrifice of the eye. The advent of the combined craniofacial approach has enabled an oncologic clearance with access to the anterior cranial fossa and orbit is of particular advantage in the management of ethmoidal adenocarcinoma. In a cohort of 42 patients treated by craniofacial resection, actuarial survival at 5 years was 43% and at 10 years 38%.[6] Of our craniofacial patients who died, 50% had local disease but a similar number developed distant metastases to lung, bone and brain, which may be the result of improved local control afforded by the craniofacial resection, as distant metastases are rarely reported in non-craniofacial cohorts (Figure 17.12).

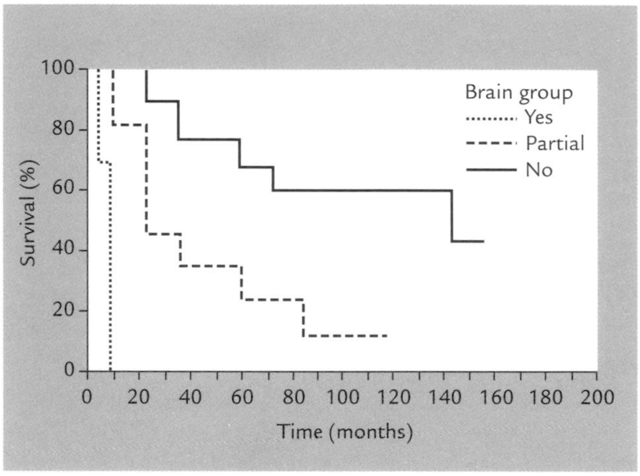

Figure 17.12 Actuarial survival Kaplan–Meier curve for patients with adenocarcinoma treated with craniofacial resection.

Adenoid cystic carcinoma

Presentation

Adenoid cystic carcinoma presents as nasal obstruction, rhinorrhoea and epistaxis. Facial pain, tingling and paraesthesia occur affecting the infraorbital division of the trigeminal nerve.[23] Orbital involvement includes proptosis and diplopia. A palpable mass may be found in the medial canthal region or on hard palate.

Incidence, sex ratio and age range

Adenoid cystic carcinoma has an incidence of 1.3% of all sinonasal tumours.[24] The sex ratio is 2:1 male to female[25] and the age ranges between 12 and 84 years with the majority occurring in the fourth to sixth decades.

Pathophysiology/modes of spread

The maxilla and hard palate are the commonest sites in the sinonasal region with spread to involve the orbit and nasolacrimal region in up to two-thirds of cases.[26] Early spread occurs by perineural infiltration along cranial nerves and there is frequent haematogenous dissemination particularly to lungs. As a consequence local 'recurrence' is the rule rather than the exception and complete local excision is rarely possible. However, pulmonary metastases do not necessarily imply a rapid demise with patients living up to 7 or 8 years. By contrast, cervical lymphadenopathy is relatively rare. The true incidence of systemic metastases varies from 20% to 50%, which may manifest up to 15–22 years after initial presentation. Consequently, 5-year survival figures are rendered meaningless.

Prognostic factors

There is no agreement on the prognostic importance of size, site, patient age, symptoms or histological classification. However, of the three histological types: tubular, cribriform and solid, solid is said by some authors to be the more aggressive.[24] Whilst two-thirds of patients are alive in most series at 5 years, this falls to 10% or less at 20 years, suggesting that the majority of patients will die of the disease if followed for long enough.[20]

Results of treatment/survival

Radical primary surgery combined with radiotherapy is rarely curative but will reduce the number and speed of local recurrence. As complete extirpation of all adjacent cranial nerves is impracticable, the patient should be offered the most radical operation, which also combines an acceptable morbidity, for example a craniofacial resection or total maxillectomy with or without orbital clearance or in the case of a localized lesion on the palate, a subtotal maxillectomy preserving the orbital floor. Neck dissection is rarely indicated.

In a cohort of 15 patients undergoing craniofacial resection 5-year actuarial survival was 51% and 10-year actuarial survival 36%.[6]

Pulmonary metastases have been managed by wedge resection or lobectomy in selected cases and the presence of pulmonary metastases does not preclude local surgery. Chemotherapy has no part to play either for cure or palliation. Carbamazepine may be used to control the associated neuralgia from perineural involvement.

Olfactory neuroblastoma

Presentation

Olfactory neuroblastoma has a non-specific presentation: nasal obstruction, epistaxis and hyposmia. The tumour is generally slow growing with 24% of patients having symptoms for longer than 1 year.[27]

Epidemiology

Experimental work with the Syrian hamster has produced olfactory neuroblastoma-type tumours with diethyl-nitrosamine.[28]

Incidence, sex ratio and age range

Approximately 5% of all sinonasal tumours are olfactory neuroblastomas with a slight male preponderance. A bimodal age distribution is seen with peaks in the second and third decades and later in the sixth and seventh decades.

Pathophysiology/modes of spread

The tumour arises almost exclusively in the superior nasal cavity corresponding to the anatomical distribution of the olfactory epithelium. Early spread occurs along olfactory fibrils to involve the olfactory bulbs and tracts as confirmed by craniofacial resection.[29]

Prognostic factors

The natural history of this malignancy is both variable and unpredictable. The anatomical location may make wide field resection on occasions impossible. The tumour can offer a range of local aggression, and the possibility of cervical lymphadenopathy and blood dissemination. Extent of disease has been classified into stages I–III[30] but prognosis does not correlate with histological appearances.[31]

Results of treatment/survival

The natural site of occurrence of the tumour makes it ideal for craniofacial resection. Several studies have demonstrated improved survival with craniofacial resection and radiotherapy as compared to extracranial resection and radiotherapy.[32,33] Most recent studies have suggested that craniofacial

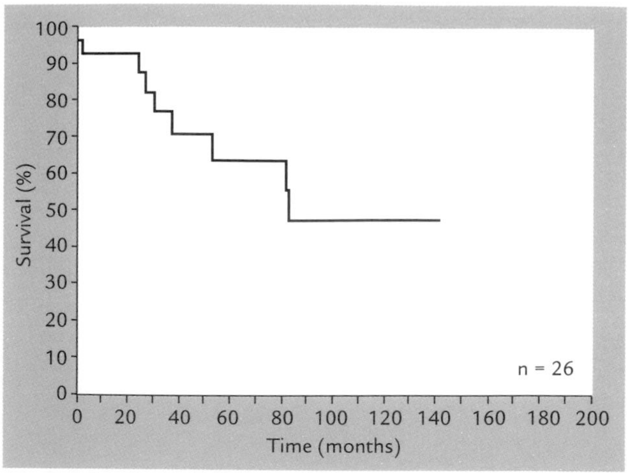

Figure 17.13 Acturial survival Kaplan–Meier curve for a olfactory neuroblastoma treated by craniofacial resection.

resection without radiotherapy for stages I and II produces satisfactory results (Figure 17.13).[34]

In a cohort of 26 patients treated by craniofacial resection (with radiotherapy for stage III disease) the 5-year actuarial survival rate was 62% and that at 10 years 47%.[6] It should be noted that local recurrence may occur after a 14-year disease-free interval.

Chemotherapy (cyclophosamide, vincristine, cisplatinum and 5-fluorouracil) has been advocated for extensive local disease and/or secondary spread.[32,35]

Malignant melanoma

Presentation

Unilateral nasal obstruction (46%), epistaxis (19%), a combination of the two (23%) or a visible mass (6%) are the common findings.[36] Lesions on the palate produce a lump that often ulcerates and bleeds.

Epidemiology

Melanocytes are derivations of neural crest and are found throughout the nasal and oral mucosa. Experimental studies have suggested that exposure to formaldehyde may increase cutaneous melanoma and in a cohort of 50 surviving patients, three had had extensive exposure to formaldehyde.[37]

Incidence

Between 15 and 20% of all malignant melanomas arise in the head and neck but the vast majority of these are cutaneous and only 0.5–2% affect the mucous membranes, and of these, the majority occur in the oral cavity. Malignant melanoma affecting the nasal cavity accounts for less than 1% of all malignant melanomas and 3% of all sinonasal neoplasia in our own cohort.

Sex ratio and age range

The ratio of men to women is roughly equal with a slight male preponderance. The age ranges from 16 to 90 years with the majority presenting in the sixth to seventh decades, maximally between 60 and 69 years.

Pathophysiology/modes of spread

The commonest site of origin is from the lateral wall particularly from the inferior and middle turbinates followed by the nasal septum. The tumour spreads along mucosal planes, is capable of producing satellite lesions but tends not to destroy adjacent cartilage or bone extensively in the early stages.

Between 10% and 18% of patients will present with cervical lymphadenopathy and 4% with lung metastases.[36] Local recurrence, cervical lymphadenopathy and metastatic disease can occur at any time with systemic metastases in the lung, liver, brain and skin usually present at the time of death from disease.

Prognostic factor

The patients live in an interesting immunological balance with the tumour that may be upset by other factors such as a viral infection. Thus some patients succumb very rapidly to overwhelming disease whereas others may live for long periods of time with local or even systemic disease that may be resected many times.

The age, sex, degree of pigmentation and mitotic activity do not directly correlate with prognosis[36] and unlike skin melanoma, correlation of depth of invasion and junction activity with outcome does not apply to mucosal disease.[38]

Results of treatment/survival

Despite the relative lack of radiosensitivity, some of the longest survivors are those receiving local surgical clearance and radiotherapy. The surgical approach of choice has been the lateral rhinotomy, which is a quick procedure in elderly patients with a low morbidity, offering good access to the common sites of origin of the disease. The incisions for a midfacial degloving are often not ideal and a craniofacial resection is contraindicated as it seems to remove the bony barrier to local intracranial spread. Localized disease, particularly recurrence, may be excised by an endonasal endoscopic approach though the surgeon should be aware of the

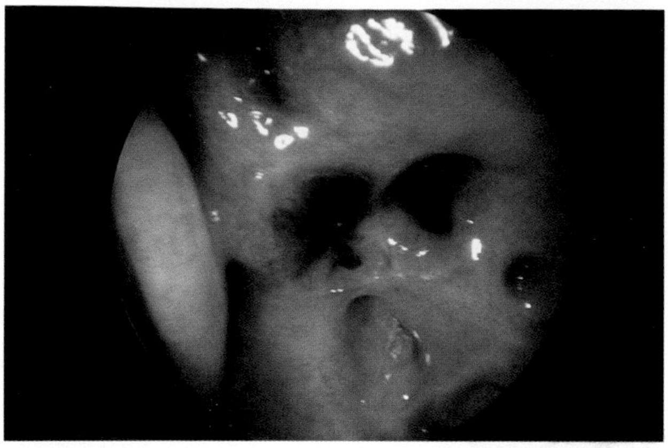

Figure 17.14 Endoscopic photograph showing recurrent malignant melanoma in posterior nasal cavity adjacent to middle turbinate.

possibility of amelanotic disease and satellite lesions (Figure 17.14). A coagulating laser such as the argon or KTP may be useful for recurrences that produce epistaxis.

Radiotherapy is now given postoperatively in all cases unless precluded by dissemination of disease or general health of the patient.

The overall prognosis is poor with more than 50% dead within 3 years and 66% dead within 5 years. Five-year survival rates of 6–31% have been quoted in the literature but again the natural history of the disease makes 5-year survival meaningless and the patient is constantly at risk of death from this condition. Palatal lesions have an even worse prognosis with the majority of patients dead within 1–2 years from presentation. At present the use of palliative interleukins, interferon and other chemotherapy are of unproven benefit in mucosal melanoma.

Staging

Although the TNM classification has been applied to sinonasal malignancy, most tumours are T4 at presention and a tumour infiltrating the skull base will inevitably have a different prognosis from one arising in the anterior floor of the maxillary sinus. The relatively low incidence of metastatic spread also limits the usefulness of the conventional TNM classification. More meaningful approaches have based classification on spread of disease[39–42] but none of these classifications takes into account information derived from modern imaging or the prognostic impact of improved oncologic resection by a craniofacial approach (Table 17.2).

Table 17.2 TNM classification systems

Lederman et al[11]	
T1	Tumour to one sinus or a tissue of origin (e.g. turbinate, septum, vestibule)
T2	Tumour limited in horizontal spread to the same region, or to adjacent vertically related regions
T3a	Tumour involving three regions, with or withour orbital involvement
T3b	Extension of the tumour beyond the upper jaw (e.g. nasopharynx, cranial cavity, pterygopalatine fossa)
Harrison[12]	
T1	Tumour limited to the antral mucosa, with no evidence of bone erosion
T2	Bony erosion without evidence of involvement of the skin, pterygopalatine fossa or ethmoidal labyrinth
T3	Bony erosion with involvement of the skin and ethmoidal labyrinth
T4	Tumour extension to the nasopharynx, sphenoid sinus, cribriform plate or pterygopalatine fossa
AJC[13] (based on Sisson[14])	
T1	Tumour confined to the antral mucosa of the infrastructure without bone erosion
T2	Tumour confined to the suprastructure and mucosa without bone destruction, or to the infrastructure with destruction of medial or inferior bony walls only
T3	Massive tumour, invading the skin of the cheek, the orbit, the posterior ethmoids, sphenoid sinus, nasopharynx, pterygoid plates or base of skull

Investigations

General guidelines

Although sinonasal malignancy is rare, persistent nasal symptoms should always be investigated particularly if unilateral. Endoscopic examination of the nose may facilitate early detection of neoplasia. Care should be taken to adequately decongest the nose and an attempt should always be made to examine beyond a septal deflection. All tissue removed during routine sinonasal procedures, for example polypectomy should be submitted for histology.

Diagnostic investigation

Adequate and representative tissue must be obtained for expert histological opinion. This is

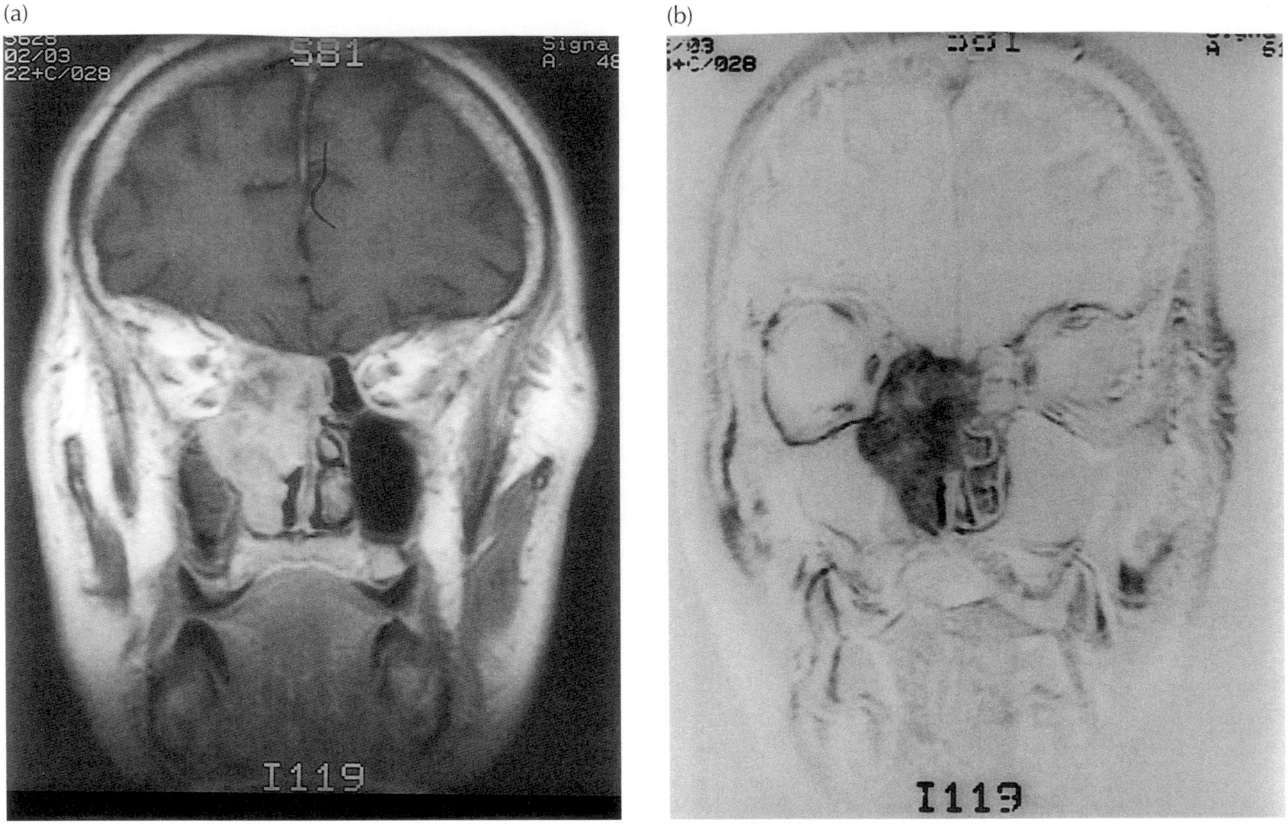

Figure 17.15 (a) Coronal MRI (T1-weighted gadolinium-DTPA) showing adenocarcinoma of the right ethmoid. (b) Same view after subtraction of T1 sequences with and without gadolinium-DTPA to define the localization of tumour.

best performed under a general anaesthetic and with the use of endoscopic techniques, it is rarely if ever necessary to transgress normal tissue planes by a sublabial or external incision. When lymphoma is suspected, fresh tissue may be required. A diagnosis of 'anaplastic' carcinoma should always be queried and tissue sent for immunohistochemistry.

Haematological investigations may be appropriate, for example HIV test for Kaposi's sarcoma or lymphoma; blood films for chloroma (granulocytic sarcoma); ANCA, ACE, ESR etc. in the differential diagnosis of midline destructive lesions such as Wegener's granulomatosis or sarcoidosis.

Localizing investigations

A combination of CT and MRI provides an accuracy of 98%[43] in determining extent of disease. Direct coronal and axial CT with contrast enhancement demonstrates bone detail and best detects early cribriform plate erosion. Magnetic resonance imaging (3 planar sections with gadolinium-DTPA) allows soft tissue differentiation between tumour, inflammation, mucus retention and fibrosis.[43]

Tumour definition may be enhanced by subtraction GdMR,[44] fat suppression and free even echo rephasing (FEER) 'angiography' (Figure 17.15).

Treatment policy

General guidelines

There are three main objectives of the treatment of sinonasal malignancy:

1. Curative resection of the tumour;
2. Reconstruction and rehabilitation;
3. Where cure cannot be achieved, a genuine attempt at palliation.

Specific guidelines: General principles of results of treatment/survival

Surgery
In choosing the correct therapeutic modality it is important to understand the natural history of each individual histology. Whilst an endonasal endoscopic approach may be possible for localized

benign lesions, it is clear that this would be inappropriate for the vast majority of malignant tumours due to the extent, site and spread of the tumour. At present one should be extremely cautious in assessing the value of a technique based on anecdotal cases with short-term follow-up. In the largest published series of malignant tumours treated endoscopically, Neubauer et al[45] emphasized the need for more radical approaches if the orbit or skull base were transgressed. However, the benefits of the rigid endoscope in the diagnosis, biopsy and long-term follow-up of patients with sinonasal malignancy is self-evident.

The vast majority of patients therefore undergo some form of surgical excision be it lateral rhinotomy (and medial maxillectomy), midfacial degloving, some form of partial or total maxillectomy, total rhinectomy, or craniofacial resection with or without orbital clearance.

The lateral rhinotomy approach, attributed to Moure in 1902[46] but described as early as 1848, gives excellent access to the nasal cavity, the entire frontoethmosphenoidal complex and medial maxilla. Limiting the superior extent of the incision to the medial canthus and careful repair of the alar margin diminishes the cosmetic problems that originally limited its popularity. It is still the approach of choice for malignant melanoma but has been superseded in many other circumstances by midfacial degloving, which offers greater bilateral access and avoids all external scars. This combines bilateral sublabial incisions with elevation of the soft tissues of the mid-third of the face via intercartilaginous incisions. Its only limitations are the time taken for careful closure to avoid vestibular stenosis and oroantral fistula and limited access to the frontal sinus. It is the procedure of choice for young patients, those with extensive benign neoplasia and for malignancy of the nasal cavity and upper jaw where the skull base has not been compromised. It was popularized by Price et al[47] and in a series of over 70 patients we have experienced minimal long-term morbidity.[48] It may of course be combined with a bicoronal incision for access to the anterior skull base.[49] The Weber–Fergusson incision is now rarely employed except in those older patients with malignancy of the upper jaw requiring conventional radical maxillectomy with or without orbital clearance and for procedures such as the maxillary swing designed for access to the nasopharynx.[50]

The craniofacial resection is now utilized for all malignant tumours that involve the anterior skull base, which allows an oncologic resection of lesions. This was hitherto impossible and was previously managed by total maxillectomy and orbital clearance. The craniofacial operation was originally described in 1954[51] and was subsequently developed by Ketcham et al[52] and Terz et al[53] and more recently by Cheeseman and others.[54] It is well recognized that the poor prognosis associated with malignant tumours of the nose and paranasal sinuses is largely a consequence of local recurrence or rather residual disease in the region of the skull base. A combined approach offers an oncologic resection with minimal morbidity and excellent cosmesis. Present experience indicates that a combination of radiotherapy and radical surgery offers the best prognosis for radiosensitive tumours with radical resection optimally performed 6 weeks following radiotherapy irrespective of response. The craniofacial resection also enables careful assessment of any extension of disease from the ethmoids into the orbit using frozen section evaluation of orbital periosteum. As a consequence of this, a proportion of eyes have been salvaged. If the orbital periosteum has been penetrated by disease, orbital clearance is performed, usually with preservation of the skin and orbicularis muscle which results in a skin-lined socket into which a prosthesis may be placed at a later date.

The craniofacial operation utilizes an extended lateral rhinotomy incision (or midfacial degloving with bicoronal incision) and provides access to the anterior cranial fossa via a shield-shaped window craniotomy, which can be replaced at the end of the procedure. Through the craniotomy, the frontal lobes and overlying dura are retracted as dissection of the dura is carried out on a wide front progressing posteriorly onto the smooth bone of the jugum sphenoidale, exposing cribriform plate, ethmoid and orbital roofs. An en bloc removal of both ethmoid complexes and cribriform plate together with the perpendicular plate of the ethmoid can then be performed with additional resection of adjacent structures as appropriate. In cases where the medial bony wall of the orbit has been breached but the periosteum is intact, the compromised area of periosteum may be resected and grafted using a split skin graft with preservation of the globe and its musculature. Similarly dura may be resected and repaired with fascia lata to which a thin fenestrated split skin graft is applied. As for other radical sinus surgery, the surgical cavity is packed with ribbon gauze soaked in Whitehead's varnish (compound iodoform paint: iodoform benzoin, prepared storax, tolu balsam and solvent ether) which is removed under a short general anaesthetic at 10 days. The standard closure can be modified using local flaps and bone grafts if required following excision of extensive anteriorly-placed disease. The incision heals remarkably well (Figure 17.16) and the patients can be followed-up with regular examination under anaesthesia combined with subtraction GdMRI (Figure 17.17).

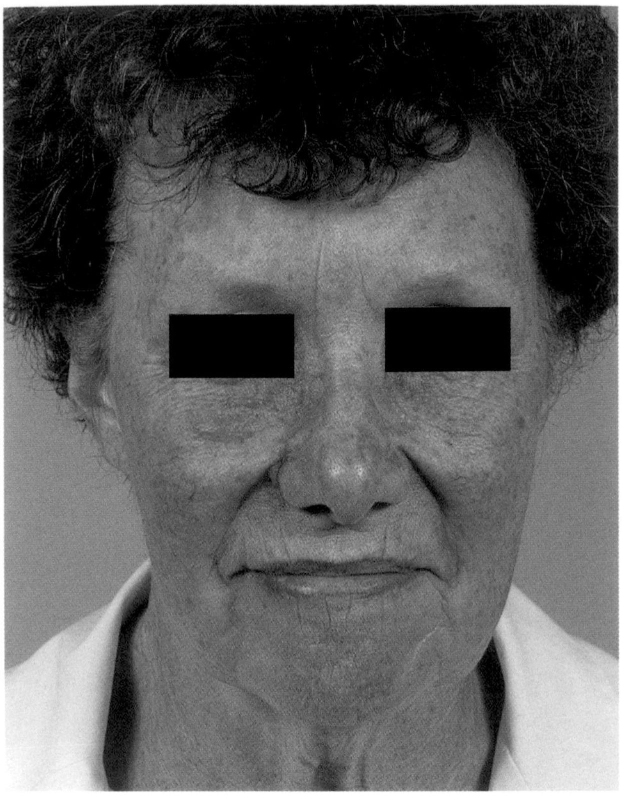

Figure 17.16 Clinical photograph of a patient showing extended lateral rhinotomy incision two years after craniofacial resection.

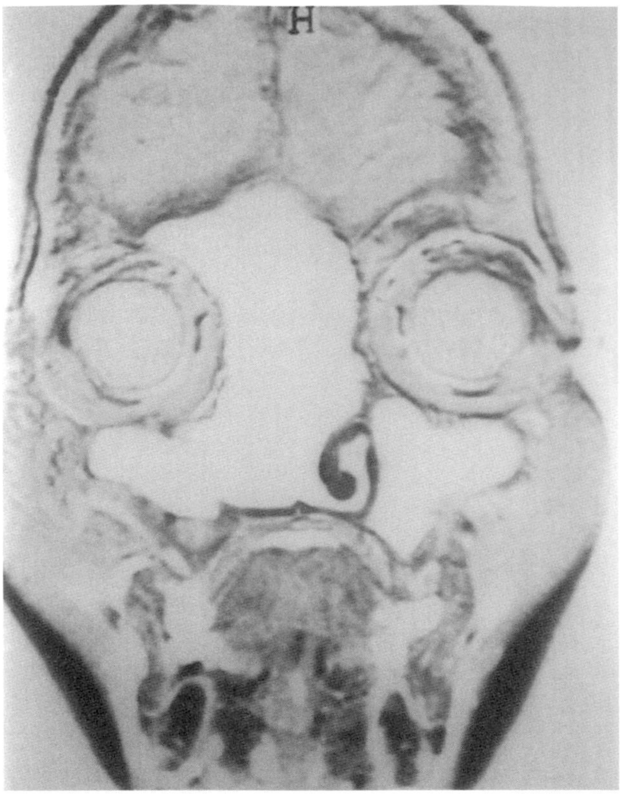

Figure 17.17 Coronal substraction MRI showing craniofacial cavity in patient with previous squamous cell carcinoma of the right antroethmoid region.

Rhinectomy is occasionally required for extensive nasal tumours and the resulting defect is most conveniently repaired with a prosthesis which may be held in place by spectacles and tissue adhesive or osseointegrated implants.

Radiotherapy

External beam radiotherapy has been used generally in combination with surgery for squamous cell carcinoma and other radiosensitive tumours.[55] Care is taken to protect the orbit, brain and pituitary fossa whilst delivering an optimum therapeutic dose of approximately 60 Gy. This is important to avoid radiation-induced cataracts, keratosis or retinal changes. Three-field external beam treatment is generally used.

Occasionally implants of radioactive gold or iodine have been used in the treatment of inoperable recurrent adenoid cystic carcinoma of the skull base, as has afterloading with irridium-192 for recurrence in the nasopharynx.

Chemotherapy

Of the three oncologic modalities, surgery, radiotherapy and chemotherapy, chemotherapy has proved least useful in the treatment of sinonasal malignancies with the exception of mesenchymal tumours such as embryonal rhabdomyosarcoma and lymphoma. In the presence of extensive poorly differentiated squamous cell carcinoma (Figure 17.5) palliative chemotherapy has been given with some good effect with a reasonable tumour response for anything up to 18 months to 2 years. Marked tumour regression has also been produced with high dose intra-arterial cis-platinum combined with intravenous sodium thiosulphate as a neutralizing agent in some selected extensive squamous cell carcinoma lesions[56] but there is no evidence that adjuvant chemotherapy has any significant effect. Remarkably good results have been published for the use of topical 5-fluorouracil in sinus cavities after surgical debulking for squamous cell carcinoma of the maxilla[18,19] though they have not been reproduced from other centres.

Specific guidelines: reconstruction and rehabilitation

Whilst the clinician's primary goal is curative eradication of the malignancy this should not be at the expense of the patient's appearance and function. Any disability consequent on major sinonasal surgery is immediately apparent and difficult to hide. In a study designed to assess perception of relative severity of 11 common facial disfigurements resulting from surgery, orbital exenteration and radical maxillectomy scored highest with rhinectomy only outweighed by mandibulectomy.[57] In a recent study using a modified EORTC questionnaire a series of 49 patients who had undergone ablative surgery for a head and neck malignancy during the preceding 2 years were studied. This included 11 craniofacial patients who reported significant problems with vision, smell, taste and headaches. High levels of fatigue were reported by this group,[58] which has also been described in other studies[59] and could represent a somatic manifestation of psychological distress.

Patients undergoing radical maxillectomy require close liaison with an expert maxillofacial prosthedontist. The patient must be assessed preoperatively to obtain dental impressions and modify existing dentures so that a temporary obturator may be placed in the surgical cavity at the end of the procedure. This can be done using gutta percha moulded to the self-retaining preprepared denture base.[60] This will allow relatively normal speech and nutrition in the immediate postoperative period. A permanent hard acrylic or soft polymer obturator can be fashioned in due course.

Osseointegration techniques have greatly facilitated the appearance and retention of both intraoral and facial prostheses, after rhinectomy or orbital clearance. The Branemark system of osseointegrated implants uses titanium screws that become integrated into the skeleton and to which the prosthesis can be firmly attached by a press-stud or magnet arrangement.[61] The screws can be implanted at the time of the resection or as a secondary procedure. They must be implanted in bone at least 3–4 mm in depth. Radiotherapy slows the process of integration, which may take up to 1 year in the orbital socket. This is much slower than in the intraoral cavity. A temporary prosthesis can be offered in the interim.

Palliation

Sinonasal malignancy, if left untreated, produces appalling disfigurement often accompanied by pain, bleeding and blindness. It could also be argued that tumours such as malignant melanoma and adenoid cystic carcinoma carry an ultimately poor prognosis and it is therefore more likely that treatment buys a symptom-free interval rather than cure. As the surgical procedures carry a minimal morbidity with good cosmesis and function there are many instances where they may be undertaken without expectation of a curative excision. This is particularly true of craniofacial resection and it is quite possible for patients to undergo several revision procedures during the course of their disease for example in chondrosarcoma of the skull base. This can provide the patient with long symptom-free periods and enable vision to be preserved by judicious orbital decompression.

Palliative radiotherapy (and chemotherapy) may also be appropriate for extensive radiosensitive tumours that have spread intradurally and/or affect the cavernous sinus and middle cranial fossa.

REFERENCES

1. Acheson ED, Cowdell RH, Hadfield E et al. Nasal cancer in woodworkers in the furniture industry. *Br Med J* 1968; **ii**: 587–596.
2. Wilhelmsson B, Drettner B. Nasal problems in wood furniture workers. A study of symptoms and physiological variables. *Acta Otolaryngol* 1984; **98**: 548–555.
3. Drettner B, Wilhelmsson B, Lundh B. Experimental studies on carcinogenesis in the nasal mucosa. *Acta Otolaryngol* 1985; **99**: 205–207.
4. Lund VJ. Malignancy of the nose and sinuses: epidemiological and aetiological considerations. *Rhinology* 1991; **29**: 57–68.
5. Roush GC. Epidemiology of cancer of the nose and paranasal sinuses, current concepts. *Head Neck Surg* 1979; **2**: 3–11.
6. Lund VJ, Howard DJ, Wei W et al. Craniofacial resection. The tumours of the nasal cavity and paranasal sinuses: a 17-year experience. *Head Neck Surg* 1998; **20**: 97–105.
7. Weber AL, Stanton AC. Malignant tumours of the paranasal sinuses: radiologic, clinical and histopathologic evaluation of 200 cases. *Head Neck Surg* 1984; **6**: 761–776.
8. Takasaka T, Kawamoto K, Nakamura K. A case-control study of nasal cancers. *Acta Otolaryngol Suppl* 1987; **435**: 136–142.
9. Doll R, Morgan IG, Speizer FE. Cancer of the lung and sinuses in nickel workers. *Br J Cancer* 1970; **12**: 32–41.
10. Harrison DFN. Snuff – its use and abuse. *Br Med J* 1964; **ii**: 1649–1652.
11. Rankow RM, Conley J, Fodor P. Carcinoma of the maxillary sinus following thorotrast instillation. *J Maxillofac Surg* 1974; **2**: 119–126.

12. Woodson GE, Robbins T, Michaels L. Inverted papilloma. Consideration in treatment. *Arch Otolaryngol* 1985; **111**: 806–811.
13. Helliwell TR, Yeoh LH, Stell PM. Anaplastic carcinoma of the nose and paranasal sinuses, light microscopy, immunohistochemistry and clinical correlation. *Cancer* 1986; **58**: 2038–2045.
14. Robin PE, Powell DJ, Stansbie JM. Carcinoma of the nasal cavity and paranasal sinuses: incidence and presentation of different histological types. *Clin Otolaryngol* 1979; **4**: 431–456.
15. Weymuller EA, Reardon EJ, Nash D. Comparison of treatment modalities in carcinoma of the maxillary sinus. *Arch Otolaryngol* 1980; **106**: 625–629.
16. Har-El G, Hadar T, Krespi YP. An analysis of staging systems for carcinoma of the maxillary sinus. *Ear Nose Throat J* 1988; **67**: 511–520.
17. Sisson GA, Toriumi DM, Atiyah RA. Paranasal sinus malignancy: a comprehensive update. *Laryngoscope* 1989; **99**: 143–150.
18. Sakai S, Honki A, Fuchihata DD et al. Multidisciplinary treatment of maxillary sinus cancer. *Cancer* 1983; **52**: 1360–1364.
19. Knegt PP, Jong PC, Andel JG. Carcinoma of the paranasal sinuses. *Cancer* 1985; **62**: 1–5.
20. Harrison DFN, Lund VJ. *Tumours of the Upper Jaw.* London: Churchill-Livingstone, 1993; 115–121.
21. Hyams VJ, Batsakis JG, Michaels L. *Tumors of the Upper Respiratory Tract and Ear.* Washington, DC: Armed Forces Institute of Pathology, 1986; 95–100, 104–106.
22. Matsuba HM, Mauney M, Simpson JR et al. Adenocarcinoma of major and minor salivary gland origin. *Laryngoscope* 1988; **98**: 784–788.
23. Conley J, Dingman DL. Adenoid cystic carcinoma in the head and neck (cylindroma). *Arch Otolaryngol* 1974; **100**: 81–90.
24. Chilla R, Schroth R, Eysholdt U et al. Adenoid cystic carcinoma of the head and neck. Controllable and uncontrollable factors in treatment and prognosis. *Otol Rhinol Laryngol* 1980; **42**: 346–367.
25. Howard DJ, Lund VJ. Reflections on the management of adenoid cystic carcinoma of the nose and paranasal sinuses. *Otolaryngol Head Neck Surg* 1985; **93**: 338–340.
26. Friedman I, Osborn DA. *Pathology of Granulomas and Neoplasms of the Nose and Paranasal Sinuses.* Edinburgh: Churchill Livingstone, 1982; 152–157.
27. Schwabb G, Micheau C, Le Guillou C. Olfactory esthesioneuroma: a report of 40 cases. *Laryngoscope* 1988; **98**: 872–876.
28. Herrold K. Induction of olfactory neuroepithelial tumours in Syrian hamsters by diethynitrosamine. *Cancer* 1964; **17**: 205–215.
29. Harrison DFN. Surgical pathology of olfactory neuroblastoma. *Head Neck Surg* 1984; **7**: 60–64.
30. Kadish, S, Goodman M, Wang CC. Olfactory neuroblastoma: a clinical analysis of 17 cases. *Cancer* 1976; **37**: 1571–1576.
31. Lund VJ, Milroy CM. Olfactory neuroblastoma; clinical and pathologic aspects. *Rhinology* 1993; **31**: 1–6.
32. Levine PA, McLean WC, Cantrell RW. Esthesioneuroblastoma: the University of Virginia experience. *Laryngoscope* 1986; **96**: 742–746.
33. Gulguerov P, Calcaterra T. Esthesioneuroblastoma: the UCLA Experience 1970–1990. *Laryngoscope* 1992; **102**: 843–849.
34. Eden BV, Debo FRF, Lamer GF. Esthesioneuroblastoma: long term outcome and patterns of failure. The University of Virginia Experience. *Cancer* 1994; **73**: 2556–2562.
35. Weiden L, Yarrington CT, Richardson GR. Olfactory neuroblastoma, chemotherapy and radiotherapy for extensive disease. *Arch Otolaryngol* 1984; **110**: 759–760.
36. Lund VJ. Malignant melanoma of the nasal cavity and paranasal sinuses. *J Laryngol Otol* 1982; **96**: 347–355.
37. Holmström M, Lund VJ. Malignant melanoma of the nasal cavity following occupational exposure to formaldehyde. *Br J Indust Med* 1991; **48**: 9–11.
38. Clark WH, From L, Bernadino EA et al. The histogenesis and histologic behaviour of primary human melanoma of the skin. *Cancer Res* 1969; **29**: 707–720.
39. Lederman M, Busby ER, Mould RF. The treatment of tumours of the upper jaw. *Br J Radiol* 1969; **42**: 561–581.
40. Harrison DFN. A critical look at the classification of maxillary sinus carcinomata. *Ann Otol Rhinol Laryngol* 1978; **87**: 3–9.
41. Chandler JR, Guillamondegui OM, Sisson GA. Clinical staging of cancer of the head and neck: a new system. *Am J Surg* 1976; **132**: 532–538.
42. Sisson GA, Johnson NE, Amir CS. Cancer of the maxillary sinus: clinical classification and management. *Ann Otol Rhinol Laryngol* 1963; **72**: 1050–1059.
43. Lund VJ, Howard DJ, Lloyd GAS, Cheesman AD. Magnetic resonance imaging of paranasal sinus tumours for craniofacial resection. *Head Neck Surg* 1989; **11**: 279–283.
44. Lund VJ, Lloyd GAS, Howard DJ et al. Enhanced magnetic resonance imaging and subtraction techniques in the post-operative evaluation of craniofacial resection for sinonasal malignancy. *Laryngoscope* 1996; **106**: 553–558.
45. Neubauer U, Fahlbusch R, Wigand ME, Weidenbecher M. Malignant tumors of the anterior skull base. *Neurosurg Rev* 1992; **15**: 187–192.
46. Moure EJ. Traitement des tumeurs malignes primitives de l'ethmoide. *Revue Hebdomadaire de Laryngologie* 1902; **2**: 401–412.
47. Price JC, Holliday MJ, Johns ME. The versatile midface degloving approach. *Laryngoscope* 1988; **98**: 291–295.
48. Howard DJ, Lund VJ. The midfacial degloving approach to sinonasal disease. *J Laryngol Otol* 1992; **106**: 1056–1062.
49. Shah J, Kraus DH, Arbit E et al. A craniofacial resection of the tumours involving the anterior skull base. *Otolaryngol Head Neck Surg* 1992; **106**: 387–393.
50. Lam KH, Wai FL, Yue CP et al. Maxillary swing approach to the orbit. *Head Neck Surg* 1991; **13**: 107–113.
51. Smith RR, Klopp CT, Williams JM. Surgical treatment of cancer of the frontal sinus and adjacent areas. *Cancer* 1954; **7**: 991–994.

52. Ketcham AS, Wilkins RH, Van Buren JM et al. A combined intracranial approach to the paranasal sinuses. *Am J Surg* 1963; **106**: 698–703.
53. Terz JJ, Young HF, Lawrence W. Combined craniofacial resection for locally advanced carcinoma of the head and neck. *Am J Surg* 1980; **140**: 613–624.
54. Cheesman AD, Lund VJ, Howard DJ. Craniofacial resection for tumours of the nasal cavity and paranasal sinuses. *Head Neck Surg* 1986; **8**: 429–435.
55. Raben A, Pfistr D, Harrison LB. Radiation therapy and chemotherapy in the management of cancers of the nasal cavity and paranasal sinuses. In: Kraus DH, Levine HL (eds). *Nasal Neoplasia*. New York: Thiema, 1997; 183–202.
56. Robbins KT, Storniolo AM, Hryniuk WM, Howell SB. 'Decadose' effects of cisplatin squamous cell carcinoma of the upper aerodigestive tract. II. Clinical Studies. *Laryngoscope* 1996; **106**: 37–42.
57. Dropkin MJ, Malgady RG, Scott DW et al. Scaling of disfigurement and dysfunction in postoperative head and neck patients. *Head Neck Surg* 1983; **6**: 559–570.
58. Jones E, Lund VJ, Howard DJ et al. Quality of life of patients treated surgically for head and neck cancer. *J Laryngol Otol* 1992; **106**: 238–242.
59. Krouse JH, Krouse HJ, Fabian RL. Adaptation to surgery for head and neck cancer. *Laryngoscope* 1989; **99**: 789–794.
60. Manderson RD. Prosthetics in head and neck surgery. In: McGregor IA, Howard DJ (eds). *Head and Neck Surgery, Part 2*. 4th edn. London: Butterworth-Heinemann, 1992; 576–592.
61. Tjellstrom A. Osseointegrated systems and their application in the head and neck. *Arch Otolaryngol Head Neck Surg* 1989; **3**: 39–70.

18 Management of tumours of the temporal bone

David A Moffat and Melville da Cruz

Introduction

Tumours involving the temporal bone are rare but present with symptoms similar to inflammatory ear disease. A high index of suspicion is required for the early diagnosis of malignant tumours. Pain, bleeding from the ear canal and facial palsy may herald the onset of malignancy. Local extension of tumour to structures surrounding the temporal bone occurs early and often silently, and as a result, most tumours present at a relatively advanced stage. The prognosis of treated squamous cell carcinoma (SCC) of the temporal bone is determined primarily by the extent of local disease at diagnosis. Combined treatment of tumours limited to the external auditory canal (EAC) can result in a moderate 5-year survival, but advanced cancer has a very poor prognosis.

The surgical management of patients with temporal bone cancer is a major undertaking involving resection of major structures and high treatment morbidity. Treatment is best carried out by a multidisciplinary team skilled in dealing with the complex regions of the temporal bone and skull base.

Surgical anatomy

The anatomy of the temporal bone and adjacent regions is complex and contains the organs of hearing and balance, the cranial nerves responsible for facial movement, speech and swallowing and the major vessels providing arterial supply and venous drainage to the cranium and brain. The temporal bone is in turn surrounded by important structures of the face and infratemporal fossa, the dura of the middle and posterior cranial fossae and underlying brain and upper neck and cervical spine. A conceptual organization of the various compartments of the temporal bone is important in understanding the spread of temporal bone cancer and forms the anatomical basis of the previously described en bloc resections of the temporal bone.

The tympanic membrane and promontory of the middle ear form the medial resection margins for tumours arising in the EAC. Small tumours limited to the lateral portion of the external canal can be excised en bloc with a sleeve resection of the external canal and adjacent conchal bowl (Figure 18.1). The tympanic membrane forms the medial limit of the resected margin.

More medially arising EAC tumours can be removed by lateral temporal bone resection (LTBR)[1] where the medial limit is formed by the promontory of the first turn of the cochlea and the bloc includes the tympanic membrane (Figure 18.1). Tumours extending into or involving the middle ear can be removed by subtotal temporal bone resection by including the otic capsule in the resection (STBR).[2–4] Total temporal bone resection (TTBR)[5,6] for tumours involving the petrous apex includes removing the complete temporal bone (Figure 18.1). Extended temporal bone resection (ETBR) with supraomohyoid neck dissection for advanced and recurrent cancer has been recently advocated.[6] Infratemporal fossa skull base approaches have been designed for resection of tumours involving the jugular foramen.[7] The normal anatomical structures contained within each compartment determine the functional deficits associated with resections of tumours arising within these regions. Excision of the external ear by sleeve resection and LTBR results in cosmetic deformity and moderate conductive hearing loss. Resection of middle ear tumours by STBR including the otic capsule results in total hearing loss, transient vertigo, facial nerve palsy and risk of CSF leak. Extension of the resection inferiorly to include the neurovascular compartments of the jugular foramen results in sacrifice of the lower

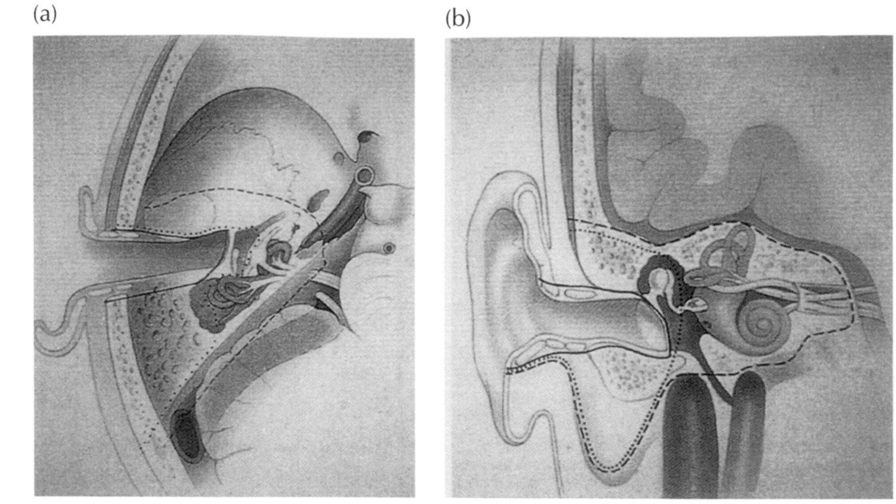

Figure 18.1 (a, b) The concept of en bloc resection of the temporal bone is illustrated in the axial and coronal planes. Sleeve resection of the external auditory canal (solid line) is rarely indicated for small lesions of the EAC. Lateral temporal bone resection (dotted line) is indicated for most cancers limited to the EAC. Total temporal bone resection (dashed line) is indicated for advanced temporal bone cancer and is performed by a combination of en bloc and piecemeal resection techniques, rather than neatly as shown in this diagram. (Reproduced from the *Atlas of Neuro-otology and Skull Base Surgery*; Robert K. Jackler MD; Mosby 1996, with kind permission of the editor).

cranial nerves and the additional deficits of dysphonia and dysphagia with risk of aspiration. Resection of the surrounding structures such as mandible and infratemporal fossa, dura and overlying brain, facial and lower cranial nerves, internal carotid artery (ICA)[6,8,9] and dural venous sinuses is possible, but the morbidity of the resection is considerably increased. Careful preoperative planning is required prior to deciding which resection is applicable and difficult intraoperative decisions may be required before extending the resection limits to surrounding anatomical regions.

General considerations

Age

Temporal bone cancer tends to affect the 50–60-year-old age group predominantly, although younger ages have been reported particularly with tumours of the middle ear.[10] A typical mean age is 72.6 within a range of 56–98.[11] Sarcomas are limited to children.

Incidence

Little information is available on the incidence of temporal bone malignancy as few centres deal with enough cases to gain a large experience with the patterns of disease. In Britain the age adjusted incidence is 1/1 000 000 per year for women, and 0.8/1 000 000 per year for men.[12] Expressed as a fraction of all otological complaints the incidence is in the region of 0.025–0.005%.[10,13,14] The prevalence has been reported as 0.006%.[15]

Gender

The gender proportion is near to equal,[16] although many studies have shown a slight female preponderance, ratio of 1:1.2.[17]

Aetiology

Aetiological factors implicated in the development of temporal bone cancer have been studied. Temporal bone cancer can be divided into two major groups: (1) laterally arising in the skin of the external ear involving the pinna and lateral third of the EAC. Exposure to ultraviolet radiation is the major aetiological factor.[18] (2) In more medially arising external auditory canal tumours and middle ear cancer, chronic inflammation is thought to be the major aetiology, as about half of these cancers are associated with a long history of chronic discharge.[17,19] Occupational factors such as radiation exposure in watch dial makers,[20,21] frost bite[18] and a possible link with aflatoxin generated by fungi in the EAC,[17] have been proposed as aetiological factors.

Classification

Sites of temporal bone cancer

To some extent this classification is artificial as advanced tumour involves multiple sites and it is difficult to identify the site of origin. (see Table 18.1).

Table 18.1 Sites of temporal bone cancer

	Lewis[13]	Nelms and Paparella[22]	Conley and Schuller[23]
Auricle (%)	60	85	60–70
External canal (%)	30	12	20–30
Middle ear (%)	10	1.5	10

Histology

The most common type of malignancy arising in the temporal bone is squamous carcinoma. Adenocarcinoma is much less common and other histopathological types are very rare (see Table 18.2).

Most malignant tumours of the temporal bone arise from the epithelial elements of the EAC and middle ear. Metastasis to the temporal bone occurs by haematogenous spread, usually to marrow-containing regions, commonly the petrous apex,[25] or by direct extension from the nasopharynx and parotid gland. Haematological malignancies such as lymphoma, leukaemia and eosinophilic granuloma can also involve the temporal bone and should be considered in multiple or bilateral lesions.

Non-neoplastic destructive temporal bone lesions and benign neoplasm need to be differentiated from malignant tumours of the temporal bone and include fibrous dysplasia,[26–28] osteoradionecrosis, necrotizing otitis externa,[29–31] sarcoid, Paget's disease and giant cell tumour of bone. Careful evaluations with multiple deep-tissue biopsies are required to avoid sampling error and confirm the tissue diagnosis prior to planning definitive treatment.

Natural history and mechanisms of spread of malignant tumours

Spread tends to occur via extension through the numerous vascular, neural and natural foramina between the temporal bone and surrounding structures (Figures 18.2 and 18.3). Extension is multidirectional such that deep local spread to surrounding areas may be present but unsuspected at the time of surgery. This may account for the high incidence of local recurrence following surgery.[11] Invasion of blood vessels in the skin of the EAC gives recurrent bloody otorrhoea, the most common presenting symptom of EAC cancer. Lateral extension along the

Table 18.2 Histology of primary temporal bone cancers. Adapted from Krespi et al[24]

	Conley (1965)*	Lewis (1982)*	Tucker (1965)*	Kuhel (1995)†
Squamous cell carcinoma	24	86	68	82.2
Adenocarcinoma	4	2	1	8.8 (including adenoid cystic carcinoma)
Basal cell carcinoma	1	8	—	5.6
Metastasis	—	—	8	— —
Sarcoma	5	2	6	—
Melanoma	—	—	—	— 0.4
Miscellaneous	2	2	6	0.4
Total no. of cases	36	100	89	> 500

*Absolute numbers; †percentages.

(a) (b)

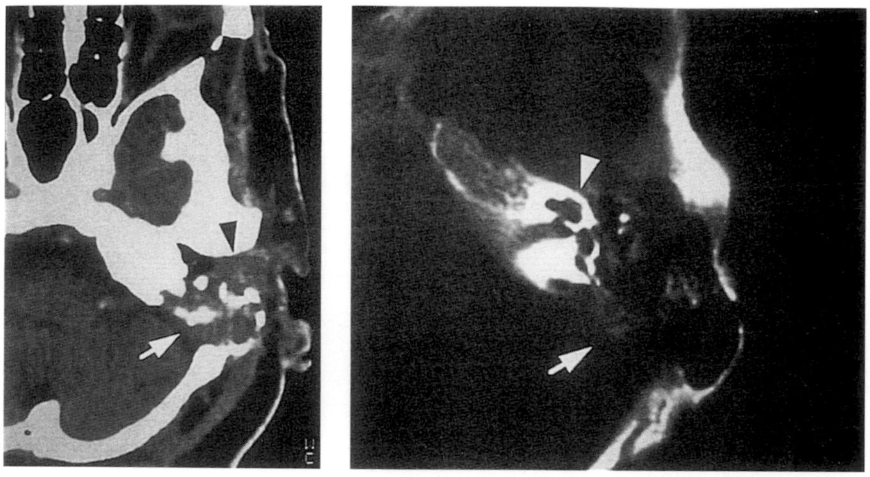

Figure 18.2 Axial CT scans of the temporal bone. (a) In the contrast-enhanced scan the apparent limits of the tumour can be seen. Involvement of the lateral temporal bone with margins extending to the pinna and periauricular skin, the temporomandibular joint (black arrow head) and the posterior fossa dura and sigmoid sinus (white arrow) is shown. (b) The posterior fossa bony plate has been destroyed (white arrow). In the bone window CT settings the otic capsule structures including the cochlea (arrow head) are well preserved. The otic capsule is highly resistant to cancerous invasion and involvement of the cochlea and semicircular canals usually occurs late in the untreated history of temporal bone malignancy. In this case the patient presented with a 60dB hearing loss and intact cochlear and vestibular function. Cancer of the temporal bone spreads primarily by direct extension and is usually found to be more extensive at operation than shown by preoperative imaging.

subcutaneous plane gives the appearance of thickened oedematous external canal skin (Figures 18.3a and 18.3d). Circumferential spread with extension to the conchal bowl may occur giving rise to an appearance similar to chronic otitis externa.

Anterior extension to the temporomandibular joint (Figure 18.2a), parotid gland and infratemporal fossa occurs via the fissures of Santorini, the petrosquamous fissure and preformed defects of the external canal (foramen of Hüschke), presenting with preauricular swelling and trismus. Involvement of the root of the zygoma with extension to the masseter muscle and subsequent downward extension to the mandible and infratemporal fossa occurs in advanced cancer. Inferior extension to the jugular foramen, foramen magnum and cervical vertebrae, and upper neck, results in fullness and lower cranial nerve palsies. Medial growth through the tympanic membrane with extension of tumour into the middle ear cleft (Figure 18.3a–f) allows spread via the pneumatized spaces of the temporal bone. Extension to the petrous apex, internal carotid artery (ICA)[32] and nasopharynx via the Eustachian tube can easily occur. The internal carotid artery and otic capsule bone are highly resistant to tumour invasion and involvement of the labyrinth occurs late resulting in sensori-neural hearing loss (SNHL) and vertigo (Figure 18.2). Extension to the internal auditory canal (IAC) may occur through the vestibule.

Superior extension to the epitympanic space and thin bone of the tegmen tympani will involve the middle fossa dura and temporal lobe and is the most common route of intracranial spread (Figure 18.3). This is suggested by persistent deep temporal headache. Posterior extension to the retroauricular sulcus and mastoid occurs through preformed defects of the EAC or direct bony erosion (Figure 18.3). Involvement of the posterior fossa dura can occur from the mastoid.

Lymphatic spread

The skin of the external ear canal has a sparse lymphatic network. Drainage is to the preauricular, mastoid, subparotid and subdigastric nodes initially, and then to deep upper cervical nodes.[33,34] Clinically evident metastatic spread to regional lymph nodes is not common at the time of presentation (10–15%)[6,35–37] and is seen only in advanced cancer. Extension via peritubal lymphatics to the nasophar-

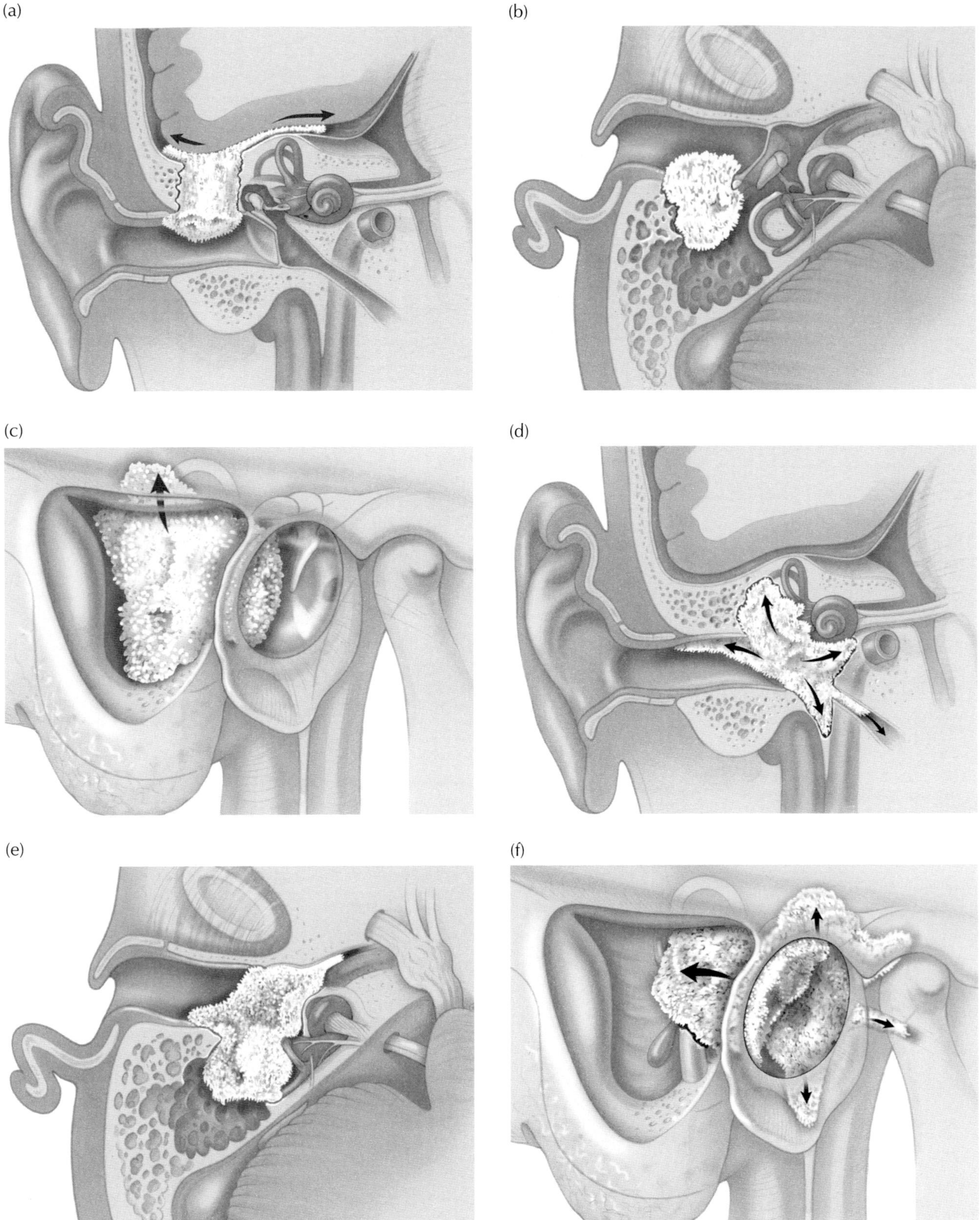

Figure 18.3 (a) Coronal section of an advanced temporal bone SCC demonstrating superior spread through the tegmen with involvement of dura and temporal lobe of the brain. (b) Axial section of the lesion showing its posterior extent in the mastoid. (c) Parasagittal section illustrating superior spread into the middle cranial fossa. (d) Coronal section of a very advanced temporal bone SCC illustrating the lines of spread within the temporal bone: superiorly, medially and laterally. (e) Axial view of the lesion demonstrating spread anteriorly, posteriorly, medially and laterally. (f) Parasagittal view showing anterior, posterior, superior and inferior spread. (Figure 18.3 'Squamous cell carcinoma', Chapter 5, page 71 in *Tumors of the Ear and Temporal Bone* – Eds: Jackler and Driscoll, 2000, Lippincott Williams and Wilkins. Reproduced with kind permission of the editors.)

ynx may occur with involvement of the retropharyngeal nodes. Lymphatic micrometastasis may be a cause for early regional treatment failure.[11] Adenoid cystic carcinoma, basal cell carcinoma (BCC) and squamous cell carcinoma (SCC) have a particular propensity for perineural spread. The predominant nerve at risk is the facial nerve. Spread distally extends to the stylomastoid foramen and to the extratemporal facial nerve. Extension to the parotid segment of the facial nerve can selectively involve branches of the facial nerve giving weakness in a particular region of facial musculature. Medial spread leads to the geniculate ganglion, intracranial portions of the facial nerve and brain stem. Spread along the greater superficial petrosal nerve (GSPN) can occur leading to involvement of the floor of the middle cranial fossa.

Haematogenous spread of temporal bone cancer to distant sites is rare at the time of presentation, and indicates incurable disease.

Metastases in the lung and bone are the most common sites and may occur with squamous cancer, adenoid cystic carcinoma, adenocarcinoma and sarcoma. Metastasis to the temporal bone by haematological spread from tumours at distant sites occurs but is uncommon The petrous apex is the most common location for metastasis due to the presence of vascular bone marrow.[25] Metastasis to the middle ear, mastoid and external canal also occurs. Presenting symptoms are pain, hearing loss, mass in the external auditory canal and facial numbness.[10,38,39] The most likely primary sites are breast, lung, kidney, prostate, salivary, pharynx or nasopharynx, gastrointestinal tract and the occult primary.[40]

Haematological malignancies such as lymphoma, leukaemia and eosinophilic granuloma can also involve the temporal bone and should be considered in multiple or bilateral lesions. Intracranial spread by direct extension of tumour from the middle ear occurs and is typical of advanced sarcoma. Meningeal spread produces multiple cranial nerve palsies.[41,42]

Clinical presentation

Pain, bleeding, discharge, facial palsy and hearing loss are the most common presenting symptoms of temporal bone cancer. A high index of suspicion is required for early diagnosis of malignancy as these symptoms are typical of inflammatory ear disease and both conditions can coexist[29,31] although the pain tends to be more severe in malignant disease and bleeding is relatively uncommon in chronic inflammatory disease. The range of symptoms and signs associated with the presentation of temporal bone cancer are shown in Table 18.3.

Table 18.3 Clinical presentation of temporal bone cancer

	Leonetti et al[43]* (*N* (%))	Kuhel et al[16]† (%)	Pensak et al[34] (%)
Symptoms			
Pain	19 (74)	51	60
Hearing loss	18 (69)	29	20
Headache	12 (46)		
Facial numbness	8 (31)		
Hoarseness	3 (12)		
Dysphagia	1 (4)		
Vertigo/tinnitus		15	
Signs			
Ear canal mass	26 (100)	37	
Bloody otorrohea	18 (69)	61	60
Facial paralysis	13 (50)	16	35
Cranial nerve defects	8 (31)		10
Parotid, neck mass	7 (27)		
Temporal mass	4 (15)	19	

*26 cases.
†442 cases.

(a) (b)

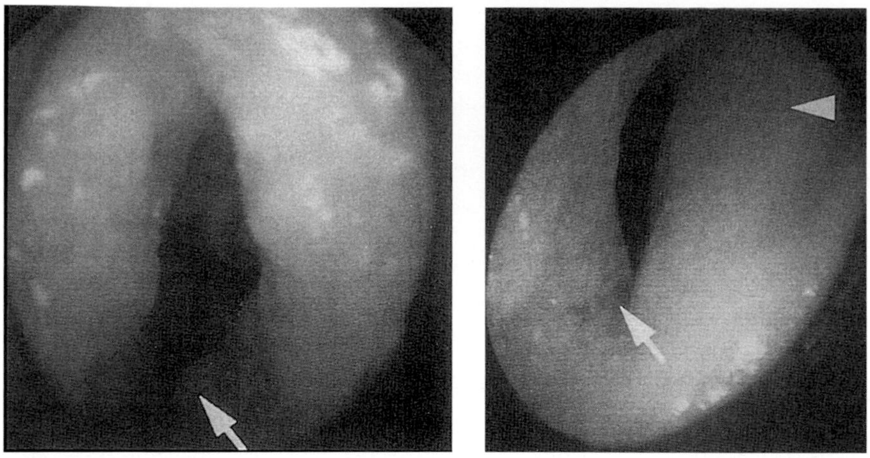

Figure 18.4 (a, b) The canal appearances of the SCC illustrated in Figure 18.3 are shown in these photographs. The presumed site of origin of the cancer is represented by the ulcerated area of the floor of the EAC (white arrow head in Figure 18.4a). The surrounding canal skin is oedematous due to carcinomatous involvement and the posterior canal wall is bulging forward due to extension of the cancer to the postauricular sulcus (white arrow head in Figure 18.4b). A high degree of suspicion is required to diagnose cancer of the EAC early as the presenting symptoms and canal appearances can easily be mistaken for ulcerating otitis externa. The two conditions may coexist.

Otoscopy reveals an exophytic lesion that is friable and bleeds to touch. Tumours can bear a similar appearance to chronic suppurative otitis media with granulation tissues but malignant tumours tend to be predominantly exophytic (Figure 18.4).

Clinical assessment

The aim of preoperative assessment is to confirm the diagnosis of malignancy, define the extent of disease and to formulate a treatment plan. This is achieved with history taking, thorough physical examination, imaging and biopsy. The length of the history and the rate at which symptoms develop give some idea of the extent of local spread and the degree of malignancy of the tumour. A long history of aural discharge suggests cancer associated with inflammatory ear disease (Marjolin's ulcer). Pulsatile tinnitus suggests a tumour of vascular origin such as a glomus tumour or a middle ear vascular anomaly or a dural arteriovenous abnormality. Deep headache raises the suspicion of dural involvement. Facial weakness indicates invasion of the facial nerve. The onset of vertigo and SNHL indicates invasion of the labyrinth, and the development of speech and swallowing problems heralds involvement of the lower cranial nerves in the jugular foramen. The onset of trismus due to involvement of the temporomandibular joint, pterygoid muscles or mandible suggests advanced disease that has spread anteriorly. The appearance of periauricular and parotid swelling is a grave sign.

Clinical examination includes careful microscopic examination of the location of tumour and its visible extent. Particular note is made of facial weakness, trismus, periauricular swellings and regional lymph node enlargement. Cranial nerve deficits are carefully recorded. Thorough assessment of hearing and balance function is recorded clinically and documented with audiometry.

General physical examination is carried out to detect distant spread. Assessment of the patient's nutritional and mental state gives some idea of the patient's general response to major surgery. Detailed assessment is made of coexisting illnesses and the patient's overall fitness for general anaesthesia.

Investigations

Biopsy

External canal lesions offer an opportunity for direct biopsy, but if a vascular tumour or vascular anomaly is suspected then biopsy is best deferred until clinical and radiographical assessments including carotid arteriography have been completed.

Multiple deep biopsies should be taken to avoid a sampling error. Results that return a report of chronic inflammation when there is suspicion of malignancy should be repeated as neoplastic and inflammatory disease commonly coexist.[29,31]

Imaging

Imaging is mandatory as part of the preoperative assessment and provides information on the nature of destructive temporal bone lesions and the extent of local and regional spread. Computerized tomography (CT) scanning and magnetic resonance imaging (MRI) are complementary in the assessment of temporal bone tumours. High-resolution CT (1 mm cuts or less) in the axial and coronal planes provides accurate delineation of the extent of the destruction of the bone since bone has a positive signal. MRI, on the other hand, where bone gives a negative signal impressively demonstrates soft tissue involvement such as dura, temporal lobe and brain or ptyeroid muscle especially when enhanced with gadolinium-DTPA. The presence of distant metastasis can be assessed with chest X-ray and skeletal survey. Accurate postoperative imaging aids in the planning of radiotherapy fields and identifies patients with recurrent disease for palliative treatment.

Computerized tomography

High-resolution CT scanning in the axial and coronal planes is excellent for identifying bony erosion of the temporal bone and adjacent skull base[36,44] since bone has a positive signal (Figure 18.5). The bony architecture of the lesion may indicate the nature of the tumour. A diffuse ground glass appearance is suggestive of fibro-osseous dysplasia, an onion skin appearance is associated with giant cell tumours of the temporal bone and Paget's disease has the specific radiological appearance of demineralized bone.

Erosion of the external canal, mastoid cortex, tegmen or petrous apex may indicate previously unsuspected deeper disease. Involvement of regional lymph nodes with tumour can be seen with ring enhancement of enlarged nodes.[45]

Magnetic resonance imaging

The high sensitivity and specificity of postcontrast MRI scanning is useful in defining the extent of intracranial and soft tissue involvement. In MRI bone has a negative signal. Involvement of the dura and brain is an important prognostic indicator and high resolution MRI scanning in the axial and coronal planes with gadolinium-DTPA enhancement is mandatory (Figure 18.6). Extension to the infratemporal fossa, and spread to regional lymph node

(a) (b)

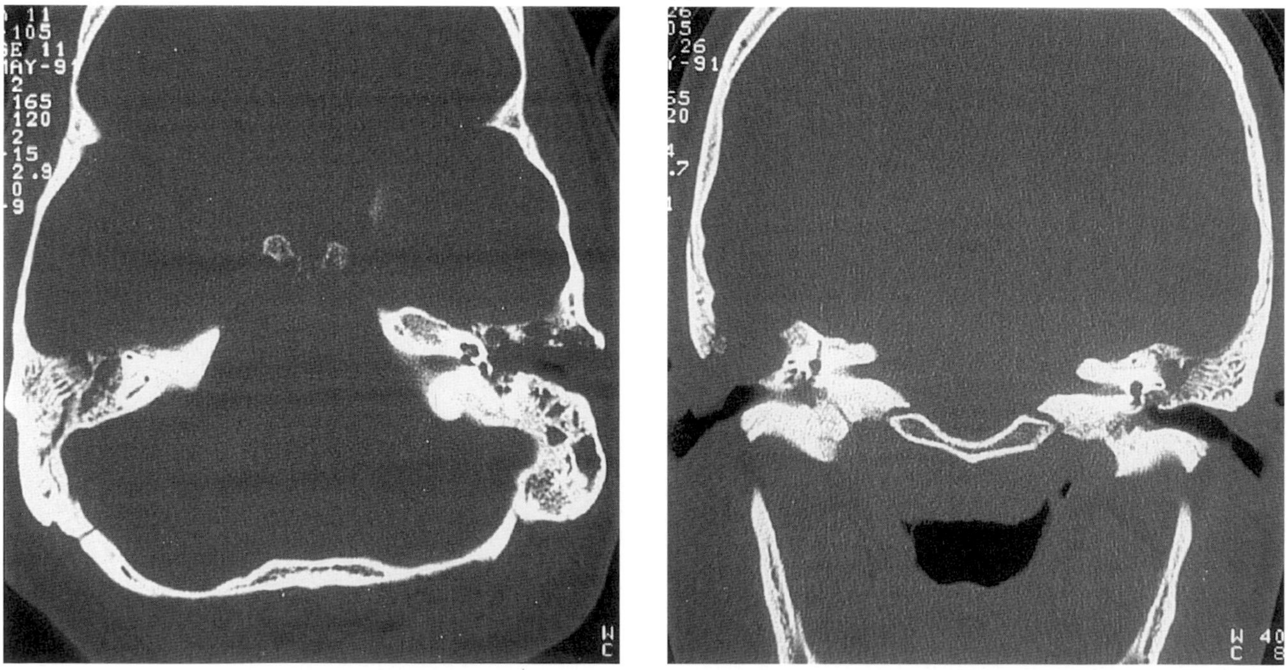

Figure 18.5 (a, b) Axial CT scan of extensive SCC of left temporal bone demonstrating marked bony erosion anteriorly and laterally (Figure 18.5a). The coronal CT in the same patient shows marked erosion of the superior surface of the temporal bone and soft tissue filling the external auditory canal (Figure 18.5b).

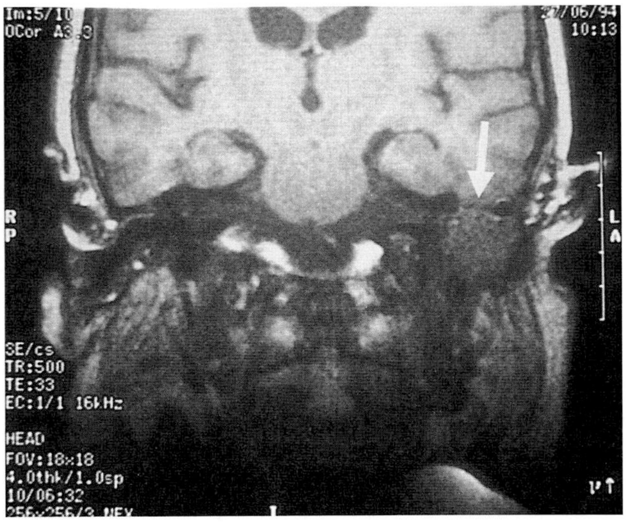

Figure 18.6 Coronal T1-weighted MRI scan demonstrating an SCC of the left temporal bone eroding the superior surface of the bone with dural involvement (white arrow). At surgery the tumour was noted to have invaded the temporal lobe of the brain.

groups can be identified,[36,44] and tissue confirmation of the nature of disease is required prior to embarking on definitive treatment.

Angiography

Advanced disease involving the petrous apex may involve the intrapetrous carotid artery[32] although this is a rare finding at surgery and the ICA is relatively resistant to invasion by temporal bone tumours. Angiography is used preoperatively to assess the internal carotid artery and delineates the vascular pattern of the cerebral arterial anatomy (Figure 18.7). Use of balloon occlusion techniques or cross-flow studies to demonstrate adequate contralateral cross-flow, suggests that safe en bloc resection of the internal carotid artery can take place.[8,9] Confirmation of contralateral venous drainage allows safe resection of the sigmoid/jugular venous complex without risk of cerebral oedema. Vascular anomalies and glomus jugular tumours can be diagnosed preoperatively, without need for biopsy and provide an opportunity for preoperative embolization with coils and feathers.

Ultrasound

The role of ultrasound is limited to the assessment of the relationship of neck masses to the great vessels and assisting in guided percutaneous biopsy of neck nodes.

Other imaging techniques

Distant spread to lung, bone and liver can be assessed preoperatively with chest X-ray and bone

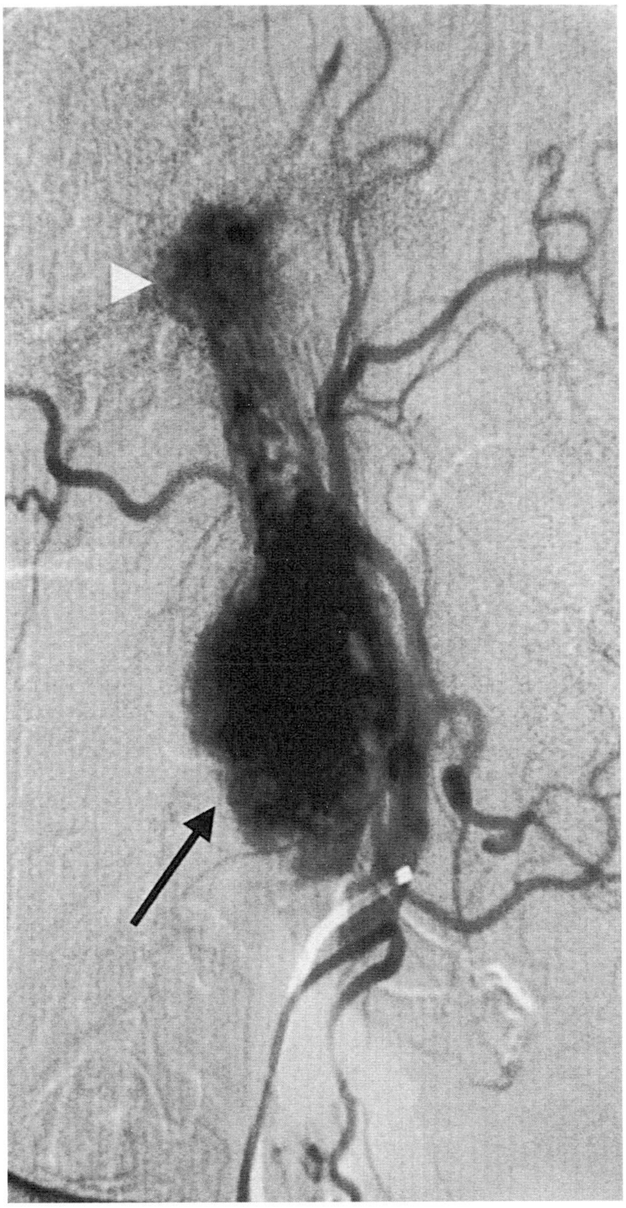

Figure 18.7 Right carotid arteriogram showing the multicentric nature of some glomus tumour types. This patient has a glomus tympanicum (white arrow head) and a carotid body tumour (black arrow) on the same side.

scan or skeletal survey. Technetium scanning is useful in excluding inflammatory conditions of the skull base as a cause of symptoms.[29,31] Indium-labelled white-cell scanning can help in the diagnosis of inflammatory disease of the temporal bone.

Staging

Several staging systems for malignancy involving the external ear have been proposed but currently no universally accepted system exists. Ideally a preoperative staging system should allow the extent of tumour to be easily categorized, aid in planning treatment and be useful as a basis for evaluating the outcomes of treatment. A widely accepted staging system would facilitate the comparison of results between centres.

Stell and McCormick[46] proposed a staging system for cancer involving the EAC and middle ear based on clinical assessment, facial nerve status and imaging, which was later revised by Clark et al (Table 18.4).[47]

More recently, Arriaga et al[48] devised a staging system based on preoperative clinical and CT findings that emphasizes the extent of local disease as the major prognostic indicator, the adverse effect of regional lymph node spread, and the need for preoperative imaging to assess the extent of local disease (Table 18.5).

N status

Involvement of lymph nodes is a poor prognostic finding and automatically places the patient in a higher category (i.e. stage III (T1, N1) or stage IV (T2, 3 and 4, N1) disease.

Table 18.4 Staging system: Clark's modification of Stell et al's proposal[47]

T1	Tumour limited to site of origin
T2	Tumour extending beyond site of origin indicated by facial paralysis or radiological evidence of bone destruction
T3	Involvement of parotid gland/temporomandibular joint/skin (i.e. extracranial)
T4	Involvement of dura/base of skull (i.e. cranial)

Table 18.5 Staging system[48]

T1	Tumour limited to the EAC without bony erosion or evidence of soft tissue extension
T2	Tumour with limited EAC erosion (not full thickness) or radiological findings consistent with limited (< 0.5 cm) soft tissue involvement
T3	Tumour eroding the osseous EAC (full thickness) with limited (< 0.5 cm) soft tissue involvement of middle ear and/or mastoid, or causing facial paralysis at presentation.
T4	Tumour eroding the cochlea, petrous apex, medial wall of middle ear, carotid canal, jugular foramen, or dura, or with extensive (> 0.5 cm) soft tissue involvement

M status

Distant metastasis indicates a very poor prognosis and immediately places a patient in the stage IV category.

Treatment policy

Treatment of temporal bone malignancy is a major undertaking. Accurate preoperative assessment and the organization of the necessary specialist resources for surgical resection and reconstruction by a multidisciplinary team, postoperative recovery and rehabilitation are necessary. Provision for delivery of radiotherapy and long-term follow-up is required.

Principles of surgical resection

Two contrasting approaches to temporal bone resection have been developed, their application being dependent on the extent of local disease and the particular preferences of different individual units.

Early lesions

The principle of en bloc resection when applied to localized, small tumours confined to the EAC allows the utilization of a lateral temporal bone resection (LTBR), which may realistically remove small EAC lesions leaving a clear margin of normal surrounding tissue. Careful preoperative assessment of the extent of tumour is required but few cancers are discovered early enough for en bloc surgical resection to be applied as the sole treatment modality especially since these tumours are so aggressive.

Advanced lesions

The feasibility of planned en bloc resections for advanced lesions has been challenged. The multidirectional spread of locally advanced cancer[43] does not allow the accurate preoperative assessment of the local extent of the tumour to take place. Preoperative imaging commonly underestimates the extent of tumour and this has a critical prognostic significance. Total temporal bone resection en bloc may lead to vascular compromise of the brain stem as a result of sacrifice of the intrapetrous internal carotid artery as well as VII, IX, X, XI and XII cranial nerve palsies and many surgeons in the field think that this may be unacceptable since there is no definitive evidence that it improves the ultimate prognosis. One technique of surgical excision that has been proposed for these lesions by many skull-base surgeons is step-wise removal of visible disease.[3,6,15,36,48,49] Initial bloc resection is followed by piecemeal removal of residual tumour and the petrous apex is removed with a high speed drill. The theoretical risk of dissemination of tumour cells has not been substantiated but most clinicians would consider it wise to recommend postoperative radiotherapy. The technique acknowledges that en bloc resection of deeper tissues is not possible in view of the anatomy and the vital structures within and adjacent to the temporal bone. Considerable intraoperative decision-making about the limits of resection is required. No comparison of the two techniques has been made as yet.

Management of the neck

Resection of regional lymph nodes as part of the en bloc principle, can be accomplished by adding a total parotidectomy and supraomohyoid neck dissection.[16]

Extended temporal bone resections

Extension of the resection to include dura, brain, parotid, ascending ramus and head of the mandible, infratemporal fossa plus or minus the ICA,[8,9] is possible but greatly increases the morbidity of the surgical procedure.[5,6,8,50] An extended resection, however, with total temporal bone removal, inclusion of the surrounding structures including parotid gland, head and ascending ramus of mandible, local venous sinuses, lower cranial nerves and supraomohyoid neck dissection followed by radiation has shown improved survival rates for recurrent and advanced de novo squamous cancer of the temporal bone[6] (Figure 18.8).[6]

(a)

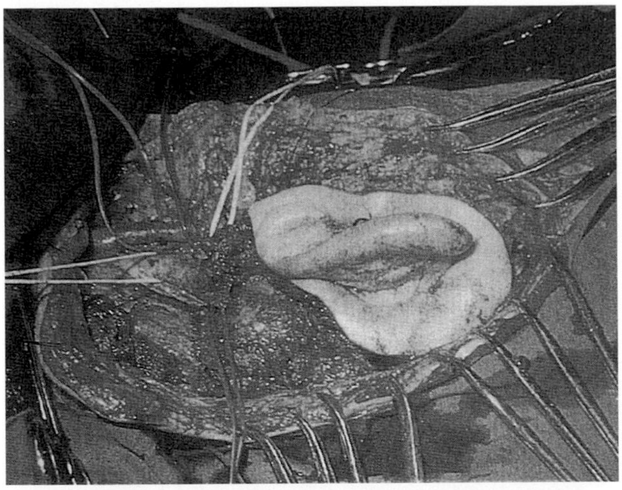

(b)

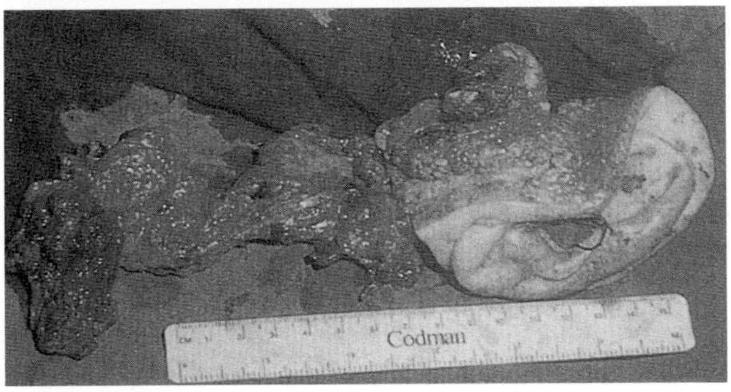

Figure 18.8 (Photographs taken during surgery showing (a) the extensive tissue defect following extended temporal bone resection for advanced squamous cell carcinoma of the EAC. Early in the procedure the major neurovascular structures of the neck are identified and controlled with coloured slings. (b) The en bloc lateral temporal bone specimen with radical neck dissection is seen. These photographs correspond to the images shown in Figures 18.1, 18.2 and 18.4.

Reconstruction

Extended temporal bone surgical resection leaves a large triangular composite defect with many different tissue types to be reconstructed. Lateral temporal bone resection will still leave a large defect in view of the necessary sacrifice of the pinna, which needs to be excised with a margin of healthy tissue in an 8 × 6-cm oval. The depth or medial extent of the defect will obviously be less than that of a total or extended temporal bone resection but nonetheless the defect to be reconstructed is considerable. Each reconstructive situation is unique and careful pre- and intraoperative consideration of the reconstructive options is needed.

Major issues of cosmesis, the durability of the repair particularly postirradiation, and the detection of recurrent tumour need to be taken into account. Watertight closure of the CSF pathways is essential to avoid meningitis. Vascularized pedicled[51,52] or revascularized free flaps[53–56] are commonly used and satisfy most of the demands for reconstruction. Commonly used flaps include local and regional rotation flaps, and free tissue flaps. The utilitarian scalp rotation (Figure 18.9) and nape flaps have a good blood supply and may be indicated in the elderly where the length of the procedure is important in reducing risk. Vascularized pedicled flaps including latissimus dorsi and trapezius flaps (Figure 18.10) have been used. The Chinese free forearm flap based on the distal radial artery has been used but the modified Chinese flap just distal to the antecubital fossa and based on the recently described anterior cubital artery (Figure 18.11) is a more useful flap since it is larger and has been

(a)

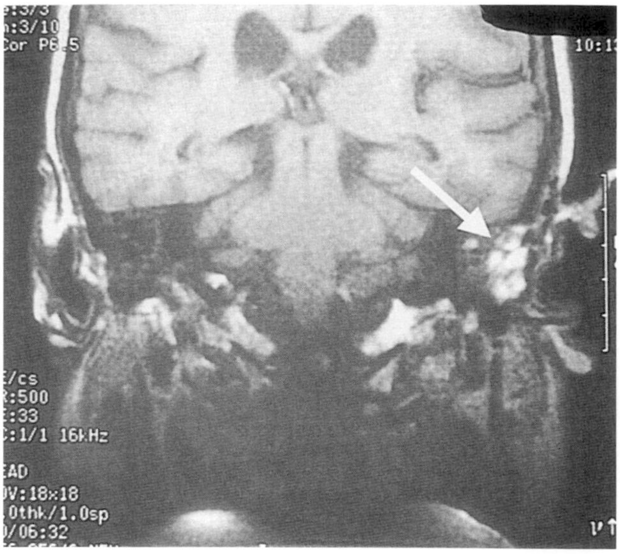

(b)

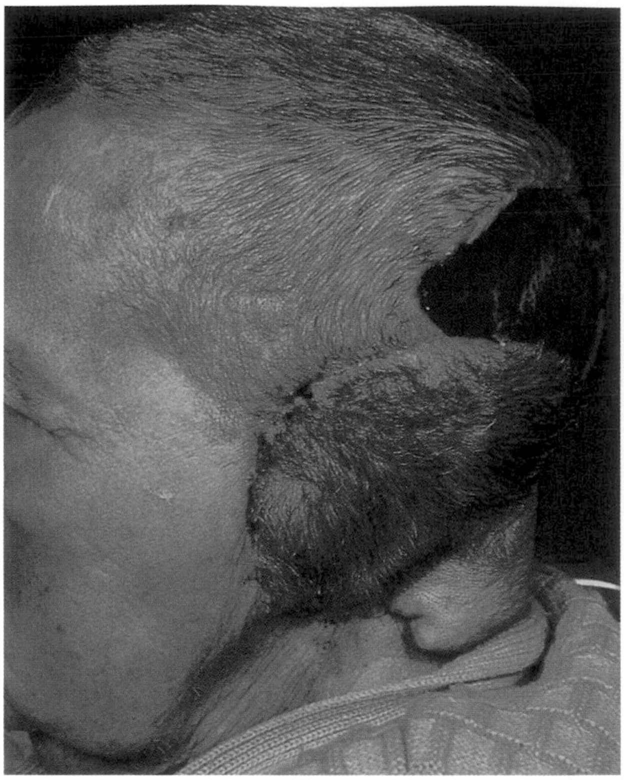

Figure 18.9 (a) Coronal T1-weighted MRI scan showing extensive SCC of left temporal bone (white arrow); (b) shows the patient postoperatively following a total temporal bone resection and scalp rotation flap.

(a)

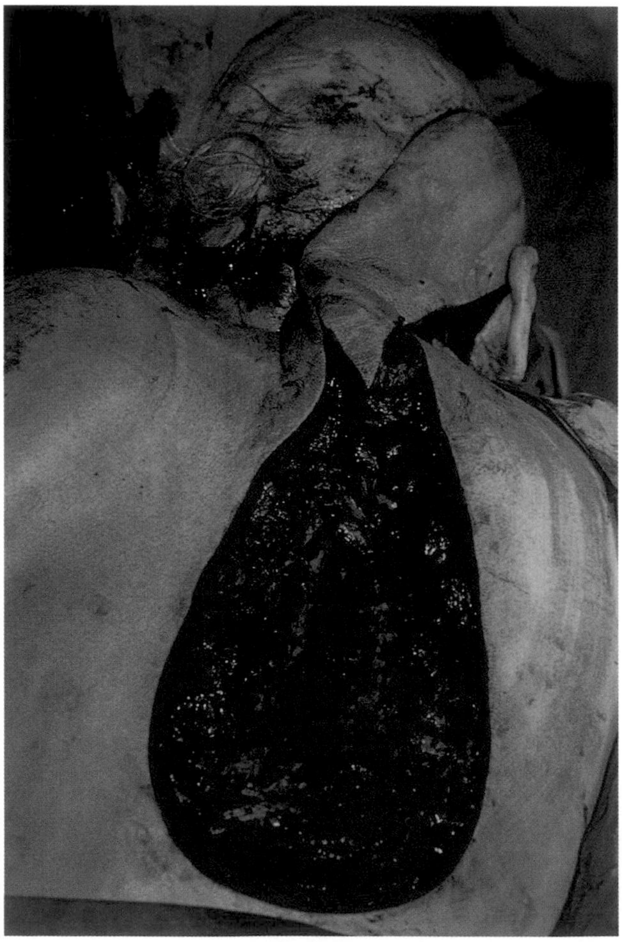

(b)

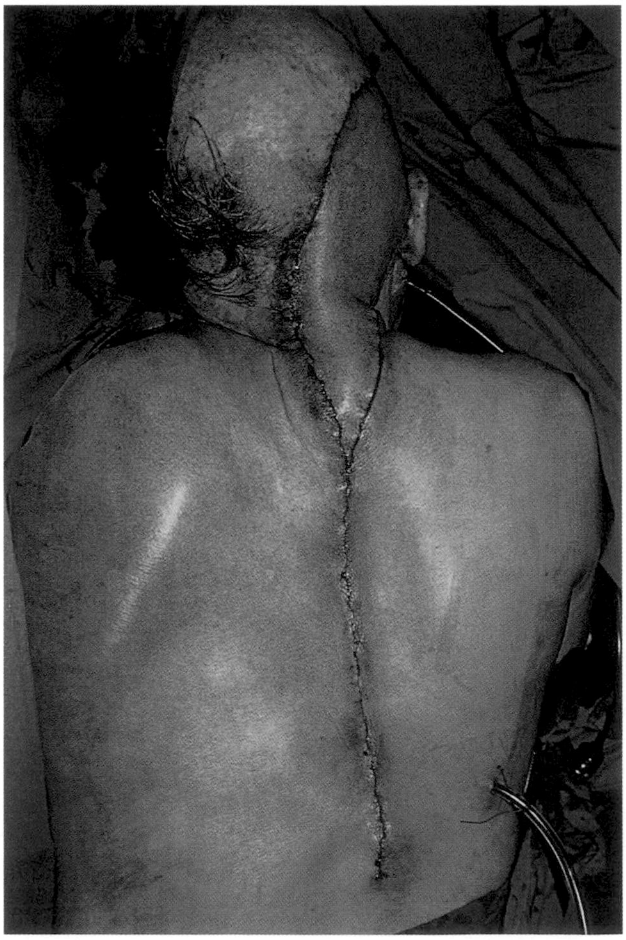

Figure 18.10 (a) Trapezius vascular pedicled flap, raised and inserted to cover defect; (b) immediately postoperatively.

(a)

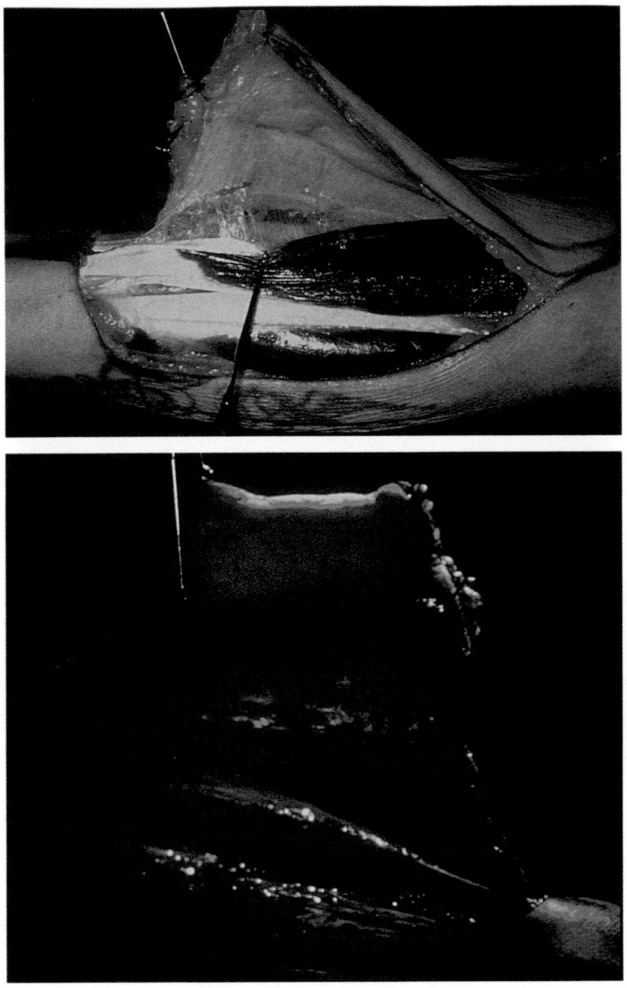

(b)

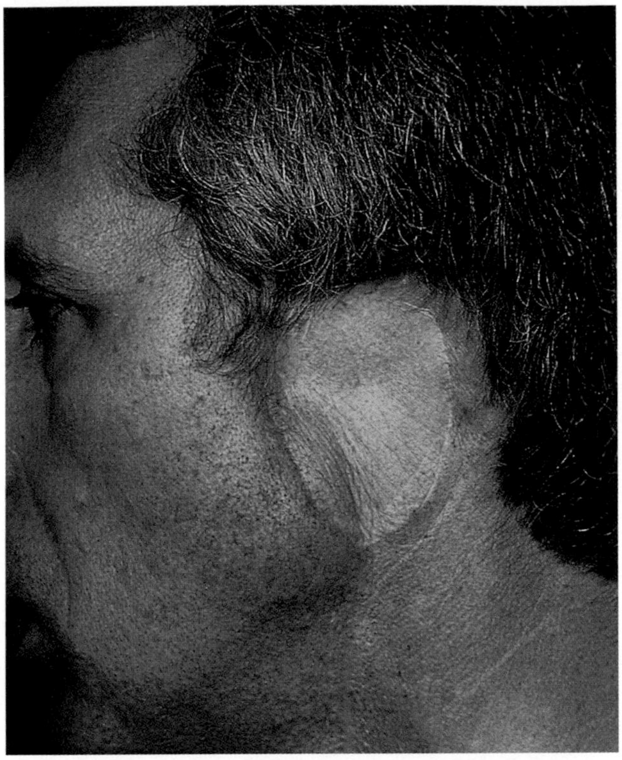

Figure 18.11 Modified Chinese free flap based on the anterior cubital artery. (a) This flap is larger and more useful than the flap based on the distal radial artery. (b) The good cosmetic result can be seen 2 years later.

employed very successfully. Free lateral upper arm and thigh flaps have also been used.

Rehabilitation

Following surgery patients may be left with several problems that require rehabilitation. The cosmetic appearance and residual neurological deficits need to be carefully assessed. Adequate consideration needs to be given to the psychological and nutritional state of the patient recovering from major surgery. Much of the management of neurological deficits is supportive as most defects become functionally compensated with time.

Vertigo resulting from labyrinthectomy is transient, with compensation occurring within a few weeks. Loss of hearing is rarely a major problem as the hearing thresholds in the contralateral ear are usually within normal limits. A CROS aid can be used with a prosthetic pinna.

Early postoperative management of facial weakness resulting from facial nerve resection aims to provide corneal protection. Initial treatment with lubricant ointment such as lacrilube and the provision of a clear eye shield at night and artificial tears during the day provides adequate corneal protection. Medium term but temporary corneal protection results from the partial ptosis produced with botulinum toxin injection to the orbicularis oculis. Tarsorrhaphy or insertion of a gold weight to the upper tarsal plate provides longer term corneal protection. For permanent facial weakness a variety of facial nerve procedures including grafting, static and dynamic muscle or nerve and tendon transfers can be used.[57,58]

Laryngeal function may be severely compromised by acute loss of the lower cranial nerves IX, X, XI and XII, and further exacerbated by facial nerve palsy causing oral incompetence, hypoglossal palsy causing poor tongue control, and mandibular resection interfering directly with mastication. Marked dysphagia due to a palsy of the glossopharygeal

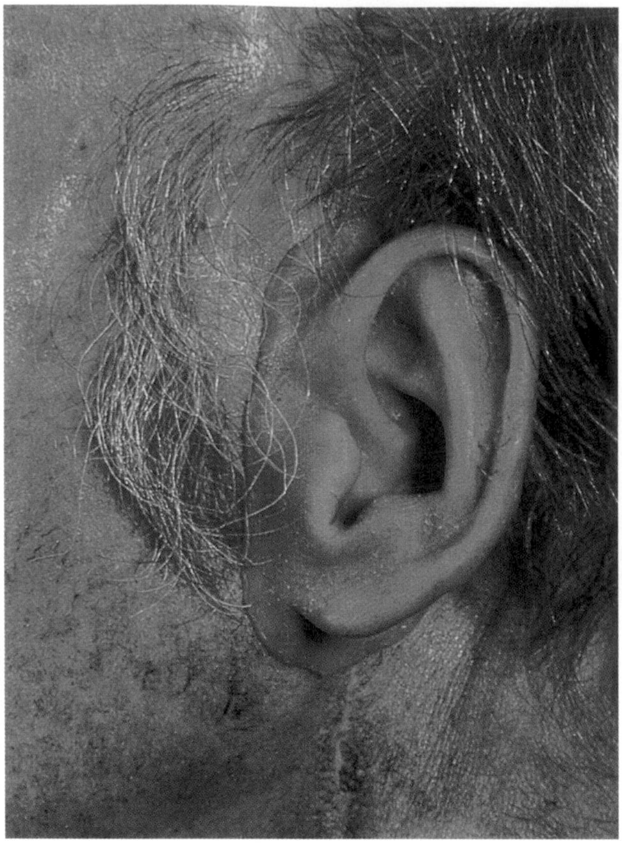

Figure 18.12 Customized prosthetic pinna attached with tissue adhesive provides good cosmesis.

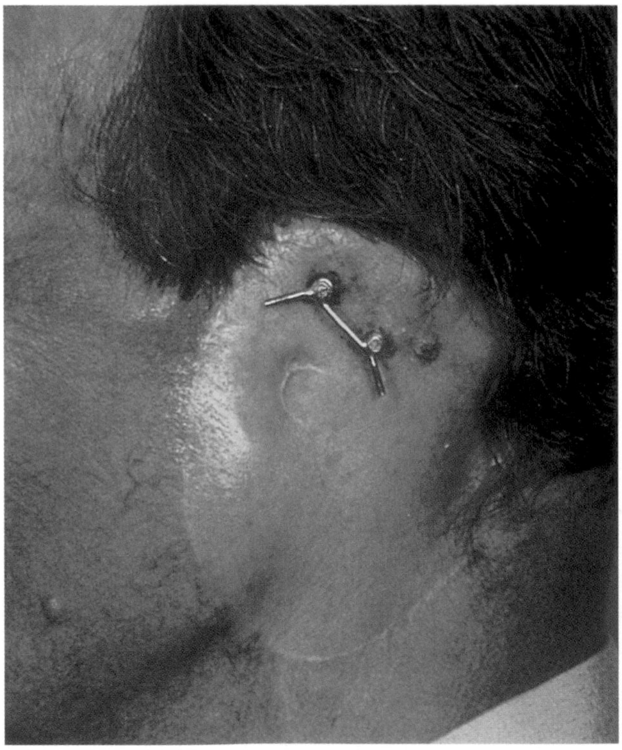

Figure 18.13 Osseointegrated titanium posts allow the fixation of a titanium bar to which a prosthetic pinna can be attached more securely. Unfortunately owing to the extensive nature of the surgery necessitated in SCC of the temporal bone this is rarely possible.

nerve will produce pooling of saliva in the ipsilateral pyriform fossa with spillover into the larynx and the concomitant risk of aspiration pneumonia. In the early postoperative phase nutrition is provided with alimentary feeds via a nasogastric tube or percutaneous endoscopic gastrostomy. As control of swallowing improves an oral diet of varying consistency can be introduced. A few patients do not gain full laryngeal compensation and aspiration continues to be a major problem. Speech improves greatly with compensation of the contralateral vocal cord, which may swing over the midline particularly in young patients. Dysphonia tends to increase during the day but vocal quality may be acceptable. In many patients, however, the dysphonia warrants microlaryngoscopy and injection of the vocal fold with fat (temporary) or teflon (permanent), or medialization of the vocal cord with thyroplasty surgery.

Consideration needs to be given to cosmesis in these patients. Provision of a hair piece may be useful in disguising the operated area particularly after scalp rotation flaps where there is a defect of the scalp which will require split skin grafting. A customized plastic pinna carefully constructed and attached to the flap with tissue adhesive has found favour with many patients in order to improve cosmesis (Figure 18.12). Rarely is there enough surrounding bone remaining to attach osseointegrated titanium posts but if there is, consideration should be given to attaching a titanium bar (Figure 18.13) to which can be fixed the plastic pinna prosthesis and this is clearly more robust than tissue adhesive.

The role of radiotherapy in temporal bone cancer

Radiotherapy can be given with one of three aims: as single-modality curative treatment, as a part of combined modality treatment; or with palliative intent.

Curative radiotherapy

Although radiotherapy alone is adequate treatment for early lesions of the pinna, it is generally accepted that radiotherapy as a definitive single modality treatment is inadequate treatment for squamous carcinoma of the external auditory canal and middle ear and advanced lesions.[10,59]

Combined treatment

In most centres radiotherapy is given as part of a planned combined treatment with surgery regardless of the extent of the tumour or the status of tumour free margins.[59,60] Commonly used regimes are planned with fields to include the local area of resection and regional nodal groups. Dosage regimes depend on the tolerance of the surrounding tissues to radiation. Total dosages vary from 5000 cGy in 20 fractions over 4 weeks, to 6000–7000 cGy in 30–35 fractions over 6–7 weeks. Complications of irradiation include otitis externa, cartilage necrosis, hearing loss, facial weakness, brain softening and osteoradionecrosis. Postoperative irradiation following an extended temporal bone resection has produced encouraging survival results in advanced and recurrent cancer.[6]

Palliation

Surgical palliation

In view of the difficulty in assessing the extent of an SCC of the temporal bone preoperatively with a likely underestimate of the size and degree of infiltration on imaging it may not be possible to completely excise the lesion even with extended temporal bone resection. Some surgeons, therefore, are of the opinion that surgery is not indicated in advanced lesions. The results which have been achieved with ETBR and postoperative radiotherapy would be justification for radical surgical treatment and indeed there is an argument for ETBR as a palliative procedure to obviate bone pain and lessen the likelihood of tumour fungation.

Palliative radiotherapy

Palliation aims to control the distressing symptoms of pain, discharge and bleeding. Debulking the tumour will increase the likelihood of successful palliation with radiotherapy. The efficacy of radiotherapy in controlling these symptoms is not known and may not be superior to simple treatments of adequate analgesics and aural toilet.

Radiotherapy given as treatment for glomus tumours decreases the vascularity of the tumours and commonly halts their growth. It is effective treatment for decreasing the pulsatile tinnitus.

Role of chemotherapy

Chemotherapy has not been used successfully in SCC of the temporal bone but topical 5-fluorouracil may have a place in the palliation of fungating tumours. Cryotherapy with a liquid nitrogen spray has also been used for palliation of fungating tumours.

Prognosis and outcome

It is difficult to meaningfully compare the treatment outcome of temporal bone malignancy for several reasons. Temporal bone malignancy is so rare that no one centre has a large experience in treatment. Lack of universally accepted staging systems and the wide variety of treatment protocols applied make comparison of results difficult. No prospective study comparing different treatment protocols has been carried out as yet. Despite these limitations, an analysis of the previously reported outcomes of 144 cases of temporal bone cancer by Prasad and Janecka[61] allows broad generalizations concerning the nature of temporal bone cancer and its treatment to be made.

The local extent of tumour at diagnosis is an important prognostic indicator. When disease is detected early and limited to the external canal a lateral temporal bone resection can be performed. More extensive disease extending into the middle ear and surrounding structures including dura, brain, pterygoids, otic capsule and carotid carries a worse prognosis and hence surgery must be tailored to the disease stage. Review of the literature by Prasad and Janecka[61] demonstrated when disease had extended into the middle ear a lateral temporal bone resection offered a 28.7% survival whereas a more extensive subtotal temporal bone resection had a 41.7% 5 year survival. This highlights the importance of aggressive en bloc resection.

Moffat[6] in 1997 reported his data on 15 patients who underwent either a lateral temporal bone resection or for more advanced disease extended temporal bone resection. He achieved an overall outcome of 47.5% 5-year survival. One more recent review of 39 patients survival for stage I and II disease was 100% and stage III and IV disease was 40%. This again demonstrated the increased survival of early stage disease and the importance of early diagnosis and aggressive surgical management.

The place of extended resections, in terms of survival, including the ICA, dural sinuses, dura and brain is unknown. Lymph node metastasis at the time of presentation is a poor prognostic sign. The addition of postoperative radiotherapy to the treatment of limited small external canal lesions resected with LTBR made little difference to the 5-year survival rate, 48% with DXT and 44.4% without DXT. At present there is insufficient information to make statements concerning the results of treatments of various histological types of temporal bone cancer, with few exceptions.

Local recurrence is the most common sequel of treatment failure (83%), followed by locoregional failure (9%), regional failure alone (5.5%) and distant metastasis associated with regional failure (2%).[62] Half the recurrences are in the first 12 months following treatment, and 85% of recurrences occur within 3 years of treatment.[63] Recent evidence suggests that salvage treatment for advanced and recurrent cancer in the form of extended temporal bone resection and postoperative radiotherapy results in improved 5-year survival rates of 47%.[6] In this study all recurrences occurred within the first 12 months after treatment implying that for salvage surgery if the patient survives a year then there is a high chance of cure.

Summary of non-scc lesions

Epithelial carcinoma

Basal cell carcinoma (BCC) is the most common cutaneous malignancy. It has a propensity for deep local invasion and perineural spread with metastases being rare. Primary melanoma of the temporal bone is extremely rare with a very poor prognosis. Glandular tumours are one of three types: adenoid cystic, adenocarcinoma or mucoepidermoid. Adenoid cystic carcinomas are the most common glandular tumours.[64,65] Adenocarcinomas are usually well-differentiated low-grade papillary cancers[66] that arise from the middle ear mucosa or possibly endolymphatic sac.[67] The long-term outcome for high grade adenocarcinoma and mucoepidermoid carcinoma is poor. In contrast, survival lengths for adenoid cystic carcinoma can be long even in the presence of metastases.[64,69–71]

Chondrosarcoma

Chondrosarcoma of the temporal bone is extremely rare. These tumours may be indolent and present late. They tend to invade locally and metastasize late. They may extend outside the temporal bone and into the cerebellopontine angle. Radical surgery and postoperative radiotherapy is the treatment of choice.

Rhabdomyosarcoma

These are rare aggressive tumours almost exclusively limited to childhood age groups. Only 100 cases of rhabdomyosarcoma (RMS) of the ear were reported to 1975.[72,73] The mean age at presentation is 5.[74] Until recently the prognosis has been extremely poor, but following the multimodality treatment (surgical resection, followed by radiotherapy and chemotherapy) protocol recommended by The Intergroup Rhabdomyosarcoma Study Committee treatment outcomes have greatly improved.[75] Mean survival from diagnosis is 2.8 years[81] and 11 of 24 patients were alive at 5 years.[76] Recurrent sarcoma tends to spread early to the lungs and bone, and intracranially to involve multiple cranial nerves.

Benign/malignant glomus tumours

The incidence of large benign glomus tumours (Fisch types B,C,D) is 1 per 1.3 million of the population.[77] Ten percent are of multicentric origin.[78] Rarely they can metastasize to local lymph nodes and to distant sites and are frankly malignant. Malignant glomus tumours are extremely rare and occur 40 times less frequently than benign lesions (1 per 52 million population).[77] Glomus jugulare tumours are twice as common in females as in males. Although they are usually non-chromaffin paragangliomata with no endocrine function there has been an increasing number of reports of vasoactive tumours and it is important to carry out a urinary assay of the metabolites dopamine and 3-methoxy-4-hydroxy mandelic acid (vanillylmandelic acid (VMA): normal up to 7 mg per 24 hours).

Surgery is the primary treatment since other modalities will not eradicate the tumour and are not curative. Standard otological approaches for glomus tumours arising in the middle ear cleft are adequate. Small glomus tympanicum tumours can be excised permeatally after raising a Rosen's flap and a KTP laser assists control of the vascular pedicle. Larger tympanicum tumours should be approached via an extended facial recess approach so that adequate control of the jugular bulb can be achieved. For larger tumours arising from the jugular bulb region, a combination of otological and skull-base techniques is necessary to gain control of the carotid artery and sigmoid-jugular complex. The trans- and infratemporal fossa approach is very satisfactory.[77] The major postoperative problems arise from possible loss of cranial nerve function, 7,9,10,11,12th may be affected in varying degrees and facial paralysis, laryngeal dysfunction, aspiration, and CSF leak are complications that can lead to considerable morbidity. Large glomus jugulare tumours in young people are more aggressive and have a propensity to recur. In this group postoperative radiotherapy is indicated. It may also be necessary if there is doubt about the totality of the surgical excision. Careful regular and prolonged follow-up is mandatory.

External beam radiation as a primary treatment modality is effective in reducing the growth rate and vascularity of glomus tumours, and can be used as palliative therapy in those unfit for surgery. It may slow down or stop the tumour from growing. Most commonly relieved symptoms are tinnitis, vertigo, bleeding and pain.[63] Hearing loss and cranial nerve function rarely change. Moderate dosages are effective, 3500 cGy over 3 weeks, with response rates being between 75 and 100%.[79–81] Osteoradionecrosis of the temporal bone in varying degrees may ensue in the longer term as a result of the endarteritis obliterans produced by the radiation. In its mildest and most common form this is just an otits externa but rarely extensive necrosis of the temporal bone can occur with sequestrum formation.

Carotid arteriography and embolization with coils and feathers is a useful adjunct to surgery and should be performed 2 or 3 days preoperatively. Substantial reduction in intraoperative blood loss can be achieved with a reduced operative risk of diffuse intravascular coagulopathy. Embolization as a stand alone procedure may be considered to control growth rate and ameliorate troublesome symptoms such as pulsatile tinnitus. The outcome of combined embolization and radiotherapy is uncertain at the present time.

Benign destructive lesions (giant cell tumours, fibro-osseous dysplasia and Paget's disease)

A wide range of benign neoplasms and non-neoplastic destructive lesions can present with symptoms mimicking temporal bone cancer. These conditions rarely involve the otic capsule and a wide margin of normal bone or soft tissue is not required. Surgical principles in these situations must be individualized but aim to preserve the otic capsule and facial nerve. Conventional surgical approaches developed for inflammatory ear disease are applicable.

Metastases

These may be asymptomatic and discovered incidentally as a solitary or multiple solid temporal bone lesions. Metastases to the EAC[10,38,39] and middle ear have been reported. They present as conductive hearing loss due to Eustachian tube dysfunction or involvement of the ossicular chain or tympanic membrane. Treatment must be individualized, generally palliative. Localized radiotherapy or chemotherapy appropriate to tumour type may be beneficial.

REFERENCES

1. Conley JJ, Novack AJ. The surgical treatment of tumour of the ear and temporal bone. *Arch Otolaryngol* 1960; **71**: 635–652.
2. Campbell E, Volk BM, Burkland CW. Total resection of the temporal bone for malignancy of the middle ear. *Ann Surg* 1951; 397–404.
3. Ward GE, Loch WE, Lawrence W. Radical operation for carcinoma of the external auditory canal and middle ear. *Am J Surg* 1951; **82**: 169.
4. Parsons H, Lewis JS. Subtotal resection of the temporal bone for malignancy of the middle ear. *Cancer* 1954; **7**: 995–1001.
5. Hilding DA, Selker R. Total resection of the temporal bone for carcinoma. *Arch Otolaryngol* 1969; **89**: 636–645.
6. Moffat DA, Grey P, Ballagh RH, Hardy DG. Extended temporal bone resection for squamous cell carcinoma. *Otolaryngol Head Neck Surg* 1997; **116**: 617–623.
7. Fisch U, Fagan P, Valavanis A. The infratemporal fossa approach for the lateral skull base. *Otolaryngol Clin North Am* 1984; **17**: 513–552.
8. Graham MD, Sataloff RT, Kemink JL et al. Total en bloc resection of the temporal bone and carotid artery for malignant tumors of the ear and temporal bone. *Laryngoscope* 1984; **94**: 528–533.
9. Sataloff RT, Myers DL, Lowry LD, Spiegel JR. Total temporal bone resection for squamous cell carcinoma. *Otolaryngol Head Neck Surg* 1987; **96**: 4–14.
10. Crabtree JA, Britton BH, Pierce MK. Carcinoma of the external auditory canal. *Laryngoscope* 1976; **86**: 405–415.
11. Spector JG. Management of temporal bone carcinomas: a therapeutic analysis of two groups of patients and long-term follow-up. *Otolaryngol Head Neck Surg* 1991; **104**: 58–66.
12. Morton RP, Stell PM, Derrick PP. Epidemiology of cancer of the middle ear cleft. *Cancer* 1984; **53**: 1612–1617.
13. Lewis JS. Cancer of the ear: A report of 150 cases. *Laryngoscope* 1960; **70**: 551–579.
14. Conley JJ. Cancer of the middle ear and temporal bone. *N Y State J Med* 1974; **74**: 1575–1579.
15. Kinney SE, Wood BG. Malignancies of the external ear canal and temporal bone: surgical techniques and results. *Laryngoscope* 1987; **97**: 158–164.
16. Kuhel WI, Hume CR, Selesnick SH. Cancer of the external auditory canal and temporal bone. *Otolaryngol Clin North Am* 1996; **29**: 827–852.
17. Johns ME, Headington JT. Squamous cell carcinoma of the external auditory canal. A clinico-pathologic study of 20 cases. *Arch Otolaryngol* 1974; **100**: 45–49.
18. Nager G. *Pathology of the Ear and Temporal Bone.* Baltimore: Williams and Wilkins, 1993; Adenocarcinoma of the middle ear.
19. Austin JR, Stewart KL, Fawzi N. Squamous cell carcinoma of the external auditory canal. Therapeutic

prognosis based on a proposed staging system. *Arch Otolaryngol Head Neck Surg* 1994; **120**: 1228–1232.

20. Beal DD, Lindsay JR, Ward PH. Radiation induced carcinoma of the mastoid. *Arch Otolaryngol* 1965; 81
21. Rubin RJ, Thaler SU, Holzer N. Radiation induced carcinoma of the temporal bone. *Laryngoscope* 1977; **87**: 1613–1621.
22. Nelms CR Jr, Paparella MM. Early external auditory canal tumors. *Laryngoscope* 1968; **78**: 986–1001.
23. Conley J, Schuller DE. Malignancies of the ear. *Laryngoscope* 1976; **86**: 1147–1163.
24. Krespi YP, Levine TM. Management of tumours of the temporal bone. In: Alberti PW, Rubin RJ (eds). *Otologic Surgery and Medicine*. New York: Churchill Livingstone, 1988; 1409–1422.
25. Procter B, Lindsay JR. Tumours involving the petrous pyramid of the temporal bone. *Arch Otolaryngol* 1947; **46**: 180–194.
26. Fries JW. The roentogen features of fibrous dysplasia of the skull and facial bones. A critical analysis. *Ther Nucl Medi* 1957; 77.
27. Nager GT, Kennedy DW, Kopstein E. Fibrous dysplasia: a review of the disease and its manifestations in the temporal bone. *Ann Otol Rhinol Laryngol Suppl* 1982; **92**: 1–52.
28. Lambert PR, Brackmann DE. Fibrous dysplasia of the temporal bone: the use of computerised tomography. *Otolaryngol Head Neck Surg* 1984; **92**: 461–467.
29. Mattucci KF, Setzen M, Galantich P. Necrotizing otitis externa occurring concurrently with epidermoid carcinoma. *Laryngoscope* 1986; **96**: 264–266.
30. al Shihabi BA. Carcinoma of temporal bone presenting as malignant otitis externa. *J Laryngol Otol* 1992; **106**: 908–910.
31. Grandis JR, Hirsch BE, Yu VL. Simultaneous presentation of malignant external otitis and temporal bone cancer. *Arch Otolaryngol Head Neck Surg* 1993; **119**: 687–689.
32. Michaels L, Wells M. Squamous cell carcinoma of the middle ear. *Clin Otolaryngol* 1980; **5**: 235–248.
33. Jesse RH, Goepfert H, Lindberg RD, Johnson RH. Combined intra-arterial infusion and radiotherapy for the treatment of advanced cancer of the head and neck. *Am J Roentgenol Radium Ther Nucl Med* 1969; **105**: 20–25.
34. Pensak ML, Willging JP. Tumours of the temporal bone. In: Jackler RK, Brackmann DE (eds). *Neurotology*. St Louis: Mosby, 1994; 1049–1057.
35. Arena S, Keen M. Carcinoma of the middle ear and temporal bone. *Am J Otol* 1988; **9**: 351–356.
36. Arriaga M, Curtin HD, Takahashi H, Kamerer DB. The role of preoperative CT scans in staging external auditory meatus carcinoma: radiologic-pathologic correlation study. *Otolaryngol Head Neck Surg* 1991; **105**: 6–11.
37. Hahn SS, Kim JA, Goodchild N, Constable WC. Carcinoma of the middle ear and external auditory canal. *Int J Radiat Oncol Biol Phys* 1983; **9**: 1003–1007.
38. Sadek SA, Dixon NW, Hardcastle PF. Metastatic carcinoma of the external auditory meatus secondary to carcinoma of the rectum. A case report. *J Laryngol Otol* 1983; **97**: 459–464.
39. Goldman NC, Hutchison RE, Goldman MS. Metastatic renal cell carcinoma of the external auditory canal. *Otolaryngol Head Neck Surg* 1992; **106**: 410–411.
40. Imamura S, Murakami Y. Secondary malignant tumors of the temporal bone. A histopathologic study and review of the world literature. *Nippon Jibiinkoka Gakkai Kaiho* 1991; **94**: 924–937.
41. Dehner LP, Chen KT. Primary tumors of the external and middle ear. III. A clinico-pathologic study of embryonal rhabdomyosarcoma. *Arch Otolaryngol* 1978; **104**: 399–403.
42. Tefft M, Fernandez C, Donaldson M et al. Incidence of meningeal involvement by rhabdomyosarcoma of the head and neck in children: a report of the Intergroup Rhabdomyosarcoma Study (IRS). *Cancer* 1978; **42**: 253–258.
43. Leonetti JP, Smith PG, Kletzker GR, Izquierdo R. Invasion patterns of advanced temporal bone malignancies. *Am J Otol* 1996; **17**: 438–442.
44. Grossman CB (ed.) The temporal region. In: *Magnetic Resonance Imaging and Computed Tomography of the Head and Spine*. Baltimore: Williams and Wilkins, 1990; 281–307.
45. Yousem DM, Som PM, Hackney DB et al. Central nodal necrosis and extracapsular neoplastic spread in cervical lymph nodes: MR imaging versus CT. *Radiology* 1992; **182**: 753–759.
46. Stell PM, McCormick MS. Carcinoma of the external auditory meatus and middle ear. Prognostic factors and a suggested staging system. *J Laryngol Otol* 1985; **99**: 847–850.
47. Clark LJ, Narula AA, Morgan DA, Bradley PJ. Squamous carcinoma of the temporal bone: a revised staging. *J Laryngol Otol* 1991; **105**: 346–348.
48. Arriaga M, Curtin H, Takahashi H. Staging proposal for external auditory meatus carcinoma based on preoperative clinical examination and computed tomography findings. *Ann Otol Rhinol Laryngol* 1990; **99**: 714–721.
49. Shih L, Crabtree JA. Carcinoma of the external auditory canal: an update. *Laryngoscope* 1990; **100**: 1215–1218.
50. Gacek RR, Goodman M. Management of malignancy of the temporal bone. *Laryngoscope* 1977; **87**: 1622–1634.
51. McGregor IA, Jackson IT. The extended role of the delto-pectoral flap. *Br J Plast Surg* 1970; **23**: 173–185.
52. Bakamijan VY, Long M, Rigg B. Experience with the medially based deltopectoral flap in reconstructive surgery of the head and neck. *Br J Plast Surg* 1971; **24**: 174–183.
53. McCraw JB, Magee WP Jr, Kalwaic H. Uses of the trapezius and sternomastoid myocutaneous flaps in head and neck reconstruction. *Plast Reconstr Surg* 1979; **63**: 49–57.
54. Ariyan S, Cuono CB. Myocutaneous flaps for head and neck reconstruction. *Head Neck Surg* 1980; **2**: 321–345.
55. Lamberty BGH, Cormack GC. The ante-cubital fasciocutaneous flap. *Br J Plast Surg* 1983; **36**: 428–433.
56. Jones NF, Schramm VL, Sekhar LN. Reconstruction of the cranial base following tumour resection. *Br J Plast Surg* 1987; **40**: 155–162.

57. May M. Facial reanimation after skull base trauma. *Am J Otol* 1985; **Suppl**: 62–67.
58. May M, Croxson GR, Klein SR. Bell's palsy: management of sequelae using EMG rehabilitation, botulinum toxin, and surgery. *Am J Otol* 1989; **10**: 220–229.
59. Lederman M. Malignant tumours of the ear. *J Laryngol Otol* 1965: 79.
60. Wang CC. Radiation therapy in the management of carcinoma of the external auditory canal, middle ear, or mastoid. *Radiology* 1975; **116**: 713–715.
61. Prasad S, Janecka IP. Efficacy of surgical treatments for squamous cell carcinoma of the temporal bone: a literature review. *Otolaryngol Head Neck Surg* 1994; **110**: 270–280.
62. Prasad S, Janecka IP. Malignancies of the temporal bone-radical temporal bone resection. In: Brackmann DE (ed.) *Otologic Surgery*. Philadelphia: WB Saunders, 1994; 49–62.
63. Harwood AR, Keane TJ. Malignant tumours of the temporal bone and external ear: medical and radiation therapy. In: Alberti PW, Rubin RJ (eds). *Otologic Surgery and Medicine*. New York: Churchill Livingston, 1988; 1389–1408.
64. Pulec JL. Glandular tumors of the external auditory canal. *Laryngoscope* 1977; **87**: 1601–1612.
65. Perzin KH, Gullane P, Conley J. Adenoid cystic carcinoma involving the external auditory canal. A clinico-pathologic study of 16 cases. *Cancer* 1982; **50**: 2873–2883.
66. Glasscock ME, 3rd, McKennan KX, Levine SC, Jackson CG. Primary adenocarcinoma of the middle ear and temporal bone. *Arch Otolaryngol Head Neck Surg* 1987; **113**: 822–824.
67. Heffner DK. Low-grade adenocarcinoma of probable endolymphatic sac origin. A clinicopathologic study of 20 cases. *Cancer* 1989; **64**: 2292–2302.
68. Wetli CV, Pardo V, Millard M, Gerston K. Tumors of ceruminous glands. *Cancer* 1972; **29**: 1169–1178.
69. Dehner LP, Chen KT. Primary tumors of the external and middle ear. Benign and malignant glandular neoplasms. *Arch Otolaryngol* 1980; **106**: 13–19.
70. Cannon CR, McLean WC. Adenoid cystic carcinoma of the middle ear and temporal bone. *Otolaryngol Head Neck Surg* 1983; **91**: 96–99.
71. Hicks GW. Tumors arising from the glandular structures of the external auditory canal. *Laryngoscope* 1983; **93**: 326–340.
72. Feldman BA. Rhabdomyosarcoma of the head and neck. *Laryngoscope* 1982; **92**: 424–440.
73. Naufal PM. Primary sarcomas of the temporal bone. *Arch Otolaryngol* 1973; **98**: 44–50.
74. Wiatrak BJ, Pensak ML. Rhabdomyosarcoma of the ear and temporal bone. *Laryngoscope* 1989; **99**: 1188–1192.
75. Raney RB Jr, Lawrence W Jr, Maurer HM et al. Rhabdomyosarcoma of the ear in childhood. A report from the Intergroup Rhabdomyosarcoma Study-I. *Cancer* 1983; **51**: 2356–2361.
76. Mandell LR. Ongoing progress in the treatment of childhood rhabdomyosarcoma [published erratum appears in *Oncology (Huntingt)* 1993 Mar; **7**(3): 104]. *Oncology Huntingt* 1993; **7**: 71–83.
77. Moffat DA, Hardy DG. Surgical management of large glomus jugulare tumours: infra- and trans-temporal approach. *J Laryngol Otol* 1989; **103**: 1167–1180.
78. Bickerstaff ER, Howell JS. The neurological importance of tumours of the glomus jugulare. *Brain* 1953 ; **76**: 576–593.
79. Tidwell TJ, Montague ED. Chemodectomas involving the temporal bone. *Radiology* 1975; **116**: 147–149.
80. Kim JA, Elkon D, Lim ML, Constable WC. Optimum dose of radiotherapy for chemodectomas of the middle ear. *Int J Radiat Oncol Biol Phys* 1980; **6**: 815–819.
81. Wang CC. Paraganglioma of the head and neck. In: *Radiation Therapy of Head and Neck Neoplasms*. Boston: John Wright, 1983; 279.

19 Tumours of the parapharyngeal space

Nigel J P Beasley, Patrick J Gullane and Saurin R Popat

Introduction

Tumours of the parapharyngeal space make up between 0.5 and 1% of all head and neck neoplasms, occurring at any age.[1] They consist of a heterogeneous group of tumours that can mimic other disease processes. Overall 80% are benign and 20% malignant.[1,2] Tumours may arise from any of the structures within the parapharyngeal space, but salivary gland neoplasms and neurogenic tumours are the most common. A thorough knowledge of the anatomy of the parapharyngeal space helps in understanding the varied pathology and surgical approaches to this region.

Anatomy

The parapharyngeal space is a potential space defined by the fascial planes of the neck. It can be visualized as an inverted five-sided pyramid or cone with its base under the temporal bone and its apex in the neck at the hyoid bone.[3] The base is located superiorly in a small area of the inferior petrous temporal bone anteromedial to the base of the styloid process and just anterior to the jugular foramen and the carotid canal openings. The apex is found at the junction of the greater cornu of the hyoid with the midpart of the digastric muscle. Laterally the parapharyngeal space is limited by the fascia overlying the pterygoid

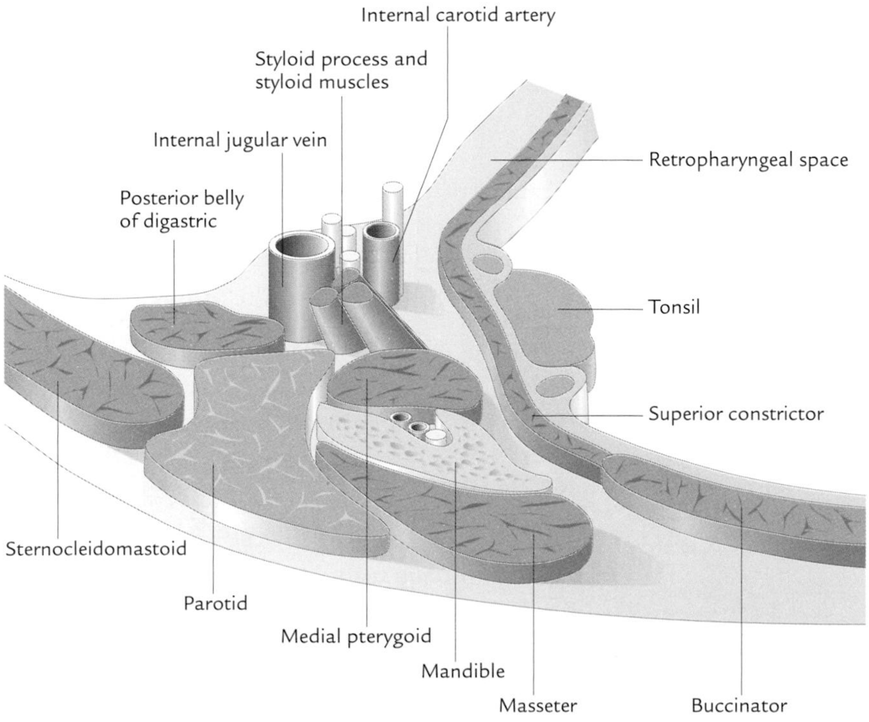

Figure 19.1 Normal anatomy of the parapharyngeal space.

Table 19.1 Normal structures within the parapharyngeal space

	Prestyloid space	Poststyloid space
Vascular	Internal maxillary artery	Internal carotid artery Internal jugular vein
Nervous	Lingual nerve Inferior alveolar nerve Auriculotemporal nerve	Cranial nerves IX, X, XI, XII Cervical sympathetic trunk
Other	Loose areolar and adipose tissue	Lymph nodes

Table 19.2 Differential diagnoses of parapharyngeal space neoplasms[2,14]

	Group	Pathology
Prestyloid (45%)	Salivary (45%)	Benign: pleomorphic adenoma Malignant: adenoid cystic carcinoma, carcinoma ex pleomorphic adenoma, acinic cell carcinoma, mucoepidermoid carcinoma
Poststyloid (45%)	Paraganglioma (20%)	Carotid body tumour Glomus vagale
	Neurogenic (15%)	Neurilemmoma Neurofibroma
	Lymph nodes (10%)	Lymphoma Metastases
Others (10%)	Vascular	Haemangiopericytoma, angiosarcoma, haemangioma
	Connective tissue	Rhabdomyosarcoma, lipoma, liposarcoma, fibrosarcoma, osteosarcoma

muscles, the medial aspect of the deep-lobe of the parotid and the ascending ramus of the mandible. Medially the space abuts the fascia overlying the pharyngeal constrictors and the tensor and levator palatini. Anteriorly the space is bounded by pterygomandibular raphe and the posterior wall is formed by the posterior part of the carotid sheath and prevertebral fascia (Figure 19.1). The parapharyngeal space communicates with the retropharyngeal and submandibular spaces, which allow spread of tumour along fascial planes with little resistance. Lymphatics from the parapharyngeal space drain to the upper deep cervical lymph nodes.

The parapharyngeal space is divided into pre- and poststyloid regions by the styloid process and the stylomandibular ligament that runs from the styloid to the angle of the mandible.[3] The contents of the pre- and poststyloid space are shown in Table 19.1. Prestyloid tumours are almost always of salivary origin and poststyloid lesions usually paragangliomas or neural in origin with occasional primary or secondary lymph node neoplasms being found (Table 19.2).

Pathology

Salivary gland neoplasms

Salivary gland tumours in the parapharyngeal space may arise from the deep-lobe of the parotid, from minor salivary glands in the lateral pharyngeal wall or ectopic salivary tissue in the parapharyngeal space.

Deep-lobe parotid tumours

About 5–10% of parotid tumours start in the deep-lobe of the gland, they are almost always benign pleomorphic adenomas. Deep-lobe tumours may extend into the parapharyngeal space either directly through the stylomandibular tunnel or below the stylomandibular ligament.[4] The stylomandibular tunnel is formed posteroinferiorly by the stylomandibular ligament and anteriorly by the ascending ramus of the mandible. Tumours passing through here have the classic 'dumbbell' and are palpable as a retromandibular mass externally while displacing the tonsil and soft palate medially. Tumours arising from the retromandibular portion of the gland tend to pass behind the stylomandibular ligament, have a more rounded appearance and become very large before causing symptoms.

Minor salivary gland tumours

A smaller number of tumours arise from minor salivary glands in the mucosa of the lateral pharyngeal wall or in ectopic salivary tissue in the parapharyngeal space. These can be distinguished from deep-lobe tumours radiologically and pathologically as there is a layer of fat separating the tumour from the deep-lobe of the parotid.

Paragangliomas

Paragangliomas are highly vascular neoplasms of neural crest origin arising in paraganglial (glomus body) cells of the neck and temporal bone. In the neck they give rise to two distinct lesions in different locations. Carotid body paragangliomas arise in the crotch between the internal and external carotid artery and tend to splay the two vessels apart. Vagal paragangliomas (glomus vagale) are usually associated with one of the vagal ganglia and displace the carotid anteriorly and laterally. Pathologically they are encapsulated brownish tumours with a firm consistency. Histologically clusters of epitheloid cells are seen separated by a highly vascular fibrous stroma. Head and neck paragangliomas rarely secrete catecholamines unlike the histologically similar phaeochromocytoma found in the adrenal medulla.

About 10% of patients with head and neck paragangliomas have a positive family history.[5] There is an autosomal dominant pattern of inheritance with incomplete penetrance as the maternally derived gene is inactivated during female oogenesis. Children of female carriers are not affected but may pass the gene onto their offspring.[6] More women than men develop non-familial paragangliomas (ratio 2:1) and about 5% of these patients have multiple lesions. The sex ratio is equal for familial paragangliomas and about 30% will have multiple lesions and are probably at increased risk of an associated phaeochromocytoma.[5] Patients living at high altitude have an increased risk of developing a paraganglioma, they have an increased female to male ratio and are less likely to have a family history or bilateral disease.[7]

About 2–5% of paragangliomas are malignant, recognized by the presence of regional or distant metastases or invasion of surrounding structures. However, the multicentric nature of these tumours can make this diagnosis difficult.

Vagal paragangliomas (glomus vagale) make up less than 5% of head and neck paragangliomas. Tumours are often interwoven with the nerve fibres and at least 50% of patients have one or more cranial nerve palsies on presentation. Often, these tumours are found high in the parapharyngeal space where the vagus enters the jugular foramen and may involve in the skull base causing multiple cranial nerve palsies (IX–XII). Up to 40% of patients have multiple tumours and a family history of paraganglioma.[8,9]

Neurogenic tumours

The parent cell of both common neurogenic tumours in the head and neck is probably the Schwann cell. They account for 20–30% of all parapharyngeal space lesions[10] and give rise to two distinct tumour types; neurilemmomas (schwannomas) and neurofibromas. The vagus and the cervical sympathetic trunk are the most commonly involved nerves. Most are asymptomatic and present as a mass in the neck.

Neurilemmomas

Neurilemmomas are the most common neurogenic tumour arising in the parapharyngeal space. They are solitary, slow-growing, well-encapsulated tumours that are almost never associated with von Reklinghausen's neurofibromatosis (NF1). The associated nerve fibres are draped over the lesion and can be dissected from the nerve at surgery. Pain and neurological dysfunction are unusual but patients may experience paraesthesia. They very rarely if ever turn malignant.

Neurofibromas

Neurofibromas are not encapsulated and nerve fibres run through the tumour making it difficult to dissect them from the nerve of origin without sacrificing fibres. These lesions are associated with NF1 and are usually multiple and subcutaneous but can be found in the parapharyngeal space. Sarcomatous change occurs in about 6–10% of lesions in patients with NF1 and is usually indicated by sudden growth or recurrence of the tumour after resection. Malignant neurofibrosarcomas invade adjacent tissues and may metastasize.

Symptoms and signs

Tumours of the parapharyngeal space give rise to symptoms and signs due to pressure on surrounding structures (Table 19.3). Owing to the location of these tumours the onset of symptoms is often insidious and may be quite subtle. Tumours must be at least 3 cm in size before they are clinically detectable.[3]

Most lesions in the parapharyngeal space present as a painless mass in the anterior neck near the angle of the mandible although in some there may be a little local or radiating tenderness (Figure 19.2). Medial displacement of the tonsil and soft palate may cause partial upper airway obstruction with snoring, obstructive sleep apnoea, dysphagia or dysarthria as the presenting symptoms (Figure 19.3). Paragangliomas and other vascular lesions may be pulsatile with audible bruits or present with pulsatile tinnitus due to the noise of turbulent vascular flow. Lesions of neural origin or glomus vagale may present with single or multiple cranial nerve palsies (IX–XII), particularly hoarseness and a vocal cord palsy or a Horner's syndrome. Large tumours may cause Eustachian tube dysfunction and otitis media with effusion. Malignancy should be suspected with symptoms of pain, trismus, and cranial nerve neuropathies particularly in the presence of a small mass.[11]

A complete examination of the head, neck and upper aerodigestive tract is required with particular attention to the function of the facial nerve, presence of bruits, and the integrity of cranial nerves IX–XII. Bimanual palpation of the oropharynx should be

Table 19.3 Presenting symptoms and signs of parapharyngeal space tumours[2]

Symptoms	Frequency (%)
Intraoral/neck mass	85
Ear pressure or pain	36
Dysphagia	13
Hearing loss	11
Hoarseness	10
Facial or jaw pain	6
Facial nerve weakness, throat pain, pulsatile tinnitus, tongue paraesthesia, aspiration, headache, hypertension, syncope	< 5
Signs	
Intraoral displacement of tonsil/soft palate	65
Neck mass (11% pulsatile)	58
Vocal cord paralysis/paresis	8
Hearing loss/ OME	9
Palatal paralysis	5
Atrophic or fasiculating tongue	5
Horner's syndrome	2
Trismus	2

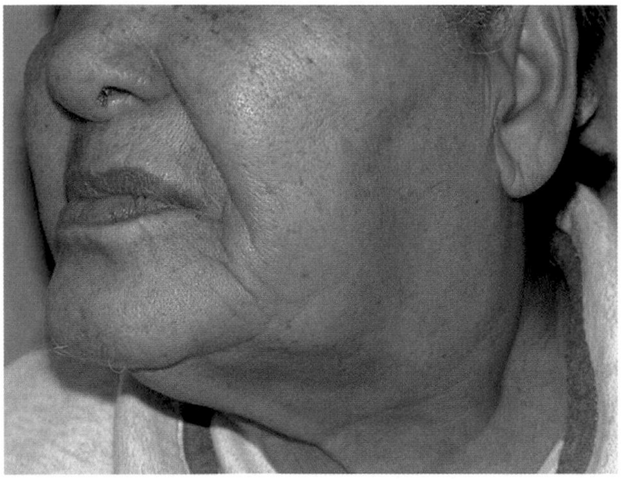

Figure 19.2 Patient with a left-sided neck mass, carotid body tumour.

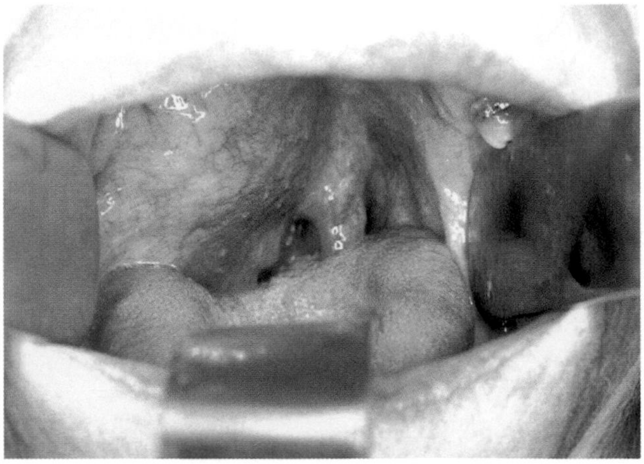

Figure 19.3 Intraoral view of a parapharyngeal tumour pushing the lateral wall of the pharynx medially (deep-lobe parotid tumour).

carried out when possible to determine the mobility and consistency of the tumour mass as well as to determine whether there is significant tenderness or a pulsatile nature to the neoplasm.

Investigation

All patients with a mass in the parapharyngeal space require either a computerized tomography (CT) scan or magnetic resonance imaging (MRI) of the neck to determine the size of the tumour and its relationship to surrounding structures. Tumours found in the prestyloid space rarely need further investigation as almost all arise from the deep-lobe of the parotid or minor salivary glands. Those arising in the post-styloid space often require angiography to help differentiate paraganglial from neural lesions and determine the vascularity of the tumour. Fine-needle aspiration (FNA) may be a valuable adjunct to these investigations while incisional biopsy is to be discouraged due to seeding of some tumours and possible massive uncontrolled bleeding.

Radiology

It is generally acknowledged that MRI is superior to CT in the evaluation of parapharyngeal space lesions. It gives a clear picture of normal structures including major vessels and their relationship to the tumour. MRI may also give some indication of the nature of the pathology and the margin of tumour can be more precisely assessed.[11] The only significant disadvantage with MRI is the lack of information about bone erosion at the skull base and in some patients where skull base involvement is suspected, CT may be necessary.

The pathology of the tumour may be evident from its inherent appearance on MRI and the way it displaces the carotid sheath and parapharyngeal fat. T1-weighted images are best for examining normal anatomy and tumour–fat interfaces while T2-weighted images are best for looking at tumour margins and the tumour–muscle interface. Prestyloid lesions tend to push the carotid posteriorly and the parapharyngeal fat medially and posteriorly (Figures 19.4 and 19.5). Deep-lobe parotid tumours in this area have a homogeneous appearance with a moderate to high signal on T2-weighted images. Minor salivary gland tumours and ectopic salivary tissue can be differentiated from deep-lobe tumours as the fat plane is preserved between the deep-lobe of the parotid and the tumour. Poststyloid lesions push the carotid anteriorly and the parapharyngeal fat pad anteriorly and laterally (Figures 19.6 and 19.7). Paragangliomas arising from the carotid body tend to splay apart the internal and external carotid artery and have a salt and pepper appearance due to vascular flow voids. Schwannomas and neurofibromas

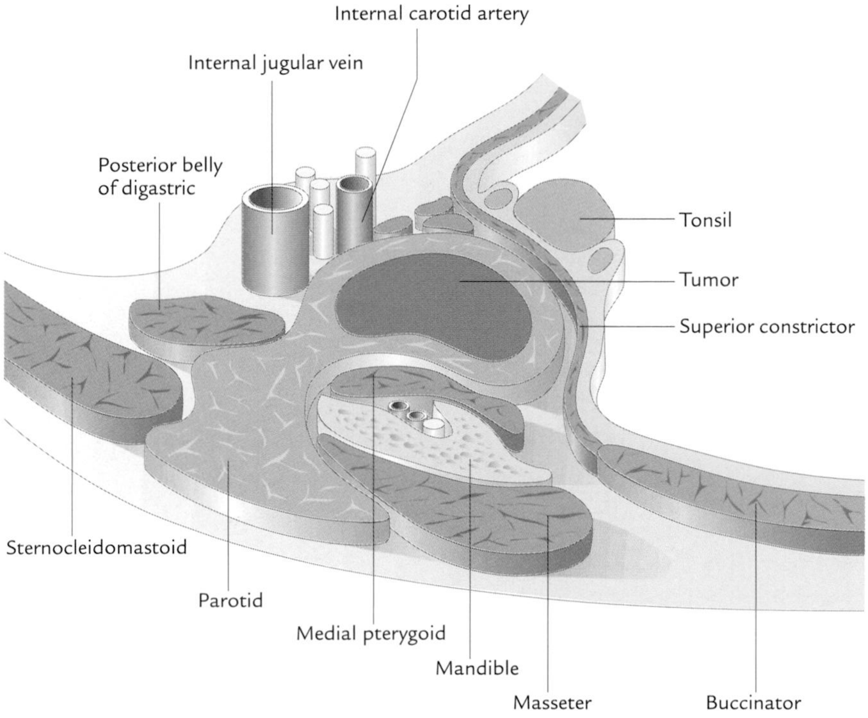

Figure 19.4 Location of a prestyloid, deep-lobe parotid tumour in relation to other structures in the neck.

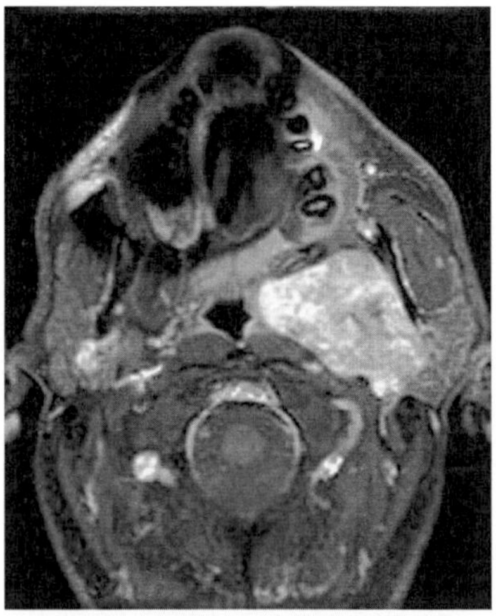

Figure 19.5 MRI of a deep-lobe parotid tumour.

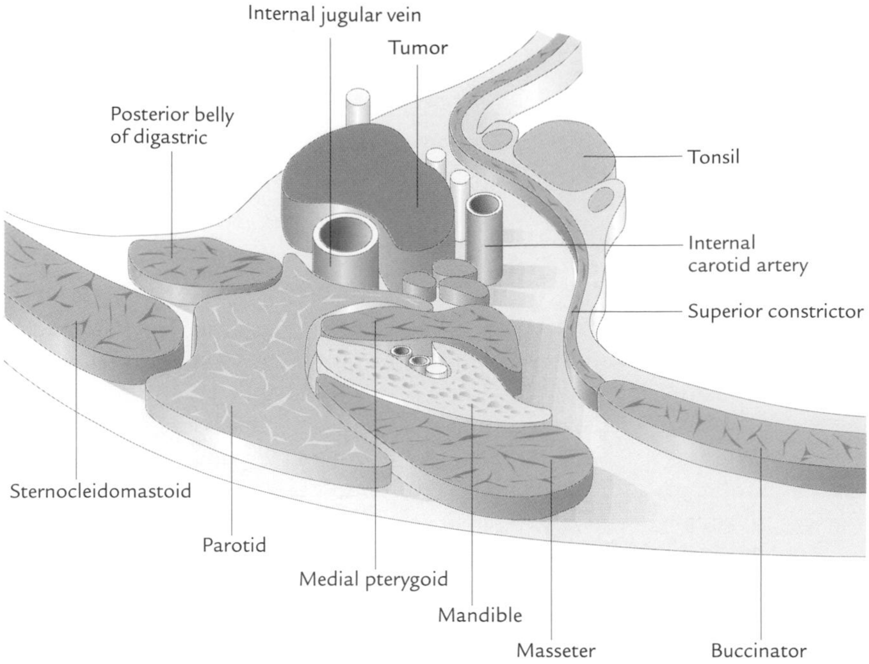

Figure 19.6 Location of a poststyloid, vagal neurilemmoma, in relation to other structures in the neck.

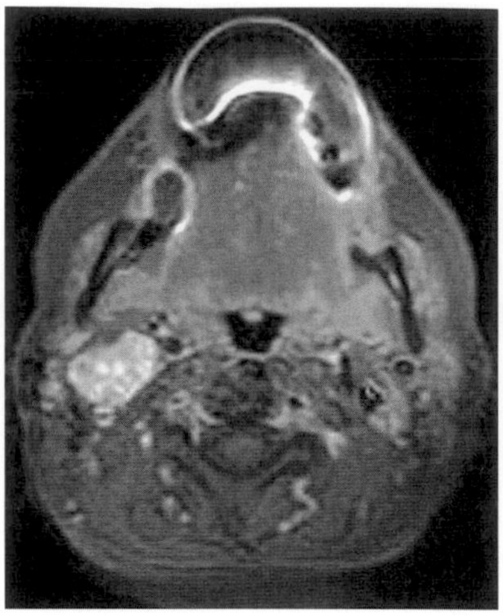

Figure 19.7 MRI of a vagal neurilemmoma.

tend to have a more homogeneous appearance with moderate to high signal on T2-weighted images. Lymph nodes have a characteristic radiological appearance. Malignancy should be suspected when there is loss of the normal tissue planes, invasion of the muscle or replacement of the normal increased fat signal of the bone marrow and skull base on T1 images by lower density tumour signal.[11]

Angiography

Angiography of all lesions suspected to be a paraganglioma in the poststyloid space is necessary to confirm the diagnosis, determine the vascularity of the tumour and examine their relationship to the great vessels of the neck. Carotid body paragangliomas splay the internal and external carotid artery apart producing the so called 'lyre' sign on angiography (Figure 19.8) while glomus vagale are found more superiorly and tend to displace the carotid artery anteriorly. Angiography in patients with paragangliomas will identify major feeding vessels for possible embolization or ligation and pick up other clinically silent vascular lesions in the neck. It will also pick up an evidence of vessel invasion in patients with malignant parapharyngeal tumours.

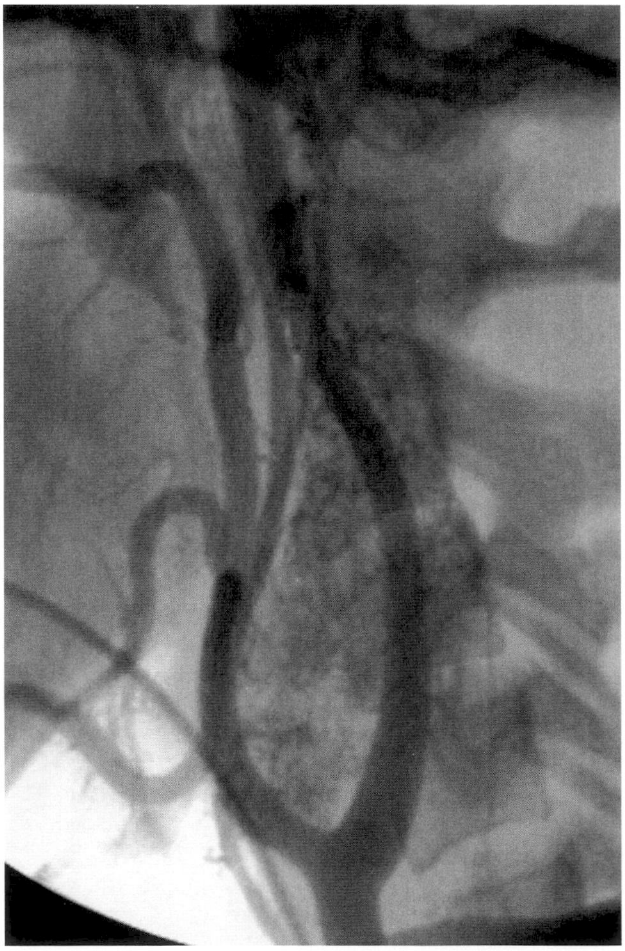

Figure 19.8 Angiogram of a carotid body tumour demonstrating the 'lyre' sign due to splaying of the internal and external carotid artery.

Cytology

Transcervical or transoral FNA cytology will aid in the diagnosis of many parapharyngeal lesions including salivary gland tumours and paragangliomas.[12] Schwannomas are often missed and other diagnoses such as spindle cell neoplasms, granulomatous inflammation or benign lesions may be mistaken.[13] It has been suggested that FNA cytology adds little to the management of parapharyngeal neoplasms as radiological investigations usually give an indication of the likely pathology.

Special investigations

Head and neck paragangliomas rarely secrete catecholamines but it is generally recommended that when the diagnosis is suspected 24-hour urinary catecholamine levels should be taken.[3,14] This is particularly important in patients with multicentric lesions, a family history of paraganglioma or with symptoms of hypertension, palpitations, flushing, tachycardia, nervousness, excessive sweating, nauseas, diarrhoea or fatigue.

There is some debate as to the best method of detecting multiple tumours in patients with paragangliomas, particularly in patients with a familial history. MRI or CT are the gold standard but usually limited to sites of clinical suspicion such as the neck and adrenals.^{111}Indium pentetreotide scans will detect paragangliomas all over the body and it has been suggested that this is a better screening tool as it is very sensitive and safe. Suspected lesions are then followed up with MRI.[15]

Management

There is general consensus in the literature that salivary gland tumours, neurilemmomas and neurofibromas should be treated surgically with postoperative radiation reserved for cases with malignant pathology.[1] The surgical approach to these tumours is discussed below. The management of paragangliomas however is more controversial as both radiation and surgery are effective.

Radiation targets the vascular stroma of paragangliomas rather than the paraganglial cells themselves, which are radioresistant. Using a regimen of 45–50 Gy in 25 fractions over 4 weeks responses range from prevention of further growth to complete resolution of the tumour with minimal morbidity (Table 19.4).[16] Under 10% of tumours fail to respond and growth of the tumour can be controlled in at least 75% aged over a 20-year period.[17] The main concern, particularly in younger patients, is the induction of second primary tumours in the long term.

Surgery is generally safe for patients with small- to moderate-sized tumours. Major neurovascular complications and mortality are low and long-term control rates high (Table 19.5). Current literature generally advocates surgery for small to moderate size paragangliomas, particularly in younger patients, or those causing compressive symptoms. Radiation is generally reserved for older patients or those with high-risk lesions where the risk of complications from surgery is unacceptably high. Radiation is also recommended for residual or recurrent tumour after surgery and for patients with multiple paragangliomas where there is a risk of causing multiple cranial nerve palsies.[1] A period of observation can also be considered in the elderly and high-risk patients, particularly those with multiple tumours. However many of these lesions eventually grow and cause significant symptoms, although not affecting long-term survival.[30]

Surgical approaches

Transoral

The transoral approach, although direct and advocated by some in the past for small salivary gland tumours of the parapharyngeal space, allows

Table 19.4 Results of radiation for paragangliomas of the head and neck, carotid body tumours and glomus vagale

Reference	Year	Number of patients	Significant complications (%)	Local control (%)	Follow-up (years)
Mitchell and Clyne[18]	1985	11	0	100	7 (median)
Mumber and Greven[19]	1995	15	0	100	11 (median)
Valdagni and Amichetti[20]	1990	7	0	100	1–19
Verniers et al[21]	1992	22	0	100	10 (median)
Cole and Beiler[16]	1994	30	0	97	3–27
Hinerman et al[22]	2001	18	0	96	9 (median)

Table 19.5 Results of surgery for paragangliomas, carotid body tumours (CBT) and glomus vagale (GV)

Reference	Year	Number of patients	Cranial nerve palsies (%)	CVA (%)	Local control (%)	Follow-up (years)
Nora et al (CBT)[23]	1988	52	21	10	94	2–21
McPherson et al (CBT + GV)[24]	1989	25	22	0	96	3 (median)
Williams et al (CBT)[25]	1992	30	13	3	100	—
Hodge et al (CBT + GV)[26]	1988	17	47	0	100	5 (minimum)
Biller et al (GV)[8]	1989	18	100	0	89	1–16
Kraus et al (CBT)[27]	1990	14	29	0	100	3 (mean)
Powell et al (CBT + GV)[17]	1992	13	64	0	54	9 (median)
Netterville et al (CBT)[28]	1995	25	12	0	100	1–9
Netterville et al (GV)[29]	1998	39	100	3	100	1–12
Urquhart et al (GV)[9]	1994	16	31	0	100	2–12

no control of major vessels and results in an unacceptably high level of seeding and recurrence. For this reason it can no longer be recommended.

Transcervical

The transcervical route gains access to the parapharyngeal space through the lateral neck. It is ideal for small- to moderate-sized poststyloid lesions such as paragangliomas and nerve sheath tumours that do not abut the skull base as there is limited exposure superiorly and vascular control at the skull base is difficult to establish. After lifting subplatysmal flaps the marginal mandibular division of the facial nerve should be identified and preserved and control of major vessels established proximally and distally. The submandibular gland can be removed or preserved. The digastric tendon and stylomandibular ligament may be divided and the mandible dislocated anteromedially to provide more superior access. Subadventitial dissection of paragangliomas is recommended to avoid excessive bleeding while taking care to avoid rupturing the carotid artery. Neurilemmomas may be shelled out from their capsule.

Transparotid-cervical

The transparotid-cervical approach is similar to above but the superficial lobe of the parotid is removed prior to resection of the tumour (Figure 19.9). This approach is best suited to deep-lobe parotid lesions that extend into the neck and the parapharyngeal space. The facial nerve is then dissected off the deep-lobe of the parotid and mobilized to allow access to the parapharyngeal space. Again the submandibular gland can be retracted or removed and the stylomandibular ligament divided and the mandible dislocated anteriorly to provide more access to the parapharyngeal

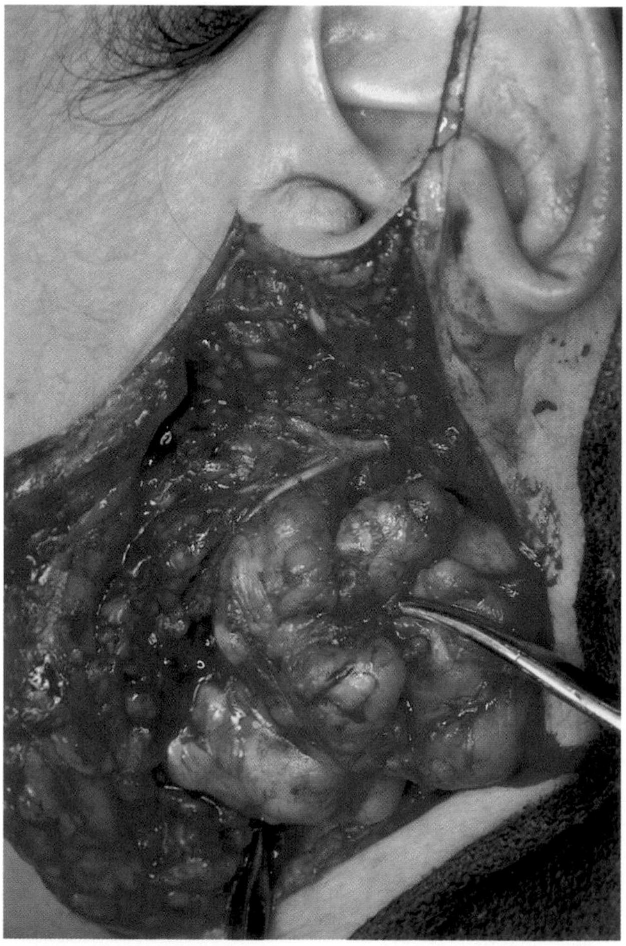

Figure 19.9 Transparotid transcervical approach to a deep-lobe parotid tumour.

space. For particularly large tumours an osteotomy can be performed at the angle of the mandible just proximal to the inferior alveolar nerve, protecting the neurovascular supply to the mandible. This manoeuvre provides additional access to the superior aspect of the parapharyngeal space. The skull base itself, however, is still not fully exposed with an angle mandibulotomy alone.

Transparotid/cervical with midline mandibulotomy

Greatly improved exposure for both of the above approaches may be gained by performing a midline mandibulotomy and retracting the mandible laterally (Figure 19.10). This is recommended for larger (> 10 cm) or recurrent tumours and those which are vascular, malignant or where carotid artery exposure at the skull base is required. For this approach, a tracheostomy is required to prevent postoperative airway obstruction from pharyngeal oedema. A midline mandibulotomy is made and the intraoral mucosa is divided along the lateral gutter between the alveolus and the tongue, taking care to identify and preserve the hypoglossal and lingual nerves. The parapharyngeal space is widely exposed and the lateral skull base can be accessed. Deep and superiorly based parapharyngeal masses can be removed.

Infratemporal fossa approaches

For lesions extending into the jugular foramen and lateral skull base such as glomus vagale an infratemporal fossa approach is required (Fisch type A). It involves extending the transparotid-cervical dissection to include a radical mastoidectomy and transposition of the facial nerve anteriorly after carefully dissecting it from its bony canal. The skin of the bony ear canal with the tympanic membrane is removed and the ear canal closed into a blind pouch. The jugular bulb and the internal carotid artery in the temporal bone can be drilled out providing distal access to the great vessels. With this exposure a tumour in the superior parapharyngeal space and the lateral skull base is readily accessed and removed. The Eustachian tube is packed off with fat, fascia and bone dust and the facial nerve repositioned at the end of the procedure. For those tumours with intracranial extension a suboccipital craniotomy will provide access to the intracranial portion of the tumour.

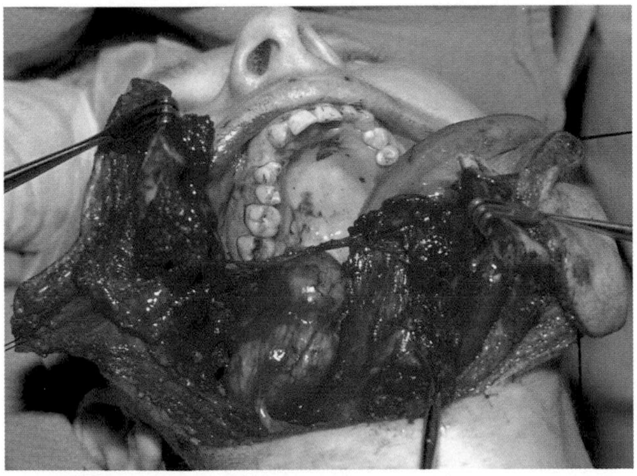

Figure 19.10 Transcervical approach with midline mandibulotomy for a large vagal neurilemmoma.

Preoperative embolization

Preoperative embolization of paragangliomas prior to surgery is thought to reduce blood loss and facilitate surgery but a recent study in patients with 4–5-cm tumours did not demonstrate any significant difference in blood loss, transfusion requirement, operative time or perioperative morbidity.[31] There is a small risk of cerebrovascular event during embolization and it should be performed within 24 hours of surgery to avoid the development of an inflammatory response.

Resection and replacement of the carotid artery

In a few patients with large vascular tumours or those invading the major vessels of the neck, resection and replacement of the common or internal carotid artery may be needed. Preoperative balloon occlusion testing and stable xenon-enhanced CT cerebral blood flow measurements will give an indication of the risk this poses to the patient and can significantly alter management.[32]

Complications of surgery

Neurovascular morbidity is the commonest complication of surgery in the parapharyngeal space. Cranial nerve palsies occur postoperatively in 20–60% of patients, some due to traction or devascularization of the nerve, others due to deliberate sacrifice of an involved nerve.[24] Cranial nerves VII, IX–XII and the sympathetic chain are at risk depending upon preoperative neural involvement by tumour, the location of the lesion, and the surgical approach. Unilateral vagal palsies are the commonest problem and occur in almost all patients with glomus vagale.[8,9] They can present with any combination of dysphonia, dysphagia or aspiration. Rehabilitation of the voice should wait until compensation from the other cord has occurred unless aspiration is a major problem. Gastrostomy feeding may be indicated prior to compensation. Resection of neurilemmomas involving the cervical sympathetic trunk may result in Horners' syndrome. Most patients can tolerate a single cranial nerve palsy but multiple palsies are often disabling. Intimal damage to the common or internal carotid artery may result in a cerebrovascular accident and vascular damage at the time of surgery may require ligation of the internal or common carotid artery. Patients having surgery of the parapharyngeal space must be counselled about the risk of neurovascular damage, which is expected in a proportion of patients.

REFERENCES

1. Carrau RL, Myers EN, Johnson JT. Management of tumors arising in the parapharyngeal space. *Laryngoscope* 1990; **100**: 583–589.
2. Hughes KV III, Olsen KD, McCaffrey TV. Parapharyngeal space neoplasms. *Head Neck* 1995; **17**: 124–130.
3. Olsen KD. Tumors and surgery of the parapharyngeal space. *Laryngoscope* 1994; **104** (Suppl 63): 1–28.
4. Batsakis JG. Deep-lobe parotid gland tumors. *Ann Otol Rhinol Laryngol* 1984; **93**: 415–416.
5. Grufferman S, Gillman MW, Pasternak LR et al. Familial carotid body tumors: case report and epidemiologic review. *Cancer* 1980; **46**: 2116–2122.
6. McCaffrey TV, Meyer FB, Michels VV et al. Familial paragangliomas of the head and neck. *Arch Otolaryngol Head Neck Surg* 1994; **120**: 1211–1216.
7. Rodriguez-Cuevas S, Lopez-Garza J, Labastida-Almendaro S. Carotid body tumors in inhabitants of altitudes higher than 2000 meters above sea level. *Head Neck* 1998; **20**: 374–378.
8. Biller HF, Lawson W, Som P, Rosenfeld R. Glomus vagale tumors. *Ann Otol Rhinol Laryngol* 1989; **98**: 21–26.
9. Urquhart AC, Johnson JT, Myers EN, Schechter GL. Glomus vagale: paraganglioma of the vagus nerve. *Laryngoscope* 1994; **104**: 440–445.
10. Hamza A, Fagan JJ, Weissman JL, Myers EN. Neurilemmomas of the parapharyngeal space. *Arch Otolaryngol Head Neck Surg* 1997; **123**: 622–626.
11. Miller FR, Wanamaker JR, Lavertu P, Wood BG. Magnetic resonance imaging and the management of parapharyngeal space tumors. *Head Neck* 1996; **18**: 67–77.
12. Rana RS, Dey P, Das A. Fine needle aspiration (FNA) cytology of extra-adrenal paragangliomas. *Cytopathology* 1997; **8**: 108–113.
13. Yu GH, Sack MJ, Baloch Z, Gupta PK. Difficulties in the fine needle aspiration (FNA) diagnosis of schwannoma. *Cytopathology* 1999; **10**: 186–194.
14. Pensak ML, Gluckman JL, Shumrick KA. Parapharyngeal space tumors: an algorithm for evaluation and management. *Laryngoscope* 1994; **104**: 1170–1173.
15. Myssiorek D. Cervical sympathetic schwannoma. *Otolaryngol Head Neck Surg* 1998; **119**: 150.
16. Cole JM, Beiler D. Long-term results of treatment for glomus jugulare and glomus vagale tumors with radiotherapy. *Laryngoscope* 1994; **104**: 1461–1465.
17. Powell S, Peters N, Harmer C. Chemodectoma of the head and neck: results of treatment in 84 patients. *Int J Radiat Oncol Biol Phys* 1992; **22**: 919–924.
18. Mitchell DC, Clyne CA. Chemodectomas of the neck: the response to radiotherapy. *Br J Surg* 1985; **72**: 903–905.
19. Mumber MP, Greven KM. Control of advanced chemodectomas of the head and neck with irradiation. *Am J Clin Oncol* 1995; **18**: 389–391.
20. Valdagni R, Amichetti M. Radiation therapy of carotid body tumors. *Am J Clin Oncol* 1990; **13**: 45–48.
21. Verniers DA, Keus RB, Schouwenburg PF, Bartelink H. Radiation therapy, an important mode of treatment for head and neck chemodectomas. *Eur J Cancer* 1992; **28A**: 1028–1033.
22. Hinerman RW, Mendenhall WM, Amdur RJ et al. Definitive radiotherapy in the management of chemodectomas arising in the temporal bone, carotid body, and glomus vagale. *Head Neck* 2001; **23**: 363–371.
23. Nora JD, Hallett JW Jr, O'Brien PC et al. Surgical resection of carotid body tumors: long-term survival, recurrence, and metastasis. *Mayo Clin Proc* 1988; **63**: 348–352.
24. McPherson GA, Halliday AW, Mansfield AO. Carotid body tumours and other cervical paragangliomas: diagnosis and management in 25 patients. *Br J Surg* 1989; **76**: 33–36.
25. Williams MD, Phillips MJ, Nelson WR, Rainer WG. Carotid body tumor. *Arch Surg* 1992; **127**: 963–967; discussion 967–968.
26. Hodge KM, Byers RM, Peters LJ. Paragangliomas of the head and neck. *Arch Otolaryngol Head Neck Surg* 1988; **114**: 872–877.
27. Kraus DH, Sterman BM, Hakaim AG et al. Carotid body tumors. *Arch Otolaryngol Head Neck Surg* 1990; **116**: 1384–1387.
28. Netterville JL, Reilly KM, Robertson D et al. Carotid body tumors: a review of 30 patients with 46 tumors. *Laryngoscope* 1995; **105**: 115–126.
29. Netterville JL, Jackson CG, Miller FR et al. Vagal paraganglioma: a review of 46 patients treated during a 20-year period. *Arch Otolaryngol Head Neck Surg* 1998; **124**: 1133–1140.
30. van der Mey AG, Frijns JH, Cornelisse CJ et al. Does intervention improve the natural course of glomus tumors? A series of 108 patients seen in a 32-year period. *Ann Otol Rhinol Laryngol* 1992; **101**: 635–642.
31. Litle VR, Reilly LM, Ramos TK. Preoperative embolization of carotid body tumors: when is it appropriate? *Ann Vasc Surg* 1996; **10**: 464–468.
32. de Vries EJ, Sekhar LN, Horton JA et al. A new method to predict safe resection of the internal carotid artery. *Laryngoscope* 1990; **100**: 85–88.

20 Salivary gland neoplasms

Jeffrey D Spiro and Ronald H Spiro

Introduction

The major and minor salivary glands of the head and neck are the site of a diverse group of both benign and malignant neoplasms. Because of the low incidence, large number of different histologic subtypes, variety of potential sites, and the need for extended follow-up, an individual clinician is unlikely to accumulate significant personal experience with most types of salivary neoplasms. In this chapter, the aetiology, incidence, pathology and presentation of salivary tumours will first be reviewed. Treatment options and results will then be discussed, in an effort to provide insight into these varied and challenging neoplasms.

Anatomic considerations

Parotid gland

The paired parotid glands are located in close proximity to the cartilage of the external auditory canal, which lies posterior to the parenchyma of the gland. Anteriorly the gland abuts both the lateral and posterior border of the ramus of the mandible and the overlying masseter muscle, while inferiorly it rests medially on the posterior belly of the digastric muscle, as well as the sternomastoid muscle laterally. Medially the parotid is adjacent to the parapharyngeal space, while superiorly it reaches the arch of the zygoma (Figure 20.1) Accessory parotid tissue is

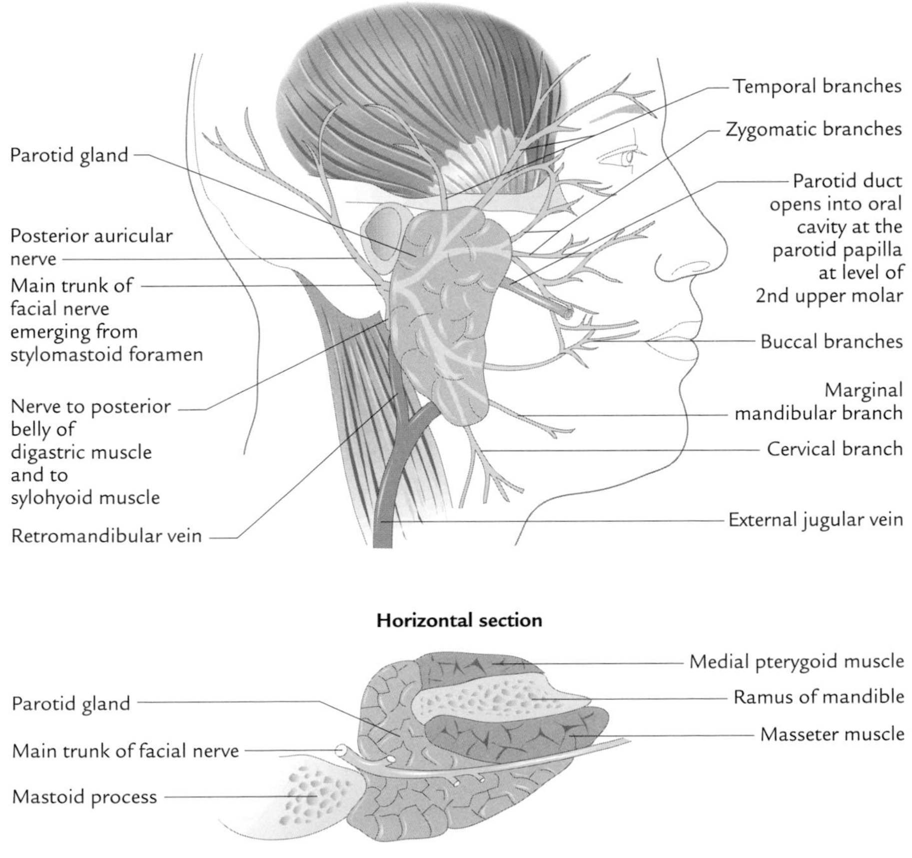

Figure 20.1 Anatomic relations of the parotid gland

usually present anterior to the body of the gland along the course of Stenson's duct.

The facial nerve courses through the parotid gland, where it divides initially into an upper and lower division. The nerve then further divides into its five principal branches, but the exact pattern of arborization varies considerably, and surgeons need to be familiar with these common variations.[1] Although there is no true anatomic separation, the parotid gland is arbitrarily divided into 'superficial' and 'deep' lobes by the plane of the facial nerve.

There are numerous lymph nodes located within, and adjacent to, the capsule of the parotid gland that serve as the first echelon of nodal drainage for the temporal scalp, portions of the cheek, the pinna, and the external auditory canal. For this reason, the parotid gland may harbour metastatic cutaneous malignancy from these sites. Efferent lymphatics from the gland communicate with lymph nodes of the upper and middle deep jugular chain.

Submandibular gland

The paired submandibular glands are located in the anterior triangle of the neck, and are bounded superiorly and laterally by the body of the mandible. The mylohyoid muscle is located anterior to the gland,

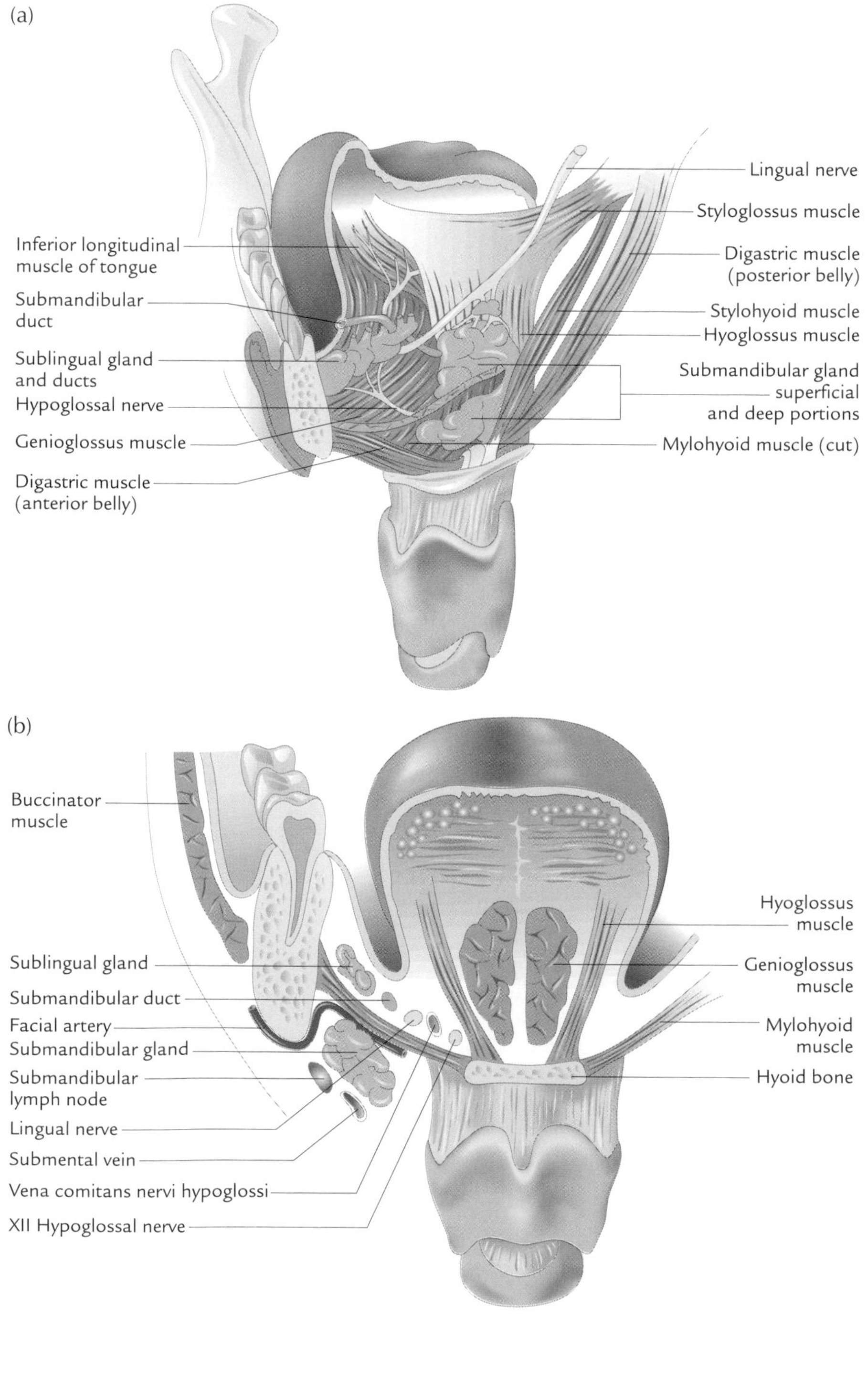

Figure 20.2 (a) and (b) Anatomic relations of the submandibular gland.

while the hyoglossus muscle lies medial to the gland. The platysma muscle overlies the lateral surface of the gland, and the hyoid bone is located inferiorly and medially. The submandibular (Wharton's) duct exits the gland medial to the mylohyoid muscle, then courses anteriorly and superiorly to empty into the anterior floor of mouth.

Several important nerves lie in close proximity to the submandibular gland. The marginal branch of the facial nerve runs just deep to the platysma along the superolateral aspect of the gland. The lingual and hypoglossal nerves are located adjacent to the deep (medial) surface of the gland, while the nerve to the mylohyoid is adjacent to the superior aspect of the gland (Figure 20.2). In addition to being at risk during surgery on the gland, these nerves provide potential pathways for perineural extension of malignant submandibular neoplasms.

Unlike the parotid gland, there are no lymph nodes within the parenchyma of the submandibular gland. There are, however, a number of lymph nodes in close proximity to the gland near the inferior border of the mandible and adjacent to the facial vessels. These nodes are the first echelon of drainage for portions of the lip and oral cavity, as well as facial skin, and drain in turn to the deep jugular chain of nodes. Pathologic enlargement of these nodes may be confused with a tumour of the submandibular gland, and metastatic cancer in these nodes may also involve the adjacent gland by direct extension.

Sublingual glands

Located beneath the mucosa of the floor of the mouth, the small paired sublingual glands drain directly into the oral cavity through numerous small ducts. Tumours arising in the sublingual glands are usually difficult to distinguish from those arising in minor salivary glands located submucosally in the floor of the mouth.

Minor salivary glands

Small submucosal glands are located throughout the upper aerodigestive tract, and may give rise to salivary-type neoplasms in locations such as the larynx, pharynx and paranasal sinuses. These glands are found in highest concentration in the palate. Small rests of heterotopic salivary tissue can also be found within cervical lymph nodes, the mandible, the thyroid gland, and the middle ear and can also give rise to salivary neoplasms in these unusual locations.[2]

Incidence and aetiology

Malignant salivary neoplasms account for about 7% of epithelial cancers of the head and neck in the United States, with an annual incidence of about 1 per 100 000 population.[3] A similar incidence is reported from both the United Kingdom and Denmark.[4,5] Benign salivary neoplasms occur more frequently, but the precise incidence is difficult to quantify as they are obviously not included in cancer registry data.

The site distribution of salivary gland tumours in several large series is summarized in Figure 20.3.[6–8] The majority of salivary neoplasms originate in the parotid gland, while minor salivary gland and submandibular gland neoplasms are much less common. True primary tumours of the sublingual gland are quite unusual.[9] The relative incidence of benign and malignant tumours in these various sites is depicted in Figure 20.4.[6–8,10–15] While most parotid neoplasms are benign, about half of submandibular tumours are malignant, and an even higher proportion

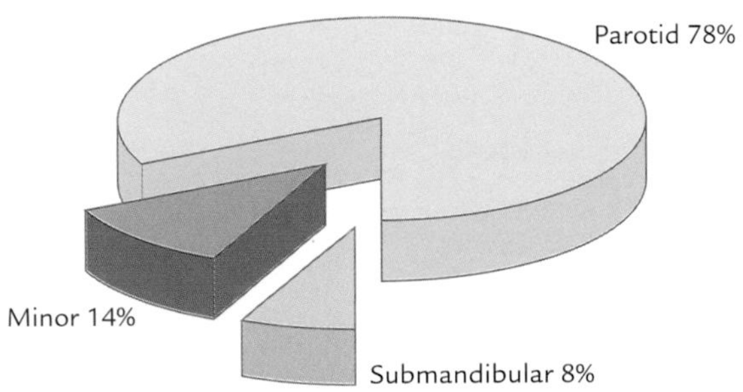

Figure 20.3 Distribution of salivary neoplasms by site (total of 8863 cases).

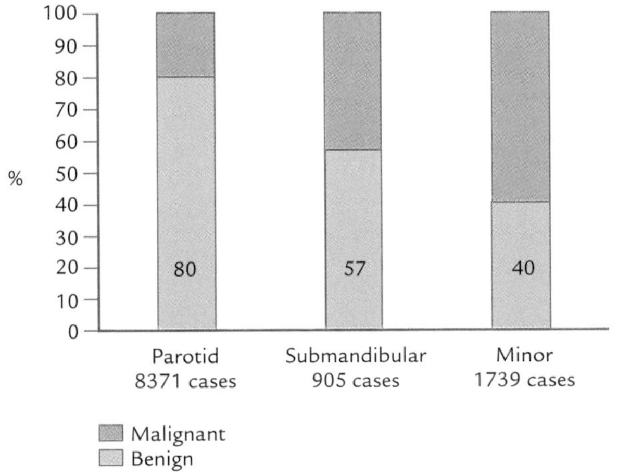

Figure 20.4 Relative proportion of benign versus malignant salivary neoplasms at various primary sites. Numbers under each site are total cases represented per site.

of minor salivary neoplasms will be malignant. In examining the statistics concerning minor salivary tumours, one must consider the site within the upper aerodigestive tract, and the source of the data. Minor salivary tumours encountered outside the oral cavity are far more likely to be malignant, and reports from tertiary referral centres are also more likely to contain a higher proportion of patients with malignant tumours.[13–15] Because the parotid gland is by far the most common site of origin, and a significant majority of parotid tumours are benign, the most common salivary neoplasm typically encountered will be a benign parotid tumour.

In most cases, the aetiology of salivary gland neoplasms remains obscure. There are, however, a number of predisposing factors that have been identified. Exposure to ionizing radiation has been implicated both in survivors of the atomic bomb explosion at Hiroshima and in individuals who received low-dose irradiation to the head and neck in childhood.[16–19] Exposure to wood dust has been associated with an increased incidence of a clear cell variant of adenocarcinoma of the nasal cavity and paranasal sinuses, but it is not clear whether these tumours arise in submucosal glands or respiratory epthelium.[20,21] Genetic factors are suggested by the increased incidence of salivary carcinoma in Eskimo families.[22] One recent report correlates Warthin's tumour with cigarette smoking,[23] while another study associates the use of aromatic amines contained in hair dye with salivary cancer.[24]

Histologic classification

One of the more challenging aspects of salivary neoplasms is their varied histologic appearance. Most centres utilize a classification scheme based on the one originally descibed by Foote and Frazell.[25] The system currently used at Memorial Sloan-Kettering Cancer Center is summarized in Table 20.1.

Table 20.1 Histologic classification of salivary neoplasms

Benign
Pleomorphic adenoma
Warthin's tumour
Lymphoepithelial lesion
Oncocytoma
Monomorphic adenoma
Malignant
Mucoepidermoid carcinoma
Adenoid cystic carcinoma
Adenocarcinoma
Malignant mixed tumour
Acinic cell carcinoma
Epidermoid carcinoma
Anaplastic carcinoma

Pleomorphic adenoma, or benign mixed tumour, is the most common salivary neoplasm overall, and the most frequently encountered benign salivary tumour in all sites. Warthin's tumour, or papillary cystadenoma lymphomatosum, is next in frequency among benign neoplasms. Other benign tumours are uncommon as a group. These include oncocytoma, monomorphic adenoma, and the benign lymphoepithelial lesion of Godwin.[6–8,26,27]

Among malignant tumours, mucoepidermoid carcinoma, adenoid cystic carcinoma, adenocarcinoma, and malignant mixed tumour are most common. Acinic cell carcinoma, primary squamous carcinoma and anaplastic carcinoma are encountered less frequently.[6–8,10–15,26] Different histologic types of salivary cancer are more prevalent in certain salivary sites than in others. The relative incidence of various malignant tumours by salivary site according to pooled data from a number of large reported series is presented in Figure 20.5 for the parotid [4–8,28–34] submandibular[5–8,35–40] and minor salivary glands.[6,8,14,41] Mucoepidermoid carcinoma is the most common malignant parotid neoplasm, while adenoid cystic carcinoma is the most frequently encountered submandibular malignancy. In minor salivary sites, these two types of salivary cancer have a similar incidence, followed closely by adenocarcinoma.

The parotid gland may also be the site of metastases from cutaneous carcinoma arising in areas of the scalp or facial skin which drain to intraparotid lymph nodes. Squamous carcinoma or melanoma arising in these sites accounts for 70–80% of metastases to the parotid gland. While metastases from infraclavicular primary sites to the parotid may also occur, they are much less common.[42–46]

Benign tumours

Pleomorphic adenoma

This neoplasm was formerly known as benign mixed tumour because it contains both epithelial and mesenchymal elements. As noted above, it is the most common salivary neoplasm encountered overall, mainly because of its high incidence in the parotid gland. Pleomorphic adenomas are

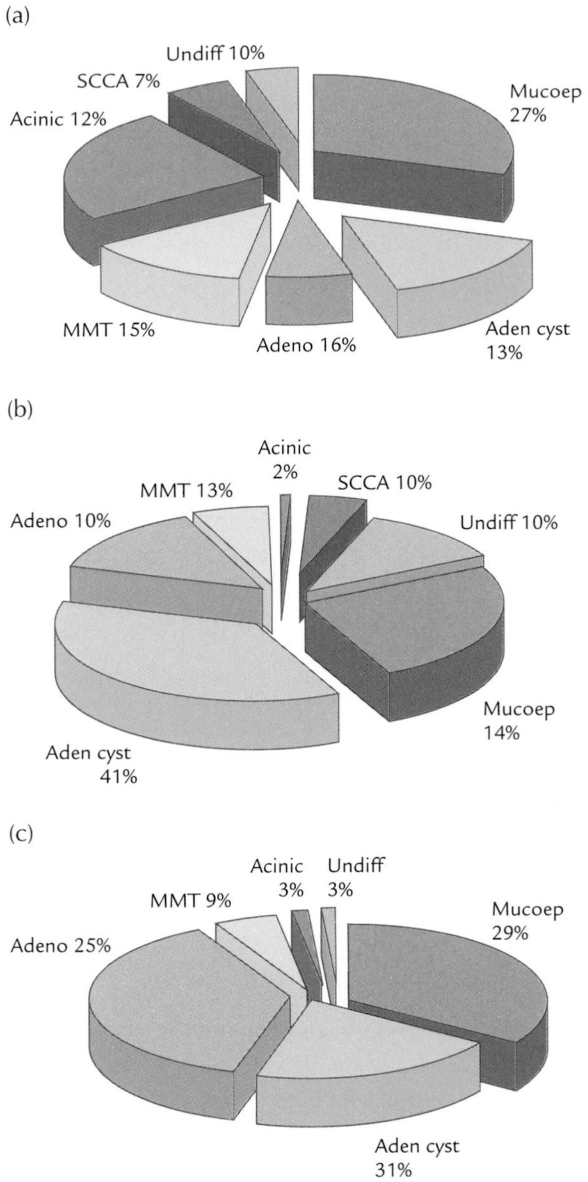

Figure 20.5 (a) Overview of malignant histology for parotid gland (total of 2331 cases). Adeno: adenocarcinoma; Aden cyst: adenoid cystic carcinoma; Mucoep: mucoepidermoid carcinoma; MMT: malignant mixed tumour; Acinic: acinic cell carcinoma; SCCA: squamous carcinoma; Undiff: undifferentiated carcinoma. (b) Overview of malignant histology for submandibular gland (total of 499 cases). (c) Overview of malignant histology for minor salivary sites (total of 1107 cases).

surrounded by a pseudocapsule, beyond which there are numerous microscopic extensions. This is one reason surgeons in the United States have avoided simple enucleation of these tumours, fearing an increase in local recurrence. Such recurrences are typically evident within 5 years of excision, but a significant proportion may occur 10 years or more following excision.[6,47]

Warthin's tumour (papillary cystadenoma lymphomatosum, adenolymphoma)

This tumour is also known as cystadenolymphoma, and is rarely encountered outside the parotid gland, where it is the second most common benign neoplasm. The tendency for this neoplasm to occur in the parotid gland is a direct result of its histologic origin within lymph nodes inside the capsule of the parotid gland. Warthin's tumour tends to occur in the tail of the parotid gland in older male patients, and is also noted to be bilateral in a small but significant number of cases.[48–50]

Oncocytoma

This is a rare benign tumour usually found in the parotid. It occurs in older women and is slow growing, attaining an average size of 3–4 cm. It is almost always solitary.

Monomorphic adenomas

These tumours are similar in clinical presentation to pleomorphic adenomas and usually arise in the parotid gland. There are various types depending on the histological pattern and the cell of origin. The commonest of these is the basal cell adenoma. Monomorphic adenomas usually arise in the lower part of the parotid gland and occur almost exclusively in males with a peak age incidence of 50–70 years.

Malignant tumours

Mucoepidermoid carcinoma

As noted above, mucoepidermoid carcinoma is the most common malignant neoplasm encountered in the parotid gland, and the most prevalent salivary cancer overall. In the past, low-grade lesions with well defined glandular elements were not considered malignant because they metastasize so infrequently. In contrast, high-grade mucoepidermoid carcinoma may be nearly devoid of glandular features under the microscope, rendering it hard to distinguish from primary squamous carcinoma without the use of special stains to identify mucin-producing cells.[51–58] High-grade lesions are aggressive and have a proclivity for regional metastases, with an incidence as high as 70% in one report.[55] Intermediate-grade lesions will display histologic and clinical features between the extremes noted above. The natural history of intermediate- and high-grade mucoepidermoid carcinoma is less protracted than that of many other types of salivary cancer, and 5-year follow-up should be indicative of long-term cure in most cases.

Adenoid cystic carcinoma

This interesting neoplasm is notable for its protracted natural history, and its tendency towards both local recurrence and pulmonary metastases. As previously noted, it is the most common malignant neoplasm of the submandibular gland, and shares this distinction with mucoepidermoid carcinoma in minor salivary sites. If patients with adenoid cystic carcinoma are followed for extended periods, disease-related deaths are noted to occur even 20 or more years after treatment.[59–61] Prolonged survival has also been observed in many patients with documented pulmonary metastases.[62]

Adenoid cystic carcinoma can present a variety of histologic appearances, with solid, tubular and cribriform patterns described. In some centres, a grading system has attempted to correlate these subtypes with outcome, demonstrating a poor prognosis for the solid pattern, and a more favourable outcome for the tubular pattern.[63–66] Other reports, including those from Memorial Hospital, demonstrate that differences in survival based on histologic grading disappear when follow-up exceeds 10 years.[60,68,69] This suggests that histologic grading may correlate with the length of the disease-free interval, but not the ultimate disease outcome in adenoid cystic carcinoma.

Adenocarcinoma

Adenocarcinoma arising in salivary glands may assume a variety of appearances on microscopic examination, including papillary, ductal (resembling breast cancer), and mucinous histologic subtypes.[70,71] In those studies where grading of salivary adenocarcinoma is performed, high-grade lesions are associated with a much worse prognosis than low grade lesions.[70–72] Survival data demonstrate a significant decline from 5 to 10 years after treatment, which indicates the need for adequate long-term follow-up when assessing the results of treatment for this type of salivary cancer.[70–72]

Malignant mixed tumour

This type of malignant salivary neoplasm is distinguished histologically by some features of pleomorphic adenoma in association with a malignant epithelial component, usually adenocarcinoma. There is some controversy as to the origin of these tumours, which are believed to arise either from a pre-existing benign mixed tumour (i.e. carcinoma-ex-pleomorphic adenoma) or to develop de novo.[73–75] As with adenocarcinoma, disease-related deaths may occur 10 or more years after treatment, and adequate long-term follow-up is needed to correctly assess treatment results.[73–75]

Acinic cell carcinoma

This uncommon salivary neoplasm is seldom encountered outside the parotid gland, and is generally associated with fairly indolent behaviour. It is considered a low-grade malignancy, but higher grade variants occur (papillocystic). It has the capability to metastasize or recur locally, particularly if extensive at diagnosis or inadequately treated initially.[76–79]

Clinical presentation and evaluation

Benign or malignant neoplasms of major salivary glands most often present as an asymptomatic swelling of the affected gland.

History

The most common presenting symptom of benign or malignant neoplasms arising in major salivary glands is an asymptomatic swelling. For minor salivary sites, the symptoms will vary according to the location, as summarized in Figure 20.6. Episodic swelling of major salivary glands accompanied by pain and related to salivary stimuli is suggestive of duct obstruction. One study estimates that 80–90%

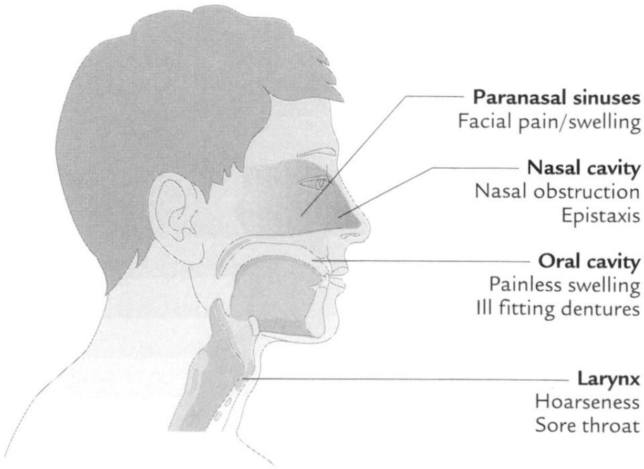

Figure 20.6 Typical symptoms of minor salivary tumours by site.

of submandibular gland enlargement is a result of inflammatory disease.[80]

Pain is reported in 2.5–4% of patients with benign parotid tumours, and 10–29% of patients with parotid cancer.[4,5,32,81,82] The same symptom is reported in a few patients with benign submandibular neoplasms, and up to 50% of patients with malignant submandibular tumours.[11,35–37] Pain is clearly more common with malignant salivary neoplasms, but it is not by itself diagnostic of malignancy. In general, the duration of symptoms tends to be shorter in those patients with malignant tumours. However, it is possible for patients with salivary cancer to present with an asymptomatic swelling that has been present for several years, or even a decade or more.[6] Therefore, the fact that a salivary gland mass has been present for an extended period of time is no guarantee that it is benign.

Physical findings

As previously noted, the location of a salivary mass is an important consideration, as the likelihood of malignancy is directly related to the site of origin. Most benign minor salivary gland tumours arise in the oral cavity, while neoplasms arising in other minor salivary sites are usually malignant.[15] The size of a salivary tumour is important to document. Malignant neoplasms tended to be larger at presentation, but about half of the major salivary cancers treated at Memorial Hospital were 3 cm or less in size at diagnosis.[6]

Although about 10% of parotid gland tumours arise medial to the plane of the facial nerve in the so-called deep 'lobe' of the gland, more than three-fourths of these tumours will present as a typical external parotid mass, similar to typical neoplasms arising lateral to the nerve. The remainder will present with palatal or pharyngeal swelling, with or without a palpable external mass, as depicted in Figure 20.7.[83] Tumours arising in accessory parotid tissue will present as a mass in the cheek, near the anterior border of the masseter muscle and separate from the main body of the parotid gland, similar to Figure 20.8.[84]

Minor salivary tumours will typically present as a submucosal mass, but ulceration of the overlying mucosa is sometimes noted, particularly after trauma from dentures or previous biopsy (Figure 20.9). If locally advanced, patients with lesions arising in the

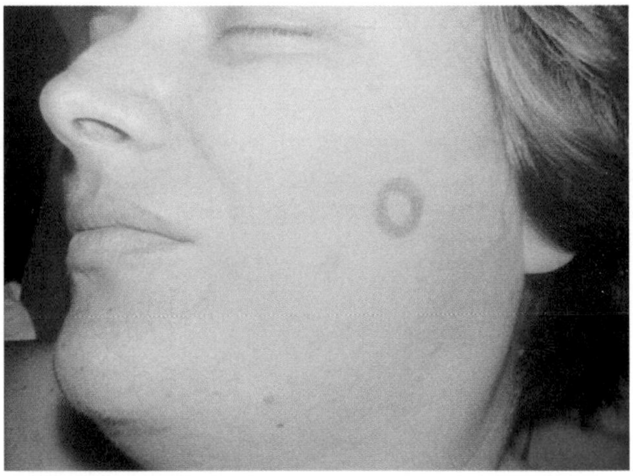

Figure 20.8 Typical location of a tumour arising in accessory parotid tissue anterior to the gland, in this instance an adenoid cystic carcinoma.

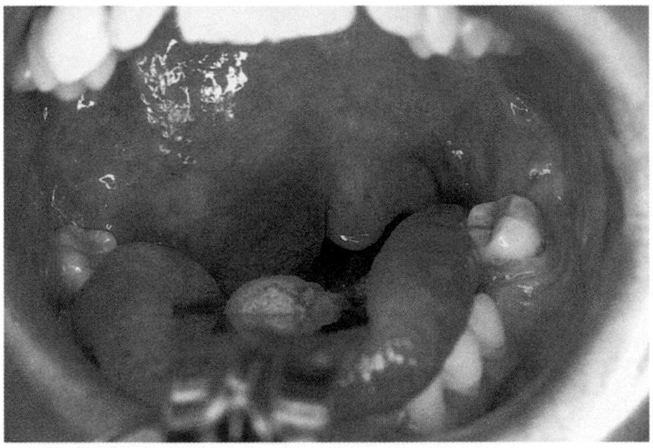

Figure 20.7 Medial displacement of the palate and tonsil seen with deep lobe parotid tumours extending into the parapharyngeal space.

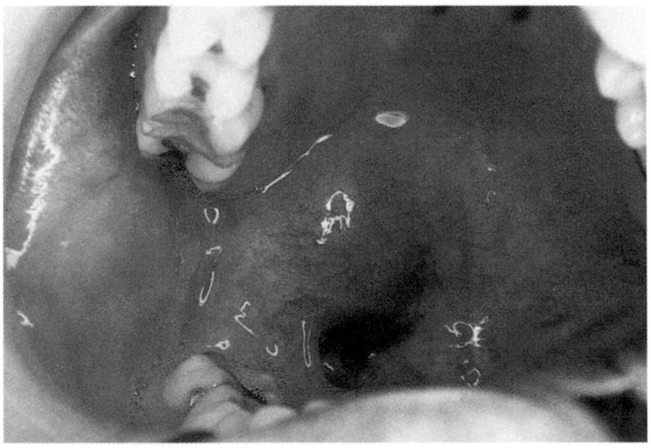

Figure 20.9 Minor salivary tumours usually present as asymptomatic swellings beneath intact mucous membranes. It is not possible clinically to distinguish this low grade mucoepidermoid carcinoma in the right soft palate just posterior to the junction with the hard palate from a benign tumour arising in the same site.

nasal cavity or paranasal sinuses may have facial swelling or displacement of the orbital contents. The true extent of minor salivary neoplasms arising in less accessible sites such as the paranasal sinuses is usually not appreciated on physical examination alone.

There are certain physical findings that help to distinguish benign from malignant major salivary neoplasms, as summarized in Figure 20.10. Fixation of the tumour to either skin or deep structures suggests extension of malignant disease outside the gland with invasion of surrounding tissues. With untreated parotid cancer, fixation to skin was noted in 9% of patients at Memorial Hospital, while fixation to deep tissues was noted in 13% of patients at the MD Anderson Hospital and 17% of patients at Memorial Hospital.[81,85]

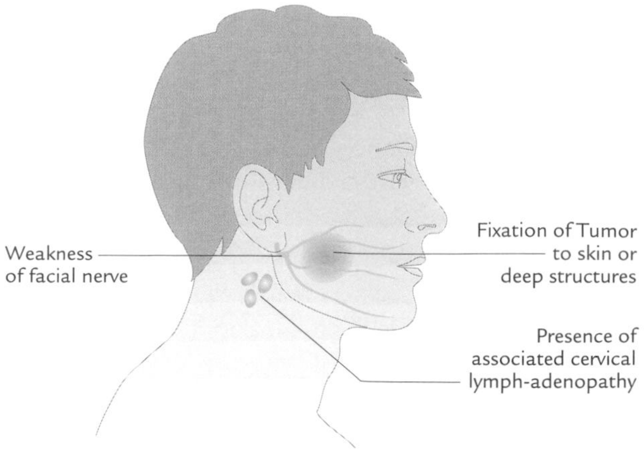

Figure 20.10 Physical findings indicative of malignancy in a major salivary neoplasm.

Weakness or paralysis of the facial nerve in a previously untreated patient almost always indicates that a tumour is malignant. While there are anecdotal reports of facial palsy in association with benign parotid neoplasms, some degree of facial nerve dysfunction has been noted in 9–25% of patients with previously untreated parotid cancer.[4,5,10,81,82,85–87] This finding is usually associated with a poor prognosis, and is most commonly encountered in patients with adenoid cystic carcinoma, undifferentiated carcinoma, and squamous carcinoma.[81,86,87]

The presence of nodal enlargement in association with a salivary tumour is another strong indicator of malignancy. Cervical node metastases are noted at presentation in 13–25% of patients with parotid cancer,[4,31,81,85] and 14–33% of patients with submandibular gland cancer.[35,40,88] In patients with malignant submandibular neoplasms one must be careful to distinguish direct extension to adjacent lymph nodes from actual lymphatic metastases. The histologic subtypes of salivary cancer most likely to metastasize to regional lymph nodes are squamous carcinoma, high-grade mucoepidermoid carcinoma, high-grade adenocarcinoma, and malignant mixed tumour.[32,35,81] In the Memorial Hospital experience with minor salivary cancer, regional node metastases were present initially in 14% of cases.[15]

Diagnostic imaging

Careful history and physical examination are often sufficient to establish the diagnosis and the extent of a tumour in the major salivary glands. If palpation of a major salivary lesion suggests fixation to adjacent structures, diagnostic imaging is indicated to better

(a) (b)

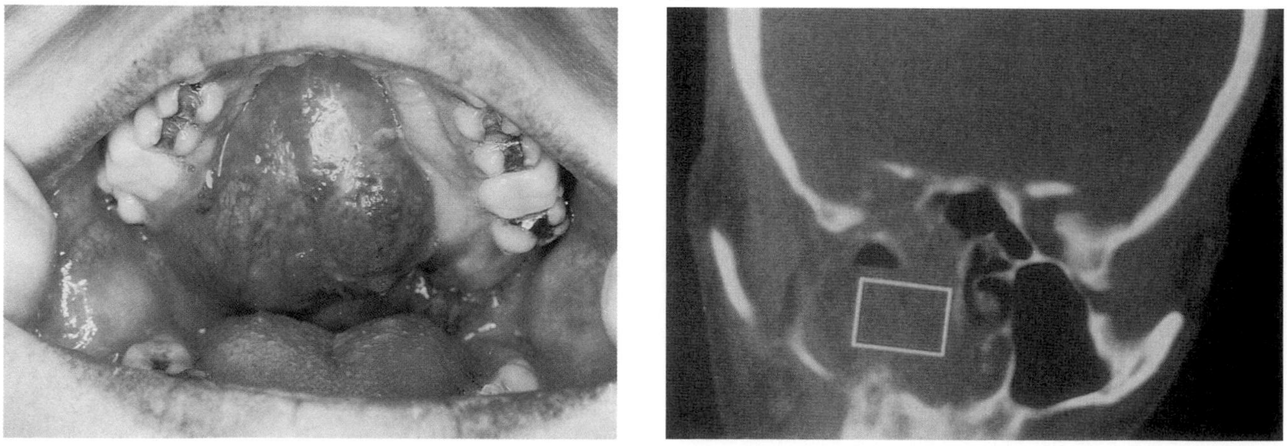

Figure 20.11 (a) Extensive adenoid cystic carcinoma presenting as a mass that replaces the entire palate in a 37-year-old woman. Radiographic imaging is essential in order to appreciate the true extent and origin of this tumour. (b) Coronal CT view shows clinically unsuspected destruction of the skull base and invasion of the anterior cranial fossa by a massive tumour that seems to have originated in the right maxillary antrum.

Table 20.2 AJCC and UICC staging systems for salivary cancer

AJCC staging system

Primary tumour (T)

TX	Primary tumour cannot be assessed
T0	No evidence of primary tumour
T1	Tumour 2 cm or less in greatest dimension
T2	Tumour > 2 cm but not > 4 cm in greatest dimension
T3	Tumour > 4 cm but not > 6 cm in greatest dimension
T4	Tumour > 6 cm in greatest dimension

All T categories are subdivided into:

(a)	No local extension
(b)	Evidence of local extension: invasion of skin, soft tissues, bone or nerve

Regional lymph nodes (N)

NX	Regional nodes cannot be assessed
N0	No regional lymph node metastasis
N1	Metastasis in single node 3 cm or less
N2a	Metastasis in single ipsilateral node > 3 cm but not > 6 cm
N2b	Metastasis in multiple ipsilateral nodes, none > 6 cm
N2c	Metatasis in bilateral or contralateral nodes, none > 6 cm
N3	Metastasis in lymph node > 6 cm

Distant metastasis (M)

MX	Distant metastasis cannot be assessed
M0	No distant metastasis
M1	Distant metastasis

Stage grouping

Stage I	T1a or T2a/N0/M0
Stage II	T1b or T2b or T3a/N0/M0
Stage III	T3b or T4a/N0/M0
	Any T (except T4b)/N1/M0
Stage IV	T4b/any N/M0
	Any T/N2 or N3/M0
	Any T/Any N/M1

UICC staging system

Primary tumour (T)

TX	Primary tumour cannot be assessed
T0	No evidence of primary tumour
T1	Primary tumour 2 cm or less in greatest dimension; no extraparenchymal extension
T2	Primary tumour > 2 cm but not > 4 cm; no extraparenchymal extension
T3	Primary tumour > 4 cm but not > 6 cm and/or extraparenchymal extension without VII nerve involvement
T4	Primary tumour > 6 cm and/or invades base of skull/VII nerve

Regional lymph nodes (N)

NX	Regional lymph nodes cannot be assessed
N0	No regional lymph node metastasis
N1	Metastasis to single ipsilateral node 3 cm or less
N2a	Metastasis to single ipsilateral node > 3 cm but not > 6 cm
N2b	Metatasis to multiple ipsilateral nodes none > 6 cm
N2c	Metastasis to bilateral/contralateral nodes none > 6 cm
N3	Metastasis to node > 6 cm

Distant metastasis (M)

MX	Distant metastasis cannot be assessed
M0	No distant metastasis
M1	Distant metastasis

Stage grouping

Stage I	T1 or T2/N0/M0
Stage II	T3/N0/M0
Stage III	T1 or T2/N1/M0
Stage IV	T4/N0/M0
	T3/N1/ M1
	T4/N1/M0
	Any T/N2 or N3/M0
	Any T/Any N/M1

delineate the extent of disease. Deep-lobe parotid tumours involving the parapharyngeal space and minor salivary tumours arising in the nasal cavity or paranasal sinuses usually require radiographic evaluation to define the full extent of disease (Figure 20.11). As a general guideline, these studies should only be obtained if they will directly impact the management of the patient.

Several imaging modalities may be useful to the clinician when evaluating a salivary gland tumour.[89] In cases of suspected inflammatory disease in the submandibular gland, plain radiographs may demonstrate a calculus in the gland or in Warthin's duct. Computed tomography (CT) scans are best for the evaluation of cortical bone involvement by neoplasms, while magnetic resonance imaging (MRI) better visualizes soft tissue details, as well as medullary bone involvement. In the paranasal sinuses, MRI may also help to distinguish tumour from opacification of an obstructed sinus by fluid.

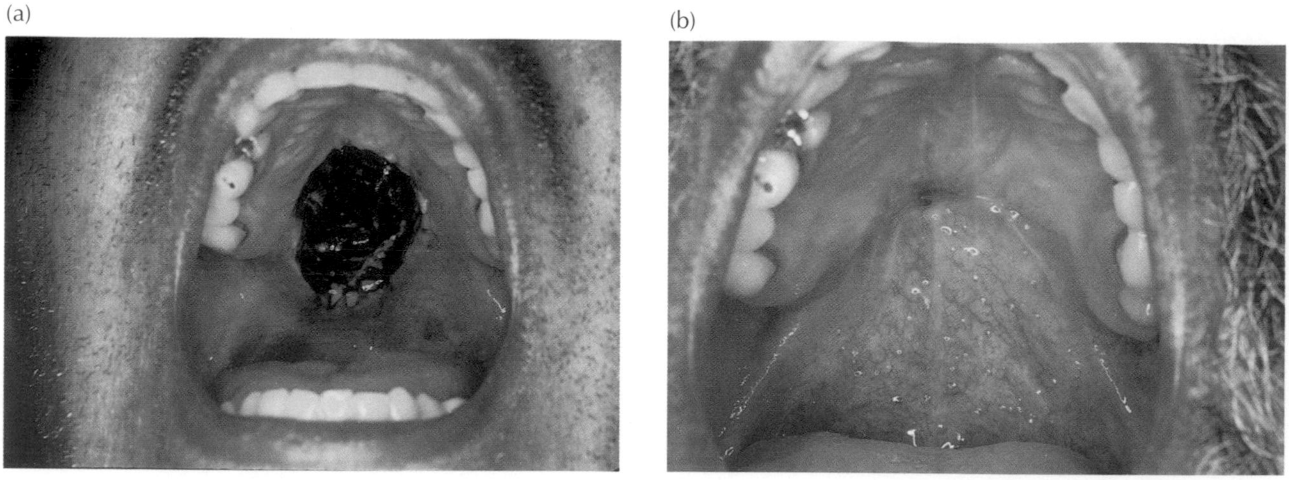

Figure 20.12 (a) Palatal defect remaining after removal of a benign pleomorphic adenoma down to the underlying bone. Wound was packed with xeroform gauze and allowed to heal by secondary intention. (b) Healed palate about 4 months later.

Fine-needle aspiration biopsy

Fine-needle aspiration biopsy (FNABx) provides an opportunity to obtain information about the histology of a salivary tumour prior to the initiation of treatment. In centres with an experienced cytopathologist, the distinction between benign and malignant neoplasms can be made with a high degree of reliability.[90–93] The ability of aspiration cytology to provide an exact diagnosis varies widely between centres, particularly when dealing with a malignant salivary neoplasm.[90–93]

FNABx is not essential for every patient. Those who have small, clinically obvious intraparotid tumours will be effectively treated by conventional subtotal parotidectomy regardless of the histologic diagnosis. Needle biopsy may have its greatest utility in the diagnosis of a submandibular mass, where it can help to distinguish neoplastic from more common inflammatory changes, which may spare the patient unnecessary surgery. Aspiration cytology may also differentiate a reactive lymph node adjacent to a salivary gland from a tumour within the gland itself. Caution must always be exercised in applying the results if the aspiration cytology is inconsistent with the clinical presentation.

Staging

Clinical staging of salivary cancer is essential when comparing treatment results and estimating prognosis. Some years ago, the senior author proposed a staging system for major salivary cancer that incorporated the size of the lesion and the presence or absence of facial nerve palsy or fixation to adjacent structures.[81] The current AJCC and UICC staging systems, while more complex, still utilize these basic elements, as documented in Tables 20.2.[94,95] While there is no separate staging system for minor salivary cancer, a study from Memorial Hospital demonstrated that the staging system used for squamous carcinoma at various primary sites has similar prognostic value for minor salivary cancer arising in the same sites.[96] This approach to minor salivary lesions has been incorporated in the current staging systems for salivary cancer.[94,95]

Treatment: surgery

Surgical resection is the principle form of treatment for both benign and malignant salivary tumours.

Benign lesions

In general, surgical treatment of benign salivary tumours at any site consists of adequate local excision. Resection of minor salivary tumours must be tailored to the specific primary site in question, which is usually the oral cavity in patients with benign tumours (Figure 20.12). Benign neoplasms arising in the submandibular gland can be resected through a simple excision of the gland itself, except in the case of the rare recurrent neoplasm in this location which may require a more extended procedure.

The most common site for a benign salivary neoplasm is the parotid gland. Most surgeons in the United States perform a resection of the superficial 'lobe' of the parotid gland with exposure and preservation of the facial nerve as minimal treatment

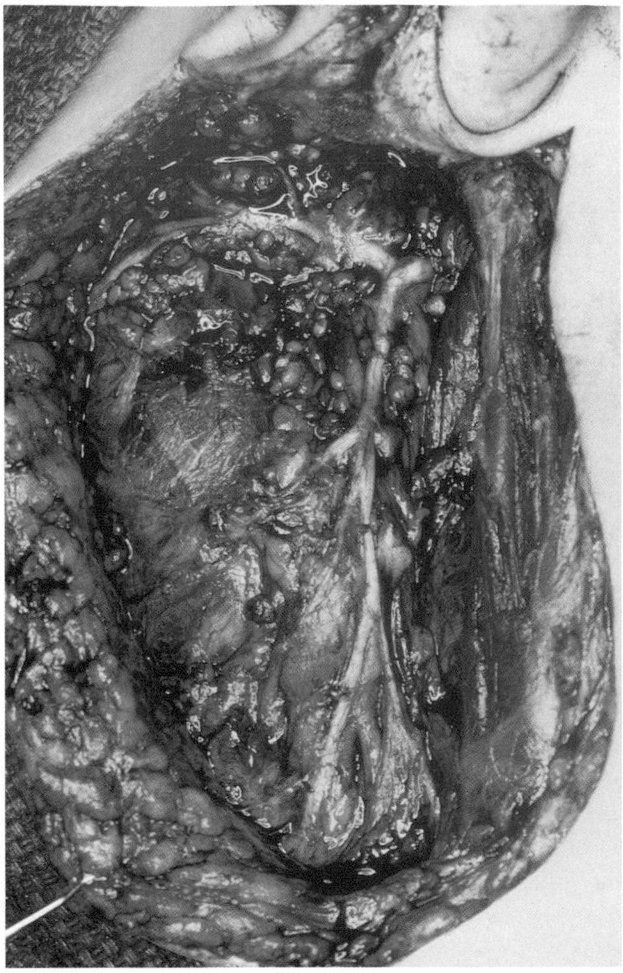

Figure 20.13 Operative field after a conventional subtotal parotidectomy that exposes the facial nerve and removes all of the gland lateral to it.

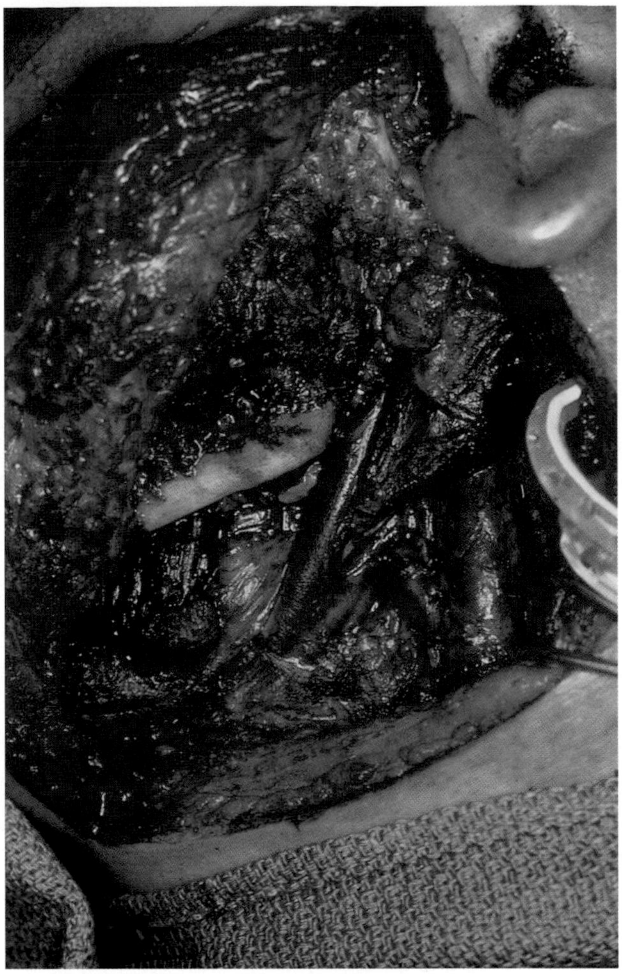

Figure 20.14 Radical parotidectomy performed in conjunction with a supraomohyoid neck dissection for a sizable, high-grade mucoepidermoid carcinoma. The resection has been extended to include the underlying masseter muscle, and the lower division of the facial nerve was included with the specimen. Nerve grafting is always performed if proximal and distal stumps can be identified.

in such cases (Figure 20.13). Surgeons in the United Kingdom have considerable experience with more limited extracapsular dissection of such lesions, which is sometimes followed by postoperative radiotherapy, and report very good results and few complications with these more conservative procedures.[97,98]

When a benign tumour arises in the 'deep' lobe of the parotid gland, initial removal of the 'superficial' lobe with identification and preservation of the facial nerve is usually required. Even sizable lesions in this location can then usually be excised through a transcervical approach, which may be facilitated by excision of the submandibular gland. Other approaches to the parapharyngeal space are described in Chapter 19. Tumours arising in accessory parotid tissue are best excised through a standard parotidectomy flap that is extended anteriorly, rather than an incision directly through the overlying cheek skin. Such an approach permits excision of the main parotid gland if the duct must be resected, and also facilitates identification of the buccal branch of the facial nerve.[84,99]

In cases of recurrent pleomorphic adenoma of the parotid gland, the choice of secondary surgical procedure will depend on the extent of the initial surgery. In patients who have not yet had a formal superficial parotidectomy with nerve dissection, this procedure remains a good option. If the nerve has been previously dissected, subsequent dissection will be technically challenging because of scar tissue, and a higher incidence of nerve dysfunction should be expected. Sacrifice of all, or a portion, of the facial nerve may be necessary if recurrent benign disease is adherent to nerve branches.

Malignant lesions: parotid gland

Surgery remains the mainstay of treatment for cancer of the parotid gland. Excision of the lateral portion of the gland with dissection of the facial nerve is the minimum procedure utilized for early-stage lesions. In the case of a more extensive parotid cancer, the resection may need to be extended to include adjacent structures such as the mandible, zygoma, or temporal bone, as well as some or all of the facial nerve (Figure 20.14). In general, these more extensive 'radical' parotidectomies are associated with a poor outcome.

There has been a trend toward conservatism in the management of the facial nerve in the surgical treatment of malignant parotid tumours, supported by the increasing use of adjuvant irradiation. The incidence of sacrifice of either the entire nerve or a portion thereof varies from 29% to 40% in reported series.[28,30,81,85] Most head and neck surgeons would currently advocate preservation of facial nerve branches unless they are adherent to or directly invaded by the tumour. This approach relies on the use of postoperative radiotherapy to control any microscopic residual disease. If major branches, or the main trunk, of the facial nerve must be sacrificed, immediate cable grafting of the facial nerve should be accomplished utilizing branches of the cervical plexus or the sural nerve.

Malignant lesions: submandibular gland

Simple excision of the submandibular gland may be sufficient in cases where the tumour is confined within the capsule of the gland. Given the high incidence of adenoid cystic carcinoma at this site, a more extensive regional resection is often required, which may include the adjacent muscles, the lingual or hypoglossal nerves, a portion of the mandible, or the floor of the mouth (Figure 20.15). One study advocates a block dissection of the submandibular triangle as the minimal procedure in cases of submandibular cancer,[36] but it is more reasonable to tailor the resection to the extent of the tumour. Depending on the histologic diagnosis, a supraomohyoid neck dissection may be appropriate as part of the initial treatment. In some reports, radical neck dissection has been employed in this setting, but the inclusion of the lowest jugular nodes, the posterior triangle lymphatics, and non-lymphatic structures remote from the gland adds little to the margins of resection adjacent to the gland itself. Moreover, any operation is not truly 'radical' in patients with larger tumours unless the bed of the gland is included with the surgical specimen.

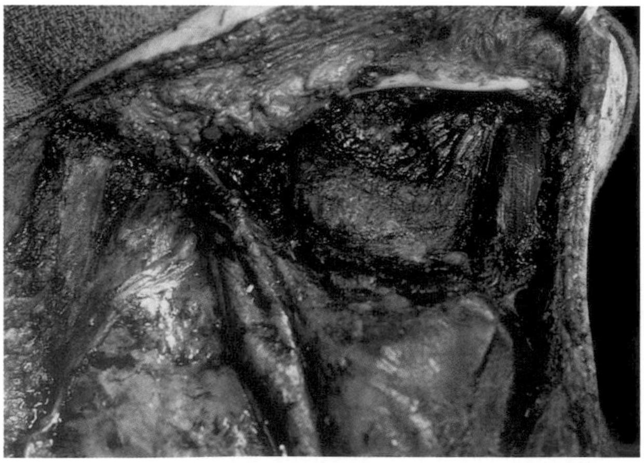

Figure 20.15 This 34-year-old man had a radical neck dissection for an adenoid cystic carcinoma of the right submandibular gland. Because the tumour involved adjacent tissues, the entire bed of the gland was removed en bloc with the neck specimen, including the mylohyoid, digastric, stylohyoid and hyoglossus muscles, lingual and hypoglossal nerves, and a portion of the overlying floor of the mouth.

Malignant lesions: minor salivary glands

Malignant minor salivary neoplasms may arise at various sites in the upper aerodigestive tract, and surgical treatment will obviously vary depending on the site of origin. In general, these lesions are resected in a manner similar to that utilized for squamous carcinoma arising at the same primary site. This may require procedures as diverse as laryngectomy for a lesion arising in the larynx and maxillectomy for a lesion arising in the maxillary antrum.

Malignant lesions: neck dissection

In those infrequent instances when a patient with salivary cancer presents with palpable nodal metastases, a comprehensive lymphadenectomy is clearly indicated, which may or may not preserve the accessory nerve. The approach to the clinically negative neck is more controversial. Because the incidence of regional metastases is relatively low for most types of salivary cancer, elective lymphadenectomy at Memorial Hospital is reserved for those patients with high-grade mucoepidermoid carcinoma or primary squamous carcinoma, which are known to have a high incidence of nodal involvement. Other approaches have been advocated, including routine sampling either of the primary tumour or of first echelon nodes at risk by frozen section.[100–102]

Malignant lesions: intraoperative frozen section analysis

As noted above, some surgeons advocate the use of intraoperative frozen section analysis of salivary neoplasms to guide decisions regarding the extent of resection, such as the need for elective regional lymphadenectomy. As with FNABx, frozen section analysis is reliable in distinguishing benign from malignant neoplams, but the ability to establish a precise histologic diagnosis depends upon the quality of the sample and the skill and experience of the pathologist.[103–106] For this reason, caution is required when using information obtained by frozen section, particularly when the pathology report appears to conflict with the clinical findings.

Table 20.3 Indications for postoperative radiotherapy

High grade malignancy/unfavourable histology
Advanced clinical stage
Positive margins of resection
Recurrent disease
Positive neck nodes following neck dissection

Treatment: radiation therapy

Salivary neoplasms were once thought to be relatively resistant to radiotherapy, but experience acquired during the past two decades demonstrates that this treatment modality does have an important role. Radiotherapy has been most frequently employed as adjunctive treatment following surgery, usually in the setting of high-grade and/or advanced-stage lesions, where there is concern about adequacy of excision. The indications for postoperative radiotherapy in the treatment of salivary cancer are summarized in Table 20.3.

In addition to the use of more conventional beam energies, there is a growing experience with fast neutron radiation therapy. This form of teletherapy appears to offer biologic advantages specific to the treatment of malignant salivary neoplasms, particularly adenoid cystic carcinoma. It has been utilized primarily in the setting of recurrent or residual disease following surgery in inaccessible locations, such as the skull base, but may be more effective as a primary treatment for tumours in these difficult locations.[107,108] Morbidity is a significant concern with neutron therapy, and more time and experience are necessary to better assess its role.

Treatment: chemotherapy

The proclivity for distant recurrence displayed by certain types of salivary cancer, particularly adenoid cystic carcinoma and high-grade adenocarcinoma, highlights the need for effective systemic chemotherapy. Unfortunately at present no consistently effective drug regimens have been identified. This is clearly an area that requires further clinical investigation in multi-institutional clinical trials. At this time, chemotherapy is hard to justify other than for palliation of patients with symptomatic unresectable or disseminated disease.

Results

Benign lesions

The results of primary surgery for benign salivary neoplasms are generally excellent. The reported recurrence rates for pleomorphic adenoma of the parotid gland are generally less than 5%.[97,98,109,110] While surgeons in the United States favour superficial parotidectomy with facial nerve dissection as a minimum procedure, recent studies suggest no significant difference between this procedure and more limited excisions, in regard to both disease control and incidence of facial nerve injury.[97,98]

When pleomorphic adenoma recurs following initial surgery, subsequent treatment is less successful and is, as expected, associated with higher morbidity. Control rates for surgery in this setting vary widely, perhaps as a result of variable follow-up;[111–115] in one-study one third of second, or subsequent, recurrences occurred 10 or more years after treatment.[115] In prior reports, permanent dysfunction of all or part of the facial nerve occurred in 12–25% of cases following treatment for recurrent pleomorphic adenoma of the parotid gland.[111–115] The use of radiotherapy has been suggested to help avoid sacrifice of facial nerve branches in this setting.[116]

Malignant lesions: general considerations

When analysing the results of treatment for salivary cancer, several important issues must be considered. The natural history of different types of malignant salivary tumours varies considerably. Five-year follow-up is adequate for most patients with intermediate or high grade mucoepidermoid carcinoma and primary squamous carcinoma. Ten-year follow-up is needed in order to appreciate the indolent behavior of some malignant salivary tumours. Disease-related deaths from adenoid cystic carcinoma, for example, may occur 20 or more years following treatment. Survival must also be distinguished from cure; prolonged survival has been observed in patients with adenoid cystic carcinoma even in the presence of documented pulmonary metastases. Finally, the relatively small number of patients with salivary cancer of any specific type, stage, and site of origin means that conclusions regarding treatment must be accepted with caution.

Malignant lesions: analysis by histology or grade

Histologic grade of salivary cancer is usually reflected in the clinical stage of the disease. When tumour grading is possible, as with mucoepidermoid, acinic cell, and adenocarcinomas, it is of definite prognostic significance. Survival by histologic grade for patients treated at Memorial Hospital is depicted in Figure 20.16. In two recent studies concerning prognostic variables in cancer of the parotid gland, histologic grade was identified as an important predictor of outcome.[4,85] It should be noted that, in general, histologic grade tends to be reflected in the clincal stage of patients with salivary cancer; those patients with microscopically high-grade lesions usually present with advanced-stage lesions.

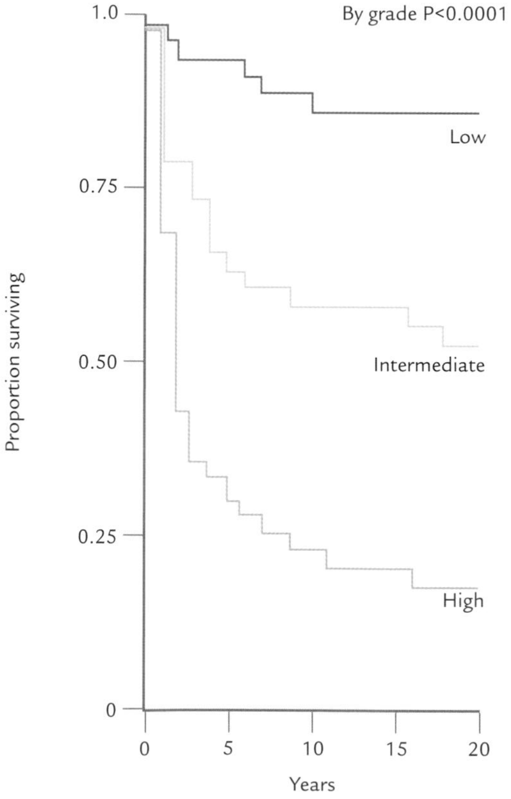

Figure 20.16 Differences in survival were significant when Memorial Hospital patients with salivary gland carcinoma were stratified according to the histologic grade of the primary tumour. Grading was possible for mucoepidermoid carcinomas, adenocarcinomas, acinic cell carcinomas, and squamous cell carcinomas.

Survival curves for various types of salivary cancer treated at Memorial Hospital show significant variation (Figure 20.17). Acinic cell carcinoma is associated with a favourable 5-year survival of 76% to 100% in various reports.[76–79] In one study, local recurrence was common in those patients with parotid lesions treated by local excision rather than formal superficial parotidectomy.[78] In patients with mucoepidermoid carcinoma, treatment results are usually reported by tumour grade, which is a highly significant prognostic indicator. Five-year survival varies from 76% to 100% in patients with low-grade lesions, but drops to 22–49% for high-grade lesions.[52–58]

Five-year survival figures for adenoid cystic carcinoma vary from 50% to over 80%, but are particularly misleading.[59–69] When follow-up is extended to 10 years, survival decreases to 29–67%, and then falls to about 25% after 15 years.[60,61] Local recurrence is common, and distant metastases (usually pulmonary) occur in about half of all patients.[62] As previously discussed, some studies suggest that grading of adenoid cystic carcinoma is of prognostic value, while other reports demonstrate that grade may correlate with disease-free interval, but not ultimate survival.[63–69]

Overall 5-year survival for patients with salivary adenocarcinoma is 76–85%, but falls to 34–71% after

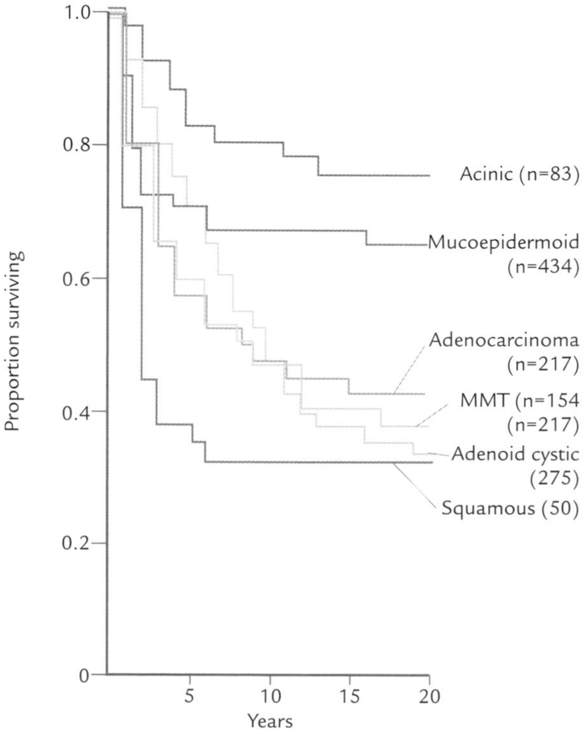

Figure 20.17 Survival in Memorial Hospital patients treated for salivary gland carcinoma according to histologic diagnosis.

10 years.[70–72] As with mucoepidermoid carcinoma, histologic grading of adenocarcinoma correlates well with outcome, with high-grade lesions carrying a poor prognosis. Patients with malignant mixed tumour have a 5-year survival of 31–65%, which diminishes to 23–36% when follow-up is extended to 10 years.[73–75]

Malignant lesions: analysis by clinical stage

The extent of disease at presentation, as documented by clinical stage, is the strongest predictor of treatment outcome in salivary cancer. Clinical staging has been demonstrated to be predictive of outcome for both major and minor salivary gland cancers. Survival by stage for patients treated at Memorial Hospital is depicted in Figure 20.18.[6] Similar results have been reported from other centres in the United States. Recent multivariate analysis of data from the United Kingdom confirmed clinical stage as the most important independent predictive factor, with 10-year survival rates of 96%, 70%, 47%, and 19% reported for AJCC stages I through IV, respectively.[5] Analysis of data on parotid cancer from Denmark revealed remarkably similar corrected survival rates of 85%, 69%, 43%, and 14% for UICC stages I through IV respectively.[4]

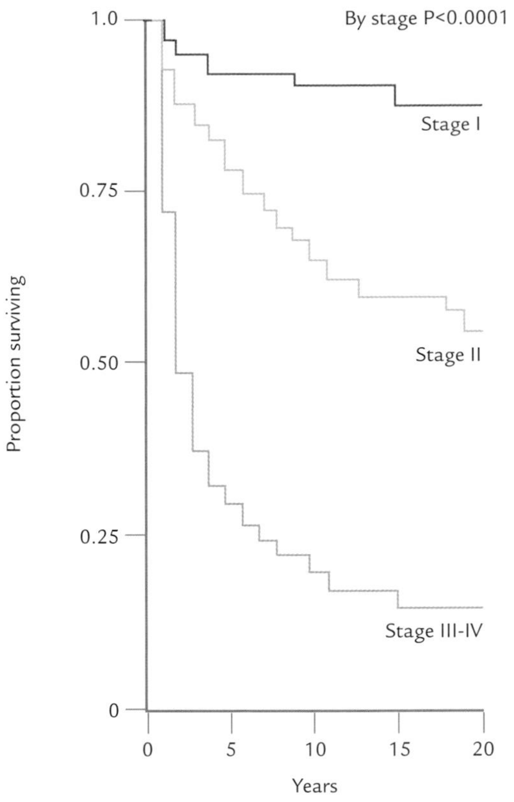

Figure 20.18 Survival in Memorial Hospital patients treated for salivary gland carcinoma according to clinical stage.

Malignant lesions: analysis by treatment

While conventional beam radiotherapy alone is relatively ineffective as a primary treatment for salivary cancer, centres that utilize fast neutron radiotherapy to treat salivary gland cancer report more encouraging short-term results. This modality is often employed in cases of inoperable disease, as well as gross residual or recurrent disease following prior surgical resection. In one report, patients treated primarily with fast neutron radiotherapy had a 92% actuarial 5-year locoregional control rate, leading the authors to suggest that surgical resection prior to neutron therapy be limited to those patients where disease-free margins can be achieved.[108]

In patients with salivary cancer treated with surgery alone, treatment failure at the primary site is a significant problem. In a report from Memorial Hospital concerning patients treated some years ago when adjuvant radiotherapy was seldom used, the locoregional recurrence rates were 39%, 60% and 65% for parotid, submandibular and minor salivary primary sites, respectively. Isolated treatment failure in cervical lymph nodes was seldom a problem.[6] In an effort to improve locoregional control rates for salivary cancer, the use of adjuvant radiotherapy has been increasing during the past two decades, particularly in those patients with advanced stage disease or other adverse prognostic findings.

Retrospective data from a number of centres suggests that the addition of postoperative radiotherapy improves the locoregional control of malignant salivary neoplasms, but prolonged survival has not been consistently demonstrated.[30,31,41,72,82,117] This probably reflects, in part, treatment failure at distant sites, as well as a tendency to select those patients with less favourable presentation for adjuvant treatment. In recent reports from the MD Anderson Hospital, improvements in local control were most evident in patients with either parotid or submandibular cancer when the disease extended beyond the confines of the gland.[85,88,118] In an attempt to overcome the selection bias inherent in retrospective studies, a matched-pair analysis of patients treated at Memorial Hospital with or without postoperative radiotherapy was performed.[119] There was a significant improvement in both local control of disease and survival in those patients with stage III and IV disease who received combination therapy, but a similar benefit was not evident for patients with early stage disease.

REFERENCES

1. Katz AD, Catalano P. The clinical significance of the various anastamotic branches of the facial nerve: report of 100 patients. *Arch Otolaryngol* 1987; **113**: 959–962.
2. Batsakis JG. Heterotopic and accessory salivary tissue. *Ann Otol Rhinol Laryngol* 1986; **95**: 434–436.
3. National Cancer Institute, Biometry Branch. The Third National Cancer Survey: Advanced Three Year Report 1969–1971 Incidence. Bethesda MD: National Cancer Institute, 1974.
4. Pedersen D, Overgaard J, Sogaard H et al. Malignant parotid tumors in 110 consecutive patients: treatment results and prognosis. *Laryngoscope* 1992; **102**: 1064–1069.
5. Renehan A, Gleave EN, Hancock BD et al. Long-term follow-up of over 1000 patients with salivary gland tumours treated in a single center. *Br J Surg* 1986; **83**: 1750–1754.
6. Spiro RH. Salivary neoplasms: overview of a 35 year experience with 2807 patients. *Head Neck Surg* 1986; **8**: 77–84.
7. Eneroth CM. Salivary gland tumors in the parotid gland, submandibular gland, and the palate region. *Cancer* 1971; **27**: 1415–1418.
8. Eveson JW, Cawson RA. Salivary gland tumours: a review of 2410 cases with particular reference to histological types, site, age and sex distribution. *J Pathol* 1985; **146**: 51–58.
9. Spiro RH. Treating tumors of the sublingual glands, including a useful technique for repair of the floor of the mouth after resection. *Am J Surg* 1995; **170**: 457–460.
10. Woods JE, Cheng GC, Beahrs OH. Experience with 1360 primary parotid tumors. *Am J Surg* 1975; **130**: 460–462.
11. Simons JN, Beahrs OH, Woolner LB. Tumors of the submaxillary gland. *Am J Surg* 1964; **108**: 485–494.
12. Conley J, Myers EN, Cole R. Analysis of 115 patients with tumors of the submandibular gland. *Ann Otol Rhinol Laryngol* 1972; **81**: 323–330.
13. Chaudry AP, Labay GR, Yamane GM et al. Clinicopathologic and histogenetic study of 189 intraoral minor salivary tumors. *J Oral Med* 1984; **39**: 58–78.
14. Waldron CA, El-Mofty SK, Gnepp DR. Tumors of the intraoral minor salivary glands: a demographic and histologic study of 426 cases. *Oral Surg Oral Med Oral Pathol* 1988; **66**: 323–333.
15. Spiro RH, Koss LG, Hajdu SI, Strong EW. Tumors of minor salivary origin: a clinicopathologic study of 492 cases. *Cancer* 1973; **31**: 117–129.
16. Takeichi N, Hirose F, Yamamoto H. Salivary gland tumors in atomic bomb survivors, Hiroshima, Japan: I. Epidemiologic observation. *Cancer* 1976; **38**: 2462–2468.
17. Saku T, Hatashi Y, Takahara O et al. Salivary gland tumors among atomic bomb survivors, 1950–1987. *Cancer* 1997; **79**: 1465–1475.
18. Maxon HR, Saenger EL, Buncher CR et al. Radiation-associated carcinoma of the salivary glands: a controlled study. *Ann Otol Rhinol Laryngol* 1981; **90**: 107–108.
19. Katz AD, Preston-Martin S. Salivary gland tumors and previous radiotherapy to the head and neck: report of a clinical series. *Am J Surg* 1984; **147**: 345–348.
20. Klintenberg C, Olofsson J, Hellquist H, Sokjer H. Adenocarcinoma of the ethmoid sinuses: a review of 28 cases with special reference to wood dust exposure. *Cancer* 1984; **54**: 482–488.
21. Hadfield EH, Macneth NG. Adenocarcinoma of the ethmoids in furniture workers. *Ann Otol Rhinol Laryngol* 1971; **80**: 699–703.
22. Merrick Y, Albeck H, Nielson NH, Hansen HS. Familial clustering of salivary gland carcinoma in Greenland. *Cancer* 1986; **57**: 2097–2102.
23. Pinkston JA, Cole P. Cigarette smoking and Warthin's tumor. *Am J Epidemiol* 1996; **144**: 183–187.
24. Spitz MR, Fueger JJ, Goepfert H et al. Salivary gland cancer: a case-control investigation of risk factors. *Arch Otolaryngol Head Neck Surg* 1990; **116**: 1163–1166.
25. Foote FW Jr, Frazell EL. Tumors of the major salivary glands. *Cancer* 1953; **6**: 1065–1133.
26. Marin VTW, Salmaso R, Onnis GL. Tumors of salivary glands: review of 479 cases with particular reference to histological types, site, age and sex distribution. *Appl Pathol* 1989; **7**: 154–160.
27. Rodriguez-Bigas MA, Sako K, Razack MS et al. Benign parotid tumors: a 24 year experience. *J Surg Oncol* 1991; **46**: 159–161.
28. Hodgkinson DJ. The influence of facial nerve sacrifice in surgery of malignant parotid tumors. *J Surg Oncol* 1976; **8**: 425–432.
29. Friedman M, Levin B, Grybauskas V et al. Malignant tumors of the major salivary glands. *Otolaryngol Clin North Am* 1986; **19**: 625–636.
30. Guillamondegui OM, Byers RM, Luna MA et al. Aggressive surgery in treatment for parotid cancer: the role of adjunctive postoperative radiotherapy. *Am J Roentgenol* 1975; **1213**: 49–54.
31. Tu G, Hu Y, Jiang P, Qin D. The superiority of combined therapy in parotid cancer. *Arch Otolaryngol* 1982; **108**: 710–713.
32. Rafla S. Malignant parotid tumors: natural history and treatment. *Cancer* 1977; **40**: 136–144.
33. Hollander L, Cunningham MP. Management of cancer of the parotid gland. *Surg Clin North Am* 1973; **53**: 113–119.
34. Hugo NE, McKinney P, Griffith BH. Management of tumors of the parotid gland. *Surg Clin North Am* 1973; **53**: 105–111.
35. Spiro RH, Hajdu SI, Strong EW. Tumors of the submaxillary gland. *Am J Surg* 1976; **132**: 463–468.
36. Byers RM, Jesse RH, Guillamondegui OM, Luna MA. Malignant tumors of the submaxillary gland. *Am J Surg* 1973; **126**: 458–463.

37. Lowe JT Jr, Farmer JC Jr. Submaxillary gland tumors. *Laryngoscope* 1974; **84**: 542–552.
38. Trial ML, Lubritz J. Tumors of the submandibular gland. *Laryngoscope* 1974; **84**: 1225–1232.
39. Pyper PL, Beverland DE, Bell DM. Tumors of the submandibular gland. *J R Coll Surg Edinb* 1987; **32**: 233–235.
40. Rafla S. Submaxillary gland tumors. *Cancer* 1970; **26**: 821–826.
41. Chou C, Zhu G, Luo M, Xue G. Carcinoma of the minor salivary glands: results of surgery and combined treatment. *J Oral Maxillofac Surg* 1996; **54**: 448–453.
42. Conley J, Arena S. Parotid gland as a focus of metastasis. *Arch Surg* 1963; **897**: 757–764.
43. Nicholas RD, Pinnock LA, Szymanowski RT. Metastases to parotid nodes. *Laryngoscope* 1980; **90**: 1324–1328.
44. Khurana VG, Mentis DH, O'Brien CJ et al. Parotid and neck metastases from cutaneous squamous cell carcinoma of the head and neck. *Am J Surg* 1995; **170**: 446–450.
45. Jecker P, Hartwein J. Metastasis to the parotid gland: is a radical surgical approach justified? *Am J Otolaryngol* 1996; **17**: 102–105.
46. Batsakis JG. Pathology consultation: metastases to major salivary glands. *Ann Otol Rhinol Laryngol* 1990; **99**: 501–503.
47. Batsakis JG, Regezi JA. The pathology of head and neck tumors: salivary glands, part 3. *Head Neck Surg* 1979; **1**: 260–271.
48. Chapnick JS. The controversy of Warthin's tumor. *Laryngoscope* 1983; **93**: 695–716.
49. Eveson JW, Cawson RA. Warthin's tumor (cystadenolymphoma) of salivary glands: a clinicopathologic investigation of 278 cases. *Oral Surg Oral Med Oral Pathol* 1986; **61**: 256–262.
50. Yoo GH, Eisele DW, Askin FB et al. Warthin's tumor: a 40 year experience at the Johns Hopkins Hospital. *Laryngoscope* 1994; **104**: 799–803.
51. Batsakis JG, Regezi JA. The pathology of head and neck tumors: salivary glands, part 2. *Head Neck Surg* 1979; **1**: 167–180.
52. Eneroth CM, Hjertman L, Moberger G, Soderberg G. Mucoepidermoid carcinomas of the salivary glands with special reference to the possible existence of a benign variety. *Acta Otolaryngol* 1972; **73**: 68–74.
53. Spiro RH, Huvos AG, Berk R, Strong EW. Mucoepidermoid carcinoma of salivary gland origin: a clinicopathologic study of 367 cases. *Am J Surg* 1978; **136**: 461–468.
54. Healey WV, Perzin KH, Smith L. Mucoepidermoid carcinoma of salivary gland origin: classification, clinicopathologic correlation and results of treatment. *Cancer* 1970; **26**: 368–388.
55. Evans HL. Mucoepidermoid carcinoma of salivary glands: a study of 69 cases with special attention to histologic grading. *Am J Clin Pathol* 1984; **81**: 696–701.
56. Nascimento AG, Amaral ALP, Prado LAF et al. Mucoepidermoid carcinoma of salivary glands: a clinicopathologic study of 46 cases. *Head Neck Surg* 1986; **8**: 409–417.
57. Hicks MJ, el-Naggar AK, Flaitz CM et al. Histocytologic grading of mucoepidermoid carcinoma of major salivary glands in prognosis and survival. *Head Neck* 1995; **17**: 89–95.
58. Plambeck K, Friedrich RE, Hellner D et al. Mucoepidermoid carcinoma of the salivary glands: clinical data and follow-up of 52 cases. *J Cancer Res Clin Oncol* 1996; **122**: 177–180.
59. Batsakis JG, Regezi JA. The pathology of head and neck tumors: salivary glands, part 4. *Head Neck Surg* 1979; **1**: 340–349.
60. Spiro RH, Huvos AG, Strong EW. Adenoid cystic carcinoma of salivary origin. *Am J Surg* 1974; **128**: 512–520.
61. Blank C, Backsoom A, Eneroth CM et al. Adenoid cystic carcinoma of the parotid gland. *Acta Radiol* 1967; **6**: 177–196.
62. Spiro RH. Distant metastasis in adenoid cystic carcinoma of salivary origin. *Am J Surg* 1997; **174**: 495–498.
63. Eby LS, Johnson DS, Baker HW. Adenoid cystic carcinoma of the head and neck. *Cancer* 1972; **29**: 1160–1168.
64. Grahne B, Lauren C, Holsti LR. Clinical and histologic malignancy of adenoid cystic carcinoma. *J Laryngol Otol* 1977; **91**: 743–749.
65. Matsuba HM, Simpson JR, Mauney M, Thawley SE. Adenoid cystic carcinoma: a clinicopathologic correlation. *Head Neck Surg* 1986; **8**: 200–204.
66. Perzin KH, Gullane P, Clairmont AC. Adenoid cystic carcinomas arising in salivary glands: a correlation of histologic features and clinical course. *Cancer* 1978; **42**: 265–282.
67. Szanto PA, Luna MA, Tortoledo E, White RA. Histologic grading of adenoid cystic carcinoma of the salivary glands. *Cancer* 1984; **54**: 1062.
68. Spiro RH, Huvos AG. Stage means more than grade in adenoid cystic carcinoma. *Am J Surg* 1992; **165**: 623–628.
69. Nasimento AG, Amaral ALP, Prado LAF et al. Adenoid cystic carcinoma of salivary glands: a study of 61 cases with clinicopathologic correlation. *Cancer* 1986; **57**: 312–319.
70. Spiro RH, Huvos AG, Strong EW. Adenocarcinoma of salivary origin: a clinicopathologic study of 204 patients. *Am J Surg* 1982; **144**: 423–431.
71. Kemp BL, Batsakis JG, el-Naggar AK et al. Terminal duct adenocarcinomas of the parotid gland. *J Laryngol Otol* 1995; **109**: 466–468.
72. Simpson JR, Matsuba HM, Thawley SE, Mauney M. Improved treatment of salivary gland adenocarcinomas: planned combined surgery and irradiation. *Laryngoscope* 1986; **96**: 904–907.
73. Spiro RH, Huvos AG, Strong EW. Malignant mixed tumors of salivary origin: a clinicopathologic study of 146 cases. *Cancer* 1977; **39**: 388–396.
74. LiVolsi VA, Perzin KH. Malignant mixed tumors arising in salivary glands: I. Carcinomas arising in benign mixed tumors: a clinicopathologic study. *Cancer* 1977; **39**: 2209–2230.

75. Gerughty RM, Scofield HH, Brown FM, Hennigar GR. Malignant mixed tumors of salivary origin. *Cancer* 1969; **24**: 471–486.
76. Spiro RH, Huvos AG, Strong EW. Acinic cell carcinoma of salivary origin: a clinicopathologic study of 67 cases. *Cancer* 1978; **41**: 924–935.
77. Batsakis JG, Chinn EK, Weimert TA et al. Acinic cell carcinoma: a clinicopathologic study of 35 cases. *J Laryngol Otol* 1979; **93**: 325–340.
78. Oliveira P, Fonseca I, Soares J. Acinic cell carcinoma of the salivary glands: a long term follow-up study of 15 cases. *Eur J Surg Oncol* 1992; **18**: 7–15.
79. Spafford PD, Mintz DR, Hay J. Acinic cell carcinoma of the parotid gland: review and management. *J Otolaryngol* 1991; **20**: 262–266.
80. Galia LJ, Johnson JT. The incidence of neoplastic versus inflammatory disease in major salivary gland masses diagnosed by surgery. *Laryngoscope* 1981; **91**: 512–516.
81. Spiro RH, Huvos AW, Strong EW. Cancer of the parotid gland: a clinicopathologic study of 288 primary cases. *Am J Surg* 1975; **130**: 452–459.
82. Borthune A, Kjellevold, Kaalhus O, Vermund H. Salivary gland malignant neoplasms: treatment and prognosis. *Int J Radiat Oncol Biol Phys* 1986; **12**: 747–754.
83. Nigro MF, Spiro RH. Deep lobe parotid tumors. *Am J Surg* 1977; **134**: 523–527.
84. Johnson FE, Spiro RH. Tumors arising in accessory parotid tissue. *Am J Surg* 1979; **138**: 576–578.
85. Frankenthaler RA, Luna MA, Lee SS et al. Prognostic variables in parotid cancer. *Arch Otolaryngol Head Neck Surg* 1991; **117**: 1251–1256.
86. Eneroth CM. Facial nerve paralysis: a criterion of malignancy in parotid tumors. *Arch Otolaryngol* 1972; **95**: 300–304.
87. Conley JJ, Hamaker RC. Prognosis of malignant tumors of the parotid gland with facial paralysis. *Arch Otolaryngol* 1975; **101**: 39–41.
88. Weber RS, Byers RM, Petit B et al. Submandibular gland tumors: adverse histologic factors and therapeutic implications. *Arch Otolaryngol Head Neck Surg* 1990; **116**: 1055.
89. Weissman JL. Imaging of the salivary glands. *Semin Ultrasound CT MR* 1995; **16**: 546–568.
90. Lindberg RD, Ackerman M. Aspiration cytology of salivary gland tumors: diagnostic experience from six years of routine laboratory work. *Laryngoscope* 1976; **86**: 584–589.
91. O'Dwyer P, Farrar WB, James AG et al. Needle aspiration biopsy of major salivary gland tumors: its value. *Cancer* 1986; **57**: 554–557.
92. Layfield LJ, Tan P, Glasgow BJ. Fine needle aspiration of salivary gland lesions: comparison with frozen sections and histologic findings. *Arch Pathol Lab Med* 1987; **111**: 346–353.
93. Atula T, Greenman R, Laippala P, Klemi PJ. Fine-needle aspiration biopsy in the diagnosis of parotid gland lesions: evaluation of 438 biopsies. *Diagn Cytopathol* 1996; **15**: 185–190.
94. American Joint Committee on Cancer. *Manual for Staging of Cancer.* 4th edn. Philadelphia: JB Lippincott, 1992.
95. International Union Against Cancer. *TNM Classification of Malignant Tumors.* 5th edn. New York, NY: Wiley-Liss, 1997.
96. Spiro RH, Thaler HT, Hicks WS et al. The importance of clinical staging of minor salivary tumors. *Am J Surg* 1991; **162**: 330–336.
97. McGurk M, Renehan A, Gleave EN, Hancock BD. Clinical significance of the tumour capsule in the treatment of parotid pleomorphic adenomas. *Br J Surg* 1996; **83**: 1747–1749.
98. Prichard AJ, Barton RP, Narula AA. Complications of superficial parotidectomy versus extracapsular lumpectomy in the treatment of benign parotid lesions. *J R Coll Surg Edinb* 1992; **37**: 155–158.
99. Afify SE, Maynard JD. Tumours of the accessory lobe of the parotid gland. *Postgrad Med J* 1992; **68**: 461–462.
100. Ball ABS, Fish S, Thomas JM. Malignant epithelial parotid tumors: a rational treatment policy. *Br J Surg* 1995; **82**: 621–623.
101. Johns ME. Parotid cancer: a rational basis for treatment. *Head Neck Surg* 1980; **3**: 132–144.
102. Krause CJ. The management of parotid neoplasms. *Head Neck Surg* 1981; **3**: 340–343.
103. Hillel AD, Fee WE. Evaluation of frozen section in parotid gland surgery. *Arch Otolaryngol* 1983; **109**: 230–232.
104. Wheelis RF, Yarrington CT Jr. Tumors of the salivary glands: comparison of frozen section diagnosis with final pathologic diagnosis. *Arch Otolaryngol* 1984; **110**: 76–77.
105. Granick MS, Erickson ER, Hanna DC. Accuracy of frozen section diagnosis in salivary gland lesions. *Head Neck Surg* 1985; **7**: 465–467.
106. Rigval NR, Miller P, Lore JM, Kaufman S. Accuracy of frozen section diagnosis in salivary gland lesions. *Head Neck Surg* 1985; **7**: 465–467.
107. Krull A, Schwarz R, Engenhart R et al. European results in neutron therapy of malignant salivary gland tumors. *Bull Cancer Radiother* 1996; **83 (Suppl)**: 125–129.
108. Buchholz TA, Laramore GE, Griffen BR et al. The role of fast neutron therapy in the management of advanced salivary gland malignant neoplasms. *Cancer* 1992; **69**: 2779–2788.
109. Leverstein H, van der Wal JE, Tiwari RM et al. Surgical management of 246 previously untreated pleomorphic adenomas of the parotid gland. *Br J Surg* 1997; **84**: 399–403.
110. Laccourreye H, Laccourreye O, Cauchois R et al. Total conservative parotidectomy for primary benign pleomorphic adenoma of the parotid gland: a 25 year experience with 229 patients. *Laryngoscope* 1994; **104**: 1487–1494.
111. O'Dwyer PJ, Farrar WB, Finkelmeier WR et al. Facial nerve sacrifice and tumor recurrences in primary and recurrent benign parotid tumors. *Am J Surg* 1986; **152**: 442–445.

112. Conley JJ, Clairmont AA. Facial nerve in recurrent benign pleomorphic adenoma. *Arch Otolaryngol* 1979; **105**: 247–251.

113. Fee WE, Goffinet DR, Calcaterra JC. Recurrent mixed tumors of the parotid gland: results of surgical therapy. *Laryngoscope* 1978; **88**: 265–273.

114. Phillips PP, Olsen KD. Recurrent pleomorphic adenoma of the parotid gland: report of 126 cases and a review of the literature. *Ann Otol Rhinol Laryngol* 1995; **104**: 100–104.

115. Niparko JK, Beauchamp ML, Krause CJ et al. Surgical treatment of recurrent pleomorphic adenoma of the parotid gland. *Arch Otolaryngol* 1986; **112**: 1180–1184.

116. Samson MJ, Metson R, Wang CC, Montgomery WW. Preservation of the facial nerve in the management of recurrent pleomorphic adenoma. *Laryngoscope* 1991; **101**: 1060–1062.

117. Fu KK, Leibel SA, Levine ML et al. Cancer of the major and minor salivary glands. *Cancer* 1977; **40**: 2882–2890.

118. Garden AS, El-Naggar AK, Morrison WH et al. Postoperative radiotherapy for malignant tumors of the parotid gland. *Int J Radiat Oncol Biol Phys* 1997; **37**: 79–85.

119. Armstrong JG, Harrison LB, Spiro RH et al. Malignant tumors of major salivary origin: a matched pair analysis of the role of combined surgery and postoperative radiotherapy. *Arch Otolaryngol Head Neck Surg* 1990; **116**: 290–293.

21 Cancer of the thyroid gland

Peter H Rhys Evans, Andrew See and Clive L Harmer

Introduction

Cancer of the thyroid is rare but includes several distinct tumour types each associated with characteristic epidemiological, clinical and prognostic features. Unlike most head and neck tumours, thyroid cancer is more common in women and often follows a protracted natural history. The majority are differentiated carcinomas with a spectrum of papillary and follicular types that are unique in their potential for target therapy with radioactive ^{131}I. Cure can be achieved with surgery and adjuvant therapy but there is controversy regarding optimal treatment necessary to eradicate the disease and yet minimize potential morbidity.

Rarer tumours include medullary carcinoma arising from the parafollicular cells which is treated surgically, and aggressive anaplastic carcinoma and thyroid lymphoma, for which external beam radiotherapy and chemotherapy are of value. The thyroid may also be the site of metastases or may be invaded directly by squamous cell carcinoma of the hypopharynx or larynx.

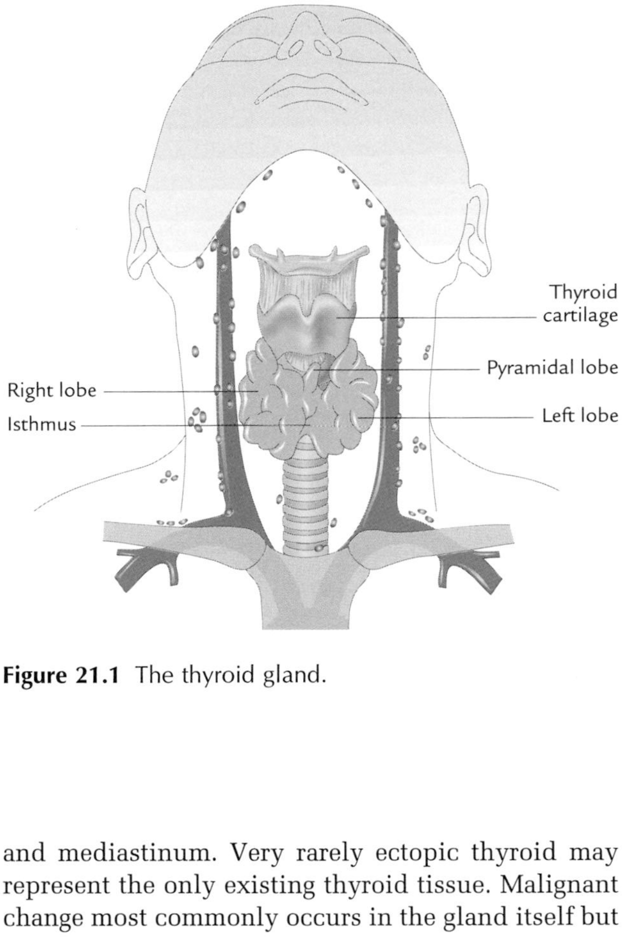

Figure 21.1 The thyroid gland.

Surgical anatomy

The thyroid gland lies within the pretracheal fascia in the front of the neck, and consists of two symmetrical pear-shaped lobes united in the midline by an isthmus that overlies the second to fourth tracheal rings (Figure 21.1). There is often a pyramidal lobe, which may extend (usually to the left) as high as the top of the thyroid cartilage.

Anatomical variations[1,2] include absence of one of the lobes (0.03%) or the isthmus (0.02%), and ectopic thyroid tissue in the posterior tongue (lingual thyroid 0.02%), anywhere along the course of the thyroglossal tract (0.01%), or in other sites (0.01%). These less common sites include the larynx, trachea[3] and mediastinum. Very rarely ectopic thyroid may represent the only existing thyroid tissue. Malignant change most commonly occurs in the gland itself but may develop in ectopic sites. Thyroid tissue found in cervical lymph nodes (lateral aberrant thyroid) is almost invariably metastatic from an occult well-differentiated thyroid carcinoma.

Vascular supply

The thyroid blood supply[2] is derived from the superior thyroid artery (arising from the external carotid artery), inferior thyroid artery (from the thyrocervical trunk of the subclavian artery) and occasionally from the thyroidea ima artery (from the brachiocephalic artery). The thyroid veins drain into the internal jugular (middle and superior thyroid)

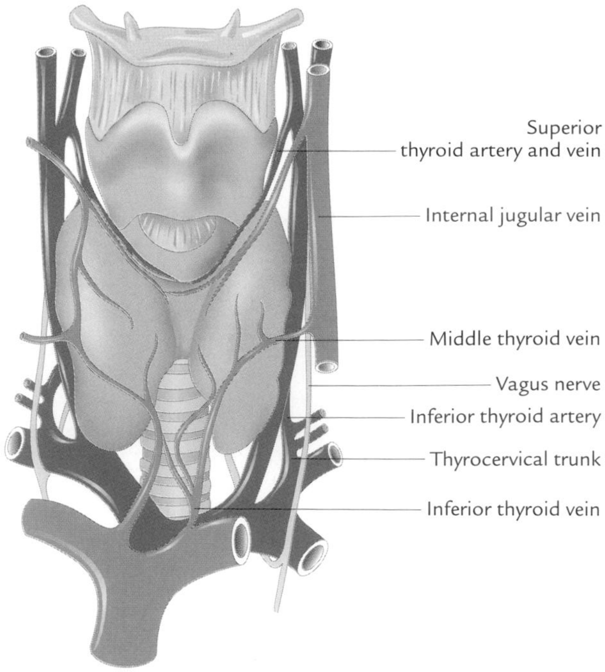

Figure 21.2 Blood supply of the thyroid gland.

and brachiocephalic (inferior thyroid) veins. An intimate knowledge of the anatomical course, relations and variations of the superior and inferior thyroid pedicles is essential for safe thyroid surgery (Figure 21.2).

Recurrent laryngeal nerve

Of particular importance is a clear understanding of the close anatomical relationship of the recurrent laryngeal nerve to the thyroid gland and its clinical significance for several reasons:

1. Potential involvement of the nerve by thyroid tumours is a useful clinical and prognostic sign; laryngoscopy should always be carried out either with a mirror or fibreoptic endoscope prior to any thyroid surgery;
2. Paralysis of the nerve may or may not cause significant voice problems;
3. The risk to the nerve during thyroid surgery depends not only on the site and pathology of the tumour but also on the experience of the surgeon.

The recurrent laryngeal nerves branch from the vagus low in the neck and descend into the superior mediastinum. On the right side the nerve loops around the subclavian artery and ascends in a medial direction towards the tracheo-oesophageal groove. At the lower pole of the thyroid gland the nerve is therefore slightly more lateral than on the left side where the nerve has looped around the ligamentum arteriosum at the level of the aortic arch and ascended in a more medial position towards the cricothyroid membrane.

On both sides the nerve lies in close relation to the branches of the inferior thyroid artery. In most cases the nerve lies posterior to the artery but several anatomical variations occur (Figure 21.3). The nerve may also be non-recurrent, more commonly on the right side in 2–3%, traversing medially in a loop directly from the vagus nerve (Figure 21.4). This anomaly is associated with a retro-oesophageal right subclavian artery.

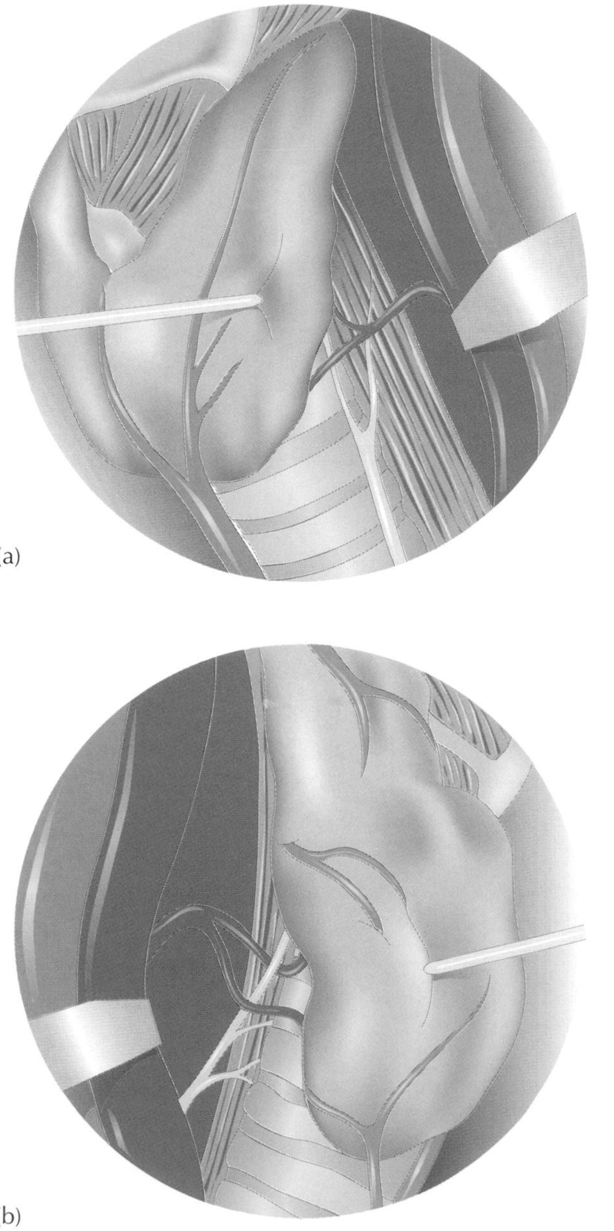

(a)

(b)

Figure 21.3 Relationship of the recurrent laryngeal nerve to the inferior thyroid artery. (a) Left side; (b) right side.

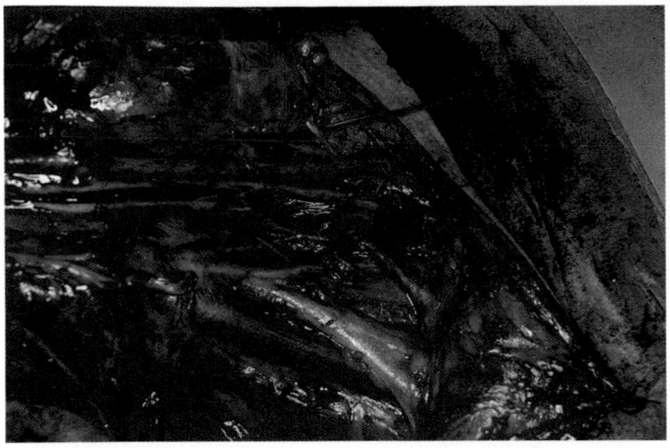

Figure 21.4 Non-recurrent recurrent laryngeal nerve (on the right side). Blue markers also identify the vagus and phrenic nerves.

Superior laryngeal nerve

The external branch of the superior laryngeal nerve, which innervates the lateral cricothyroid muscle lies in close relationship with the superior laryngeal pedicle and should be carefully identified and preserved when tying off the superior laryngeal artery and vein. It is particularly vunerable with mass ligation of the superior pole. Damage to the nerve will cause alteration of the voice typically with loss of high registers and deepening of tone due to loss of vocal cord tension control.

Parathyroid glands

The relationship of the parathyroid glands to the thyroid is important (Figure 21.5). Every attempt should be made during surgery to identify and preserve some functioning parathyroid tissue. The anatomical relations are discussed in more detail in Chapter 22.

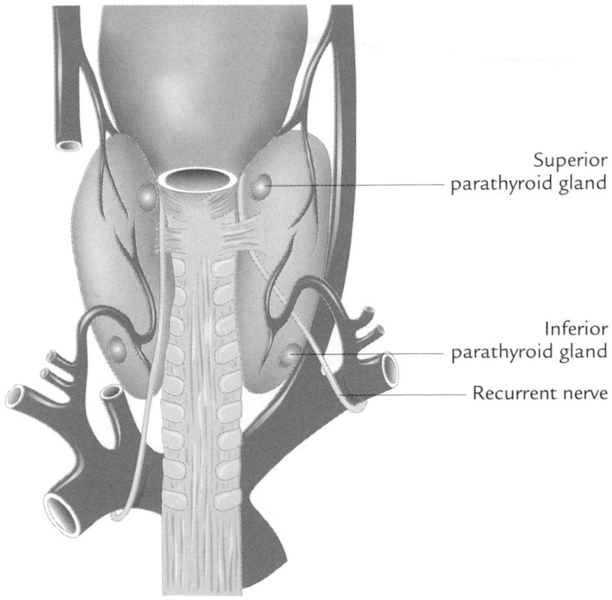

Figure 21.5 Common positions of the parathyroid glands.

Lymphatic drainage

The gland has a rich lymphatic network,[2] which connects freely between both lobes and drains into the following lymph node groups: pericapsular, pretracheal (delphian), tracheo-oesophageal (paratracheal, level VI), deep cervical chain (levels II, III and IV), posterior triangle (level V, occipital and supraclavicular), retropharyngeal and retro-oesophageal (Figure 21.6).

Molecular biology

Hormone production

The production of the hormones thyroxine (T_4) and tri-iodothyronine (T_3) by the thyroid gland is regulated by the secretion of thyroid-stimulating hormone (TSH, thyrotropin) from the pituitary gland, which in turn is influenced by thyrotropin-releasing hormone (TRH) from the hypothalamus. T_3 and T_4 are incorporated and stored as thyroglobulin (Tg) in the colloid and the secretion of these three substances can be measured by radioimmunoassay, as can calcitonin, which is secreted by the parafollicular cells of the thyroid gland.

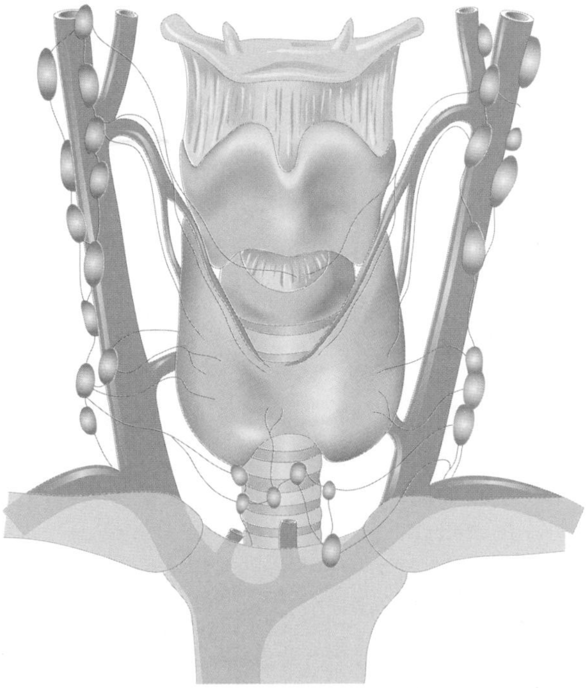

Figure 21.6 Lymphatic drainage of the thyroid gland.

Table 21.1 Thyroid growth factors

Stimulators	Inhibitors
Thyroid stimulating hormone (TSH)	Iodine
Growth hormone (GH)	Lithium
Iodine deficiency	Vitamin A
Vitamin C	Transforming growth factor beta (TGF-beta)
Epidermal growth factor (EGF)	
Fibroblastic growth factors (FGF 1 and 2)	
Interleukin 1	
Prostaglandin E2	

Tumour markers

Thyroglobulin is also secreted by well-differentiated carcinoma cells and following total thyroidectomy, subsequent radioiodine ablation and T4 suppression therapy, the Tg level should be unrecordable. Tg assay during follow-up is therefore a helpful tumour marker and measurable levels are associated with tumour recurrence or metastases. In medullary thyroid carcinoma (MTC), which arises from the parafollicular cells, calcitonin is similarly a tumour marker following total thyroidectomy.

Growth factors

Under normal conditions thyroid follicular cell activity is regulated by a number of extracellular growth factors that either stimulate or inhibit growth. They mediate their effects through receptors on the cell surface and also via a number of intracellular signal transduction pathways. Each step in the pathway is controlled genetically by a number of growth-promoting proto-oncogenes and growth-inhibiting tumour suppressor genes.[4] The principle factors influencing thyroid growth are listed in Table 21.1.

Thyroid cancer

It is now possible to describe a sequential set of molecular events that lead to the development of thyroid cancer.[5] The *RET* proto-oncogene encodes a protein receptor tyrosine kinase and *RET* gene alterations have been identified in papillary carcinoma.[6] The lower incidence and associated poorer prognosis in men and in postmenopausal as compared with premenopausal women, are compatible with a major role for sex hormones in thyroid carcinogenesis.[7]

Table 21.2 Classification of malignant thyroid tumours

Tumour type	Incidence (%)
Differentiated follicular cell-derived carcinomas	
Papillary carcinoma	60–65
Follicular carcinoma	15–20
Hurthle cell carcinoma	2–5
Parafollicular cell-derived carcinomas	
Medullary carcinoma	
Sporadic	4–6
Familial	2–3
Anaplastic (undifferentiated) carcinoma	
Giant cell, small cell and spindle cell variants	5–10
Other primary thyroid tumours	
Lymphoma	1
Others (squamous cell carcinoma, sarcoma)	
Secondary cancer to the thyroid from kidney, breast, colon, melanoma	1

Classification

The vast majority of thyroid swellings are due to cystic degenerative changes but there are a number of benign tumours, the commonest being follicular cell adenoma, then Hurthle cell adenoma and the rare teratoma. Malignant tumours may arise from the follicular cells (papillary, follicular, anaplastic), the parafollicular cells (medullary) or the stroma (lymphoma, sarcoma). Papillary carcinoma is by far the commonest type of malignant thyroid tumour, representing about 60–65%, followed by follicular (15–20%) and medullary types, particularly in the younger age groups. In older patients anaplastic carcinoma is more prevalent (5–10%) and carries a much worse prognosis. Rarer tumours include Hurthle cell carcinoma (2–5%), lymphoma and metastases (Table 21.2).

Natural history

Presentation

Differentiated thyroid carcinoma most commonly presents in a euthyroid patient as a 'solitary thyroid nodule' identified on examination or scan, of which 10–50% may be malignant. It may be small and asymptomatic but larger swellings usually cause discomfort in the anterior lower neck with 'globus-

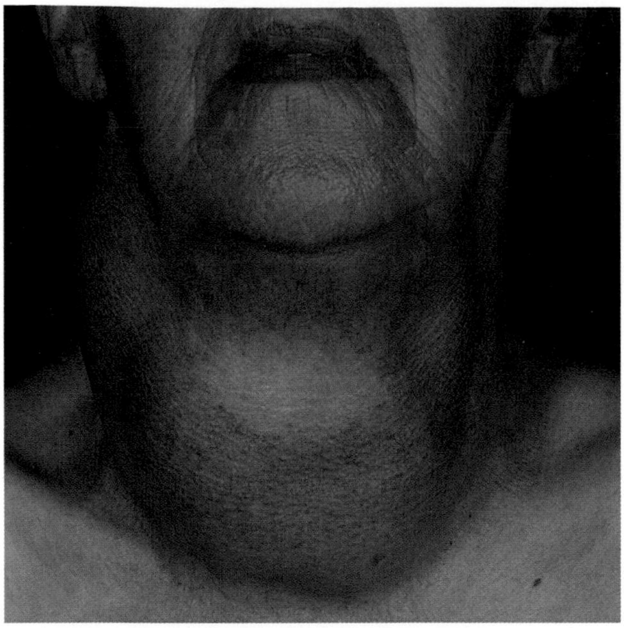
Figure 21.7 Nodes with a longstanding goitre.

type' symptoms and, less commonly, tracheal and/or oesophageal compression. Anaplastic carcinoma and lymphoma usually present with more rapid onset of swelling.

The other frequent presentation is of cervical lymphadenopathy (which may be cystic in up to 30%) associated with an occult or asymptomatic primary. Nodes may also appear in someone with a long-standing goitre (Figure 21.7). Less commonly tumours may present with a vocal cord palsy, dysphagia, or in rare instances with haemoptysis.[3] Thyroid carcinoma may be associated with hyperthyroidism in up to 20% of patients.[8] In patients with medullary carcinoma symptoms such as diarrhoea may be present (Table 21.3).

Age at presentation is important in someone with a thyroid nodule, 50% being malignant under 14 years and 45% in the over 50 year age group (Table 21.4). Malignant nodules are also much more likely on fine-needle aspiration in males (29%) than females (4%). A history of irradiation or other malignant

Table 21.3 Symptoms of thyroid cancer

Thyroid nodule (10–50% of solitary nodules)
Cervical lymphadenopathy
Hoarseness
Haemoptysis
Stridor
Dysphagia/'globus'
Hyperthyroidism
Diarrhoea (MTC)

Table 21.4 Associated factors in thyroid cancer

Clinical presentation		
Age: nodules	< 14 yrs – 50% malignant	
	> 50 yrs – 45% malignant	
Sex: nodules (FNA)	M – 29% malignant	
	F – 4% malignant	
Previous irradiation		
Genetic factors –	Gardner's syndrome (FCP)	
	Cowden's disease	
Papillary Ca and breast, ovarian and CNS malignancies		

tumours (breast or ovarian) may be significant. A family history of thyroid cancer is found in 5% of patients with papillary carcinoma and 30% of patients with medullary tumours. Genetic factors are also associated with Gardner's syndrome (familial colonic polyposis) and Cowden's disease.

Incidence

The prevalence of occult thyroid carcinoma in some adult populations may be as high as 5–10%[9] but the incidence of clinically evident thyroid carcinoma is only 0.05%. In a European population the incidence varies between 1.75 per 100 000 population (0.00175%) for males and 6.38 (0.00638%) for females.[10] This implies that only 1–2% of occult carcinomas evolve into overt tumour during life, similar to the situation in prostatic carcinoma. The world-wide incidence[2] is in the region of 4 per 100 000 population per annum, although this does vary widely, with the highest being in Iceland and Hawaii (15 per 100 000 per annum). The UK incidence of 1.2 per 100 000 is one of the lowest in the world.

Mortality rate

The overall figure for thyroid carcinoma is 4 per million per annum, giving an average mortality rate of 10%[2] but this does vary widely depending on many factors.

Sex ratio

This varies with histological type[2] but in general, unlike squamous cell carcinoma of the head and neck, tumours are more common in females. For differentiated and anaplastic thyroid carcinomas the female to male ratio is 3:1 and for medullary carcinoma the ratio is 4:3.

Aetiological factors

The most important risk factor in differentiated thyroid carcinoma is previous irradiation[11,12] especially before the age of 16. Therapeutic irradiation may have been given previously for thymic enlargement or other benign conditions in childhood, for example haemangioma, keloid, tinea infection and acne. The increase in thyroid carcinoma in Belarussian children after the Chernobyl disaster in 1986 is well documented.[13–15] This has been characterized by a high incidence in boys giving an almost equal sex ratio, increased aggressiveness with intraglandular tumour dissemination (92%), capsular and soft tissue invasion (89%) and cervical node metastases (88%).[13] Papillary carcinoma was diagnosed in 99% of cases. The short latent period of 4–6 years (mean 5.8) is similar to that seen in the USA 5 years after large releases of ^{131}I from nuclear plants and atomic weapons tests.[16] Diagnostic and therapeutic use of ^{131}I, on the other hand, has not been shown to be carcinogenic.[20]

Other factors include genetic predisposition,[2,17] geographical distribution,[2] Hashimoto's disease[2,18,19] and iodine content of the diet. In several surveys a positive correlation has also been found between increasing parity and incidence of differentiated thyroid carcinoma.[20]

Prognostic factors

The significance of various prognostic factors such as age in differentiated thyroid cancer was recognized by Sloan in 1954[21] and later by the EORTC group in 1979.[22] Since then a number of staging systems have been proposed in an attempt to predict outcome and to help tailor treatment and extent of surgery (Table 21.5). These schemes are based on multivariate analysis of retrospective data[21–25] which have resulted in identification of important prognostic factors that include gender, histology, size, grade, presence of nodal and distant metastases, extent of tumour and completeness of resection. Five of the most widely used are summarized below.

Table 21.5 Staging systems for thyroid cancer

Age (Sloan, 1954)
Age, sex, histology, size, mets (EORTC, 79)
Age, grade, extent, size (AGES, Hay, 1987)
Age, mets, extent, size (AMES, Cady, 1988)
Grade, age, mets, extent, size (GAMES, Shah, 1996)
Mets, age, completeness of resection, invasion, size (MACIS, Hay, 1993)
TNM system (UICC, 1992)

AGES (Mayo Clinic,1987)

Age >40; histological **G**rade >1; **E**xtrathyroid extension; **S**ize >3cm

Hay et al[23] proposed this prognostic system in which patients were divided into four groups that correlate with progressively shorter survival, according to their prognostic score (PS) which was calculated from a formula based on these four risk factors (Table 21.6). Eighty-five percent of the total cohort were in group I whose 20-year cause-specific mortality was only 1% (Table 21.7).

Table 21.6 AGES prognostic system

PS = 0.05 × age (in years if > 40)
+ 1 (if grade is 2), or + 3 (if grade is 3 or 4)
+ 1 (for extrathyroid extension), or + 3 (for distant metastases)
+ 0.02 × tumour size (in cm)

Table 21.7 Mortality for AGES groups

Group	PS	Mortality (%)
I	< 3.99	1
II	4–4.99	20
III	5–5.99	67
IV	6 +	87

AMES (Lahey Clinic 1988)

Age > 40 for males or > 50 for females; **M**etastasis; **E**xtrathyroid extension; **S**ize > 5 cm

Cady introduced this simpler scheme[23] dividing patients into high risk (AMES factors present) and low risk (AMES factors absent) groups. Those who are over the age limit and who have any of the other adverse risk factors are classified as high risk, while all others including all patients below the age limit are classified as low risk. Only 5% of patients in the low-risk group but 55% in the high-risk group developed recurrent disease, with a cause specific mortality of 1.8% and 46%, respectively. It was calculated that the 40-year survival was 95% for the low-risk group and 45% for the high-risk group of patients.

GAMES (Memorial Sloan Kettering Cancer Centre 1992)

histological **G**rade >2; **A**ge > 45 years; distant **M**etastasis; **E**xtension beyond the thyroid capsule; **S**ize > 4cm

The controversy over extent of thyroid surgery was addressed by Shah et al.[25–27] In low-risk groups total thyroidectomy offered no survival advantage over lobectomy. Staging of patients into high- and low-risk patient and tumour-risk groups provides criteria for justifying partial rather than total thyroidectomy (Tables 21.8 and 21.9).

Table 21.8 High- and low-risk prognostic factors

High risk	Low risk
Females > 45 yrs	Females < 45 yrs
Males	Small size T1
Size: Papillary > 1.5 cm	Complete excision
Size: Follicular > 1 cm	No nodes/mets
Incomplete resection	Low grade histology
Extrathyroid spread	Papillary
Local and distant mets	
High-grade follicular	

Table 21.9 Conservation surgery

Low-risk pt + low-risk tumour – lobectomy
High-risk pt + low-risk tumour – ?lobectomy
Low-risk pt + high-risk tumour } Total
High-risk pt + high-risk tumour } Thyroidectomy
Total thyroidectomy for all tumours > 1.5 cm

MACIS (Mayo Clinic 1993)

Metastasis; **A**ge > 40; **C**ompleteness of resection; extrathyroid **I**nvasion; **S**ize

Hay et al[28] revised their earlier staging system because grading of tumours was not universally used. Patients were similarly divided into four risk groups and the prognostic score calculated (Table 21.10). Using the MACIS scoring system the 20-year mortality ranged from 1% in group I to 76% in group IV (Table 21.11).

Table 21.10 MACIS scoring system

PS = 0 (if no metastases) or + 3 (if metastases present)
+ 3.1(if age is < 40) or 0.08 × age (if age 40 +)
+ 1 (if incomplete resection)
+ 1 (if extrathyroid invasion)
+ 0.3 × tumour size (in cm)

Table 21.11 Mortality for MACIS groups

Group	PS	Mortality (%)
I	< 6	1
II	6–6.99	11
III	7–7.99	44
IV	8 +	76

DAMES (Karolinska Institute 1992)

DNA ploidy; **A**ge > 40 for females and > 50 for males; **M**etastasis; **E**xtension beyond the thyroid capsule; **S**ize > 5cm.

This was based on a study[29] which showed that the assessment of tumour nuclear DNA content added prognostic value to the existing AMES risk group system (Table 21.12)

Table 21.12 DAMES scoring system

Ploidy	AMES	DAMES	Recurrence or metastases (%)
Euploid +	AMES low risk =	DAMES low risk	8
Euploid +	AMES high risk =	DAMES intermediate risk	55
Aneu-ploid +	AMES high risk =	DAMES high risk	100

TNM staging systems

Various staging systems have been devised for thyroid carcinoma, based primarily on the TNM classification (Table 21.13)[30] but also taking account of their diverse histology and age at presentation. The T stage depends on tumour size and whether or not growth is confined within the gland capsule. Each T stage is further subdivided depending on whether the tumour is unifocal or multifocal, which can be determined accurately only on histological examination. For this reason staging is usually described as a

Table 21.13 TNM staging for thyroid carcinoma

Primary tumour	
Tx	Primary tumour cannot be assessed
T0	No evidence of primary tumour
T1	Tumour 1cm or less in greatest dimension, limited to the thyroid
T1a	Unifocal
T1b	Multifocal
T2	Tumour 1–4cm in greatest dimension, limited to the thyroid
T2a	Unifocal
T2b	Multifocal
T3	Tumour > 4cm in greatest dimension, limited to the thyroid
T3a	Unifocal
T3b	Multifocal
T4	Tumour of any size, extending beyond the thyroid capsule
T4a	Unifocal
T4b	Multifocal
Regional lymph nodes	
Nx	Regional lymph nodes cannot be assessed
N0	No regional lymph node metastasis
N1a	Metastasis in ipsilateral cervical lymph node(s)
N1b	Metastasis in midline, contralateral or bilateral cervical lymph node(s) or metastasis in mediastinal lymph node(s)
Metastases	
M0	No metastases
M1	Metastases present

Table 21.14 Stage grouping for thyroid carcinoma

(a) Papillary or follicular carcinoma in patients aged 45 years or older			
Stage I	T1	N0	M0
Stage II	T2–3	N0	M0
Stage III	T4	N0	M0
	T1–3	N1	M0
Stage IV	T1–4	any N	M1
(b) Papillary or follicular carcinoma in patients under 45 years of age			
Stage I	T1–4	N0	M0
Stage II	T1–4	any N	M1
(No stage III or IV)			
(c) Medullary carcinoma, any age			
Stage I	T1	N0	M0
Stage II	T2–4	N0	M0
Stage III	T1–4	N1	M0
Stage IV	T1–4	any N	M1
(d) Anaplastic carcinoma, any age			
Stage IV	T1–4	any N	M0–1
(No stage I, II or III; all cases are stage IV)			

Table 21.15 Histological grade

I	Minimal pleomorphism, encapsulated and circumscribed tumour
II	Some cellular pleomorphism, often with intraglandular invasion
III	Dedifferentiated and pleomorphic tumour, often with extracapsular invasion

pathological stage (e.g. pT2b N1a). Unlike squamous carcinoma staging in the head and neck, nodal disease in the superior mediastinum is classified by N stage rather than as metastatic spread (M stage).

Taking into account the histology and age factors, thyroid carcinomas can be staged into various prognostic groups as shown in Table 21.14.

The histological grading of thyroid carcinoma is also an influential factor and is summarized in Table 21.15. Lymphomas have a complex grading system and classification;[31] in the thyroid they are predominantly of non-Hodgkin's B cell type.

Clinicopathological features

Solitary thyroid nodule

A solitary thyroid nodule is defined as 'any discrete macroscopic intrathyroidal lesion that is clearly distinguishable from the adjacent normal thyroid parenchyma'.[32] This is usually diagnosed on ultrasound or scan; its clinical significance and management is based on the principle of confirmation or exclusion of cancer.[32,33] Solitary thyroid nodules comprise two histological groups:

1. Degenerative lesions: cysts, degenerative colloid nodules;
2. Neoplastic lesions: (a) benign: follicular adenoma (90%), Hurthle cell adenoma (10%), teratoma; (b) malignant: papillary, follicular, medullary or anaplastic carcinoma.

The frequency of thyroid nodules compared with the relative scarcity of thyroid cancer makes it a priority to reduce the number of thyroid explorations for benign disease.[32–34] However, the overall incidence of

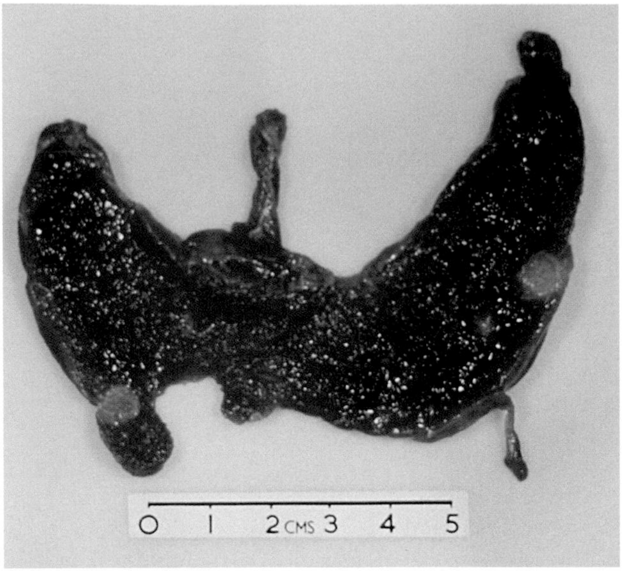

Figure 21.8 Multiple papillary carcinomas of the thyroid.

malignancy in patients presenting with thyroid nodules is 10%. This is increased when stratified for age and sex.[2,34,35] (Females under 50 years: 10%; and over 50 years: 30%; males under 50 years: 15%; and over 50 years: 45%.) It is also important clinically to distinguish a true solitary thyroid nodule from the dominant nodule in a multinodular goitre,[2,35] since the latter carry a much lower risk of malignancy of <1%.

Papillary carcinoma

The entity of benign papillary adenoma was previously argued[2,36] but the World Health Organization has stipulated that any tumour containing papillary structures will be designated as papillary carcinoma, with no existing benign counterpart.[2,37] Papillary carcinoma typically affects the young female, with a mean age of diagnosis of 35–45 yrs. The overall sex ratio is three females to one male but is 9:1 in Japan.[2] There is a high incidence of multifocality and bilateralism,[2] reported as 30–87.5% (Figure 21.8).[38]

Papillary carcinoma can be divided into pure papillary carcinoma (3%) and mixed papillary follicular carcinoma (97%). This distinction is not important clinically, as the mixed tumours are similar in biological behaviour and clinical outcome irrespective of the proportion of the papillary component. However, a 'tall cell' variant is also recognized, which has a poorer prognosis (Figure 21.9).

Spread of disease is usually to paratracheal and cervical lymph nodes initially, and much later to the mediastinal lymph nodes. Distant metastasis usually occurs late and is limited to the lungs and rarely the bones.[2] Although the disease often follows an indolent course, with an overall 20-year survival of 90–95%,[32] it tends to be more aggressive in later life and may progress rapidly after remaining localized for years.[32,34] The main features are summarized in Table 21.16.

Table 21.16 Features of papillary carcinoma

Commonest type – 80%
Typically females 35–45 years
Sex ratio F:M 3:1 (Japan 9:1)
Multifocality and bilateralism 30–87%
Pure papillary 3%: mixed pap/foll 97%
Lymph node metastases in 50%
Late distant metastases to lungs (+ bones)
20 year survival 90–95%

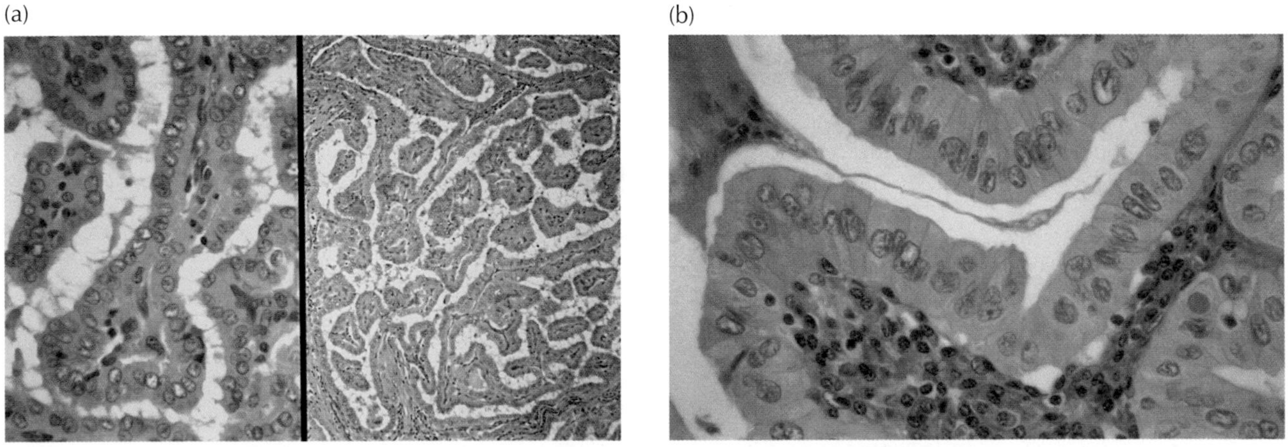

Figure 21.9 Histological features of papillary carcinoma. (a) Papillary; (b) tall cell variant.

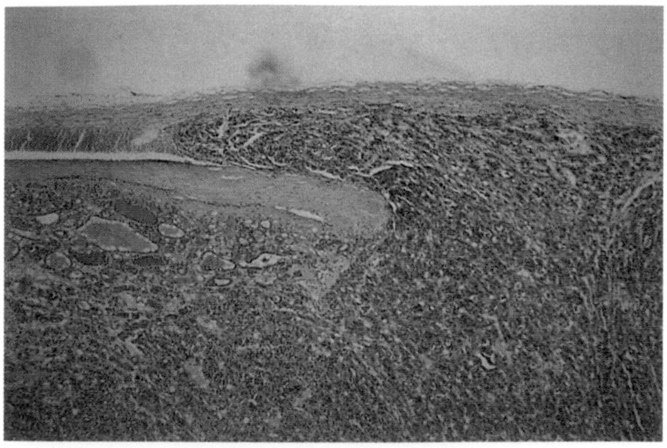

Figure 21.10 Histological features of follicular carcinoma showing capsular invasion.

Follicular carcinoma

Follicular carcinoma is defined as a malignant thyroid tumour with features of follicular cell differentiation.[2] Mixed papillary/follicular tumours should be excluded. The disease is usually unifocal, with less than 2% of cases bilateral. There is often a pre-existing history of multinodular goitre and geographically occurrence is more frequent in iodine deficient areas. However, it is almost always a solitary tumour and rarely may be clinically occult. Follicular carcinoma affects a slightly older age group (mean 40–50 years) with a sex ratio similar to that of papillary carcinoma of three females to one male.

Often it is very well differentiated, with minimal or even non-existent cellular pleomorphism; histological recognition is dependent on the identification of capsular or vascular invasion (Figure 21.10).[2,32–34] This makes differentiation from follicular adenoma, which often has some degree of cellular pleomorphism, unreliable by needle biopsy and even by frozen section.[32,34]

Prognosis is still good with adequate treatment but not as good as papillary carcinoma, with a mean 10-year survival of 80–85%, and 20-year survival of 70–75%.[2,24] Spread is blood borne to the lungs, bones and rarely the brain or liver. Lymphatic spread is unusual (Table 21.17).

Hurthle cell carcinoma

Hurthle cell carcinoma is the malignant counterpart of Hurthle cell adenoma, also known as oncocytoma.[39] It is characterized by plump cells with intensely eosinophilic cytoplasm and large vesicular nuclei. It carries a distinctly poorer prognosis,[2,39] partly because it is unable to take up radioactive iodine. The WHO recommends that it be included as the oxyphilic variant of follicular carcinoma.[30,37]

Table 21.17 Features of follicular carcinoma

10% thyroid tumours
Older age group 40–50 years
Sex ratio F:M 3:1
Solitary and unifocal – bilateral cases in 2%
Pre-existing MNG or iodine deficient area
Vascular invasion (lungs, bones, brain)
Survival 80–85% at 10 years, 70–75% at 20 years

Medullary carcinoma

Medullary carcinoma of the thyroid (MCT) arises from parafollicular or calcitonin secreting C cells. It comprises 5–10% of thyroid malignancies and the cells usually contain *calcitonin* granules.[2] There is no benign counterpart but C cell hyperplasia may have the potential of malignant transformation.

MCT was first described as a sporadic form in 1959 and its association with familial multiple endocrine neoplasia (MEN) syndromes was recognized by Sipple in 1961. In MEN 2A syndrome MCT is associated with hyperparathyroidism and/or phaeochromocytoma, being transmitted by an autosomal dominant gene (Table 21.18). The medullary carcinoma is present in all affected family members, although a palpable thyroid swelling may not become evident before the age of 40 years.[40]

MEN 2B syndrome is less common but the carcinoma is more aggressive, being associated with phaeochromocytoma and a marfanoid appearance. There are also multiple mucosal neuromas affecting the lips, tongue (Figure 21.11), oropharynx and large bowel. Approximately 20% of MCT are familial (FMCT) inherited as an autosomal dominant condition with no associated endocrinopathy.[41]

Fifty to seventy percent of MEN-associated tumours are multifocal but the sporadic form is more often unifocal. Familial forms of the disease are usually more indolent than the sporadic type, with the exception of MEN.[2,30,42,43]

Table 21.18 MEN syndromes

	2a	2b	FMTC
MTC	+	+	+
Phaeo	+	+	–
Parathyroid	+	–	–

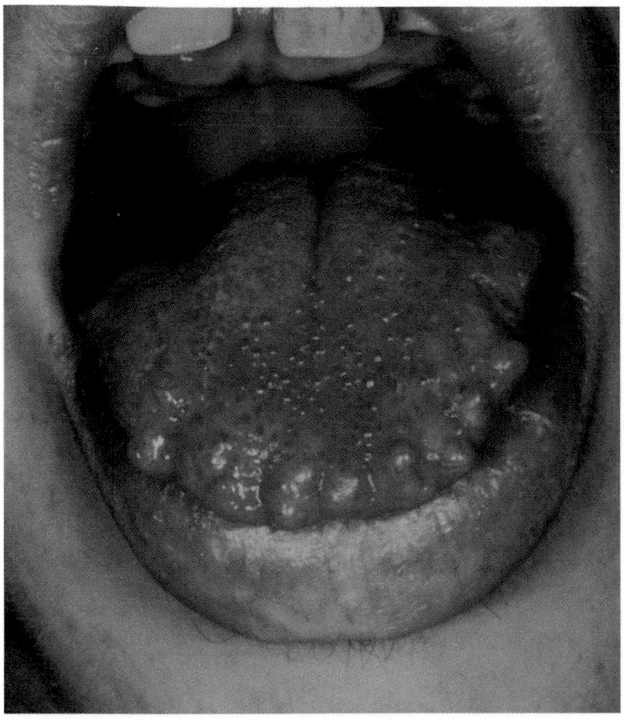

Figure 21.11 MEN syndrome showing neuromas of the tongue.

The mean age at presentation is 40–60 years for sporadic disease but 15–20 years for MEN-associated medullary carcinoma.[2] Lymph node metastases (often bilateral) are frequently present at diagnosis. Distant metastases may also be present in the lungs, bones or liver.[2]

Prognosis is worse than that of follicular carcinoma. It is dependent on tumour subtype (non-MEN familial > MEN-associated > sporadic > MEN) and stage at presentation, being worse if lymph node metastases are present. With adequate treatment the overall mean 10-year survival is 75–80% and 20-year survival is 60–65%.[2,42,43]

Anaplastic carcinoma

Anaplastic carcinoma is a highly malignant tumour that appears partially or totally undifferentiated on light microscopy but has epithelial differentiation on ultrastructural or immunohistochemical grounds.[2] It is a highly lethal form of thyroid cancer, which is rapidly progressive and presents late, typically with respiratory obstruction. There are three histological variants: small cell, spindle cell and giant cell, with increasingly poor prognosis. However many previously labelled small cell carcinomas have been subsequently proven on histochemical staining to be malignant lymphomas,[2] which corresponds with the better prognosis.

Anaplastic carcinoma can arise from a pre-existing papillary or follicular carcinoma[2,44] or multinodular thyroid. There is early spread to the cervical and mediastinal lymph nodes, lungs, liver and bones. Typically elderly females are affected, with a mean age at presentation of 60–75. The sex ratio is three females to one male.[2] Prognosis is dismal, with a mean overall survival of 3–6 months from time of diagnosis.

Thyroid lymphoma

Primary thyroid lymphoma constitutes less than 1% of all thyroid malignancies. Almost all are non-Hodgkin's lymphomas, usually of B cell phenotype and of large cell morphology.[2,45] Secondary lymphoma to the thyroid is five times more common. Systemic 'B' symptoms are rare.

Thyroid lymphoma spreads within the gland initially, replacing most or all of it. It is usually of diffuse pattern but may be nodular. Regional lymphatic spread is common to the cervical and mediastinal nodes. Eighty percent arise in pre-existing Hashimoto's disease. However, only a very small percentage of patients with Hashimoto's thyroiditis develop malignant lymphoma.[2]

Similarly to anaplastic carcinoma it typically affects the elderly female, with the mean age at presentation of 65–75 years and a sex ratio of three females to one male.[2] It is of great importance to distinguish thyroid lymphoma from anaplastic carcinoma due to their somewhat similar presentation yet different treatment and prognosis. Stage I involves the thyroid gland only; any regional lymph node involvement above the diaphragm becomes stage II.[80]

Clinical evaluation

The clinical presentation of a patient with thyroid carcinoma has been discussed earlier in this chapter. The suspicious symptoms and associated features are summarized in Tables 21.3 and 21.4. In addition, careful examination of the patient may reveal signs that further increase the suspicion of malignancy (Table 21.19).

Table 21.19 Clinical signs of malignancy

Hard, fixed or irregular thyroid swelling
Cervical lymphadenopathy
Recurrent laryngeal nerve palsy

Investigations

Fine-needle aspiration cytology

Fine-needle aspiration cytology (FNAC) has become the key investigation in the work-up of thyroid nodules[32,33,46–48] and is indicated in the evaluation of all thyroid nodules. It is a safe, easy, cheap and reliable test that will effectively distinguish between neoplastic (potentially malignant) lesions and degenerative (probably benign) disease with an accuracy of up to 95%. Since its introduction the incidence of malignancy in patients undergoing surgery for nodular disease has increased from 10% to 50% because of increased accuracy of preoperative diagnosis. The number of patients subjected to thyroid surgery has also fallen from 67% to 43%.[46] Even in experienced hands 10–15% of aspirations are inadequate or non-diagnostic, but this may be reduced by half by repeated aspirations or by ultrasound-guided FNAC. Typical results of FNAC are shown in Table 21.20.

A strategy for evaluation of a solitary or dominant thyroid nodule is given in Figure 21.12.[33,34] FNAC is also invaluable in assessing any associated cervical lymphadenopathy.

Table 21.20 Results of thyroid FNAC

Degenerative conditions (75%)
Thyroid cyst
Fluid should be sent for cytological assessment
Degenerative or colloid nodule
<1% risk of malignancy
Neoplastic conditions (4% positive; 11% suspicious)
Papillary neoplasm
99% accuracy in positive reports
60% accuracy in suspicious reports
Follicular neoplasm
Unreliable for distinguishing between follicular adenoma and well-differentiated follicular carcinoma: excision required
Medullary carcinoma
Reliable diagnosis when combined with calcitonin staining
Anaplastic carcinoma
Usually diagnostic but may not distinguish from lymphoma or metastatic carcinoma
Lymphoma
Open biopsy required for immunocytochemistry
Other specific tumours
Inconclusive (10%)
FNAC should be repeated (under ultrasound guidance)

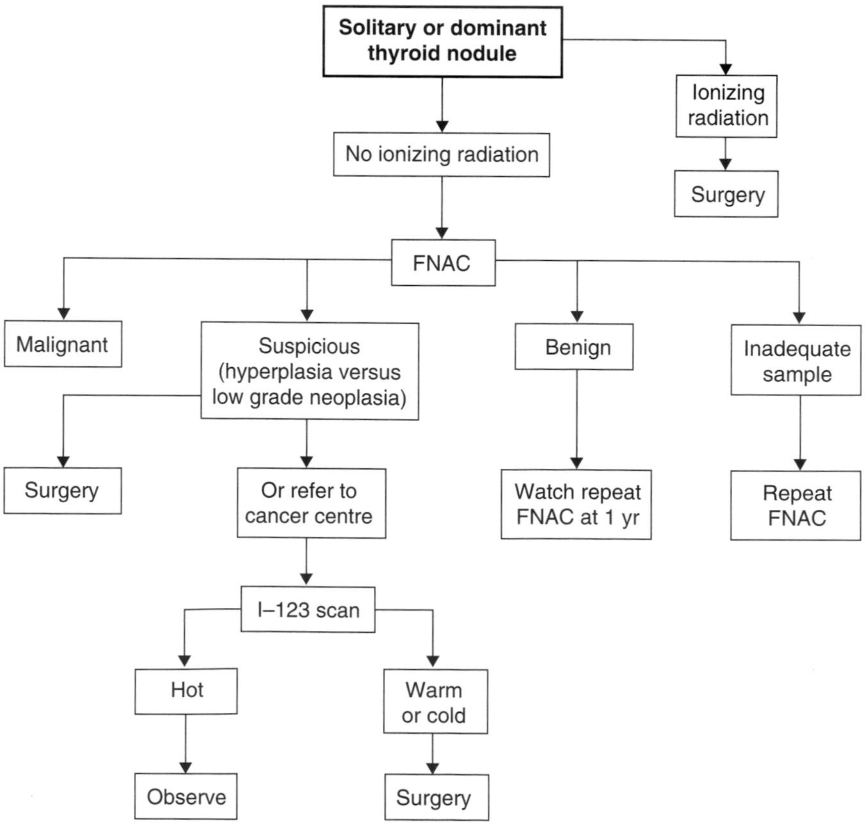

Figure 21.12 Evaluation of a solitary or dominant thyroid nodule.

Ultrasonography

High-frequency real-time high-resolution ultrasonography (up to 3 mm resolution with 7 MHz or 10 MHz probe) is currently the most sensitive method for evaluating thyroid nodules,[49] and is ideally used in combination with FNAC in preliminary assessment. It effectively distinguishes a solitary thyroid nodule from the dominant nodule in a multinodular goitre. It is effective in assessing the size and position of cervical lymphadenopathy.[49,50] It is also useful in identifying and sampling an apparently occult primary tumour in patients presenting with metastatic nodes.

Radionuclide scanning

Thyroid scintigraphy was previously the most commonly used investigation for thyroid nodules. Technetium 99m is taken up by the thyroid and is readily available but uptake is low and scans are neither sensitive nor specific, although the information provided in terms of 'hot' or 'cold' nodules may be helpful (Figure 21.13). Iodine-123 is ideal but its cost and availability restrict its use. These scans are no longer used as first-line investigation of thyroid nodules but remain invaluable for whole-body imaging following total thyroidectomy for well-differentiated carcinoma.

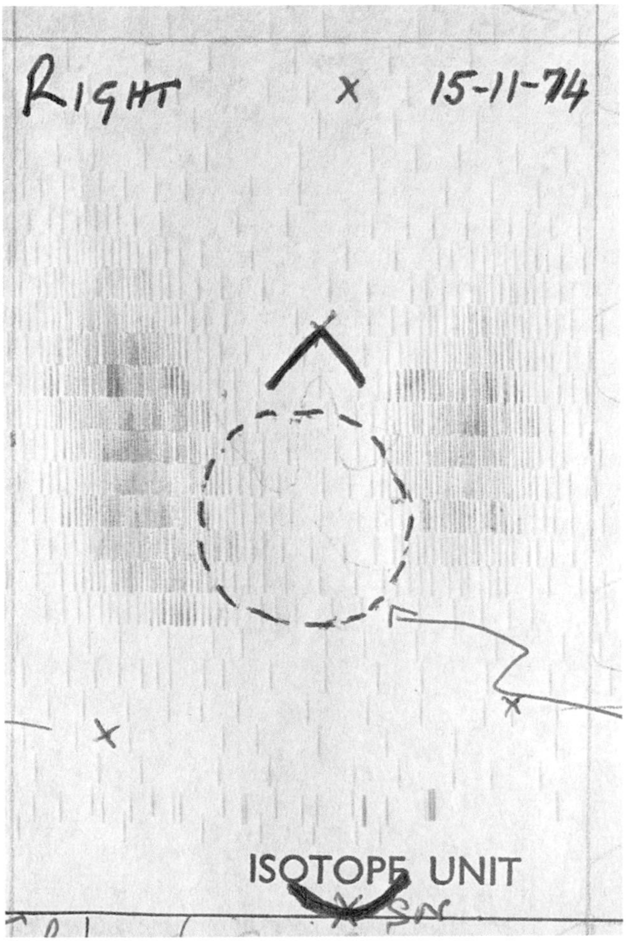

Figure 21.13 'Cold' nodule on thyroid scan.

In medullary carcinoma a variety of scanning agents including pentavalent dimercaptosuccinic acid (DMSA) and metaiodobenzylguanidine (mIBG) may locate in recurrent or metastatic disease (Figure 21.14). However, they are not taken up by tumour cells as readily as ^{131}I in differentiated carcinoma and positive scans occur in only 30% of tumours.

Computerized tomography and magnetic resonance imaging

CT and MR scanning do not have a role in the routine diagnosis of thyroid malignancy[32,34] but once the diagnosis is made can provide invaluable information to assess extrathyroid involvement of the larynx, trachea, oesophagus and carotid sheath. They may also help to identify possible neck disease and to assess the superior mediastinum for retrosternal spread or nodal metastases. They are essential for evaluation of recurrent thyroid tumours and possible metastases. In MCT and lymphoma they are indicated for exclusion of phaeochromocytoma and staging respectively (Table 21.21).

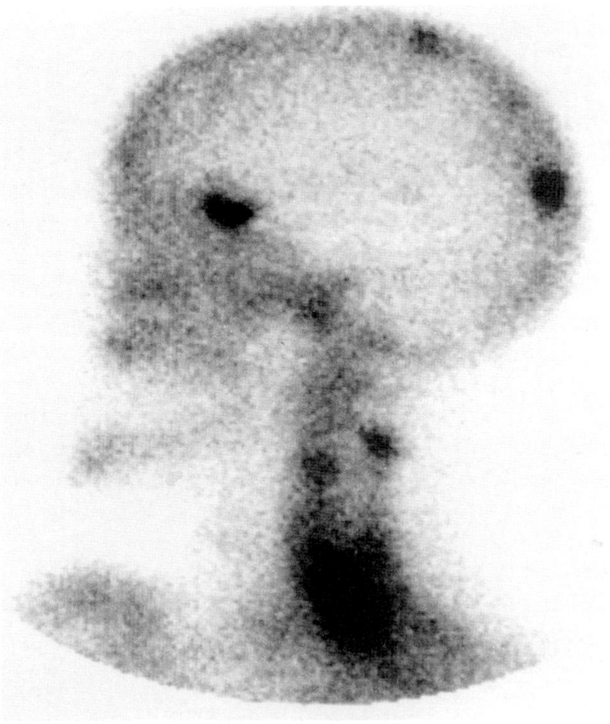

Figure 21.14 Metastases from MTC shown on mIBG scan.

Table 21.21 Indications for CT/MR scanning

Neck	Possible bilateral lobe involvement
	Extrathyroid invasion of trachea, larynx, oesophagus, carotid
	Lymph node involvement
Thorax	Retrosternal spread
	Superior mediastinal nodes
	Pulmonary metastases in MTC/anaplastic carcinoma
Abdomen	Exclusion of phaeochromocytoma in MTC
	Liver metastases in MTC/anaplastic carcinoma
	Lymphoma staging

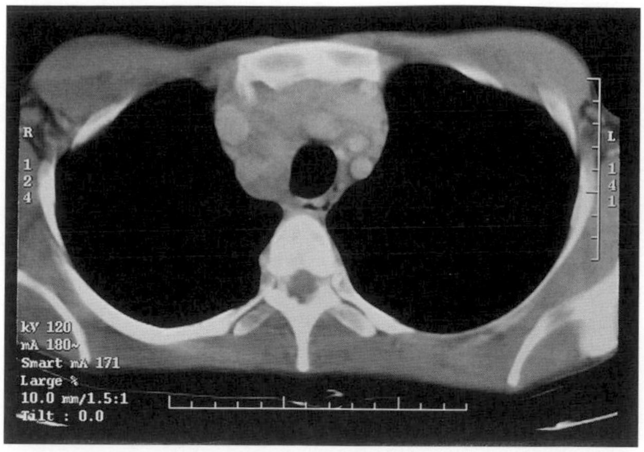

Figure 21.15 Large papillary carcinoma mediastinal nodes resected by thoracocervical approach.

The main disadvantage of CT scanning is the necessary administration of iodine contrast, which can block subsequent use of diagnostic or therapeutic radioiodine for 6 months. MRI involves neither radiation nor iodine and with increasing diagnostic ability is the investigation of choice in differentiated carcinoma.

CT or MR scanning of the mediastinum is indicated when mediastinal lymphadenopathy is suspected. A plain chest radiograph is adequate as preoperative screening for pulmonary metastases, which may need confirmation by whole thoracic CT.

CT scanning of the abdomen is part of the metastatic screen for medullary and anaplastic carcinoma as well as lymphoma[42,43] but not indicated for papillary or follicular carcinoma.

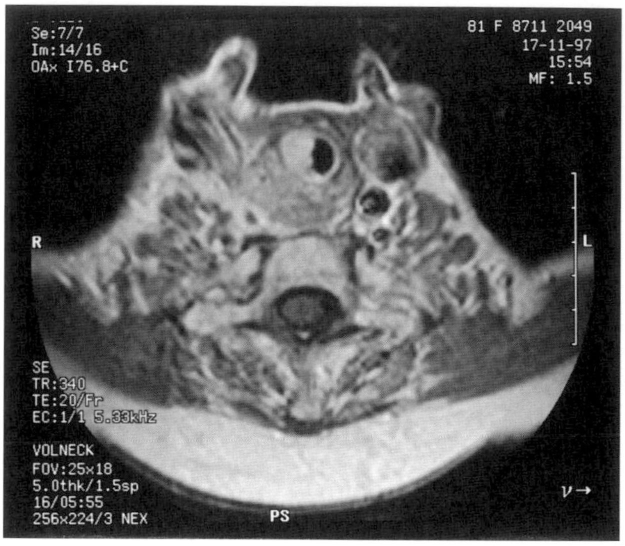

Figure 21.16 Intratracheal papillary carcinoma.

Blood tests

Thyroid function tests (i.e. serum free thyroxine (T4) and thyroid stimulating hormone (TSH)) should be requested for all patients with thyroid disease. Thyroid autoantibodies (anti-microsomal and anti-thyroglobulin) are indicated if Hashimoto's disease or thyroid lymphoma is suspected.

Tumour markers, thyroglobulin[51] for papillary/follicular carcinoma and calcitonin and carcinoembryonic antigen (CEA) for medullary carcinoma, should be measured preoperatively in all cases. They have a proven role in monitoring and follow-up[52] and calcitonin is also helpful in initial diagnosis.

Other screening investigations

Indirect or fibreoptic laryngoscopy to assess vocal cord mobility and/or intratracheal disease is indicated for all patients with suspected thyroid malignancy. It is mandatory for both preoperative and postoperative assessment.

Serum calcium and 24-hour urinary catecholamines are indicated in all patients with medullary carcinoma to screen for MEN 2.[42,43,53] Indium-111 octreotide scanning is reliable in excluding an associated phaeochromocytoma. Serum calcium should also be measured prior to any thyroid surgery and postoperatively to monitor possible parathyroid deficiency.

Previously, if MEN 2 was diagnosed, all first degree relatives were screened by clinical examination, thyroid ultrasound, serum calcitonin with pentagastrin stimulation, serum calcium and 24-hour urinary catecholamines.[42,43,53,54] Since the identification of the chromosomal abnormality, it is now preferable to refer the index case to a clinical geneticist.

Treatment

The general management of a patient presenting with a thyroid swelling is outlined in Figure 21.17. If malignancy is proven the subsequent management is governed by appropriate specific protocols depending on the histology (Figures 21.18–21.21). Surgery remains the optimal initial treatment for papillary, follicular and medullary carcinoma, providing the best chance of cure. Radiotherapy is the main option for anaplastic carcinoma and thyroid lymphoma, preceded by open biopsy if FNAC is not conclusive.

There remain two important challenges in the surgical management of thyroid lesions.

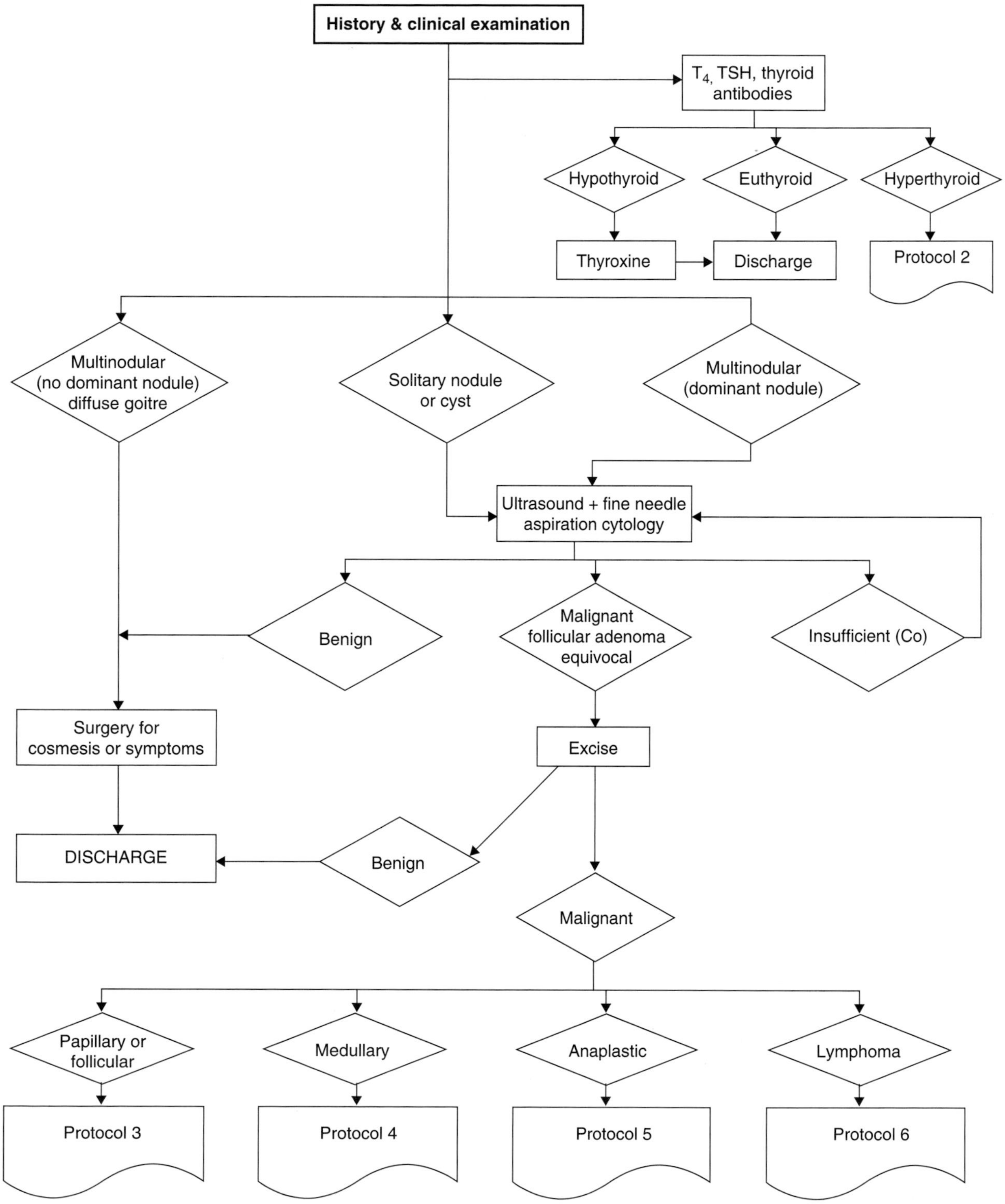

Figure 21.17 Protocol for management of a thyroid swelling.

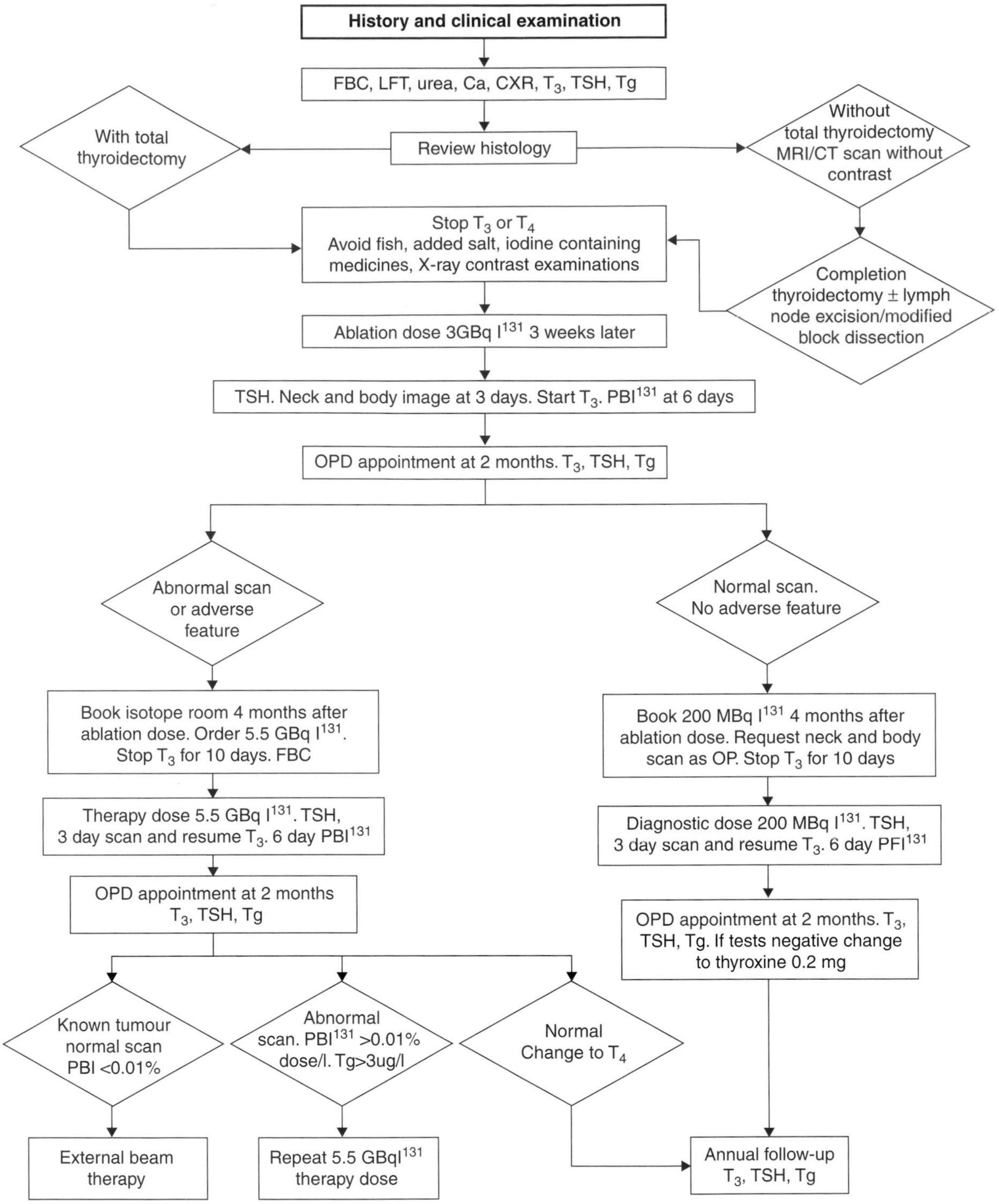

Figure 21.18 Protocol for differentiated thyroid carcinoma.

1. Reducing the benign to malignant ratio for thyroid operations. Palpable thyroid nodules are found in 3–8% of adults, the incidence increasing with age and 50% have nodules on ultrasonic or CT imaging. In contrast, thyroid carcinoma is designated as a rare cancer (less than 1% of all cancers), with a low mortality rate. There is therefore a need to identify the minority of patients with nodules who carry a significant risk of malignancy.
2. Fine tuning the extent of surgery according to prognostic indices. With the different tumour types and the wide variation in natural history and biological behaviour, treatment must be tailored so that, whilst ensuring the best chance of cure, it is not so aggressive as to cause unnecessary morbidity in those patients with better prognosis.

There are also other controversial aspects of management that continue to be debated.

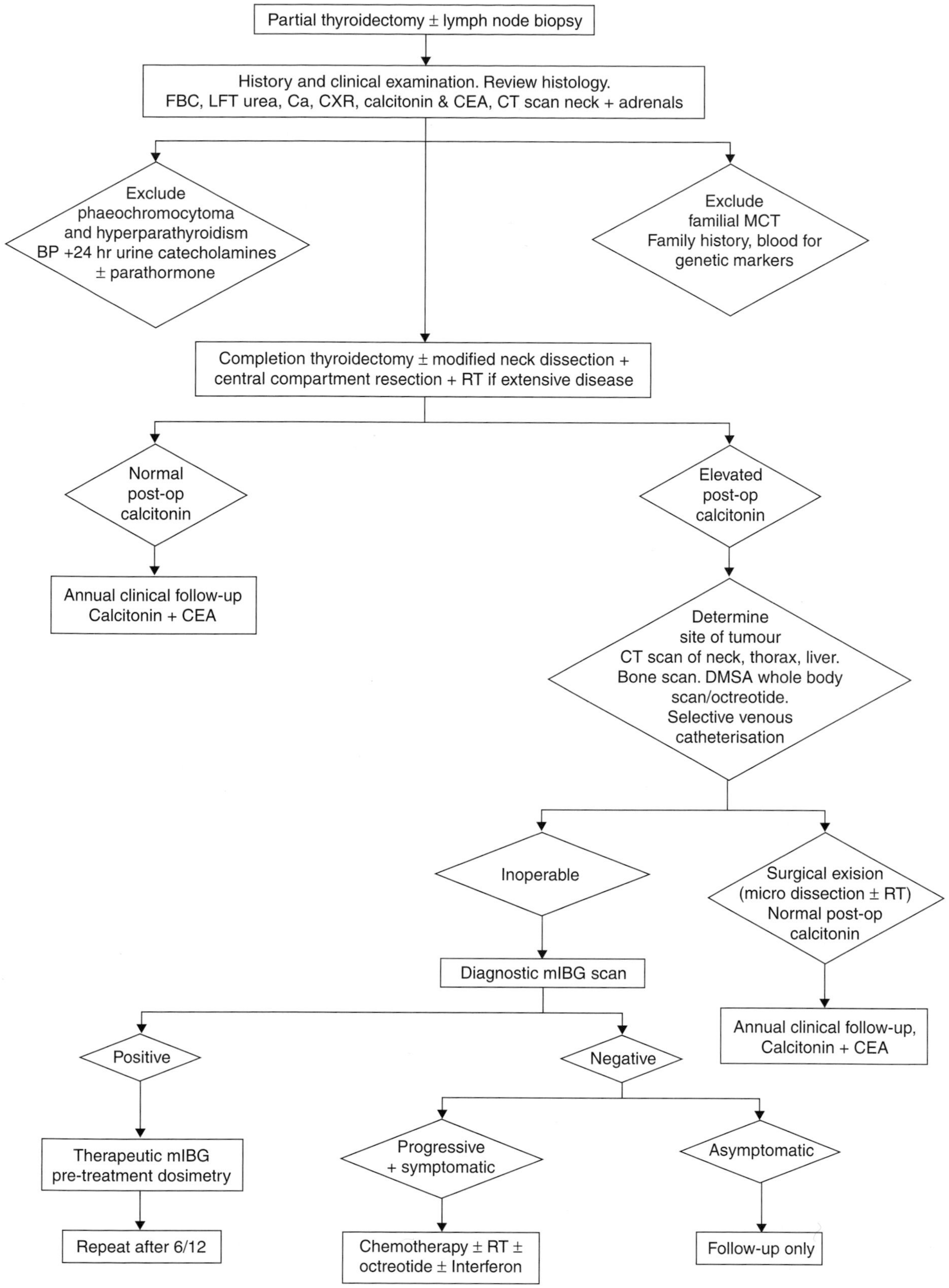

Figure 21.19 Protocol for medullary thyroid carcinoma.

1. Lobectomy or total thyroidectomy? The extent of surgical resection remains controversial. Lobectomy with isthmusectomy is advocated for early papillary and follicular carcinoma with good prognostic indices[26] but others favour a minimum of total or near-total thyroidectomy.[32,34,36]
2. Node picking or proper node dissection? The extent of neck dissection is also still debated.

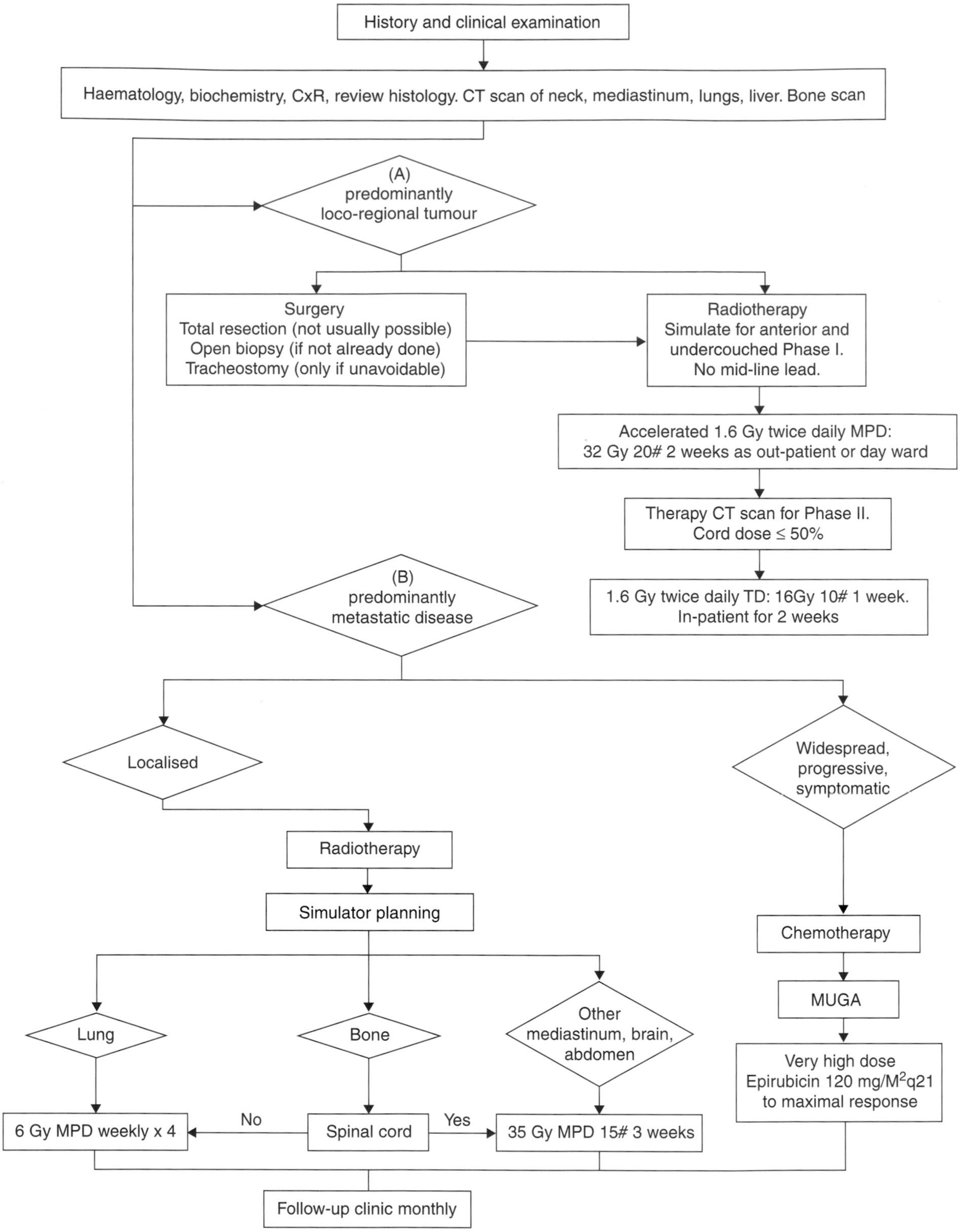

Figure 21.20 Protocol for anaplastic thyroid carcinoma.

'Node plucking' or 'berry picking' operations are almost certainly inadequate, such that the minimum operation should be some form of modified radical or selective neck dissection[32,34] depending on node status.

3. TSH suppression? Postoperative TSH suppression therapy is indicated in all patients with well-differentiated thyroid malignancy.[32,34] For patients with other tumours, physiological thyroid hormone replacement is required to achieve a normal TSH level.
4. Radioactive iodine? Radioiodine has played an important role in the management of differentiated thyroid carcinoma for over 50 years.[55] In

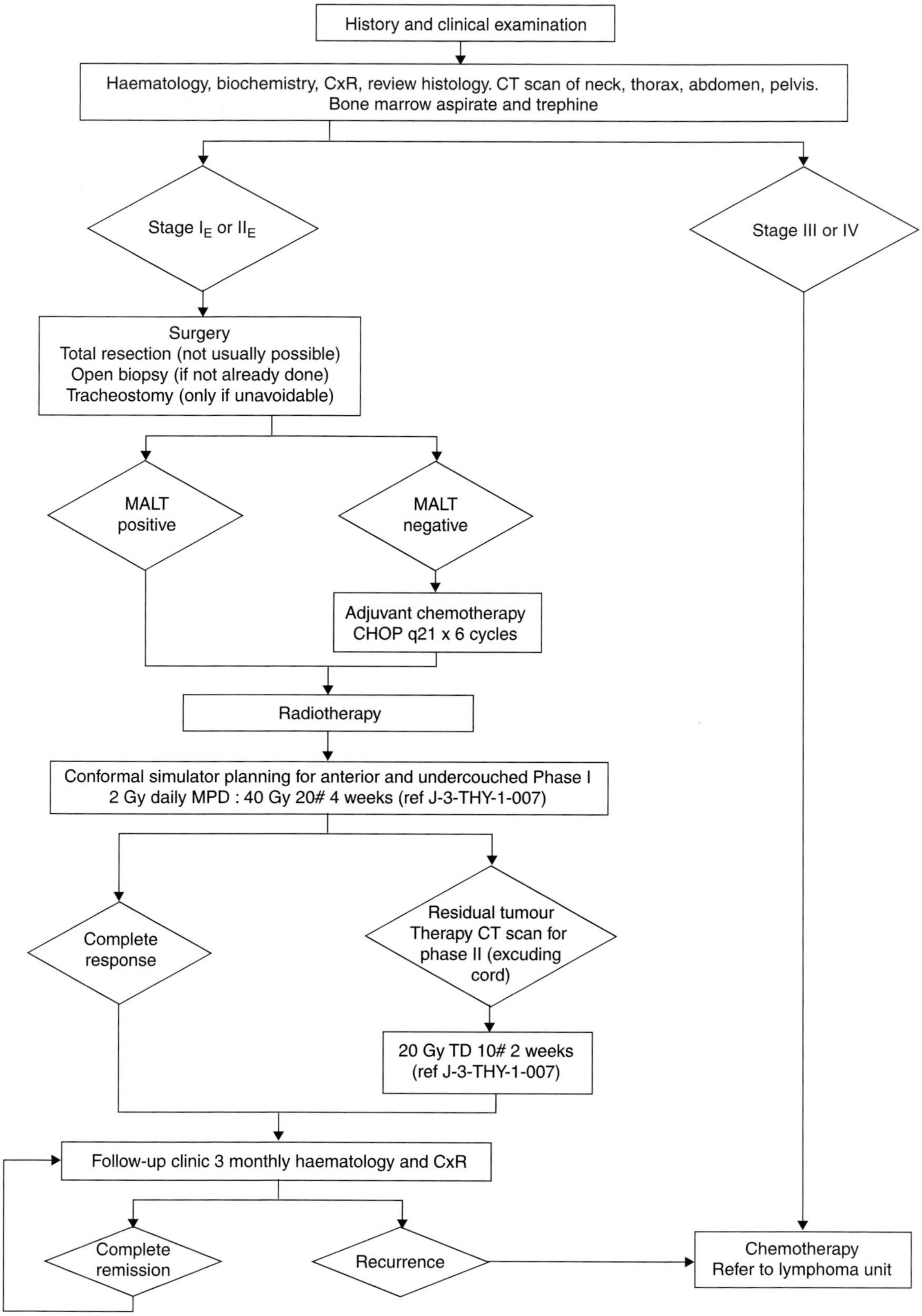

Figure 21.21 Protocol for primary lymphoma of the thyroid.

addition to its use as a diagnostic aid to assess possible sites of residual thyroid tissue or tumour, it can be used in a therapeutic role for the treatment of known inoperable residual or metastatic cancer, or in an ablative setting to destroy normal residual thyroid tissue after thyroid surgery. The rationale for radioiodine ablation[56,57] includes subsequent iodine treatment of any residual cancer as well as improvement in the sensitivity of subsequent radionuclide scanning and thyroglobulin monitoring.

5. External beam radiotherapy? External beam radiotherapy has a proven adjuvant role in the treatment of differentiated as well as medullary thyroid carcinoma.[58–60] It is used, when indicated, in addition to radioiodine therapy. It is also the main therapeutic modality for anaplastic carcinoma and thyroid lymphoma.
6. Chemotherapy? Cytotoxic chemotherapy has shown little potential in thyroid cancer apart from thyroid lymphoma. Medullary carcinoma is the only other thyroid tumour to demonstrate significant response to chemotherapy[61] where it has a palliative role.

Papillary carcinoma

Partial thyroidectomy versus total thyroidectomy?

There is continued controversy concerning the extent of thyroid resection, some advocating a more conservative approach for low-risk groups[26] whilst others would recommend total thyroidectomy for all patients who are diagnosed preoperatively for the reasons given in Table 21.21. In a disease where at least 80% of patients are cured whatever the extent of surgery, the higher potential morbidity rates associated with total thyroidectomy must be weighed against the small increase in cure rate and reduction in recurrence. Retrospective studies have shown some value in separating patients into high- and low-risk groups[23,24,26,27] whilst others have recommended total (or near-total) thyroidectomy for tumours over 1.5 cm in size (Table 21.9).[32,34,36]

Preoperative diagnosis of carcinoma

Patients with preoperatively diagnosed cancer from cytology may initially have lobectomy and isthmusectomy; if frozen section confirms malignancy the other lobe is resected at the same operation, completing the total thyroidectomy (Figure 21.18). If thyroid carcinoma has been diagnosed from biopsy or cytology of a lymph node, it is appropriate to carry out total thyroidectomy and neck dissection (+/– superior mediastinal dissection as indicated by preoperative scan)

Postoperative diagnosis of papillary carcinoma

When the diagnosis of papillary carcinoma is made postoperatively after lobectomy in a patient with good prognostic indices, it is acceptable to adopt a 'wait and see' policy with TSH suppression and close clinical follow-up provided that:

Table 21.22 Advantages of total thyroidectomy

Multifocal disease exists histologically in up to 87.5% of cases[38]
Locoregional recurrence is higher after unilateral lobectomy (25%) compared with bilateral lobectomy (6%)[62]
Any residual tumour has the potential to transform to anaplastic carcinoma[2,44]
Although differentiated thyroid carcinoma tends to follow an indolent course irrespective of the extent of treatment, this slow progression of disease is deceptive and survival after 15 years has been shown to be significantly lower in patients treated non-radically, with cause-specific mortality occuring up to 40 years after initial treatment[63]
Follow-up with thyroglobulin and radioiodine scans are easier to interpret after total thyroidectomy[32]
Complications of hypoparathyroidism and recurrent laryngeal nerve injury are minimal in experienced hands

1. There is no evidence of multifocal tumour in the resected specimen;
2. There is good histological tumour clearance;
3. The tumour is small (< 1.5cm).

Central compartment dissection

The role of elective unilateral tracheo-oesophageal groove clearance of nodes down to the level of the thymus awaits clarification.[34,42,43] Those who favour the procedure quote that this is the commonest site of lymph node metastases, that the potential morbidity associated with reoperating at a later date is much greater, and that without it there is an increased risk of subsequently finding inoperable disease or tracheal infiltration. Against it is an increased incidence of postoperative hypoparathyroidism and recurrent laryngeal nerve damage but these should be minimal in experienced hands.

Our policy is to carry out an elective tracheo-oesophageal groove clearance on the ipsilateral side down to the level of the thymus. The contralateral side is cleared if there is multifocal or bilateral disease. When paratracheal nodal disease is demonstrated clinically or radiologically, or palpable disease is found at operation, therapeutic dissection is carried out as far down the mediastinum as required so that all palpable disease is removed. If superior mediastinal disease is detected (Figure 21.15) preoperatively or at the primary operation it is preferable to resect this down to the arch of the aorta with a combined thoracocervical approach,[64,65] preserving the recurrent laryngeal nerves rather than risk the inevitable recurrence, which will be almost impossible to resect completely (Figure 21.22).

Cervical lymph node dissection

For clinical N0 disease there is no proven benefit for elective deep cervical chain dissection[66] although it is mandatory to palpate potential node sites at operation and proceed to modified neck dissection if frozen section is positive. For clinical N+ disease it is our policy to carry out a selective neck dissection (levels II-VI) with preservation of the internal jugular vein, the sternomastoid, cervical sensory plexus (C2,3,4) and accessory nerve if not clinically involved at operation. If disease is present in level II it is preferable to include level I in the dissection. If previous nodectomy has been performed with positive histology, a completion modified radical neck dissection is carried out to clear all potentially involved nodes.

Locally advanced papillary cancer

For more extensive tumour involving the larynx, trachea, oesophagus or common carotid artery, there is controversy concerning potential functional morbidity associated with wide radical excision against likelihood of cure. For unresectable disease initial therapy consists of total thyroidectomy with maximal debulking of tumour followed by radioiodine therapy +/- external beam radiotherapy.[5,58] Occasionally iodine-negative progressive or recurrent disease may demand more radical surgery comprising partial or total laryngectomy, oesophagectomy, tracheal or carotid artery resection with appropriate reconstruction. Long-term disease control and prolonged survival may be achieved.[67–69]

Postoperative radioiodine ablation

A single ablation dose of 3 GBq of radioiodine-131 is routinely given.[5] It has been shown that recurrence is significantly reduced by postoperative iodine in combination with thyroid suppression[70,71] as well as the likelihood of cancer death. In one series the cumulative recurrence rate was 6% in patients receiving radioiodine in addition to TSH suppression compared with 12% in patients who underwent TSH suppression alone.[71]

Subsequent radioiodine therapy

Residual inoperable disease can be treated by repeated therapeutic doses of 5.5 GBq of radioiodine every 6 months until all tumour has been eradicated.[5] This regime has been shown to be safe with no significant increased incidence of pulmonary

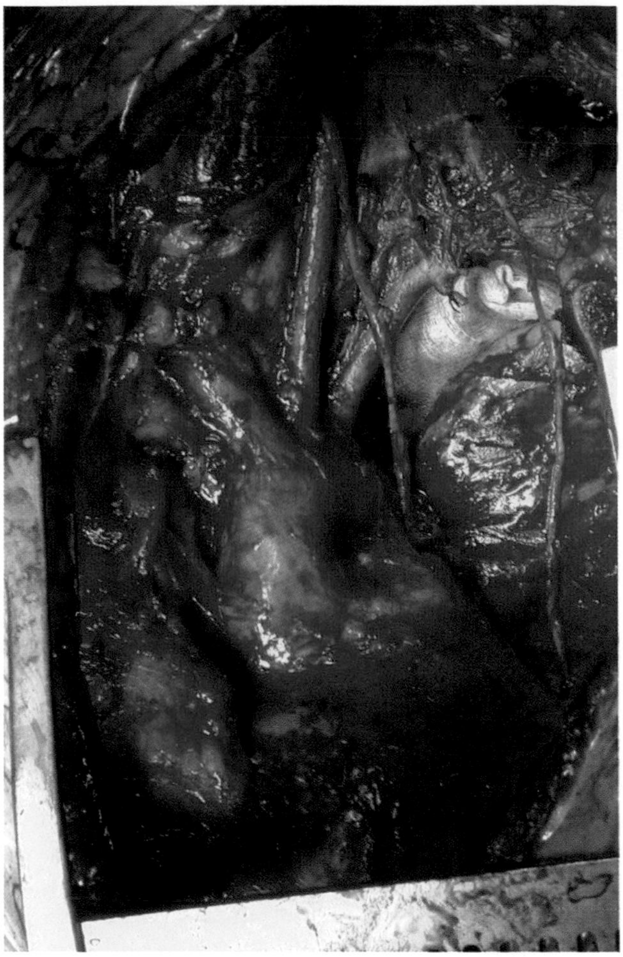

Figure 21.22 Thoraco-cervical resection for superior mediastinal disease.

fibrosis, subfertility, abnormal birth history, or secondary malignancy,[5,72,73] provided that the following precautions are taken.

1. All patients undergoing radioiodine therapy should have undergone total or near-total thyroidectomy so as to reduce the dose of radioactivity to the minimum.
2. Existing pregnancy must be excluded at the time of iodine administration. Conception should be delayed for both male and female patients for 6 months thereafter.
3. Liberal fluid intake and frequent micturition during isotope therapy achieve rapid renal excretion of surplus radioactivity. A laxative should routinely be prescribed to reduce dose to the bowel.
4. Iodine-rich foods as well as iodine-based contrast radiography should be avoided for 3 weeks prior to radioiodine therapy to make it more effective.
5. Lemon drops or bitter sweets will stimulate secretion of saliva and reduce dose to the salivary glands, minimizing subsequent xerostomia.
6. Repeat doses should be prescribed only when therapeutic benefit can be demonstrated.

External beam radiotherapy

External beam radiotherapy using megavoltage photons to a dose of 60 Gy over 6 weeks can be given in addition if there is incomplete surgical resection of tumour due to extrathyroidal or extranodal disease.[74] This has been shown to significantly decrease the locoregional recurrence rate in such patients from 23% to 11% at 5 years.

Follow-up

The serum thyroglobulin level should be measured and the patient is put on TSH suppression for life. Follow-up includes annual clinical examination and thyroglobulin assay for life. If thyroglobulin levels rise above 3 ng/ml a diagnostic radioiodine scan would be indicated.

Recurrent papillary carcinoma

Recurrence of differentiated thyroid carcinoma occurs in up to 25% of patients and in many instances this is due to incomplete or inadequate primary treatment. Historically many patients have been treated with less than total thyroidectomy and 'node picking', with reliance on postoperative radioactive iodine to eradicate microscopic or even macroscopic cervical, paratracheal or mediastinal nodal disease which is present in up to 80% of patients. Appropriate head and neck training in selective and modified radical neck dissection techniques is essential. Referral to an appropriate specialist should be considered before a patient's disease is deemed inoperable.

At initial presentation potential nodal disease and upper aerodigestive tract involvement should be properly assessed by a thorough ENT examination with MR of the neck and mediastinum so that optimal complete eradication of disease can be achieved at the first operation. Recurrent papillary carcinoma should be reassessed by clinical examination, indirect laryngoscopy and MR. All locoregional disease should be excised where possible followed by repeat radioiodine treatment +/– external beam radiotherapy. In the older patient with intralaryngotracheal disease (Figure 21.16) satisfactory prolonged palliation may be achieved with endoscopic resection rather than recourse to total laryngectomy.[3] Radical locoregional surgery may occasionally be necessary.[32,34,67–69]

Follicular carcinoma

Differences from papillary carcinoma

The management of follicular carcinoma is similar to that of papillary carcinoma, including radioiodine ablation, with minor differences:

1. Although there are proponents for lobectomy only for early follicular carcinoma with good prognostic indices, the consensus is for total thyroidectomy due to the poorer prognosis for this tumour.
2. All follicular neoplasms diagnosed on FNAC should be regarded as potential follicular carcinomas and subjected to lobectomy and isthmusectomy with frozen section, proceeding to total thyroidectomy if malignancy is confirmed. It is, however, very difficult to diagnose carcinoma on frozen section because this can be determined only on demonstration of capsular or vascular invasion (Figure 21.10). In most cases the procedure is terminated and paraffin section awaited. If cancer is subsequenly confirmed we would usually advocate completion thyroidectomy followed by radioactive iodine ablation.

Medullary carcinoma

Surgical management

The minimum initial treatment for medullary carcinoma is total thyroidectomy and bilateral central compartment (level VI) lymph node dissection (Figure 21.19).[32,34,42,74] For clinically positive necks selective neck dissection (levels II-V) should be included with addition of level I if level II nodes are involved. Limited superior mediastinal disease can be resected through the neck incision but occasionally a thoracocervical approach with upper median sternotomy[64] is required. The aim is surgical clearance of all macroscopic and microscopic disease.[34,42,74]

Postoperative work-up

Postoperative calcitonin and carcinoembryonic antigen (CEA) levels should be measured[42,61,75] and if normal or undetectable, usually indicate a good chance of cure. False positives do occur, and a frequent scenario is that of a calcitonin level which, although lower than it was preoperatively, remains elevated[76] without any obvious macroscopic disease.

DMSA and mIBG scanning

A pentavalent DMSA whole-body scan may localize tumour suitable for surgical resection. Postoperative mIBG scanning[77] is sometimes useful. If this isotope is taken up by tumour a therapeutic dose of radioiodine-131-labelled mIBG can be given to treat metastatic disease. If the tumour does not take up mIBG, conventional methods of investigation including CT of the thorax and abdomen plus bone scanning will be necessary. Not infrequently no site of tumour can be documented and such patients should be simply followed up annually and considered for surgery if a resectable metastasis subsequently becomes apparent.

External beam radiotherapy

This modality is reasonably effective for treating surgically unresectable residual or recurrent disease, in which case a high dose of at least 60 Gy over 6 weeks is required.[42,43,59,60,75] Adjuvant irradiation is recommended for extensive resected disease, multiple node involvement, or extracapsular spread, similar to squamous cell carcinoma at other head and neck sites.

Cytotoxic chemotherapy

Apart from lymphoma, medullary carcinoma is the only thyroid cancer to show any significant response to cytotoxic chemotherapy, with a partial response rate of up to 60%.[61] However, response is short-lived and toxicity from drugs such as doxorubicin is severe. With no demonstrable survival benefit, its role is palliative, used in the context of unresectable, progressive and symptomatic disease. Other active drugs include cisplatin, carboplatin and etoposide but combination chemotherapy has not been shown to be of benefit.[61] A less toxic agent can be selected initially, escalating to a more toxic drug when a previously responsive tumour develops resistance.

Follow-up

Routine follow-up consists of 6 monthly clinical examination together with measurement of calcitonin and CEA levels for the first 5 years, and annually thereafter.[42,76]

Anaplastic carcinoma

Surgical management

The vast majority of cases present at an advanced inoperable state. It is important to differentiate this from thyroid lymphoma, which can present similarly but which has a different prognosis and management. Occasionally isthmuthectomy may relieve respiratory obstruction but open biopsy and tracheostomy are preferably avoided in order to minimize the risk of fungation (Figure 21.20).[44]

External beam radiotherapy

This is the only worthwhile modality of treatment.[59] Survival is not prolonged but airway and swallowing obstruction can be relieved or avoided. Radiotherapy is given using wide fields extending from both mastoids down to the carina, including both sides of the neck and supraclavicular fossae. A dose of 50–60 Gy over 5–6 weeks is necessary to achieve worthwhile regression.[44,59] Accelerated treatment comprising two fractions each day over a shorter period of time may be more effective.

Cytotoxic chemotherapy

Although radiotherapy response usually follows high-dose treatment most patients die from widespread metastases within 6 months. No effective systemic therapy exists. In a series of 29 patients at the Royal Marsden Hospital, 18 evaluable courses of chemotherapy were given for anaplastic carcinoma and only three showed a partial response.[61]

Combination therapy

A recent study reported good results with combined modality treatment involving aggressive surgical debulking, postoperative accelerated radiotherapy and combination chemotherapy,[78] but this regimen requires further evaluation.

Thyroid lymphoma

Surgical management

The only surgical management for primary lymphoma of the thyroid is a generous open biopsy to determine accurate diagnosis by immunocytochemistry. Mucosa-associated lymphoid tissue (MALT) status should also be assessed by the histological pattern .[45,59]

Stage I and II disease

The principles of treatment are similar to that of other non-Hodgkin lymphomas.[79,80] For stage I and MALT-positive disease this consists of a dose of 40 Gy external beam radiotherapy, given over 4 weeks to both sides of the neck and mediastinum. For stage I MALT negative and all stage II patients this should be preceeded by combination cytotoxic chemotherapy such as the CHOP regime (cyclophosphamide, doxorubicin, vincristine and prednisolone).[45,61]

Stage III and IV disease

Patients with stage III and IV disease are treated with more intensive primary chemotherapy followed by radiotherapy to sites of initial bulk disease.[45]

REFERENCES

1. Williams ED, Toyn CE, Harach HR. The ultimobranchial gland and congenital thyroid abnormalities in man. *J Pathol* 1989; **159**: 135–141.
2. Rosai J, Carcanjiu ML, DeLellis RA. Tumours of the thyroid gland. In: *Atlas of Tumour Pathology*. Washington DC: Armed Forces Institute of Pathology, 1992.
3. See ACH, Patel SG, Montgomery PQ et al. Intralaryngotracheal thyroid: ectopic thyroid disease or invasive carcinoma? *J Laryngol Otol* 1998; **112**: 673–676.
4. Wynford-Thomas D. Thyroid cancer. In: Nemoine N, Neoptolemus J, Cooke T (eds). *Cancer: A Molecular Approach*. Oxford: Blackwell Scientific, 1994; 192–222.
5. Harmer CL, McCready VR. Thyroid cancer: differentiated carcinoma. *Cancer Treat Rev* 1996; **22**: 161–177.
6. Goodfellow PJ, Wells SA Jr. RET gene and its implications for cancer. *J Natl Cancer Inst* 1995; **87**: 1515–1523.
7. Harach HR, Williams ED. Childhood thyroid cancer in England and Wales. *Br J Cancer* 1995; **72**: 777–783.
8. Rosler H, Wimpfheimer C, Ruchti C et al. Hyperthyroidism in thyroid cancer. Retrospective study of 53 cases. *Nuklearmedizin* 1984; **23**: 293–300.
9. Pelzzo MR, Piotto A, Rubello D et al. High prevalence of occult papillary thyroid carcinoma in a surgical series for benign thryoid disease. *Tumori* 1990; **76**: 255–257.
10. Delisle MJ, Schvartz C, Theobald S et al. Cancers of the thyroid. Value of a regional registry on 627 patients diagnosed, treated and followed by a multidisciplinary team. *Ann Endocrinol Paris* 1996; **57**: 41–19.
11. Calandra DB, Shah KH, Lawrence AM et al. Total thyroidectomy on irradiated patients. A 20 year experience in 206 patients. *Ann Surg* 1985; **202**: 356–360.
12. Schneider AB, Pinsky S, Bekerman C et al. Characteristics of 108 thyroid cancers detected by screening in a population with a history of head and neck irradiation. *Cancer* 1980; **46**: 1291–1297.
13. Abelin T, Averkin JI, Egger M et al. Thyroid cancer in Belarus post-Chernobyl: improved detection or increased incidence? *Soz-Praventivmed* 1994; **39**: 189–197.
14. Nikiforov Y, Gnepp DR. Pediatric thyroid cancer after the Chernobyl disaster. Pathomorphologic study of 84 cases (1991–1992) from the Republic of Belarus. *Cancer* 1994; **74**: 748–766.
15. Buglova EE, Kenigsberg JE, Sergeeva NV. Cancer risk estimation in Belarussian children due to thyroid irradiation as a consequence of the Chernobyl nuclear accident. *Health-Physics* 1996; **71**: 45–49.
16. Mangano JJ. A post-Chernobyl rise in thyroid cancer in Connecticut, USA. *Eur J Cancer Prev* 1996; **5**: 75–81.
17. Lote K, Anderson K, Nordal E et al. Familial occurrence of papillary thyroid carcinoma. *Cancer* 1980; **46**: 1291–1297.
18. Chesky VE, Hellwig CA, Welch JW. Cancer of the thyroid associated with Hashimoto's disease: an analysis of 48 cases. *Am J Surg* 1962; **28**: 678–685.
19. Ott RA, Calandra DB, McCall A et al. The incidence of thyroid carcinoma in patients with Hashimoto's thyroiditis and solitary cold nodules. *Surgery* 1985; **98**: 1202–1206
20. Salabe GB. Aetiology of thyroid cancer: an epidemiological overview. *Thyroidology* 1994; **6**: 11–19.
21. Sloan W. Of the origin, characteristics and behaviour of thyroid carcinoma. *J Clin Endocrinol Metab* 1954; **14**: 1309–1335
22. Byar DP, Green SB, Dor P et al. A prognostic index for thyroid carcinoma: a study of the EORTC thyroid cancer co-operative group. *Eur J Cancer* 1979; **15**: 1033–1041.
23. Hay ID, Grant CS, Taylor WF, McConahey WM. Ipsilateral lobectomy versus bilateral lobar resection in papillary thyroid carcinoma: a retrospective analysis of surgical outcome using a novel prognostic scoring system. *Surgery* 1987; **102**: 1088–1095.
24. Cady B, Rossi R. An expanded view of risk group definition in differentiated thyroid carcinoma. *Surgery* 1988; **104**: 947–953.
25. Shah JP, Loree TR, Dharker D et al. Prognostic factors in differentiated carcinoma of the thyroid gland. *Am J Surg* 1992; **164**: 658–661.
26. Shah JP, Loree TR, Dharker D, Strong EW. Lobectomy versus total thyroidectomy for differentiated carcinoma of the thyroid gland: a matched-pair analysis. *Am J Surg* 1993; **166**: 331–334.
27. Shah JP. Thyroid and parathyroids. In: Shah JP (ed.) *Head and Neck Surgery*, 2nd edn. New York: Mosby Wolfe, 1996; 393–429.
28. Hay ID, Bergstralh EJ, Goellner JR et al. Predicting outcome in papillary thyroid carcinoma: development of a reliable prognostic scoring system in a cohort of 1779 patients treated surgically at one institution during 1940 through 1989. *Surgery* 1993; **114**: 1088–1097.
29. Pasieka JL, Zedenius J, Auer G et al. Addition of nuclear DNA content to the AMES risk group classification for papillary thyroid carcinoma. *Surgery* 1992; **112**: 1154–1159.
30. Hernenak P, Sobin LH. Thyroid carcinoma. In: *TNM Classification of Malignant Tumours: International Union against Cancer*, 4th edn. New York: Springer-Verlag, 1987.
31. Rhys Evans PH. Tumours of the oropharynx and lymphomas of the head and neck. In: Kerr A (ed.) *Scott Brown's Disease of the Ear, Nose and Throat*. London: Butterworth, 1996; 14.
32. Hay ID, Klee GG. Thyroid cancer diagnosis and management. *Clin Lab Med* 1993; 725–734.
33. Mazzaferri EL. Management of a solitary thyroid nodule. *New Engl J Med* 1993; **328**: 553–559.
34. Tezelman S, Clark OH. Current management of thyroid cancer. *Adv Surg* 1995; **28**: 191–221.
35. Belfiore A, Sava L, Runello F et al. Solitary automatously functioning thyroid nodules and iodine deficiency. *J Clin Endocrinol Metab* 1983; **56**: 283–287.

36. Vickery JL. Thyroid papillary carcinoma: pathological and philosophical controversies. *Am J Surg Pathol* 1983; **7**: 797–807.
37. Hedinger C, Williams ED, Sobin LH. Histological typing of thyroid tumours. In: *International Classification of Tumours*, 2nd edn. World Health Organization, New York: Springer-Verlag, 1988; 11.
38. Russel WO, Ibanez ML, Clark LR et al. Thyroid carcinoma: classification, intraglandular dissemination and clinicopathological study based on whole organ sections of 80 glands. *Cancer* 1968; **16**: 1425–1460.
39. Tallini G, Carcangio ML, Rosai J. Oncocytic neoplasm of the thyroid gland. *Acta Pathol* 1992; **42**: 305–311.
40. Dunn JM, Farndon JR. Medullary thyroid carcinoma. *Br J Surg* 1993; **80**: 6–9.
41. Watkinson J. The management of thyroid tumours. Personal communication.
42. Moley JF. Medullary thyroid cancer. *Surg Clin North Am* 1995; **75**: 405–420.
43. Gautvik KM. Medullary carcinoma of the thyroid: an update of diagnostic and prognostic factors. *Scand J Clin Lab Invest* 1991; **51**: 85–89.
44. Tan RK, Finley RK, Driscoll D et al. Anaplastic carcinoma of the thyroid: a 24 year experience. *Head Neck* 1995; **17**: 41–47.
45. Tupchong L, Hughes F, Harmer CL. Primary lymphoma of the thyroid: clinical features, prognostic factors and results of treatment. *Int J Radiat Oncol Biol Phys* 1986; **12**: 1813–1821.
46. Hamburger JI, Hussain M, Nishiyama R et al. Increasing the accuracy of fine needle biopsy for thyroid nodules. *Arch Pathol Lab Med* 1989; **113**: 1035–1039.
47. Gharib H, Goellner JR, Johnson DA. Fine needle aspiration biopsy of the thyroid: a 12 year experience with 11,000 biopsies. *Clin Lab Med* 1993; **13**: 3.
48. Goellner JR, Gharib H, Melton LJ III et al. Fine needle aspiration cytology of the thyroid. *Acta Cytol* 1987; **31**: 587–590.
49. Solbiati L, Clioffi V, Ballerati E. Ultrasonography of the neck. *Radiol Clin North Am* 1992; **30**: 941–954.
50. Katz JF, Kane RA, Reyes J et al. Thyroid nodules: sonographic pathologic correlation. *Radiology* 1984; **151**: 741–745.
51. Lindegard MW, Paus E. Thyroglobulin in patients with differentiated thyroid carcinoma. *Scand J Clin Lab Invest* 1991; **51**: 79–84.
52. Palmer BV, Harmer CL, Shaw HJ. Calcitonin and carcinoembryonic antigen in the follow up of patients with medullary carcinoma of the thyroid. *Br J Surg* 1984; **71**: 101–104.
53. Gagel RF, Tashjian AH, Cummings T et al. The clinical outcome of prospective screening for multiple endocrine neoplasia. *N Engl J Med* 1988; **318**: 478–484.
54. Ponder BAJ, Finer N, Coffrey R et al. Family screening in medullary thyroid carcinoma without a family history. *Quart J Med* 1988; **252**: 299–308.
55. Seidlin SM, Marinelli LD, Oshry E. Radioactive iodine therapy: effect on functioning metastases of adenocarcinoma of the thyroid. *JAMA* 1946; 132: 838–845.
56. Wong JB, Kaplan MM, Meyer KB et al. Ablative radioiodine therapy for apparently localised thyroid carcinoma: a decision analytic perspestive. *Endocrinol Metab Clin North Am* 1990; **19**: 635–644.
57. Harmer CL, McCready VR. Thyroid cancer: differentiated carcinoma. *Cancer Treat Rev* 1996; **22**: 161–177.
58. Tubiana M, Haddad E, Schlumberger M et al. External radiotherapy in thyroid cancers. *Cancer* 1985; **55**: 2062–2071.
59. Harmer CL. External beam therapy for thyroid cancer. *Ann Radiol* 1977; **20**: 791–800.
60. Steinfield AD. The role of radiation therapy in medullary cancer of the thyroid. *Radiology* 1977; **123**: 745–749.
61. Hoskin PJ, Harmer CL. Chemotherapy for thyroid cancer. *Radiother Oncol* **1987**; 187–194.
62. Hay ID, Bergstralh EJ, Ebdersold JR et al. Papillary thyroid carcinoma, <1.5 cm: Woolner's 'occult' tumour revisited. *J Endocrinol Invest* 1992; **15**: 32.
63. Powell S, Harmer CL. Death from thyroid cancer after 40 years: rationale for intensive surgical treatment. *Eur J Surg Oncol* 1990; **16**: 457–461.
64. Ladas G, Rhys Evans PH., Goldstraw P. Anterior cervical transsternal approach for the resection of neural tumours of the thoracic inlet. *Ann Thorac Surg* 1999; **67**: 785–789.
65. Rhys Evans PH, Rees P, Goldstraw P. Thoraco-cervical approach for resection of superior mediastinal tumours. *Ann R Coll Surg* 1999 (in press)
66. Hutter RUP, Frazell EL, Foote FW. Elective radical neck dissection: an assessment of its use in the management of papillary thyroid cancer. *Cancer* 1970; **20**: 86–91.
67. Breaux E, Guillamondegui OM. Treatment of locally invasive carcinoma of the thyroid: how radical? *Am J Surg* 1980; **140**: 514–518.
68. Ballantyne AJ. Resections of the upper aerodigestive tract for locally invasive thyroid cancer. *Am J Surg* 1994; **168**: 636–639.
69. Friedman M, Shelton VK, Skolnick GM et al. Laryngotracheal invasion by thyroid carcinoma. *Ann Otol Rhinol Laryngol* 1982; **91**: 363–367.
70. Mazzaferri EL, Jhiang SM. Long term impact of initial surgical and medical therapy on papillary and follicular thyroid cancer. *Am J Med* 1994; **97**: 418–428.
71. Young RL, Mazzaferri EL, Rahe AJ et al. Pure follicular thyroid carcinoma: impact of therapy in 214 patients. *J Nucl Med* 1977; **21**: 733–737.
72. Sarker SD, Beierwaltes WH, Gill SP et al. Subsequent fertility and birth histories of children and adolescents treated with iodine 131 for thyroid cancer. *J Nucl Med* 1976; **17**: 460–464.
73. Edmonds CJ, Smith T. The long term hazards of the treatment of thyroid cancer with radioiodine. *Br J Radiol* 1985; **59**: 45–51.
74. Harmer CL, Bidmead M, Shepherd S, Sharp A, Vini L. Radiotherapy planning techniques for thyroid cancer. *Br J Radiol* 1998; **71**: 1069–1075.
75. Tissel LE, Hansson G, Jansson S et al. Reoperation in the surgical treatment of asymptomatic metastasizing medullary thyroid carcinoma. *Surgery* 1986; **99**: 60– 66.

76. Van Heeden JA, Grant CS, Gharig H et al. Long term course of patients with persistent hypercalcitoninemia after apparent curative primary surgery for medullary thyroid carcinoma. *Ann Surg* 1990; **212**: 395–399.
77. Ball ABS, Tait DM, Fisher C et al. Treatment of metastatic para-aortic paraganglioma by surgery, radiotherapy and iodine 131 mIBG. *Eur J Surg Oncol* 1991; **17**: 543–546.
78. Tennvall J, Lundell G, Hallgust P et al. Combined doxorubicin, hyperfractionated radiotherapy and surgery in thyroid carcinoma: report on 2 protocols, the Swedish Anaplastic Thyroid Carcinoma Group. *Cancer* 1994; **74** 1348–1354.
79. Harmer CL. Radiotherapy in the management of thyroid cancers. *Ann Acad Med Singapore* 1996; **25**: 413–419.
80. Harmer CL. Thyroid cancer. In: Horwich A (ed.) *Oncology: A Multidisciplinary Textbook.* London: Chapman and Hall, 1995; 565–583.

22 Tumours of the parathyroid glands

Peter H Rhys Evans and Andrew See

Introduction

Parathyroid tumours are uncommon and only account for a small percentage of head and neck neoplasms. The overwhelming majority are benign adenomas that present as primary hyperparathyroidism. Parathyroid carcinomas are extremely rare and usually are associated with a florid history of severe hypercalcaemia. Patients with a malignant tumour are also more likely to have a palpable mass in the neck.

Until 20 years ago hyperparathyroidism was considered a rare condition whose surgical management was fraught with difficulties. The availability of routine serum calcium assay and plasma intact parathyroid hormone (PTH) levels has resulted in more frequent diagnosis even in asymptomatic cases.[1,2] The importance of diagnosis is highlighted by increasing evidence of higher mortality from cardiovascular disease in patients with few symptoms and only marginally raised serum calcium.[3] It is now recognized as the third most common endocrine disorder after diabetes and thyroid disease.[4]

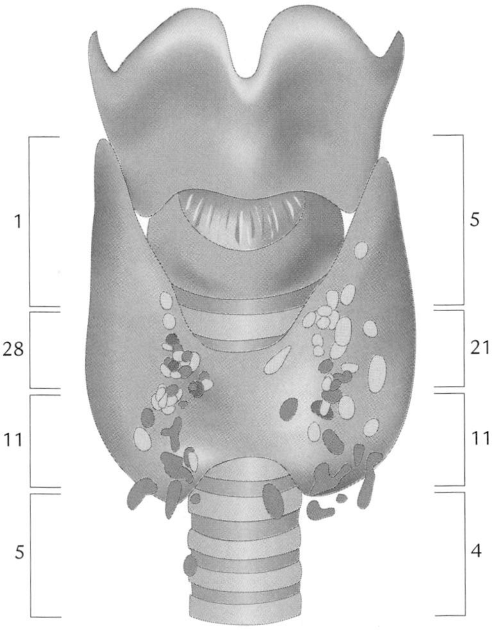

Figure 22.1 Composite diagram indicating the positions of all the parathyroid glands found in 25 bodies. (Modified from Heinbach WF Jnr. (1933) *Anat Rec* 57; 251.) (Superior, yellow; inferior, green.)

Since the early 1980s there have also been significant advances in diagnosis with more sophisticated and accurate preoperative localization techniques. Together with more experienced surgical management this has been the key to successful treatment in 92.7% of cases in a large multicentre study[5] to over 95% in specialized centres.[6,7]

Surgical anatomy

Embryology and position

The four parathyroid glands arise embryologically from the 3rd and 4th branchial pouches and in the adult human occupy a rather variable position in the anterior neck and mediastinum (Figure 22.1).

The superior parathyroids arise together with the lateral thyroid gland from the fourth branchial pouch and in the adult occupy a relatively constant position, usually adjacent to the upper pole of the thyroid gland. Seventy-seven percent are in a juxtacricoidal position behind the thyroid gland, 22% are just behind the upper thyroid pole and 1% in the undescended retropharyngeal position.[8,9] Fifty percent of superior parathyroids lie beneath the capsule of the thyroid glands, but true intrathyroid parathyroids are very rare.

The inferior parathyroids paradoxically arise from the third branchial pouch together with the thymus gland and descend to a much more variable position. Forty-two percent lie adjacent to the lower thyroid pole near the point of entry of the inferior thyroid artery (i.e. 'normal' position) and a further 15% are juxtathyroidal and can lie in any position near the thyroid gland. A further 41% are intrathymic and 2% are ectopic, lying anywhere up to and including the hyoid superiorly, the pulmonary hilum in the posterior mediastinum inferiorly and the carotid sheaths bilaterally. Although 41% of inferior parathyroid glands are intrathymic, the vast majority of these (95%) lie in the superior thymic tongue, which is almost always accessible from the neck.[8,9]

The inferior glands usually lie in close proximity to the recurrent laryngeal nerve and the inferior thyroid artery. Wang also found 1% to be in the retropharyngeal or retrooesophageal area.[8]

Table 22.1 Classification of parathyroid tumours

	Incidence (%)
Neoplastic conditions	
Solitary parathyroid adenoma	80–85
Multiple parathyroid adenomas	0.5–1
Parathyroid carcinoma	2–3
Hyperplastic conditions	
Chief cell (nodular) hyperplasia	10–12
Clear cell (water cell) hyperplasia	2–4
Other conditions	
Parathyroid cysts	< 0.1
Secondary cancer of the parathyroids (breast, renal, pulmonary)	< 0.1

Number

Reports of missing parathyroid glands are probably more likely to be due to occult than truly missing glands, but supernumerary parathyroid glands have been reported in 2–6.5% of adults.[9] Anatomical studies of parathyroid glands have typically shown an incidence of 0.2–0.6% with two glands, 5–13% with three glands, 80–91% with four glands, 4–5% with five glands and 0.5% with six glands.[10,11] Cases with seven and even eight glands have been reported.

Macroscopic appearance

Sir Richard Owen, conservator of the Hunterian Museum of the Royal College of Surgeons of England was the first to describe the parathyroid gland in an Indian rhinoceros as a 'small compact yellow glandular body attached to the thyroid at the point where the veins emerge'.[12] In humans the orange-yellow glands are sometimes difficult to distinguish from adjacent fat lobules; they typically measure 6 × 3 × 2 mm in size and weigh 30–40 mg.[10]

Clinicopathological features

General considerations

Presentaion

The vast majority of parathyroid tumours are functional adenomas and therefore present with primary hyperparathyroidism (HPT). An increasing proportion of these are now being identified on general screening of asymptomatic patients. Very few grow sufficiently to actually present as a lump in the neck (Table 22.1).

Carcinomas on the other hand are extremely rare and 50% have a palpable neck mass or cervical lymphadenopathy. The presence of a recurrent laryngeal nerve palsy is also suspicious of carcinoma. Nevertheless it is usually difficult to clinically distinguish the different tumour types, and since the preoperative management is similar, parathyroid tumours tend to be considered and managed together as a group at this stage (Table 22.1).

Secondary hyperparathyroidism is a compensatory condition in response to the hypocalcaemic state seen in a multitude of conditions like vitamin D deficiency, severe chronic intestinal malabsorbtion and chronic renal failure. It can sometimes progress to tertiary hyperparathyroidism in which the parathyroid glands become automatously funtioning, hyperplastic or adenomatous. This is most commonly seen in patients with end-stage renal failure, and results in a hypercalcaemic syndrome similar to primary hyperparathroidism, requiring surgical treatment for the parathyroid glands.

Epidemiology

The annual incidence of primary HPT is about 400 per million population per year, of which 2–3% are carcinomas.[9,13] The average age at presentation is 44 years, but ranges from 12 to 72 years. Adenomas are three times more common in females and affect 1 in 500 women over 40 years of age[14] and 3% of postmenopausal females.[15] The incidence of carcinoma is equal in both sexes.

Genetic predisposition

No discernible aetiological factor has been identified in over 90% of cases of parathyroid neoplasia, but multiple endocrine neoplasia (MEN) types 1 and 2 are associated with an inherited genetic predisposition for parathyroid hyperplasia. Loss of alleles on chromosome 11 results in parathyroid tumours in some patients with MEN1 and also in some cases of solitary adenomata.[16–18]

The normal gene appears to inhibit tumour formation and parathyroid glands from patients with gene depletion are unusually large. Primary hyperparathyroidism affects up to 90% of the MEN1 gene carriers and it appears to be a multiglandular disorder with a high propensity for recurrence after parathyroid surgery.[19] Seventy percent of excised glands show nodular hyperplasia, which appears to be more commonly associated with recurrence and 30% have diffuse hyperplasia. Autotransplantation of the diffusely hyperplastic glands into the arm is an alternative to total parathyroidectomy and if there is recurrence it will not necessitate re-exploration of the neck with its associated high morbidity risk.

Pathology

Parathyroid hyperplasia is invariably of chief cell origin as are the majority of parathyroid adenomas and carcinomas. Tumours of oxyphil cell origin do exist but they are rare and do not produce hyperparathyroidism.[9]

Prognostic factors

Successful excision of the parathyroid adenoma(s) is the definitive curative treatment in primary HPT with resolution in well over 90% in experienced hands. In a multivariate analysis of 95 patients, good prognostic factors in parathyroid carcinoma in order of importance were found to be en bloc resection of the tumour, age of patient, histopathology and DNA ploidy.[14] Other prognostic factors include time to recurrence and the presence of metastatic disease.[20,21]

Parathyroid adenoma

Parathyroid adenoma is the most common cause of primary HPT. The vast majority of adenomas are solitary, but multiple adenomas do exist and it is important to be able to distinguish these from parathyroid hyperplasia intraoperatively. The size of a parathyroid adenoma is typically 1–1.5 g but varies from less than 0.5 g to over 10 g (Figure 22.2). They

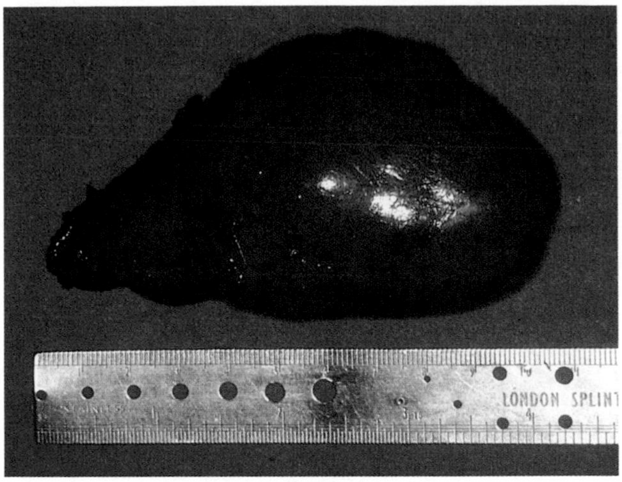

Figure 22.2 Parathyroid adenoma.

tend to be much larger in secondary or tertiary hyperparathyroidism. The typical gross appearance is that of a soft reddish-brown or tan coloured gland, often embedded in fat, The surgeon should be able to visually distinguish it not only from lobules of fat, which are yellow and float in saline (Wang's test), but also from thyroid nodules, which are firmer and redder in colour, and lymph nodes, which are a greyish pink and intermediate in consistency. Adenomas are more commonly found in the inferior glands.

Microscopically most consist of large chief cells arranged in sheets or in a pseudoglandular pattern, with absent or minimal intracellular or intercellular fat.[9] Often the nuclei may be pyknotic or pleomorphic which should not be mistaken for mitoses that are the hallmark of carcinoma.[9,22]

Chief cell hyperplasia

Chief cell or nodular hyperperplasia accounts for 80–85% of parathyroid hyperplasia which involves all four (or more) glands. The glands are smaller than those in parathyroid adenomas and are typically 0.5–1 g in size, but can range up to 10 g. There is often marked variation in size of the individual glands[9] and not infrequently patients can present confusingly with one markedly enlarged gland and three slightly enlarged or almost normal-sized glands.

Microscopically they consist of cords, sheets or follicular arrangements of chief cells not unlike adenomas.[9] There is also minimal intracellular fat as seen in adenomas, but there is a variable amount of intercellular stromal fat cells. The classical method of distinguishing hyperplasia from adenoma by the presence of intercellular fat is nowadays considered to be unreliable, and the current criterion for diagnosing adenoma during frozen section intraoperatively is the finding of a normal parathyroid gland (recognized from both adenoma and hyperplasia by the presence of abundant intracellular fat granules), which is not seen in parathyroid hyperplasia.[8,9]

Either form of MEN (type 1 or 2) can be associated with chief cell hyperplasia of the parathyroids. Although it was previously thought that MEN was not associated with other forms of parathyroid conditions, it is now known to be also associated with single and multiple adenomas, but to a much lesser extent.[8,9]

Clear cell hyperplasia

This is a relatively uncommon form of parathyroid hyperplasia. The clear cell form of parathyroid hyperplasia also originates from the parathyroid chief cell and presents with hyperparathyroidism, but usually to a lesser degree.

Macroscopically they tend to be very large, usually 5–10 g but ranging up to 50–60 g in size. Microscopically they consist of sheets of large pale vacuolated clear or 'water' cells. They are not known to be associated with MEN.[9]

Parathyroid carcinoma

These are rare tumours, and are usually functional and present with marked hyperparathyroidism. Non-functioning tumours account for only a small proportion and tend to be far more aggressive and are usually incurable. This is probably because they are not associated with hypercalcemia and therefore escape early clinical detection, presenting in an advanced state.

The preoperative clinical differentiation between parathyroid carcinoma and adenoma is often difficult but clinical features suggesting carcinoma include: (a) severely elevated serum calcium levels (usually > 3.5 mmol/l);[13,21] (b) grossly elevated serum PTH levels (usually greater than 4 times normal)[21]; (c) palpable tumour (> 2 cm in 50% of cases);[21] and (d) voice change suggestive of vocal cord palsy. However they are not totally reliable, and the possibility of malignancy may only arise intraoperatively. Clinicopathological features of malignancy are summarized in Table 22.2.

Table 22.2 Clinicopathological features of parathyroid carcinoma

Clinical
Severe HPT
Grossly elevated PTH
Palpable neck mass
Recurrent laryngeal nerve palsy
Metastases
Intraoperative appearance
Hard white tumour
Irregular contour
Local invasion
Thick capsule
Histology
Mitoses
Necrosis
Capsular invasion
Vascular invasion

Carcinomas are hard, grey-white and large with an average weight of about 10 g.[13] They are often adherent to adjacent structures and sometimes are encased within a fibrous or inflammatory-like reaction.[9] More advanced tumours may invade surrounding structures such as the thyroid, larynx, pharynx, trachea, oesophagus, or carotid sheath. If malignancy is suspected an adequate en bloc resection should be carried out to give optimum chance of cure.[13,20,21]

Histological features of malignancy include a trabecular pattern, nuclear palisading, mitotic figures, capsular and vascular invasion. Although the majority of these features is present in most carcinomas, needle biopsy is usually unreliable and even frozen section confirmation is often difficult, and final diagnosis usually rests on the postoperative paraffin section and the histological report.[9,22]

Parathyroid carcinoma spreads both via the lymphatics and haematogenously. About 35% of patients have evidence of metastases in the cervical lymph nodes at the time of presentation, and of these about a third have associated blood-borne distant metastases, usually in the lungs, but sometimes in the liver or bones.[9,22]

Local recurrence occurs in 28–50% and if within 2 years of initial treatment the long-term prognosis is very poor.[9,13] Overall 5-year survival is reported as 50–60%, but is better in patients in whom en bloc resection of the tumour is achieved.[7,13]

Most patients who die from disease succumb to complications of hypercalcaemia rather than to local disease progression.[9]

Investigations

General guidelines

Parathyroid tumours most commonly present with primary HPT, manifested by hypercalcaemia together with an elevated parathyroid hormone (PTH) level. This is often associated with diseases of the respective target organs, usually renal (urinary calculi) and less often skeletal (osteitis cystica) or pancreatic (acute or chronic pancreatitis) disorders. The other common presentation is that of tertiary hyperparathyroidism, usually in patients with end-stage renal disease.

Patient evaluation should begin with a careful and thorough history and physical examination including the assesment of the evidence of target organ involvement, previous history of thyroid or parathyroid surgery, voice change and the presence of a neck mass or cervical lymphadenopathy or both.

The subsequent investigation of a patient with a parathyroid tumour is best divided into three categories:

1. Confirmation of diagnosis and assessment of target organ involvement;
2. Tumour localization (preoperative and intraoperative);
3. Staging and screening investigations (where appropriate).

Diagnostic investigations

Serum levels

The basic investigations for the diagnosis of primary or tertiary hyperparathyroidism are serum levels of calcium phosphate and parathyroid hormone (PTH). Primary HPT would show hypercalcaemia associated with a low serum phosphorus and an elevated PTH level, a combination that would in most cases be practically diagnostic. However, in some patients there may be an ectopic source of PTH that needs to be excluded, the most common source being lung and renal carcinoma, which in some cases may be occult.[9] Lack of specificity may lead to difficulty distinguishing hypercalcaemia due to HPT and that resulting from malignancy. The latter is often due to a PTH-related peptide (PTHrP) but the development of a more sensitive immunoassay technique[23] now gives excellent discrimination between the two related disorders.[4]

There is at present no good tumour marker for parathyroid carcinoma. The use of alpha or beta human chorionic gonadotrophin (HCG) is still under evaluation as a marker. It has been shown to be elevated in the majority of patients with parathyroid carcinoma but not demonstrated with benign parathyroid lesions. PTH is a good marker for detecting parathyroid tumours, and for postsurgical monitoring and follow-up, but it does not distinguish well between carcinoma and other parathyroid tumours. Although it has been said that serum PTH levels are usually greater than four times the normal range in carcinoma patients[21] and rarely so in other tumours, this is not invariably the case.

DNA cytometry

Levin et al[25] have suggested the use of DNA cytometry to help identify suspected cases of parathyroid carcinoma. They found that analysis of a variety of parathyroid tissue showed only carcinomas (4/9) to have an aneuploid DNA pattern. They recommended that patients with marked hypercalcaemia or a palpable parathyroid tumour should be considered for fine-needle aspiration cytology. If aneuploid DNA is identified an en bloc resection should be carried out.[18]

Screening tests

Screening for target organ involvement may be required, depending on how the patient had presented, and would include: chest X-ray; KUB X-ray; and serum amylase and alkaline phosphatase.

Preoperative localizing investigations

Surgeons experienced in parathyroid surgery generally agree that localization investigations are indicated for recurrent or persistent primary HPT,[24–29] but the use of these studies to identify parathyroid adenomas before initial neck exploration remains controversial.[30–32] There is also some dispute as to whether unilateral (UND) or bilateral neck exploration (BNE)[25,26,28] is the optimal surgical approach. Preoperative localization studies often fail to identify multiple adenomata, asymmetric hyperplasia or ectopic glands and therefore identification of all four glands at operation is considered the 'gold standard'.[18] However, permanent postoperative hypoparathyroidism is a potential problem in up to 8%, particularly if routine biopsy of normal glands is undertaken.

The most frequent causes of failure to successfully treat primary HPT are an inadequate initial exploration and the presence of ectopic glands. A significant correlation between the chances of success and the experience of the surgeon has been documented and it is suggested that a minimum of 10 procedures per year is necessary to achieve acceptable results.[33]

Table 22.3 Distribution of parathyroid disease in 72 patients with sporadic PHP

Parathyroid disease	Type of neck exploration			
	Preoperative US		No US	
	UNE	BNE	BNE	Total (%)
Single adenoma	25	32	7	64 (88.8)
Double adenoma	2*	0	1	3 (4.2)
Hyperplasia (1 PG)	1	1	1	3 (4.2)
Hyperplasia (4 PG)	0	2†	0	2 (2.8)
Carcinoma	0	0	0	0
Total	28	35	9	72

*Contralateral adenoma detected at re-exploration in one patient, and at relocalization studies in the other patient.
†In one patient a UNE was converted to BNE as two enlarged ipsilateral glands were detected.

The endocrine radiologist Dr J Doppman has put it more succinctly, suggesting that 'the only localization study needed by a patient undergoing initial parathyroid surgery is to locate an experienced parathyroid surgeon'.[34]

Ultrasonography
High-resolution real-time ultrasound (US) using high-frequency probes (7 MHz or 10 Mhz) provides an excellent non-invasive and cost-effective method for detecting parathyroid tumours. Reported accuracy of preoperative US varies from 43% to 92% largely depending on the presence of bilateral adenomata and the experience of the radiologist.[35,36] A high cure rate of 93% can be achieved in patients undergoing a US-guided UNE compared with 97% when bilateral exploration was performed with similar morbidity.[37] The two failures in the UNE group were due to the presence of contralateral adenomas (Table 22.3). US can also be combined with more specific imaging techniques such as radionuclide scanning.

CT scanning
This has not been shown to be as sensitive as ultrasound in detecting neck lesions and is more costly. It is more successful in detecting adenomas in ectopic sites such as the superior mediastinum and tracheo-oesophageal groove and in patients who have undergone previous surgical exploration. CT may also help to identify pulmonary and hepatic metastases in patients with malignant disease. Sensitivity ranges from 41% to 86% with an average of 63%.[34]

Magnetic resonance imaging
This has shown considerable promise in imaging parathyroid tumours but costs are prohibitive and as such it is not used as a first-line investigation. As with CT scanning it gives good resolution for tumours in the superior mediastinum and paratracheal area and in patients with persistent hypercalcaemia after surgical parathyroid exploration. A review of six recent studies showed an average sensitivity of 74%, which is better than other modalities.[34]

Radionuclide scanning
The classical technique of thallium technitium subtraction scanning (Tl-201/Tc99m) has proven to be a useful and relatively non-invasive method for localizing parathyroid tumours in both the neck and the mediastinum (Figure 22.3), with a reported sensitivity of over 80%.[38] Others have been less optimistic with sensitivities averaging 55%.[34] There is also a size limitation and this technique does not identify tumours under 1 cm.

Recent studies have shown even better results with MIBI scanning,[39,40] a new method of subtraction scanning using sestamibi iodine-123 and technetium-99m, with a sensitivity rate of over 95%. Another radionuclide scan, using gallium (Ga-67) scintiscanning,[41] has been demonstrated to be taken up by parathyroid carcinoma, but not by parathyroid adenomas. However the validity of this scan requires further evaluation.

Although preoperative localization studies are being used with increasing frequency the four commonly used techniques (US, CT, MRI and RI scanning) are

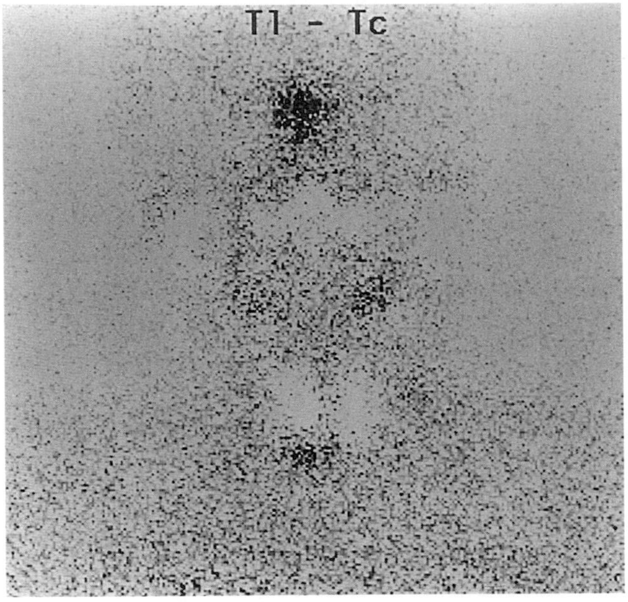

Figure 22.3 Technitium subtraction scan localizing parathyroid adenoma.

limited to a sensitivity of between 50% and 65% and a false-positive rate of 15–20%. This compares with the success rate of about 95% achieved with bilateral neck exploration carried out by an experienced surgeon.

The potential advantages and disadvantages of using these tests are summarized in Table 22.4 and overall it would seem that there is little justification for their routine use before initial surgery. Doppman and Miller[32] have eloquently argued this case but point out that for the 5–8% of patients destined to have an unsuccessful initial exploration, the medicolegal consequences of failed initial surgery may force the issue so that non-invasive localizing techniques may be required as part of the 'standard of care'.

Intraoperative techniques

Localization

Intraoperative localization is becoming less frequently necessary, due to the range of sophisticated preoperative studies that have become available, and the increasing experience of parathyroid surgeons. The use of intraoperative intravenous dyes such as methylene blue to selectively stain the parathyroid glands has largely fallen out of favour because of poor specificity of the dyes and occasional toxic reactions. The role of intraoperative ultrasound is still being evaluated.

Highly selective venous sampling for PTH levels has also been advocated[3] with exposure and sampling of bilateral superior, middle and inferior thyroid veins prior to exploration but this is also rarely used as it is expensive, complicated and time consuming.

Confirmatory

A simpler method is the quick intraoperative assay of the biologically active N-terminal fragment of PTH,[42] which has a half-life of only 3–6 minutes. A fall in levels intraoperatively will confirm the removal of the offending parathyroid lesion. However the level of laboratory support for this technique is not widely available. Another recently developed technique measures urinary cyclic AMP levels, which have been shown to fall within 20 minutes of removal of the parathyroid tumour.

Staging and screening investigations

Patients who are suspected preoperatively to have parathyroid carcinoma should be screened for metastatic disease with a chest X-ray, liver ultrasound and a bone scan. Those who have confirmed carcinoma whose PTH levels fall to within normal levels postoperatively require no further investigation. However if this is not the case, appropriate staging investigations[43–45] would include CT or MRI scans of the neck, thorax and abdomen and, if not already done, a bone scan. Radionuclide subtraction scans have not been shown to be effective in detecting metastatic parathyroid carcinoma. All patients with parathyroid hyperplasia should undergo additional screening for MEN syndrome.

Table 22.4 Localization techniques for parathyroid tumours

Advantages	Disadvantages
Improvement in surgical results	Low sensitivity (65%) compared with an experienced surgeon (95%)
Only one side of neck explored	A high false-positive rate of 15–20%
Reduced operating time	Multiple adenomas and hyperplastic glands missed
Medicolegal	Substantial costs

Treatment of parathyroid tumours

General guidelines

Surgery is the principal modality of treatment for all parathyroid tumours. This involves exploration in previously unoperated cases with three main objectives: adequate resection of the parathyroid tumour(s); cure of the hypercalcaemia; and prevention of recurrence of disease. Current controversies in the management of parathyroid tumours include the following.

Role and timing of localizing tests

As previously discussed (Table 22.4), the role of preoperative localization in previously unoperated patients is controversial. There are many who consider this to be unnecessary[46,47] as successful intraoperative localization by experienced surgeons is usually in the region of 90–96%. However, it seems reasonable to carry out a preoperative ultrasound scan, usually in combination with a radionucleide subtraction scan, for several reasons. These are noninvasive and comparatively inexpensive investigations. In the majority of patients with successful preoperative localization a unilateral exploration is adequate, and bilateral exploration becomes unnecessary.[48–50] This can decrease operative exploration time by 30–50% in the majority of patients, converting a prolonged exploration into a brief, curative procedure with minimal morbidity. Preoperative imaging of the parathyroid tumour may increase the chance of detecting a parathyroid carcinoma. Also, there are medicolegal advantages as discussed previously.

Indications for primary parathyroid surgery

Patients presenting with classical hyperparathyroid symptoms of 'painful bones, renal stones, psychic moans, abdominal groans and fatigue overtones' are likely to be already developing complications of hypercalcaemia and surgery is plainly indicated. However, an increasing number of asymptomatic patients are being picked up with minimally elevated levels of calcium and there is debate as to whether these patients should be carefully followed-up or should undergo surgery. Persistent hypercalcaemia due to HPT is undoubtedly associated with higher risk of cardiovascular disease,[3,51] but restoration of normal calcium does not necessarily improve hypertension. Psychiatric symptoms affect almost two-thirds of patients with HPT and many of these are reversed following surgery.[52] There is also some evidence that the associated bone disease may be improved by surgery.

Unilateral versus bilateral exploration

Surgical identification of all four glands remains the 'gold standard' because unilateral exploration may miss multiglandular disease and ectopic adenomas as well as asymmetric hyperplasia. Unilateral exploration may be advocated[31] because of reduced operating time and morbidity as well as avoidance of obliterative scarring of the contralateral neck.

Surgical principles of parathyroid exploration

1. Meticulous operative technique with a bloodless field.
2. Mobilization of the ipsilateral thyroid lobe including division of the superior pedicle.
3. Demonstration of the recurrent laryngeal nerve along the tracheo-oesophageal groove down to the level of the thymus gland.
4. Histological confirmation by frozen section biopsy and radiopaque tagging (usually with a small metal clip) of all parathyroid glands encountered.

Parathyroid adenoma and hyperplasia

Surgical management of parathyroid adenoma

When preoperative localization has been used and identified a suspicious lesion, that side is explored and more often than not an adenoma is easily found (Figure 22.4). If not immediately apparent, exploration deep to the recurrent laryngeal nerve may successfully reveal the abnormal gland (Figure 22.5). Removal of that gland and biopsy of the other normal ipsilateral gland is usually sufficient and exploration of the other side can be avoided. Multiple adenomas are rare but are more common in the elderly.

Surgical management of parathyroid hyperplasia

If the second gland is found to be abnormal as well, further exploration is indicated. The standard

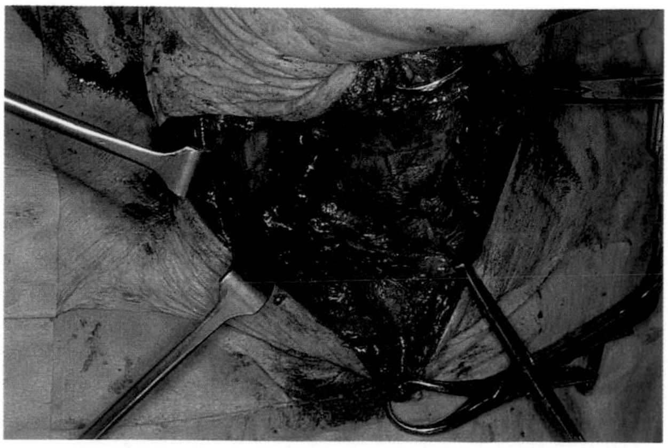

Figure 22.4 Intraoperative localization of a parathyroid adenoma adjacent to the thyroid.

management of parathyroid hyperplasia is subtotal parathyroidectomy which consists of the total removal of three glands and the partial removal of the most normal looking gland, preserving its blood supply intact.

Parathyroid carcinoma

Surgical management

The only effective and potentially curative treatment for parathyroid carcinoma is surgery. Whenever possible the side of the neck to be explored initially should be directed by preoperative localization or by intraoperative palpation. On locating an abnormal gland, the first objective is the gross recognition of a parathyroid carcinoma.[9,13] Any lesion vaguely suspicious of a carcinoma should be treated as one and requires an en bloc resection[13,20,21] including the ipsilateral thyroid lobe and isthmus and any adherent structure. Clearance of the ipsilateral tracheo-oesophageal groove lymph nodes (level VI) is also necessary. Frozen section can be utilized but this is not definitive in the majority of cases.[9,22]

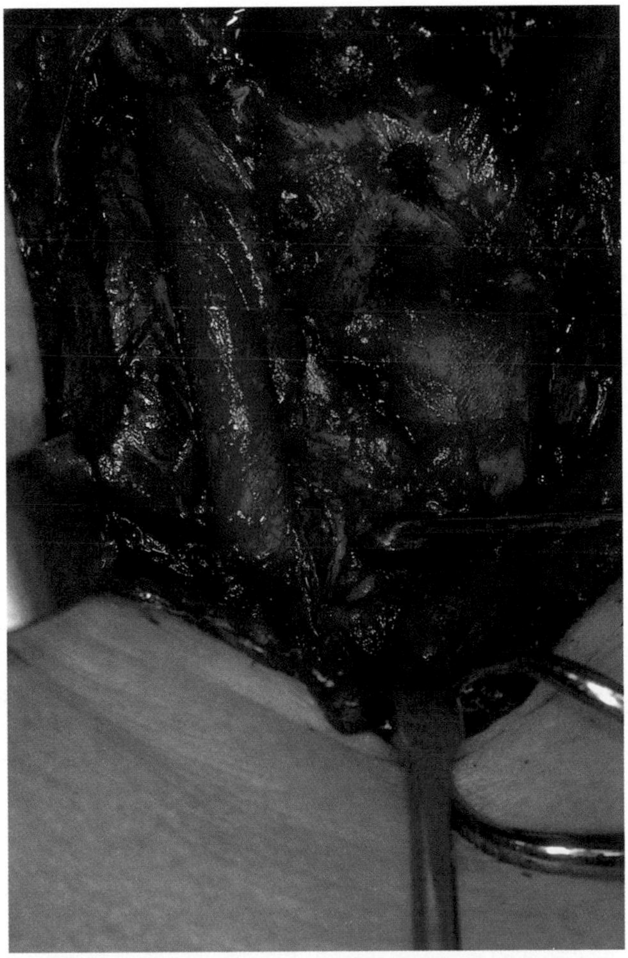

Figure 22.5 A more deeply situated adenoma lying on the deep aspect of the recurrent laryngeal nerve.

Locally advanced parathyroid carcinoma

When this is encountered the lesion should be resected as thoroughly as possible despite the extent of involvement,[43,44] even at the expense of the integrity of the recurrent laryngeal nerve, larynx, trachea, oesophagus or carotid artery.[20,21,24,44] This is because an incompletely resected carcinoma will inevitably result in early recurrence, and complete resection will not be possible in recurrent cases.[45] Needless to say, radical surgery should only be carried out after histological confirmation, and if frozen section is not definitive resection should be delayed until a confirmatory paraffin section report is obtained.

Cervical lymph node dissection

The role of elective cervical lymph node clearance is controversial and some advocate a routine radical neck dissection at the time of parathyroid surgery for carcinoma. We would advocate a selective neck dissection (level VI) for N0 disease and a modified radical neck dissection only in the presence of gross cervical node involvement.[13,24]

Radiotherapy

Radiotherapy has no place in the management of parathyroid carcinoma except perhaps in the postoperative setting if resection has been incomplete. Occasional response has been reported.[21]

Chemotherapy

There has been no established routine role for chemotherapy in the management of parathyroid carcinoma and rarely has it been of benefit.[21,53]

Postoperative follow-up

Patients after surgery for parathyroid carcinoma should have serum calcium and PTH levels measured in the immediate postoperative period to confirm that they have fallen to within normal levels. Subsequently they should be monitored 3 monthly for the first 2 years, 6 monthly for the next 3 years and yearly thereafter.

Survival

If surgical resection has been successful the 5-year survival is in the region of 50–70%. The great majority of patients, however, die from their disease mainly from the effects of hypercalcaemia. Thirty percent develop metastases to the neck (15%), the lungs (12%), liver (8%) and bone (8%).

Metastatic parathyroid carcinoma

The principle of aggressive debulking should apply equally to metastatic parathyroid carcinoma[20,21,43–45] for two important reasons.

1. Parathyroid carcinoma even at an advanced stage behaves in an indolent, slowly progressive fashion, and meaningful palliation for prolonged duration, often many years, can be achieved by aggressive tumour debulking.
2. Patients who succumb to advanced parathyroid carcinoma almost invariably do so as a result of the metabolic consequences of uncontrolled hypercalcaemia than from an invasive carcinoma. All surgically resectable disease should be removed or debulked as thoroughly as possible, to the extent of a thoracotomy[54] for lung metastasis or hepatic resection[43,44] for liver metastasis.

Recurrent parathyroid carcinoma

Recurrence of parathyroid carcinoma is usually heralded by the reappearance of hypercalcaemia and an elevated PTH. A complete reassesment would then be required, including a radionuclide subtraction scan to look for locoregional recurrence in the neck, as well as CT or MRI scans of the neck, thorax and abdomen, and a bone scan. Although recurrent disease is essentially incurable, agressive debulking[20,21,43–45] remains the rule of the day, for the reasons given above. However it is important that localization should precede surgical intervention, and 'blind' neck explorations should never be attempted. When necessary, the patient should be temporized with medical management until the serum calcium can be reduced to around 3.5 mmol/l when the imaging investigations are more likely to be successful.

Complications

Hungry bone syndrome

This temporary but troublesome postoperative condition is due to the reversal of parathyroid osteodystrophy, and must be anticipated in every case of parathyroid resection. It should be preempted by preoperative calcium loading where possible, and if not possible rapid and effective treatment in the early postoperative period.

Hypoparathyroidism

The risk of permanent hypoparathyroidism following bilateral exploration and biopsy of normal parathyroids is in the region of 8% but may not be detected for up to 4 years after surgery.[42]

Failed parathyroid exploration

Occasionally, routine exploration fails to reveal the tumour and all four parathyroids within the normal boundaries of a cervical parathyroid exploration, which are the hyoid superiorly, the carotid sheaths bilaterally and the thymus gland inferiorly. In this situation it is acceptable to close up and resort to further localizing investigations. If three glands are identified, as is most often the case, they should be biopsied and tagged, and an ipsilateral thymectomy and thyroid lobectomy (on the side of the missing parathyroid) carried out in the hope that the occult gland is within one of these glands.

Even in experienced hands, about 5% of patients have persistent or recurrent hypercalcaemia following primary parathyroid surgery, due to occult or ectopic disease. However this figure can sometimes be significantly higher, due to missed glands by inexperienced or occasional parathyroid surgeons.

As far as possible preoperative localization should be established by imaging investigations prior to surgery. All available modalities should be attempted, beginning with the most non-invasive, until this can be achieved.[40,46]

Cervical thymectomy

The commonest location of an occult gland is intrathymic[9] usually in the superior thymic tongue, which is easily accessible from a standard cervical incision. The other common location is within the thyroid gland. In the event that preoperative localization prior to re-exploration is unsuccessful, a meticulous search within the normal boundaries of a cervical parathyroid exploration should be carried out. If this is still not successful, the superior thymic tongue, or the entire thymus gland[20] if this can be safely performed, should be resected for histological examination. An ipsilateral hemithyroidectomy on the side of the missing parathyroid, if not already performed should also be carried out.

Mediastinal exploration

Open mediastinal exploration for middle mediastinal parathyroid disease is carried out usually via an anterior median sternotomy approach, or less commonly via an anterolateral thoracotomy approach. This should only very rarely be indicated, apart from metastatic malignant disease, and preoperative localization is essential.[33,40,44,46]

Management of hypercalcaemia

Intractable severe hypercalcaemia, as seen in uncontrolled metastatic parathyroid carcinoma, is often the terminal event in these patients, with death resulting from cardiac arrythmias, renal failure or coma due to central nervous system depression. The most effective management for these patients is surgical debulking of the tumour. However this may not always be feasible, and outlined below are the main medical approaches[20] to control of severe hypercalcaemia.

1. Systemic corticosteroids are usually effective, but prolonged treatment and high doses will result in severe osteoporosis and other unacceptable side-effects.
2. Oral or parenteral phosphates are effective and often used in combination with steroid therapy, and can achieve long-term control, but side-effects include soft tissue calcification with long-term use.
3. Calcitonin specifically antagonizes the effects of PTH, but the effect is short-term. It is also usually used in combination with steroid therapy.
4. Loop diuretics such as frusemide in combination with adequate hydration can be an effective short-term measure.
5. Chelating agents like ethylene diamine tetra-acetate (EDTA) bond with calcium to form soluble excretable complexes, and can also be very effective in the short term. The disadvantage is that they must be administered intravenously, and long-term use will result in renal damage.
6. Peritoneal dialysis and haemodialysis can be effectively used to quickly lower the serum calcium level, but the effect is also transient.
7. Other agents such as oestrogen therapy and chemotherapeutic agents (e.g. mithramicin) have been described, but their potential benefits are minimal.

REFERENCES

1. Heath H, Hodgson SF, Kennedy MA. Primary hyperparathyroidism. Incidence, morbidity and potential economic impact in a community. *N Engl J Med* 1980; **302**: 189–193.
2. Mundy GR, Cove DH, Fisken R. Primary hyperparathyroidism: changes in the pattern of clinical presentation. *Lancet* 1980; **i**: 1317–1320.
3. Saharay M, Farooqui A, Farrow S et al. Intraoperative parathyroid hormone assay for simplified localization of parathyroid adenomas. *J R Soc Med* 1996; **89**: 261–264.
4. Wheeler MH. Primary hyperparathyroidism: a surgical perspective. *Ann R Coll Surg Engl* 1998; **80**: 305–312.
5. Barbier J, Kraimps JL, Denizot A, Henry JF. Current surgical aspect of primary hyperparathyroidism (100 years after F D von Recklinghausen). *Chirurgie* 1992; **118**: 439–447.
6. Irvin GL, Dembrow VD, Prudhomme DL. Operative monitoring of parathyriod gland hyperfunction. *Am J Surg* 1991; **162**: 299–302.
7. Van-Heerden JA, Grant CS. Surgical treatment of primary hyperparathyroidism: an institutional perspective. *World J Surg* 1991; **15**: 688–692.
8. Wang CA. The anatomical basis of parathyroid surgery. *Ann Surg* 1976; **183**: 271–275.
9. Castleman B, Roth SI. Tumours of the parathyroid gland. In: *Atlas of Tumour Pathology*. Washington, DC: Armed Forces Institute of Pathology, 1978.
10. Gilmour IR. The gross anatomy of the parathyroid glands. *J Pathol* 1938; **46**: 133–148.
11. Graney DE. Thyroid and parathyroid anatomy. In: Cumming CW, Fredrickson JM, Harker LA et al (eds). *Otolaryngology—Head and Neck Surgery*. St Louis: CV Mosby, 1986; 2469–2473.
12. Owen R. On the anatomy of the Indian rhinoceros (*Rh. Unicornis*, L) *Trans Zoo Soc Lond* 1862; **iv**: 31–58.
13. Grandberg PO, Cedermark B, Farnebo LO et al. Parathyroid tumours. *Curr Probl Cancer* 1985; **9**: 1.
14. Sandelin K, Auer G, Bondeson L et al. Prognostic factors in parathyroid cancer: a review of 95 cases. *World J Surg* 1992; **16**: 724–731.
15. Palmer M, Jacobsson S, Ackerstrom G et al. Prevalence of hypercalcaemia in a health survey: a 14 year follow-up of serum calcium values. *Eur J Clin Invest* 1998; **118**: 39–46.
16. Friedman E, Sakaguchi K, Bale AE et al. Clonality of parathyroid tumours in familial multiple endocrine neoplasia type 1. *N Engl J Med* 1989; **321**: 213–218.
17. Thakker RV, Bouloux P, Wooding C et al. Association of parathyroid tumours in multiple endocrine neoplasia type 1 with loss of alleles on chromosome 11. *N Engl J Med* 1989; **321**: 218–224.
18. Mowschenson PM, Silen W. Developments in hyperparathyroidism. *Curr Opin Oncol* 1990; **2**: 95–100.
19. Hellman P, Skogseid B, Juhlin C, Akerstrom G. Findings and long- term results of parathyroid surgery in multiple endocrine neoplasia. *World J Surg* 1992; **16**: 718–723.
20. Van Heerden JA, Weiland LH, ReMine K et al. Cancer of the parathyroid glands. *Arch Surg* 1979; **114**: 475–80.
21. Anderson BJ, Samaan NA, Vassilopoulou-Sellin R et al. Parathyroid carcinoma: features and difficulties in diagnosis and management. *Surgery* 1983; **94**: 906–15.
22. Schantz A, Castleman B. Parathyroid carcinoma. A study of 70 cases. *Cancer* 1973; **31**: 600–5.
23. Dekker A, Watson CG, Barnes EL. The pathological assessment of primary hyperparathyroidism and its impact on therapy. *Ann Surg* 1979; **190**: 671–677.
24. Wang CA, Gaz RD. Natural history of parathyroid carcinoma. *Am J Surg* 1985; **193**: 522.
25. Levin KE, Clark OH. The reasons for failure in parathyroid operations. *Arch Surg* 1989; **124**: 911–915.

26. Clark OH, Okerlund MD, Moss AA et al. Localization studies in patients with persistent or recurrent hyperparathyroidism. *Surgery* 1985; **98**: 1083–1194.
27. Shen W, Duren M, Morita E et al. Reoperation for persistent or recurrent primary hyperparathyroidism. *Arch Surg* 1996; **131**: 861–867.
28. Cheung PS, Borgstrom A, Thompson NW. Strategy in re-operative surgery for hyperparathyroidism. *Arch Surg* 1989; **124**: 676–680.
29. Rodriquez JM, Tezelman S, Siperstein AE et al. Localization procedures in patients with persistent or recurrent hyperparathyroidism. *Arch Surg* 1994; **129**: 870–875.
30. Whelan PJ, Rotsein LE, Rosen IB et al. Do we really need another localizing technique for parathyroid glands? *Am J Surg* 1989; **158**: 382–384.
31. Tibblin S, Bondesson A-G, Uden P. Current trends in the surgical treatment of solitary parathyroid adenoma; a questionnaire study from 53 surgical departments in 14 countries. *Eur J Surg* 1991; **157**: 103–107.
32. Doppman JL, Miller DL. Localization of parathyroid tumours in patients with asymptomatic hyperparathyroidism and no previous surgery. *J Bone Miner Res* 1991; **6**: 153–159.
33. Malmaeus J, Granberg PO, Halvorsen J et al. Parathyroid surgery in Scandinavia. *Acta Chirurg Scand* 1988; **154**: 409–413.
34. Doppman J. Pre-operative localization of parathyroid tissue. In: Belezikan J (ed.) *Parathyroid.* York Press: 1994; 553–566.
35. Lucas RJ, Welsh RJ, Glover JL. Unilateral neck exploration for primary hyperparathyroidism. *Arch Surg* 1990; **125**: 982–984.
36. Lloyd MN, Lees WR, Milroy EJ. Pre-operative localization in primary hyperparathyroidism. *Clin Radiol* 1990; **41**: 239–243.
37. Ammori BJ, Madan M, Gopichandran TD et al. Ultrasound-guided unilateral neck exploration for sporadic primary hyperparathyroidism: is it worthwhile? *Ann R Coll Surg* 1998; **80**: 433–437.
38. Okerland MD, Sheldon K, Corpuz S et al. A new method with high sensitivity and specificity for localization of abnormal parathyroid glands. *Ann Surg* 1984; **200**: 381–399.
39. Wei JP, Burke GJ, Mansberger AR. Prospective evaluation of technitium 99m sestamibi and iodine 123 radionuclide imaging of abnormal parathyroid glands. *Surgery* 1992; **121**: 1111–1117.
40. Weber CJ, Vansant J, Alazraki N. Value of technitium 99m sestamibi iodine 123 imaging in reoperative parathyroid surgery. *Surgery* 1993; **114**: 1011–1018.
41. Iwase M, Shimizu Y, Kitahara H et al. Parathyroid carcinoma visualised by gallium 67 citrate scintigraphy. *J Nucl Med* 1986; **27**: 63–5.
42. Irvin GL, Dembrow VD, Prudhomme DL. Clinical usefulness of an intraoperative 'quick PTH' assay. *Surgery* 1993; **114**: 1019–1023.
43. Flye MW, Brennan MF. Surgical resection of metastatic parathyroid carcinoma. *Ann Surg* 1981; **193**: 425–432.
44. Fujimoto Y, Obara T, Ito Y et al. Localization and resection of metastatic parathyroid carcinoma. *World J Surg* 1986; **10**: 539–547.
45. Sandelin K, Tullgren O, Farnebo LO. Clinical course of metastatic parathyroid cancer. *World J Surg* 1994; **18**: 594–598.
46. Miller DL. Preoperative localization and interventional treatment of parathyroid tumours: when and how? *World J Surg* 1991; **15**: 706–715.
47. Shaha AR, Jaffe BM. Cervical exploration for primary hyperparathyroidism. *Surg Oncol* 1993; **52**: 14–17.
48. Billingsley KG, Fraker DL, Doppman JL et al. Localization and operative management of undescended parathyroid adenomas in patients with persistent primary hyperparathyroidism. *Surgery* 1995; **116**: 982–989.
49. Tibblin S, Bondeson AG, Ljungberg O. Unilateral parathyroidectomy in hyperparathyroidism due to single adenoma. *Ann Surg* 1982; **195**: 245–250.
50. Worsey MJ, Carty SE, Watson CG. Success of unilateral neck exploration for sporadic primary hyperparathyroidism. *Surgery* 1993; **114**: 1024–1029.
51. Palmer M, Adami HO, Bergstrom R et al. Mortality after operation for primary hyperparathyroidism. A follow-up of 441 patients operated on from 1956–1979. *Surgery* 1987; **102**: 1–7.
52. Carty SE, Norton JA. Management of patients with persistent or recurrent primary hyperparathryoidism. *World J Surg* 1991; **15**: 716–723.
53. Chahinian AP, Holland JF, Marinescu A et al. Case report. Metastatic non-functioning parathyroid carcinoma: ultrastructural evidence of secretory granules and response to chemotherapy. *Am J Med Sci* 1981; **282**: 80–84.
54. Dubost C, Jehanno C, Lavergne A et al. Successful resection of intrathoracic metastases from two patients with parathyroid carcinoma. *World J Surg* 1984; **8**: 547–556.

23 Cutaneous melanoma of the head and neck

Christopher J O'Brien, Irvin Pathak and Jeremy McMahon

Epidemiology

In countries with substantially caucasian populations, the incidence of cutaneous melanoma has risen sharply over recent decades.[1–5] Epidemiological investigations suggest that increasing melanoma rates are real and due primarily to increased exposure to ultraviolet radiation, rather than a consequence of more complete reporting. Mortality trends in white populations have also been increasing but less steeply than incidence rates[1] and, on a cohort basis, mortality appears to have stabilized or started to decline.[1,6–8]

Approximately 10–20% of cutaneous malignant melanomas arise on the skin of the head and neck.[4,9] In a series of 998 patients with cutaneous melanoma of the head and neck treated at the Sydney Melanoma Unit, the male to female ratio was 3:2 and the age incidence fairly evenly distributed through the adult decades.[10] Melanoma rarely occurs during childhood and adolescence. Table 23.1 shows the distribution of head and neck cutaneous melanoma by subsite with the face being the commonest individual primary site in the report from the Sydney Melanoma Unit. Other workers have also found a similar preponderance of facial melanoma on subsite analysis.[10–12]

Table 23.1 Distribution of head and neck melanoma according to subsite

Subsite	Primary melanomas (%)
Face	47
Neck	29
Scalp	15
Ear	10

Data from O'Brien et al.[10]

Etiology and risk factors

Melanoma is predominantly a disease of people whose origins are European[13] and the major cause of melanoma is sun exposure. The incidence of melanoma is highest in the white population of Australia and even within this population the incidence of melanoma increases with proximity to the equator.[14] Interestingly, indoor workers are more frequently affected than outdoor workers, as are people of higher socioeconomic status.[15] This is not consistent with a simple dose-response relationship between sun exposure and melanoma. Instead, intermittent intense exposure on a recreational basis is associated with the development of melanoma.[16–18] Overall, the greatest risk appears to be associated with sunburn in childhood or adolescence.[16] Clearly, eliminating excessive exposure to sunlight is important along with the need for sunscreens. Whether or not the use of even broad spectrum sunscreens reduces the risk of melanoma is unclear however.[19]

The presence of large numbers of pigmented naevi is also known to be a risk factor for the development of melanoma. In a survey of over 4500 melanoma patients, 81% reported a change in the appearance of a pre-existing mole as the initial manifestation.[20] Furthermore, numbers of both common and atypical naevi have been found to correlate with individual melanoma risk.[21] Large congenital naevi, in particular those greater than 19 cm in diameter, are also predisposed to malignant change and transition to melanoma.[22] The presence of atypical or dysplastic naevi is associated with increased risk of melanoma. These may be familial and individuals with multiple atypical naevi, also called dysplastic naevus syndrome, should be closely monitored.[23] However, individual atypical naevi should not be regarded as being high risk precursors since the likelihood of transformation for any given lesion is low.[23]

Clinicopathological factors and prognosis

Cutaneous melanoma of the head and neck may be classified into three main histological categories: nodular melanoma; superficial spreading melanoma; and lentigo maligna melanoma (see Figures 23.1–23.4). Nodular malignant melanoma has a predominantly vertical growth phase. Superficial spreading and lentigo maligna melanoma have a prolonged radial (or lateral) growth phase but may develop nodules over time. Lentigo maligna melanoma occurs particularly on the sun-exposed skin of elderly patients.[24] The clinical utility of this classification is doubtful however since the histological types tend to have similar prognoses after correcting for tumour thickness.[25] While the Sydney Melanoma Unit series demonstrated lentigo maligna melanoma has a significantly better prognosis when all other factors were adjusted for,[10] this has not been confirmed by other workers.[9]

Desmoplastic melanoma and neurotropic melanoma are variant forms that comprise less than 1% of all

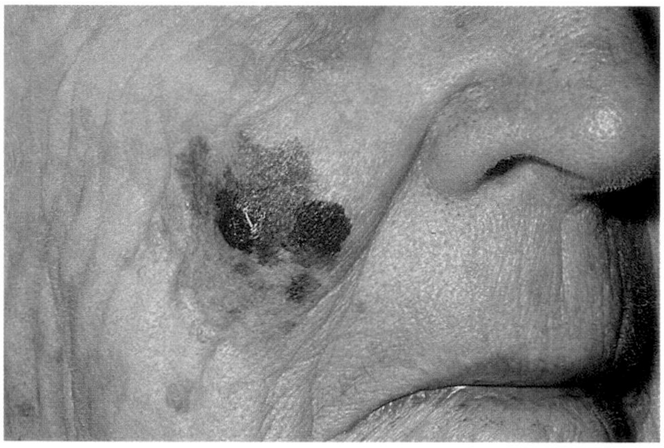

Figure 23.1 Malignant melanoma of right cheek in a 73-year-old woman.

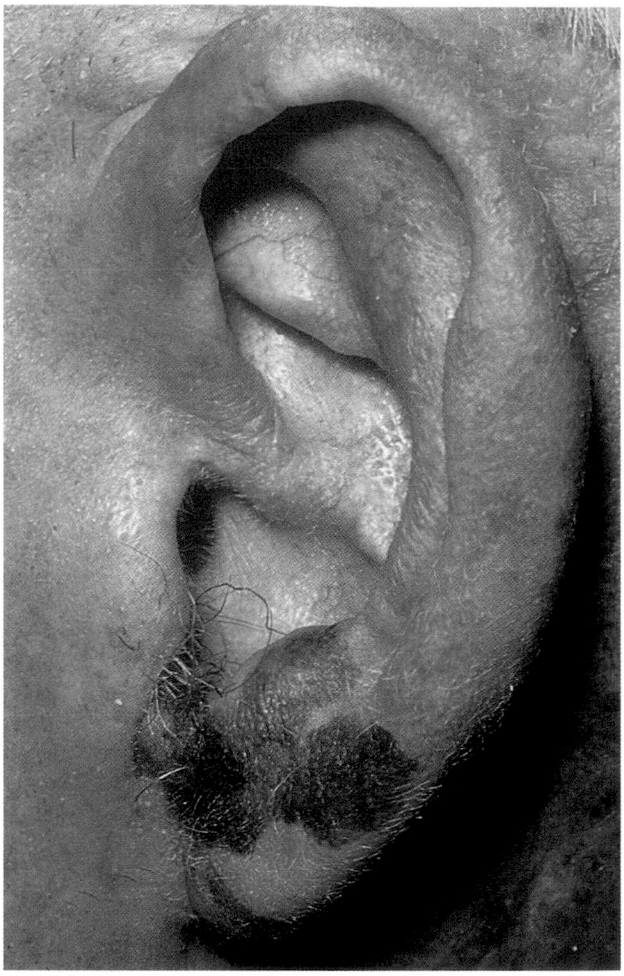

Figure 23.3 Superficial spreading melanoma of the left ear.

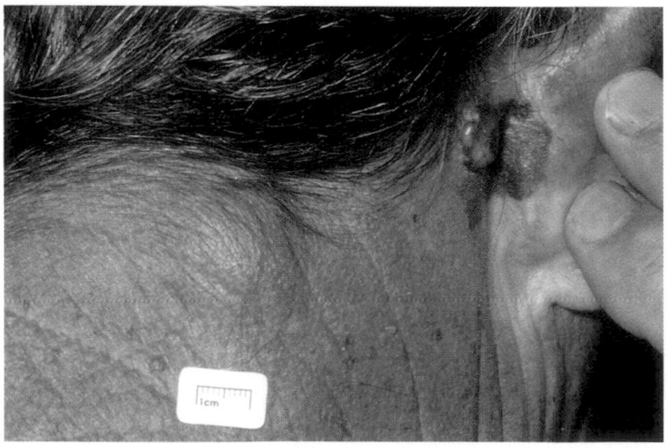

Figure 23.2 Nodular melanoma in the right postauricular area, metastatic involvement of the right occipital node.

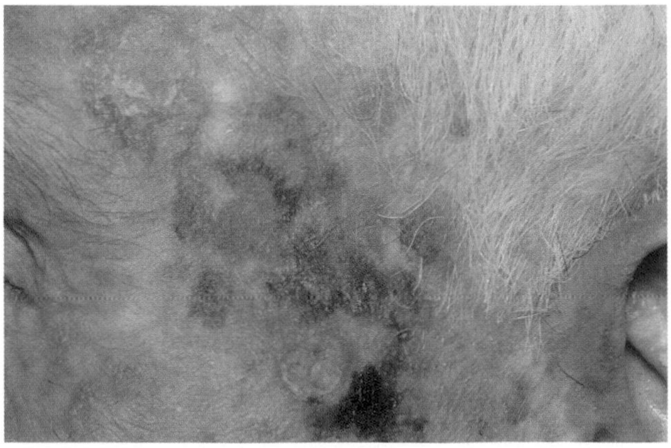

Figure 23.4 Lentigo maligna melanoma of the temple in an elderly male.

melanoma[26] and have a propensity to occur in the head and neck.[27] The majority of these are not pigmented and have the appearance of a slowly enlarging, scar-like lesion. Histologically the usual appearance is one of proliferating spindle cells within a dense collagenous stroma. The neurotropic variant has a marked propensity for perineural and endoneural invasion.[27]

The likelihood of regional metastasis, distant metastasis, and therefore survival is influenced by a number of clinical and pathological characteristics of the primary melanoma. These are summarized in Table 23.2, where the chi-squared increment gives the relative importance of each prognostic factor, whilst simultaneously accounting for the contribution of the other listed factors.

Table 23.2 Prognostic factors in localized (stage I and II) cutaneous malignant melanoma

Factor	χ^2 increment
Tumour thickness	123.13
Ulceration	54.24
Site	37.20
Surgical treatment	24.03
Clark level of invasion	18.17
Sex	14.54
Age	3.89

Data from Balch et al[26]

Tumour thickness and level of invasion

In the absence of distant and regional node metastases, tumour thickness is the most important pathological prognostic indicator in cutaneous melanoma (Table 23.2), and this applies equally in the head and neck as it does elsewhere.[10–13] Breslow first identified the significance of this third tumour dimension, in 1970. The upper reference point is the superficial aspect of the granular cell layer of the epidermis and, in the case of ulceration, the base of the ulcer. The lower reference point is the deepest point of tumour invasion.[28] A typically inverse relationship between tumour thickness and survival was found in evaluating 998 patients with cutaneous melanoma of the head and neck treated at the Sydney Melanoma Unit (Table 23.3).[10] Thicker lesions are more likely to be associated with lymph node and distant metastases on presentation and subsequently thereafter.[29] Clark level of invasion also has prognostic significance but is a less important indicator than Breslow tumour thickness.[25,30,31]

Table 23.3 Tumour thickness and disease-specific survival in 998 patients with cutaneous melanoma of the head and neck

Thickness (mm)	5-year survival (%)	10-year survival (%)
< 0.76	91	87
0.76–1.49	87	75
1.5–3.99	71	59
> 4.0	57	48

Data from O'Brien et al[10]

Tumour ulceration

Tumour ulceration has been shown to be independently associated with a worse prognosis in a number of studies.[9–12,25] O'Brien at al found the 10-year survival in patients with head and neck melanoma with ulcerated lesions was 52%, compared with 72% in non-ulcerated melanomas.[10]

Table 23.4 Survival according to anatomical subsite in 998 patients with cutaneous melanoma of the head and neck

Site	5-year survival (%)	10-year survival (%)
Face	80	69
Scalp	59*	45*
Ear	81	61
Neck	80	72

*$P < 0.001$.
Data from O'Brien et al.[10]

Anatomical site

Patients with scalp melanoma have been found to have an especially poor prognosis by some workers.[10,32] In the Sydney Melanoma Unit series patients with scalp melanoma had a 10-year survival of 45%, significantly worse than patients with lesions at other sites. This difference was confirmed on multivariate analysis (Table 23.4). Fisher[9] and Andersson et al[12] however, found no significant difference in outlook for the head and neck subsites when depth and presence of ulceration were adjusted for.

Regional lymph node involvement

Involvement of regional lymph nodes by melanoma leads to a significant decrease in 5- and 10-year survival.[9,10] Also, the number of involved nodes appears to significantly influence the likelihood of distant dissemination and death from disease.[30,33] In a series of patients undergoing neck dissection for cutaneous melanoma at the Sydney Melanoma Unit, patients with histologically positive nodes (clinically apparent or occult) had 5- and 10-year survival rates of 48% and 34%, respectively, whereas those with histologically negative nodes had survival rates of 75% and 67%.[34] A single involved node carries a 5-year survival of 50% while involvement of two to four nodes worsens the prognosis significantly.[33] Figure 23.5 demonstrates the influence of the number of involved nodes on survival. Furthermore, in a series of patients treated at Duke University, those with pathologically proven regional disease, following elective lymph node dissection (clinically negative, pathologically positive), had no better survival than those with clinically apparent regional disease (clinically positive, pathologically positive).[9]

Distant metastases

There is currently no effective treatment for distant metastatic disease. Balch et al reported a median survival of only 6 months for patients with distant spread.[26] The location of distant metastases was also of prognostic importance in that study. Skin, subcutaneous tissues, and distant lymph nodes were common sites of relapse. In greater than 20% these non-visceral sites were the sole manifestation of distant metastases, and a quarter of such patients were alive at 1 year, with a small number of long-term survivors. Visceral sites of metastases were most commonly lung, brain, liver and bone. The median survival for this group was 2–6 months and the 1-year survival was less than 10%.[26]

Age

In general, younger patients who have melanoma have a better prognosis than their older counterparts.[9–11,33] Advancing age also correlates with increased tumour thickness.[33]

Gender

Virtually all studies have demonstrated a better prognosis in melanoma for women than their male counterparts.[1,9,11] Part of the reason for better survival rates is that melanoma is more commonly observed on the extremities in women and these tumours have a better survival rate than lesions on the trunk or head and neck.[33] Furthermore, in a study of cutaneous melanoma of the head and neck women had less melanoma of the scalp than men.[9]

Staging

Staging of melanoma (Tables 23.5 and 23.6) should be according to the new AJCC system.[35] The 'length by width' classification of the primary tumour, which correlates with prognosis in most tumour types, is replaced with thickness, which is more predictive of outcome. Clinical 'T' classification is not therefore possible. Excisional biopsy and histopathological examination are necessary for proper staging.

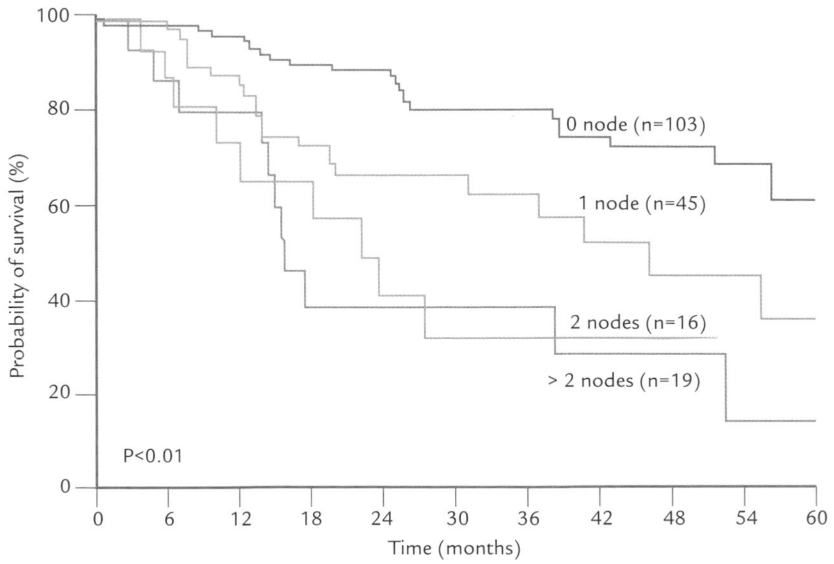

Figure 23.5 Influence of number of nodes involved with melanoma on survival. (Data from O'Brien et al[53]).

Table 23.5 Melanoma staging

Primary Tumour (T)	
TX	Primary tumour cannot be assessed (eg. Shave biopsy or regressed melanoma)
T0	No evidence of primary tumour
Tis	Melanoma *in situ*
T1	Melanoma ≤ 1.0 mm in thickness with or without ulceration
T1a	Melanoma ≤ 1.0 mm in thickness and level II or III, no ulceration
T1b	Melanoma ≤ 1.0 mm in thickness and level IV or V or with ulceration
T2	Melanoma 1.01–2.0 mm in thickness with or without ulceration
T2a	Melanoma 1.01–2.0 mm in thickness, without ulceration
T2b	Melanoma 1.01–2.0 mm in thickness, with ulceration
T3	Melanoma 2.01–4.0 mm in thickness with or without ulceration
T3a	Melanoma 2.01–4.0 mm in thickness, without ulceration
T3b	Melanoma 2.01–4.0 mm in thickness, with ulceration
T4	Melanoma > 4.0 mm in thickness with or without ulceration
T4a	Melanoma > 4.0 mm in thickness, no ulceration
T4b	Melanoma > 4.0 mm in thickness, with ulceration
Regional Lymph Nodes (N)	
NX	Regional lymph nodes cannot be assessed
N0	No regional lymph nodes
N1	Metastasis in one lymph node
N1a	Clinically occult (microscopic) metastases
N1b	Clinically apparent (macroscopic) metastases
N2	Metastasis in two to three regional nodes or intra-lymphatic regional metastasis *without* nodal metastases.
N2a	Clinically occult (microscopic) metastases
N2b	Clinically apparent (macroscopic) metastases
N2c	Satellite or in-transit metastasis *without* nodal metastasis
N3	Metastasis in four or more regional nodes, or matted metastatic nodes, or in-transit metastasis or satellite(s) *with* metastasis in regional node(s)
Distant Metastasis (M)	
MX	Distant metastasis cannot be assessed
M0	No distant metastasis
M1	Distant metastasis
M1a	Metastasis to skin, subcutaneous tissues or distant lymph nodes
M1b	Metastasis to lung
M1c	Metastasis to all other visceral or distant metastasis at any site associated with an elevated serum lactic dehydrogenase (LDH)

Table 23.6 Clinical stage grouping

Stage 0	Tis	N0	M0
Stage IA	T1a	N0	M0
Stage IB	T1b	N0	M0
	T2a	N0	M0
Stage IIA	T2b	N0	M0
	T3a	N0	M0
Stage IIB	T3b	N0	M0
	T4a	N0	M0
Stage IIC	T4b	N0	M0
Stage III	Any T	N1	M0
	Any T	N2	M0
	Any T	N3	M0
Stage IV	Any T	Any N	M1

Satellite lesions and subcutaneous nodules within 2 cm of the primary tumour are considered extensions of the primary mass and coded pT4b. Those occurring more than 2 cm from the primary are coded in-transit metastases (N2b).

For the purposes of staging two 'M' categories are included. This is justified by the more favourable therapeutic response of patients who have skin, subcutaneous, or distant nodal involvement as the sole site of distant metastatic disease.

Diagnosis

Clinical diagnosis

The aim in clinical diagnosis is to identify malignant melanoma in its earliest stage of development when it is readily curable. Generally, small malignant melanomas are asymmetrical, poorly circumscribed, with notched, scalloped or jagged borders and dark pigmentation with variable shades of brown. There may also be black, blue, and pink areas. The so-called 'ABCDE' (Asymmetry, Border irregularity, Colour variegation, Diameter > 6 mm, and Elevation) is a useful aid in clinical diagnosis.[36,37] Bleeding and ulceration are however late signs of malignancy.[36]

Distinguishing atypical nevi from early melanoma can be difficult. The use of dermatoscopy and photographic baseline records may be useful.[36] Only lesions that have acquired the clinical features of malignant melanoma or have changed 'out of step' with other pigmented lesions are considered for removal and histological assessment.

Biopsy

The technique of choice is a total excisional biopsy with narrow margins, incorporating subcutaneous fat. This allows assessment of the whole lesion and accurate microstaging. Following excision, primary closure is preferable to local flaps or skin grafting. Incisional or punch biopsy should be reserved for larger lesions, or where the lesion is located in a functionally and aesthetically sensitive area.

Diagnostic work-up

Careful clinical assessment of the regional lymph nodes is essential for management planning. The parotid region nodes deserve particular attention. These nodes drain the face, anterior scalp, and ear. The occipital and postauricular nodes also require careful palpation along with the other levels of the neck. Where level IV and level V nodes are involved the axilla should also be examined.[38]

Because of the low return from anatomical imaging techniques for the detection of disseminated disease in patients who have clinical stage I or II disease, extensive diagnostic testing has not been proven cost-effective.[39] All patients should have liver function tests and a chest X-ray but CT scanning should be reserved for symptomatic or high-risk patients. Recent studies have focused on positron emission tomography (PET) in the evaluation of high-risk patients.[40,41] PET has greater sensitivity than whole body CT in the detection of metastatic disease but false-positive scans do occur with PET in association with acute inflammatory processes, including that associated with surgical wound healing.

Treatment of melanoma

The objectives of treatment for patients with melanoma include the control of local disease and prevention, where possible, of distant spread. Unfortunately, the absence of an effective means of preventing and treating distant metastases continues to limit our ability to improve outcomes in high-risk patients. Early diagnosis and adequate primary surgery are the mainstays of therapy.

Treatment of the primary melanoma

Cutaneous melanomas of all sites, including the head and neck, require surgical excision but the extent of excisional margins continues to engender debate.[42,43] The current recommendations, however, are based on thickness of the primary melanoma. In general a 1-cm clearance for thin melanomas (< 1 mm), 2 cm for intermediate thickness (1–4 mm) and 2–3 cm for thick melanomas (> 4 mm) are adequate. These margins are based on the National Institutes of Health Consensus Development Panel[43] and several randomized trials.[44–46] For example, Veronesi et al[44] compared 1-cm versus 3-cm margins in 612 patients with primary tumours less than 2 mm in thickness. Only four patients in the entire study group developed local recurrence as the first relapse, and all four of these had received a 1-cm excision margin for tumours between 1 and 2 mm thickness. The disease-free and overall survival rates at a mean follow-up of 55 months were similar in both groups at 96%. The Intergroup Melanoma Trial[45] compared 2 and 4 cm margins in 486 patients with intermediate thickness melanomas (1–4 mm). The local recurrence rate was the same for both groups and there was no survival difference between the two groups.

A current randomized trial, being carried out by the British Association of Plastic Surgeons comparing 1 cm versus 3 cm margins for melanomas greater than 2 mm thickness, should provide further useful data as it is the first study to examine the efficacy of 1 cm margins for thicker depths of melanoma.

Surgery for melanoma of the head and neck is complicated by functional and cosmetic considerations. About half of all head and neck melanomas occur on the face.[10] Excision of these lesions requires the preservation of appearance and function, without compromising the oncologic result. In practice, a 1-cm margin usually proves to be adequate.[10] Every attempt should be made to achieve primary closure using local tissues in order to avoid skin grafts on the face or neck. If primary closure is not possible or desirable, local flaps provide the best cosmetic and functional result for facial cutaneous defects without compromising survival.[47] Skin grafts are both cosmetically acceptable and effective on the scalp.

Desmoplastic neurotropic melanoma may be associated with a higher rate of local recurrence than other forms of the disease. In a study of 280 patients accrued over a 10-year period at the Sydney Melanoma Unit,[48] it was found that the rate of local recurrence for desmoplastic neurotropic melanoma was 20%, while desmoplastic melanomas which did not display neurotropism were found to have a recurrence rate of only 6.8%. Wider margins are therefore justifiable for the desmoplastic variant especially if neurotropism is present. The current treatment philosophy at the Sydney Melanoma Unit is to excise with at least a 1-cm margin and then follow with radiotherapy to the area. If a named nerve is involved, the radiotherapy is extended to the skull base to encompass the nerve in question.

Management of the N0 neck

This issue continues to provoke controversy. The rationale for treating clinically negative lymph nodes among patients with cutaneous melanoma is that elective lymphadenectomy may remove subclinical micrometastases from the lymphatic basin at risk, and thereby prevent spread to the rest of the body. This theoretical benefit however does not translate into clinical reality. Elective neck dissection can improve regional control of disease and identify patients at risk of distant failure but unfortunately no useful adjuvant therapy exists for the high-risk group.

A number of studies have been performed to evaluate the efficacy of elective lymphadenectomy but the results have almost invariably been negative.[49–51] A retrospective review of 534 patients with clinical stage I melanoma of the head and neck treated at the Sydney Melanoma Unit and University of Alabama did reveal a significant benefit for elective lymphadenectomy in patients with intermediate tumour thickness.[52] However, this study included patients referred from outside these two institutions, creating a bias in favour of elective lymphadenectomy. In 1991 the Sydney Melanoma Unit published the largest single institution experience of head and neck melanoma, and analysed its own patient population to evaluate the benefits of elective lymph node dissection. There were 998 patients in this series and a total of 234 patients with melanomas greater than 1.5-mm thickness received prophylactic neck dissection, consistent with the philosophy of the SMU at the time. Retrospective univariate analysis of patients treated only at the SMU indicated a small survival advantage to patients with intermediate thickness melanoma treated by elective neck dissection.[10] However, when multivariate analysis was carried out, no benefit could be demonstrated for elective neck dissection.

Three prospective randomized trials have been unable to demonstrate the efficacy of elective lymphadenectomy. Veronesi et al[49] carried out a study of 267 patients with extremity melanomas. Patients were randomized to receive elective lymphadenectomy or observation only, but there were no differences found in survival between the two groups or in any subset analysed. The Mayo clinic in 1986 published a prospective, randomized study of 171 patients who received immediate elective lymphadenectomy, delayed elective lymphadenectomy at 3 months or observation only. All patients had localized (stage I) melanoma restricted to the extremities or lateral trunk. Results indicated no improvement in disease-free survival in the elective lymphadenectomy group; however, almost two-thirds of the patients in this study had thin lesions and therefore would have been at low risk for nodal metastases.[50]

Many of the methodological problems of earlier studies were taken into account in the design of the Intergroup study.[51] The Intergroup Melanoma Surgical Program enrolled 740 patients with stages I and II melanoma. Patients were randomized to observation of the regional lymph node basin or elective lymphadenectomy. All patients with trunk melanomas had cutaneous lymphoscintigraphy in order to identify the lymph node basins at risk and to direct lymphadenectomy. There was no difference in overall 5-year survival between the observation and elective lymphadenectomy groups (86% versus 82%; $P = 0.25$). However, there was a subgroup of patients 60 years of age or younger with tumours 1–2 mm in thickness and no ulceration who had an increased survival with elective lymphadenectomy (88% versus 81%; $P = 0.04$). More than 90% of patients with regional recurrence had clinical evidence of their relapse within 5 years, and distant relapses were still occurring after 9 years.[51] The small benefit found only on subgroup analysis in this study has failed to convince surgeons of the efficacy of elective lymphadenectomy in cutaneous melanoma. In fact, this analysis has been criticized because the subgroup that appeared to benefit from elective dissection was manufactured and was not part of the original stratification process.

When a decision is made to carry out an elective lymphadenectomy, a selective neck dissection based on site of the primary melanoma is most appropriate. Melanomas of the anterior scalp and face tend to drain to the parotid gland and node levels I, II and III, while those lying on the scalp through the coronal plane and those involving the ear drain to the parotid gland and levels I–V. Melanomas arising on the posterior scalp tend to drain to levels II–V including the occipital group of nodes.[54] In a series of 106 patients having elective neck dissection based on these clinically predicted lymph drainage pathways, O'Brien et al[53] described a rate of geographic miss of 3%, indicating that clinical prediction of which nodes are at risk, based on the site of the primary, can be very accurate. The incidence of pathologically positive nodes in the clinically negative neck however was only 8%. Overall the benefits of elective neck dissection have not been demonstrated and furthermore, length of hospital stay, cost and morbidity can be significant. A common complication, for example, is paresis of the marginal mandibular nerve after parotidectomy combined with neck dissection.[52]

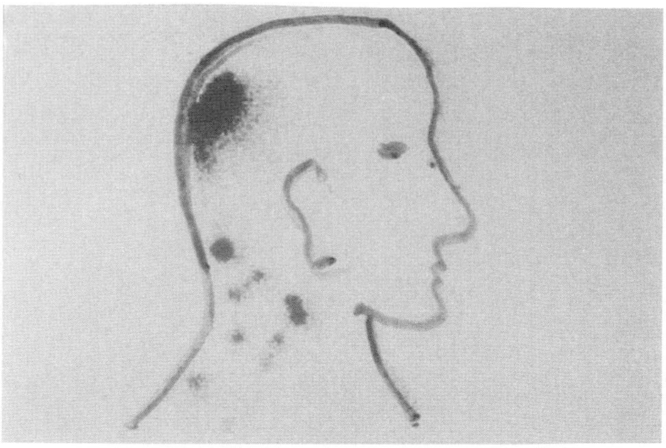

Figure 23.6 Lymphoscintigram of right posterior parietal melanoma with multiple nodes seen.

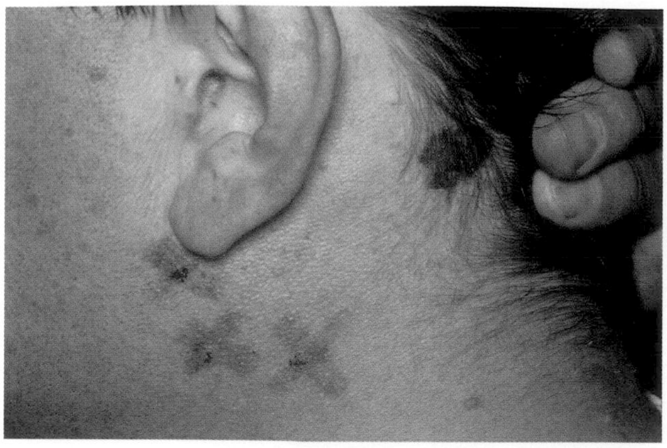

Figure 23.7 Left post-auricular melanoma with three marked sentinel nodes.

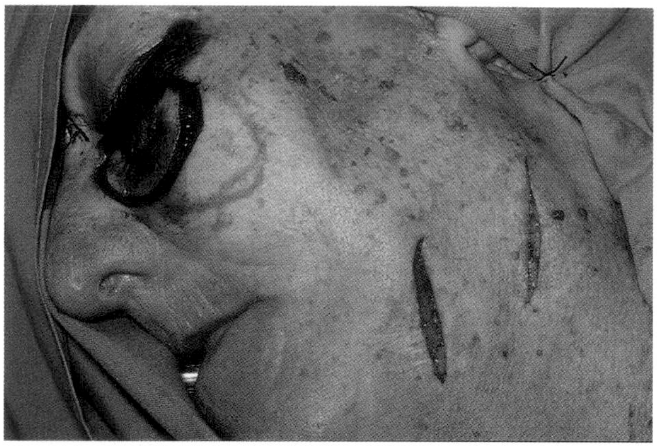

Figure 23.8 Primary infraorbital melanoma being resected following injection of blue dye. Two left neck sentinel nodes also biopsied.

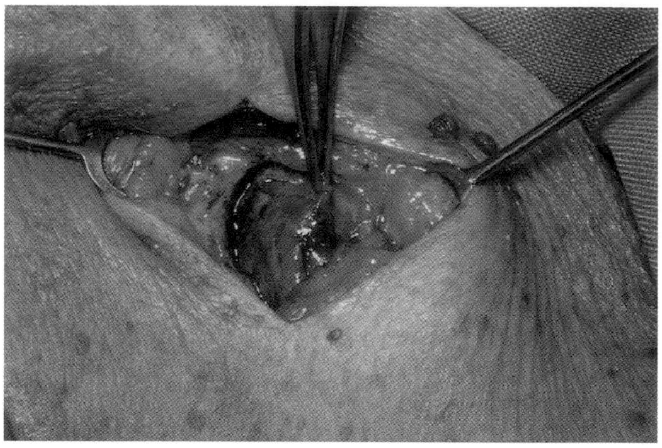

Figure 23.9 Blue-stained sentinel node, identified in the submandibular region in the patient shown in Figure 23.8.

Sentinel node biopsy

The unproven benefits of elective lymphadenectomy combined with the potential cost and morbidity of the procedure have led to the development of the technique of sentinel node biopsy. This method is based on the theory that there is a 'sentinel' node, or nodes, in each lymphatic basin and that this node(s) is the first node to be involved with metastatic disease.[55] A sentinel node is defined as a lymph node or nodes having direct and independent drainage from the primary tumour site, as identified on the preoperative lymphoscintigram. Sentinel nodes can be identified preoperatively by lymphoscintigraphy and intraoperatively by the injection of vital dye and hand-held gamma probe. At the Sydney Melanoma Unit a combination of all three methods is used to identify the sentinel node. Four to six injections of technetium 99m antimony trisulfide colloid are placed intradermally in volumes of 0.05–0.1 ml around the site of the primary melanoma. This material has a small particle size of 3–12 μm that facilitates its delivery through the lymphatic network. The study must be performed prior to wide excision of the primary since wide excision, beyond simple biopsy, is likely to alter normal lymphatic drainage. Scanning is carried out immediately and in a delayed fashion 2.5 hours later (Figure 23.6). The sentinel node or nodes are then marked with a dermal tattoo (Figure 23.7). The surgical procedure is performed ideally within 24 hours of lymphoscintigraphy, while there is still radioactivity in the node, to take advantage of intraoperative localization with the hand-held gamma probe. At the time of surgery, the primary site is injected (Figure 23.8) with 0.5–1 ml of patent blue-V dye (Rhone–Poulec–Rhorer, Sydney, Australia). An incision is made over the marked node and dissection is performed in order to identify the blue-stained lymphatic that is then traced to the blue-stained sentinel node (Figure 23.9). Exploration around this may identify other blue-stained nodes. The hand-held gamma probe is used to confirm the sentinel node by its high counts

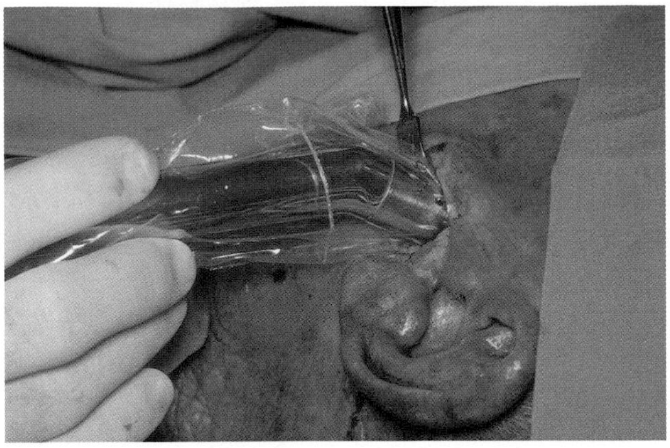

Figure 23.10 Gamma probe searching for left preauricular sentinel node.

(Figure 23.10) and the subsequent presence of only background radiation once the node or nodes have been removed. The sentinel node is removed and sent for histological analysis.[55–58]

Sentinel node biopsy in the head and neck presents special problems. There are several reasons for this. There may be difficulty in recognizing which of the many nodes demonstrated on lymphoscintigraphy are actually sentinel nodes (Figures 23.10). Also, if the primary site overlies the sentinel node, both the radiopharmaceutical injection and the blue dye injection are likely to obscure the sentinel node. In addition, the actual nodes may be small and difficult to find at the time of surgery. The potential for damage to important anatomic structures such as the facial nerve when dissecting for parotid sentinel nodes must also be considered. A superficial parotidectomy or selective neck dissection may be more appropriate in some circumstances. In a study of 97 patients with head and neck melanoma, sentinel nodes were identified by lymphoscintigraphy in 95 patients. Of these patients, 50% had three or more sentinel nodes identified on lymphoscintigraphy.[50] Finding these nodes at operation is not straightforward, for the reasons presented, however some authors claim very high rates of success in identifying sentinel nodes at surgery. Wells et al[59] indicate that they were able to identify the sentinel nodes in 55 of 58 patients (95%) in the head and neck.

The clinical benefit from sentinel node biopsy remains unclear. Certainly, sentinel node biopsy returns a higher rate of positivity for clinically negative nodes, around 20%, when compared with the node-positive rate for elective neck dissection, about 8%. This increased accuracy in staging is presumably because only a single or few nodes are examined pathologically and immunohistochemical stains are done. An advantage is that patients without microscopic disease can avoid unnecessary lymphadenectomy.

Management of the clinically positive neck

Our current state of knowledge indicates that treatment of the clinically positive neck probably requires comprehensive neck dissection. This is because any lymph node level can be involved with disease once metastatic lymphadenopathy is present in the neck. Shah et al[60] analysed the distribution of pathologically positive nodes in 111 radical neck dissection specimens. Levels II–IV were most commonly involved, but 23% also had level I disease and 19% had level V involvement. In addition, patients with ear, face and anterior scalp lesions were at high risk for parotid involvement. O'Brien et al[52] evaluated 175 patients undergoing various forms of neck dissection for cutaneous melanoma and confirmed that there was a recurrence rate of 23% with selective neck dissection, that is dissection of only certain node groups, and 0% for modified radical neck dissection, a comprehensive dissection, for clinically positive neck disease. In that study, patients having radical neck dissection had a 14% recurrence rate but they were also the group that had more advanced disease. Superficial parotidectomy should be included for lesions of the face, ear or anterior scalp that have metastasized to the neck even in the absence of clinical parotid involvement.[61]

Patients with clinical metastatic melanoma have a poor prognosis overall, however the outlook is not hopeless. The 5- and 10-year survival rates for patients treated by neck dissection at the Sydney Melanoma Unit were 48% and 34%, respectively.[10] Therefore, therapeutic neck dissection is a worthwhile procedure.

Radiotherapy for melanoma

Most patients who die of melanoma do so with disseminated disease, while the primary site remains controlled. Because of this, the problem of regional recurrence after lymphadenectomy has received little attention. However, recurrence in the parotid bed or neck can cause severe morbidity and worsen prognosis.[62] Therapeutic neck dissection may fail in up to 30% of cases.[10] Singletary et al[61] reported even higher rates of regional recurrence with increasing number of nodes involved, noting up to 44% rates of recurrence after dissection of matted nodes. These results indicate a potential need for adjuvant therapy after therapeutic neck dissection in order to improve locoregional control for this group of patients.

Unfortunately, melanoma has carried a reputation for resistance to radiotherapy for much of this

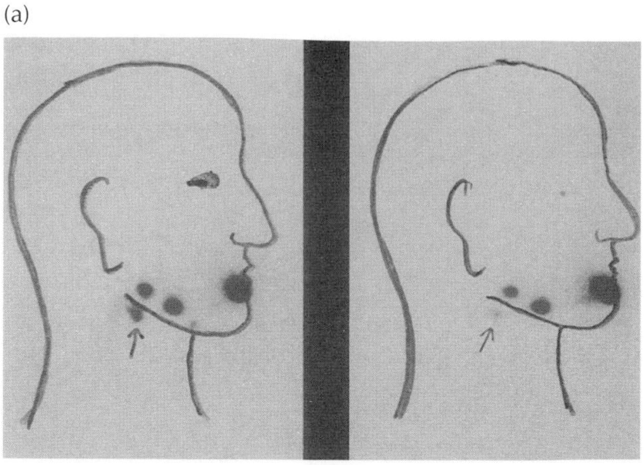

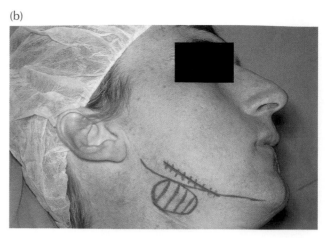

Figure 23.11 (a) These lymphoscintigrams are from a young man with melanoma of the right side of the lower lip. These are two brightly enhancing nodes seen on the initial scan (right) with a faint node below the line of the jaw. This latter node enhances more brightly on the delayed scan (left) but was thought to be a second tier node rather than a sentinel node. (b) Sentinel node biopsy of the two nodes seen on the initial scan was attempted through an incision marked by the blue line. The nodes were not identified. Six months later, the patient returned with an enlarged node, just below the jaw. This was shown to be the node that enhanced only faintly on the initial scan.

century.[63,64] However, over the last decade, radiotherapy has been applied successfully in a number of settings for the treatment of melanoma. In part this has been due to an improved understanding of the radiobiology of this disease.

The remarkable ability of melanoma cells to repair sublethal damage has led to the development of high dose per fraction radiotherapy in an effort to overcome this phenomenon. This technique delivers the total amount of radiation in a hypofractionated course with each fraction containing a greater dose. High dose per fraction therapy aims to overcome the ability of melanoma cells to repair sublethal damage, but late radiation effects in normal tissue may be increased.

The Sydney Melanoma Unit published a non-randomized study of 152 dissected necks or parotids comparing neck dissection alone with neck dissection and adjuvant radiotherapy for pathologically positive disease. The adjuvant radiotherapy regimen used consisted of six fractions of 5.5 Gy delivered twice weekly for 3 weeks. The group of 45 dissected necks or parotids that received adjuvant radiotherapy demonstrated a 6.5% regional recurrence rate while the group that received neck dissection only, recurred in the neck 18.7% of the time.[65]

Although the clear benefits of high dose per fraction radiotherapy have not been definitively demonstrated for melanoma, the adjuvant use of radiotherapy for patients with nodal metastases does appear to improve the locoregional control of disease.[66]

Adjuvant therapy in melanoma

Immunotherapy

Following the publication of a randomized controlled trial demonstrating improved relapse free and overall survival in patients with high-risk resected melanoma, treated with interferon alpha, there was considerable optimism about the efficacy of this immunotherapy agent.[67] In this study, high-dose interferon alpha was employed with considerable treatment-related toxicity. A follow-up study (Intergroup 1690) was designed to compare high-dose with low-dose interferon alpha. However, the results of Intergroup 1690, published in abstract form, failed to confirm any beneficial effect of interferon alpha either in high or low dosage. Interferon alpha, in combination with other agents, has not proven beneficial in patients with advanced (stage III and IV) disease.[68] Until there is clarification of the benefit or otherwise of interferon alpha, its use, outside the context of a clinical trial, cannot be recommended in the adjuvant treatment of melanoma.

A substantial number of melanoma-associated antigens have been identified, and the antibody and cellular responses to these targets characterized. Clinical trials have been, and continue to be, conducted utilizing a number of different vaccine approaches. Allogeneic, autologous, whole cell, cell lysate, and purified antigens have all been the subject of investigation.[69] Although no phase III clinical trial has demonstrated a significant improvement in survival of patients receiving vaccine therapy, phase II trials have shown enhanced survival for patients who develop a humoral and/or cellular response to a melanoma vaccine. On-going research seeks to determine which aspects of enhanced immunoresponsiveness improve clinical outcome.[70]

Chemotherapy

Adjuvant chemotherapy regimens for the treatment of metastatic melanoma have been extensively evaluated and none has been demonstrated to improve survival. Multiagent regimens have proven to be no more effective than single-agent dacarbazine which produces response rates of approximately 20%.[71] Recent work has focused on combinations of chemotherapy and immunotherapy, although a recent phase III trial demonstrated no associated benefit from the addition of tamoxifen and interferon alpha to dacarbazine.[68]

REFERENCES

1. Wingo PA, Ries LAG, Risenberg HM *et al.* Cancer incidence and mortality 1973–1995 – A report card for the US. *Cancer* 1998; **82**: 1197–1207.
2. Armstrong BK, Kricker A. Cutaneous melanoma. *Cancer Surv* 1994; **19/20**: 219–240.
3. Giles GG, Thursfield VJ, Staples MP. The bottom line: cancer mortality trends in Australia 1950–1991. *Cancer Forum* 1994; **18**: 18–23.
4. Mackie RM, Hole D, Hunter JA *et al.* Cutaneous malignant melanoma in Scotland: incidence, survival, and mortality 1979–94. *Br Med J* 1997; **315**: 1117–1121.
5. Elwood JM, Gallagher RP. Body site distribution of cutaneous malignant melanoma in relationship to sun exposure. *Int J Cancer* 1998; **78**: 276–280.
6. Swerdlow AJ, dos Santos Silva I, Reid A *et al.* Trends in cancer incidence and mortality in Scotland: description and possible explanations. *Br J Cancer* 1998; **77 (Suppl 3)**: 1–54.
7. Giles GG, Armstrong BK, Burton RC *et al.* Has mortality stopped rising in Australia. Analysis of trends between 1931 and 1994. *Br Med J* 1996; **312**: 1121–1125.
8. Melia J. Changing incidence and mortality from cutaneous malignant melanoma. *Br Med J* 1997; **315**: 1106–1107.
9. Fisher S. Cutaneous malignant melanoma of the head and neck. *Laryngoscope* 1989; **99**: 822–836.
10. O'Brien CJ, Coates AS, Pettersen-Schaeffer K *et al.* Experience with 998 cutaneous melanomas of the head and neck over 30 years. *Am J Surg* 1991; **162**: 310–314.
11. Ringborg U, Afzelius LE, Lagerlof B *et al.* Cutaneous malignant melanoma of the head and neck. *Cancer* 1993; **71**: 751–758
12. Andersson AP, Gottlieb J, Drzewiecki KT *et al.* Skin melanoma of the head and neck. *Cancer* 1992; **69**: 1153–1156.
13. Parkin DM, Muir CS, Whelan SC *et al.* Cancer incidence in five continents. Lyon, France: International Agency for Research on Cancer, 1992; IARC Scientific Publication No. 120.
14. Bulliard JL, Cox B, Elwood JM. Latitude gradients in melanoma incidence and mortality in the non-Maori population of New Zealand. *Cancer Causes Control* 1994; **5**: 234–40.
15. Lee JA, Strickland D. Malignant melanoma: social status, indoor and outdoor work. *Br J Cancer* 1980; **41**: 757–763.
16. Cooke KE, Skegg DC, Fraser J. Socio-economic status, indoor and outdoor work, and malignant melanoma. *Int J Cancer* 1984; **34**: 57–62.
17. Autier P, Dore J-F. Influence of sun exposure during childhood and adulthood on melanoma risk. *Int J Cancer* 1998; **77**: 533–537.
18. Westerdahl J, Olsson H, Ingvar C. At what age do sunburn episodes play a crucial role for the development of malignant melanoma? *Eur J Cancer* 1994; **30A**: 1647–1654.
19. International Agency for Research on Cancer. IARC Monographs on the evaluation of carcinogenic risks to humans. Ultraviolet Radiation; Vol 55 Lyon, France, IARC 1992.
20. Autier P, Dore JF, Schiffers E *et al.* Melanoma and use of sunscreens: an EORTC case-control study in Germany, Belgium, and France. *Int J Cancer* 1995; **61**: 749–755.
21. Balch CM, Karakosis C, Mettlin C. Management of cutaneous melanoma in the United States. *Surg Gynecol Obstet* 1984; **158**: 311–319.
22. Bataille V, Grulich A, Saseini P *et al.* The association between naevi and melanoma in populations with different levels of sun exposure: a joint case-control study of melanoma in the UK and Australia. *Br J Cancer* 1998; **77**: 505–510.
23. Kaplan EN. The risk of malignancy in large congenital nevi. *Plast Reconstr Surg* 1974; **53**: 421–428.
24. Seykora J, Elder D. Dysplastic nevi and other risk factors for melanoma. *Semin Oncol* 1996; **23**: 682–687.
25. Clark WH Jr, Ainsworth AM, Bernardino EH *et al.* The development biology of primary human malignant melanomas. *Semin Oncol* 1975; **2**: 83–93.
26. Balch CM, Soong HJ, Shaw HM *et al.* An analysis of prognostic factors in 8500 patients with cutaneous melanoma. In: Balch CM, Houghton AN, Milton GW *et al* (eds). *Cutaneous Melanoma.* Philadelphia: Lippincott, 1992; 165–187.
27. Sagebiel RW. Unusual variants of melanoma: fact or fiction? *Semin Oncol* 1996; **23**: 703–708.
28. Jain S, Allen PW. Desmoplastic malignant melanoma and its variants: a study of 45 cases. *Am J Surg Pathol* 1989; **13**: 358–363.

29. Breslow A. Thickness, cross-sectional area and depth of invasion in the prognosis of cutaneous melanoma. *Ann Surg* 1970; **170**: 902–908.
30. Berdeaux DH, Meyskens FL, Parks B *et al.* Cutaneous malignant melanoma: the natural history and prognostic factors influencing the development of stage II disease. *Cancer* 1989; **63**: 1430–1436.
31. Clark WH, From L, Bernardino EA *et al.* The histogenesis and biological behaviour of primary human malignant melanomas of the skin. *Cancer Res* 1969; **29**: 705–726.
32. Morton DL, Davtayan DG, Wanek LA *et al.* Multivaraite analysis of the relationship between survival and microstage of primary melanoma by Clark level and Breslow thickness. *Cancer* 1993; **71**: 3737–3743.
33. Wanebo HJ, Cooper PH, Young DV *et al.* Prognostic factors in head and neck melanoma: effect of lesion location. *Cancer* 1988; **62**: 831–837.
34. O'Brien CJ, Gianoutsos MP, Morgan MJ. Neck dissection for cutaneous malignant melanoma. *World J Surg* 1992; **16**: 222–226.
35. Balch CM, Buzaid AC, Soong SJ et al. Final version of the American Joint Committee on Cancer staging system for cutaneous melanoma. *J Clin Oncol* 2001; **19**: 3635–48.
36. Steiner A, Pehamberger H, Wolff K. In vivo epiluminescence microscopy of pigmented lesions. II. Diagnosis of small pigmented skin lesions and early detection of melanoma. *J Am Acad Dermatol* 1987; **17**: 584–589.
37. Menzies SW, Crotty KA, Ingver C, McCarthy WH. *An Atlas of Surface Microscopy of Pigmented Skin Lesions.* Sydney: McGraw-Hill, 1996.
38. Shah JP, Kraus DH, Dubner S et al. Patterns of regional lymph node metastases from cutaneous melanoma of the head and neck. *Am J Surg* 1991; **162**: 320–323.
39. Iscoe N, Kersey P, Gapski J et al. Predictive value of staging investigations in patients with clinical stage I malignant melanoma. *Plast Reconstr Surg* 1987; **80**: 233–237.
40. Rinne D, Baum RP, Hor G, Kaufman R. Primary staging and follow-up of high risk patients with whole-body 18F-Fluorodeoxyglucose positron emission tomography. *Cancer* 1998; **82**: 1664–1671.
41. Holder WP, White RL, Zuger JH et al. Effectiveness of positron emission tomography for the detection of melanoma metastases. *Ann Surg* 1998; **227**: 764–771.
42. Handley WS. The pathology of melanotic growths in relation to their operative treatment. *Lancet* 1907; **i**: 927.
43. National Institutes of Health Consensus Development Panel on Early Melanoma. *JAMA* 1992; **268**: 1314.
44. Veronesi U, Cascinelli N. Narrow excision: a safe procedure for thin cutaneous melanoma. *Arch Surg* 1991; **126**: 438–41.
45. Balch C, Urist M, Karakousis C et al. Efficacy of 2 cm surgical margins for intermediate thickness melanomas 1–4 mm: results of a multi-institutional randomized surgical trial. *Ann Surg* 1993; **218**: 262.
46. Ringborg U, Andersson R, Eldh J et al. Resection margins of 2 versus 5 cm for cutaneous malignant melanoma with a tumour thickness of 0.8–2.0 mm. *Cancer* 1996; **77**: 1809.
47. Ariyan S. Plastic and reconstructive surgery in melanoma patients. In: Balch C (ed.) *Surgical Approaches to Cutaneous Melanoma.* Basel: S Karger, 1985.
48. Quinn M, Crotty K, Thompson J et al. Desmoplastic and desmoplastic neurotropic melanoma: experience with 280 patients. *Cancer* 1998; **83**: 1128–1135.
49. Veronesi U, Adamus J, Bandiera D et al. Inefficacy of immediate node dissection in stage I melanoma of the limbs. *N Engl J Med* 1977; **297**: 627–630.
50. Sim F, Taylor W, Pritchard D et al. Lymphadenectomy in the management of stage I malignant melanoma: a prospective randomized study. *Mayo Clin Proc* 1986; **61**: 697–705.
51. Balch C, Soong SJ, Bartolucci A et al. Efficacy of an elective regional lymph node dissection of 1–4 mm thick melanomas for patients 60 years of age and younger. *Ann Surg* 1996; **224**: 255–266.
52. Urist MM, Balch CM, Soong SJ et al. Head and neck melanoma in 534 clinical stage 1 patients: a prognostic factors analysis and results of surgical treatment. *Ann Surg* 1984; **200**: 769–775.
53. O'Brien CJ, Petersen-Schaefer K, Ruark D et al. Radical, modified and selective neck dissection for cutaneous malignant melanoma. *Head Neck* 1995; **17**: 232–41.
54. O'Brien CJ, Uren R, Thompson J et al. Prediction of potential metastatic sites in cutaneous head and neck melanoma using lymphoscintigraphy. *Am J Surg* 1995; **170**: 461–6.
55. Morton D, Wen DR, Wong J et al. Technical details of intraoperative lymphatic mapping for early stage melanoma. *Arch Surg* 1992; **127**: 392–399.
56. Uren R, Howman G, Shaw H et al. Lymphoscintigraphy in high risk melanoma of the trunk: predicting draining node groups, defining lymphatic channels and locating the sentinel node. *J Nucl Med* 1993; **34**: 1435–1440.
57. Thompson J, McCarthy W, Bosch C et al. Sentinel lymph node status as an indicator of the presence of metastatic melanoma in regional lymph nodes. *Melanoma Res* 1995; **5**: 255–260.
58. Reintgen D, Cruse W, Wells K et al. The orderly progression of melanoma nodal metastases. *Ann Surg* 1994; **220**: 759–767.
59. Wells K, Rapaport D, Cruse W et al. Sentinel lymph node biopsy in melanoma of the head and neck. *Plast Reconstr Surg* 1997; **100**: 591–594.
60. Shah J, Kraus D, Dubner S et al. Patterns of regional lymph node metastases from cutaneous melanoma of the head and neck. *Am J Surg* 1991; **162**: 320–323.
61. O'Brien C, Petersen-Schafer K, Papadopoulos T et al. Evaluation of 107 therapeutic and elective parotidectomies for cutaneous melanoma. *Am J Surg* 1994; **168**: 400–403.
62. Singletary S, Byers R, Shallenberger R et al. Prognostic factors in patients with regional cervical node metastases from cutaneous malignant melanoma. *Am J Surg* 1986; **152**: 371–376.
63. Adair F. Treatment of melanomas. *Surg Gynecol Obstet* 1936; **62**: 406–409.

64. Del Regato J, Spjut H. *Cancer: Diagnosis, Treatment and Diagnosis.* St. Louis: CV Mosby, 1977.
65. O'Brien C, Petersen-Schaefer K, Stevens G et al. Adjuvant radiotherapy following neck dissection and parotidectomy for metastatic malignant melanoma. *Head Neck* 1997; **19**: 589–594.
66. Cooper J. The evolution of the role of radiation therapy in the management of mucocutaneous melanoma. *Hematol/Oncol Clin North Am* 1998; **12**: 849–862.
67. Kirkwood JM, Strawderman MH, Ernstoff MS et al. Interferon alfa-2b adjuvant therapy of high-risk resected cutaneous melanoma: the Eastern Cooperative Oncology Group Trial EST 1685. *J Clin Oncol* 1996; **14**: 7–17.
68. Falkson CI, Ibrahim J, Kirkwood J et al. Phase III trial of dacarbazine versus dacarbazine with interferon alpha-2b versus dacarbazine with tamoxifen versus dacarbazine with interferon alpha-2b and tamoxifen in patients with metastatic malignant melanoma: an Eastern Cooperative Oncology Group study. *J Clin Oncol* 1998; **16**: 1743–1751.
69. Ollila DW, Kelley MC, Gammon G et al. Overview of melanoma vaccines: active specific immunotherapy for melanoma patients. *Semin Surg Oncol* 1998; **14**: 328–336.
70. Chan AD, Morton DL. Active immunotherapy with allogeneic tumour cell vaccines: present status. *Semin Oncol* 1998; **25**: 611–622.
71. McClay EF, McClay M-ET. Systemic chemotherapy for the treatment of metastatic melanoma. *Semin Oncol* 1996; **23**: 744–753.

24 Sarcomas of the head and neck

Irvin Pathak, Camilla MA Carroll, Brian O'Sullivan, Peter C Neligan and Patrick J Gullane

Introduction

Sarcomas of the head and neck constitute less than 1% of head and neck malignancies. The rarity of these tumours may lead to a delay in diagnosis or improper initial management that may have untoward consequences. Multidisciplinary management of these patients is essential in order to facilitate diagnosis, formulate a treatment plan and optimize outcome. The literature on head and neck sarcoma is sparse. Fortunately, the treatment of these tumours has been studied more extensively in other parts of the body. Concepts of pathogenesis and treatment may be borrowed from other sites and applied to the head and neck. This is especially true of soft tissue sarcomas of the extremities and superficial areas of the trunk. In these sites, randomized trials on treatment have been carried out. Published series in the literature of head and neck sarcoma are available. However, these reports often mix paediatric and adult cases, various histology and a wide range of time periods. This makes interpretation of data for the care of the individual patient more difficult.

These tumours tend to afflict people in the most productive time years of their lives. The resultant disability and morbidity can be staggering. The prognosis for sarcomas varies according to histology, grade, location and size of the primary. Tumours with higher grade of histology and those greater than 5 cm carry a poor prognosis. Gross residual tumour also carries an unfavourable outcome.[1–3] In the Princess Margaret series, the 5-year cause-specific survival was 62%, with a local relapse rate of 41% and distant relapse rate of 31%.[1] Significant progress has been made in the last 20 years in the management and outcomes of these patients. Much of this has been related to the implementation of specialized multidisciplinary teams for the care of these patients. Despite this, many of these patients continue to suffer from the ravages of recurrent disease and mortality.

The multidisciplinary sarcoma team

The single-most important improvement in the care of the sarcoma patient has been the implementation of multidisciplinary teams consisting of surgeons, radiation oncologists, medical oncologists, pathologists, radiologists and clinical nurse specialists. Prior to this, the radiation oncologist would often see the patient for the first time after surgery had already been performed making planning difficult. With a multidisciplinary team, all members see the patient and formulate a treatment plan prior to implementation of any of the portions of the therapy. Part of this approach must also include review of all pathology by an experienced pathologist. The initial biopsy often is performed in an outside centre. This needs to be obtained and reviewed in the host institution. Pathology is essential for clarification of the diagnosis, tumour grading as well as for the determination of margins. Adherence to protocols in diagnosis and treatment of these patients produces consistency in the approach to this disease. This should allow comparison of treatment approaches from centre to centre as well as ensuring quality of care. Finally, this approach lends itself to audit of outcomes of particular therapeutic approaches. This multidisciplinary approach allows for the optimal care of patients with these difficult problems.[4]

Molecular biology of sarcomas

There appear to be two types of genes involved in regulating cell growth and whose malfunction can lead to neoplastic growth, oncogenes and tumour suppressor genes. Oncogenes promote growth and inhibit differentiation. Mutations in these genes are dominant over the wild type gene and result in the overexpression of a protein product leading to unchecked cell division. Examples of this in sarcomas include mdm2 and c-myc.

The protein product of the *c-myc* oncogene is a 65 000 molecular weight molecule found in the nucleus of cells, binding to DNA. It has been implicated in the regulation of the G1/S transition of the cell cycle. Overexpression of *c-myc* has been demonstrated in a number of soft tissue sarcomas including synovial sarcoma, liposarcoma and chondrosarcoma. The murine double minute (*mdm2*) oncogene encodes a nuclear phosphoprotein that interacts with the tumour supressor gene *p53* to inhibit *p53*-mediated gene transcription.

A subgroup of oncogenes undergo translocations such that the regulatory region from one gene is joined to the functional region of another gene. This produces a chimeric gene producing a protein that is inappropriately expressed, such as the PAX3–FKHD translocation in alveolar rhabdomyosarcoma. These genes are balanced by the tumour suppressor genes that inhibit growth and promote differentiation. Mutations of these genes are recessive to the wild type gene and their complete absence is required for tumourigenesis. The retinoblastoma susceptibility gene (*RB1*) and *p53* gene are prototypic of tumour suppressor genes.

The tumour suppressor gene *p53* is a 20-kb gene localized to 17p13 and encodes a 393-amino-acid protein that arrests the cell cycle at G1 in response to DNA damage. Cells with mutant *p53* do not arrest at G1 in response to DNA damage allowing the division of abnormal cells.

Inactivation of both *RB1* and *p53* is required for the initiation of an osteosarcoma. Nearly all synovial sarcomas exhibit a translocation at t(X;18)(p11.2;q11.2). This can be used to distinguish this tumour from other histologically similar sarcomas.[5] Genetic abnormalities have been identified in other sarcomas[6] (see Table 24.1).

Classification of head and neck sarcomas

Sarcomas of the head and neck can be divided into two principle categories, those tumours arising from soft tissue and those arising from bone. Tumours arising from the soft tissues of the head and neck comprise a heterogeneous group with varied histology, location and behaviour. Classification of sarcomas has traditionally been based on morphologic similarities between neoplastic cells and normal tissues. The tumour may not necessarily arise from the tissue type from which it derives its name. More recently, the techniques of electron microscopy, immunohistochemistry and cytogenctics have been

Table 24.1 Cytogenetic and molecular abnormalities in soft tissue sarcoma[5]

Histology	Cytogenetic abnormality	Molecular abnormality	Diagnostic utility
Chondrosarcoma	t(9;22)(q31;q12)	CHN-EWS fusion	Yes
Clear cell sarcoma	t(12;22)(q13;q12)	ATF1-EWS fusion	Yes
DFSP	Ring form of chromosome 17 and 22		Yes
Ewing's sarcoma	t(11;22)(q24;q12)	FL11 fusion	Yes
	t(21;22)(q12;q22)	ERG-EWS fusion	Yes
	t(7;22)(22;12)	ETV1-EWS fusion	Yes
Hemangiopericytoma	Translocation at 12q13		No
Leiomyosarcoma	Deletion of 1p		No
Liposarcoma			
Myxoid	t(12;16)(q13;p11)	CHOP-TLS fusion	Yes
Well differentiated	Ring chromosome 12		Yes
MFH	Complex		No
MPNST	Complex		No
Rhabdomyosarcoma			
Alveolar	t(2;13)(q35q14)	PAX3-FKHR fusion	Yes
	t(1;13)(p36;q14)	PAX3-FKHR fusion	Yes
Embryonal	+2q,+8,+20	Deletion 11p15	Yes
Synovial sarcoma	t(X;18)(p11;q11)	SSXT-SSX fusion	Yes

applied in the diagnosis and classification of these tumours. The techniques of molecular biology are also being used in the pathologic evaluation of sarcomas of the head and neck.

In many instances, electron microscopy can be useful in the diagnosis of soft tissue sarcoma. Specifically, it allows recognition of cellular details such as cross striations for rhabdomyosarcoma even in many poorly differentiated lesions. Immunohistochemistry allows the recognition of epithelial cells, muscle cells, Schwann cells, endothelial cells and others. This technique does have limitations. As neoplastic cells transform, they express epitopes that are not present on cells for which the tumour is named. Thus a rhabdomyosarcoma may at times express cytokeratin or S100. Despite its shortcomings, immunohistochemistry is extremely helpful in confirming the diagnosis of head and neck sarcomas. Specific chromosomal aberrations have been found in association with certain types of sarcoma. These features can be exploited for the diagnosis of certain sarcomas. Table 24.1 outlines the cytogenetic and molecular aberrations found in soft tissue sarcomas and their potential diagnostic utility.[5]

Staging of soft tissue sarcoma is outlined in Table 24.2. The rarity of lymph node involvement in sarcoma makes the NX designation less appropriate than in epithelial malignancy of the head and neck. The N0 designation is more appropriate for situations in which lymph node involvement is not clinically evident.

Table 24.2 Staging for soft tissue sarcoma (American Joint Committee on Cancer)

Primary tumour	
TX	Primary tumour cannot be assessed
T0	No evidence of primary tumour
T1	Tumour less than 5 cm in greatest dimension
T1a	Superficial tumour
T1b	Deep tumour
T2	Tumour more than 5 cm in greatest dimension
T2a	Superficial tumour
T2b	Deep tumour
Regional lymph nodes	
NX	Regional nodes cannot be assessed
N0	No regional lymph node metastases
N1	Regional lymph node metastases
Distant metastases	
MX	Distant metastases cannot be assessed
M0	No distant metastases
M1	Distant metastases

Sarcomas of striated muscle origin in children

Rhabdomyosarcoma (RMS) of the head and neck in adults is an uncommon entity. However, it is the most common soft tissue sarcoma in children under the age of 15. Thirty-four percent of all paediatric rhabdomyosarcomas occur in the head and neck.[7] These are divided by location into parameningeal (16%), orbital (9%) and non-orbital non-parameningeal (10%). The initial signs and symptoms vary according to the site and size of the lesion. These initial manifestations, such as aural discharge or nasal obstruction, may mimic other more common conditions of the head and neck in children leading to a delay in diagnosis.

Histologically, RMS appears similar to fetal skeletal muscle prior to innervation. The classification of RMS was adopted by the Intergroup Rhabdomyosarcoma Study (IRS) Committee and World Health Organization based on recommendations by Horn and Enterline.[7,8] This classification recognizes embryonal, botryoid, alveolar and pleomorphic subtypes. Sixty percent of RMS can be classified as embryonal and 20% alveolar. Electron microscopy has been particularly helpful in these tumours as the presence of sarcomeres with Z bands, actin, and myosin filaments are all diagnostic. The immunohistochemical profile of RMS includes positive reactions for desmin, myoglobin, MyoD1 and HHF-35. Embryonal RMS has variable amounts of primitive spindle or round cells in a myxoid background. These rhabdomyoblasts appear in a variety of unusual shapes termed ‘tadpole’ or ‘strap’ cells. Cross striations on light microscopy can be seen in half of these cells. The botryoid RMS is felt to be a variant of embryonal RMS and only accounts for 5% of cases. It is defined as a tumour having polypoid morphology with the presence of subepithelial aggregates of malignant cells, which is referred to as the cambium layer. Botryoid tumours have a particularly favourable prognosis.[9] A diagnosis of alveolar RMS is made if the tumour has alveolar-like spaces that are filled with round malignant, eosinophilic cells. Presence of any amount of alveolar morphology in the lesion qualifies it to be alveolar RMS. The presence of alveolar morphology has been identified as a poor prognosticator.[10] There is also a solid variant of this tumour that lacks alveolar spaces but is still included in this subtype. The presence of sheets of anaplastic cells warrants a diagnosis of pleomorphic RMS. Over the last 10–15 years, many of the lesions that would have been previously described as pleomorphic RMS are now being classified as malignant fibrous histiocytoma of the pleomorphic-storiform subtype,[11] decreasing the incidence of this variant of RMS.

Table 24.3 Clinical grouping used by the IRS

Group I	Localized disease, completely resected A. Confined to organ or muscle of origin B. Infiltration outside organ or muscle of origin; regional nodes not involved
Group II	Compromised or regional resection including A. Grossly resected tumours with microscopic residual tumour B. Regional disease, completely resected, nodes involved, tumour extension into adjacent organ or both C. Regional disease with involved nodes, grossly resected, but with evidence of microscopic residual tumour
Group III	Incomplete resection or biopsy with gross residual disease remaining
Group IV	Distant metastases at onset of disease

Staging of paediatric RMS is based on a modification of the TNM system that relies on pretreatment assessment of tumour extent. The Intergroup Rhabdomyosarcoma Study Committee grouping recognizes four major categories based upon amount of tumour remaining after initial surgery and degree of dissemination at the time of initial diagnosis (Table 24.3). With multimodality therapy, paediatric RMS has achieved a 70% 5-year rate of survival.

Sarcomas of striated muscle origin in adults

As previously mentioned, RMS is a rare condition in the adult patient. The primary site of origin in adults is the craniofacial skeleton with the majority occurring in the ethmoid sinuses. The median age at initial presentation is in the mid-twenties. The majority of lesions are in the IRS groups III or IV. Most patients with ethmoidal rhabdomyosarcoma have extension into the orbit or anterior cranial fossa as well as distant metastases, at presentation.[12] Prior irradiation is the most significant risk factor for the development of sarcomas in adults.[13] The histologic classification of adult RMS is identical to that of paediatric RMS: embryonal, botryoid, alveolar and pleomorphic. This condition is much more aggressive in adults than children and results in a higher overall mortality rate.[14] Survival in one study was 7.6% at 5 years.[12]

Sarcomas of fibrous tissue

Sarcomas of fibrous tissue are often referred to as fibrohistiocytic tumours. These lesions are composed of neoplastic spindle cells but also often harbour histiocytic cells containing phagocytosed material such as iron. These cells represent wandering monocytes that act as scavengers but do not contribute to the cellular population of fibrohistiocytic tumours. Tumours of fibrous tissue form a spectrum of malignant behaviour, from the benign fibrous histiocytoma (dermatofibroma), to dermatofibrosarcoma protuburans to the malignant fibrous histiocytoma.

The dermatofibroma is considered a benign tumour of fibrous tissue that usually presents as a subcutaneous nodule consisting of fibroblast-like spindle cells, histiocytes and blood vessels separated from a hyperplastic epidermis by a clear (Grenz) zone.[15] These tumours may rarely be associated with basal cell carcinoma.

Dermatofibrosarcoma protuburans (DFSP) is a rare tumour of the dermis that has a high recurrence rate and the potential to transform into other sarcomas. The DFSP is composed of densely packed spindle cells arranged in a storiform or cartwheel pattern. DFSP subtypes include the Bednar tumour, which has melanin-containing cells along with the standard spindle cells of this neoplasm. At the periphery of the DFSP, there is diffuse infiltration of the dermal stroma extending to the subcutaneous tissue, resulting in a honeycomb pattern. The peripheral aspects of the lesion have a very bland appearance that melds into the normal dermis imperceptibly. This creates difficulties in determining adequacy of excision with resulting recurrence after presumed adequate resection (see Figures 24.1–24.4). Recurrence rates of up to 40% have been reported even with 2-cm margins and 20% with 3-cm margins.[16,17] Resection margins are the primary determinant of recurrence, with most recommendations being for 3-cm margins.

Malignant fibrous histiocytoma (MFH) is the most common soft tissue sarcoma of middle and late adulthood. Most of these sarcomas occur in striated

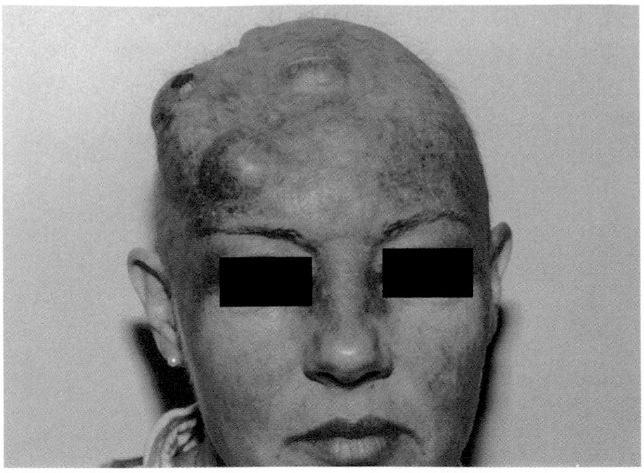

Figure 24.1 Young woman with a recurrent scalp dermatofibrosarcoma protuburans following preoperative irradiation.

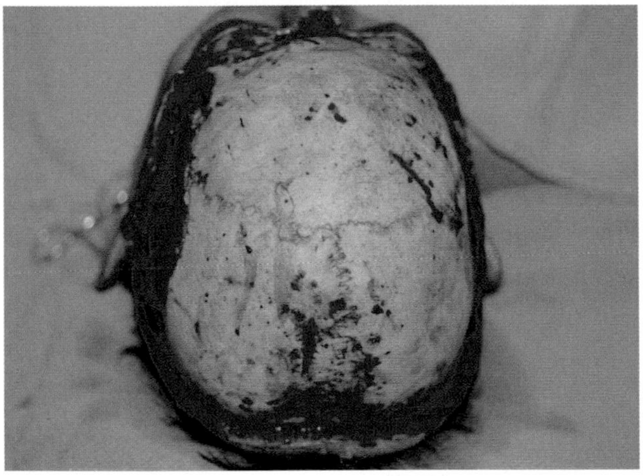

Figure 24.2 Wide excision of scalp dermatofibrosarcoma protuburans.

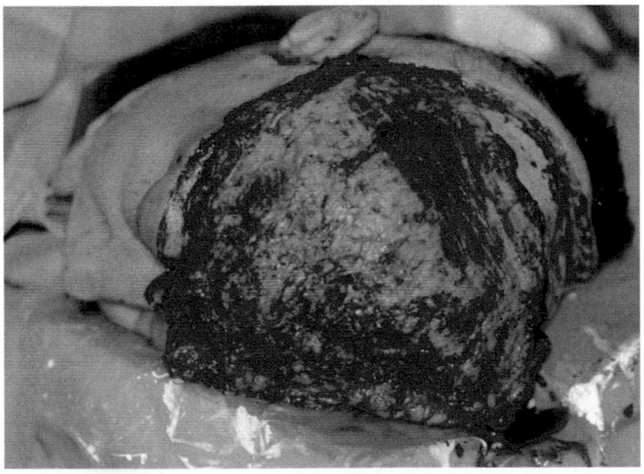

Figure 24.3 Reconstruction of near total scalp defect with bilateral latissimus dorsi muscle only free tissue transfers which will be resurfaced with split thickness skin grafts.

(a)

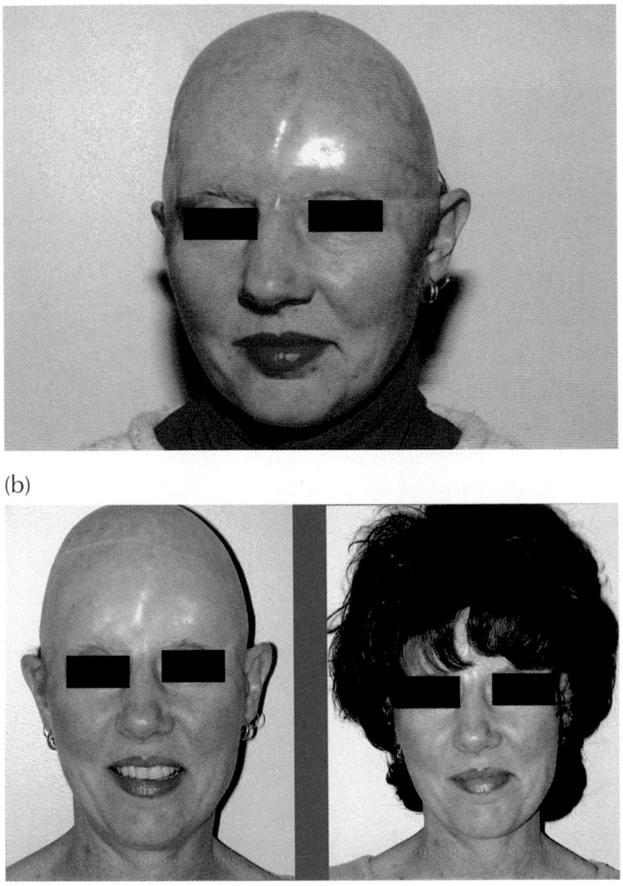

(b)

Figure 24.4 (a) Postoperative result 3 months later. (b) 2 years postoperatively without/with camouflage.

muscle with less than 10% being restricted to the subcutaneous tissues. The diagnosis of fibrosarcoma has largely been supplanted by MFH. The term fibrosarcoma is restricted to a small number of tumours having a herring-bone pattern of interwoven fascicles on histologic examination. Cells other then fibroblasts may take on a histiocyte-like appearance such as smooth muscle, striated muscle and Schwann cells. Thus, poorly differentiated sarcomas of many different cell origins may take on the appearance of MFH. Like the fibrosarcoma, the diagnosis of pleomorphic rhabdomyosarcoma has become a rarity with most of these neoplasms now being diagnosed as pleomorphic-storiform MFH. The pleomorphic-storiform subtype is the most common form of MFH. Other subtypes include giant cell, angiomatoid, myxoid, and inflammatory. The giant cell MFH contains histiocytic giant cells and used to be known as giant cell tumour of soft parts but is now classified as a subtype of MFH. The majority of MFH are found in deep tissues but the angiomatoid variety is found in the subcutaneous tissues of patients in the first or second decade of life. This subtype of MFH consists of uniform histiocytic cells with blood-filled pseudocysts that are not lined by endothelial cells. Fat-containing histiocytes in association with inflammatory cells are the hallmark of the inflammatory subtype of MFH. Metastasis of MFH is related to size, depth and grade. A local recurrence rate of 25%, metastatic rate of 34% and survival of 50% is reported with MFH treated surgically.[15]

Sarcomas of vascular tissue

Angiosarcoma

Angiosarcomas are tumours of vascular tissue that can arise in any area of the body but most frequently occur in the head and neck. These neoplasms commonly present as purple lesions on the skin of the head and neck in elderly men. The estimated male preponderance is 3:1. Half of these lesions occur on the scalp, and many of the remainder, on the upper face. Many of the lesions of the scalp are multifocal.[18] The bruise-like, macular appearance of these lesions often delays intervention due to misdiagnosis. The cause of angiosarcoma is not known, although it has been associated in other sites with chronic lymphoedema, previous irradiation, and environmental toxins such as Thorotrast and vinyl chloride.[19] The pathologic features of this tumour are diverse. This lesion consists of areas of vascular channels, sheets of cells and cells of undifferentiated morphology. Most tumours contain one of these three patterns, however, some lesions may consist of all three. Vascular anastamosing channels are lined by atypical cells, several cell layers thick. Highly cellular tumours appear solid as the vascular channels are effaced by the crowding of cells. Low-grade tumours are more likely to show recognizable areas of vascular channels, where high-grade tumours show disordered architecture, haemorrhage, and large pleomorphic cells with frequent mitoses. Immunohistochemistry can aid in the diagnosis. Factor VIII-related antigen is positive in tumours of vascular differentiation. UEA 1 (*Ulex europaeus 1*) is another marker which may have increased sensitivity.[18] Cutaneous epithelioid angiosarcoma is a variant of angiosarcoma that can be confused with carcinoma and requires electron microscopy for diagnosis. Angiosarcoma is treated with wide local excision and postoperative radiotherapy. Despite aggressive treatment, this disease is marked by a tendency for local recurrence, multifocality and poor survival. Lateral extension through the dermis makes assessment of surgical margins difficult. Size appears to be the most important prognostic factor as lesions smaller than 7 cm in size may do well, while lesions greater than 10 cm in size have a uniformly poor prognosis.[20] Neck metastases are found in 10–15% of patients.[20] Elective neck dissection is not recommended except in large tumours greater than 7 cm. Distant metastases are common with rates up to 63% at 5 years being reported.[21] Overall disease-free survival at 3 years is 13–33%.[19–21]

Hemangiopericytoma

The most common sites of hemangiopericytoma are the lower extremities and pelvis. The head and neck is the third most common site. The neck, perioral soft tissues (see Figures 24.5–24.9), and sinonasal tract are the sites of occurrence in the head and neck. Presenting symptoms include a painless mass in the neck or soft tissues of the face. Sinonasal hemangiopericytoma presents with nasal obstruction and epistaxis and appears as a grey polypoid mass that bleeds briskly on manipulation. Hemangiopericytoma is a tumour of blood vessels, which is felt to arise from Zimmerman's pericyte. These lesions consist of wide open blood vessels lined by normal endothelial cells. Tightly packed tumour cells occupy the space between these vessels. The vessels form a 'staghorn pattern' and contain perivascular hyalinization termed the grenz zone. The immunohistochemical profile includes positivity for vimentin and factor XIIIa. Wide local excision is the treatment of choice with some authorities advocating preoperative embolization. Although this is a low-grade malignancy, metastases have been reported in 3% of cases with a 3.3% incidence of death. Metastases are to locoregional lymph nodes. This tumour lacks encapsulation and has infiltrating margins, which may account for the high rate of recurrence, reported to be as high as 18–50%.[22–24]

Kaposi's sarcoma

Kaposi's sarcoma (KS) is the most frequent malignant lesion in patients infected with HIV. As many as 95% of all patients with AIDS have KS in the cutaneous or visceral forms. In the United States, KS is 10 times more common in homosexual men with HIV than in other subgroups with HIV and is in fact the most common initial complication of HIV infection in homosexual men. This is a multifocal, systemic disease which often involves the skin and mucosal surfaces. Lesions of the hard palate are the most common intraoral manifestation. Visceral involvement is not rare. Lesions may vary in appearance from red to violaceous nodules, macules or plaques. Cutaneous lesions are divided into patch, plaque or nodular stages.[25] Severity of KS has been graded as 1: limited cutaneous; 2: disseminated cutaneous; and 3: cutaneous and visceral.[26] KS consists of spindle-shaped cells associated with endothelial cells, fibroblasts, inflammatory cells, and the formation of new blood vessels. Treatment must be individualized for

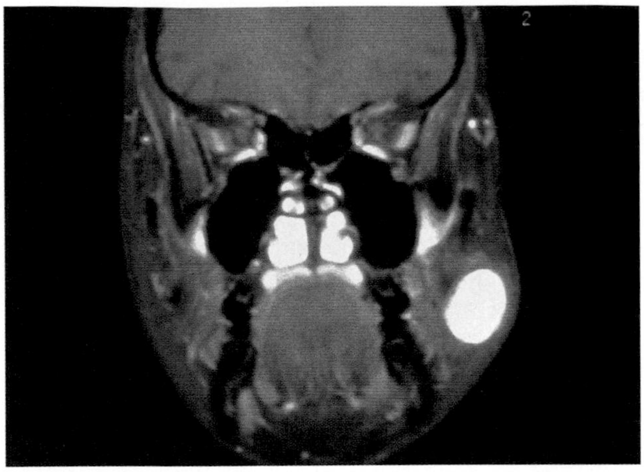

Figure 24.5 Enhanced coronal MRI scan showing a haemangiopericytoma lateral to the masseter muscle.

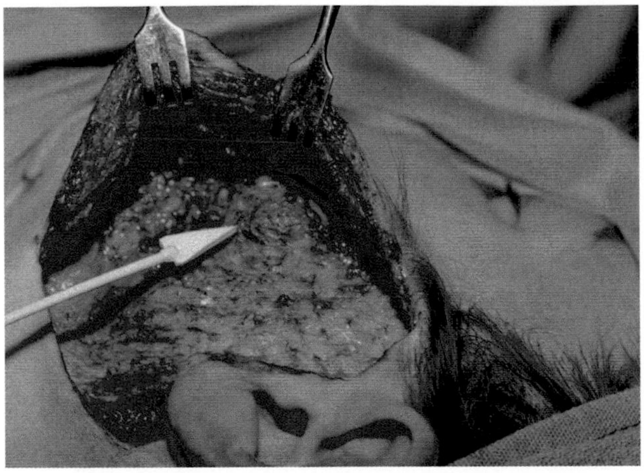

Figure 24.6 Exposure of haemangiopericytoma anterior to the parotid gland (pointer) by using a modified Blair incision and raising a SMAS layer flap.

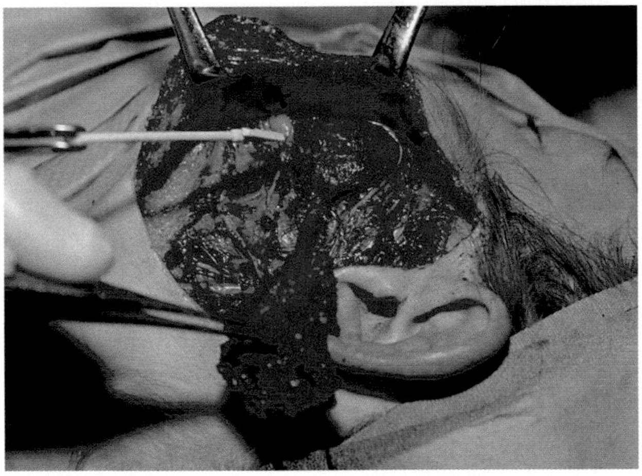

Figure 24.7 Superficial parotidectomy performed in order to identify the facial nerve prior to tumour (pointer) removal.

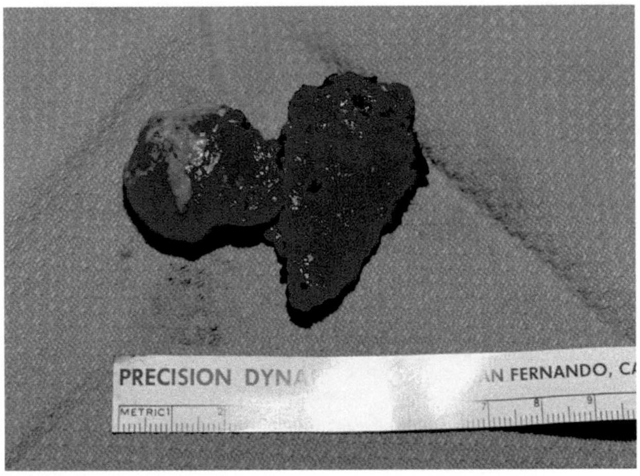

Figure 24.8 Pathology specimen showing superficial lobe of parotid and attached haemangiopericytoma.

(a) (b)

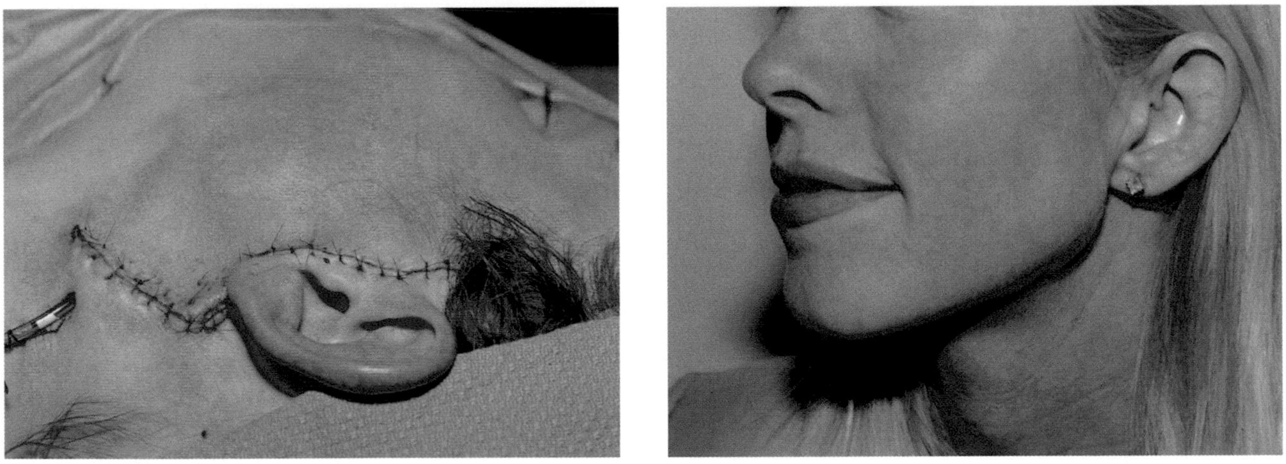

Figure 24.9 (a) Immediate postoperative appearance after closure of incision. (b) Final postoperative appearance.

patients with KS. Local disease can often be treated with observation or cosmetic make up. Surgical excision, liquid nitrogen cryotherapy, intralesional chemotherapy have all been used for local disease. Radiation therapy for early cutaneous or oral KS is beneficial. Systemic chemotherapy is often limited by intolerance to drugs but may be required in rapidly progressive disease, symptomatic visceral disease or pulmonary KS. Interferon alpha has also shown promise in this setting.[25,27]

Sarcomas of adipose tissue

The head and neck is a rare site for liposarcoma, comprising 4% of all liposarcomas. In this site, the neck is the single-most common location, although 38% involve the larynx/pharynx. The supraglottis is the most common subsite in the larynx. Liposarcomas are comprosed of cells termed lipoblasts in which the cytoplasm contains one or more fat vacoules deforming the nucleus. There are four types of liposarcoma described. The well-differentiated liposarcoma is a neoplasm of borderline malignancy, which is usually easy to remove. Myxoid liposarcomas contain an abundant mucinous stroma with a network of capillaries. This subtype is also of low-grade and rarely metastasizes. Round cell and pleomorphic subtypes have a high rate of metastases, in the range of 80%.[11] Histologic grade appears to have the most bearing on prognosis. Treatment with surgical excision offers the best control rate. Radiation has not been well studied in this condition. Overall survival is 67% at 5 years.[28]

Sarcomas of smooth muscle

Leiomyosarcoma of the head and neck is a rare lesion. These tumours range from well-differentiated lesions mimicking normal smooth muscle to highly malignant sarcomas, the diagnosis of which depends mainly upon immunohistochemistry and electron microscopy. Leiomyosarcomas may occur in superficial or deep parts of the body. Smooth muscle is sparse in the head and neck and is found mainly in the walls of blood vessels and the erector pili musculature of the skin. The lesion is usually circumscribed and made up of elongated cells growing in interlacing cords. Most commonly, the tumour is a discrete, painless, subcutaneous or submucosal mass. There does not appear to be a characteristic location for these sarcomas in the head and neck. Surgery followed by radiotherapy appears to offer the most reasonable chance of control of these tumours.[29–31]

Sarcomas of synovial differentiation

Synovial sarcomas tend to occur in young patients between the second to fifth decades of life. They arise in relation to the prevertebral areas from the skull base to the hypopharynx, with most of them involving the parapharyngeal space. The presentation is usually that of a painless, slowly enlarging neck mass.[32] Radiology reveals calcification in up to one-third of cases with very high signal intensity on T2 MRI. Synovial sarcomas are tumours of pluripotential mesenchymal cells and not of synovial tissue as the name would imply. Synovial tissue is a modified connective tissue formed from mesenchyme that differentiates into an epithelioid cell layer and an outer connective tissue layer. There is little resemblance between synovial membranes and synovial sarcoma. Synovial sarcoma exists in a biphasic and uniphasic form. The classic biphasic form has a dual differentiation of epithelial nests in glandular configuration in a fibrosarcoma-like matrix of spindle cells arranged in fascicles. The uniphasic form contains only the sarcomatous elements or very rarely, the epithelial elements of this tumour. Dystrophic calcification and calcospherites may be prominent. Synovial sarcoma is relatively unique in its expression of epithelial cytokeratin antigens 7, 18 and 19 and epithelial membrane antigen. This can be helpful in confirming the light microscopic impression.[33] Despite its slow growth, the 5-year survival is 55% and 38% at 10 years. The late drop off is due to delayed distant metastases, usually to the lungs.[32] Wide local excision remains the mainstay of therapy. Lymphatogenous metastases are uncommon, but distant spread by the hematogenous route does occur and is the harbinger of death.[32]

Sarcomas of cartilage

The most common sites of head and neck involvement by chondrosarcoma include larynx, maxilla and skull base.[34] Chondrosarcomas are slow growing, locally aggressive tumours with a propensity for local recurrence. They arise from bone or superimposed upon benign cartilaginous tumours. Most occur in the age range from 30–60. Predisposing conditions include multiple hereditary exostoses, Ollier's disease and Maffucci's syndrome.[35] This is the most frequent mesenchymal neoplasm of the larynx. The most common site of origin in the larynx is the posterior lamina of the cricoid (75%). Hoarseness, dysphagia and dyspnoea are the presenting symptoms. Vocal cord paralysis is frequently found in association with cricoid chondrosarcoma due to involvement of the recurrent laryngeal nerve or cricoarytenoid joint. Examination usually reveals a mass covered by intact mucosa. Radiologic evaluation reveals a lobulated lesion, which has high signal on T2 MRI and a cartilaginous cap. CT may be more sensitive in demonstrating fine calcifications associated with chondrosarcomas. Tumours can be divided into low, medium or high grade. Abundant basophilic cartilaginous matrices make up the stroma of the neoplasm with the cellular component composed of binucleate or multinucleate cells. The high-grade tumours show more pronounced cellularity, increased mitoses and higher nuclear-cytoplasmic ratio. A variant called dedifferentiated chondrosarcoma contains a spindle cell component in association with the cartilaginous component of the neoplasm. This variant has a worse prognosis than the usual histologic type. Immunohistochemical studies are positive for vimentin and S-100. Surgical excision with a wide margin including the external perichondrium is the treatment of choice, with radiation reserved for recurrence and for high-grade lesions. Partial excision of the cricoid cartilage requires reconstruction with vascularized or non-vascularized tissue in order to maintain airway patency. Despite attempts at laryngeal preservation, 34% of patients eventually come to laryngectomy. Metastases are reported in only 8.5% of cases.[36] The majority of reported instances of metastases have been haematogenous, especially to the lung. Overall survival for laryngeal chondrosarcoma is in the 80% range.[37] Survival for patients with chondrosarcoma in other head and neck sites may not be as high. Lesions of the skull base have a higher rate of recurrence due to the difficulties in obtaining wide resection margins. Although chondrosarcoma is felt by some to be a radioresistant tumour, proton beam therapy has been shown to be helpful for disease at the skull base.[38,39]

Ewing's sarcoma and peripheral primitive neuroectodermal tumour

Ewing's sarcoma (ES) and primitive neuroectodermal tumours (PNET) probably share a common histogenesis and form opposite ends of a spectrum of tumours. The most compelling evidence for the linking of Ewing's sarcoma and PNET is the cytogenetic features shared by the two. Ninety percent of the tumours analysed have the t(11,22)(q24;q11.2–12) translocation. This results in the formation of chimeric genes which have the properties of transcriptional regulators. The ES-PNET group of tumours includes osseous and non-osseous ES, malignant PNET, pigmented neuroectodermal tumour, ectomesenchymoma and the Askin's tumour which is a PNET of the thoracopulmonary region. Ewing's sarcoma comprises 4–7% of all primary bone tumours. Only 3% of these arise in the craniofacial skeleton. The mandible has a 2:1 ratio over the maxilla. There is no sex preponderance. Swelling and pain of the jaw is the most common presentation. Radiology reveals an osteolytic lesion with sun-ray spicules of periosteal bone. It may also appear as a permeative lesion with an aggressive onion-skin type of periosteal reaction. Pathologic features of this small, blue, round cell tumour include nuclei with smooth contour and small nuclei with electron-lucent zones in the cytoplasm, which are lakes of glycogen. The ES-PNET group of tumours is positive for the p30–32 antigen, which is the glycoprotein product of the MIC-2 gene. Location of ES is the most important prognosticator, with gnathic bone having a low rate of mortality. With multimodality therapy including surgery, radiation and multiagent chemotherapy, survival rates have improved from 16% to 54–74%.[40–42] Extraosseous ES occurs in the head and neck in 15% of cases. These are usually involved with large nerves. Like osseous ES, this should be considered a systemic disease at outset and requires treatment with multimodality therapy. The overall 5-year survival is 48% in the Mayo clinic series.[43] It is possible that up to one half of cases previously diagnosed as ES are actually PNETs. Peripheral PNETs peak in adolescence. These are aggressive neoplasms with systemic metastases noted in 30% at presentation.[40] The prognosis for these tumours is poor despite aggressive treatment.

Sarcomas of peripheral nerve sheath origin

Malignant peripheral nerve sheath tumours (MPNST) are extremely rare lesions in the general population but occur in patients with neurofibromatosis type 1 with a reported incidence of 2–29%. Patients with NF-1 account for half of the cases with MPNST. These tumours tend to recur locally and spread haematogenously. These lesions infiltrate the fascicles of the parent nerve freely. Histologically, they are made up of tightly packed fascicles woven into a herring-bone pattern, resembling fibrosarcoma.[44] Most of these tumours are highly cellular and mitotically active. Criteria for diagnosis include tumour origin from a nerve or association with contiguous neurofibroma. Treatment with wide surgical margins followed by radiation is advocated as MPNST is the sarcoma with the highest local recurrence rate of all sarcomas. Adjuvant chemotherapy has not been shown to alter survival in this disease. MPNST associated with NF-1 may carry a worse prognosis, but reported series are not consistent in this respect.[45] This tumour portends a poor prognosis especially when the size exceeds 5 cm.[45]

Sarcomas of osseous origin

Osteogenic sarcoma is a rare, highly malignant tumour that occurs with an incidence of 1 per 100 000. Seven percent of these can occur in the head and neck. The majority of these occur in the mandible, usually involving the body or symphisis (see Figures 24.10–24.15). The alveolar ridge is the most common site in the maxilla. Head and neck osteosarcoma occurs in the third and fourth decades of life, where long bone osteosarcoma predominates in the teenage years. Painless swelling is the most frequent presentation of head and neck osteosarcoma, where pain is usually the primary symptom in long bone osteosarcoma. Patients with involvement

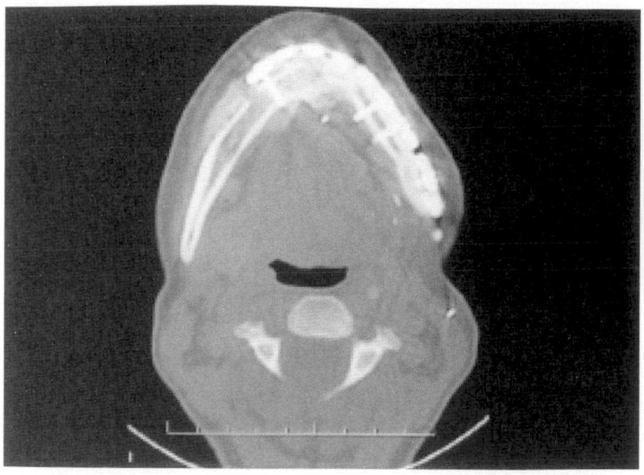

Figure 24.10 CT scan of a young woman with previously resected osteosarcoma mandible reconstructed with free fibula and plate, now presenting with recurrent osteosarcoma of right mandibular parasymphisis and body.

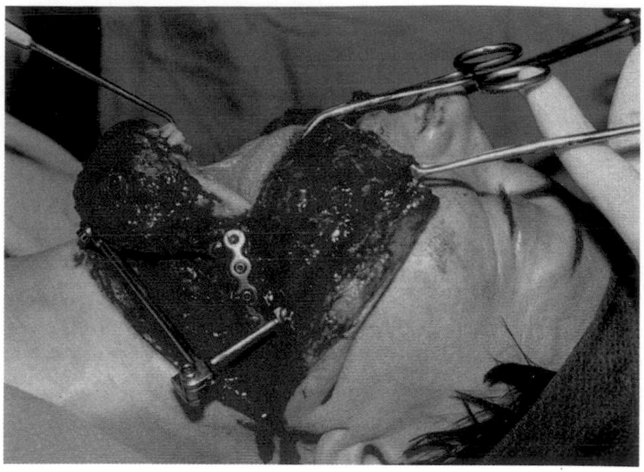

Figure 24.11 Intraoperative photograph showing tumour resection (towel clip on tongue, external fixator device in situ) with old plate transected.

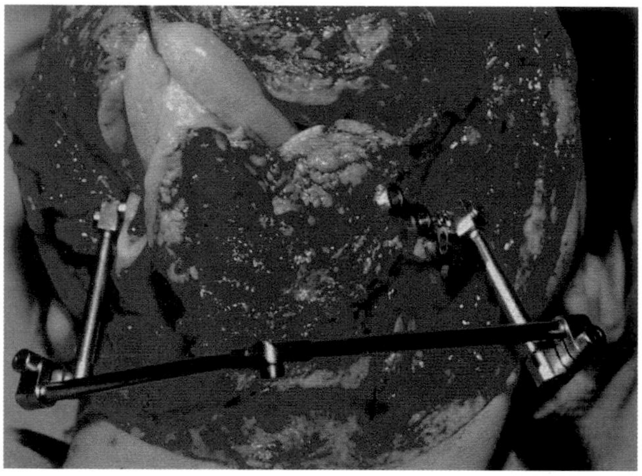

Figure 24.12 Intraoperative photograph of subsequent defect with external fixator in place.

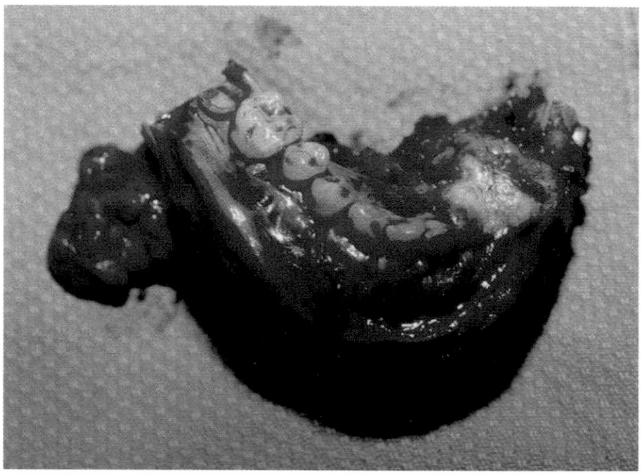

Figure 24.13 Pathology specimen of mandibular osteosarcoma.

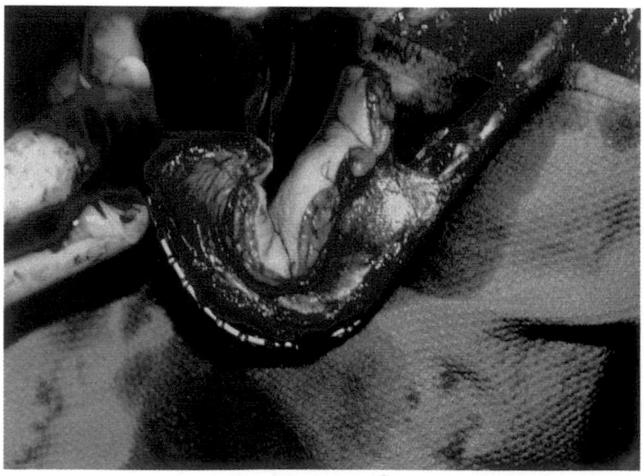

Figure 24.14 Free fibula osteocutaneous flap being contoured to a new reconstruction plate while still attached to the leg.

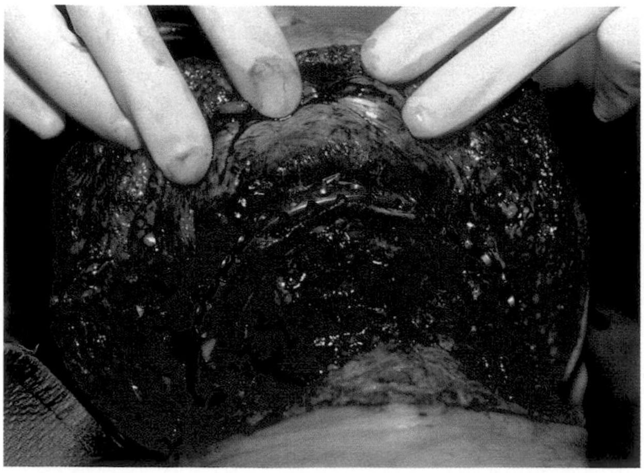

Figure 24.15 Free fibula osteocutaneous free flap inset into defect.

of the jaw are often first seen by the dentist for loosening of teeth. The major risk factors for development of osteosarcoma include prior irradiation and Paget's disease with the skull being the favoured site for the development of Paget's disease-associated osteosarcoma.[46,47] The most common radiologic appearance is that of an osteolytic lesion. Alkaline phosphatase levels are often raised, and can be very helpful in the posttreatment setting for the detection of residual or recurrent disease. To be classified as an osteosarcoma, the tumour must consist of malignant stromal cells with the production of osteoid substance. Conventional osteosarcomas make up 90% of all tumours and are divided into osteoblastic, chondroblastic and fibroblastic depending upon the predominant histologic pattern. Other subtypes include periosteal, paraosteal, low-grade central, high-grade peripheral, small cell and telengiectatic. Fibroblastic and paraosteal subtypes appear to have a more favourable prognosis. Although surgical therapy remains the mainstay of treatment, adjuvant chemotherapy has had a major impact on attaining metastases-free survival in long bone osteosarcoma. Chemotherapy usually consists of cisplatin/adriamycin/dacarbazine regimens with cisplatin being delivered intra-arterially by some centres. In long bone osteosarcoma, this also has increased rates of limb salvage. It is recognized that there is an 80–90% rate of micrometastases at presentation in long bone osteosarcoma. Thus, chemotherapy is required not only to control the local problem, but also to eradicate systemic disease. The combined approach of surgery and chemotherapy has increased cure rates from 20% to rates of 65–75%.[47] It appears likely that head and neck osteosarcoma is quite similar to long bone osteosarcoma in behaviour. Radiotherapy is more likely to be applied in head and neck osteosarcoma especially in cases where wide surgical margins cannot be obtained.[46] Osteosarcoma is relatively radioresistant, with doses of 6000 cGy required for effectiveness. Otherwise, head and neck osteosarcoma is treated in a similar manner to long bone osteosarcoma with combined surgery and chemotherapy.

Radiation-induced sarcoma

Radiation therapy is an important modality in the treatment of cancer patients. However, the long-term risks of radiotherapy do include the risk of sarcomagenesis. This risk is only in the order of 0.03–0.8% on long-term follow-up. The criteria for radiation-induced sarcoma first described by Cahan et al[48] include prior history of irradiation, latency period of several years, development of sarcoma in the irradiated field and the histologic confirmation of sarcoma. Minimum doses of 1000 cGy appear to be necessary for the induction of sarcoma. The latency period for the development of sarcoma after radiotherapy may range up to 50 years with a median of 14 years.[49] Radiation-induced sarcomas include a wide range of histology. Malignant fibrous histiocytoma and angiosarcoma are amongst the most common sarcomas induced by radiotherapy.[50,51] The overall prognosis for radiation-induced sarcoma is poor with most series reporting 5-year survival rates of 10–30%.[48]

Diagnostic approach to head and neck sarcomas

The evaluation of the patient with head and neck sarcoma must include biopsy and imaging of the primary with investigation for systemic metastases. This includes a CT chest, CT abdomen and also a bone marrow biopsy in the case of rhabdomyosarcoma.

Radiologic evaluation of head and neck sarcomas

Modern treatment of head and neck sarcomas emphasizes a multidisciplinary, multimodality approach to this disease. This requires accurate, highly sophisticated imaging in order to delineate tumour extent for surgical and radiotherapeutic planning. Plain radiography remains a useful means of establishing an appropriate differential diagnosis for primary bone tumours but is of less value in the diagnosis of soft tissue sarcomas. In fact, no other modality has been more specific for the prospective diagnosis of primary bone tumours than plain radiography. Radiographic features to be evaluated include location, pattern of destruction, tumour matrix, margins, periosteal reaction and adjacent soft tissue mass. Benign tumours are characterized by homogeneous appearance with a well-defined smooth or sclerotic transition from lesion to normal bone. There is little periosteal reaction and no associated soft tissue mass. Malignant lesions often are marked by permeative bone destruction, ill-defined transition to normal bone, aggressive periosteal reaction and an accompanying soft tissue mass.[52]

Computerized tomography continues to play an important role in evaluation of sarcomas. Particularly important is the ability of CT to accurately delineate bony anatomy surrounding the tumour. This is crucial in preoperative planning for ablation and reconstruction. CT is also important in assisting in differential diagnosis, as MRI is insensitive to certain features such as calcification. Unfortunately, only axial images can be obtained directly by CT with sagittal and coronal reformatted images losing fine detail.

The multiplanar imaging and soft tissue detail rendered by MRI makes this modality ideal for staging and treatment planning of sarcomas of the head and neck. Although MRI is highly accurate in delineating the extent of a soft tissue or bony abnormality, it continues to be non-specific. The majority of soft tissue sarcomas will appear as low signal intensity on T1-weighted images and high on T2. These features are non-specific and require a biopsy for diagnosis.

Contrast enhancement for CT or MRI reflects blood flow, vascular permeability and the size of the extracellular fluid compartment. These features make contrast enhancement relatively non-specific. However, it can be helpful in delineating tumour extent.[53]

Nuclear medicine imaging varies fundamentally from conventional imaging techniques, as it examines function in an anatomic context as opposed to anatomy. Thallium-201 chloride has a significant affinity for bone and soft tissue sarcomas and reflects viable tumour activity. Agents such as this can be used to follow tumour response to radiation or chemotherapy, as well as monitor for the presence of residual or recurrent disease. Thallium-201 has also been proposed as an alternative to F18 FDG glucose to distinguish radiation necrosis from tumour recurrence. Other agents such as technetium MIBI, FDG PET and SPECT scanning have also been used for these purposes.[54]

Role of biopsy in head and neck sarcoma

Open biopsy remains the gold standard in the diagnosis of bone and soft tissue sarcomas. The biopsy should be carefully designed in order to facilitate subsequent surgical removal and adjuvant therapy. In the ideal circumstance, the surgeon performing the biopsy should also be the one performing the definitive surgical procedure in the context of a multidisciplinary setting. Unplanned excisional biopsy without the benefit of preoperative imaging and regard for margins has been shown to increase the rate of local recurrence in sarcomas of the extremities.[55] The biopsy should be accomplished through the smallest incision possible with absolute haemostasis. Tumour cells are capable of spreading along tissue planes along with any extravasated blood. Postbiopsy haematomas may be responsible for tumour spread and implantation in this manner. The advancing border of the tumour is the area most likely to be the least differentiated and may prohibit correct subclassification. Open surgical biopsy provides sufficient tissue for traditional histologic analysis as well as providing tissue for flow cytometry, immunohistochemistry, electron microscopy, molecular genetics and cytogenetics.

Aspiration needle biopsy can be a useful technique but these tumours are rare, complex and difficult to diagnose even in experienced hands. Despite this, there is a growing experience in diagnosis of sarcomas with core-needle biopsy or fine-needle aspiration biopsy. Certain European centres use these techniques preferentially for diagnosis.[56,57]

Treatment issues in head and neck sarcomas

Over the past two decades, numerous advances have been made in the treatment of sarcomas. Many of these advances have come from refinements in the treatment of extremity and trunk sarcomas. A collaborative approach between ablative surgeons, reconstructive surgeons, radiation oncologists, medical oncologists and pathologists has been essential in improving treatment results.

Soft tissue sarcomas

Excision

The approach to soft tissue sarcomas in the extremities and trunk was initially that of marginal excision. This resulted in an unacceptable failure rate with local recurrences in the 80–90% range. Attempts to reduce this rate led to more radical resections in the 1960s. This did reduce local disease recurrence but only at the expense of increased morbidity. A National Cancer Institute study in 1982 evaluated limb-sparing surgery with postoperative radiation versus amputation for high-grade extremity sarcomas. This randomized prospective study showed a 75% 10-year survival in both groups.[58] The combination of radiotherapy with limb-sparing conservative surgery produces survival rates equivalent to more mutilating surgery for extremity soft tissue sarcoma.[59,60] The use of radiation at moderate doses is felt to inactivate the microscopic extensions of tumour beyond the capsule of the grossly evident tumour.

Radiotherapy

The sequencing of radiation remains an unresolved issue. Preoperative radiotherapy allows for the use of smaller fields. This may become particularly important in the head and neck where vital structures such as the optic chiasm or spinal cord may be in close proximity to the tumour mass. Other advantages of preoperative radiotherapy include the ability to plan radiotherapy based on imaging of the original tumour, an oxygen-rich environment and the ability to assess the situation in a multidisciplinary environment prior to definitive management.

Both of the groups at Massachusetts General Hospital and Princess Margaret Hospital have shown that preoperative radiotherapy at doses of 50 Gy provides excellent control without the need for postoperative radiotherapy as long as the surgical margins are clear.[61,62] Preoperative radiotherapy does have the disadvantage of delaying surgery and increasing wound complications.[63] A 30% wound complication rate has been reported in extremity sarcomas with a preoperative radiation schedule.[64] Postoperative radiotherapy does allow for accurate pathologic verification of the status of surgical margins. This may alter the way in which radiotherapy is applied. However, postoperative radiotherapy may delay the initiation of treatment if surgery results in impaired wound healing. This may be particularly worrisome as the postoperative wound is known to harbour microscopic disease. Currently, the results of a phase III study of preoperative external beam radiotherapy compared to postoperative therapy funded by the National Cancer Institute of Canada (SR2) is being completed and will probably be able to answer these questions. Treatment of small, low-grade tumours in locations where wide margins are possible may consist of surgery alone. This is particularly true of lesions that can be excised with a minimum of 2 cm of normal tissue in all planes. Lesions presenting superficial to fascia can generally be managed by surgery alone. In the head and neck, wide excision may be difficult to carry out due to anatomic constraints. This makes the role of radiotherapy even more important in order to achieve local control.[65] Radiotherapy is also required for the patient that presents from the referring centre having undergone prior excisional biopsy or other inadequate surgery.

Brachytherapy

Brachytherapy has several advantages over external beam radiotherapy including reduced scatter to normal tissues, lesser delay between surgery and radiation therapy and a much shorter time required to deliver a tumouricidal dose. For the delivery of brachytherapy, afterloading catheters are placed in the tissue bed 1 cm apart, to cover the tumour bed and an additional 2 cm around the margins. Five days after the surgery, the catheters are loaded with iridium-192 wires and a total dose of 4500 cGy is delivered in 5 days. A 5-day delay is required to minimize wound complications. The catheters are removed after treatment and the patient is discharged. Brennan et al[66] examined the efficacy of brachytherapy in extremity soft tissue sarcoma and reported the results in 1992. This study showed a statistically significant improvement in local control rates for surgery with brachytherapy versus surgery alone. However, there was no difference in overall survival. Local control was 90% with brachytherapy versus 69% for no brachytherapy in high-grade tumours. Another approach is to use adjuvant external beam radiotherapy with brachytherapy as a boost. This technique may be especially helpful in the case of positive surgical margins.[66] Brachytherapy is technically more complex with most institutions not being able to deliver this form of radiotherapy to complex lesions. Most recently, Yang et al[67] have shown similar results to Brennan's with the use of external beam radiotherapy in a randomized controlled trial of patients with extremity sarcoma.

Chemotherapy

Neoadjuvant chemotherapy has gained popularity in the treatment of osteogenic sarcomas as a powerful prognosticator of survival. In extremity osteosarcoma, chemotherapy has also allowed less radical resections in order to preserve limb function. Although early studies were encouraging, subsequent randomized prospective trials have failed to show a benefit to adjuvant chemotherapy in adult soft tissue sarcomas. The largest study of this subject showed no increase in overall survival but did increase the disease-free survival exclusively due to decreases in local relapse rates.[68] The use of adjuvant chemotherapy in Ewing's sarcoma, osteosarcoma and rhabdomyosarcoma is accepted but its benefits in adult soft tissue sarcoma have not been clearly established.[69,70]

Paediatric sarcoma

The modern treatment of paediatric rhabdomyosarcoma has improved survival rates from 30% to 70%. The demonstration of activity of vincristine, actinomycin D and cyclophosphamide against rhabdomyosarcoma led to pioneering studies of chemotherapy combined with surgery and radiation. The IRS committee has completed three national studies to answer major therapeutic questions in this disease. In patients with completely resected tumours it was shown that irradiation can be omitted from treatment protocols and that VA chemotherapy was as effective as VAC. Non-alveolar residual microscopic disease (group II) can be controlled in 90% of patients with irradiation and cyclic-sequential VA chemotherapy. Patients with gross residual disease have been treated with irradiation and chemotherapy with VAC yields a 52% survival. There has not been significant improvement of outcomes for patients with gross residual disease with the use of more aggressive protocols. Metastatic disease has not been shown to be better controlled with more aggressive chemotherapeutic regimens than VAC. The overall survival remains at 20%. The dire prognosis of patients with alveolar histology has been largely abolished due to the use of aggressive chemotherapeutic regimens. Specifically, VAC with doxorubicin and cisplatin results in 80% 5-year survival.[11]

Sarcomas of osseous origin

As previously stated, adjuvant chemotherapy has an established role in the treatment of osteosarcomas of the extremities and trunk. Prior to the use of chemotherapy, the survival of patients with single bone osteosarcoma was 20%. Pulmonary micrometastases were probably present in 80% of cases. These would appear as metastases subsequent to local treatment, leading to the patient's demise within 9 months of the appearance of pulmonary metastases. Subsequently, chemotherapeutic agents were found to be active in this disease, which was at one time felt to be chemoresistant. Methotrexate, cisplatin, adriamycin, and later ifosfamide and cyclophosphamide were all found to be efficacious. There have been two randomized trials of extremity osteosarcoma that have shown a significant increase in disease-free survival. An assessment of the role of chemotherapy in 114 patients showed a 2-year disease-free survival in 56% treated with surgery and chemotherapy and only 18% in the surgery alone arm. Eilber et al[71] showed similar findings in a subsequent study. Thus, craniofacial osteosarcoma is treated with surgery and radiation postoperatively with chemotherapy for adjuvant treatment of micrometastases.

Salvage for recurrent disease

Salvage treatment for recurrent disease in the extremities may mean amputation. However, attempts have been made to preserve limb function by the use of wide local excision and radiotherapy, either in the form of brachytherapy[72] or external beam irradiation.[73] The groups from Booth Memorial Medical Centre and Memorial Sloan-Kettering report a 5-year local control of 68%.[72] In the head and neck, further surgery for local recurrence may be even more problematic due to the anatomic proximity of major neurovascular structures. Recurrence after treatment of soft tissue sarcoma may often occur in the form of a single focus. In a study of 307 patients treated at the National Cancer Institute, isolated pulmonary metastatic disease was the most common pattern of initial recurrence (52%), followed by isolated local recurrence (20%). In this series, 45% of patients remained disease free after surgical treatment of the first recurrence.[74] As sarcomas commonly metastasize to lung, the issue of pulmonary metastasectomy is an important one in head and neck sarcomas. Pulmonary metastases do not necessarily indicate diffuse systemic metastases or untreatable spread of the primary. Seventy percent of patients with metastases will only have it in the lungs. Eighty percent of these will be in the periphery, allowing for wedge excision. In a multicentre EORTC study of 255 patients undergoing resection of pulmonary metastases for soft tissue sarcoma, a 38% 5-year survival was achieved postmetastasectomy.[75] Favourable prognosticators in this group included low-grade histology, negative margins and age less than 40. CT has replaced other modalities for the detection of pulmonary metastases. Patients are selected for metastasectomy in the context of a controlled primary, in the absence of uncontrolled extrathoracic metastases if the pulmonary lesion is deemed amenable to surgery in the face of adequate pulmonary reserve.[76] In the setting of osteogenic sarcoma, chemotherapy can be helpful in treating micrometastases although it offers no survival benefit for bulky metastases.[77] Aggressive surgical approach to pulmonary metastases in this setting has produced 5-year survivorship of 24%.[78]

Conclusions

The treatment of patients with sarcomas of the head and neck remains challenging due to the diverse histology, variable sites of presentation and the requirements of multimodality therapy. Improvements in the care of these patients have come from the collaborative efforts of multidisciplinary teams working in centralized cancer care facilities. These teams are then able to accrue the numbers of patients required to put together programmes for the appropriate investigation and treatment of these complex problems. The head and neck offers the additional challenges of anatomic constraints unique to this area. The close proximity of vital structures makes the resection of sarcomas in the head and neck extremely difficult in many situations. The importance of adjuvant treatment for this disease cannot be overstated because of these anatomic constraints. The psychological and functional problems associated with major resections in the head and neck create additional challenges. Reconstructive efforts with the use of free tissue transfer have significantly improved the cosmetic, functional and psychological outcomes of these patients. All of these approaches in combination with each other have led to the improved outcomes of these patients.

REFERENCES

1. Le Vay J, O'Sullivan B, Catton C et al. An assessment of prognostic factors in soft tissue sarcoma of the head and neck. *Arch Otolaryngol Head Neck Surg* 1994; **120**: 981–986.
2. Tran L, Mark R, Meier R et al. Sarcomas of the head and neck. *Cancer* 1992; **70**: 169–176.
3. Farhood A, Hajdu S, Shiu M, Strong E. Soft tissue sarcomas of the head and neck in adults. *Am J Surg* 1990; **160**: 365–369.
4. Wiklund T, Huuhtanen R, Blomqvist C et al. The importance of a multidisciplinary group in the treatment of soft tissue sarcomas. *Eur J Cancer* 1996; **32A**: 269–273.
5. Fletcher J. Cytogenetics of soft tissue tumours. *Cancer Treat Res* 1997; **91**: 31–50.
6. Kruzelock R, Hansen M. Molecular genetics and cytogenetics of sarcomas. *Hematol Oncol Clin North Am* 1995; **9**: 513–540.
7. Pappo A, Shapiro D, Crist W et al. Biology and therapy of paediatric rhabdomyosarcoma. *J Clin Oncol* 1995; **13**: 2123–2139.
8. Horn R, Enterline H. Rhabdomyosarcoma: a clinicopathologic study and classification of 39 cases. *Cancer* 1958; **11**: 181–199.
9. Newton W, Gehan E, Webber B et al. Classification of rhabdomyosarcoma and related sarcomas. *Cancer* 1995; **76**: 1073–1084.
10. Newton W, Soule E, Hamoudi A et al. Histopathology of childhood sarcomas, Intergroup rhabdomyosarcoma studies I and II: clinicopathologic correlation. *J Clin Oncol* 1988; **6**: 67–75.
11. Pappo A, Shapiro D, Crist W. Rhabdomyosarcoma, biology and treatment. *Pediatr Clin North Am* 1997; **44**: 953–972.
12. Unnik J. Classification and grading of soft tissue sarcomas. *Hematol Oncol Clin North Am* 1995; **9**: 677–697.
13. Nayar R, Prudhomme F, Parise O et al. Rhabdomyosarcoma of the head and neck in adults: a study of 26 patients. *Laryngoscope* 1993; **103**: 1326–1366.
14. Sercarz J, Mark R, Storper I et al. Sarcomas of the nasal cavity and paranasal sinuses. *Ann Otol Rhinol Laryngol* 1994; **103**: 699–704.
15. Quaglia M, Heller G, Ghauimi F et al. The effect of age at diagnosis in the outcome of rhabdomyosarcoma. *Cancer* 1994; **73**: 109–117.
16. Heenan P. Tumours of fibrous tissue involving the skin. In: Elder D (ed.) *Lever's Histopathology of the Skin.* Philadelphia: Lippincott-Raven Publishers. 1997.
17. Arnaud E, Perrault M, Revol M et al. Surgical treatment of dermatofibrosarcoma protuburans. *Plast Reconst Surg* 1997; **100**: 884–895.
18. Gayner S, Lewis J, McCaffrey T. Effects of resection margins on dermatofibrosarcoma of the head and neck. *Arch Otolaryngol Head Neck Surg* 1997; **123**: 430–433.
19. Mark R, Tran L, Sercarz J et al. Angiosarcoma of the head and neck. *Arch Otolaryngol Head Neck Surg* 1993; **119**: 973–978.
20. Aust M, Olsen K, Lewis J et al. Angiosarcoma of the head and neck. *Ann Otol Rhinol Laryngol* 1997; **106**: 943–951.
21. Holden C, Spittle M, Wilson-Jones E. Angiosarcoma of the face and scalp: prognosis and treatment. *Cancer* 1987; **119**: 973–978.
22. Morrison W, Byers R, Garden A et al. Cutaneous angiosarcoma of the head and neck. *Cancer* 1995; **76**: 319–327.
23. Catalano P, Brandwein M, Shah D et al. Sinonasal hemangiopericytoma: a clinicopathologic and immunohistochemical study of seven cases. *Head Neck* 1996; **18**: 42–48.
24. El-Naggar, Batsakis J, Garcia G et al. Sinonasal hemangiopericytomas. Clinicopathologic and DNA content study. *Arch Otolaryngol Head Neck Surg* 1992; **118**: 134–137.
25. Chawla O, Oswal V. Hemangiopericytoma of the nose and paranasal sinuses. *J Laryngol Otol* 1987; **101**: 727–737.
26. Wang C, Schroeter A, Suen J. AIDS related kaposi's sarcoma. *Mayo Clin Proceed* 1995; **70**: 869–879.
27. Bauman S, Geier S, Thoma-Gerber E et al. Conjuctival microvasculopathy and kaposi's sarcoma in patients with AIDS. *AIDS* 1994; **8**: 134–135.
28. Colledge J, Fisher C, Rhys-Evans P. Head and neck liposarcoma. *Cancer* 1995; **76**: 1051–1058.
29. Mindell R, Calcaterra T, Ward P. Leiomyosarcoma of the head and neck: a review of the literature and report of two cases. *Laryngoscope* 1994; **85**: 904–910.
30. Schenberg M, Slootweg P, Koole R. Leiomyosarcoma of the oral cavity. *J Craniomaxillofac Surg* 1993; **21**: 342–347.
31. Branford R, Reaume C, Wesley R. Leiomyosarcoma of the floor of the mouth. *J Oral Surg* 1977; **35**: 590–594.
32. Carillo R, Rodriguez-Peralto J, Batsakis J. Synovial sarcoma of the head and neck. *Ann Otol Rhinol Laryngol* 1992; **101**: 367–370.
33. Bukachevsky R, Pincus R, Scectman F et al. Synovial sarcoma of the head and neck. *Head Neck* 1992; **14**: 44–48.
34. Ruark D, Schlehaider U, Shah J. Chondrosarcoma of the head and neck. *World J Surg* 1992; **16**: 1010–1016.
35. Burkey B, Hoffman H, Baker S et al. Chondrosarcoma of the head and neck. *Laryngoscope* 1990; **100**: 1301–1305.
36. Nicolai P, Ferlito A, Sasaki C, Kirchner J. Laryngeal chondrosarcoma: incidence, pathology, biological behavior and treatment. *Ann Otol Rhinol Laryngol* 1990; **99**: 515–523.
37. Lewis J, Olsen K, Inwards C. Cartilagenous tumours of the larynx: clinicopathologic review of 47 cases. *Ann Otol Rhinol Laryngol* 1997; **106**: 94–100.
38. Mark R, Tran L, Sercarz J, Fu Y, Calcaterra T, Parker R. Chondrosarcoma of the head and neck. *Am J Clin Oncol* 1993; **16**: 232–237.
39. Rassekh C, Nuss D, Kapadia S et al. Chondrosarcoma of the nasal septum: skull base imaging and clinicopathologic correlation. *Otolaryngol Head Neck Surg* 1996; **115**: 29–37.

40. Batsakis J, Mackay B, El-Naggar A. Ewing's sarcoma and peripheral primitive neuroectodermal tumour: an interim report. *Ann Otol Rhinol Laryngol* 1996; **105**: 838–843.
41. Mamede R, Mello F, Barbieri J. Prognosis of Ewings sarcoma in the head and neck. *Otolaryngol Head Neck Surg* 1990; **102**: 650–653.
42. Wood R, Nortje C, Hesseling P, Grotepass F. Ewings tumour of the jaw. *Oral Surg, Oral Medicine, Oral Pathol* 1990; **69**: 120–127.
43. Rud N, Reiman H, Pritchard D et al. Extraosseous Ewings sarcoma. *Cancer* 1989; **64**: 1540–1553.
44. Wanebo J, Malik J, Vandenberg S et al. Malignant peripheral nerve sheath tumours. *Cancer* 1993; **71**: 1247–1253.
45. Ducatman B, Scheithauer B, Piepgras D et al. Malignant peripheral nerve sheath tumours. *Cancer* 1986; **57**: 2006–2021.
46. Oda D, Bavisotto L, Schmidt R et al. Head and neck osteosarcoma at the University of Washington. *Head Neck* 1997; **19**: 513–523.
47. Kassir R, Rassekh C, Kinsella J et al. Osteosarcoma of the head and neck: meta analysis of non randomized studies. *Laryngoscope* 1997; **107**: 56–61.
48. Cahan W, Woodward H, Higinbothan N et al. Sarcoma arising in irradiated bone: Report of eleven cases. *Cancer* 1948; **1**: 3–29.
49. Mark R, Poen J, Tran L et al. Postirradiation sarcoma. *Cancer* 1994; **73**: 2653–2659.
50. Brady M, Garfein C, Petrek J, Brennan M. Post radiation sarcoma in breast cancer patients. *Ann Surg Oncol* 1994; **1**: 66–72.
51. Taghian A, deVathar E, Terrier P et al. Long-term risk of sarcoma following radiotherapy for breast cancer. *Int J Radiat Oncol Biol Phys* 1991; **21**: 361–367.
52. Jaffe N, Patel S, Benjamin R. Chemotherapy in osteosarcoma. *Hematol Oncol Clin North Am* 1995; **9**: 825–837.
53. Massengill A, Seeger L, Eckardt J. Role of plain radiography, CT and MRI in sarcoma evaluation. *Hematol Oncol Clin North Am* 1995; **9**: 571–605.
54. Podoloff D. The role of radionuclide scans in sarcoma. *Hematol Oncol Clin North Am* 1995; **9**: 605–626.
55. Noria S, Davis A, Kandel R et al. Residual disease following unplanned excision of soft tissue sarcoma of an extremity. *J Bone Joint Surg* 1996; **78**: 650–655.
56. Ball A, Ficher C, Pittan M. Diagnosis of soft tissue tumours by Tru Cut biopsy. *Br J Surg* 1990; **77**: 756–758.
57. Ayala A, Zornoza J. Primary bone tumours: percutaneous needle biopsy, radiologic and pathologic study of 222 biopsies. *Radiology* 1983; **149**: 675–679.
58. Rosenberg S, Kent H, Costa J. Prospective randomized evaluation of the role of limb sparing surgery, radiation therapy and adjuvant chemoimmunotherapy in the treatment of adult soft tissue sarcoma. *Surgery* 1978; **84**: 62–69.
59. Harrison L, Franzese F, Gaynor J, Brennan M. Long term results of a prospective randomized trial of adjuvant brachytherapy in the management of completely resected soft tissue sarcomas of the extremity and superficial trunk. *Int J Radiat Oncol Biol Phys* 1993; **27**: 259–265.
60. Sadoski C, Suit H, Rosenberg A et al. Preoperative radiation, surgical margins and local control of extremity sarcomas of soft tissues. *J Surg Oncol* 1993; **52**: 223–230.
61. Wilson A, Davis A, Bell R et al. Local control of soft tissue sarcoma of the extremity: the experience of a multidisciplinary sarcoma group with definitive surgery and radiotherapy. *Eur J Cancer* 1994; **30A**: 746–751.
62. Saddegh M, Bauer C. Wound complications in surgery of soft tissue sarcoma. *Clin Orthoped* 1993; **289**: 247–253.
63. Bujko K, Suit H, Springfield D, Convery K. Wound healing after preoperative radiation for sarcoma of the soft tissue. *Surg Gynecol Obstet* 1993; **176**: 124–134.
64. Rosenberg S, Tepper J, Glatstein E et al. The treatment of soft tissue sarcoma of the extremities. Prospective randomized evaluation of (1) limb sparing surgery plus radiation therapy compared with amputation and (2) the role of adjuvant chemotherapy. *Ann Surg* 1982; **196**: 305–315.
65. Eeles R, Fisher C, A'Hern R et al. Head and neck sarcoma: prognostic factors and implications for treatment. *Br J Cancer* 1993; **68**: 201–207.
66. Brennan M, Casper E, Harrison C et al. The role of multimodality therapy in soft tissue sarcomas. *Ann Surg* 1991; **214**: 328–338.
67. Yang J, Chang A, Baker A et al. Randomized prospective study of the benefit of adjuvant radiotherapy in the treatment of soft tissue sarcoma of the extremity. *J Clin Oncol* 1998; **16**: 197–203.
68. Schram M, Gunderson L, Sim F et al. Soft tissue sarcoma – integration of brachytherapy, resection and external irradiation. *Cancer* 1990; **66**: 451–456.
69. Bramwell V, Rouesse J, Steward W. Adjuvant CYVADIC chemotherapy for adult soft tissue sarcoma – reduced local recurrence but no improvement in survival: a study of the European Organization for Research and Treatment of Cancer. *J Clin Oncol* 1994; **12**: 1137–1149.
70. Mertens W, Bramwell V. Adjuvant chemotherapy for soft tissue sarcomas. *Hematol Oncol Clin North Am* 1995; **9**: 801–815.
71. Eilber F, Giuliano A, Eckardt J. Adjuvant chemotherapy for osteosarcoma: a randomized prospective trial. *J Clin Oncol* 1987; **5**: 21–26.
72. Nori D, Shupak K, Shiu M, Brennan M. Role of brachytherapy in recurrent extremity sarcoma in patients treated with prior surgery and irradiation. *Int J Radiat Oncol Biol Phys* 1991; **20**: 1229–1233.
73. Essner R, Selch M, Eilber F. Reirradiation for extremity soft tissue sarcomas. *Cancer* 1991; **11**: 2813–2817.
74. Potter D, Glenn J, Kinsella T et al. Patterns of recurrence in patients with high-grade soft tissue sarcoma. *J Clin Oncol* 1985; **3**: 353–366.
75. van Geel A, Pastorino U, Jauch K et al. Surgical treatment of lung metastases. *Cancer* 1996; **77**: 675–682.
76. Rusch VW. Pulmonary metastasectomy. Current indications. *Chest* 1995; **107 (Suppl 6)**: 322–331.
77. Putnam J, Roth J. Surgical treatment for pulmonary metastases from sarcoma. *Hematol Oncol Clin North Am* 1995; **9**: 869–888.
78. Saltzman D, Snyder C, Ferrell K et al. Aggressive metastasectomy for pulmonic sarcomatous metastases: a follow up study. *Am J Surg* 1993; **166**: 543–547.

25 Juvenile angiofibroma

Camilla MA Carroll, Irving Pathak and Patrick J Gullane

Definition and historical background

Juvenile angiofibroma is a rare benign but locally aggressive tumour originating in the region of the sphenopalatine foramen and presenting almost exclusively in adolescent males.[1–7] Early descriptions of nasal masses by Hippocrates are believed to have included cases of angiofibromas.[8] Chelius in 1847 described the presence of a fibrous nasal mass in the pubertal male.[9] Chaveau writing in 1906 believed the site of origin of these lesions to be in the nasopharynx and coined the term juvenile nasopharyngeal angioma. Friedberg's histological analysis of these tumours in the 1940s demonstrated them to be composed of connective tissue and vascular elements and he amended the term to juvenile nasopharyngeal angiofibroma.[10] The introduction of modern radiological techniques however further refined the understanding of the origin and growth patterns of these lesions and it is currently believed that the site of origin is not within the nasopharynx but from the region of the sphenopalatine foramen.[11,12] Hence nasopharyngeal has been dropped from the nomenclature and these lesions are currently known as juvenile angiofibromas.

Incidence

The true incidence of these lesions is unknown, but a figure of 0.05% of all head and neck tumours is often quoted.[1,2] Some authors allude to a higher incidence in the Asian subcontinent, specifically India and Egypt.[1] However Harrison believes that this can be explained on the grounds of local referral patterns to a few centres of expertise, rather than as a result of a definitive ethnic susceptibility.[4]

The overwhelming majority of angiofibromas have been documented in adolescent males[2,13–15] with only a handful of histologically documented cases described in females.[16–21] The mean age at presentation is 13 years with a range from 5 to 50 years.[2,4,5,13]

Aetiology

The aetiological background of this tumour remains unresolved. Over the decades several authors have investigated the possibility of a tumour site in the nasopharynx whose growth patterns are under the influence of fluxes in circulating levels of sexual hormones. Brunner is credited with the identification of the site of origin of this tumour, based on the work he carried out in 1942 on full-term embryos.[22] He identified a region of endothelially lined vascular spaces in the fascia basilis of the sphenoid. These findings were later to be confirmed by Harrisons's work in 1987.[4] He demonstrated similar endothelial tissue in the region of the sphenopalatine foramen and the base of the pterygoid plates in both male and female 24-week-old human fetuses. Investigators then hypothesized that growth of this vascular tissue was secondary to hormonal fluctuations taking place in the male during puberty. Martin in 1948 suggested that growth of the tumour tissue was due to a relative overproduction of oestrogens or a lack of androgens.[23] Schiff suggested tumour growth was due to an alteration in the pituitary androgen–oestrogen axis.[24] Walike and Mackay demonstrated that diethylstilboestrol decreased the growth potential of endothelial cells and stimulated the growth of fibrous tissue.[25] They suggested therefore that this oestrogen might cause regression of the angiofibroma. Maurice and Milad further subscribed to this theory in 1981.[26] They concluded that the angiofibroma arose from ectopic genital tissue, which grew under the influence of male sex hormones during puberty. Farag and coworkers studied tumour samples from seven males and presented their findings in 1987.[27] The results of their analysis led to the following observations, that the angiofibromatous tissue was not in fact ectopic sequestered genital tissue, but normal nasal mucosa that had an excess of androgen receptors and grew during puberty as a result of fluctuations in circulating levels of male sex hormones. To date however no definitive study is available that has quantified angiofibroma growth rates with changes in oestrogen and androgen levels.

Clinical presentation

The clinical presentation is usually dependent on tumour site and local extension at the time of diagnosis (Table 25.1). Neel detailed the patterns of tumour spread, which takes place by submucosal extension and through local tissue planes of least resistance.[11] The tumour can extend anteriorly into the nasal cavity, superiorly into the sphenoid sinus and the sella, laterally via the sphenopalatine foramen into the pterygomaxillary fossa, the infratemporal fossa and the inferior orbital fissure. Tumour spread intracranially is via the sella or the foramen lacerum into the middle cranial fossa. The majority of patients present with unilateral nasal obstruction and spontaneous epistaxis.[2–5,13,16,21,28] Patients with more extensive tumour spread may also present with hypernasal speech, proptosis, conductive hearing loss, cheek swelling and cranial nerve deficits of III–VI.[28] Clinical examination should consist of endoscopic examination of the nasal cavity and the nasopharynx. The appearance of the tumour mass tends to reflect its vascularity and may appear as pale white if predominantly composed of fibrous tissue or dark red and fleshy if vascular. Nasendoscopy usually reveals a polypoid or submucosal mass filling the nasopharynx or obstructing the posterior nares. More extensive tumours may prolapse below the soft palate, cause diffuse swelling over the maxillary antrum and extend into the upper neck and infratemporal fossa.

Table 25.1 Presenting complaints
Unilateral epistaxis
Nasal obstruction
Rhinorrhoea
Hypernasal speech
Serous otitis media
Maxillary swelling
Anosmia
Proptosis
Exophthalmos
Diplopia
Headaches
Neck mass
Cranial nerves III–VI deficits

Once clinical evaluation is complete diagnosis is currently established using dual radiological imaging with contrast-enhanced high-resolution CT scanning and gadolinium-enhanced MRI.[29–32] The diagnosis is based on the location of the tumour and its pattern of spread, which can be accurately mapped out using contrast enhanced CT scanning.[2,3,30,31] As the tumour originates in the region of the sphenopalatine foramen there is usually enlargement of this foramen on CT imaging (Figure 25.1).[4] Tumour vascularity is demonstrated by the presence of signal voids on MRI (Figure 25.2).[32] Gadolinium-enhanced MRI clearly distinguishes tumour from surrounding tissue and is very sensitive in delineating intracranial extension; CT is also valuable in this context (Figure 25.3). Biopsy of the mass continues to be contraindicated because of the risk of intractable haemorrhage and the fact that an accurate diagnosis can be safely established using current imaging modalities. The introduction of CT and MRI has eliminated the need to establish a diagnosis using angiography. Currently the role of angiography is in preoperative embolization to reduce tumour blood supply prior to surgery (Figure 25.4).

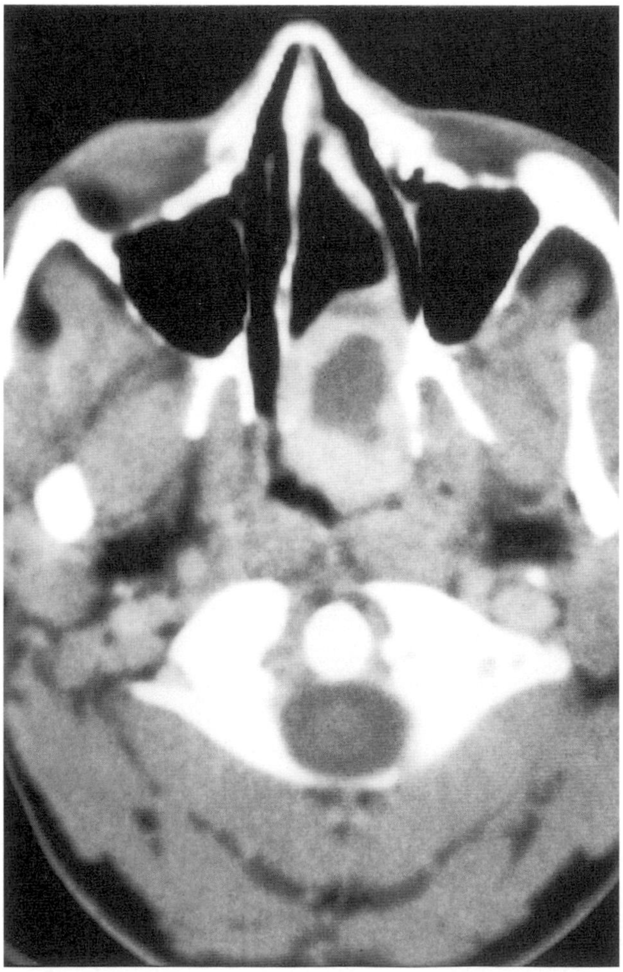

Figure 25.1 CT image of angiofibroma in the region of the pterygopalatine foramen.

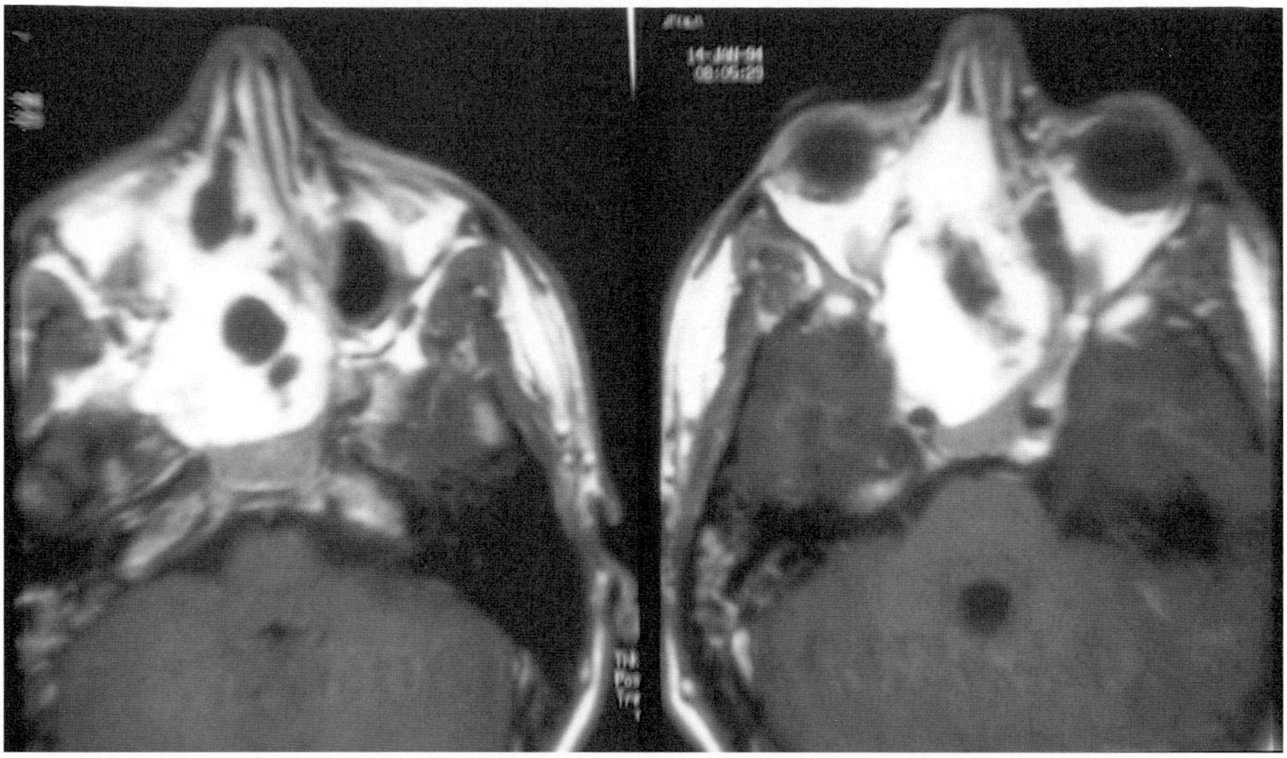

Figure 25.2 MRI with gadolinium enhancement demonstrating the highly vascular tumour with signal voids.

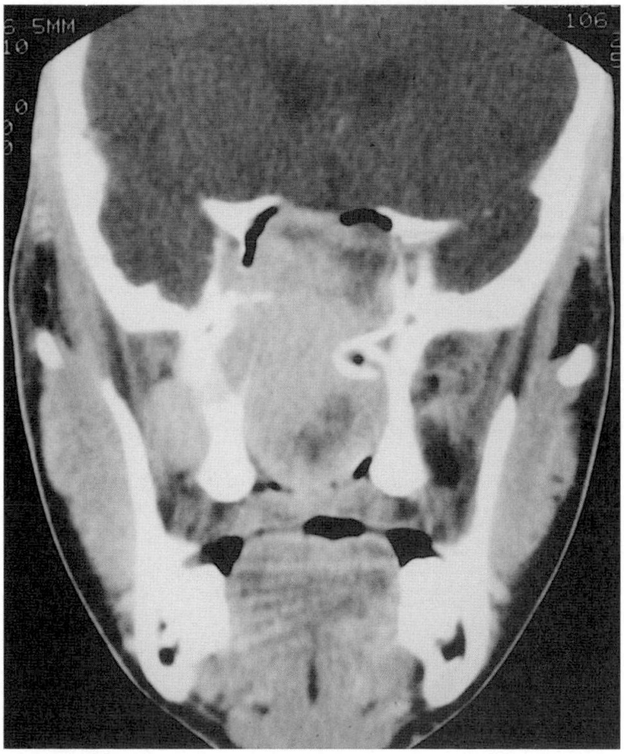

Figure 25.3 CT image demonstrating intracranial extension of angiofibroma.

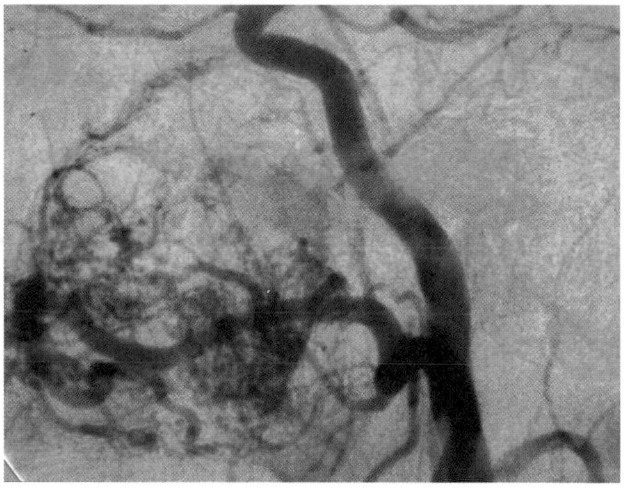

Figure 25.4 Angiogram demonstrating the blood supply of the angiofibroma.

Staging of the disease is based on the CT findings. The three established staging systems are those of Sessions (1981),[3] Fisch (1983)[33] and Chandler (1984),[2] (Table 25.2). Each system is based on the well-recognized patterns of tumour spread and the higher the stage the more extensive the disease. Staging assists in planning management strategies and in the reporting of results, therefore the universal adoption of one staging system would allow for easier transfer of information and comparison of results between centres.

Table 25.2 Staging systems for juvenile angiofibroma

Sessions et al[3]	
Ia	Tumour limited to the nasopharynx and/or nares
Ib	Extension to one or more sinuses
IIa	Minimal extension into the pterygomaxillary fossa
IIb	Full occupation of the pterygomaxillary fossa
III	Intracranial extension
Fisch[33]	
I	Tumour limited to nasal cavity and nasopharynx with no bone erosion
II	Tumour invading the pterygomaxillary fossa and all sinuses, with bony destruction
III	Tumour invading the infratemporal fossa, orbit and parasellar region, remaining lateral to the cavernous sinus
IV	Tumours with extensive invasion of the cavernous sinus, optic chiasmal region or pituitary fossa
Chandler et al[2]	
I	Tumour confined to the nasopharynx
II	Tumour extension to the nasopharynx and/or sphenoid sinus
III	Tumour extension into one or more of the following sites: maxillary antrum, ethmoid sinus, pterygomaxillary or infratemporal fossae, orbit, cheek
IV	Intracranial extension

Differential diagnosis

The diagnosis of juvenile angiofibroma is made on the basis of the clinical presentation, physical examination and pattern of spread on CT imaging. However other lesions do present in the nasal cavity and nasopharynx, which give rise to nasal obstruction and epistaxis in this age group. Benign lesions such as simple nasal polyps can cause nasal obstruction and an antrochoanal polyp can prolapse into the nasopharynx. Tumours that expand within the pterygopalatine fossa and cause bowing of the posterior maxillary wall, such as rhabdomyosarcoma, haemangiopericytoma and neurilemmomas must be differentiated from juvenile angiofibroma. Some of these lesions are also vascular with signal voids seen on MRI making the differential from juvenile angiofibroma difficult and on occasion a tissue diagnosis may be necessary.

Pathological appearance

The macroscopic appearance of the angiofibroma is in part dependent on the varying amounts of fibrous to vascular elements within it. The mass can vary in appearance from pale white to red and fleshy with visible overlying vessels, which bleed on contact (Figure 25.5). These tumours are non-encapsulated and spread by submucosal extension and local infiltration.[11] The gross specimen is usually a lobulated mass with a base of varying width. The microscopic features of this tumour were defined by Sternberg in1954.[34] He suggested that the tumour was a variant of an angioma because of the presence of vascular elements dispersed throughout a dense connective tissue network (Figure 25.6). Electron microscopic studies carried out by McGavern and Taxy led them to conclude that the stromal cells may arise from fibroblasts or myofibroblasts, which are frequently seen in other fibroproliferative disorders.[35,36] It has been suggested by certain authors that tumours with a predominantly fibrous composition on serial sectioning may represent the end stage of tumour involution.

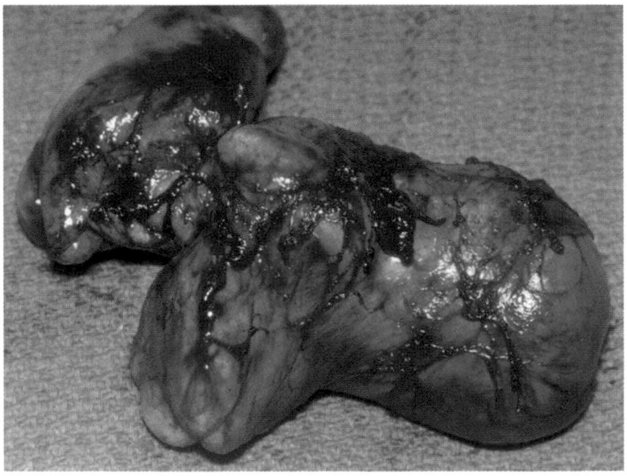

Figure 25.5 Macroscopic pathological specimen.

Natural history of the disease

Controversy still exists as to the natural progression of this disease.[4] The literature supports the fact that angiofibroma is a disease predominantly of males[2,13–15] with only a handful of reported cases occurring in females.[16–21] Patients tend to present when the tumour has grown to sufficient size to cause symptoms, which is usually during the adolescent years. The mean age at presentation is 13 years with a range from 5 to 50 years.[2,4,5,13] There are no significant numbers of untreated control cases in the

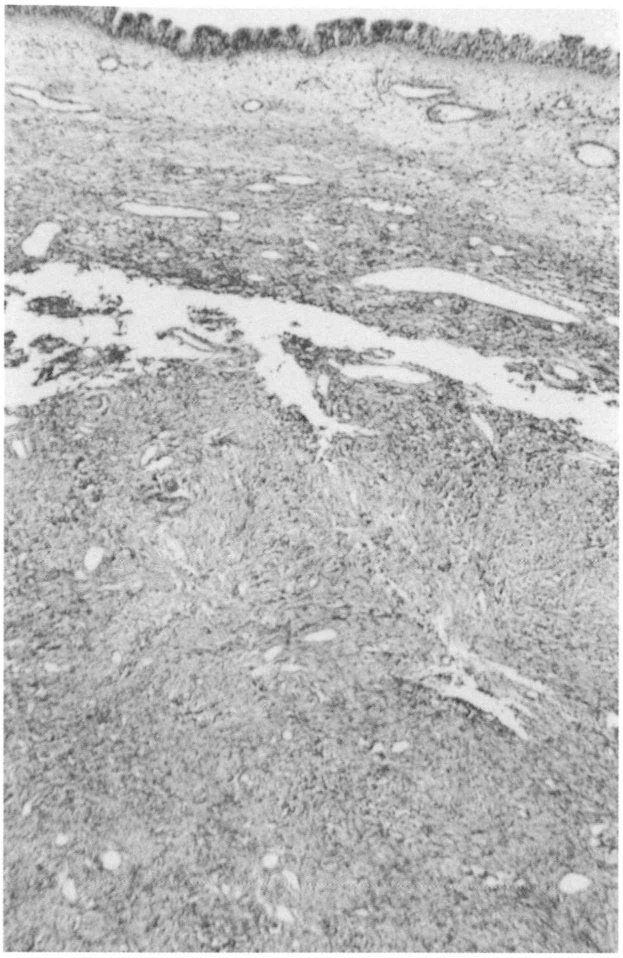

Figure 25.6 Microscopic pathological specimen.

literature, that have been serially followed with radiological imaging to support the theory that these tumours will eventually undergo involution and cease to grow. Despite this however there is a belief that tumour involution does in fact take place.[37,38] Stansbie and Phelps,[39] reported radiological documentation of intracranial tumour growth cessation in a patient who had undergone previous surgery. Weprin and Siemers,[40] reported a single case of an 11-year-old boy with biopsy-proven angiofibroma who received no treatment but was followed with serial radiological imaging over an 11-year period. The patient was followed between 1978 and 1989 and during this period there was progressive involution of an originally extensive intracranial angiofibroma. A CT scan carried out in 1989 showed no evidence of tumour, thus confirming complete and spontaneous tumour resolution. These authors suggest that this case report adds weight to the theory that angiofibromas are hormone dependent and post-pubertal stabilization of sex hormone fluctuations can lead to involution of these tumours. However the overwhelming evidence suggests that these are locally aggressive tumours that will continue to grow and spread in the absence of adequate treatment, with a tendency to recur if incompletely excised.[41,42]

The potential for malignant transformation of the benign angiofibroma has also been alluded to in the literature. Makek et al[43] reported a case of fibrosarcoma developing in a previously benign angiofibroma. However this patient had undergone four previous surgical resections and two courses of radiation treatment. They reviewed other case reports of malignant transformation and noted that all patients had received radiation treatment varying from 11 months to 21 years prior to malignant transformation. The majority of these lesions were reported as fibrosarcomas, which led Makek's group to conclude that the fibrous elements of the angiofibroma appeared to be the tissue most likely to undergo malignant transformation when exposed to radiation in the form of treatment. Of note is the fact that the Toronto group, which treated 55 patients with primary radiation, demonstrated no cases of malignant transformation within the tumour with a follow-up period ranging from 3 to 26 years.[21]

Management

Surgery with preoperative embolization and postoperative radiotherapy for residual disease is currently practised by most centres treating patients with angiofibromas. Historically numerous methods of treatment were employed in the management of this tumour, including cryosurgery,[44] sclerotherapy and electrocoagulation.[24] Medical treatment using oestrogen analogues had been in vogue in the 1970s and 1980s as a result of the various theories suggesting that tumour growth occurred in response to androgen stimulation.[28,45–47] This form of therapy has now been largely abandoned.

Chemotherapeutic agents have been used by one centre. Goepfert in 1985 treated five patients with two chemotherapeutic regimens. The first regimen was a combination of doxorubicin and dacarbazine. The second regimen was vincristine, dactinomycin and cyclophosphamide. Tumour regression was recorded in all patients.[48] Goepfert suggested that chemotherapeutic agents should be used in the management of residual disease where surgery or radiotherapy were not indicated. He also suggested that chemotherapeutic agents should be used in the setting of controlled trials.

Embolization

Angiofibromas are highly vascular lesions that derive their main blood supply from the external

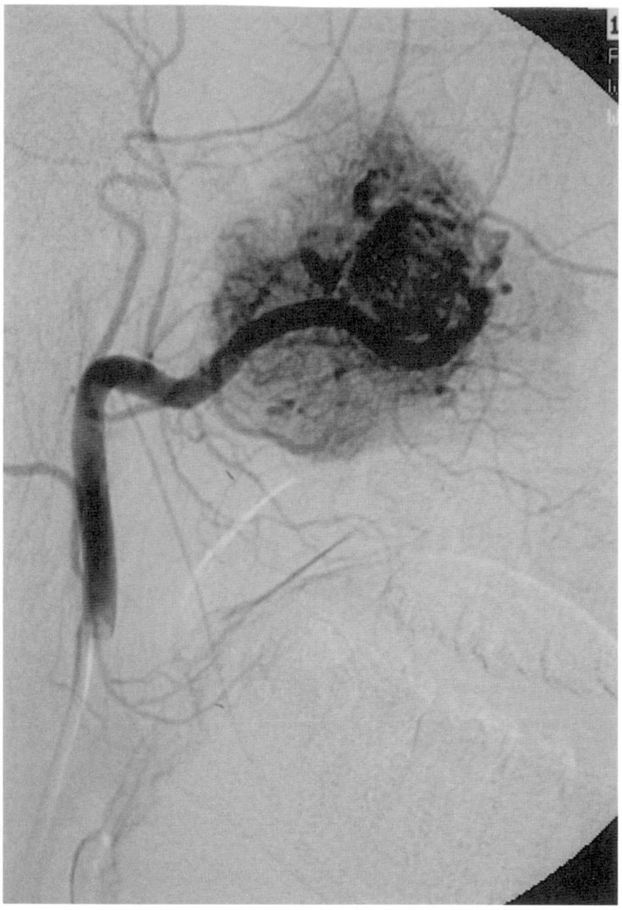

Figure 25.7 Pre-embolization angiogram.

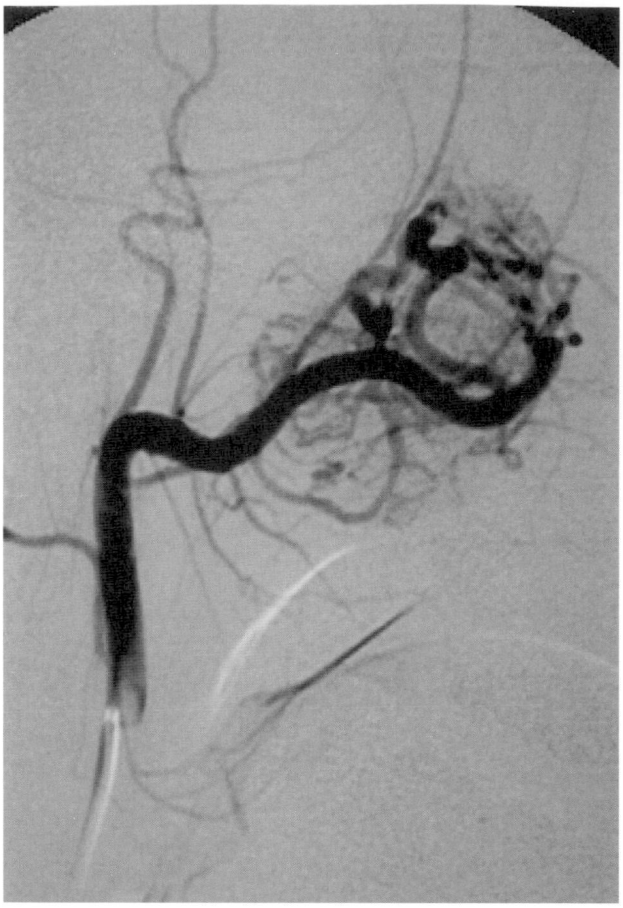

Figure 25.8 Postembolization angiogram.

carotid system via the internal maxillary artery (Figures 25.7 and 25.8). Additional supplies may be derived from the anterior branch of the ascending pharyngeal artery and the palatal branches of the external carotid system.[49–51] As the tumour expands and spreads it picks up blood supplies from the internal carotid system through the sphenoidal artery and the ophthalmic artery. Large tumours tend to receive a substantial blood supply from the arteries on the contralateral side.

Tumour removal without prior embolization has been reported to be associated with significant intraoperative blood loss and there are reports of intraoperative mortalities secondary to haemorrhage.[15,50] Robertson was the first to advocate preoperative embolization in the early 1970s.[52] He proposed that occluding the vessels supplying the tumour would lead to less blood loss at the time of surgery. Since then many authors have published their results suggesting that preoperative embolization reduces blood loss and assists in the ease of surgical resection as a result of a drier operative field.[14,53–57]

Angiography with a view to embolization is recommended 48–72 hours prior to planned surgery.[57] The material used to embolize the feeding vessels is either Gelfoam particles[51,53–54] of 1 mm in diameter or polyvinyl alcohol.[58] Gelfoam is usually resorbed within a few weeks allowing the internal maxillary artery to recanalize partially or completely. Polyvinyl alcohol causes more permanent occlusion. Delay in performing surgery or the use of large particle size will adversely effect the success of embolization.[57] Selective catheterization of the tumour feeding vessels requires the skill of an experienced interventional radiologist who is familiar with the blood supply to the face. Complications arising from embolization occur when there has been accidental embolization of cerebral vessels, ophthalmic vessels and facial vessels, resulting in hemiparesis, blindness and facial soft tissue and skin necrosis.[51,59,60] However most reported series have few or no cases of permanent complications.

Radiation

The majority of centres treating angiofibromas will use adjunctive radiotherapy in the management of residual tumour following surgery or inoperable intracranial disease. The group from the Princess Margaret Hospital in Toronto has the largest experience of treating angiofibromas with primary radiotherapy.[61–65]

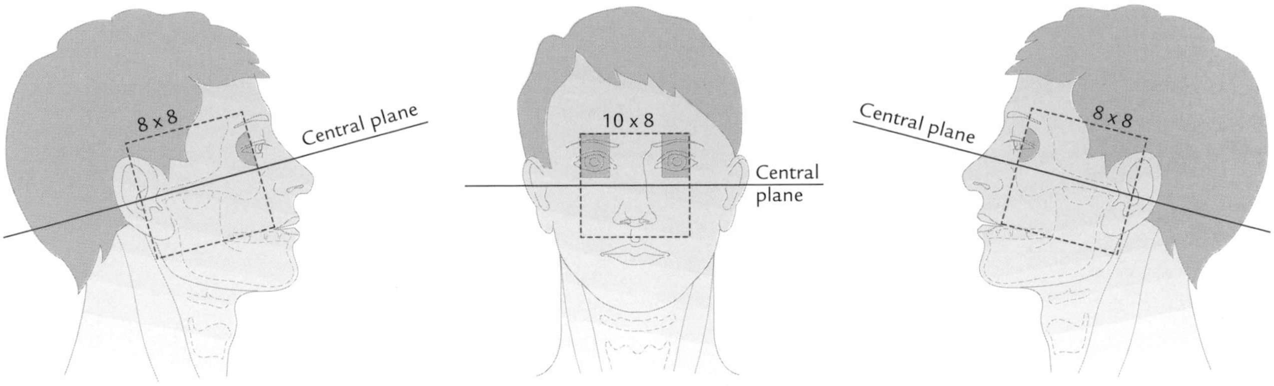

Figure 25.9 Radiation fields as graphically demonstrated by Cummings.

They suggest that primary radiotherapy is as effective as primary surgery and poses no greater threat of serious morbidity. Their most recent paper was published in 1984.[21] The outcome of 55 patients treated with primary radiotherapy, with a follow-up ranging from 3 to 26 years was reviewed in this paper. They state that with accurate CT imaging of the disease extent and using adequate radiation fields, control rates in excess of 80% could be achieved (Figure 25.9). Their treatment protocol consists of external beam radiation of 3000–3500 cGy delivered over 3 weeks. Cummings emphasizes that tumour regression following radiation treatment takes place slowly, over a period of 12–20 months. Complete tumour regression, as demonstrated by clinical examination can be used as an index of control, as these patients rarely presented with recurrences.

Acute or late complications as a result of radiotherapy were infrequently encountered. Facial skeletal growth was not interfered with and there were no cases of hypopituitorism. Two patients developed cataracts, as the orbit was involved with disease and therefore was in the field of radiation. Late tumour induction was recorded in two patients, with one case of radiation-induced thyroid cancer and one facial basal cell carcinoma.

Surgery

Primary surgical extirpation of angiofibromas is generally recognized as the mainstay of treatment. The surgical approach used will be determined by the stage of the disease as detailed from the clinical and radiological work-up. The approach used must provide adequate exposure for tumour visualization and removal.[28] However other factors must also be taken into account when planning the surgical approach such as the patient's age and the future growth of the facial skeleton and the need therefore to limit the functional and aesthetic deformity of the craniofacial skeleton.

The surgical approaches can be defined as transfacial approaches and transbasal approaches where there is an indication to expose or remove part of the skull base. The transfacial approaches can be further subdivided into transoral, transnasoethmoidal and transmaxillary.[66] The skull base approaches can be subdivided into the anterior and lateral approaches. Small lesions confined to the nasal cavity and paranasal sinuses with minimal extension into the pterygopalatine fossa can be removed using endoscopic techniques. Mitskavich et al[67] have reported such a case with a 2-year follow-up where the patient remains disease free.

Tumours involving the nasal cavity and extending anteriorly and inferiorly into the maxillary sinus can be approached through a midfacial degloving incision (Figure 25.10).[68,69] This transoral approach described by Conley in 1979 sites an incision in the gingivobuccal sulcus spanning from one maxillary tuberosity to the other and extended into the pyriform aperture down to the periosteum.[68] An osteotomy in the anterior maxillary wall is then performed to gain access to the tumour mass. Complete reconstruction of the facial skeleton is achieved at the end of the resection by fixation of the

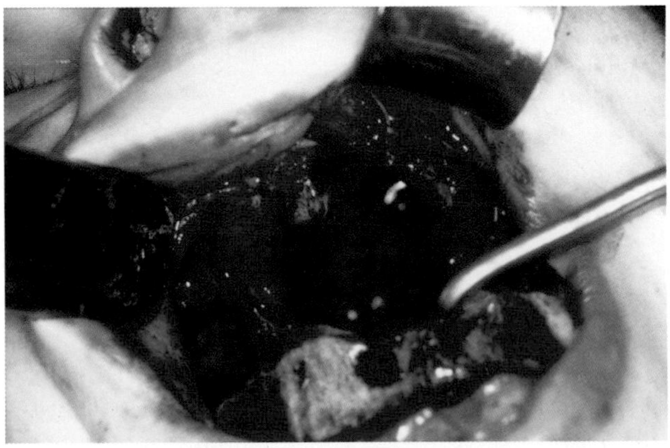

Figure 25.10 Facial degloving approach.

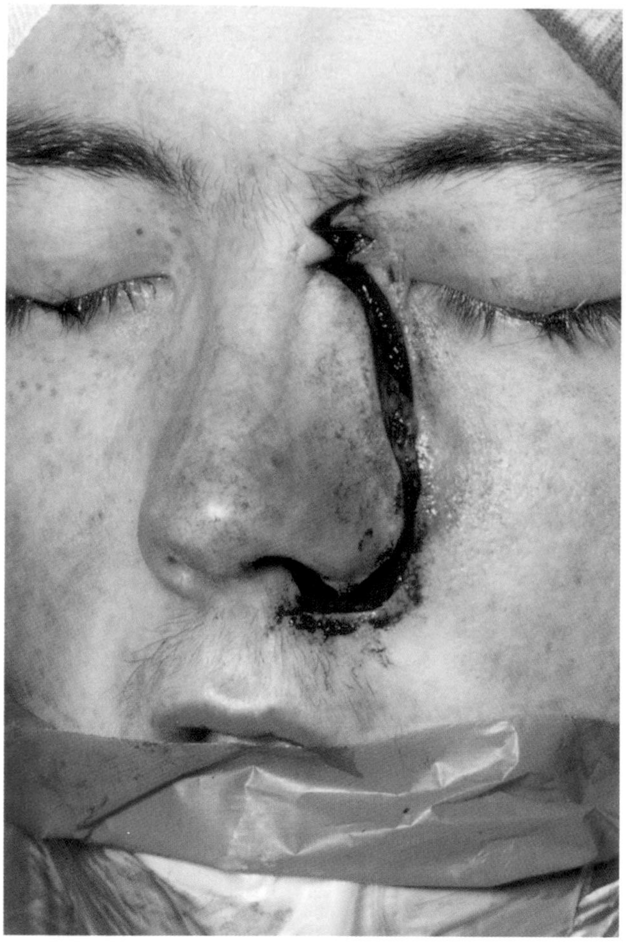

Figure 25.11 Approach via a lateral rhinotomy incision.

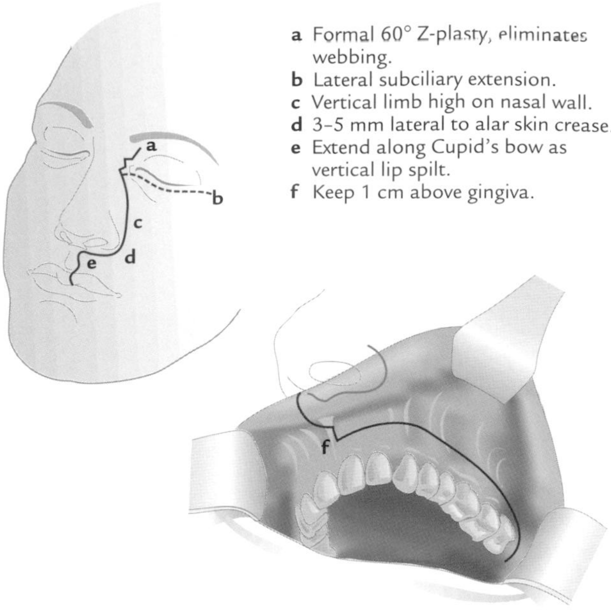

a Formal 60° Z-plasty, eliminates webbing.
b Lateral subciliary extension.
c Vertical limb high on nasal wall.
d 3–5 mm lateral to alar skin crease.
e Extend along Cupid's bow as vertical lip spilt.
f Keep 1 cm above gingiva.

Figure 25.12 Approach via a Weber-Ferguson incision.

osteotomized bone segments. Minimal disruption of facial growth has been reported with this approach and the main complication is that of nasal aperture stenosis. This can be overcome by the judicious incorporation of Z-plasties into the rim incision.

Tumours that extend to involve the ethmoid sinus and the nasopharynx can be approached using a lateral rhinotomy incision with a mono or bilateral reflection of the nasal pyramid depending on the extent of the tumour (Figure 25.11).[5,28,70,71] Again meticulous repositioning of the bony nasal pyramid is essential to achieve long-term satisfactory aesthetic results. Tumour that extends to involve the entire nasal cavity and the maxillary sinus with erosion of the posterior wall of the sinus is best approached through a Weber-Ferguson incision (Figure 25.12).[5,28] Wide exposure of the tumour is gained by complete removal of the frontal process of the maxilla, nasoantral wall below the inferior turbinate, lacrimal bone, lamina papyracea and the anterior and posterior ethmoid cells up to the level of the cribriform plate. During this dissection care is taken to preserve the lacrimal sac and duct and the periosteum of the medial wall of the orbit.

Tumours where the main ethmoidal-sphenoidal extension involves the anterior skull base are approached through a bicoronal incision and an anterior craniofacial resection.[72]

The incidence of tumour extension into the infratemporal fossa and the orbital apex and middle cranial fossa is quoted as being 10–20%.[71,36] The treatment of intracranial extension is controversial.[71] Fisch advocates a lateral skull base approach in the management of Fisch type III and type IV tumours, with a single lateral extradural approach to the middle cranial fossa.[33] The frontal branch of the facial nerve, temporalis muscle, zygomatic arch and masseter muscle are all displaced inferiorly to allow access to the infratemporal fossa. During tumour resection the internal carotid artery is visible at all times using this approach. Fisch states that with a lateral skull base approach it is possible to radically remove Fisch type III tumours, with subtotal removal of type IV tumours and postoperative radiotherapy used in the treatment of symptomatic intracranial residual disease.[33] Some authors suggest that these type IV tumours are best managed with primary radiotherapy because of the greater morbidity and mortality associated with this type of surgical approach.[28,71]

The recurrence rates following surgery in recent series range from 6% to 24% (Figure 25.13).[73–77] This is in comparison to rates of 61% recorded by Biller[78] in 1978 and 45% by Boles and Dedo[79] in 1976. The significant reduction in recurrence rates has been attributed to a better understanding of the disease process in combination with accurate preoperative staging with CT imaging.

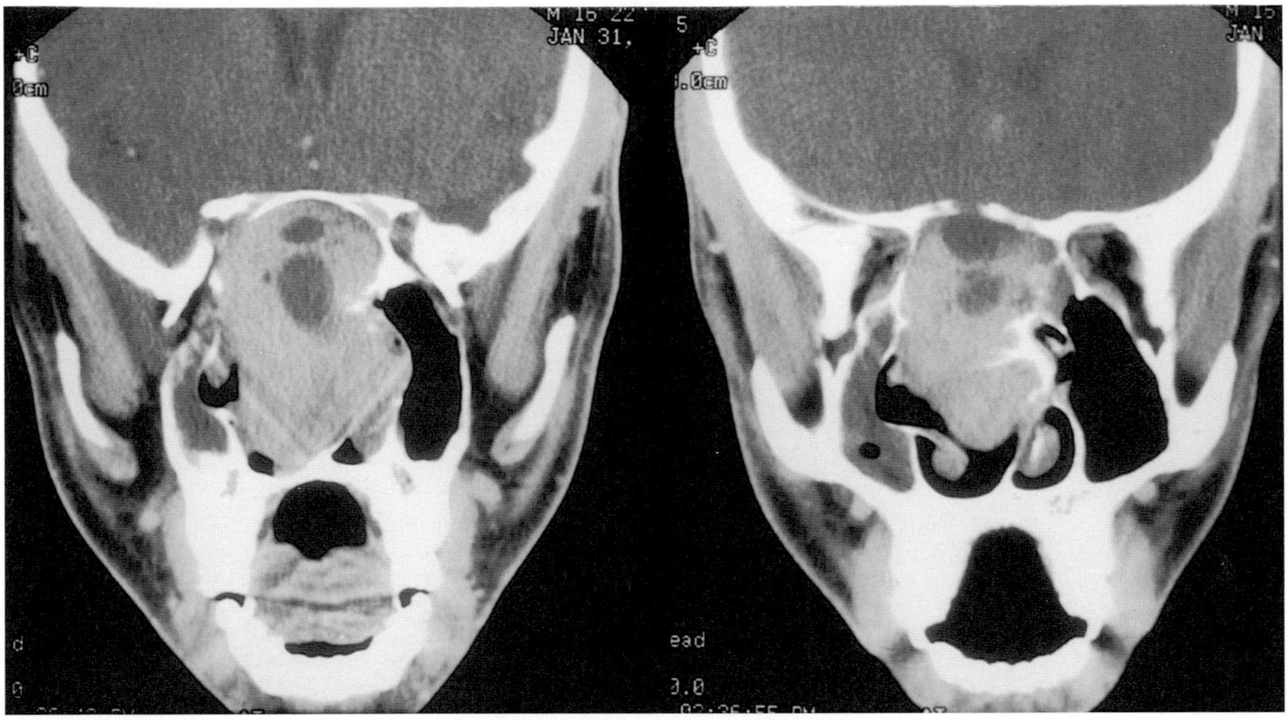

Figure 25.13 CT images demonstrating recurrence following treatment.

Future developments

The fact that angiofibromas are highly vascular tumours has led several authors to investigate if their growth is regulated by angiogenic growth factors. Basic fibroblast growth factor, an angiogenic growth factor which stimulates endothelial cells, smooth muscle cells and fibroblasts[80–82] has been identified in angiofibromas.[83]

Nagai et al[84] localized transforming growth factor-β_1 (TGF-β_1) in the endothelial and fibroblast cells of angiofibromatous tissue. TGF-β_1[85] induces various extracellular matrix proteins and vascular endothelial growth factor (VEGF). VEGF has been demonstrated to be involved in the regulation of normal and pathological angiogenesis.[86–88] Nagai et al concluded that TGF-β_1 may be involved in the development of fibrosis in angiofibromas and stimulate the production of VEGF leading to new blood vessel formation within the tumour. Platelet-derived growth factor B (PDGF-B),[89] a direct-acting angiogenic growth factor, has been identified by immunohistochemical analysis in angiofibromatous tumour tissue.[84] This again suggests that PDGF-B may contribute to the development of new blood vessel formation and fibrosis within the angiofibroma.

Inhibition of the expression of angiogenic growth factors by angiofibromas may lead to a reduction in tumour growth, or indeed tumour involution. The delivery of an anti-angiogenic agent to the tumour bed, for example by selective angiography has potential for future use in the clinical setting.

REFERENCES

1. Batsakis JG. *Tumours of the Head and Neck.* 2nd edn. Baltimore: Williams and Wilkins, 1979; 296–300.
2. Chandler JR, Goulding R, Moskowitz et al. Nasopharyngeal angiofibromas: staging and management. *Ann Otol Rhinol Laryngol* 1984; **93**: 322–329.
3. Sessions RB, Bryan RN, Naclerio RM et al. Radiographic staging of juvenile angiofibroma. *Head Neck Surg* 1981; **3**: 279–283.
4. Harrison DFN. The natural history, pathogenesis and treatment of juvenile angiofibroma. *Arch Otolaryngol Head Neck Surg* 1987; **113**: 936–942.

5. Iannetti G, Belli E, De Ponte F et al. The surgical approaches to nasopharyngeal angiofibroma. *J Craniomaxillofac Surg* 1994; **22**: 311–316.
6. Jacobsson MB, Petruson B, Svendsen P et al. Juvenile nasopharyngeal angiofibroma: a report of eighteen cases. *Acta Otolaryngol* 1988; **105**: 132–139.
7. Mishra SC, Shukla GK, Bhatia N et al. A rational classification of angiofibroma of the post nasal space. *J Laryngol Otol* 1989; **103**: 912–916.
8. Hippocrates. *Oeuvres Completes.* Vol 10. (Traduction nouvelle par E. Littre) Paris: JB Baillière, 1839–1861.
9. Chelius JM. *System of Surgery.* Vol 2. London: Henry Renshaw, 1847.
10. Friedberg SA. Vascular fibromas of the nasopharynx. *Arch Otolaryngol* 1940; **13**: 313–326.
11. Neel HB, Whicker JH, Devine KD et al. Juvenile angiofibroma: review of 120 cases. *Am J Surg* 1973; **126**: 547–556.
12. Lund VJ, Lloyd GAS, Howard DJ. Juvenile angiofibroma: imaging technigues in diagnosis. *Rhinology* 1989; **28**: 97–102.
13. Antonelli AR, Cappiello J, Di Lorenzo D et al. Diagnosis, staging and treatment of juvenile nasopharyngeal angiofibroma (JNA). *Laryngoscope* 1987; **97**: 1319–1325.
14. Economou TS, Abermayor E, Ward PH. Juvenile nasopharyngeal angiofibroma: an update of the UCLA experience, 1960–1985. *Laryngoscope* 1988; **98**: 170–175.
15. Ward PH. The evolving management of juvenile nasopharyngeal angiofibroma. *J Laryngol Otol* 1983; **8** (Suppl): 103–104.
16. Witt TR, Shah JR, Sternberg SS. Juvenile nasopharyngeal angiofibroma. A 30 year clinical review. *Am J Surg* 1983; **146**: 521–525.
17. Finnerman WB. Juvenile nasopharyngeal angiofibroma in the female. *Arch Otolaryngol* 1951; **54**: 620–623.
18. Parchet V. L'Angiofibrome nasopharingien chez la femme. *Ann Otolaryngol* 1951; **68**: 60–69.
19. Handousa A, Farig H, Elwi AM. Nasopharyngeal fibroma: clinico-pathological study of 70 cases. *J Laryngol Otol* 1954; **68**: 647–666.
20. Osborn DA, Sokolovski A. Juvenile nasopharyngeal angiofibroma in an elderly female. *Arch Otolaryngol* 1981; **89**: 602–603.
21. Cummings BJ, Blend R, Keane T et al. Primary radiation therapy for juvenile nasopharyngeal angiofibroma. *Laryngoscope* 1984; **94**: 1599–1605.
22. Brunner H. Nasopharyngeal fibroma. *Ann Otol Rhinol Laryngol* 1942; **51**: 29–63.
23. Martin H, Ehrlich HE, Abels JC. Juvenile nasopharyngeal angiofibroma. *Ann Surg* 1948; **129**: 513–536.
24. Schiff M. Juvenile nasopharyngeal angiofibroma: a theory of pathogenesis. *Laryngoscope* 1959; **69**: 981–1016.
25. Walike JW, Mackay B. Nasopharyngeal angiofibroma: light and electron miscrscopic changes after stilbesterol therapy. *Laryngoscope* 1970; **79**: 1108–1113.
26. Maurice M, Milad M. Pathogenesis of juvenile nasopharyngeal fibroma. *J Laryngol Otol* 1981; **95**: 1121–1126.
27. Farag NM, Ghanimah SE, Ragie A et al. Hormone receptors in nasopharyngeal angiofibroma. *Laryngoscope* 1987; **97**: 208–211.
28. Gullane PJ, Davidson J, O'Dwyer T, Forte V. Juvenile angiofibroma: a review of the literature and a case series report. *Laryngoscope* 1992; **102**: 928–933.
29. Davis KR. Embolization of epistaxis and juvenile nasopharyngeal angiofibromas. *Am J Roentgenol* 1987; **148**: 209–218.
30. Weinstein MA, Levine H, Duchesneau PM et al. Diagnosis of juvenile angiofibroma by computed tomography. *Radiology* 1978; **126**: 703–705.
31. Levine HL, Weinstein MA, Tucker HM et al. Diagnosis of juvenile nasopharyngeal angiofibroma by computed tomography. *Otolaryngol Head Neck Surg* 1979; **87**: 304–310.
32. Lloyd GAS, Phelps PD. Juvenile angiofibroma: imaging by magnetic resonance, CT and conventional techniques. *Clin Otolaryngol* 1986; **59**: 675–683.
33. Fisch U. The infratemporal fossa approach for nasopharyngeal tumours. *Laryngoscope* 1983; **93**: 36–44.
34. Sternberg SS. Pathology of juvenile nasopharyngeal angiofibroma. A lesion of adolescent males. *Cancer* 1954; **7**: 15–28.
35. McGavern MH, Sessions DG, Dorfman RF et al. Nasopharyngeal angiofibroma. *Arch Otolaryngol* 1969; **90**: 94–104.
36. Taxy JB. Juvenile nasopharyngeal angiofibroma: an ultrastructural study. *Cancer* 1977; **39**: 1044–1054.
37. Bahtia ML. Intracranial extensions of juvenile angiofibroma of the nasopharynx. *J Laryngol Otol* 1967; **81**: 1395–1403.
38. Jacobsson M, Petruson B, Ruth M et al. Involution of juvenile angiofibroma with intracranial extension. *Arch Otolaryngol Head Neck Surg* 1989; **115**: 238–239.
39. Stansbie JM, Phelps PD. Involution of residual juvenile nasopharyngeal angiofibroma. *J Laryngol Otol* 1986; **100**: 599–603.
40. Weprin LS, Siemers PT. Spontaneous regression of juvenile nasopharyngeal angiofibroma. *Arch Otolaryngol Head Neck Surg* 1991; **117**: 796–799.
41. Bryan RN, Sessions RB, Horowitz BL. Radiographic management of juvenile angiofibromas. *Am J Neuroradiology* 1984; **93**: 322–329.
42. McCombe A, Lund VJ, Howard DJ. Recurrence in juvenile angiofibroma. *Rhinology* 1990; **28**: 97–102.
43. Makek MS, Andrews JC, Fisch U. Malignant transformation of a nasopharyngeal angiofibroma. *Laryngoscope* 1989; **99**: 1088–1092.
44. Maniglia AJ, Mazzarella LA, Minkowitz S et al. Maxillary sinus angiofibroma treated with cryosurgery. *Arch Otolaryngol* 1969; **89**: 111–116.
45. Lee DA, Rao BR, Meyer JS et al. Hormonal receptor determination in juvenile nasopharyngeal angiofibromas. *Cancer* 1980; **46**: 547–551.
46. Johns ME, MacLeod RM, Cantrell RW. Estrogen receptors in nasopharyngeal angiofibromas. *Laryngosope* 1980; **90**: 628–634.

47. Johnson S, Kloster JH, Schiff M. The action of hormones on juvenile nasopharyngeal angiofibroma. *Acta Otolaryngol* 1966; **61**: 143–159.
48. Goepfert H, Cangir A, Lee YY. Chemotherapy for aggressive juvenile nasopharyngeal angiofibroma. *Arch Otolaryngol Head Neck Surg* 1985; **111**: 285–289.
49. Rosen L, Hanafee W, Nahum A. Nasopharyngeal angiofibroma, an angiographic evaluation. *Radiology* 1966; **86**: 103–107.
50. Wilson GH, Hanafee WN. Angiographic findings in 16 patients with juvenile nasopharyngeal angiofibroma. *Radiology* 1969; **92**: 279–284.
51. Lasjaunias P, Picard L, Manelfe C et al. Angiofibroma of the nasopharynx. *J Neuroradiology* 1980; **7**: 73–95.
52. Roberson GH, Biller H, Sessions DG et al. Presurgical embolization of the internal maxillary artery in juvenile angiofibroma. *Laryngoscope* 1972; **82**: 1524–1532.
53. Roberson GH, Price AC, Davis JM et al. Therapeutic embolization of juvenile angiofibroma. *Am J Roentgenol* 1979; **133**: 657–663.
54. Pletcher JD, Newton TH, Deho HN et al. Preoperative embolization of juvenile nasopharyngeal angiofibromas of the nasopharynx. *Ann Otol Rhinol Laryngol* 1975; **84**: 740–746.
55. Waldman SR, Levine HL, Astor F et al. Surgical experience with nasopharyngeal angiofibroma. *Arch Otolaryngol* 1983; **107**: 677–682.
56. Steinberger SJ, Wetmore RF. Current management of juvenile nasopharyngeal angiofibroma. *Trans Pa Acad Ophthalmol Otolaryngol* 1984; **37**: 65–70.
57. Siniluoto TMJ, Luotonen JP, Tikkakoski TA et al. Value of preoperative embolization in surgery for nasopharyngeal angiofibroma. *J Laryngol Otol* 1993; **107**: 514–521.
58. Jacobsson M, Petruson B, Svendsen P et al. Juvenile nasopharyngeal angiofibroma. A report of eighteen cases. *Acta Oto-Laryngol* 1988; **105**: 132–139.
59. Gay I, Elidan J, Gordon R. Oronasal fistula: a possible complication of preoperative embolization in the management of juvenile nasopharyngeal angiofibroma. *J Laryngol Otol* 1983; **97**: 651–656.
60. Soong HK, Newman SA, Kumar AAJ. Branch artery occlusion. An unusual complication of external carotid embolization. *Arch Ophthalmol* 1982; **100**: 1909–1911.
61. Briant TDR, Fitzpatrick PJ, Book H. The radiological treatment of juvenile nasopharyngeal angiofibromas. *Ann Otol Rhinol Laryngol* 1973; **79**: 1108–1113.
62. Fitzpatrick PJ, Rider WD. The radiotherapy for nasopharyngeal angiofibroma. *Radiology* 1973; **109**: 171–178.
63. Briant TDR, Fitzpatrick PJ, Berman J. Nasopharyngeal angiofibroma: a twenty year study. *Laryngoscope* 1978; **88**: 1247–1251.
64. Fitzpatrick PJ, Briant DR, Berman JM. The nasopharyngeal angiofibroma. *Arch Otolaryngol* 1980; **106**: 234–246.
65. Cummings BJ. Relative risk factors in the treatment of juvenile nasopharyngeal angiofibroma. *Head Neck Surg* 1980; **3**: 21–26.
66. Belmont J. The Le Fort osteotomy approach for nasopharyngeal and nasal fossa tumours. *Arch Otolaryngol Head Neck Surg* 1988; **114**: 751–754.
67. Mitskavich MT, Carrau RL, Snyderman CH et al. Intranasal endoscopic excision of a juvenile angiofibroma. *Auris Nasus Larynx* 1998; **25**: 39–44.
68. Conley J, Price J. Sublabial approach to the nasal and nasopharyngeal cavities. *Am J Surg* 1979; **138**: 615–618.
69. Casson PR, Bonnano PC et al. The midfacial degloving procedure. *Plast Reconstr Surg* 1974; **53**: 102–113.
70. Pope T. Surgical approach to tumours of the nasal cavity. *Laryngoscope* 1989; **88**: 912–916.
71. Bremer JW, Neel HB, De Santo LW et al. Angiofibroma treatment trends in 150 patients in 40 years. *Laryngoscope* 1986; **96**: 1321–1329.
72. Standefer J, Holt GR, Brown W E et al. Combined intracranial and extracranial excision of nasopharyngeal angiofibroma. *Laryngoscope* 1983; **93**: 772–778.
73. Jafek BW, Krekorian EA, Kirsch WM et al. Juvenile nasopharyngeal angiofibroma: management of intracranial extension. *Head Neck Surg* 1979; **2**: 119–128.
74. Krekorian EA, Kato RH. Surgical management of nasopharyngeal angiofibroma with intracranial extension. *Laryngoscope* 1977; **87**: 154–164.
75. Andrews C, Fisch U, Valavanis A et al. The surgical management of extensive nasopharyngeal angiofibromas with the infratemporal fossa approach. *Laryngoscope* 1989; **99**: 429–437.
76. Tandon DA, Bahadur S, Kacker SK et al. Nasopharyngeal angiofibroma: a nine year experience. *J Laryngol Otol* 1988; **102**: 805–809.
77. Maharaj D, Fernandes CMC. Surgical experience with juvenile nasopharyngeal angiofibroma. *Acta Otolaryngol (Stockh)* 1988; **105**: 132–139.
78. Biller H.F. Juvenile nasopharyngeal angiofibroma. *Ann Otol Rhinol Laryngol* 1978; **87**: 630–632.
79. Boles R, Deedo H. Nasopharyngeal angiofibroma. *Laryngoscope* 1976; **86**: 364–370.
80. Folkman J, Klagsbrun M. Angiogenic factors. (Review). *Science* 1987; **235**: 442.
81. Moscatelli D, Presta M, Rifkin DB. Purification of a factor from human placenta that stimulates capillary endothelial cell protease production, DNA synthesis and migration. *Proc Natl Acad Sci USA* 1986; **83**: 2091.
82. Gospodarowicz D, Neufeld G, Schweigerer L. Fibroblast growth factor. (Review). *Mol Cell Endocrinol* 1986; **46**: 187.
83. Schiff M, Gonzalez AM, Ong M et al. Juvenile nasopharyngeal angiofibromas contain an angiogenic growth factor: basic FGF. *Laryngoscope* **102**: 1992; 940–945.
84. Nagai MA, Butugan O, Logullo A et al. Expression of growth factors, proto-oncogenes, and p53 in nasopharyngeal angiofibromas. *Laryngoscope* 1996; **106**: 190–195.
85. Folkman J, Ling Y. Angiogenesis. *J Biol Chem* 1992; **267**: 10931–10934.
86. Ferrara N, Houck K, Jakeman L et al. Molecular and biological properties of the vascular endothelial growth factor family of proteins. *Endocrinol Rev* 1992; **13**: 18–32.

87. Pertovaara L, Kaipainen A, Mustone T et al. Vascular endothelial growth factor is induced in response to transforming growth factor-β in fibroblastic and epithelial cells. *J Biol Chem* 1994; **269**: 6271–6274.

88. Rissau W. Angiogenesis is coming of age. *Circ Res* 1998; **82**: 926–928.

89. Ross R, Raines EW, Bowen-Pope DF. The biology of platelet-derived growth factor. (Review). *Cell* 1986; **46**: 155.

PART IV

Rehabilitation and reconstruction

26 Complications in head and neck cancer surgery

Aongus J Curran, Jonathan Irish and Patrick J Gullane

Introduction

Despite the best preoperative care, meticulous surgical technique and attentive postoperative management complications frequently arise in the head and neck cancer patient. Many of these individuals are elderly with concomitant medical problems and pose a constant challenge for those involved in their care. Early recognition of the symptoms and signs of complications can prevent amplification of existing problems. The purpose of this chapter is to focus on the major surgical complications and how they are best avoided or treated once they occur.

The neck

Vascular

Before embarking on any type of neck surgery the surgeon must have a thorough knowledge of the anatomy of the region. An understanding of vascular instruments and their use coupled with an ability to dissect and/or repair vessels will be beneficial when bleeding occurs.

Internal jugular vein

Bleeding. The internal jugular (IJV) is associated with severe haemorrhage when torn during surgery. This usually occurs at the upper or lower ends as the vein is mobilized prior to ligation. Occasionally a tear extends from a tributary to the main vessel. It is best to achieve vessel control by mobilizing with blunt clamps. Use of a spreading motion perpendicular to the wall of the vein avoids trauma. Once the vein is mobilized circumferentially, two clamps are applied proximally and distally avoiding injury to the vagus nerve prior to vessel ligation.

Uncontrolled bleeding at the skull base is first controlled with tamponade. When the vein can be identified and clamped it is ligated. In situations where the vessel retracts into the temporal bone Surgicel is packed into the area and may control the bleeding. At times it is necessary to skeletonize the jugular vein or sigmoid sinus to obtain control over the proximal bleeding point and rotate a local muscle flap into the area. Normally at the skull base, the vein should be divided at the level of the transverse process of the atlas taking care to identify and preserve the vagus, hypoglossal and accessory nerves.

Some surgeons do not tie the lower aspect of the vein until most of the neck dissection is completed as back-pressure on the venous system results in troublesome intraoperative bleeding. In this situation, leaving loose silk sutures around a well-exposed vein is necessary.

Excessive bleeding from the stump of the vein as a result of a slipped ligature may be controlled by direct pressure, which prevents air embolism and controls bleeding temporarily. No blind attempts should be made to control bleeding as this may extend a tear. With good light and exposure pressure is gradually removed and the vein rent is ligated as before. Rarely the stump plunges into the superior mediastinum necessitating a sternal split to access the internal jugular or brachiocephalic trunk.

With large venous tears, placing the patient in the Trendelenberg position is employed to reduce the risk of air embolus. In cases where the IJV is being preserved a running 6-0 vascular suture can be used to repair a tear while holding the vessel with a DeBakey vascular forceps. Its non-crushing serrated tip avoids tissue trauma. Also when the vessel is to be preserved tributaries should be ligated away from the main vessel. This avoids eddy currents and thrombosis formation of the IJ that can result in loss of a free flap when one of the venous anastomoses is into this system.[1] Postoperative facial edema and raised intracranial pressure, which are typically seen following radical neck dissection, may be avoided.

Air embolism. This may present as a sucking noise being heard over the torn vein which is usually the IJ. This rare complication occurs when a large neck vein is inadvertently opened causing air to be sucked into the negatively pressured venous system. A loud churning noise over the precordial area may result in hypotension and cardiac arrest when air embolism is not recognized and effectively managed.[8] The involved vein should be immediately compressed and the patient placed in the Trendelenberg position on the operative table. Aspiration of air from the tip of a CVP catheter is often diagnostic as well as therapeutic. In the absence of a CVP catheter discontinuation of nitrous oxide from the anaesthetic circuit and increasing airway pressures to raise venous pressure should be performed. A 'millwheel' murmur and cardiovascular collapse are usually late clinical features. Turning the patient into the left lateral Trendelenberg position may move air from the pulmonary valve and re-establish cardiac output in the event of cardiovascular collapse.

Carotid artery

Stell reported a 3% incidence of carotid artery rupture in a series of 280 patients undergoing major head and neck surgery.[2] The majority died (77%) and 11% had neurological sequelae such as hemiplegia/aphasia. Factors that contribute to this complication include prior radiation, atheromatous disease, stripping of the carotid adventitia due to tumour adherence on the vessel wall and scar formation. A mortality rate of 17% and an incidence of neurological sequelae of 28% is reported after elective ligation[3] compared with a 38% mortality and 88% incidence of neurological complications following non-elective resection.

Modern CT and gadolinium-enhanced MRI provide tumour-artery detail that helps predict the need for resection in cases of suspected invasion. To determine the effects of carotid artery resection in the setting of tumour invasion conventional angiography, dynamic brain scans and balloon-occlusion techniques with somatosensory cortical evoked potentials (SCEP) are used to assess the risks of ICA occlusion.[4–6]

Preoperative evaluation of clinical responses and SCEPs can be performed using balloon-occlusion angiography. A non-detachable balloon is introduced on a double-lumen Swan–Ganz catheter and the patient's responses are recorded for 20 minutes post occlusion. Neurological symptoms or alterations on SCEPs indicate that complete ICA resection without prior bypass surgery would be contraindicated. In 10% of patients permanent neurological deficit will be experienced following resection of the ICA despite negative findings.[6] When a tear occurs in the carotid artery during a resection a decision has to be made whether to ligate or repair the vessel. In a haemodynamically and neurologically stable patient primary repair may be feasible using a 5/0 or 6/0 nylon suture with or without shunting. When tumour invades the vessel, ligation and continuation of the resection are usually indicated. A graft using saphenous vein, Gore-Tex or Dacron may be possible in a clean, non-contaminated neck.[7]

When a tear occurs close to the skull base, ligation or packing may be the only option. If ligation is impossible, reverse bleeding from the circle of Willis can be controlled by oversewing of the vessel ends. Currently, a balloon catheter fed up into the vessel and left in an occluded position to arrest bleeding is the approach of choice. If this fails, craniotomy and trans-temporal ligation of the internal carotid may be required.

Postoperative carotid blow-out. Risk factors include prior irradiation, necrotic cervical flaps (Figure 26.1), or an orocutaneous fistula/pharyngocutaneous fistula. The patient may have undergone a surgical resection of a malignant mucosal lesion involving the oral cavity, pharynx or larynx with a radical neck dissection. Prevention may be possible by excising necrotic tissue and wound toilet with anti-septic dressings and antibiotics. A sentinel bleed may

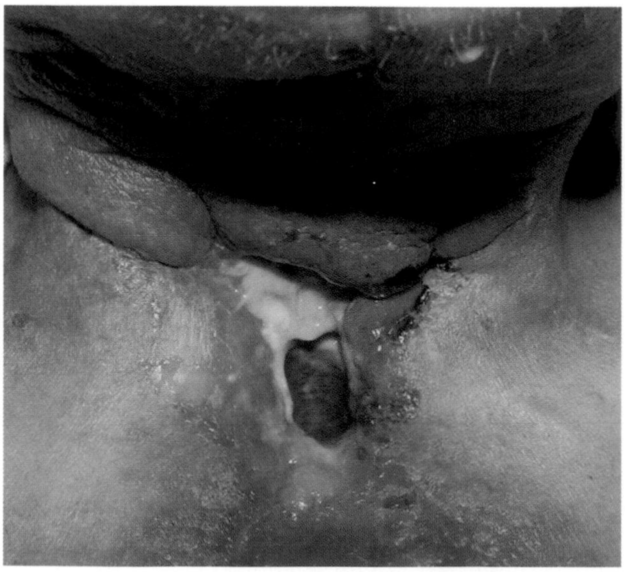

Figure 26.1 8 hours prior to a right carotid blow-out in a patient with a necrotic jejunal reconstruction.

precede the eventual blow-out and allow time to cover the exposed area with well vascularized tissue. When a massive rupture occurs on the ward direct pressure is applied to the site of bleeding, the patient is placed in the Trendelenberg position, immediate fluid replacement instituted and the airway secured. The patient is transferred to the operative room for definitive exploration and management. The vessel stumps are exposed to healthy tissue, ligated and transfixed. After appropriate debridement, the stumps are buried in healthy tissue and the area covered with a vascularized regional flap. Angiography with embolization offers a safe and rapid alternative method of achieving vascular control in patients with spontaneous rupture of the common carotid, carotid bulb or external carotid system once the patient has been stabilized. Recent advances in imaging combined with more successful embolizing techniques have made this possible.

Postoperative hematoma

Haematoma is avoided by meticulous intraoperative haemostasis. It is our practice to attach closed suction drains to a Pleuro-Vac pump or wall suction at –40 cmH_2O for the first 24 hours postoperatively. The source of bleeding is often from the skin edges, from small anterior cervical veins, the external jugular or transverse cervical arterial branches. Occasionally aspiration and application of a pressure dressing is sufficient to manage this problem; however, if bleeding is brisk the source of bleeding needs to be identified and controlled. Returning the patient to the operating room, re-exploring the wound, securing the bleeding point, irrigating the wound thoroughly and placing appropriate drains is mandatory.

Neural complications

General considerations

Gentle handling of soft tissues in the neck and avoiding traction on nerves once identified are central to preventing injuries. Direct neural transection is often due to scar tissue or a failure to identify normal/abnormal anatomy. Scarring may also impede dissection and obscure tissue planes predisposing to injury. Careful use of cautery, suction, and ties helps prevent neural trauma. Nerve monitoring may also help to reduce neural injury.

Marginal mandibular nerve

This branch of the facial nerve emerges from the parotid fascia and descends between the platysma and fascia overlying the submandibular gland. Injury results in a deformity of the lower lip, which is most noticeable when smiling. Feeding may be disrupted due to loss of oral competence. Injury is less likely by: (1) dividing the fascia low over the submandibular and reflecting it superiorly with the dissection. (2) Ligating the posterior facial vein at the lower border of the submandibular gland and dissecting deep to this plane. (3) Identifying the nerve deep to the platysma (with or without a nerve stimulator) and directly following its course. Inadvertent cutting of the nerve should be repaired with perineural 9-0 or 10-0 monofilament nylon.

Accessory nerve (cranial nerve XI)

This emerges from the jugular foramen anterolateral to the IJ. The nerve supplies motor function to the sternocleidomastoid and trapezius muscles. Sacrifice is indicated when gross metastatic disease is present in the posterior triangle, in the high jugulodigastric region or skull base. Inadvertent injury may result in an inability to abduct the shoulder beyond 90 degrees, associated with pain and discomfort in the shoulder joint. In up to 40% of patients no symptoms are experienced after radical neck dissection despite sacrificing the nerve.[9] Recent years have witnessed a trend towards a less radical approach to neck dissection with every attempt to preserve the nerve where possible. Most injuries occur during neck dissections yet simple excision of a node within the posterior triangle or in removal of a branchial cyst may result in inadvertent damage to the nerve. Injury is less likely by: (1) Finding the nerve 1 cm above Erb's point (where the cervical roots course behind the posterior border of the SCM) or as it enters the trapezius (4–6 cm above the clavicle) (Figure 26.2).

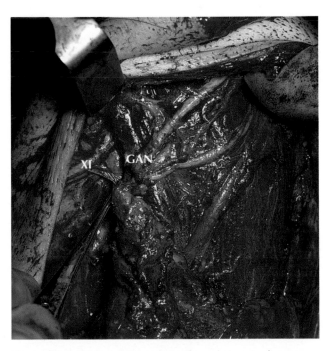

Figure 26.2 Erb's point is where the great auricular nerve (GAN) comes forward over the posterior border of the sternomastoid muscle. The accessory nerve (XI) emerges approximately 1 cm above Erb's point.

(2) Ensuring that the main trunk has been followed towards the jugular foramen. Often a branch enters the SCM and must not be confused with the true course of the nerve. (3) Dissecting along the anterior border of the SCM during selective neck dissection and identifying the nerve posterior to the IJV.

Once identified the accessory nerve should be cleared from surrounding muscle and handled gently, avoiding traction at all times. Complete disruption may be repaired by epineural or perineural repair with 9-0 or 10-0 monofilament suture. Shoulder function after cable grafting results in a level of function intermediary between sacrifice and preservation of the nerve[10]. Intensive physiotherapy and home exercise are beneficial in relieving symptoms and avoiding a permanent 'frozen shoulder'. Improved shoulder function can be achieved by anastomosing the distal transected end of the spinal accessory nerve to the proximal cervical trunk at the time of neck dissection.

Vagus nerve (cranial nerve X)

This emerges at the mid-point of the jugular foramen and courses through the neck between the IJV and carotid within the carotid sheath. Ipsilateral laryngeal and pharyngeal paralysis with loss of sensation at and below the glottis occurs when the nerve is transected low in the neck. Skull base transection results in a more severe form of injury with associated loss of sensation in the supraglottis, paralysis of the pharyngeal musculature and the vocal cord. Dysphagia and aspiration are likely sequelae following this type of damage. Injury is usually avoided by clearly identifying the nerve before ligating the internal jugular vein high in the neck. Vagal injuries as a result of crushing are usually temporary and will improve or recover over several months. When the nerve has been transected nasogastric or gastrostomy tube feeding may be necessary because of dysphagia and aspiration. Improvement in speech and swallowing may be gained by immediate or delayed vocal cord injection of teflon, glycerine or gelfoam. A Type 1 thyroplasty[11] is a worthwhile option when no recovery of a paralysed cord is apparent after 6 months. Cricopharyngeal myotomy may assist swallowing following a high vagal transection, although this is controversial. No real benefit is gained by immediate neurorraphy in cases where the nerve is transected. When the nerve is sacrificed cardiovascular and gastrointestinal symptoms are usually not apparent.

Hypoglossal nerve (cranial nerve XII)

This exits the hypoglossal foramen at the skull base and lies deep to the styloid muscles and posterior belly of the digastric before running deep to the mylohyoid muscle to supply the musculature of the tongue. The nerve is particularly prone to injury where it lies deep to the belly of the digastric muscle just anterosuperior to the carotid bifurcation. Attempts made to control bleeding from a complex of venae comitantes in this area may traumatize the nerve. Time spent cauterizing or ligating small vessels in this region is worthwhile as these vessels tend to retract deep to the nerve once transected. Cautery tips must be visualized at all times with no blind attempts to control bleeding.

Dysarthria and dysphagia usually compensate to an acceptable physiological level after a period of time when one hypoglossal nerve is resected. Bilateral hypoglossal nerve resection renders the patient an oral cripple. Primary neurroraphy is recommended when the nerve is inadvertently cut.

Brachial plexus and the phrenic nerve

The brachial plexus lies within the posterior triangle of the neck between the anterior and middle scalene muscles. It is protected by developing a plane between the deep cervical fascia and the overlying fat pad. Visualization of the plexus prior to clamping the posterior triangle fat pad should prevent injury. The phrenic courses over the anterior scalene muscles running from a lateral to medial direction. Injury results in an immobile elevated diaphragm which can cause postoperative pulmonary atelectasis and pulmonary sepsis. As dissection precedes across the posterior triangle any cervical sensory branches should be divided high thereby avoiding injury to the contributions to the phrenic from C3–5.

Sympathetic plexus

A Horner's syndrome (ptosis, miosis, enopthalmos and anhydrosis) results when the sympathetic plexus is damaged. When dissecting posterior or around the carotid sheath the trunk or the superior cervical ganglion may be inadvertently injured. The middle cervical ganglion lies in close proximity to the inferior thyroid artery. The inferior ganglion lies behind the subclavian on the first thoracic vertebra.

Greater auricular nerve

Derived from C2, C3 and loops behind the sternocleidomastoid muscle to pass superficially on its surface and supply the pinna, parotid region and skin over the mastoid bone, this nerve is easily divided when elevating the upper cervical flaps. Injury results in paraesthesia of the pinna and on occasion the development of a painful neuroma. The nerve should be visualized on the sternocleidomastoid muscle during cervical flap elevation. A decision to preserve or sacrifice the nerve can be made once the status of the upper cervical nodes is identified.

Chylous leaks

Chylous fistulae occur in 1–3% of neck dissections and mostly on the left side (75% of cases).[12] Since chyle consists of the products of fat digestion (chylomicrons) continuous loss may result in significant electrolyte disturbance, impaired wound healing and nutritional imbalance. A leak is recognized intraoperatively by the presence of a collection of clear/milky fluid in the lower neck or by a greasy feel to the surgical gloves (Figure 26.3). No routine attempt is made to identify the thoracic duct during neck dissection.

Intraoperative management

A suspected leak should be confirmed by asking the anaesthetist to apply continuous positive airway pressure (i.e. Valsalva). This increases the flow of chyle by raising the venous and lymphatic pressures. Ligation of the thinned-walled thoracic duct in isolation is not recommended and it is better to include the surrounding tissue with the duct using a non-absorbable suture. The scalene muscle can be included with this suture ligature. Surgical glues and sclerosing agents such as tetracycline have been used with some reported success.[13]

Postoperative management

The presence of fluid with a milky appearance or continuous fluid from the neck drains once feeding begins is likely to be due to a chylous fistula. An intense inflammatory response due to chyle may cause flap compromise or loss of the overlying skin. The presence of triglycerides in this fluid confirms the diagnosis when in doubt. The goal is to optimize the patient's nutritional status and reduce the volume of chyle production. Generally two types of leak arise. The low output leak can usually be managed with aspiration, a pressure dressing and dietary manipulation. Vivonex is a 98% fat-free solution which fulfils these requirements. Collaboration with a dietician and careful monitoring of electrolytes are necessary. A high output leak (> 500 ml/day) for 3 days or longer despite conservative management warrants surgical management. Persistence of this output volume necessitates neck re-exploration on the fourth or fifth postoperative day.[14] Feeding the patient 100–200 ml of cream 2–3 hours preoperatively will improve the chances of identifying the leak at the time or re-exploration. Placing the patient in the Trendelenberg position with the use of continuous positive pressure also helps in localization. The application of a sclerosing agent such as tetracycline after ligating the duct may be beneficial at this stage[13]. Closed suction drainage is used and the patient is managed postoperatively with a medium chain triglyceride diet and careful electrolytic monitoring. A thoracoscopic ligation of the thoracic duct is an effective method of controlling a leak if neck re-exploration fails or in the rare clinical situation of a chylothorax.[15]

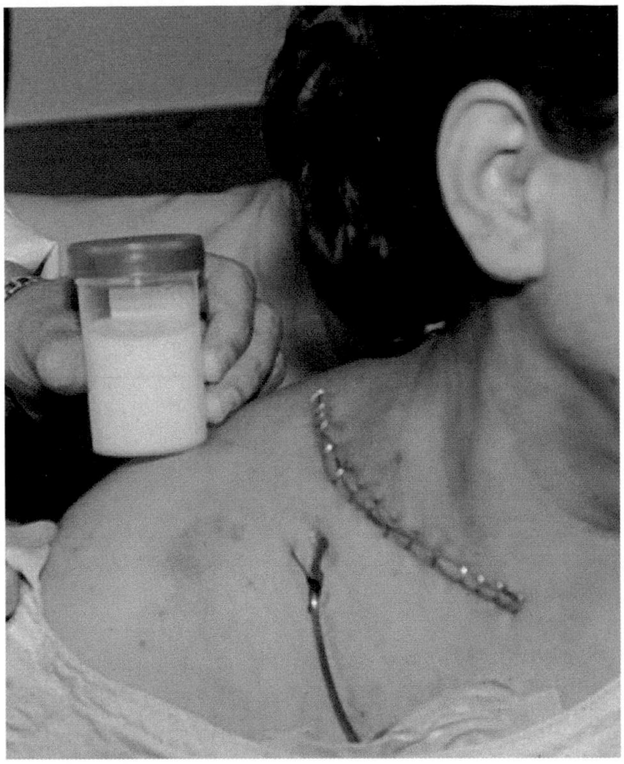

Figure 26.3 Chylous leak.

Pharyngocutaneous fistula

Occurring in 7–38% of patients, usually following oncologic resection of laryngeal or hypopharyngeal tumours,[16] pharyngocutaneous fistula is a serious and relatively common complication associated with major head and neck surgery especially in the irradiated patient. As saliva accumulates in the neck, flap necrosis, carotid exposure and rupture are likely. Risk factors include poor nutritional status, prior irradiation, poor surgical technique and any factor that impairs wound healing.[17] Technical factors such as gentle atraumatic handling of the soft tissues, achieving a watertight anastomosis, ensuring complete haemostasis and using closed suction drains to eliminate dead space are key factors in its prevention. A pharyngocutaneous fistula initially presents with erythema and tenderness in the lower neck incision or skin flap. There may be an associated pyrexia and leukocytosis. The extent of the fistula will become apparent over a number of days and is primarily dependent on the degree of mucosal separation at the site of closure. With massive fistulas the entire neck skin may slough, exposing major neural and vascular structures. The management may be conservative or surgical, which is dictated by size and location of the fistula. Two groups are generally seen.

Group 1

Small fistulas often heal spontaneously with meticulous wound care. This consists of antiseptic dressings, minimal debridement and antibiotics. The patient is fed by nasogastric/gastrostomy tube or parenterally with careful monitoring of nutritional and biochemical status. With this form of management the majority of fistulae heal by secondary intention. Every attempt is made to divert the flow of saliva medial to the carotid artery and to minimize tracheal aspiration. Oral feeding is commenced once the integrity of the upper aerodigestive tract is ensured by contrast medium or methylene blue dye swallow. Small fistulas may take up to 1 month or more to close by a conservative approach.

Group 2

Massive fistulas are associated with extensive overlying skin loss and mucosal dehiscence (Figure 26.4). Initial management consists of controlled exteriorization after surgical debridement. Residual or recurrent disease must be considered a possibility when a large fistula fails to close by secondary intention. The conservative measures described in group 1 also apply to this group of patients and once clean and fresh granulation tissue appears, the wound is usually ready for closure. The exception is the patient with major vessel exposure where urgent cover with vascularized tissue is needed to prevent carotid artery blow-out. Local, pedicled and free flaps may inititally be employed to cover exposed vascular structures.

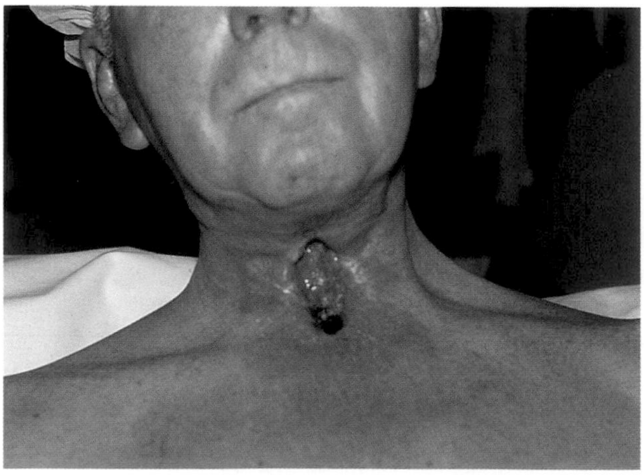

Figure 26.4 A pharyngocutanous fistula following a laryngectomy. Acknowledgements: Mr TJ O'Neill.

With respect to the fistula, the goal is to ensure that mucosal continuity is maintained and adequate skin cover is established. This is typically provided by a myocutaneous pedicled flap, e.g., pectoralis major.

Tracheostomy

General considerations

Complications may be divided into: (1) intraoperative; (2) immediate postoperative; and (3) late postoperative. Anatomical factors such as an enlarged thyroid, a short fat neck, inability to extend the neck due to arthritis, or other causes may render the procedure technically difficult.

When a tracheostomy is to be performed for airway control in a head and neck cancer patient it is advisable to try to secure the airway initially with an endotracheal tube. A flexible bronchoscope will facilitate intubation in a patient with a compromised airway. Alternatively a rigid bronchoscopy can be attempted to establish an airway as complications are increased when the operation is performed on an air-hungry struggling patient. Dexamethasone in the immediate preoperative period may be useful by reducing oedema.

Intraoperative complications

Haemorrhage during tracheostomy is usually from the anterior cervical veins or thyroid gland. In an emergency, the goal is to secure the airway and bleeding can be controlled once this is established. A vertical midline incision is best in an acute airway emergency. This reduces the risk to the local vascular structures. In an elective setting damage to major vascular structures is avoided by dissecting in the mid-line. The suprasternal region should always be palpated to exclude a high-placed innominate artery. The thyroid isthmus is usually retracted superiorly and if obstructing access to the trachea is divided and oversewn. Prior to entering the airway in the elective tracheotomy haemostasis must be complete. In the rare instance where inadvertent injury to the common carotid or innominate occurs, immediate digital pressure is necessary. The wound is opened and the clavicle/sternum split for access. The vessel injury is then sutured, patched, grafted or ligated. Other potential intraoperative complications include development of a false passage, pneumomediastinum, pneumothorax, oesophageal perforation and recurrent laryngeal nerve injury.

Early postoperative complications

Minor bleeding can often be controlled with light packing. If not successful, the patient is returned to the operating room for adequate haemostasis.

Subcutaneous emphysema may indicate partial tube dislodgement or simply be due to a tight wound closure. Correct tube position needs to be established by fibreoptic endoscopic evaluation of the airway or by chest X-ray. All patients should undergo a postoperative chest X-ray, to exclude a pneumothorax and pneumomediastinum.

Airway obstruction due to clots, secretions or tube displacement may occur especially in the first 24 hours following tracheostomy. Close monitoring of vital signs, regular suctioning, humidification and inner cannula cleaning will reduce the possibility of this complication.

Accidental decannulation may occur from an inappropriately sized tube or an incorrect tracheostomy incision. Securing the tracheotomy with sutures and ties will minimize the risks of dislodgement. Ties must be loose enough to allow two fingers to slip beneath them and are best secured when the patient's neck is flexed or in the neutral position. A stay suture at the level of the second tracheal ring will help to pull the trachea forwards and facilitate recannulation in case of early accidental decannulation.

Early tracheostomy tube change or replacement of a dislodged tube can result in pneumothorax or even death. No attempt should be made to change a tracheostomy tube without good light, suction, a range of tracheostomy tubes and a tracheal dilator. Passing a catheter into the airway prior to removing the tracheostomy tube will serve as a guide to locating the airway in the event of tissue collapse into the wound.

Late postoperative complications

Innominate artery erosion or major vessel haemorrhage occurs in approximately 0.4–4.5% of cases.[18] Correct tube placement between the second and third tracheal rings should prevent this complication. Visible pulsations of the tracheostomy tube with each heart beat may signal an impending innominate artery erosion. A sentinel bleed may precede the massive event and should prompt early evaluation of the wound often combined with angiography. In the event of a massive acute haemorrhage, immediate inflation of the tube with digital pressure on the anterior tracheal wall may control the bleed while the patient is urgently taken to the operating area.[19] A sternotomy is performed and the vessel repaired or ligated. In some cases the bleeding may come from the inferior thyroid artery, which should be accessible once the cervical incision is explored.

Subglottic or tracheal stenosis is likely in patients following prolonged endotracheal intubation, a high tracheostomy or cricothyroidotomy.[20] Inappropriate tube size, traumatic intubation, diabetes, and any factor that impairs wound healing are other aetiological factors. In select cases laser excision, dilatation or stenting may be definitive forms of therapy depending on the site, degree of the stenosis and the medical condition of the patient. Resection of the stenotic segment with a primary end-to-end anastomosis may be feasible for stenotic segments up to 4 cm in length.[21]

Tracheo-oesophageal fistula is a rare occurrence (0.01%) and is caused by pressure necrosis from an overinflated and often malpositioned tube.[22] A nasogastric tube often contributes to the development of a fistula by causing post-cricoid ulceration.[23] Diagnosis is confirmed with methylene blue swallow and fibreoptic examination. Conservative management, with enteral or parenteral nutrition may be an adequate form of therapy if aspiration is minimal. The principles of surgical repair involve closing the oesophagus in two layers, excising the necrotic trachea and performing an end-to-end anastomosis via a cervical incision. A local regional or free flap may be needed for tissue cover.

Wound infections

General considerations

The head and neck cancer patient is predisposed to the development of wound infection due to a number of preoperative factors such as malnutrition, prior radiation, anaemia, chronic infection, advanced age, extensive tumour mass and medical factors such as diabetes.[24]

Careful preoperative planning is essential to try to minimize the risk of infection. Adequate nutritional support, attention to dental hygeine, and elimination of any foci of infection in the head and neck region, respiratory system or elsewhere are important preoperative measures.

Preventative measures

Careful skin preparation, draping and maintenance of sterility at all times should reduce the risk of wound infection. Incisons must be placed along relaxed skin tension lines or creases where possible. A number of surgical principles helps to minimize infection such as atraumatic tissue handling, judicious use of cautery, maintaining viability of skin flaps by regular moistening with saline or water, wound irrigation and careful placement of wound drains.

Planning incisions. A knowledge of the vascular supply of the neck is fundamental to avoiding flap ischaemia or loss.[25] A curvilinear incision, which can be extended by dropping a vertical limb provides excellent exposure and cosmesis. A knowledge of the dose and fields of any prior radiation therapy will facilitate a prudent choice of skin incision. It is vital to include the platysma in the skin flap as it carries the blood supply to the overlying skin. A trifurcation point should be placed well posterior to the carotid reducing the risk of vessel exposure in the event of flap necrosis (Figure 26.5).

Prophylactic antibiotics. Prophylactic antibiotics in adequate dosage and at the appropriate time should diminish the likelihood of sepsis. Best results are achieved when administered immediately before, during and for 24–48 hours after surgery.[26] A number of studies have demonstrated the non-efficacy of perioperative antibiotics in clean head and neck surgery. Many surgeons continue to use prophylactic antibiotics in this setting as the cost benefit of preventing even a small number of wound infections is enormous. It is our practice to routinely use prophylactic antibiotics (a third generation cephalosporin) in clean wounds that have been previously irradiated or when dealing with malignant disease. There is a 20–30% risk of developing a wound infection when the upper aerodigestive tract is breached (clean-contaminated wound) justifying the use of antibiotics during this period.[27] It is our practice to use a cephalosporin combined with metronidazole, which provides broad spectrum anaerobic cover in this setting.

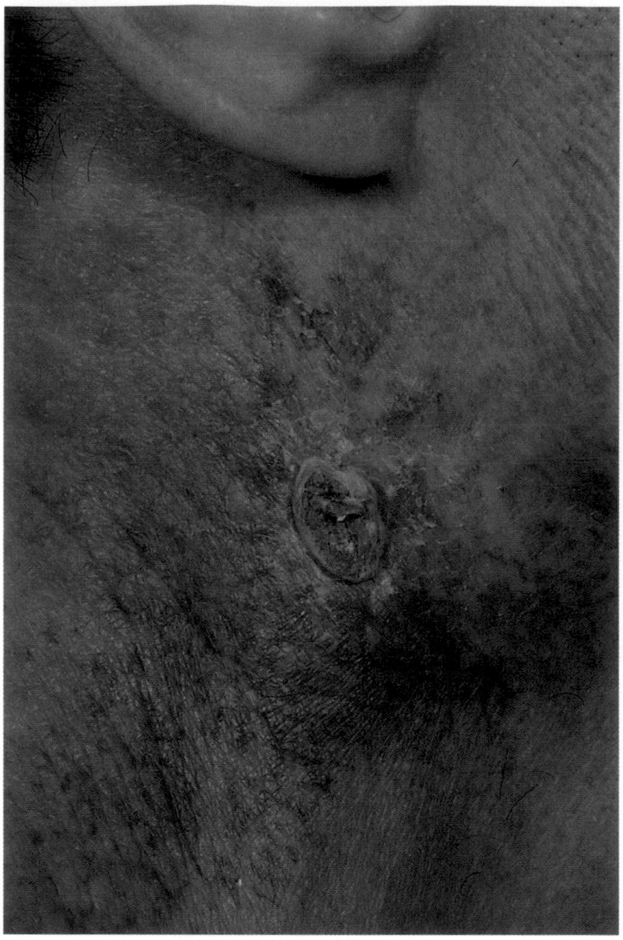

Figure 26.5 Radionecrotic breakdown of skin incision overlying the carotid artery after a radical neck dissection and post-operative radiotherapy.

Management

Many patients develop erythema and induration of the skin especially when previous radiation has been administered. Often this resolves over a number of days and does not progress to wound dehiscence. When the latter arises the principles of care involve regular sterile dressings, wound culture, appropriate antibiotic therapy and attention to nutritional support. Extensive tissue loss may require a skin graft, myocutaneous or free flap for cover.

Oral cavity

General considerations

Cancer of the oral cavity accounts for approximately 30% of head and neck carcinomas. Surgical intervention ranges from simple excision with minimal morbidity to composite resection with its attendant complications. With large resections loss of tongue mobility, intraoral sensation and mandibular support speech and swallowing problems are common.

Mandibular osteotomy has become the preferred method of access for the majority of large oral cavity and oropharyngeal tumours.[28,29] The improved exposure provided by this technique greatly facilitates surgical resection from these sites. Previous reports from our institution have described the complications following this procedure and outlined possible technical aspects to avoid or reduce their incidence.[30,31]

Fistula formation and wound dehiscence continue to prolong hospital stay, occasionally leading to plate exposure and subsequent surgical intervention. Postoperative sepsis related to the osteotomy site is reported to be from 13% to 21%.[32,33]

Previous authors have attempted to identify factors that may predispose to mandibulotomy sepsis although no consensus has been reached as to the precise cause. Preoperative irradiation and type of fixation (wire or plate) does not appear to influence the incidence of sepsis although most studies have been retrospective in nature.[36,39] Patients who undergo step osteotomy as opposed to linear cuts and those who have a marginal mandibulectomy in combination with the resection are not at an increased risk of infection.[34]

A failure to achieve a watertight mucosal closure adjacent to the mandibulotomy site even when utilizing a free flap to reconstruct the defect is an important factor. Midline or parasymphyseal osteotomy is preferred to a more lateral osteotomy.

Orocutaneous fistula

Management is similiar to that of a pharyngocutaneous fistula. The majority respond to conservative measures except those extending over the carotid artery or when wound healing fails, especially in previously irradiated wounds (Figure 26.6). Fresh vascularized tissue is needed in these situations. Other complications associated with mandibulotomy are dental injury, malunion, delayed union or non-union and neural injuries.

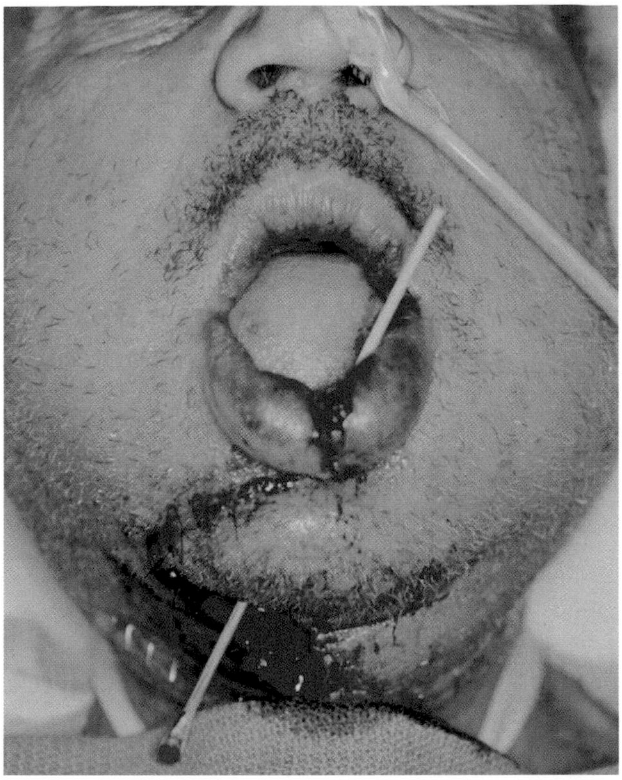

Figure 26.6 Orocutaneous fistula following composite resection and free flap repair in a previously irradiated patient.

Dental injury

Osteotomy through a tooth root predisposes to infection, tooth loss and instability of the mandibulotomy site. A tooth extraction intraoperatively may be necessary when teeth are too close together. The osteotomy can be performed through the gap to prevent these complications. Care must be taken to ensure the plate is positioned below the tooth roots to avoid injury with screws. Any patient who may require radiotherapy as part of their management must have a dental assessment. Dental prophylaxis before surgery will reduce the likelihood of dental sepsis contributing to postoperative problems.

Problems with union

A failure to accurately oppose the mandibular fragments or inadequate immobilization may predispose to a failure of bony union. This may lead to plate or mandible exposure. It is our practice to use an eight-hole 2.4-mm titanium reconstruction plate and tension band splint with wire to ensure immobilization of the mandibular fragments, following a midline mandibulotomy. Patients are fed by gastrostomy or nasogastric tube until the oral mucosa is well healed. This may take 10 days or more to prevent wound dehiscence.

Paraesthesia

Osteotomy lateral to the mental foramen causes anaesthesia to the ipsilateral lower lip and gums. When the mandible is well realigned many patients recover sensation after 3–6 months.

Osteoradionecrosis

The reported incidence of osteoradionecrosis is 2–22% following radiation to the mandible or maxilla.[35] Osteoradionecrosis is a serious complication of radiotherapy when used for head and neck cancer with considerable variation in severity (Figure 26.7). No single treatment modality has been entirely successful.

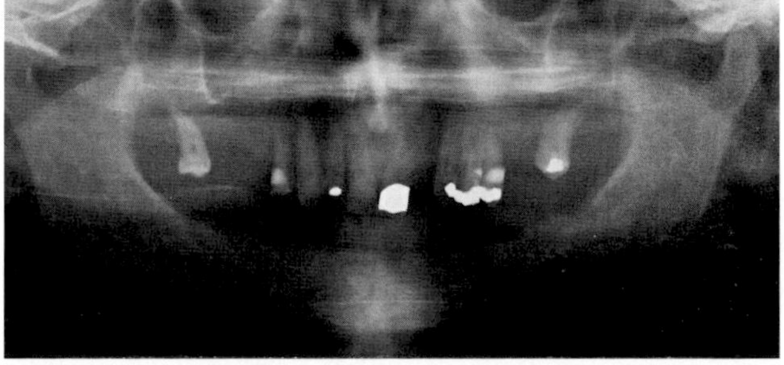

Figure 26.7 Osteoradionecrosis of the mandible.

Prevention

Patients must undergo a dental evaluation prior to therapy. It is controversial as to whether preradiation extraction reduces the risk of osteoradionecrosis conclusively.[36] Generally, teeth in the primary field of radiation that show periapical or periodontal disease and that are unlikely to be viable following radiotherapy are extracted.[37]

Management

Acute infection is treated with broad spectrum antibiotics, analgesia, oral hygiene, and by avoiding irritants such as tobacco smoke and alcohol. Sequestrectomy and hyperbaric oxygen may benefit some patients with less extensive symptoms and/or disease state. Patients with intractable pain, trismus and persisting infection are candidates for major surgical resection. This involves resecting the affected segment and using a vascularized bone graft such as fibula or iliac crest to reconstruct the mandible.

Salivary glands

Parotidectomy

Facial nerve paralysis

The reported incidence of temporary paralysis is approximately 30% and permanent paralysis less than 0.5% following superficial parotidectomy.[38] The risk to the nerve is increased when total parotidectomy is performed for large tumours or for malignant disease. Over 90% of temporary injuries resolve within 12 months. Apart from the severe psychological sequelae associated with total paralysis, eye function, mastication and emotional response are also impaired.

Prevention

The anaesthetist should avoid using a long-acting muscle relaxant to allow stimulation of neural tissue as the dissection proceeds. A wide surgical exposure using a modified 'Blair' incision is used. Tissue landmarks for the nerve are employed to avoid inadvertent injury and include: (1) the tragal pointer: the nerve is located 1 cm below and medial to this cartilaginous pointer; (2) the posterior belly of the digastric serves as a guide to the plane of the nerve; (3) the mastoid bone and tympanomastoid suture: the nerve is 6–8 mm medial to this landmark; (4) when the nerve cannot be identified by an antegrade approach, it may be possible to find a peripheral branch and trace it back to the main trunk.

Technical considerations

Once the nerve is identified it diverges laterally to the midgland region and the surgeon must be cognizant of this as dissection proceeds in the plane above the nerve. A nerve stimulator, set at 0.5 mA initially, is used to confirm identification. Repeated stimulation increases the likelihood of neuropraxia postoperatively. During mobilization bipolar cautery tips must be visualized at all times to avoid thermal trauma. No blind attempts are made to control bleeding and no undue pressure or traction must be placed on the nerve. Continuous facial nerve monitoring may be beneficial for large tumours, revision procedures and malignant lesions. Operating loupes are used by some surgeons and may help preserve smaller peripheral branches.

Management

Unintentional division of any portion of the nerve should be followed by immediate microsurgical reanastomosis with 9/0 or 10/0 monofilament suture. Coaption must be precise and free from tension. An interposition nerve graft with sural, greater auricular or lateral cutaneous nerve should be considered in cases where the nerve has to be sacrificed and primary reanastomosis is not an option.

All patients with facial paralysis must have appropriate eye care when the branch to the orbicularis oris has been damaged. Eye moisturizers, lubricants and taping the eye at night will prevent corneal desiccation. An ophthalmology consultation should be obtained if any complication such as keratitis or corneal ulceration is suspected. The management of permanent facial nerve paralysis may require dynamic procedures such as interposition nerve graft, facial hypoglossal anastomosis, cross-face nerve transfer, masseter or temporalis muscle transfer to improve facial function. Adynamic procedures using gold-weighted implants for ocular rehabilitation, Goretex implants, facial slings, rhytidectomy and blepharoplasty may also be helpful. The patient must be aware that it is not possible to restore complete facial function and the goal should be to improve the existing situation.

Other complications following parotidectomy include haemorrhage, infection, and flap necrosis. Others include commonly symptomatic Frey's syndrome and rarely salivary fistula.

Submandibular gland

Haemorrhage

Intraoperative haemorrhage from the facial artery and veins can be troublesome unless care is taken during identification and ligation. Postoperatively haematoma formation can lead to displacement of the tongue and airway compromise. Injury to the marginal mandibular branch of the facial nerve can be avoided by planning the incision 2 cm below the angle of the mandible and preserving the nerve as previously described.

Lingual nerve trauma is fortunately rare and results in loss of sensation to the anterior two-thirds of the tongue. The nerve lies deep to the mylohyoid muscle and can be identified once the muscle is retracted anteriorly. When dividing the submandibular ganglion the ligature should be placed away from the nerve to avoid injury. Hypoglossal nerve injury is rare and is best avoided by careful dissection and identification during mobilization.

Skull base

Over the past two decades a multidisciplinary approach involving otolaryngologists, neurosurgeons and plastic surgeons has evolved in the management of skull-base tumours. This has resulted in a reduction in postoperative morbidity and an increase in the number of these procedures being performed world-wide. Central to this development has been the introduction of improved, safer methods of access to the skull base coupled with an ability to reconstruct large defects with microvascular free flaps.

Complications involving these procedures may be catastrophic for the patient intraoperatively or postoperatively. The overall complication rate may be as high as 33% and may be infectious, neurovascular or related to cranial nerve trauma. Cerebrospinal fluid (CSF) leakage and meningitis are the commonest complications to arise.

Cerebrospinal fluid leakage

Cerebrospinal fluid leakage may arise following anterior skull base resection, lateral skull base resection, post transsphenoidal hypophysectomy or maxillectomy. The identification of the anatomical site of CSF rhinorrhoea may be difficult especially when intermittent in nature.[39] Unrecognized CSF leakage can result in meningitis and possibly death.[40]

Diagnosis

When the leak is profuse and clear the diagnosis is obvious. Often a small and intermittent leak may be overlooked or misinterpreted when mixed throughout nasal secretions. Collection of nasal discharge for a 'halo sign' on a cotton sheet or glucose content of greater than 30 mg/ml has traditionally been regarded as diagnostic of cerebrospinal fluid.[41] There is a high incidence of false positive results due to contamination of fluid with lacrimal secretions and blood. Recent reports have indicated that analysis of secretions for β2 transferrin provides a highly sensitive, selective, rapid and non-invasive test for the detection of CSF leakage.[42–44] Equally important is the demonstration of an absence of beta-transferrin, which obviates the need for further investigation and/or surgical intervention.

Investigations

Intrathecal tracers, fluorescein, metrizamide, and gamma cameras with a radioisotope tracer (radioactive cisternography, RIC) have been utilized to detect the source of the leak when not obvious.[45,46] Contrast CT cisternography (CCTC) has now replaced RIC yet both are invasive, time consuming and often insensitive. Recently MRI cisternography has been used to locate the precise site of CSF fistulae.[47] By comparison with other techniques MRI cisternography is fast, non-invasive and carries no apparent risk to the patient. The demonstration of a high signal through the cribriform plate and paranasal sinuses, which is continuous and similar to that of CSF in the basal cisterns is considered to be diagnostic of a fistula.

Prevention

Prevention of leaks may be difficult especially when dura is deliberately resected. In such circumstances the area must be carefully repaired primarily or with local or distant tissue as contamination with bacteria from the nasal cavity or sinonasal tract will result in meningitis.

Management

Conservative treatment consists of bed rest, laxatives, avoiding raising intracranial pressure by nose blowing or straining, and antibiotics. CSF-penetrating antibiotics are widely used although it is controversial whether the risk of meningitis is reduced.[48] A lumbar drain may also be beneficial particularly when dealing with a vigorous leak. The patient is kept supine and CSF pressure maintained between 10 and 15 cmH_2O.

Persistence of leakage beyond 7–10 days necessitates surgical intervention. Leaks occurring from the pneumatized temporal bone are best managed by obliterating the mastoid space with fascia, abdominal fat or a local temporalis muscle flap. To prevent CSF entering the Eustachian tube the middle ear should be sealed from the mastoid antrum.

Clivus leaks may require a free vascularized flap (e.g. rectus abdominis) to adequately seal the defect. Anterior skull-base leaks may be repaired via an extracranial or intracranial approach. A leak accessible through the nose may be repaired transnasally either under direct vision or endoscopically.

Fibrin glue, fat, fascia lata and local flaps may be used to seal the defect. A successful closure in 70–80% of patients can be achieved with a transnasal repair. Despite these excellent results it is estimated that 30–40% of all fistulas will recur after initial therapy. This failure may be due to an inadequate initial repair, a true recurrence at the original site and/or leakage from another site on the skull base.

Meningitis

Meningitis is a major cause of postoperative morbidity. Prolonged surgery, CSF leakage, and contamination with the bacterial flora of the upper aerodigestive tract are contributing factors. The use of broad spectrum antibiotics, a watertight reconstruction of the dura when feasible, and surgical precautions to minimize the potential for contaminating the operative field are vital preventative measures. Any patient with alteration in mental status, progressive headache and persistent pyrexia not attributable to other sources should have this diagnosis suspected. Cerbrospinal fluid must be sampled by a lumbar puncture to confirm the diagnosis.

Pneumocephalus

Pneumocephalus is more commonly seen after anterior skull-base resection and becomes significant when air becomes trapped and continues to accumulate resulting in raised intracranial pressure and displacement of intracranial contents.

Prevention

Preventative measures include complete sealing of breached dura, avoiding lumbar drains and performing a tracheostomy to prevent air being diverted intracranially with coughing or sneezing.

Management

Needle aspiration via a frontal burr hole may suffice. Re-exploration of the wound and tacking the pericranial flap forwards and/or resuturing the dura may be necessary if the patient continues to deteriorate.

Cranial nerve injury

The location of the tumour dictates which nerves are likely to be injured. Olfaction is lost when the frontal lobes are retracted during anterior skull-base approaches. Surgery in proximity to the cavernous sinus and petrous apex is likely to damage the III–IV, V and VI cranial nerves.

The facial nerve is injured typically in lateral skull base and posterior fossa surgery. Manipulation should be minimal when preservation of neural function is the goal. Cranial nerves IX, X and XII are at risk during dissection of tumours near the lower clivus and foramen magnum. With benign tumours it is usually possible to dissect and preserve the nerve. Advances in intraoperative monitoring have resulted in increased neural preservation. The most devasting neuropathies occur following lateral skull-base surgery involving the lower cranial nerves IX, X and XII.

Cerebral oedema, infarction and haemorrhage

These are other potential causes of deterioration in mental status postoperatively. Carotid artery vasospasm may occur especially with lateral skull-base surgery leading to a fatal cerebrovascular accident. Significant oedema and infarction are best avoided by minimal brain retraction. Epidural or subdural bleeds are evacuated unless collections are small.

Epidural abscess formation

This may occur in the early postoperative period or several weeks later. Acute neurological deficit is the usual presentation. Infected bone may be a contributing factor and exploration with removal is indicated. Other infectious complications include osteomyelitis and frontal sinusitis.

Reconstructive complications

Skin grafts

The principal complications of skin grafts are caused by haematoma formation or inadequate stabilization, which may lead to graft failure or infection. It is important to ensure adequate haemostasis and applying a graft of suitable thickness helps to prevent these complications. Adaptic gauze with saline/acroflavin-soaked cotton wool secured with a tie over dressing will minimize graft movement.

Local flaps

Errors in design or technical factors are responsible for most local flap failures. Blood supply entering the base of the flap may be altered by previous surgery or radiation (Figure 26.8). Use of skin hooks, avoiding compression and introducing the flap into a dry recipient bed are technical points that help maintain viability. Basing a flap inferiorly is worthwhile for facial flaps as this facilitates venous drainage. When rotation or transposition flaps require cut-backs, enough width must be preserved to avoid flap ischaemia. Excessive tension on the distal aspect of the flap must also be avoided.

Postoperatively the wound should be kept moist with a topical antibiotic that helps remove non-viable tissue and uncovers healthy tissue.

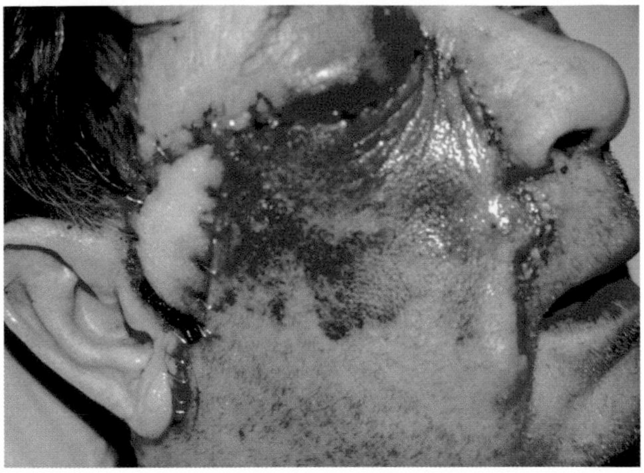

Figure 26.8 Failed transposition flap in a previously irradiated patient.

Myocutaneous flaps

A thorough knowledge of the vascular supply of any myocutaneous flap is essential prior to elevation. Partial or complete flap necrosis may occur. Generally complete flap loss occurs in less than 10% of most series (Figure 26.9).[49,50]

Prevention of complications

Separating the loosely attached skin and subcutaneous tissue from the underlying muscle by shearing can avulse an already tenuous blood supply. Avoid inwardly bevelled skin incisions, which tend to compromise the skin paddle. The vascular pedicle must be identified and preserved. Kinking must be avoided and there should be no undue compression from skin flaps, tracheostomy ties or other factors such as the mandible or reconstruction plates when insetting the flap.

In the postoperative period, the patient should be nursed head-up without compressive dressings. Wound drains help to prevent haematoma and flap compromise. Prompt debridement of any areas of skin necrosis prevents infection and potential loss to the underlying muscle. Bleeding, seroma, and fistulization are other potential sequelae.

(a) (b)

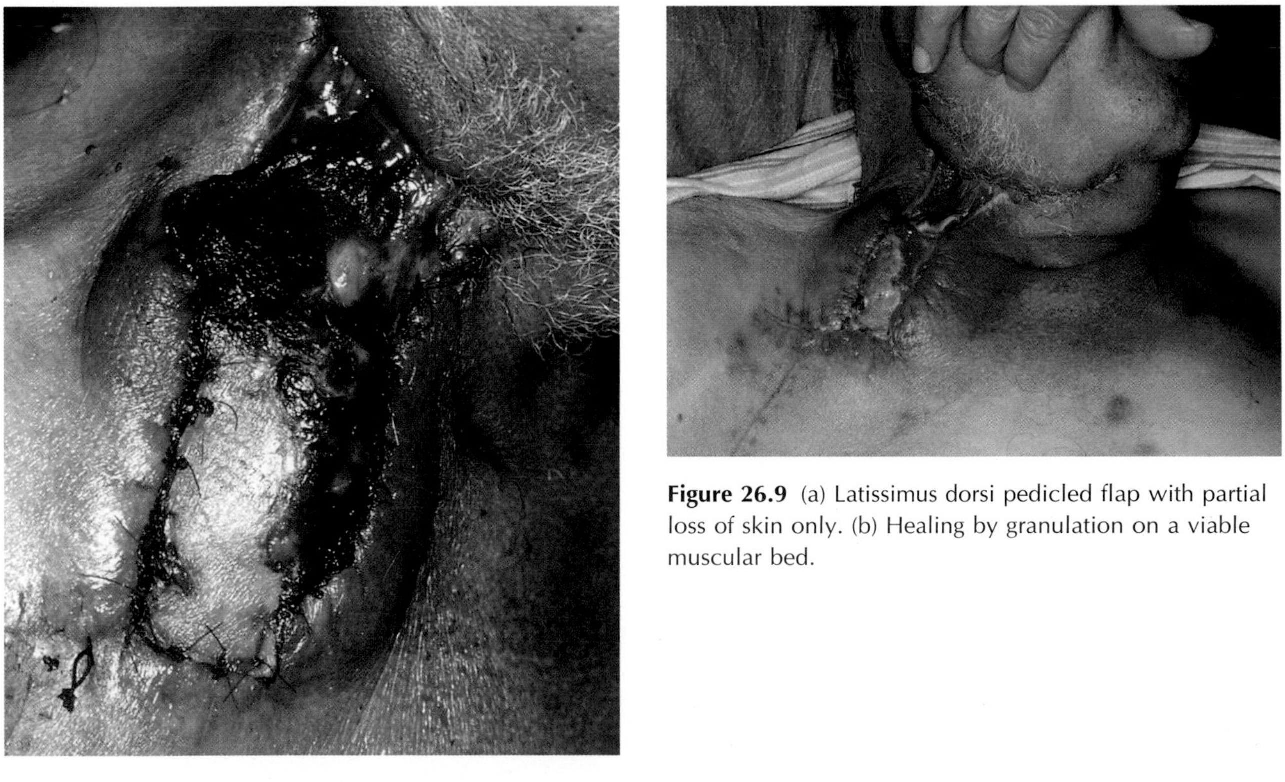

Figure 26.9 (a) Latissimus dorsi pedicled flap with partial loss of skin only. (b) Healing by granulation on a viable muscular bed.

Free flaps

Over the past decade microvascular free flaps have become widely utilized in head and neck surgery. Presently, cosmetic and functional restoration is the goal following major ablative resection. Certain flaps such as the radial forearm, the rectus abdominis and free jejunal flap have reasonably reliable vascular pedicles and are valuable tools in reconstructive head and neck surgery. Factors known to impair flap survival other than technique include prior radiation, smoking, atherosclerosis, diabetes, advanced age, and sepsis.[51]

Technical considerations

Loss of vascular perfusion is the main complication associated with free flaps. Donor and recipient vessels must be adequate prior to flap transfer as reanastomosis has to be speedy to prevent flap loss due to ischaemia. Free jejunal flaps are particularly sensitive to ischaemia (see Figure 26.1). When a vein graft is needed it should be prepared prior to dividing the vascular pedicle. Once revascularized considerable bleeding may arise from the flap and haematoma formation must be avoided.

Checking viability

In the postoperative period flap viability is checked visually and with doppler. Colour, bleeding to pin-prick and capillary refill are inexpensive, simple and reliable methods of flap monitoring. Other objective methods include measuring heat, pH, intraflap BP, light absorbancy, CO_2/O_2 content and fluorescein dye inspection with a Wood's light.[52,53] General flap viability can be determined by visual inspection by an experienced observer. Arterial insufficiency is recognized clinically by a flap that is cool to touch, white and non-blanching. Venous insufficiency is commoner and gives the flap a bluish appearance, and causes swelling and dark bleeding on pin-prick testing. Vasodilators and low-molecular-weight dextrans have been used with little evidence of success in a case of impending flap compromise. Prompt re-exploration and revision is crucial as most flaps fail to recover after 10–12 hours of ischaemia. Revision has a quoted success rate of 60–83%[53] although a more realistic figure is approximately 50%.

Thrombosed vessels require resection on either side of the anastomosis.[54] Once normal vessel wall is reached and good blood flow is re-established a reanastomosis can be performed. Flushing the arterial or venous ends with heparinized saline helps to remove thrombus. Occasionally, an interpositional vein graft or cephalic vein mobilization is necessary to avoid excessive anastomotic tension.

REFERENCES

1. Brown DH, Mulholland S, Yoo JH et al. Internal jugular vein thrombosis following modified neck dissection. In press.
2. Stell PK. Catastrophic haemorrhage after major neck surgery. *Br J Surg* 1969; **56**: 525.
3. Moore OS, Baker HW. Carotid artery ligation in surgery of the head and neck. *Cancer* 1955; **8**: 712.
4. Erba S, Horton J, Latchaw R et al. Balloon test occlusion of the internal carotid artery with stable xenon/CT cerebral flow imaging. *AJNR* 1989; **9**: 533–538.
5. Sekhar L, Sen C, Jho H. Saphenous vein graft bypass of the cavernous carotid artery. *J Neurosurg* 1990; **72**: 35–41.
6. Atkinson D, Jacobs L, Weaver A. Elective carotid resection for squamous cell carcinoma of the head and neck. *Am J Surg* 1984; **148**: 483–488.
7. Oleott C, Fee WE, Enzmenn DR et al. Planned approach to the management of malignant invasion of the carotid artery. *Am J Surg* 1981; **142**: 123–125.
8. Havas TE, Gullane PJ. *Prevention of Complications in Head and Neck Surgery. A Self-Instructional Package.* American Academy of Otolaryngology-Head and Neck Surgery Foundation, 1987.
9. Leipzig B, Suen JY, English JL et al. Functional evaluation of the spinal accessory nerve after neck dissection. *Am J Surg* 1983; **146**: 526–530.
10. Weisberger EC, Lingemen RE. Cable grafting of the spinal accessory nerve for rehabilitation of shoulder function after radical neck dissection. *Laryngoscope* 1987; **97**: 915–918.
11. Isshiki N, Taira T, Kojima H et al. Recent modifications in thyroplasty type I. *Ann Otol Rhinol Laryngol* 1989; **98**: 777–779.
12. Conley JJ. Operative complications. In: *Complications in Head and Neck Surgery.* Philadelphia: WB Saunders. 1977; 25–36.
13. Kassel RN, Havas TE, Gullane PJ. The use of topical tetracycline in the management of persistent chylous fistulae. *J Otolaryngol* 1987; **16**: 174–178.
14. Crumley RL, Smith JD. Postoperative chylous fistula prevention and management. *Laryngoscope* 1976; **86**: 804–813.
15. Kent RB, Pinson TW. Thorascopic ligation of the thoracic duct. *Surg Endosc* 1993; **7**: 52–55.

16. Giordano AM, Adams GL. Pharyngocutaneous fistula after laryngeal surgery. *Otolaryngol Head Neck Surg* 1984; **92**: 19–23.
17. Gullane PJ, Jabbour JN, Conley JJ et al. Correlation of pharyngeal fistulization with preoperative radiotherapy, reduced serum albumin and dietary obstruction. *Otolaryngol Head Neck Surg* 1979; **87**: 311–317.
18. Schlaepfer K. Fatal haemorrhage following tracheostomy for laryngeal diphtheria. *JAMA* 1924; **82**: 1581–1582.
19. Myers WO, Lawton BR, Santter RD. An operation for tracheal-innominate fistula. *Arch Surg* 1972; **105**: 269–274.
20. Esses BA, Jakek BW. Cricothyroidotomy: a decade of experience in Denver. *Ann Otol Rhinol Laryngol* 1987; **96**: 519–524.
21. Maddaus MA, Toth JL, Gullane PJ et al. Subglottic tracheal resection and synchronous laryngeal reconstruction. *J Thorac Cardiovasc Surg* 1992; **104**: 1443–1450.
22. Thomas AN. Management of tracheoesophageal fistula caused by cuffed tracheal tubes. *Am J Surg* 1972; **124**: 181–187.
23. Freidman M, Bairn H, Shelton V et al. Laryngeal injuries secondary to nasogastric tubes. *Ann Otol* 1981; **90**: 469–474.
24. Hooley R, Levine H, Flores TC et al. Predicting postoperative head and neck complications using nutritional assessment: the prognostic nutritional index. *Arch Otolaryngol* 1983; **107**: 725–729.
25. Freeland AP, Rogers JH. The vascular supply of the cervical skin with reference to incision planning. *Laryngoscope* 1975; **85**: 714.
26. Burke JF. The effective period of preventive antibiotic action in experimental incisions and dermal lesions. *Surgery* 1961; **50**: 161.
27. Johnson J, Myers EN, Thearle PB et al. Antimicrobial prophylaxis for contaminated head and neck surgery. *Laryngoscope* 1984; **94**: 46–51.
28. MacGregor IA, McDonald DG. Mandibular osteotomy in the surgical approach to the oral cavity. *Head Neck Surg* 1983; **5**: 457–462.
29. Spiro RH, Gerold FP, Shah JP, Sessions RB, Strong EW. Mandibulotomy approach to oropharyngeal tumours. *Am J Surg* 1985; **150**: 466–469.
30. Davidson J, Freeman J, Gullane P et al. Mandibulotomy and radical radiotherapy: compatible or not? *J Otolaryngol* 1988; **17**: 279–281.
31. McCann K, Irish J, Gullane P et al. Complications associated with rigid fixation of mandibulotomies. *J Otolaryngology* 1994; **23**: 210–215.
32. Christopoulos E, Carrau R, Segas J et al. Transmandibular approaches to the oral cavity and oropharynx. *Arch Otolaryngol* 1992; **118**: 1164–1167.
33. DeSanto LW, Whicker JH, Devine KD. Mandibular osteotomy and lingual flaps. *Arch Otolaryngol* 1975; **101**: 652–655.
34. Dubner S, Spiro R. Median mandibulotomy: a critical assessment. *Head Neck* 1991; **13**: 389–393.
35. Epstein JB, Wong FLW, Stevenson-Moore P. Osteoradionecrosis: clinical experience and a proposal for classification. *J Oral Maxillofac Surg* 1987; **45**: 104–110.
36. Bedwinek JM, Shukovsky LJ, Fletcher GH et al. Osteoradionecrosis in patients treated with definitive radiotherapy for squamous cell carcinomas of the oral cavity and naso- and oropharynx. *Radiology* 1976; **119**: 665–667.
37. Breumer JP, Curtis TA, Firtell DN. Radiation therapy of head and neck tumours. In: *Maxillofacial Rehabilitation: Prosthodontic and Surgical Considerations*. St Louis: Mosby Year Book, 1979; 56–60.
38. MeGurt M, Renahan A, Gleave EM. Clinical significance of the tumour capsule in the treatment of parotid pleomorphic adenomas. *Br J Surg* 1996; **83**: 1747–1749.
39. Walsh MA, Curran AJ. Cerbrospinal fluid rhinnorrhoea. *Br J Neurosurg* 1997; **11**: 189–190.
40. Park J, Streizow VV, Freidman WH. Current management of cerbrospinal fluid rhinorrhoea. *Laryngoscope* 1983; **93**: 1294–1300.
41. Ornmaya AK. Spinal fluid fistulae. *Clin Neurosurg* 1975; **23**: 363–392.
42. Meurman O, Irjala K, Juonpaa J, Laurent B. A new method of identification of cerebrospinal fluid leakage. *Acta Otolaryngol* 1979; **87**: 366–369.
43. Ryall RG, Peacock MK, Simpson DA. Usefulness of beta-2 transferrin assay in the detection of cerebrospinal fluid leaks following head injury. *J Neurosurg* 1992; **77**: 737–739.
44. Skedros DG, Cass SP, Hirsch BE, Kelly RH. Beta-2 transferrin assay in the clinical management of cerebrospinal fluid and perilymphatic leaks. *J Otolaryngol* 1993; **22**: 341–344.
45. Nicklaus P, Dutcher PO, Kido DK et al. New imaging techniques in the diagnosis of cerebrospinal fluid fistula. *Laryngoscope* 1988; **98**: 1065–1068.
46. Crowe HJ, Keogh C. The localization of cerebrospinal fluid fistulae. *Lancet* 1956; **ii**: 325–327.
47. Eljamel MS, Pidgeon CN, Toland J et al. MRI cisternography, localization of CSF fistulae. *Br J Neurol* 1994; **8**: 433–437.
48. Eljamel MS. Fractures of the middle third of the face and cerebrospinal fluid rhinorrhoea. *Br J Neurol* 1994; **8**: 289–293.
49. Shah JP, Haribhakti V, Loree TR et al. Complications of the pectoralis major myocutaneous flap in head and neck reconstruction. *Am J Surg* 1990; **160**: 352.
50. Biller HF, Baek SM, Lawson W. Pectoralis major myocutaneous island flap in head and neck surgery. *Arch Otolaryngol* 1981; **107**: 23.
51. Leonard A, Brennan M, Colville J. The use of continuous temperature monitoring in the postoperative management of microvascular cases. *Br J Plast Surg* 1982; **35**: 337–342.
52. Dingwall JA, Lord JW. The fluorescein test in the management of tubed flaps. *Bull Johns Hopkins Hosp* 1943; **73**: 129.
53. Goldberg J, Sepka R, Perona B. Laser doppler flow measurements of common cutaneous donor sites for reconstructive surgery. *Plast Reconstr Surg* 1990; **85**: 58.
54. Tsai TM, Bennett D, Pedersen W. Complications and vascular salvage of free-tissue transfers to the extremities. *Plast Reconstr Surg* 1988; **82**: 1022–1026.

27 Principles of head and neck reconstruction following cancer surgery

David Ross and Nicholas K James

Introduction

Resection of a head and neck cancer confronts the patient with several major problems in addition to the impact of their diagnosis; the concentration of anatomical structures intrinsic to eating, breathing and speech ensures these functions may be severely compromised. In addition, surgery may greatly alter an individual's appearance, thereby affecting their ability to function in society. The effects of tumour excision on the patient's physiological function and self-esteem cannot be overestimated and, where possible, considerable effort should be made to minimize the impact of both the diagnosis and treatment. By definition this requires the contribution of a multidisciplinary team, each contributing to help restore the patient to some degree of their premorbid state.

Over the last three decades considerable advances have been made in head and neck surgery. Amongst the most significant of these have been developments in reconstructive surgery of the patient following tumour ablation. The aim of reconstruction is therefore two-fold as it attempts to correct both functional and anatomical deficit.

In the formative years of plastic surgery, when contemplating the underlying principles of reconstruction, Sir Harold Gillies noted that losses must be replaced in kind.[1] In keeping with this dictum, where possible resected tissues are replaced with tissues that approximate in terms of type, thickness, texture, mobility, sensation and function. However, this is rarely achieved. To this end the reconstructive surgeon has at his or her disposal a number of flaps that may be regularly called upon to replace the constituent elements of the resected part, that is provide cover, support or lining. The challenge and reward of this aspect of surgery come in successfully matching and selecting one of a number of methods to the patient's needs and physical capabilities. Results are never optimal if the patient is tailored to a single method of repair. Appearance and function may be further enhanced by application of prosthetics and osseointegrated implants.

Thus in the first instance, it is essential to evaluate the patient preoperatively, to comprehend the extent of resection and the potential size of the resultant defect. It is equally important to appreciate the patient's concerns and expectations. By this process the possible methods of reconstruction may be discussed with the patient, giving a realistic picture of the expected function and appearance.

This chapter is divided into three sections. In the first, basic principles of reconstruction are discussed with particular reference to both patient and technique selection. The second section describes several methods of reconstruction. It is not intended to provide an exhaustive description of all known flaps, but rather to present the principles and methods that govern selection of a particular method and that experience has shown to be reliable and practical. Other chapters will discuss reconstruction of the mandible, the skull base, and intraoral region in greater detail. The final section will consider the application of these methods to reconstruction of specific sites within the head and neck.

Principles of head and neck reconstruction

Patients undergoing surgery for head and neck cancer should, ideally, be treated by a multidisciplinary team, that includes a plastic surgeon. Selection of the appropriate method of reconstruction depends on several factors of equal importance.

The patient

In developed countries, patients presenting with head and neck malignancies are usually over 60 years of age and may have other intercurrent illness, including malnutrition, cardiorespiratory disease or diabetes. Furthermore, patients may be referred for surgery following radiotherapy, which may affect the access to vascular pedicles, or the availability of local tissues as potential flaps. An integral part of the patient's assessment must include identifying their concerns and expectations of surgery. It is essential to provide the patient with a comprehensive discussion of potential reconstructive methods, paying particular attention to the expected outcome, functional result and appearance. It is also important to outline the donor site morbidity and any associated scarring or pain.

Preoperatively, the patient's suitability for prolonged anaesthesia is assessed and any anaemia corrected. Particular attention should be directed to the patient's nutritional status; involvement of a dietician and speech therapist is essential to not only advise on nutritional intake and assess swallowing capability, but also to inform and prepare the patient with regard to their postoperative rehabilitation programme. Percutaneous gastrostomy or nasogastric feeding should be considered if nutritional status is poor and oral feeding is not going to be possible in the postoperative recovery period.

The defect

Assessment of the defect includes consideration of the location and size of the resection. As elsewhere, when considering reconstruction of complex three-dimensional structures, they need to be analysed in terms of cover, support and lining.

Function

The aim of reconstruction is not to simply fill a defect, but rather to restore physiological and social function. These can be separated into several specific objectives;

1. Ensure primary wound closure and healing;
2. Restoration of lip-seal and oral continence;
3. Maintenance of oral and pharyngeal swallowing mechanisms;
4. Protection of the airway;
5. Maintain speech;
6. Protect important neurovascular structures;
7. Conserve appearance.

The surgeon

The method of reconstruction will be dependent on the experience of the surgeon and allied staff. Microsurgical experience and equipment allow use of free tissue transfer for complex one-stage reconstructions.

Instruments

Careful handling of soft tissues is particularly important as it limits bruising and necrosis, thereby preventing postoperative pain, edge necrosis and infection. Correct instrumentation is mandatory in performing microsurgical anastomoses including the use of microscopes. The judicious use of bipolar diathermy is recommended near critical vascular supplies.

Reconstructive options in the head and neck

Once the resection is complete, attention focuses on analysis of the component parts of the defect. These are broadly classified into cover, support and lining. Reconstruction of each component requires careful consideration in order to select the appropriate tissue replacement. In this way the optimal result can be achieved at least expense, in terms of patient and donor site morbidity. In addition, thought should also be given to a 'back-up' method in the event of failure.

The complexity of the methods of reconstruction follow a 'reconstructive ladder', beginning with simple split-thickness skin grafts at one end, proceeding to free tissue transfer at the other (Figure 27.1). Ascent of this ladder does not always imply a superior result as in the appropriate circumstances, a skin graft may provide the best functional and cosmetic result.

Reconstruction and tissue selection

Selecting the method of closure in head and neck reconstruction abides by the same principles as

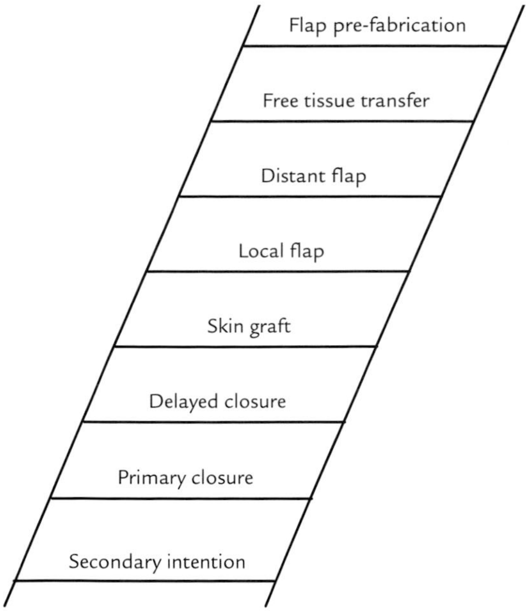

Figure 27.1 The reconstructive ladder. The point of ascent on the ladder depends on several factors. These include the patient, their defect and the surgical capabilities available.

elsewhere; the initial objective is to achieve uncomplicated primary wound healing. This is essential to protect large vessels, prevent salivary fistulae and minimize the interval before postoperative radiotherapy can be commenced. Primary closure is limited to small defects, usually in the floor of the mouth, buccal mucosa, lateral tongue and larynx/pharynx. However, it should not be achieved at the expense of tethering or limiting movement of otherwise mobile structures, that is the tongue or mandible, as these are likely to result in further functional morbidity.

Split thickness skin grafts

Split thickness skin grafts (STSGs) can be used to provide lining, and more rarely, cover at several sites in the head and neck. STSGs are relatively plentiful (Figures 27.2 and 27.3) and easy to harvest using a power dermatome or handknife. They may be used for lining defects following maxillectomy, in the floor of mouth, posterior tongue and orbit.[2,3] It is unusual to use STSGs for cover, but they may be of value for large superficial defects (Figure 27.3) and are applied as a sheet graft (meshed grafts should not be used as cover to avoid the unsatisfactory final appearance). Split thickness grafts may also be used to provide lining, following resection of buccal or lingual mucosa. This is not without difficulty though, as the graft is liable to trauma and movement and therefore requires quilting, or use of a stent.

As noted above, the use of STSGs in head and neck reconstruction has a number of limitations; they are thin, vulnerable to trauma and prone to contraction. In addition, STSGs for cover are susceptible to hypertrophic scarring at their margins. With these limitations in mind, skin grafts may provide a less than optimal source of tissue. STSG 'take' is dependent on the vascularity of the bed onto which it is placed. Accordingly STSGs will not survive on bare bone, or sloughy, infected wounds. STSGs are unlikely to take well on a previously irradiated bed. In addition colour match and texture are dissimilar from that of facial skin. If a large area requires resurfacing, a thick STSG may be harvested from the thigh or buttock, but care should be taken with the frail or malnutritioned patient as the donor site may prove difficult to heal. In these instances it is worthwhile reapplying some of the harvested skin

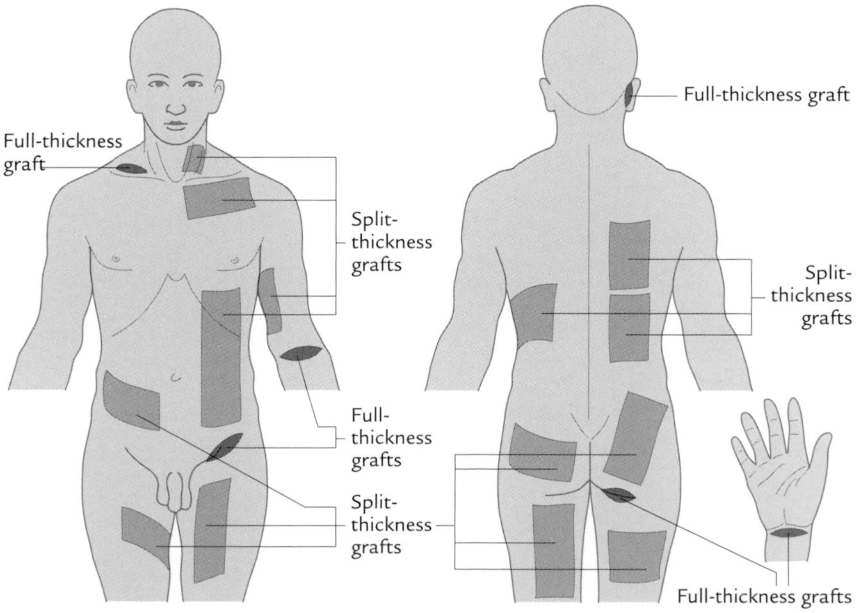

Figure 27.2 Split thickness skin grafts are relatively plentiful and may be harvested from several sites. Full thickness grafts are only available in limited sites and quantity.

(a) (b) (c)

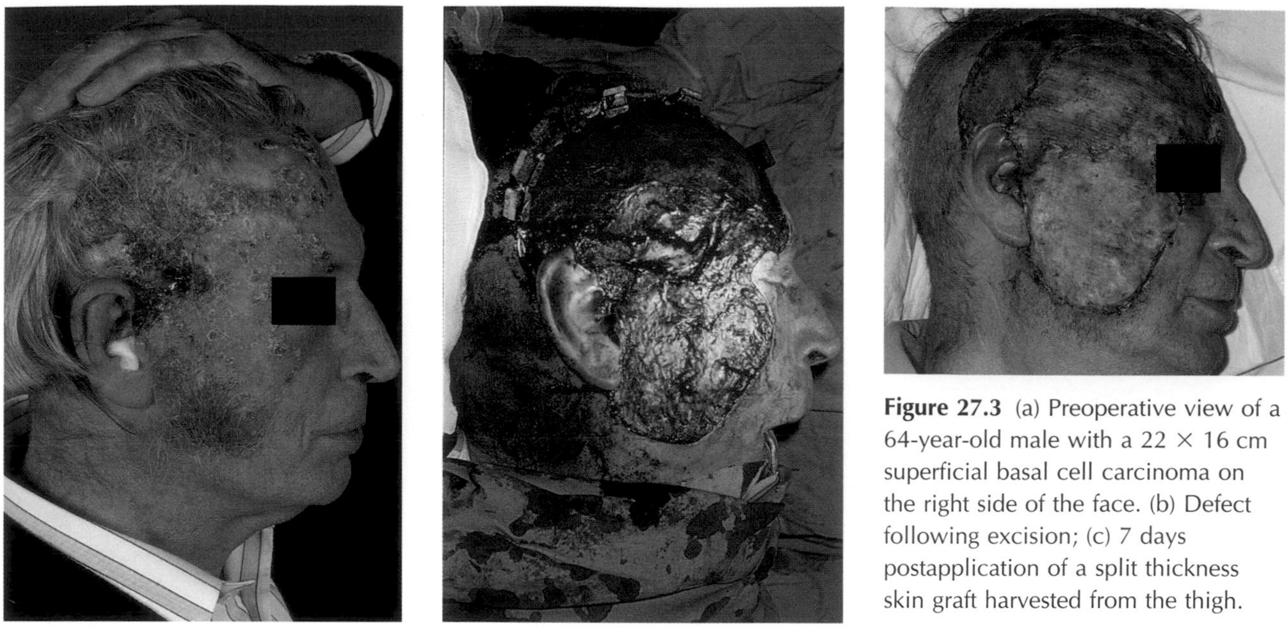

Figure 27.3 (a) Preoperative view of a 64-year-old male with a 22 × 16 cm superficial basal cell carcinoma on the right side of the face. (b) Defect following excision; (c) 7 days postapplication of a split thickness skin graft harvested from the thigh.

as a 1:6 meshed-graft on the donor site to promote healing.

Full thickness skin grafts

Full thickness skin grafts (FTSGs) are better suited to provide skin of similar quality to that of the face. However, FTSGs are only available in limited quantities, and are usually harvested from the pre- or post-auricular regions, supraclavicular area and upper eyelids (Figure 27.3). Compared to STSGs they provide better colour and texture match as well as being less susceptible to contraction. With these benefits, FTSGs are ideal for resurfacing small defects, such as following excision of basal cell or squamous cell carcinomas. However, due to their thickness, the recipient bed must be non-infected and well vascularized.

In view of the limitations noted above, skin grafts may provide a less than optimal source of tissue when attempting to reconstruct a larger, mobile structure. More robust, malleable tissues are only obtained using thicker, vascularized tissues, i.e., flaps.

Flaps and reconstructive surgery

A surgical flap, traditionally referred to as a skin flap, comprises an area of skin and subcutaneous tissue that is moved to the defect from a donor site while surviving on its own blood supply. In actuality, flaps may comprise any tissue or combination of tissues, to include skin, fat, muscle, fascia, bone and tendon. These are to be distinguished from grafts that are detached from their blood supply and rely on a recipient source and neovascularization for survival.

Classification of flaps

Many flap classifications have been proposed each dependent on varying defining principles. One of the most commonly utilized classifications is that of Daniel and Kerrigan,[4] who divide flaps according to their route and type of vascularity, the method of transfer and the tissues composing the flap (Table 27.1).

Table 27.1 Flap classification

Type (vascularity)	Random (cutaneous)
	Pedicled/axial
Technique (movement)	
Advancement	V–Y, Y–V
	Single pedicle
	Bipedicle
Pivot	Rotation
	Transposition
	Interpolation/island
Distant	Direct
	Tubed
Free	
Tissue (composition)	Cutaneous
	Fasciocutaneous
	Musculocutaneous
	Muscle
	Osseocutaneous
	Sensory

Flap vascularity

Skin flaps are perfused by either a *random* or *axial* vascular pattern. *Random* pattern flaps have no discernible dominant blood supply and are usually fed by a dermal-subdermal plexus supplied by direct cutaneous, musculocutaneous or fasciocutaneous vessels. The relevance of this distribution is that the length of random pattern flaps is usually limited to the width of the flap base. It may only be modified by a 'delay' procedure.

Axial pattern flaps are perfused by an identifiable, single arteriovenous system that proceeds along the longitudinal axis of the flap. These vessels originate as septocutaneous arteries, supplying muscles and fascia en-route to the skin. Musculocutaneous flaps consist of skin, subcutaneous fat and muscle. Arteries penetrate and supply the muscle in a defined pattern before supplying the skin via arterial perforators.

Other flap variants include island flaps, which are axial flaps raised on a pedicle consisting of the artery and vein alone. Fasciocutaneous flaps can be further defined on the basis of where perforators lie, that is subfascial, intermuscular etc.

Flap transfer

Skin flaps may be further defined by their method of transfer and the distance between donor and recipient sites and are divided into local, regional and distant.

Reconstruction aims to match the reconstructed tissues to the resection as closely as possible and therefore, flaps are chosen to match thickness, texture, colour and function. Local flaps utilize tissues adjacent to the defect that may be advanced along the long axis of the flap (i.e. V–Y). Alternatively they may be rotated, transposed or interpolated (i.e. passed over or under an intervening tissue to reach the defect). They are usually suitable for closure of small covering defects, following excision of skin lesions, though they also include mucosal flaps and tongue flaps. Larger local rotation flaps include cervicofacial and cheek rotation flaps (Figure 27.4).

Blood enters local flaps by a 'random' subdermal plexus, and therefore, the base of the flap needs to be broad. The principles of wound closure are particularly important in the raising and insetting of flaps in that they should be handled carefully, grasping the dermis with skin hooks or fine toothed forceps. Flaps should be moved and closed without tension and drains used where appropriate.

'Delaying' a flap is a staged technique to extend the axial vascular supply. This is achieved by dividing the axial supply to the distal portion of the proposed flap thereby inducing partial ischaemia. At a later date the whole flap is raised.

The blood supply of the skin and muscle has now been described in detail, particularly following Taylor's concepts of angiosomes.[5] Large cutaneous flaps may be perfused by a number of routes, though the most common involve perforators arising from fascia or underlying muscle.

Distant flaps, as their name implies, are raised from sites away from the resection and may be transferred either by use of a pedicle (i.e. the deltopectoral flap and the pectoralis major flap) or by disconnection and

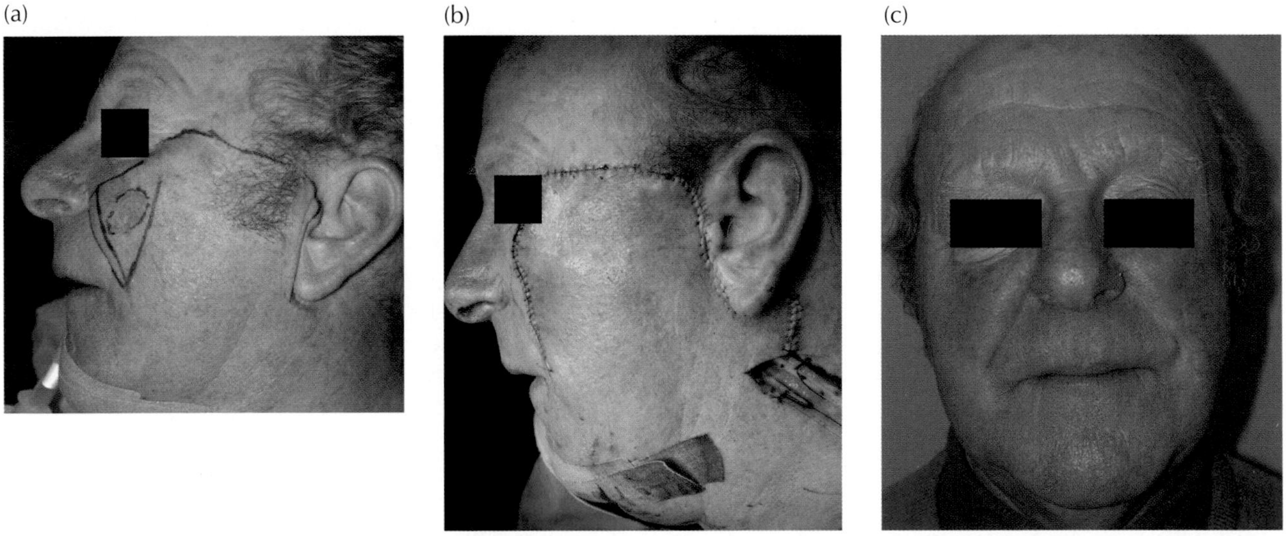

Figure 27.4 (a) Morpheic BCC on left cheek. The proposed excision defect and flap are shown. (b)The flap has been elevated and rotated into the triangular defect, insetting the flap into the nasolabial fold and side of nose. (c) Frontal view at 4 months post-surgery.

revascularization using microsurgical techniques: a free flap. Anatomically, these flaps depend on an axial flow, being fed by a named vessel, or group of vessels. The discovery of this flap type was to revolutionize head and neck surgery, for it allowed the transfer of large composite flaps from distant sites to achieve one-stage reconstruction. Further modifications have included flap prefabrication, to include skin grafts for lining or modifications to fashion tubes.[6,7] More recent advances have included innervating flaps to regenerate sensation within a cutaneous paddle. This is of obvious relevance to restoration of intraoral sensation and speech.

Microsurgery

Microsurgery is a technically demanding discipline that requires adequate expertise and experience by the surgeon, anaesthetist and nursing staff. It is expensive in terms of instrumentation, magnification and monitoring. Flap survival depends on adequate perfusion. Therefore, close collaboration between the surgeon and the anaesthetic staff is required to ensure the patient is well resuscitated, warm and pain free. Furthermore, suitable facilities should be available to monitor both the patient and flap in the early postoperative period.

Routine flaps for head and neck reconstruction

General considerations

Flaps usually provide the best method of reconstructing head and neck defects; composed of robust, well-vascularized tissues, they can be used to cover or line exposed bone. Where needed, they can include vascularized bone or tendon. Having examined the patient and their defect, it is beneficial to consider reconstructive options at different levels of the reconstructive ladder. The most appropriate methods can then be selected for the patient in an effort to produce the optimal functional and cosmetic reconstruction with the least morbidity.

This section aims to describe several established methods of reconstruction. Each flap type will be considered in terms of its surgical anatomy, application and how to raise it. Problems associated with the flap will also be considered.

Local flaps

Nasolabial flap

The nasolabial flap is an axial cutaneous flap

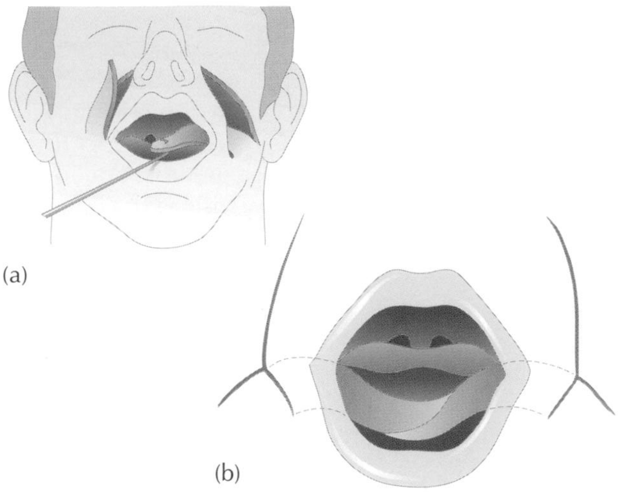

Figure 27.5 The nasolabial flap can be inset intraorally to cover small floor defects.

supplied by branches of the facial artery (Figure 27.5). It is a versatile flap that may used to reconstruct small defects in the anterior floor of the mouth anterior to the molar teeth,[8] the alar of the nose, columella and upper lip. The flap is proximally based, using excess skin of the nasolabial fold, which can be used singly or bilaterally. Distally the length is limited by the medial canthus of the eye. The proximal width of the flap depends on the excess tissue available, up to 3 cm at most.

Raising the flap

The medial and lateral borders are marked and then incised, joining them distally. Elevation then proceeds from the tip, superficial to the underlying facial muscles. When used for intraoral reconstruction, the flap is tunnelled through the cheek and inset into the floor of the mouth leaving a small mucous fistula. The donor site is closed directly in the edentulous patient, but a splint may be required to protect the pedicle if dentate. The pedicle is divided usually at about 3 weeks and the flap inset.

Problems

The height of the dentition can prevent adequate insetting of the flap and, as intimated above, patients have been known to bite through the pedicle. Tunnelling of the flap may result in a salivary fistula for up to 3 weeks. Following insetting, this may require a secondary procedure to correct it.

Forehead flap

The forehead is a versatile source of thin, robust skin that may be used to provide both cover and lining of complex facial and intraoral defects.[9] Blood supply to the forehead is derived laterally from the frontal branch of the superficial temporal vessels and medially from a vascular complex derived from the supraorbital and supratrochlear arteries. Axial pattern flaps can be based on either of these two systems for specific and varied application. The frontal branch of the superficial temporal artery passes in front of the ear and is usually palpable before it pierces the deep fascia 4–5 mm in front of the tragus. The vessel then crosses the base of the zygomatic arch to supply the flap. The laterally based forehead flap can be used to provide facial skin to cover and reconstruct the cheek, nose or lower lip. It is also of considerable use as a source of lining. The thinness of the flap makes it ideal for reconstruction within the mouth and the pharynx, particularly for salvage or where microsurgery is contraindicated or unavailable.

Raising the flap

Planning the flap is essential, as often only the distal aspect of the flap is required. If a larger flap is necessary then the whole forehead can be elevated and the donor site grafted with a thick sheet split skin graft to resurface the cosmetic unit. The flap is raised by incising through the marked upper and lower margins. The distal end of the flap is incised and the flap raised from distal to proximal superficial or deep to frontalis. The vessels may be seen on the undersurface of the flap and care must be taken with haemostasis and to include and preserve the accompanying veins. If the flap is being used for intraoral or pharyngeal reconstruction, it is then tunnelled into the oral cavity either beneath or over the zygomatic arch (Figure 27.6), taking particular care to avoid the frontal branch of the facial nerve. The donor site is closed with a split skin graft and the pedicle divided at 3 weeks.

Problems

The facial nerve is at risk when tunnelling into the oral cavity. The flap is infrequently used due to extremely poor donor site cosmesis, and for intraoral reconstruction has been largely replaced by the radial forearm free flap.

Galeofrontalis flap

The galeofrontalis flap[10] is based on the musculo-aponeurotic system of the scalp with blood supply from the superficial temporal, supraorbital and supratrochlear arteries. The flap is raised following elevation of a bicoronal or coronal scalp flap, by dividing the aponeurotic layer from the overlying skin and subcutaneous layers. The whole width of the forehead can be raised or restricted to thin strips but is limited to a maximum of about 8 cm in height. The flap provides a good source of vascularized tissue that has several applications. It may act as a barrier between the nasal and cranial cavities, particularly in the presence of CSF leaks following trauma or intracranial surgery. Other applications include covering or wrapping of bone grafts used in craniofacial reconstruction.

Temporalis flaps

The temporal area provides two flaps, supplied by separate arterial systems, which are useful in head and neck reconstruction[11] and can be raised independently (Figure 27.7).

(a) Superficial temporal fascial flap

The superficial temporal artery fascial flap is supplied by the temporal branch of the superficial temporal artery and is classified as an axial pattern fascial flap (Figure 27.7a). It can be used to line the orbit following exenteration, and may be of application in reconstruction of the upper part of the oral cavity.

Raising of the flap

The fascia can be accessed via a T-shaped or Z-shaped incision over the temporal area. The scalp is elevated immediately below the hair follicles to expose the superficial fascia. The size of the flap required is marked out and the fascia elevated, ensuring the vessels and the frontal branch of the facial nerve are preserved.

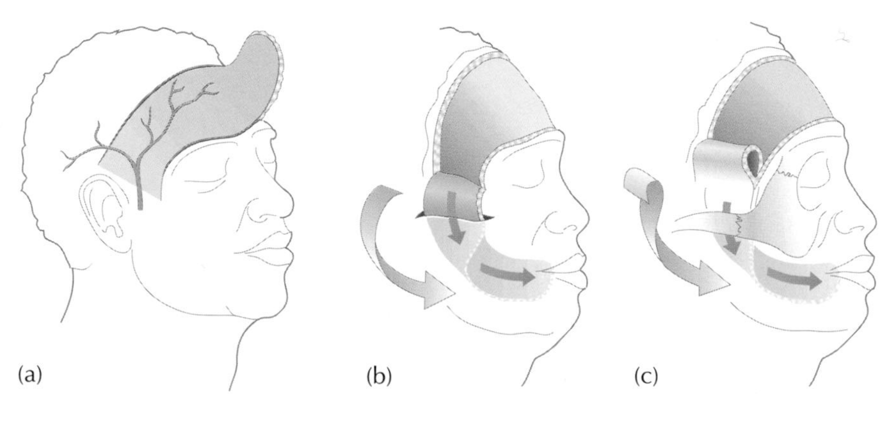

Figure 27.6 The forehead is a valuable source of thin, pliable tissue, particularly for salvage reconstruction. The whole forehead may be raised on either superficial temporal artery and the donor site sheet-grafted as a single cosmetic unit.

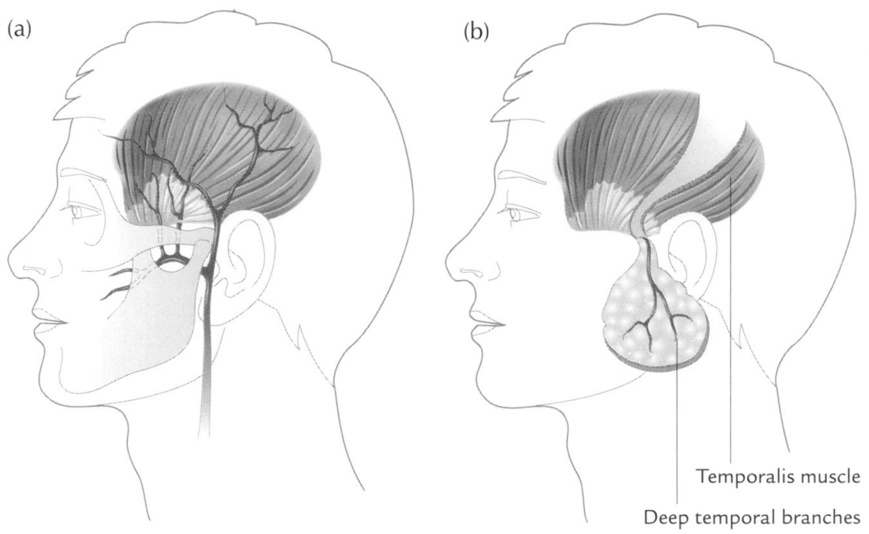

Figure 27.7 (a) The temporo-parietal fascia is supplied by the superficial temporal artery. (b) The temporalis muscle derives its blood supply from both the anterior and posterior deep temporal branches of the internal maxillary artery.

Problems

If the flap is elevated too superficially, patchy alopecia may result. The frontal branch of the VII nerve is at risk.

(b) Temporalis muscle flap

The temporalis muscle flap is a muscle flap supplied by the deep temporal artery system, which arises from the terminal branches of the maxillary artery (Figure 27.7b). The flap can be used to fill defects around the orbit and upper part of the oral cavity and the available length of the flap extended by incorporating the overlying fascia.

Raising of the flap

The muscle flap is raised in a similar fashion to the superficial temporal fascial flap. A T-shaped incision is made in the scalp over the temporal area and the superficial fascia incised to expose the underlying muscle. The pericranium is incised distally and the muscle flap raised. All or part of the muscle can be raised depending on the requirements, whilst the superficial fascia can remain attached distally to lengthen the flap. Dividing the zygomatic arch can extend the arc of rotation of the flap. This allows the flap to reach further into the oral cavity.

Problems

Raising the flap can leave the patient with a temporal hollow. If only the anterior part of the flap is being used in the reconstruction the posterior element can be transposed anteriorly to mask any contour deficit.

Distant pedicled flaps

Deltopectoral flap

The deltopectoral flap is a fasciocutaneous flap, first described by Bakamjian in 1965.[12] It represented a historic landmark in head and neck surgery as it facilitated oropharyngeal reconstruction without recourse to multistaged tubed-pedicle flaps. The flap is supplied by the intercostal perforating branches of the internal mammary artery lying at the lateral edge of the sternum between the second to fourth intercostal space. It reaches laterally over the anterior surface of the deltoid, but can be extended a further 3–5 cm using a delay procedure. In this way defects can be reconstructed in the floor of mouth, pharynx and for resurfacing the neck (Figure 27.8). With an initial delay, the flap

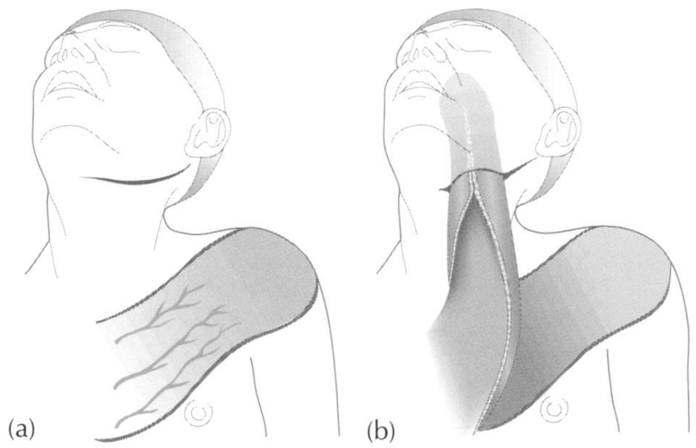

Figure 27.8 The deltopectoral flap. This flap provides an important reconstructive option for cover or lining where microsurgical facilities are unavailable or contraindicated. It is also used to resurface the neck following excision of recurrent disease under previously irradiated skin and prior to brachytherapy.

can reach as high as the zygomatic arch but attempts to extend beyond this are likely to result in distal necrosis.

In centres where microsurgery is available this flap is usually reserved for salvage surgery. However, it remains the flap of choice where free tissue transfer is contraindicated or where neck skin is involved and requires resurfacing prior to brachytherapy.

Raising of the flap

The axis of the flap is centred over the third intercostal perforator. The upper margin is marked just below the clavicle and the lower border of the flap is drawn inline with the lower border of the anterior axillary fold, approximately two fingerbreadths above the male nipple. The flap extends to the anterior deltoid region, but can be extended following a delay procedure to the thoracoacromial axis. Maximal possible flap length is approximately 45 cm.

The flap is raised from distal to proximal in a plane just beneath the fascia. Care is taken when approaching the deltopectoral groove to avoid the cephalic vein lying within it. The donor site may close directly, but often requires a split skin graft, particularly if the flap is extended onto the upper arm. The pedicle may be de-epithelialized but is otherwise divided at 2–3 weeks.

Problems

A two-stage procedure is required if the flap is used in intraoral reconstruction, increasing the risk of fistula formation. The donor site is unsightly.

Latissimus dorsi flap

The latissimus dorsi flap is a musculocutaneous flap supplied by the thoracodorsal artery plus segmental perforators from posteromedial intercostal arteries. It may be raised as muscle alone, or with a skin paddle and transferred either on its pedicle or as a free flap (Figure 27.9). This flap is selected where bulk is required, or muscle is needed to cover bone graft. When raising a pedicled flap it is important to orientate the skin paddle on the muscle in order to ensure it comes to lie in the desired location. It can be tunnelled anteriorly through the axilla and up across the clavicle to the head and neck. If a skin paddle is used, it should be limited to 8 cm in width, allowing primary closure of the back; skin grafts in this region are always unsightly and may take several weeks to heal.

Once mobilized it can be used to resurface the cheek, or supply the necessary bulk following glossectomy. The long pedicle of this flap also makes it suitable for microsurgical transfer, usually to vessels in the ipsilateral neck, giving greater freedom in the positioning of the flap.

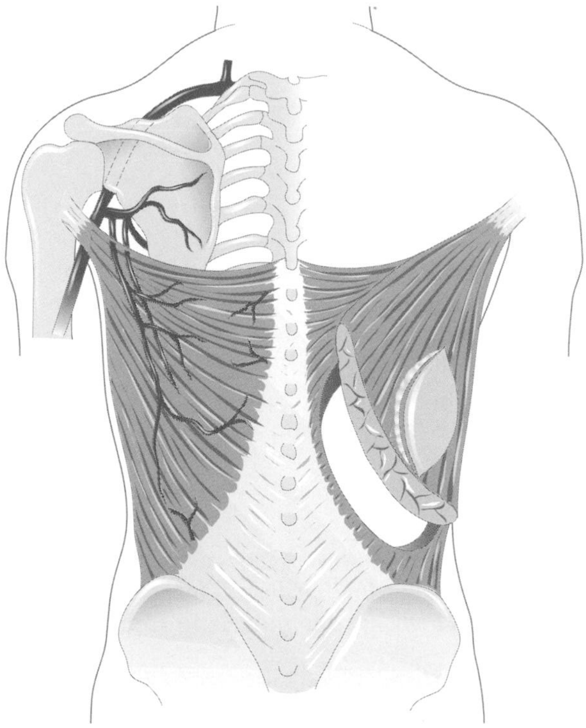

Figure 27.9 The latissimus dorsi is a robust muscle flap that may be raised alone or with a skin paddle. Due to the relatively long vascular pedicle, the flap may be advanced intraorally or to the side of the head as a pedicled flap. Microvascular transfer allows greater flexibility of positioning.

Raising of the flap

The patient is usually positioned on their side, with the flap side uppermost and the arm draped separately. The anterior border of the muscle is marked on the patient, followed by design of the skin paddle if necessary. The skin paddle should be sized to allow primary closure, and orientated to allow correct positioning with respect to the pedicle. The skin flap is marked out so that the majority lies over the muscle but can overlap the anterior edge by up to 3 cm.

The skin paddle is incised down to fascia overlying the muscle and, using a cutting diathermy, the surrounding skin elevated off the muscle. The anterior border of the muscle is then identified and dissected off the chest wall. The medial and inferior margins of the muscle dissection depend on the amount of muscle required to correct any volume deficiency.

The flap is then lifted to identify the pedicle on the underside of the muscle. The thoracodorsal vessels enter the muscle approximately 10 cm below the axilla. The artery to serratus anterior is initially seen first, 1–3 cm below the main thoracodorsal vessels.

When the flap is raised as a pedicled transfer, the humeral attachment of the muscle is divided to increase the arc of rotation. Delivery is aided into the head and neck region by a transverse incision just below the clavicle. It is essential to divide completely the humeral insertion of the pectoralis major to allow tension-free passage of the flap.

Variations

If a flap of small volume is required it is possible to raise just the anterior border of the muscle. Blood supply divides within the muscle to supply anterior and posterior division skin paddles that can be raised separately.[13]

Problems

The major practical problem with this flap is that the patient needs to be turned during the operation.

Trapezius flap

Two flaps can be raised from the region of the trapezius (Figure 27.10). Both flaps are useful for reconstructing defects in the lower part of the head and neck region and in the temporal area.

Lateral trapezius flap

The lateral trapezius flap is a type II musculocutaneous flap, supplied by the transverse cervical artery.[14] Vascularized bone can be harvested with the flap by including the acromion or spine of scapula.

Raising of the flap

The flap is marked out with its centre over the acromion. The transverse cervical artery can be identified at the time of resection in the lower part of the neck. The anterior part of the flap is raised off the deltoid muscle up to the acromoclavicular joint and raising the flap is completed by detaching the trapezius from the spine of the scapula. The fibres of the trapezius muscle are split to form the pedicle.

Upper trapezius flap

The upper trapezius flap is a musculocutaneous flap supplied by the occipital artery.[15]

Raising of the flap

The anterior border of the flap is defined by the anterior border of the trapezius muscle, from the superior nuchal line to the lateral part of the acromion process. The posterior border of the flap

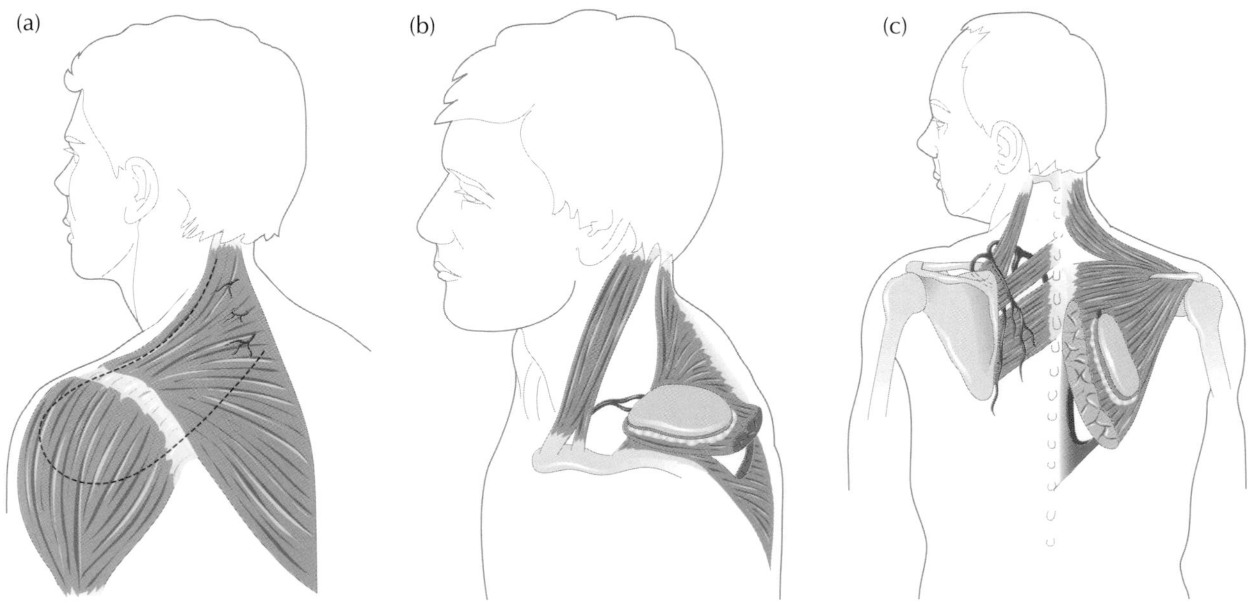

Figure 27.10 The trapezius provides three potential flaps for use in head and neck reconstructions. (a) The superiorly based trapezius flap, supplied from paraspinous perforators. (b) The lateral island trapezius flap, supplied by the transverse cervical artery. (c) The lower island trapezius flap, supplied by superficial branches of the transverse cervical artery and, lower down, the dorsal scapular artery.

extends from the dorsal spine, parallel to the anterior marking down to the spine of the scapula. A flap with a width of about 7 cm and 30 cm in length can be raised from this area. Muscle is only included in the proximal part of the flap, the distal part comprises only skin and deep fascia. The division of the superior part of the muscle takes place just above the junction of the upper two-thirds and lower one-third of the muscle; this preserves the nerve supply.

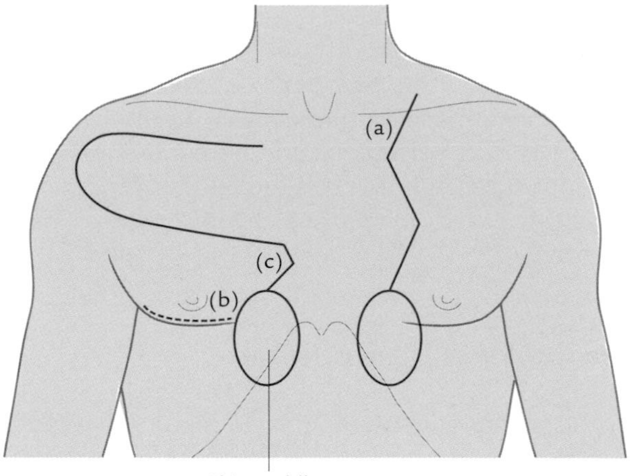

Figure 27.12 The pectoralis major myocutaneous flap may be raised by several routes. (a) Directly: this route allows flap harvest under direct vision but leaves an unsightly scar. (b) Using a submammary route and closure with a rotation flap, this gives an excellent cosmetic result. (c) 'Defensively' to preserve the deltopectoral flap.

Pectoralis major muscle flap

The pectoralis major is a musculocutaneous flap, supplied by the pectoral branch of the thoraco-acromial axis.[16] This flap is the 'workhorse' of many head and neck reconstructive surgeons as it is simple and quick to raise, mobile and can provide muscle alone or include a cutaneous paddle. The flap can reach the pharynx, floor of the mouth, and the retromolar trigone. The orientation of the flap on the chest wall can be varied depending on the size and shape of the flap required (Figure 27.11).

Raising of the flap

The pedicle of the flap runs vertically downwards from a point halfway along the clavicle until it meets a line drawn from the acromion process to the xiphisternum (though the pedicle can lie lateral to both these lines). The skin flap is usually drawn in an inferomedial position but to maximize the length of the flap, the skin paddle can be positioned parasternally. The skin paddle is outlined and incised down to the underlying pectoralis fascia and the skin edges tacked to the muscle to prevent shearing of paddle.

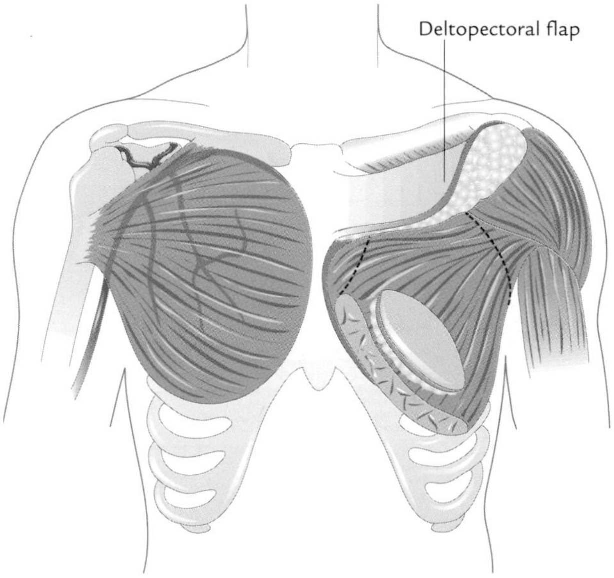

Figure 27.11 The pectoralis major flap. This muscle is mainly supplied by the pectoral branch of the thoracoacromial artery that runs along its deep surface.

The paddle and its muscle pedicle can be isolated by one of several routes (Figure 27.12) and the incision extended directly up towards the neck. Alternatively, and more aesthetically pleasing, the incision continues to skirt the inferior aspect of the pectoralis, up the side of the chest. This allows excellent exposure of the muscle and its pedicle. The final scar is also very acceptable. The muscle can then be incised to include the pedicle and as much muscle as is required. Just below the clavicle the muscle can be divided along the clavicular axis to island the flap on its vascular pedicle and tunnelled into the neck; care must be taken to prevent twisting or compression of the vessels. Finally, the flap may be raised in a 'defensive' manner so that the deltopectoral flap can be preserved for later use if necessary.

The donor site can be closed directly if the skin paddle is small but can lead to distortion of the nipple position, which is a particular limitation, especially in females. The lateral approach noted above allows rotation of tissue into the defect and further aids closure, causing less deformity.

Problems

Despite the considerable popularity of this flap, it is associated with certain problems that may affect its selection in certain patients. The myocutaneous flap is thick, even in the thin patient, with much of the bulk due to subcutaneous fat. The skin paddle is unreliable if taken too distally beyond the pectoralis major muscle for the purpose of extending the range. If a very small skin paddle is used it may not incorporate vascular perforators and be liable to necrosis. Rotation of the flap above the clavicle produces an unsightly bulge over the clavicle unless it is 'islanded'..

Sternocleidomastoid muscle flap

The sternocleidomastoid muscle flap is a type III musculocutaneous flap. It has a segmental arterial supply from the occipital artery, the superior thyroid artery and the suprascapular artery or transverse cervical artery. The muscle may be raised with an overlying skin paddle at the inferior pole (Figure 27.13). Similarly, part of the medial clavicle may be included to provide bone. However, it is rarely used as a composite flap or as a first-line reconstructive method due to the unreliability of its blood supply once raised. It can be raised either as a pedicled or island flap.[17]

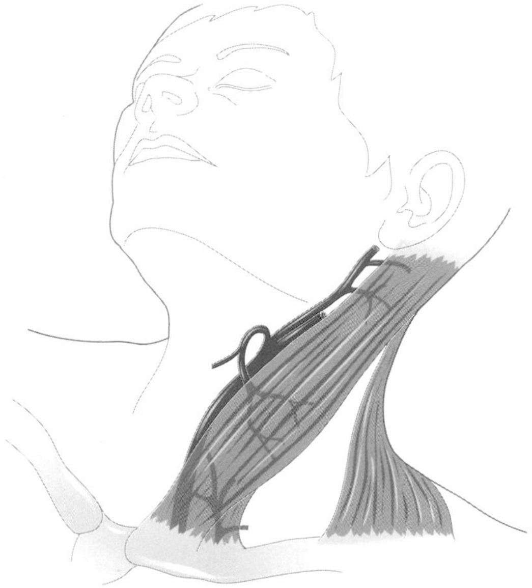

Figure 27.13 The sternomastoid flap. This may be raised with or without clavicle to provide bone for mandibular defects. However, as with the distal portion of the myocutaneous flap, blood supply is unpredictable.

The standard size of the pedicled flap is 6 × 24 cm. This allows the donor site to be closed directly. The flap extends down to the clavicle but can be extended beyond this with the addition of a delay procedure. In an island flap the skin paddle is marked out over the lower end of the muscle; the donor site can be closed directly.

Raising of the flap

Raising the sternocleidomastoid flap is very similar for both types of flap. The skin margins are incised down to the muscle. The muscle is divided inferiorly and elevated superiorly leaving the deep layer of fascia in continuity with the rest of the deep investing fascia of the neck. The lower vascular pedicle is divided, as may the middle pedicle, making blood supply to the lower end of the flap less than adequate.

Problems

As noted, these flaps have a tenuous blood supply and can be unreliable. Up to 20% of flaps suffer complete failure, whilst 50% suffer partial loss of the skin paddle.

Microvascular flaps

Microsurgery has further refined head and neck reconstruction by providing an increased repertoire of flaps, and tissues that facilitate one-stage repair. With this palette of tissues the reconstructive surgeon is able to more closely select those that match the resection specimen in composition, size and form, often producing a more refined and improved result. However, when compared to pedicled loco-regional flaps, these procedures prove more complex and demanding in terms of equipment, cost and surgical experience.

Radial artery forearm flap

The radial forearm flap is a fasciocutaneous flap,[18–20] supplied by the radial artery, with perforators travelling vertically upwards in the intermuscular septum, and others descending to the underlying radius (Figure 27.14). The latter provide access to vasularized bone. As a result of these components, the radial forearm flap provides a flexible source of tissue that is extensively used in head and neck reconstruction. It supplies thin pliable skin suitable for intraoral lining (almost the whole of the skin of the forearm can be raised). In addition, including bone or tendon may increase reconstructive options.

The radial artery is relatively large and easy to anastamose. The venous drainage of the flap is by either the venae commitantes or the superficial venous system with some surgeons incorporating the cephalic vein to increase drainage. Due to the vascular arrangement of the forearm it is possible to design double or triple skin paddles on the radial artery, enabling reconstruction of complex defects.

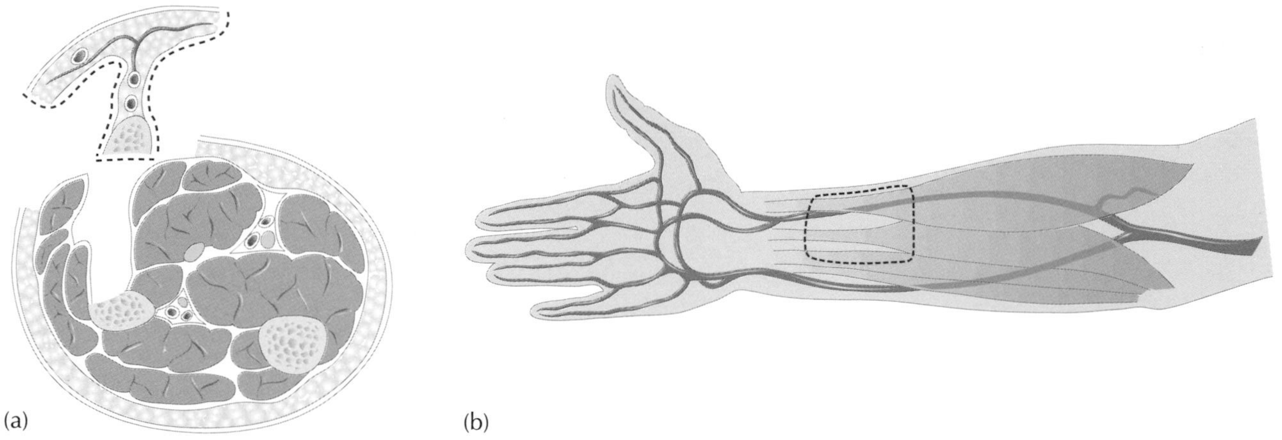

Figure 27.14 The radial forearm flap. (a) Vascular perforators ascend through the intermuscular septum from the radial artery to the forearm fascia and skin. Deep perforators descend to the radius, allowing harvesting of vascularized bone. (b) If required, the skin paddle may comprise almost the whole circumference of the forearm. Larger donor sites are covered with split skin graft, though smaller defects can be directly closed using a variety of local flaps.

Raising of the flap

The axis of the flap is marked by drawing a line between the palpable brachial pulse in the antecubital fossa and the radial artery pulse at the wrist. The site and size of the skin paddle depends on size of defect, hairiness of skin, length of pedicle required and superficial venous system. The flap is raised using a tourniquet without exsanguination, to identify necessary veins. The skin is incised down to and through deep fascia, and raised, preserving the paratenon over the flexor tendons. The dissection proceeds from both ulnar and radial sides to leave the skin paddle attached to the artery and vein alone (Figure 27.15).

Lateral retraction of brachioradialis muscle reveals the perforators and the radial artery. The vessels are divided distally and the flap raised in a proximal direction dividing the deep perforators. The donor site can be closed with either a split skin or full thickness skin graft. If a small paddle is used the defect can be closed directly by using an ulnar-based rotation flap.

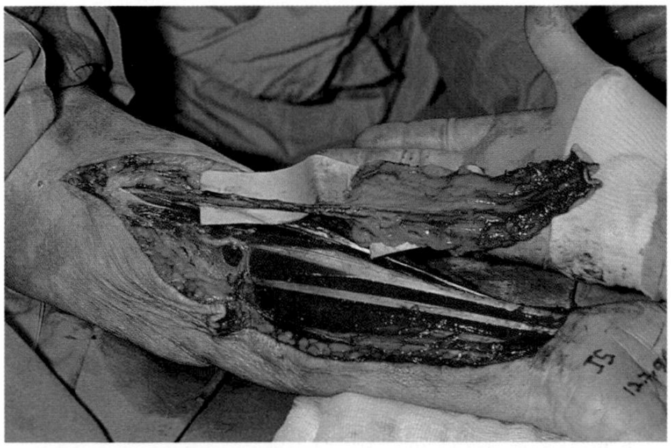

Figure 27.15 This view shows the underside of a radial forearm flap elevated on its vascular pedicle.

Radial artery free flap with bone

The radial forearm flap with bone[21] is classified as a osseofasciocutaneous flap. The perforators from the radial artery supply the radius via vessels passing through flexor pollicis longus and fascial perforators running between pronator teres and brachioradialis.

Raising of the flap

The flap is marked out as above. However the flexor pollicis longus is incised to leave a small cuff attached to the radius. The osteotomy should aim to remove approximately one-third of the cross-section of radius, with a maximum length of 12 cm. The bone cut should be boat-shaped to prevent potential weak spots in the radius and subsequent fracture. Postoperatively, the patient is placed in a protective above-elbow plaster cast for up to 6 weeks.

Variations

The flap can be raised with the palmaris longus or brachioradialis tendon, to provide sling-like support to the reconstructions. When used for intraoral reconstruction, flaps may be innervated using either the medial or lateral antebrachial nerve, usually performing a neurorraphy with the ipsilateral lingual nerve. As another variant, if minimal bulk is required, the flap may consist of fascia alone and the surface covered with a split skin graft (though this would not be indicated for intraoral reconstruction).

Problems

Skin grafts are required to cover the donor site defect in the majority of patients. This can be conspicuous, and tendons are vulnerable to rupture if the paratenon is not preserved. There is a significant danger of radial fracture when bone is harvested.

Lateral arm flap

The lateral arm flap is a type C fasciocutaneous flap, and is supplied by the posterior radial collateral artery, a terminal branch of the profunda brachii artery. The vessel passes downwards in the lateral intermuscular septum of the upper arm posterior to the brachioradialis muscle (Figure 27.16). As with the radial forearm flap, the flap may be raised as either a fasciocutaneous flap or with fascia alone. If the donor site is to be closed directly, a skin paddle of about 12 × 6 cm may be used.

Raising of the flap

The axis of the flap runs from the deltoid insertion vertically down to the lateral epicondyle. The skin paddle is centred on this line, can extend anteriorly and posteriorly up to 6 cm and is raised with the deep fascia from both a posterior and anterior direction. The cephalic vein is divided if present within the field. It is important to raise the deep fascia over biceps and triceps as well as the intermuscular septum.

The vessels supplying the flap are identified proximally in space between the deltoid insertion and triceps. The flap is raised in a proximal direction, being careful to identify and preserve the radial nerve adjacent to the upper part of the pedicle, which is then ligated as high as possible. The donor site should be designed to be closed directly, as split skin grafts leave an unsightly donor defect.

Variations

The lateral arm flap can be raised as an osseofasciocutaneous flap by incorporating a portion of the lateral supracondylar ridge. The flap can also be used as a fascial flap or as an innervated flap by incorporating the lower lateral cutaneous nerve of the arm.

Problems

Compared with the radial forearm flap, the major limitations of this flap are the relatively short pedicle and the bulk of the fasciocutaneous flap. There is troublesome numbness in the distribution of the posterior cutaneous nerve of the forearm.

Scapular and parascapular flaps

The scapular and parascapular flaps[22,23] are type B fasciocutaneous flaps, supplied by the circumflex scapular artery that divides into two branches, a horizontal (transverse) branch and a parascapular branch. Once through the triangular space, a branch of the circumflex scapular artery supplies the lateral portion of the scapula. The flap provides a large skin paddle 10–12 cm in width and up to 35 cm long, which can be raised with a bone segment up to 14 cm long for mandibular reconstruction.

As the scapular and parascapular flaps have an extensive blood supply, three types of flap with bone can be raised.[24]

1. The lateral scapular element, supplied by a branch directly from the circumflex scapular artery.
2. A combined lateral scapular bone and fascial flap (scapular or parascapular) both supplied by the circumflex scapular vessels.

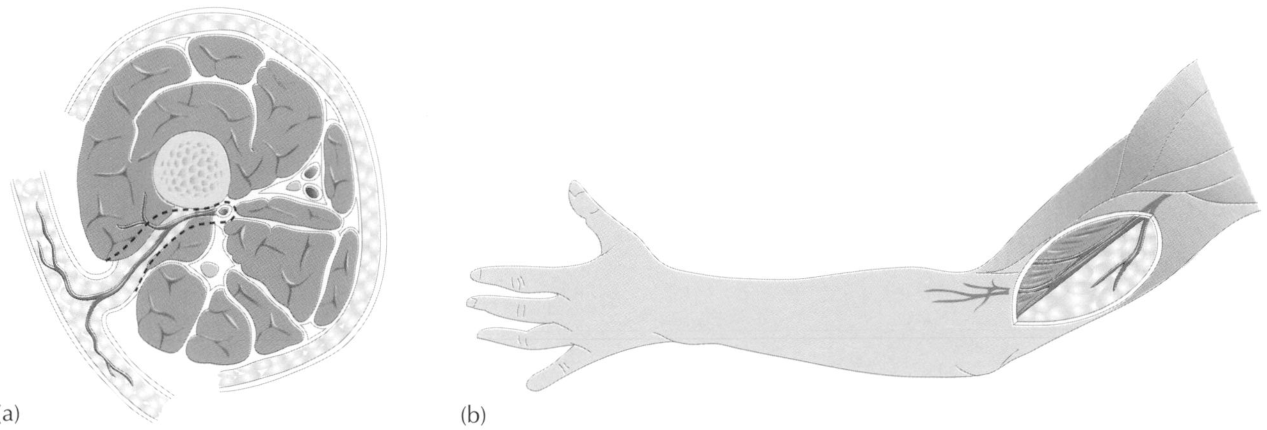

(a) (b)

Figure 27.16 The lateral arm flap is supplied by the posterior radial collateral artery and vein lying in the lateral intermuscular septum. The pedicle can be extended by careful, proximal dissection to 8–10 cm. Flaps below 6 cm in width can be directly closed minimizing donor site morbidity.

3. Lateral scapular bone segment, plus a fascial flap, plus the ipsilateral thoracodorsal pedicle, to include latissimus dorsi/serratus anterior/rib. This highly versatile complex of flaps can be orientated independently of each other and vascularized by a single, subscapular pedicle.

In all the above, the lateral bone element can be extended medially along the tip of the scapula to provide additional bone. This can be utilized to reconstruct the ascending ramus of the mandible.

Raising of the flap

The scapular flap is marked out using Urbaniak's rule of 2s.[23] With the arm at the patient's side the medial end of the flap lies 2 cm from the spinous processes, the lateral edge lies 2 cm above the posterior axillary crease. The inferior border is 2 cm above the lower pole of the scapula whilst the superior border is 2 cm inferior to the spine of the scapula. These markings produce a flap size of around 10 × 16 cm. The pedicle is identified first within the triangular space by incising the superolateral edge of the marked flap. The flap is then raised medially to laterally by incising the skin paddle down to the fascia overlying infraspinatus muscle.

Deeper dissection of the pedicle requires muscular branches to be identified and ligated. If an osseocutaneous flap is being raised the musculoperiosteal branch needs to be identified, which arises from the circumflex scapular artery 2–3 cm within the triangular space. To raise the bone element of the flap the muscles overlying the scapula are incised and the relevant osteotomies performed. This produces a segment 10–14 cm long and 1.5 cm wide.

To raise the bone on the angular artery, the vessel is exposed in the plane between teres major and latissimus dorsi, this vessel will support a bone strut of 8 cm in length or a triangle from the angle of the scapula 6 cm long. The donor site is closed directly if no bone is taken; if bone is taken the muscles need reattachment to the scapula.

The parascapular flap is raised in a similar way to the scapular flap, with the paddle orientated vertically. The surface marking of the pedicle is D = 0.5(L–2) where D is the distance below the spine of the scapula and L, the distance from the spine to the angle. The lower pole of the flap lies 25–30 cm below the marked pedicle and the flap width is up to 12 cm.

Problems

The patient needs to be turned prone or on their side in order to raise the flap. The skin paddle is often quite bulky as the subcutaneous tissue on the back can be thick, though this is amenable to thinning at a later stage. If the angular artery is used to raise a bone flap, part of teres major may be devascularized due to loss of blood supply from this same vessel. Therefore the muscle may need debridement before closure of the wound.

Deep circumflex iliac artery flap

The deep circumflex iliac artery (DCIA) flap (Figure 27.17) is supplied by the deep circumflex iliac artery that arises from the external iliac artery, opposite the exit of the deep inferior epigastric artery, just above the inguinal ligament. The major application of this

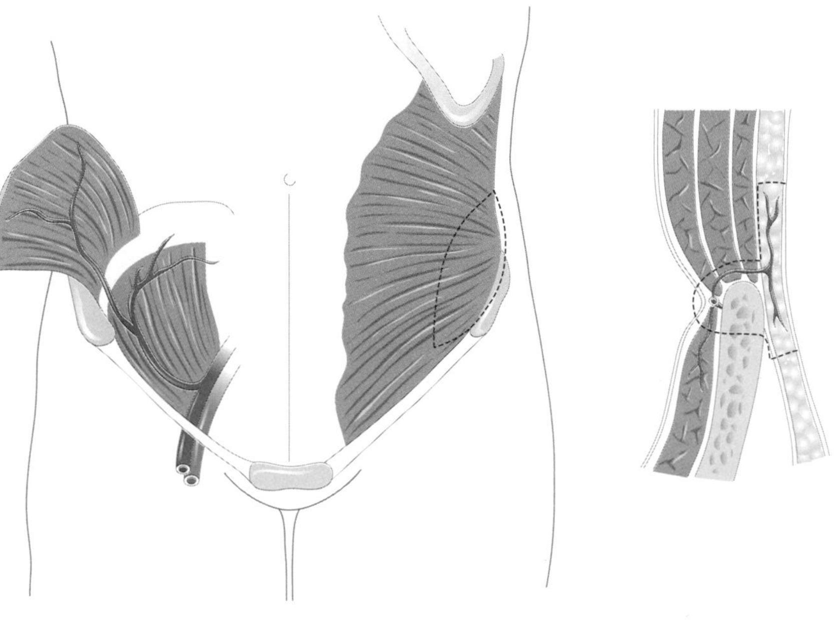

Figure 27.17 The deep circumflex iliac artery flap provides a valuable source of vascularized bone for mandibular reconstruction. Perforators extend to overlying skin allowing harvesting of an accompanying skin paddle. However, care must be taken with the closure to limit risk of a hernia.

flap is as a source of bone for mandibular reconstruction. However, it provides three different options for reconstruction depending on which tissues are required:

1. A free vascularized bone flap
2. An osseomusculocutaneous flap
3. A musculocutaneous flap

The first two options are most commonly used. The flap is extremely useful for mandibular reconstruction[25] and provides a large amount of bone as well as pliable skin for intraoral mucosal reconstruction, though vascularity to the skin paddle is not always reliable.

Raising of the flap

Either the ipsilateral or contralateral flaps may be used, depending on the amount and shape of the bone required. If a skin paddle is used, it is marked along the iliac crest with approximately two-thirds of its area above the crest and one-third below. The medial end of the skin paddle overlies or is just medial to the anterior superior iliac spine (ASIS).

The pedicle is initially identified, by either dividing through all layers above the inguinal ligament or using a transinguinal route. Once identified, the pedicle is followed laterally, taking care to preserve the veins. As the ASIS is approached the ascending branch of the deep circumflex iliac artery is identified and ligated; this can be mistaken for the main pedicle. The transversalis fascia is then incised and the deep surface of the ilium exposed. The lower part of the flap is then incised and the iliac crest split to yield an adequate amount of bone. The donor site is closed carefully in layers to prevent risk of incisional hernia.

Problems

This is a complex flap to raise and it is easy to damage the accompanying veins. Donor-site hernia can occur if a meticulous repair is not performed and the lateral cutaneous nerve of the thigh is vulnerable to injury. The skin paddle has an unreliable vascularity.

Fibula flap

The fibula flap is a type C osseofasciocutaneous flap supplied by the peroneal artery with septocutaneous and musculocutaneous perforators;[26,27] the nutrient artery to the fibula is approximately 17 cm from the fibula styloid. It is the method of choice and major source of vascularized bone for mandibular reconstruction, and can include a skin paddle. The bone stock is suitable for osseointegrated implants and can be osteotomized to recreate the mentum. The flap provides a large amount of cortical bone up to 25 cm long (Figure 27.18). It leaves an excellent donor defect, though the distal 5 cm of fibula must be left to maintain ankle stability. The skin paddle can be orientated longitudinally or transversely depending on reconstructive requirements.

The peroneal vessels provide a relatively limited pedicle, but they remain large throughout their length. As a result, they are suitable for use as recipient vessels if it is necessary to add an additional free flap in series (i.e. radial forearm flap for intraoral lining).

Raising of the flap

For an osteocutaneous flap the skin and fascia are incised posteriorly and soleus exposed, the muscle is incised to leave a small cuff on the bone to protect the musculocutaneous perforators. The skin and fascia are incised anteriorly and reflected to expose the posterior peroneal septum.

Leaving a small cuff of muscle on the bone, the interosseous membrane is incised and posteriorly incised through flexor hallucis longus to expose the peroneal vessels (the anterior tibial vessels lie anterior to the interosseous membrane). Once the vessels have been identified the superior and inferior osteotomies can be performed; the inferior pole of bone to be rotated outwards so that the vessels can be divided inferiorly. Dissection now proceeds in a proximal direction taking care not to damage the pedicle as it crosses the muscular raphe. A skin graft is usually required to close the defect.

To raise the fibula alone, the dissection is performed through a longitudinal incision lying just posterior to the lateral axis. There is no need to preserve the peroneal septum and the dissection just leaves a small amount of muscle on the bone. The fibula is identified both anteriorly and posteriorly and the osteotomies made as described above. The donor site is closed directly.

Problems

The peroneal nerve can be damaged during the dissection as it passes around the neck of the fibula. The donor site is conspicuous if skin grafted. The skin paddle is not ideal for intraoral reconstruction because it is rather thick and orientation of the skin on the bone can make reconstruction difficult.

Rectus abdominus flap

The rectus abdominus flap[28] is a type III muscle flap supplied by the deep superior epigastric artery and the deep inferior epigastric artery (Figure 27.19), with some contribution from the lower intercostal vessels. The muscle can be raised alone, or more commonly, with an accompanying skin paddle that may be orientated vertically (vertical rectus abdominis, VRAM flap) or transversly (TRAM flap).

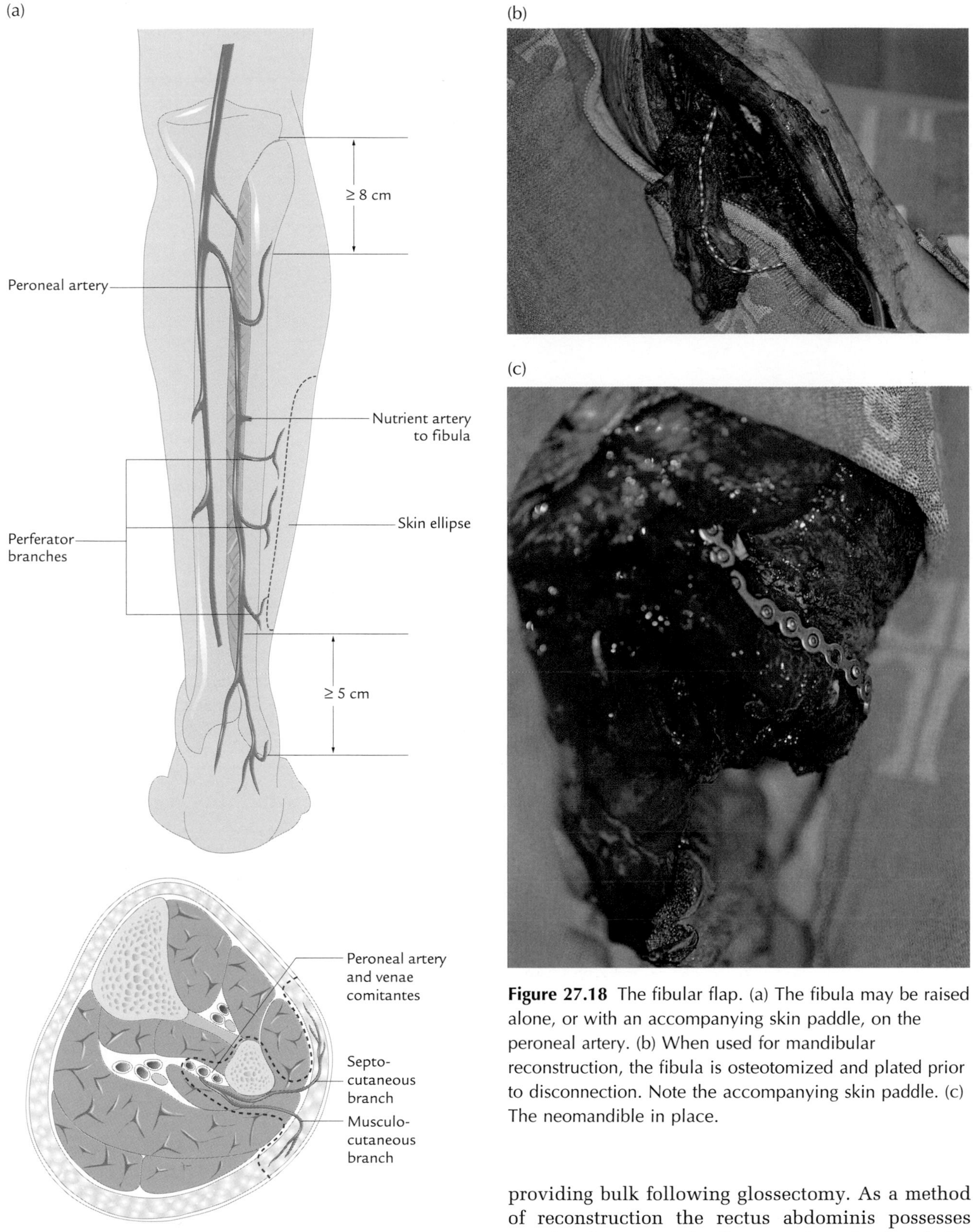

Figure 27.18 The fibular flap. (a) The fibula may be raised alone, or with an accompanying skin paddle, on the peroneal artery. (b) When used for mandibular reconstruction, the fibula is osteotomized and plated prior to disconnection. Note the accompanying skin paddle. (c) The neomandible in place.

The rectus abdominus flap is commonly used in head and neck reconstruction as it provides a large amount of tissue suitable for volume replacement that may be resurfaced with a split skin graft. Alternatively, it may be raised as a musculocutaneous flap, suitable for resurfacing the cheek, or providing bulk following glossectomy. As a method of reconstruction the rectus abdominis possesses certain advantages: the flap may be raised with the patient supine and thus simultaneously with the resection; and the pedicle is relatively long and reliable.

Raising of a muscle-only flap

Using a paramedian incision, the rectus sheath is longitudinally incised and the lateral and medial

(a)

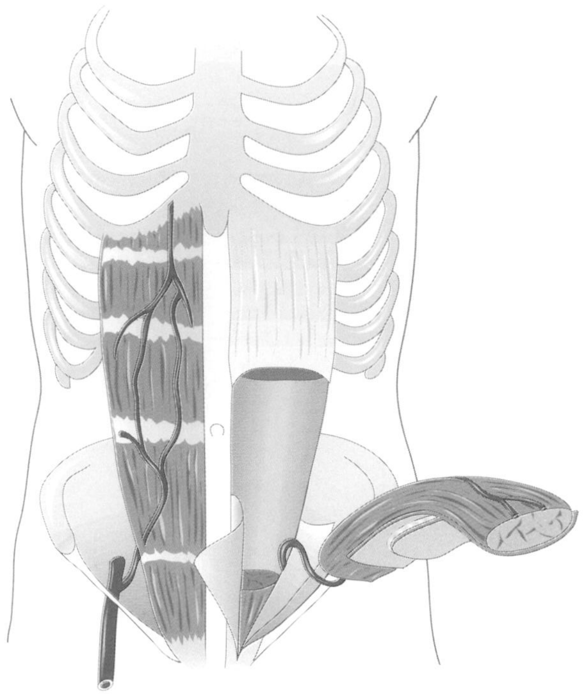

Figure 27.19 The rectus abdominis. (a) When used as a free flap, the rectus abdominis is raised on the deep inferior epigastric artery. It may be raised with a vertical (VRAM) or transverse (TRAM) skin paddle. (b) 1. This patient developed osteoradionecrosis following radiotherapy, for a squamous cell carcinoma of the mastoid. 2. The wound was thoroughly debrided and the cervical vessels exposed. 3. A free rectus muscle was laid into and over the defect and covered with a meshed split skin graft.

(b1)

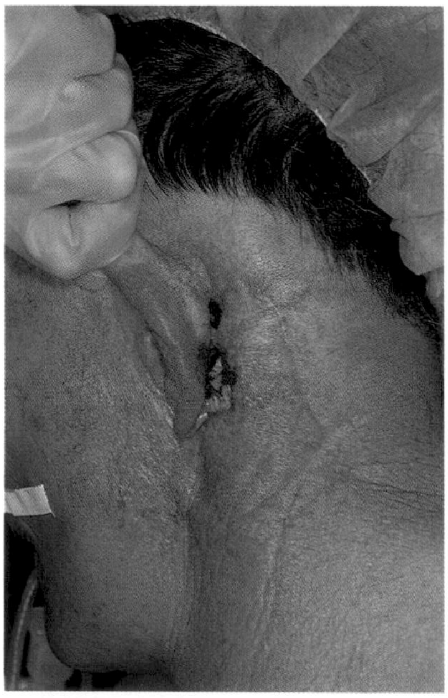

(b2)

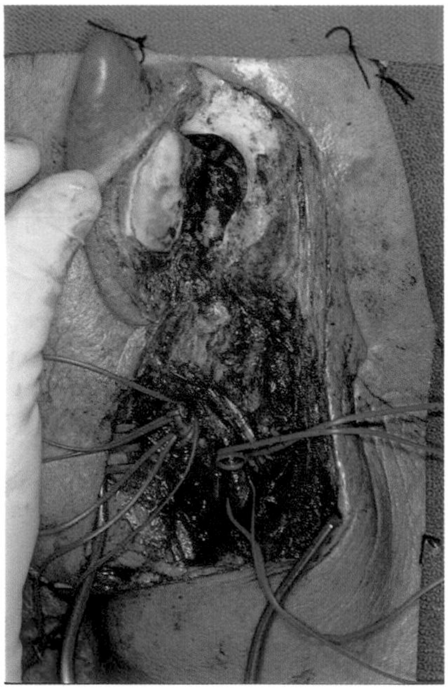

(b3)

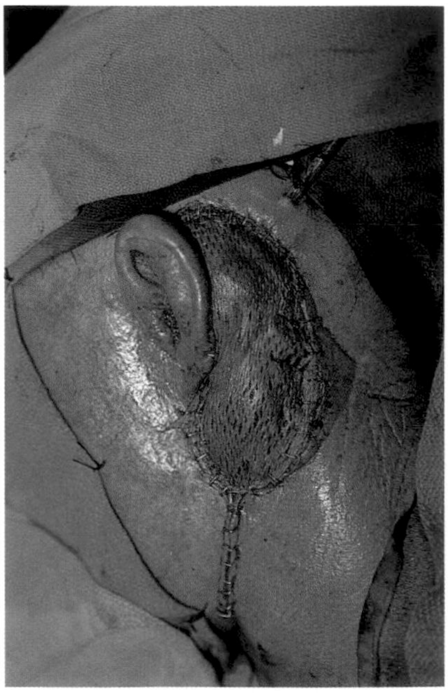

borders of the muscle identified. The pedicle is identified as it emerges from the lateral border of the lower third of the muscle. The muscle is divided at its upper and lower limits and reflected to reveal the pedicle, which is then traced to its origin and divided.

Raising of a VRAM musculocutaneous flap

The skin paddle of the flap is designed to overlie the muscle and is orientated vertically. The skin is incised down to the fascia overlying the muscle of the anterior abdominal wall including a small area of rectus sheath surrounding the periumbilical perforators. The muscle is exposed and the pedicle isolated as above. The donor site is closed in layers with the rectus sheath being closed directly or reinforced with a synthetic mesh to prevent abdominal herniae.

Raising of a TRAM flap

The TRAM flap is not routinely used in head and neck reconstruction as it provides a large, bulky flap that is rarely required. The skin paddle is positioned to lie transversely just below the umbilicus and is only suitable for harvest in patients with adequate abdominal skin folds. The contralateral side of the flap (to the pedicle) is elevated to identify the position of large perforators and these are noted when elevating the ipsilateral side. The muscle is divided above and below the flap and the pedicle identified and divided as for the VRAM flap.

Problems

Myocutaneous flaps may be excessively bulky and aesthetically suboptimal. However, this may be remedied with thinning procedures if necessary.

Reconstructive options at specific sites

General considerations

Owing to the complexity of the upper aerodigestive tract, some degree of function is nearly always lost following extirpation. The decision-making process regarding the reconstruction of any defect should be made by the reconstructive surgeon in consultation with the surgical oncologist. All the realistic options need to be considered and a compromise struck between that which produces the best function and cosmesis and least donor site morbidity.

Different sites within the head and neck present different problems for reconstruction and therefore require a variety of techniques. These methods have improved with developments in surgical skills and knowledge of the vascularity of flaps, to provide better reconstruction but it is not possible to achieve truly functional repairs because of complex:

1. Muscle structures within the upper aerodigestive tract;
2. Co-ordination of structures necessary for speech;
3. Co-ordination of structures required for swallowing.

Tissues used to fill the resection defect must be appropriately sized both in terms of area and volume. Too much bulk can hamper function by preventing co-ordinated movement. Lack of bulk, especially in the oral cavity can lead to pooling of saliva and food, poor oral hygiene and inadequate passage of food into the pharynx. Furthermore, techniques that cause tethering due to either lack of volume or because of the orientation of the flap pedicle (as in inferiorly based flaps) will prevent adequate movement of mobile structures and hinder function.

The majority of reconstructive techniques used in the head and neck region produce insensate and non-functioning cover or lining. If the surrounding normal structures have relatively normal function the deficit will not be great. However, if function is impaired, the ability to achieve full rehabilitation may prove almost impossible.

Cosmesis

Anatomical deformity, especially facial, can produce both physical and psychological problems. Counselling may help patients cope to a certain extent but prevention and correction of the deformity must be the priority of the reconstructive surgeon. The bony skeleton is the main element in dictating facial form. Accordingly, important consideration needs to be given to preserving bone where possible, and replacing it if required. To this end, maintenance of facial form has benefited from improved understanding of tumour biology and how tumours invade the mandible; mandibular conservation acts to maintain both cosmesis and function.[29,30]

Developments in prosthetics, prosthodontics and osseointegration have all played an important role in improving and maintaining cosmetic appearance following ablative surgery.[31,32]

Patient selection

In the developed world, the majority of patients with head and neck cancer are elderly, smokers and often consume a large amount of alcohol. Physically they may be malnourished, anaemic and with little cardiorespiratory reserve. Optimal treatment requires full assessment of their physical status, histological diagnosis and accurate staging, the feasibility of resection and finally, consideration of the appropriate reconstructive options.

Larynx and hypopharynx

Laryngeal reconstruction

Reconstruction following laryngectomy has to address the laryngeal defect and secondly, the extent of any accompanying pharyngeal resection. The majority of simple laryngectomies require no formal reconstruction as an adequate pharyngeal remnant remains for closure. However, when partial laryngectomy or vertical hemilaryngectomy is performed, speech preservation may be facilitated by reconstruction of these defects using local or distant tissues.[33,34]

Laryngectomy plus partial pharyngectomy

Direct closure of the larynx can be achieved primarily following laryngectomy and partial pharyngectomy. Primary closure of the pharynx requires at least 5 cm of the circumference of the pharynx to produce an adequate conduit. Primary closure is usually achieved vertically, but if this is not possible a T-shaped closure can be used. If an inadequate conduit is likely, additional lining will be required. In this instance the aim is to replace and augment the lining with thin, mobile tissue.

Reconstructive options

The optimum methods of pharyngeal reconstruction consist of regional and distant flaps. The most useful of these include the: pectoralis major;[35] latissimus dorsi;[36] radial forearm;[37] jejunal patch[38] and deltopectoral flaps.[39] Flap selection depends on the size of the defect, the patient's physical status and access to microsurgical facilities. The pectoralis major flap is the most commonly used flap in this instance as it is relatively simple to raise, robust and brings in a good blood supply to the wound.

Where microsurgical skills are available, the free radial forearm flap and jejunal patch flap are useful options for reconstruction, either as the primary procedure or as secondary techniques to salvage failed primary closure. The radial forearm provides thin, mobile skin well suited to resurface lost pharyngeal wall. Motile, mucosalized lining can be provided by using a free jejunum patch graft, particularly for extensive pharyngeal resection. The deltopectoral flap is only used as a salvage procedure, or when other options are not available.

Laryngopharyngectomy

Laryngopharyngectomy involves complete circumferential resection of the pharynx. The aim of the reconstruction is to recreate the tube of the pharynx and to maintain the ability to swallow.

Reconstructive options

As noted above, reconstruction following laryngopharyngectomy aims to provide a conduit, replace lining and, of most difficulty, maintain motility. The amount of tissue required to recreate the pharyngeal conduit cannot be derived from local tissues and, traditionally, distant myocutaneous or fasciocutaneous flaps[40] noted above have been used. The choice of flap may also be affected by the position and height of the defect,[41] its relation to the tongue base and the microsurgical abilities within the reconstructive team. However, the majority of those flaps listed above can only be tubed to create an immotile passage that is vulnerable along three suture lines.[42]

Free jejunal flap provides a tubed reconstruction with active peristalsis.[43] This is a labour-intensive method, requiring a laparotomy to harvest the jejunum and microsurgical skills to revascularize it (Figure 27.20). Considerable care needs to be taken to ensure siting the chosen segment of jejunum in relation to the selected vascular pedicle, and to avoid bruising the bowel when raising the flap and performing the bowel anastomosis. The chosen length is inset along its peristaltic axis and with slight tension, preventing redundant bowel folds. A distal segment of the transferred bowel can be exteriorized to act as a monitor and tied off after 5 days.

Gastric transposition has the advantage of one bowel anastomosis, no microvascular anastomoses and is oncologically preferable due to the whole oesophagus being removed. It requires a thoraco-abdominal approach which is associated with cardio-respiratory complications.

Oropharynx

General considerations

The oropharynx is essential to initiation of the involuntary swallow. Resection within any part of the oropharynx can alter speech or swallowing.

Reconstruction is with insensate flaps with resulting impairment of the swallow reflex and risk of aspiration especially in the elderly with pre-existing chest disease.

Pharyngeal walls

The pharyngeal walls may be subdivided into the tonsillar fossa and the posterior pharyngeal wall. Defects following excision of small lesions (T1 and small T2) within the lateral pharyngeal wall may be either closed primarily or left to granulate. Larger defects require flap reconstruction to reconstitute lining.

Reconstructive options

The following flaps can be used to reconstruct the lateral pharyngeal wall: pectoralis major; latissimus dorsi; free radial forearm; temporalis muscle/fascial;[44] forehead; sternomastoid;[45] free jejunal patch; gastro-omental; and masseter flaps.[46]

The free radial forearm flap is the method of choice, providing thin, pliable lining. The pectoralis myocutaneous flap[47] is also commonly used, but

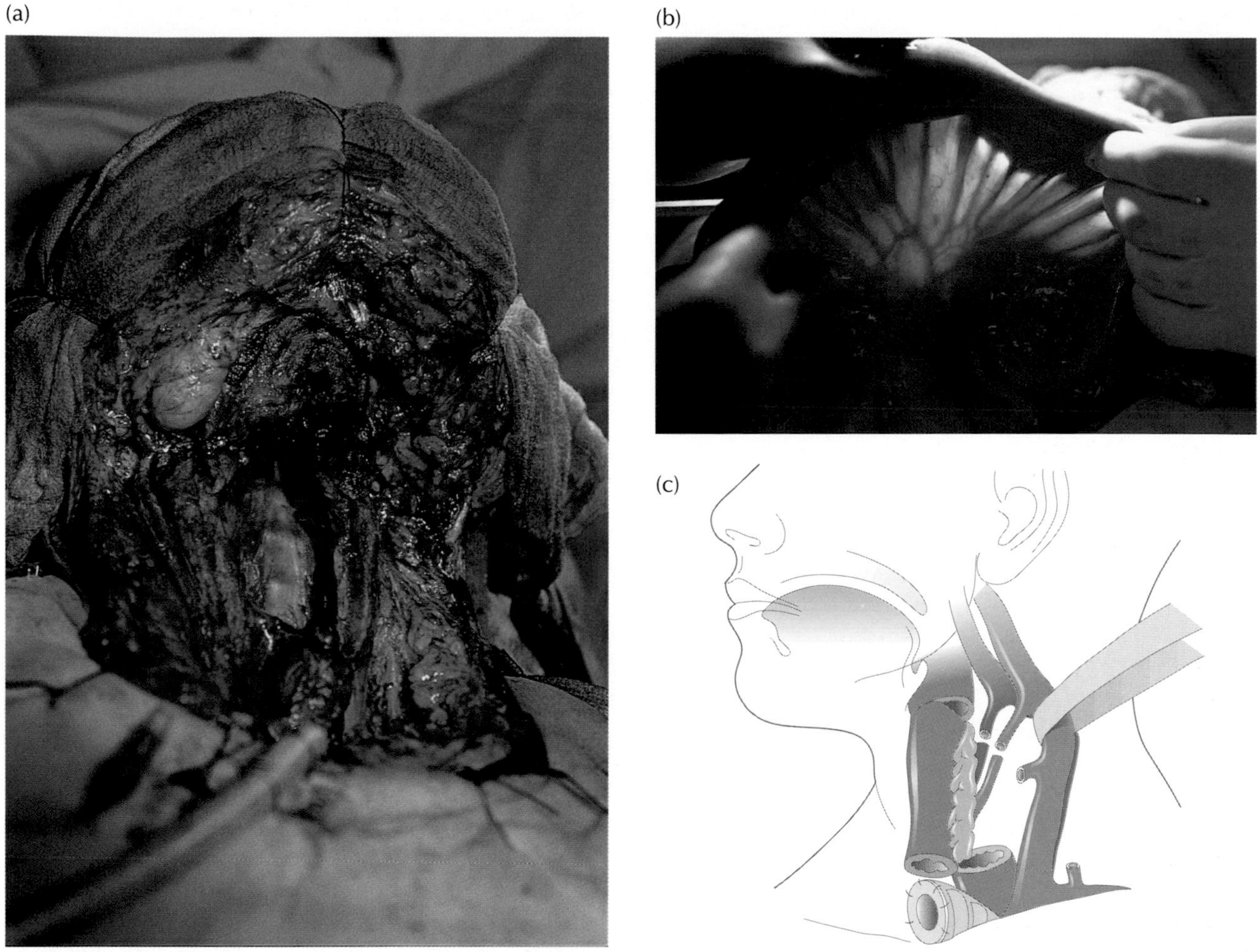

Figure 27.20 Free jejunum. (a) Defect following laryngopharyngectomy. (b) Transillumination of the jejunal vascular arcade allows selection of an appropriate vascular pedicle. (c) Diagrammatic representation of the jejunum in the neck. (d) The jejunal flap has been inset prior to revascularization; note the tension of the segment to avoid redundant bowel.

may introduce too much bulk, though this can be minimized by using the muscle or myofascial flap alone.[48]

The free jejunal patch flap also provides a good alternative where little bulk is required.[49] The temporalis muscle flap can be rotated to reach the oropharynx. The flap can then be covered with a split skin graft or left to granulate.

The base of tongue

Reconstruction of the tongue base may prove especially problematic as adequate clearance may be gained only at the expense of innervation to the remaining tongue.

Reconstructive options

The following flaps are commonly used to reconstruct the tongue base: pectoralis major; latissimus dorsi; free radial forearm; trapezius;[50] and tongue setback flaps.

Microvascular tissue transfers provide the optimal reconstruction for this area, with the radial forearm free flap as the method of choice. Resection of large lesions from the tongue base may result in loss of the hypoglossal nerves and usually leads to total or near total glossectomy, producing severe speech and swallowing difficulties. The aim of reconstruction is to fill the defect with bulky tissue using either the latissimus dorsi flap or the pectoralis major flap.[51] The rectus abdominis myocutaneous flap is also of use in this location. As stated previously, reconstruction with insensate flaps in this region result in a poor swallow and risk of aspiration especially in elderly patients with chest disease.

Total glossectomy can be complicated by aspiration, due to removal of the suprahyoid and extrinsic tongue muscles. This may be ameliorated by laryngoplasty or laryngeal suspension.[52] If aspiration is severe or persists, laryngectomy may be needed to protect the lungs and airway.

Soft palate

Resection of tumours within the oropharynx may involve removal of part or all of the soft palate that may severely compromise competence of the velopharyngeal sphincter. Incompetence leads to nasal escape during speech and regurgitation of food during swallowing. The aim of reconstruction, therefore, is to produce a functioning palate, which prevents these sequelae. Most reconstructions fail in this respect as they produce an atonic curtain-like flap. Alternative methods of preventing regurgitation and nasal escape include a variety of pharyngoplasties and obturators.

Small defects

Posterior wall pharyngoplasties in combination with local flaps can produce acceptable results both for speech and swallowing. Small free tissue transfers, such as the radial forearm flap have also been used with good effect to close palatal defects.[53]

Large defects

Myocutaneous flaps used for lateral reconstructions can produce good palatal function, though they may prove too bulky to be effective. Where total palatectomy has been performed, dental obturators provide satisfactory velopharyngeal competence.

Oral cavity

The oral cavity extends from the lips to the anterior faucial pillars. The major structures that lie within this area are the anterior two-thirds of the tongue and the upper and lower jaw. The cavity is lined with thin pliable mucous membrane that is mobile where it covers the floor of the mouth and the buccal sulcus. Over the hard palate and alveolar processes the mucosa is adherent to the underlying bone. The aim of reconstruction in this region is to restore the defect using a thin and pliable mucosal substitute that conforms to the contour of the defect.

The reconstructive problems of the oral cavity can be divided into three areas: the tongue; the buccal mucosa; and the mandible. These three areas will be dealt with separately.

Reconstructive options

Small defects throughout the oral cavity can be left to heal by granulation and re-epithelialization. The resulting scar is usually small, causes little deformity and preserves function.

Direct closure

Small defects, up to 1.5 cm in diameter, can be closed directly. For lesions lying on or near the alveolus, this may be made easier if a mandibular rim excision resection has been performed.

Split skin graft

As the mucosa in the oral cavity is thin, small areas may be resurfaced using a split skin graft. The graft can be secured by quilting the graft in place with sutures.[3] However, skin grafts are likely to contract and do not withstand trauma well.

Flaps

Ideally, local oral mucosal flaps should not be used for reconstruction of defects following resection of malignant tumours as they lie within the field of potential malignant change. Local flaps that lie outside the immediate area of mucosa include the nasolabial[8] and submental artery flaps.[54] Distant flaps include the temporalis;[55] forehead; pectoralis major; latissimus dorsi; deltopectoral; and trapezius flaps. Microvascular flaps include the following: the radial forearm; ulnar artery;[56] lateral arm flap;[57] and free jejunal patch flaps.

The tongue

The part of the tongue within the oral cavity is very mobile. Accordingly, reconstruction must not tether the tongue and limit speech, mastication and swallowing. Small lesions can be excised and the defect primarily closed. Alternatively, they may be left to epithelialize or covered with a quilted split skin graft. Defects, which extend to the floor of the mouth, may require more elaborate reconstruction. The free radial forearm flap is the method of choice in this instance, as it will provide adequate, thin pliable skin to drape over the varying contours of the oral cavity.[19]

Larger defects, such as after hemiglossectomy, may be restored using the free radial forearm flap; the radial forearm flap can be used to tailor and restore the contour of the tongue very accurately (Figure 27.21). Pedicled flaps, for example the pectoralis major myocutaneous flap, do have a role to play in partial tongue reconstruction but the inferior axis of

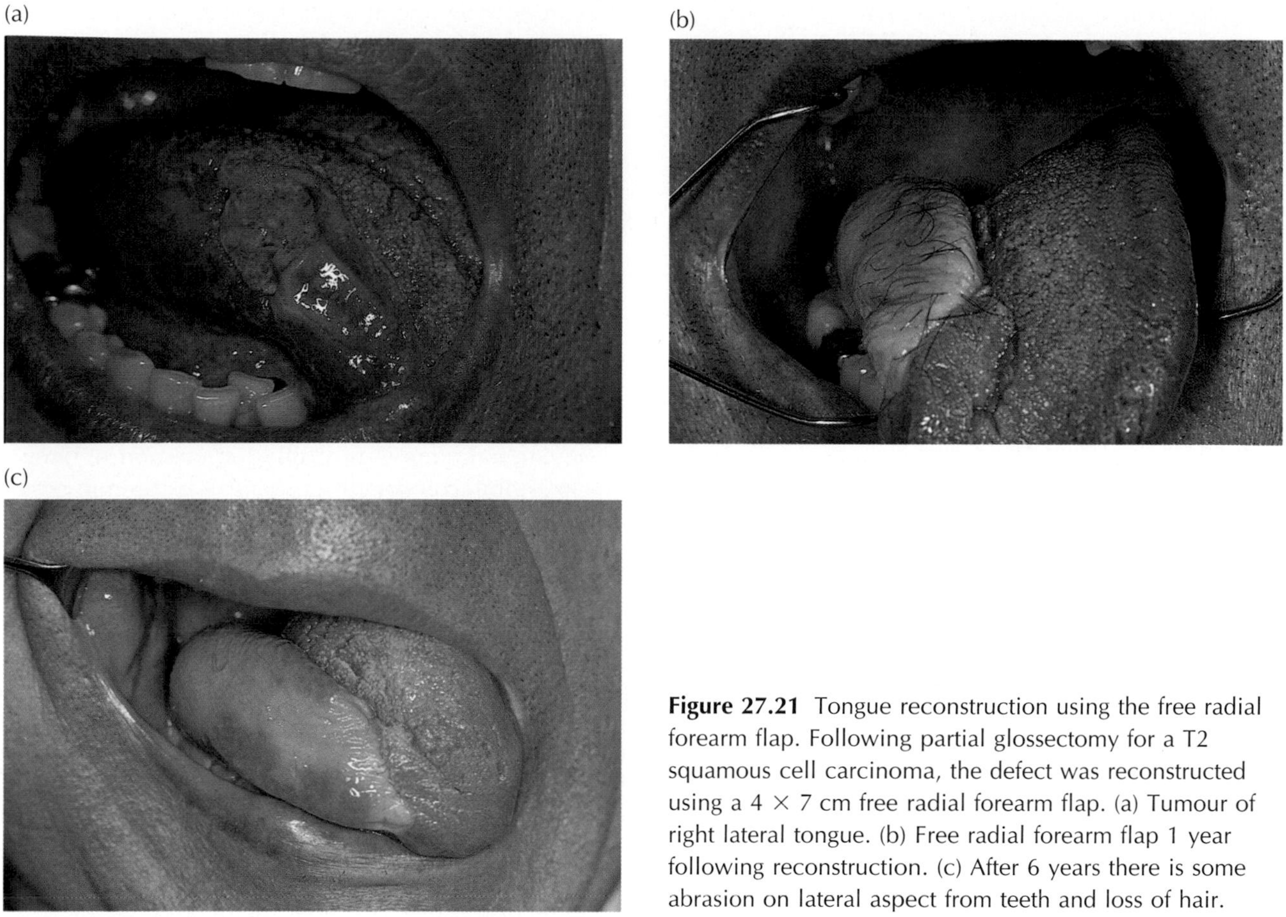

Figure 27.21 Tongue reconstruction using the free radial forearm flap. Following partial glossectomy for a T2 squamous cell carcinoma, the defect was reconstructed using a 4 × 7 cm free radial forearm flap. (a) Tumour of right lateral tongue. (b) Free radial forearm flap 1 year following reconstruction. (c) After 6 years there is some abrasion on lateral aspect from teeth and loss of hair.

the pedicle often subjects the flap, and by association the tongue, to some degree of tethering and functional limitation.

Total glossectomy leaves the patient with a considerable anatomical and functional deficit. Reconstruction aims to provide bulk that acts as a platform upon which pharyngeal swallowing may be initiated. The pectoralis major and latissimus dorsi myocutaneous flaps are usually employed in this instance, though if inset within the lingual cavity may tend to sink, even with a hyoid hitch. In the edentulous patient, this can be avoided by positioning a latissimus dorsi myocutaneous flap over the mandibular rim and suturing it to the buccal margin of the gingiva.

Oral cavity plus buccal mucosa

The method of reconstruction within the oral cavity and floor of the mouth depends on whether there is exposed bone. In cases where there is a good soft tissue cover the defects can be left to granulate and heal or be resurfaced with split skin grafts. However, where additional tissue is required or bone is exposed, the radial forearm flap is used. This flap provides a large amount of thin pliable skin, which can drape over the varying contours of the oral cavity. The ulnar artery and lateral arm flaps may also be of use here. Myocutaneous flaps tend to be too bulky for the oral cavity unless a large amount of the tongue has been removed.

The nasolabial flap and submental flap have a small, but definite role to play in oral reconstruction. The nasolabial flap can be used for small defects in the anterior floor of the mouth. The submental flap can provide a quite larger skin paddle, though its vascularity may be compromised following neck dissection.

Reconstruction of the oral cavity, including external skin cover

Advanced intraoral carcinomas may infiltrate the cheek and require excision. The reconstructive goals are to provide both lining and cover using thin pliable skin that has an acceptable colour match. In the elderly, cover may be provided by rotating cervical skin up onto the cheek. However, if a large amount of lining has been lost alternative sources will need to be sought. Bipaddled skin flaps with an intermediate de-epithelialized bridge allow use of a single flap to achieve both cover and lining. The pedicled or free latissimus dorsi can be used in this way, as can the rectus abdominis, though, both these flaps may prove bulky.

The radial forearm microvascular free flap provides enough skin to have single, double or triple skin paddles to reconstruct complex three-dimensional defects around the face. The flap can be raised with palmaris longus tendon to act as a sling to support the angle of the mouth following the reconstruction.[58]

Other options for defects requiring flaps for both surface and lining reconstruction include the subscapular artery system, which can supply all the elements required.[59]

Reconstruction of the oral cavity involving the mandible

Anterior mandibulectomy produces a dramatic retrognathic 'Andy Gump' appearance. The physical and psychological hardship for those with such a deformity is immense, and is further exacerbated by the inability to speak and eat properly. Consideration must be given to conserving and/or reconstructing the mandible.

Advances in the knowledge of tumour biology and the way tumours invade the mandible, in non-irradiated cases, have meant fewer radical bone resections. Tumour control can be achieved by performing rim resections or partial (segmental) resections of the mandible. However there are still cases where mandibulectomy is required. The aim of mandibular reconstruction is to maintain the dental arch, dental occlusion and provide a platform for prosthetic rehabilitation.

The ideal mandibular reconstruction provides bone continuity with adequate alveolar height, good facial cosmesis and arch form, and adequate osseous bulk. There may also be a need for intraoral lining. The reconstruction must be robust enough to enable radiotherapy to be used as part of the treatment regimen. Reconstruction of the mandible requires good bone stock and thin pliable skin for soft tissue cover. No single flap can provide this; the radial forearm flap has thin reliable skin but poor bone stock, whereas the fibula flap has very good bone stock but a relatively unreliable skin paddle.

Reconstructive options

Small segmental mandibulectomies posterior to the mental foramen can be left without reconstruction and myocutaneous flaps used to fill the mucosal defect.

The following techniques have all been used to reconstruct the mandible. Non-vascularized bone grafts include non-vascularized bone graft +/– reconstruction plates; titanium trays plus bone graft; allogenic bone cribs plus autogenous bone graft;[60] and myocutaneous flap plus bone graft.[61] Rib grafts harvested with both pectoralis major[62,63] and latissimus dorsi derive minimal blood supply from the accompanying muscle and are, in effect, free grafts.

Vascularized bone flaps include the radial forearm; fibula;[64] scapula;[65] and deep circumflex iliac artery flap.[66,67]

Vascularized bone is probably the method of choice for mandibular reconstruction. The technique is not so environment-dependent as non-vascularized bone grafting techniques, and has the ability to incorporate soft tissue for reconstruction within the flap and osseointegrated implants for dental restoration. The choice of flap depends on the length of the mandibular defect and the size of any accompanying soft tissue defect. Defects less than 6 cm in length may be restored using the radial forearm osseofasciocutaneous flap.[68] Defects, which are longer than 6 cm in length can be replaced with bone derived from the scapula flap, deep circumflex iliac artery (DCIA) flap or the fibula flap.

Both the DCIA flap and the fibula flap have enough bone stock to enable osseointegration implants to be inserted whereas the radial forearm flap probably does not.[69] The scapular flap can produce a section of bone up to 12 cm in length with a large skin paddle but the soft tissue is rather bulky for intraoral use. The subscapular artery complex can produce multi-component flaps that can provide lining, bone reconstruction and skin cover to fit complex defects.[70]

Conclusion

Head and neck surgery is a demanding discipline that confronts both the patient and clinician with considerable challenges. These are best managed by a multidisciplinary team, each member contributing their particular skills to provide the patient with the benefit of 'joint best practice'. Planning the preoperative and postoperative care of the patient is important, as patients must be physically and psychologically prepared.

Successful reconstruction is dependent upon suitable specialist training in a range of techniques; selecting the most appropriate treatment for a given patient, and not attempting to make one method applicable to all. Reconstructive planning should also consider what to do in the event of failure, whether it is a flap complication, or the management of recurrent disease. Patients can only be optimally managed by considering these and other factors in concert with the management of the tumour itself.

As treatment data continues to accrue, reconstructive surgeons will need to assess their work and critically assess the effect a given method has on patients. It is being increasingly recognized that quality of life analyses and outcome measures need to be investigated to allow comparison of techniques from the most important perspective of all, that of the patient. These studies will provide essential information to determine the future direction and techniques of head and neck reconstruction.

REFERENCES

1. Gillies H, Millard R. Principles. In: *Principles and Art of Plastic Surgery*. Vol 1. London: Butterworth, 1957; 48.
2. Rush BF Jr, Swaminathan A, Knightly JJ. Use of split thickness grafts in repair of excisions of the oropharynx, base of tongue and larynx. *Am J Surg* 1974; **128**: 553.
3. Schramm VL, Myers EN. Skin grafts in oral cavity reconstruction. *Arch Otolaryngol* 1980; **106**: 528.
4. Daniel RK, Kerrigan CL. Principles and physiology of flap surgery. In: McCarthy JG (ed.) *Plastic Surgery*. Philadelphia: WB Saunders, 1990.
5. Taylor GI, Palmer JH. The vascular territories (angiosomes) of the body: experimental study and clinical applications. *Br J Plast Surg* 1987; **40**: 113.
6. Khouri RK, Upton J, Shaw WW. Principles of flap prefabrication. *Clin Plast Surg* 1992; **15**: 155.
7. Pribaz JJ, Fine N, Orgill DP. Flap prefabrication in the head and neck: a 10-year experience. *Plast Reconstr Surg* 1999; **103**: 808–820.
8. Gerwitz HS, Eilber FR, Zarem HA. Use of the nasolabial flap for reconstruction of the floor of the mouth. *Am J Surg* 1978; **136**: 508–511.
9. Lewis MB, Remensnyder JP. Forehead flap for reconstruction after ablative surgery for oral and oropharyngeal malignancy. *Plast Reconstr Surg* 1978; **62**: 59.
10. Jackson IT, Adham MN, Marsh WR. Use of the galeofrontalis myofascial flap in craniofacial surgery. *Plast Reconstr Surg* 1986; **77**: 905.
11. Bradley P, Brockbank J. The temporalis muscle flap in oral reconstruction. A cadaveric, animal and clinical study. *J Maxillofac Surg* 1981; **9**: 139–145.
12. Bakamjian VY. A two stage method for pharyngo-oesophageal reconstruction with a primary pectoral skin flap. *Plast Reconstr Surg* 1965; **36**: 173.
13. Tobin GR, Schusterman M, Peterson GH et al. The intramuscular neurovascular anatomy of the latissimus dorsi muscle: the basis for splitting the muscle. *Plast Reconstr Surg* 1981; **67**: 637–641.
14. Demergasso F, Piazza MV. Trapezius myocutaneous flap in reconstructive surgery for head and neck cancer: an original technique. *Am J Surg* 1979; **138**: 533–536.
15. McGraw J, Magee WP, Kaliviac H. Uses of the trapezius and sternomastoid myocutaneous flaps in head and neck reconstruction. *Plast Reconstr Surg* 1979; **63**: 49–57.
16. Reid CD, Taylor GI. The vascular territory of the acromiothoracic axis. *B J Plast Surg* 1984; **37**: 194–212.
17. Ariyan S. The sternocleidomastoid myocutaneous flap. *Laryngoscope* 1980; **90**: 676–679.
18. Song R, Gao Y, Song Y et al. The forearm flap. *Clin Plast Surg* 1982; **9**: 21.
19. Soutar DS, Shecker LR Tanner NSB, McGregor IA. The radial forearm flap : a versatile method of intraoral reconstruction. *Br J Plast Surg* 1983; **36**: 1.
20. Soutar DS, Widdowson PW. Immediate reconstruction of the mandible using vascularised segments of radius. *Head Neck Surg* 1986; **8**: 232.
21. Cormack GC, Duncan MJ, Lamberty BGH. The blood supply of the bone component of the compound osseocutaneous radial forearm flap: an anatomical study. *Br J Plast Surg* 1986; **39**: 173–175.
22. Mayou BJ, Whitby D, Jones BM. The scapular flap: an anatomical and clinical study. *Br J Plast Surg* 1982; **35**: 8–13.
23. Urbaniak JR, Koman LA, Goldner RD. The vascularised cutaneous scapular flap. *Plast Reconstr Surg* 1982; **69**: 772–777.
24. Swartz WM, Banis JC, Newton ED et al. Osteocutaneous scapular flap for mandibular reconstruction. *Plast Reconstr Surg* 1986; **77**: 530–545.
25. Taylor GI, Townsend P, Corlett R. Superiority of the deep circumflex iliac vessels as the supply for the free groin flaps. Experimental work. *Plast Reconstr Surg* 1979; **64**: 594–604.
26. Gilbert A. Surgical technique – vascularised transfer of the fibula. *Int J Microsurg* 1979; **1**: 100–102.
27. Wei FC, Chen H, Chuang C, Noordhoff MS. Fibular osseocutaneous flap – anatomic study and clinical applications. *Plast Reconstr Surg* 1986; **78**: 191–197.
28. Taylor GI, Corlett R, Boyd JB. The versatile deep inferior epigastric artery (inferior rectus abdominus) flap. *Br J Plast Surg* 1984; **37**: 330–350.
29. McGregor AD, MacDonald DG. Routes of entry of squamous cell carcinoma to the mandible. *Head Neck Surg* 1988; **10**: 294.
30. McGregor AD, MacDonald DG. Pattern of spread of squamous cell carcinoma within the mandible. *Head Neck Surg* 1989; **11**: 457.

31. Finlay PM. Prosthodontics. In: Soutar DS, Tiwari R (eds). *Excision and Reconstruction in Head and Neck Cancer.* London: Churchill Livingstone, 1994; 103–116.
32. Branemark PI. Osseointegration and experimental background. *Am J Prosthet Dentistr* 1983; **50**: 399–410.
33. McCaffery TV. Head and neck cancer surgery. *Curr Opin Oncol* 1992; **4**: 499–503.
34. Calceterra TC. Sternohyoid myofascial flap reconstruction of the larynx for vertical partial laryngectomy. *Laryngoscope* 1983; **93**: 422–424.
35. Aryian S. The pectoralis major myocutaneous flap. A versatile flap for reconstruction in the head and neck. *Plast Reconstr Surg* 1979; **63**: 173.
36. Olivari N. The latissimus flap. *Br J Plast Surg* 1976; **29**: 126.
37. Takato T et al. Oral and pharyngeal reconstruction using the free radial forearm flap. *Arch Otol Head Neck Surg* 1987; **113**: 873.
38. Cocks HC, Kumar BN, Das Gupta AR et al. Free jejunal patch flaps in oral and oro-pharyngeal reconstruction. *J Laryngol Otol* 1999; **113**: 680–2.
39. McGregor IA, Jackson IT. The extended role of the deltopectoral flap. *Br J Plast Surg* 1970; **23**; 173.
40. Anthony JP, Singer MI, Mathes SJ. Pharyngoesophageal reconstruction using the tubed free radial forearm flap. *Clin Plast Surg* 1994; **21**: 137.
41. Lam K, Ho C, Lau W, Wei W, Wong J. Immediate reconstruction of pharyngo-oesophageal defects. *Arch Otolaryngol Head Neck Surg* 1989; **115**: 608–612.
42. Coleman JJ III. Reconstruction of the pharynx after resection for cancer. A comparison of methods. *Ann Surg* 1989; **209**: 554–560.
43. Reece GJ. Bengston BP, Schustermann MA. Reconstruction of the pharynx and cervical oesophagus using free jejunal transfer. *Clin Plast Surg* 1994; **21**: 125–136.
44. Shagets FW, Panje WR, Shore JW. Use of temporalis muscle in composite defects of the head and neck. *Arch Otolaryngol Head Neck Surg* 1986; **112**: 60–65.
45. Charles GA, Hamaker RC et al. Sternocleidomastoid myocutaneous flap. *Laryngoscope* 1989; **97**: 970–974.
46. Tiwari RM, Snow GB. Role of masseter cross-over flap in oropharyngeal reconstruction. *J Laryngol Otolaryngol* 1989; **103**: 298–301.
47. Shemen LJ, Freeman JL, Young S, Noyek AM. Pectoralis major myocutaneous flap in orophayngeal reconstruction. *Ear Nose Throat J* 1986; **65**: 61–72.
48. Shindo NL, Costantino PD, Freidman CD et al. The pectoralis major myofascial flap for intraoral and pharyngeal reconstruction. *Arch Otolaryngol Head Neck Surg* 1992; **118**: 707–711.
49. Stern JR, Keller AJ, Wernig BL. Evaluation of reconstructive techniques of oropharyngeal defects. *Ann Plast Surg* 1989; **22**: 332–336.
50. Netterville JL, Panje WR, Maves MD. The trapezius myocutaneous flap. *Arch Otolaryngol Head Neck Surg* 1987; **113**: 271–281.
51. Quillen CG, Sherwin JC, Georgiade NC. Use of latissimus dorsi myocutaneous flap for reconstruction in the head and neck. *Plast Reconstr Surg* 1978; **62**: 113.
52. Goode RL. Laryngeal suspension in head and neck surgery. *Laryngoscope* 1975; **85**: 349–355.
53. Batchelor AG, Palmer JP. A novel method of closing a palatal fistula: the free fascial flap. *Br J Plast Surg* 1990; **43**: 354.
54. Faltaous AA, Yetman RJ. The submental artery flap: an anatomic study. *Plast Reconstr Surg* 1996; **97**: 56–60.
55. McGregor IA. The temporal flap in intraoral cancer: its use in repairing the post-excisional defect. *Br J Plast Surg* 1963; **16**: 318–335.
56. Lovie MJ, Duncan GM, Glasson DW. The ulnar artery forearm free flap. *Br J Plast Surg* 1984; **37**: 486.
57. Katsaros J, Shusterman M, Beppin M et al. The lateral arm flap: anatomy and clinical applications. *Ann Plast Surg* 1984; **12**: 489.
58. Niranjan NS, Watson DP. Reconstruction of the cheek using a 'suspended' radial forearm free flap. *Br J Plast Surg* 1990; **43**: 365–366.
59. Aviv JE, Urken ML, Vickery C et al. The combined latissimus dorsi – scapular free flap in head and neck reconstruction. *Arch Otolaryngol Head Neck Surg* 1991; **117**: 1242–50.
60. Marx RE. Mandibular reconstruction, bone transplants and implants. In: Soutar DS, Tiwari R (eds). *Excision and Reconstruction in Head and Neck Cancer.* London: Churchill Livingstone, 1994; 87–102.
61. Pearlman NW, Albin RE, O'Donnell RS. Mandibular reconstruction in irradiated patient utilising osteomyocutaneous flaps. *Am J Surg* 1983; **146**: 474–7.
62. Bell MSG, Barron PT. The rib pectoralis major osteomyocutaneous flap. *Ann Plas Surg* 1981; **6**: 347–53.
63. Bhathena A, Karavana NM. One-stage total mandibular reconstruction with rib, pectoralis major osteomyocutaneous flap. *Head Neck Surg* 1986; **8**: 211–3.
64. Hidalgo DA. Free fibula flap: A new method of mandible reconstruction. *Plast Reconstr Surg* 1989; **84**: 71–9.
65. Sullivan MJ, Baker SR, Crompton R et al. Free scapular osteocutaneous flap for mandibular reconstruction. *Arch Otolaryngol Head Neck Surg* 1985; **115**: 1334–40.
66. David DJ, Tan E, Katsaros J, Sheen R. Mandibular reconstruction with vascularised iliac crest: a 10-year experience. *Plast Reconstr Surg* 1988; **82**: 792–803.
67. Taylor GI, Townsend P, Corlett R. Superiority of the deep circumflex iliac vessels as the supply for the free groin flaps: clinical work. *Plast Reconstr Surg* 1979; **64**: 745–59.
68. Boyd JB, Rosen IB, Freeman J et al. The iliac crest and the radial forearm flap in vascularised oral mandibular reconstruction. *Am J Surg* 1990; **159**: 301–8.
69. Hidalgo DA. Free fibula mandibular reconstruction. *Clin Plast Surg* 1994; **21**: 25–35.
70. Robb GL. Free scapular flap reconstruction of the head and neck. *Clin Plast Surg* 1994; **21**: 45–58.

28 Reconstruction of the oral cavity and oropharynx

Peter C Neligan and Patrick J Gullane

Introduction

The oral cavity is a unique structure that serves a multitude of functions. It is the gateway to the aerodigestive tract and is vital in the production of normal speech. It houses many specific and highly specialized structures: the mandible, the teeth, the tongue, the palate and the oropharynx. It is lined by mucosa, which is lubricated by saliva. This mucosa covers muscles that provide the motor functions that facilitate speech and swallowing. Furthermore, it is rich in nerve endings, which provide us with the special sense of taste as well as exquisite sensation that converts eating from a daily task necessary for survival to one of the most pleasurable activities.

When planning reconstruction of the oral cavity there are several considerations that must be contemplated. Issues such as prognosis, the general medical condition of the patient, and the use or planned use of radiation are important in selecting the type of reconstruction. Furthermore, the extent of the resection will help ascertain which type of reconstruction is most suitable. The fundamental question that must be answered is what tissues are being excised and consequently, which tissues need to be replaced?

Reconstructive technique

The reconstructive technique chosen can include multiple modalities but the reconstructive ladder that applies to all defects is also applied in the oral cavity. These principles have been extensively discussed in Chapter 27. In terms of reconstruction it is important to be cognizant of the fact that different reconstructive requirements exist for different areas within the mouth. These will be discussed individually.

Floor of mouth

Reconstruction of the floor of the mouth requires thin pliable tissue. The extent of the defect will determine which technique is most appropriate. Very small defects can be allowed to granulate and remucosalize or may be covered with a split thickness skin graft. Local flaps may be used effectively in moderate-sized defects. These techniques include buccal mucosal flaps, including the facial artery musculomucosal flap,[1] tongue flaps, palatal flaps[2] and nasolabial flaps. For larger defects the radial forearm flap has become the workhorse within the oral cavity. It has the advantage of being thin and pliable and has the potential for reinnervation. The flap may be raised synchronously with the ablation, which reduces operative time. Access to the floor of the mouth for ablation and reconstruction is generally achieved, except for the smaller lesions, by the use of a mandibulotomy approach. A midline mandibulotomy is preferred because it provides excellent exposure and ensures maximal bone contact to the healing segments. It is important to ensure that the mandibulotomy is accurately repaired. This is achieved either with a plate or with lag screws.[3–5] Accuracy is assured by applying the fixation prior to the mandibulotomy: the mandible is predrilled either at the site of plate hole placement or lag screw placement. The fixation device is then removed and the mandibulotomy is performed. At the end of the procedure the screws are merely inserted in the predrilled holes to give a perfect reduction and rigid fixation (Figures 28.1–28.4).

When planning the reconstruction it is important to ensure that adequate tissue is provided to cover the defect and avoid any potential tethering of the tongue, which can increase the morbidity and compromise the functional result. The defect should be carefully measured to ensure harvest of an

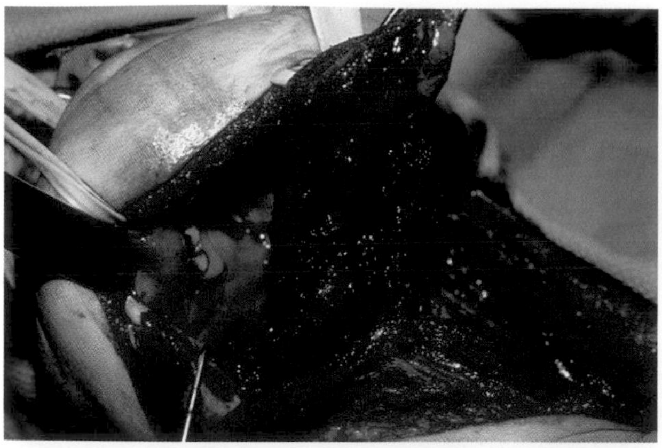

Figure 28.1 Mandibulotomy using degloving approach.

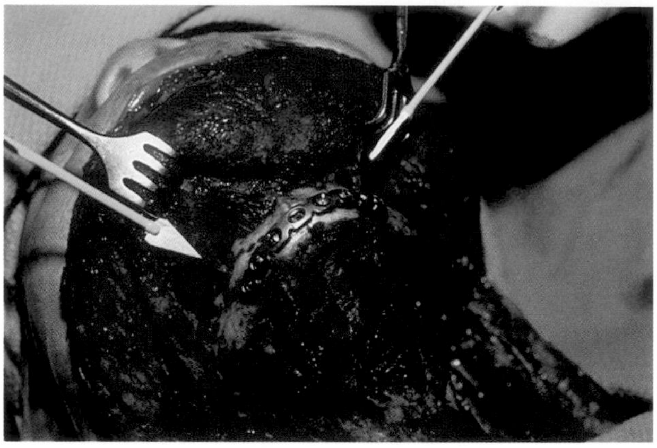

Figure 28.2 Application of fixation plate.

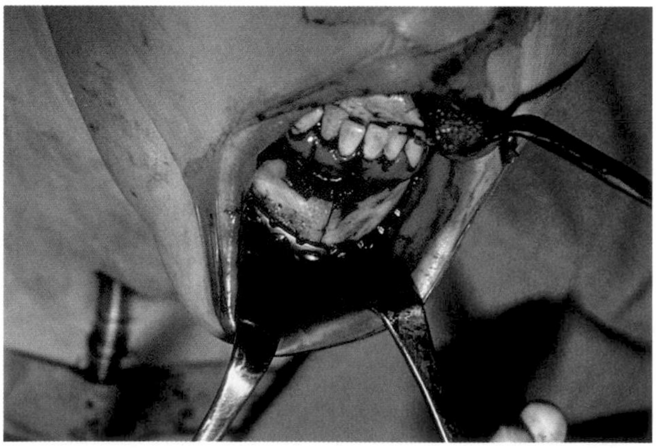

Figure 28.3 Intraoral view of plate fixation.

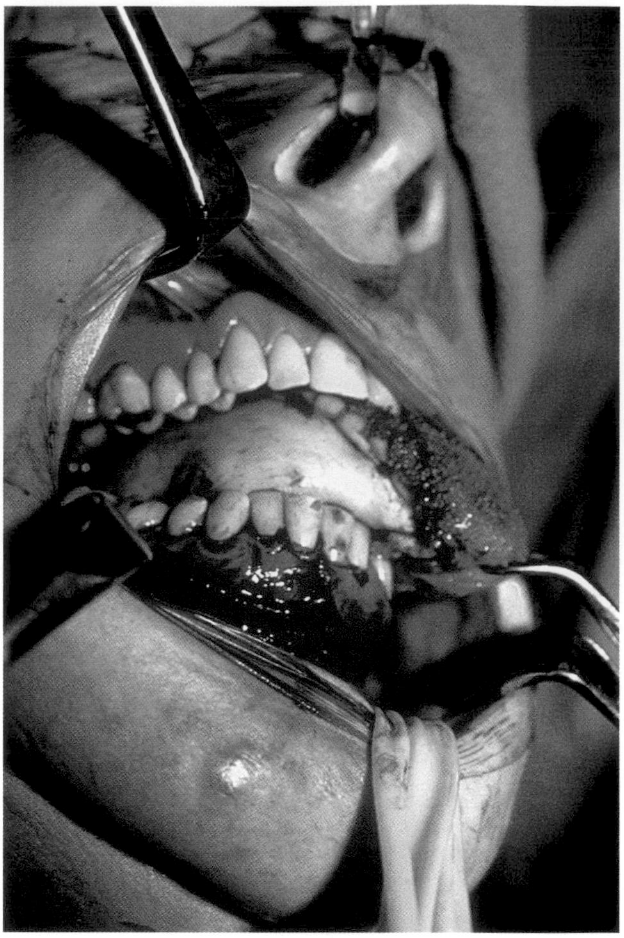

Figure 28.4 Flap inset completed.

adequately sized flap. Our flap of choice is the innervated radial forearm flap. The lateral antebrachial cutaneous nerve is harvested with the flap. It has previously been shown that reinnervation of this flap is very effective and it is thought to improve oral function by permitting the patient to sense food in the reconstructed segment of the oral cavity, which not only makes eating more comfortable but allows for improved oral hygiene.[6] Studies are currently underway to document the functional outcome of reinnervation within the oral cavity. The technique of raising the flap is critical. We have found it important to raise the flap in a suprafascial plane. This is well described and helps to significantly reduce donor site morbidity.[6–9]

Xerostomia is one of the problems encountered by many oral cavity patients following radiation. In an effort to address this particular symptom a patch of bowel can be used to reconstruct the floor of mouth.[10–13] Both colon and jejunal patches have been used for this purpose. These vascularized patches have the advantage of providing thin pliable cover as well as the potential to produce saliva. While they work well in producing mucus, the major disadvantage of this technique is that both of these tissues tolerate radiation poorly.

Tongue

The tongue is a unique muscular organ which fills the oral cavity and without which normal oral function cannot occur. The priorities for tongue

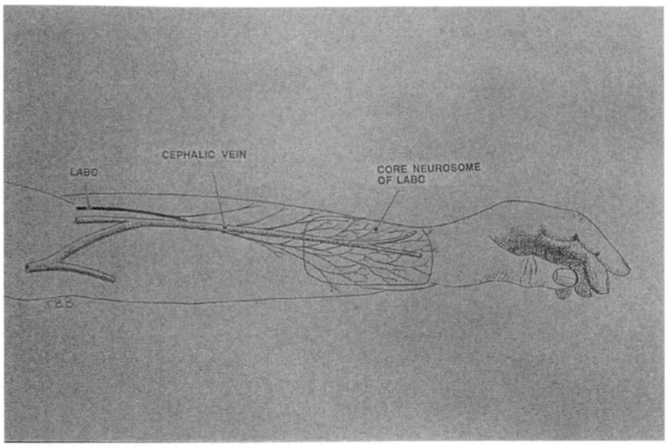

Figure 28.5 Schematic outline of innervated radial forearm flap.

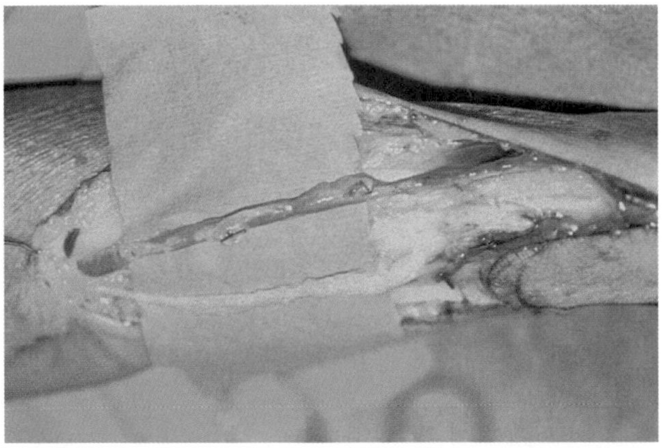

Figure 28.6 Vascular pedicle with lateral antebrachial cutaneous nerve in view.

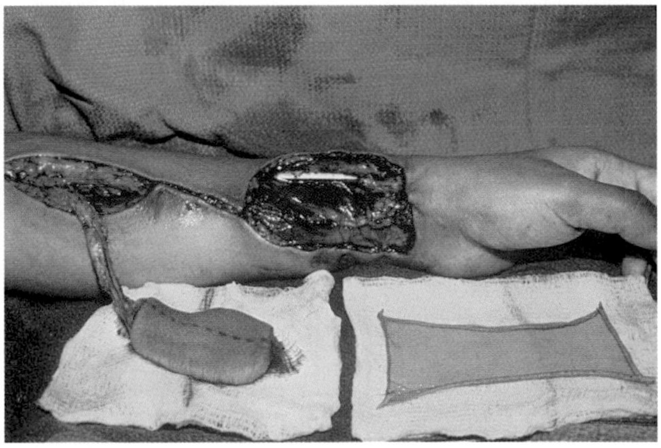

Figure 28.7 Innervated flap elevated.

reconstruction include restoration of swallowing, articulation and airway protection.[14] Normal or near-normal tongue mobility is vital for intelligible speech. As well as this the tongue plays an important role in the initiation of swallowing by propelling the food bolus posteriorly into the pharynx. Functional reconstruction of such a vital and dynamic structure is very difficult to achieve. The result of the reconstruction as well as the most

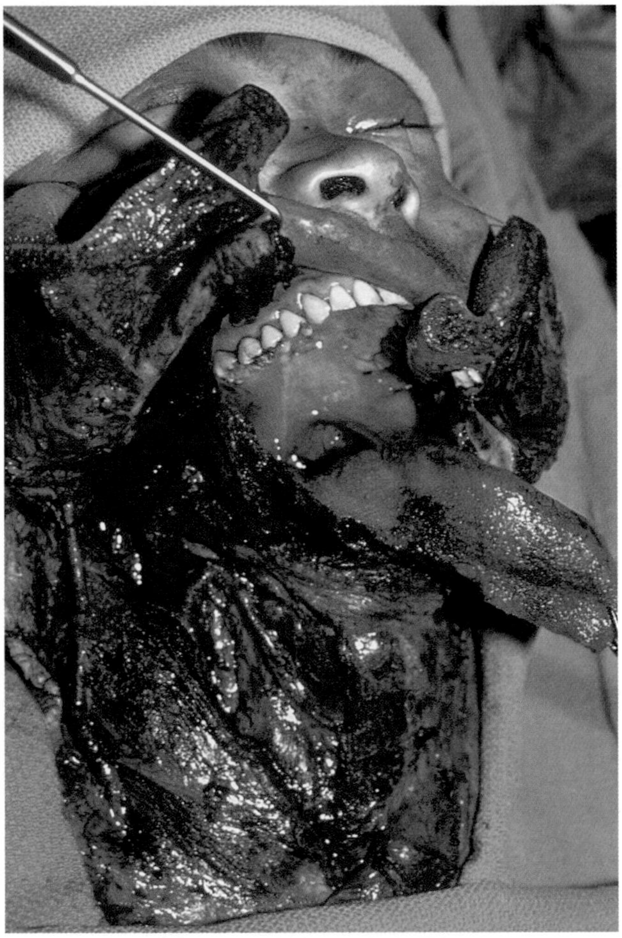

Figure 28.8 Tongue defect, mandibulotomy approach.

appropriate reconstructive choice depends on the size of the tongue defect. As more tongue is resected normal functional restoration becomes less likely and greater bulk is required in the reconstruction. For more minor resections, a thin pliable flap such as the radial forearm flap is ideal and is the flap of choice. It is important when insetting the flap to ensure that the remaining normal tongue is in no way tethered and is allowed to move optimally. The reconstruction can best be achieved by folding the flap along the lateral border of the tongue and insetting it in such a way that the part of the flap covering the resected surface of the tongue is functionally separate from the portion of the flap covering the adjacent floor of mouth (Figures 28.5–28.11). Yousif et al[15] propose a modification of the radial forearm flap for this indication, that is the combination of lateral tongue, lateral floor of mouth and alveolar ridge defect. They divide the flap into skin and fascia and fascia-only components. The skin component can be used to reconstruct the tongue, providing bulk, sensation and mobility while the fascia-only component can be used to cover the exposed alveolus. This can subsequently be skin grafted, and usually results in a resilient, thin, non-mobile tissue that does not require secondary

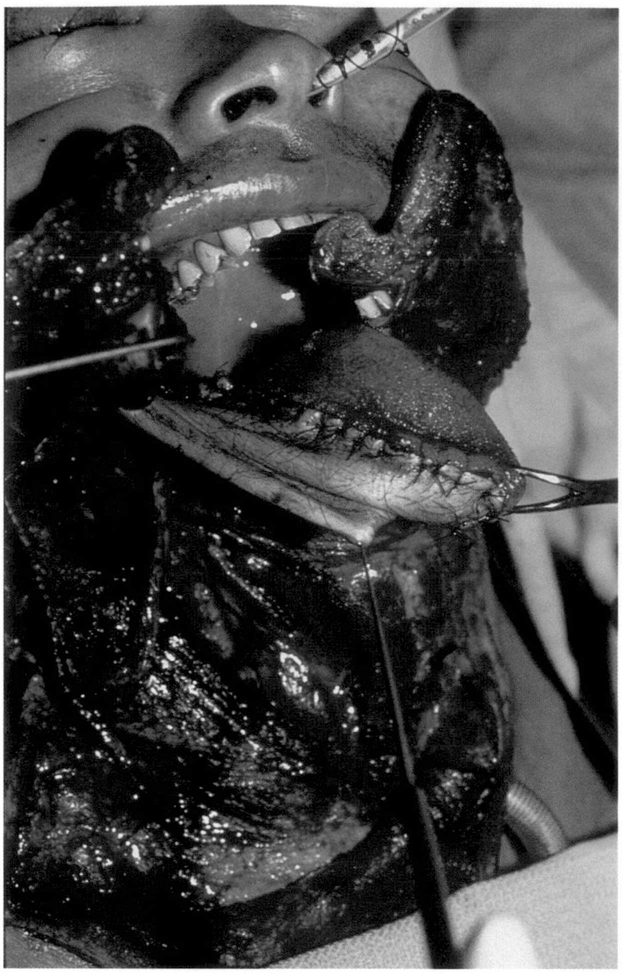

Figure 28.9 Flap folded and inset along lateral surface of tongue defect.

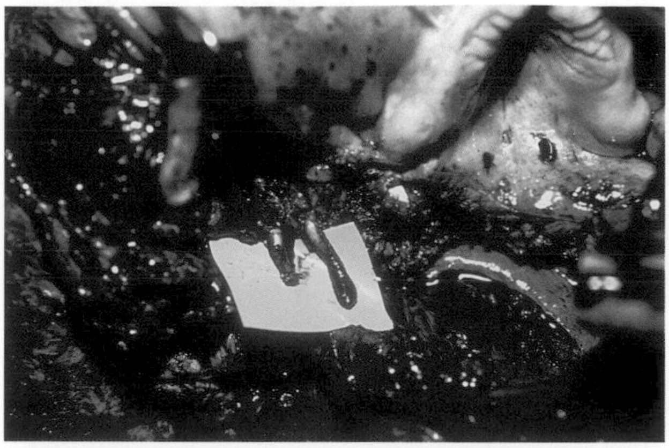

Figure 28.10 Lingual and inferior alveolar nerves prepared for interposition graft.

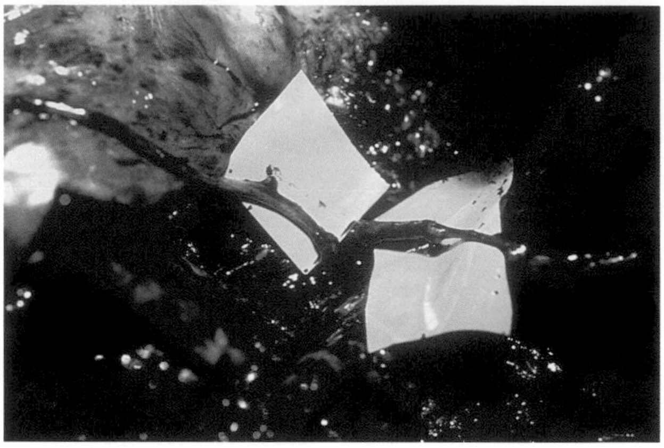

Figure 28.11 Reinnervation of radial forearm flap with lingual nerve to lateral antebrachial cutaneous nerve and inferior alveolar nerve to mentalis nerve for lip innervation.

revision to permit subsequent oral rehabilitation.[15] When more than a hemiglossectomy is performed, the results of reconstruction become less and less rewarding. As more tongue is removed, more and more muscle tissue is sacrificed thereby reducing the chances of normal tongue movement on that side.

The defect produced by subtotal glossectomy with laryngeal preservation is associated with a high incidence of significant permanent swallowing problems. However, when the bulk of the tongue is removed a bulky flap is needed. In our estimation this is the ideal situation in which to use a rectus abdominus flap[16] and is one of the few situations when this flap is used intraorally. This has the advantage of providing bulk to minimize the funnel effect and reduce the risk of inhalation (Figures 28.12–28.14). Regional flaps such as the pectoralis major provide good initial results but do not stand the test of time.[17,18] Functioning muscle flaps have been advocated in order to obliterate the space between floor of mouth and palate during swallowing but the results have been disappointing.[19,20]

The lateral oropharynx

This area adjacent to the oropharyngeal structure is considered as it is frequently involved in oral malignancies and as with areas within the oral cavity it demands thin pliable cover. Again, in our practice, the radial forearm flap is the workhorse in this area. Other thin flaps such as ulnar artery flap,[21] the lateral arm[22–24] and anterolateral thigh flap have been used successfully and the selection, again will be dictated by the size of the defect.

The palate

Soft palate

The soft palate is such a dynamic structure that reconstruction is difficult and its repair has traditionally been non-surgical, a prosthesis being frequently used to obturate the palatal defect. Fitting such a

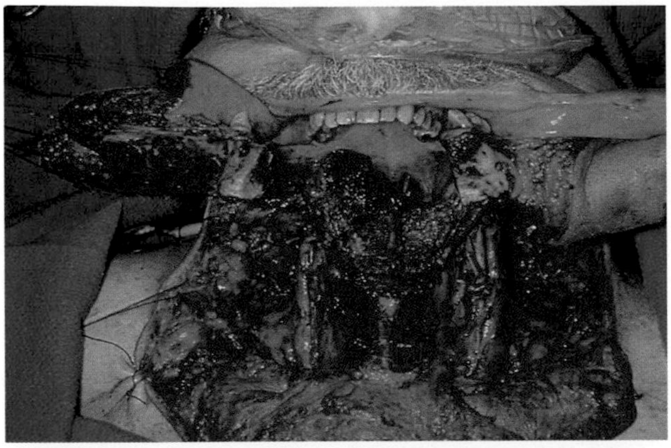

Figure 28.12 Mandibulotomy with near total glossectomy.

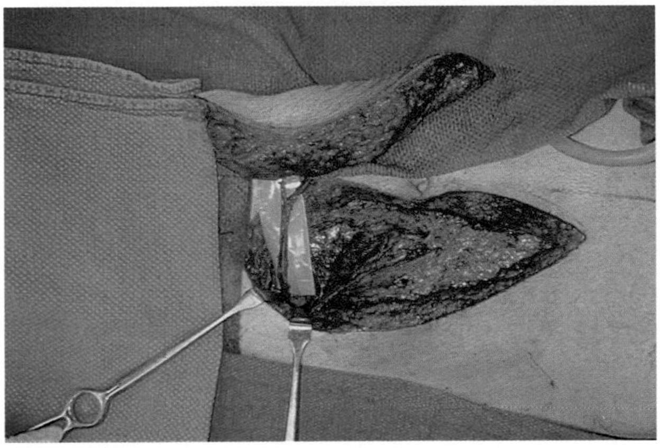

Figure 28.13 Elevation of free rectus cutaneous perforator flap on the inferior epigastric artery.

prosthesis is frequently troublesome and the prosthesis may be difficult to wear because of mucositis. Thin sensate flaps such as the radial forearm are best suited to this area.[15] Because the flap is non-dynamic however, velopharyngeal competence cannot be achieved unless the flap touches the posterior pharyngeal wall. Urken achieves this by fashioning a pharyngoplasty incorporated within his flap.[25]

Hard palate

Reconstruction is frequently achieved with the use of prostheses, an obturator being attached to the dental prosthesis in order to plug the palatal hole. While this technique works extremely well in most circumstances, there are certain situations where the patient cannot wear a denture when reconstruction incorporating bone and soft tissue such as the fibular flap is used.

The mandible

Mandibular reconstruction has evolved over the past two decades from a complex and often unsuccessful

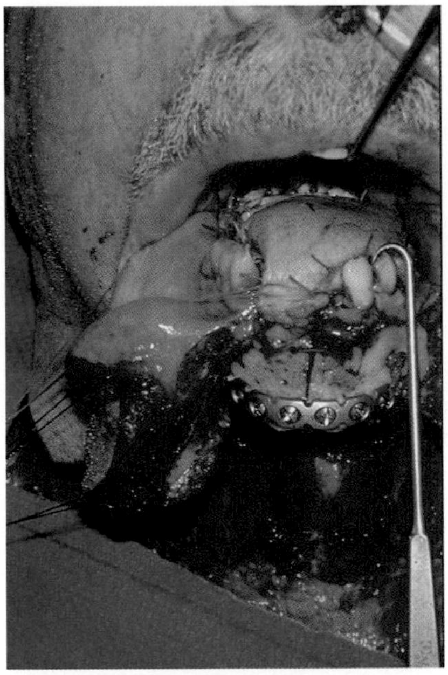

Figure 28.14 Flap inset and closure.

venture to a very reliable but still complex technique. The main reason for this advance has been the incorporation of microsurgical techniques and the development of reliable flaps for reconstruction. The concept of maintaining quality of life has become particularly important in the overall care and treatment of cancer patients.[26,27] Thus, patients with even a very limited life expectancy are routinely reconstructed if it is expected that their quality of remaining life would be significantly enhanced.[28] The high success rate of head and neck reconstructive procedures has allowed for significant improvement in both functional and aesthetic results and has completely changed the conceptual approach to mandibular reconstruction. Only patients who are medically unfit to tolerate a prolonged operation or have a poor prognosis are excluded as candidates for resection and immediate reconstruction.

The ideal tissue for mandibular reconstruction incorporating soft tissue and bone does not exist. What we seek is a combination of the best bone stock with the best skin paddle combined in a package that produces the least morbidity at both the donor and recipient sites. Repair of a mandibular defect frequently includes bone and soft tissue with which to replace either intraoral lining, external skin or both. It is also desirable that skin used to reconstruct the inside of the mouth be innervated. While such flaps do exist, each reconstruction is a compromise. The price paid for reconstruction is measured in terms of donor site morbidity, functional loss and days of life lost. This latter concept was introduced by Boyd et al in 1995 and is a valid one.[28] Given that the overall prognosis for many of these patients is limited, we must be sure that whatever intervention is performed is likely to succeed without complication. This surgery is technically demanding and technical expertise is required

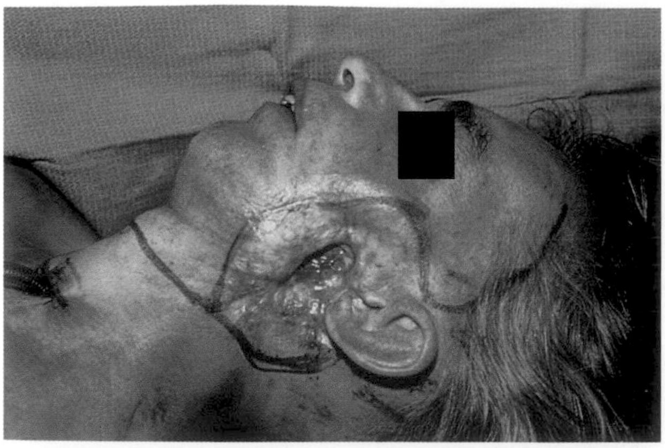

Figure 28.15 Extensive osteoradionecrosis with recurrent adenoid cystic carcinoma of the left skull base.

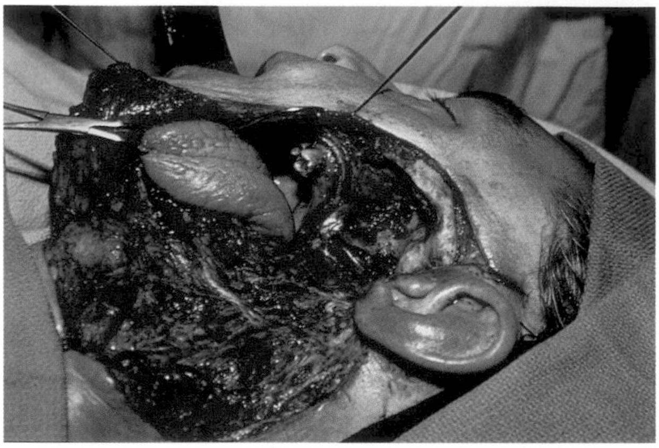

Figure 28.16 Extensive defect, bone and soft tissue.

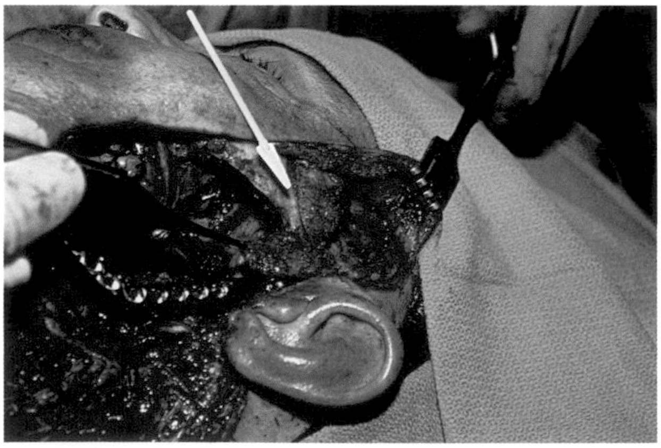

Figure 28.17 Reconstruction of hemimandible with plate. Note temporalis fascia cushion for the glenoid fossa.

that may not be universally available. It is not for the occasional surgeon and requires a critical volume of work to maintain competence. Furthermore, these operations are resource-intensive and postoperative care is demanding on nursing staff.

The choice of reconstruction depends on factors such as the bone and soft tissue requirements and the site of the defect (Figures 28.15–28.22). Donor site availability and morbidity, ease of flap dissection and

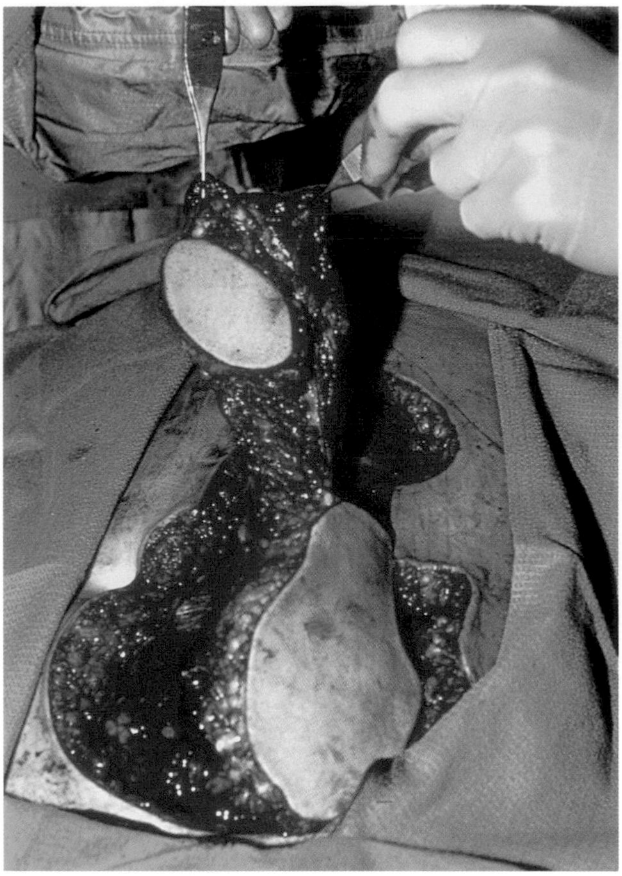

Figure 28.18 Elevation of double paddle free myocutaneous rectus flap.

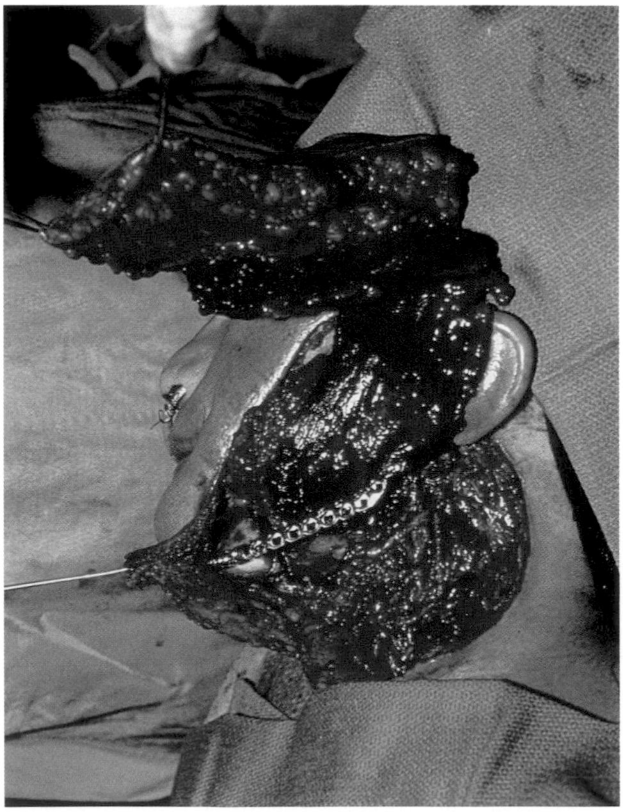

Figure 28.19 Flap inset, one paddle for lining and one for resurfacing.

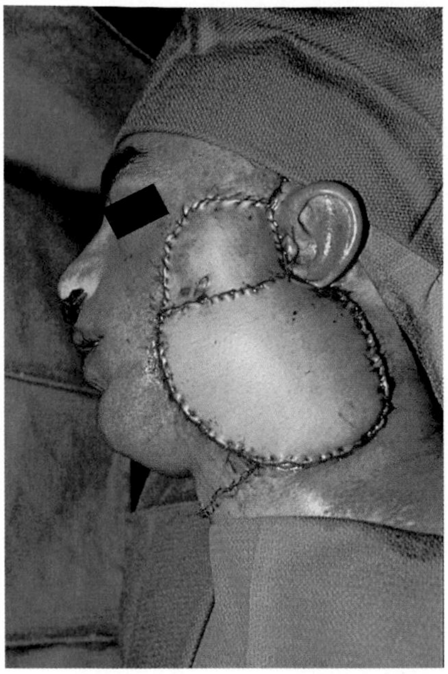

Figure 28.20 Inset and closure. Note skin graft on muscle.

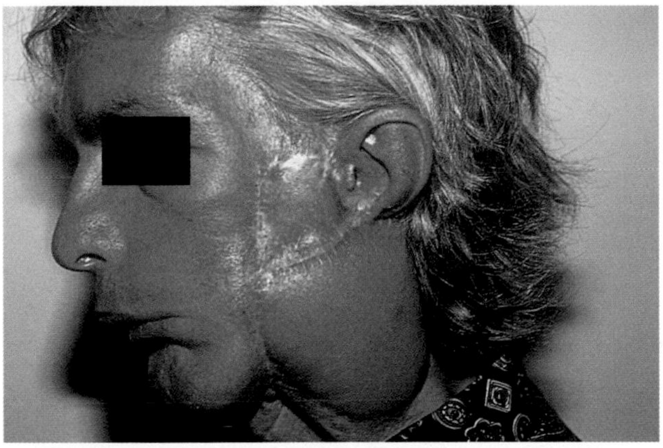

Figure 28.21 One year postoperative.

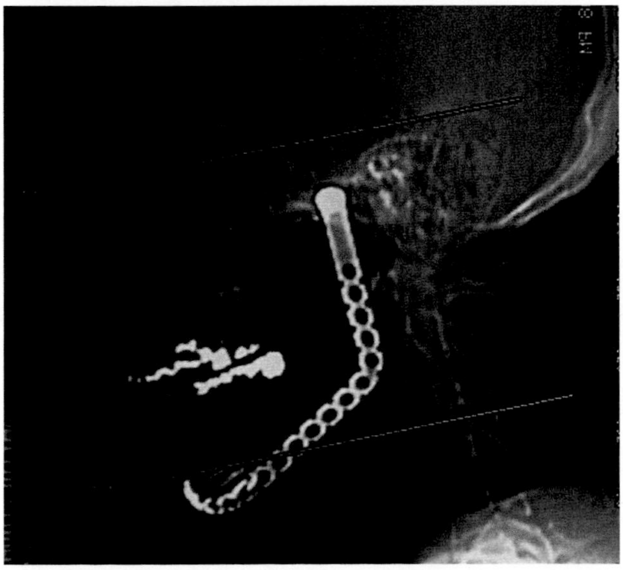

Figure 28.22 Plate at 1 year.

status of the recipient vessels in the neck as well as the patient's overall medical condition may also influence the final decision. However, while microsurgery has revolutionized mandibular reconstruction, there is still also a place for more traditional techniques. Smaller defects can sometimes be reconstructed with reconstruction plates alone, and in certain circumstances the use of non-vascularized bone is still a reasonable approach.[29] It may even be acceptable not to reconstruct the bony defect in a small subset of patients with posterolateral defects. There is one absolute indication for vascularized bony mandibular reconstruction. That is in the central anterior mandibular defect, the C defect according to the HCL classification.[30] Using any other technique results in an unacceptable functional and cosmetic result.

While rib,[31–33], metatarsal bone,[34–36] humerus[37] and clavicle[38–39] all have been used in mandibular repair, the most widely used current donor sites include the fibula,[40,41] iliac crest,[42–44] scapula[45–47] and radius.[48] Of these the fibula is by far the most popular.

The fibular osseocutaneous free flap

The fibula can provide up to 25 cm of uniform-shaped bicortical bone. It can tolerate multiple osteotomies because of its profuse periosteal blood supply. The bone stock is adequate to support osseointegrated implants, however the height of the neomandible is limited relative to that of the native dentate mandible. The skin island, based on the septocutaneous blood supply is adequate in size and reliable in more than 90% of patients.[49,50] The skin has the potential for innervation but its quality is intermediate in thickness and pliability and therefore ranks behind that of the radial forearm flap. The vascular pedicle is adequate in length and can effectively be lengthened by dissecting it off the proximal fibula. The flap can include the flexor hallucis longus muscle to provide soft-tissue bulk where needed. Donor leg morbidity, with or without skin grafting following fibula free flap harvest is minimal (Figures 28.23–28.29).[51]

The iliac crest osseocutaneous flap

The ileum, based on the deep circumflex iliac artery (DCIA) and vein has a natural curvature not unlike that of the mandible. A total of 14–16 cm of bone can be harvested by extending the resection posteriorly to the sacroiliac joint.[52] This bone can be contoured to reconstruct the anterior mandibular arch with osteotomies through the outer cortex and is well suited for placement of osseointegrated implants.[53–55] The blood supply of the skin paddle of this osseocutaneous flap comes from an array of perforators that

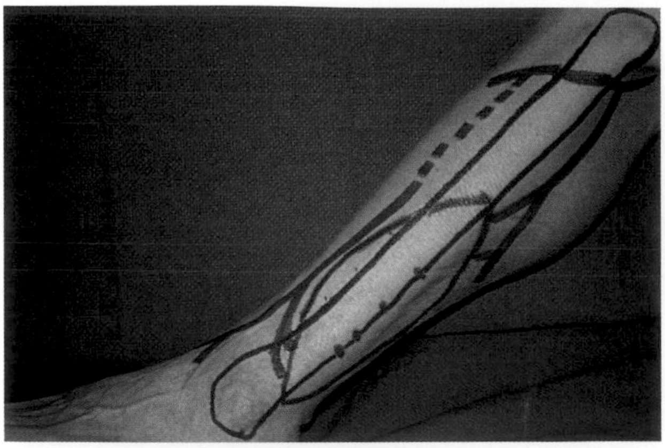

Figure 28.23 Outline of planned osseocutaneous free fibular flap. Note skin paddle designed low on the leg.

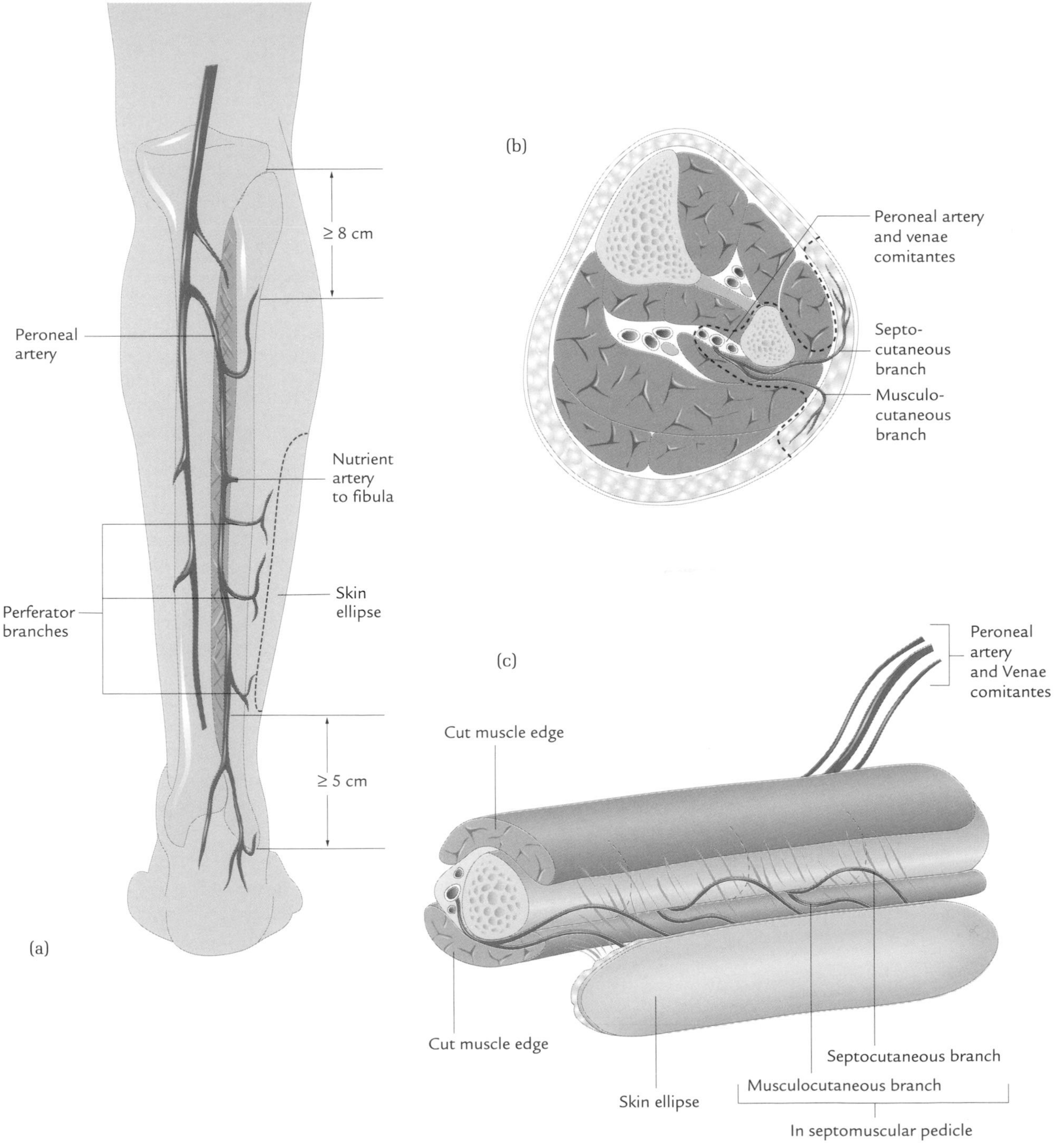

Figure 28.24 Schematic outline of fibular graft and opening osteotomies (- - - - - - - -).

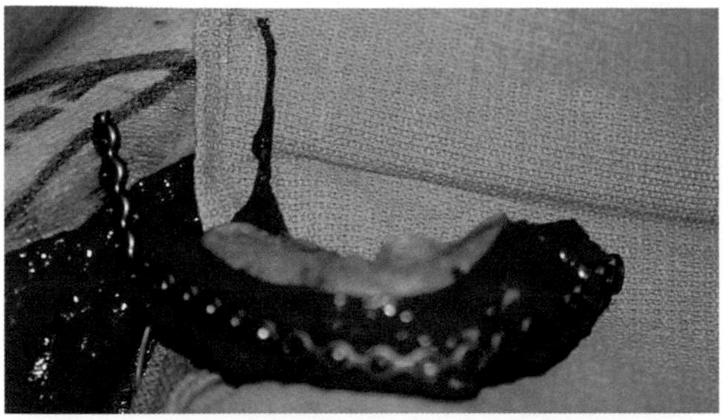

Figure 28.25 Plate contoured and then transferred to the leg where bony osteotomies are performed and then vascular pedicle divided and tissue transferred. This reduces ischaemia time.

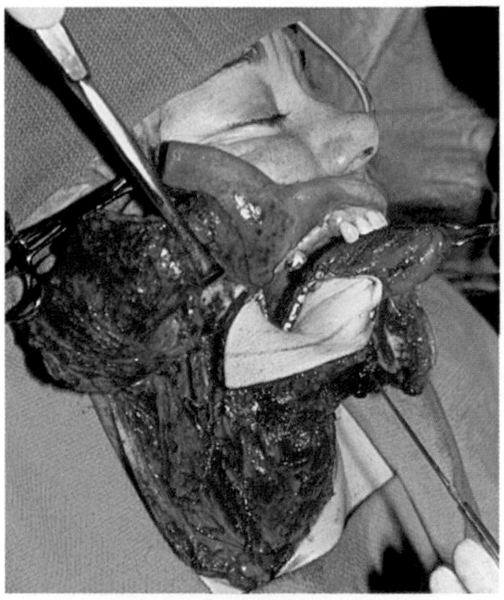

Figure 28.28 On occasion two flaps are employed. Radial forearm for soft tissue lining which provides thinner skin with innervation combined with free fibular bone graft.

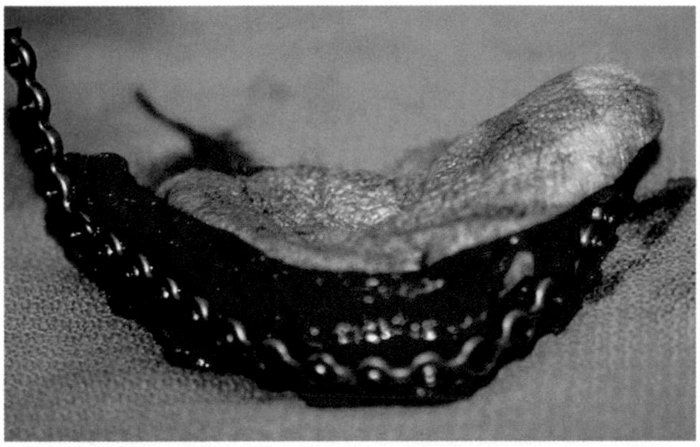

Figure 28.26 Flap transfer.

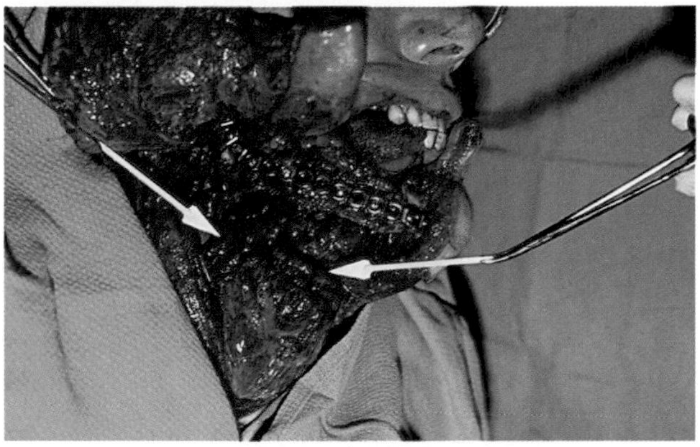

Figure 28.29 Fibula fixed with low profile titanium plate.

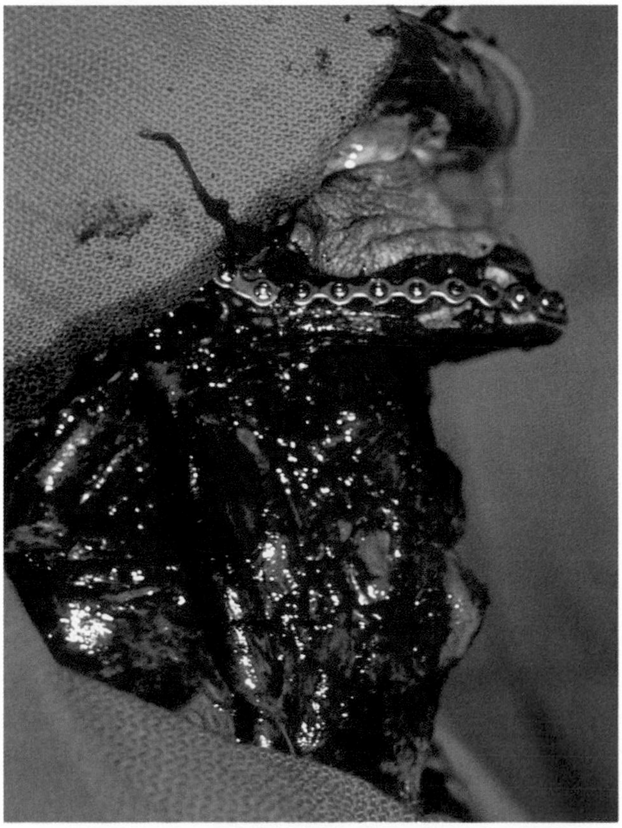

Figure 28.27 Flap inset completed.

are located in a zone along the medial aspect of the iliac crest. It is important when insetting the skin paddle to maintain the relationship of skin to bone so as not to torque the perforators. Furthermore, the skin is bulky and not particularly pliable so that it is usually less than the optimal choice for intra-oral reconstruction. Donor site morbidity also can be substantial. Patients frequently are slow to ambulate because of pain. Moreover, abdominal wall weakness, frank herniation and occasional gait disturbances can occur.[55,56] The donor defect of the DCIA can be minimized by splitting the ileum and taking only the inner table of the bone with the flap.[57] In this manner, the crest itself is left and the abdominal repair is much more secure. Holes are drilled in the remaining crest to which the three layers of abdominal musculature are attached. Furthermore, the muscles on the lateral side of the crest are undisturbed thereby minimizing donor site morbidity. Finally, the cosmetic defect of this manoeuvre is significantly less than when the traditional flap is used. The only disadvantage to this technique is that the thickness of bone harvested by this means is generally inadequate to facilitate use of osseointegrated implants for dental rehabilitation. The traditional criticism of this flap has been the

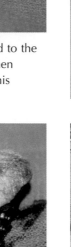

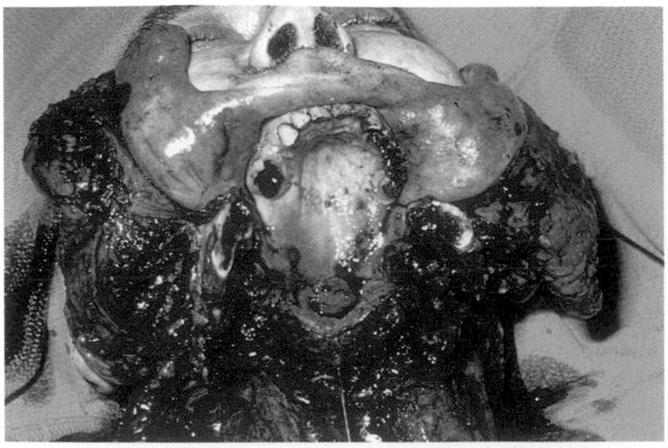

Figure 28.30 Total glossectomy and mandibulectomy.

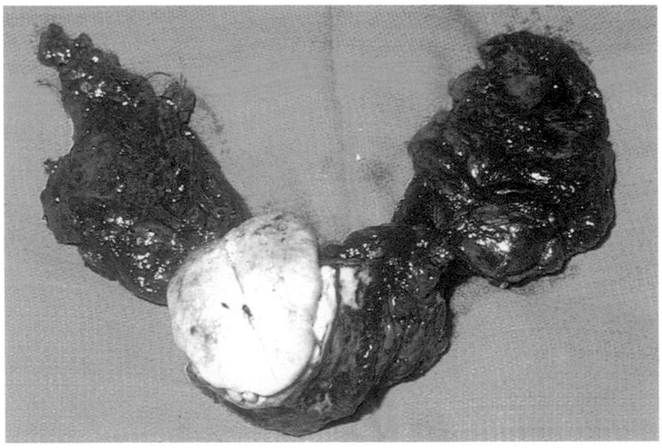

Figure 28.31 Total glossectomy specimen.

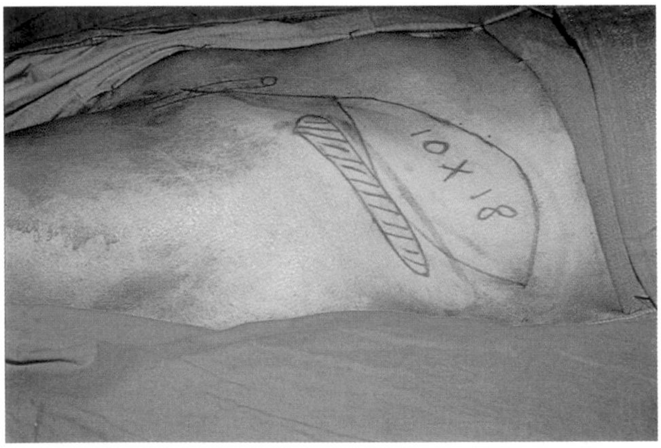

Figure 28.32 Outline of flap.

bulk of the associated skin paddle. Using muscle instead of skin has become a popular alternative, which not only minimizes bulk but provides adequate muscle to cover most defects. This modification using the internal oblique, vascularized by the ascending branch of the DCIA has rekindled interest in this flap for both mandibular and maxillary reconstruction (Figures 28.30–28.37).[58–60]

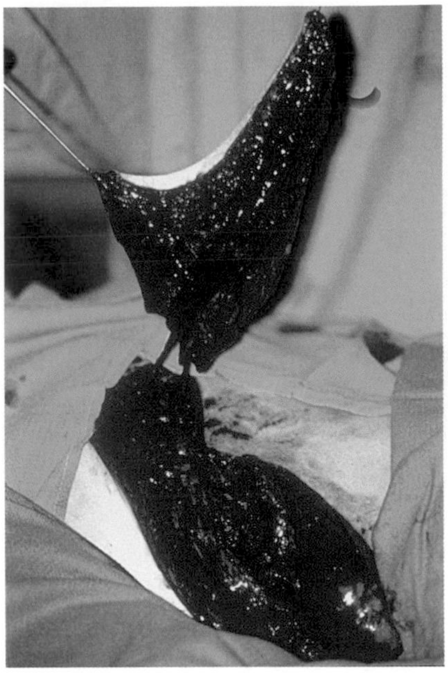

Figure 28.33 Elevation of flap.

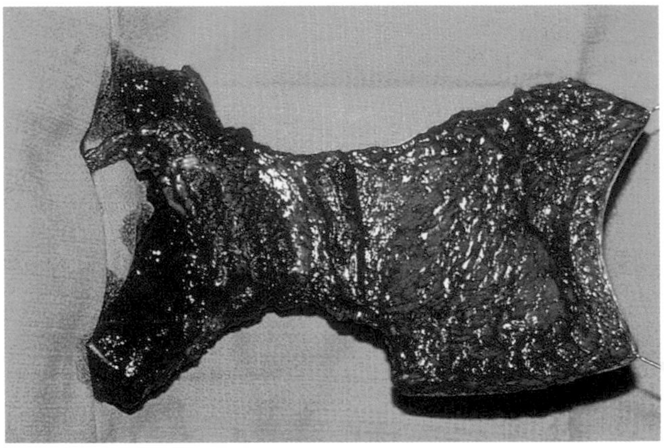

Figure 28.34 Osseocutaneous free iliac graft. Note thick skin paddle.

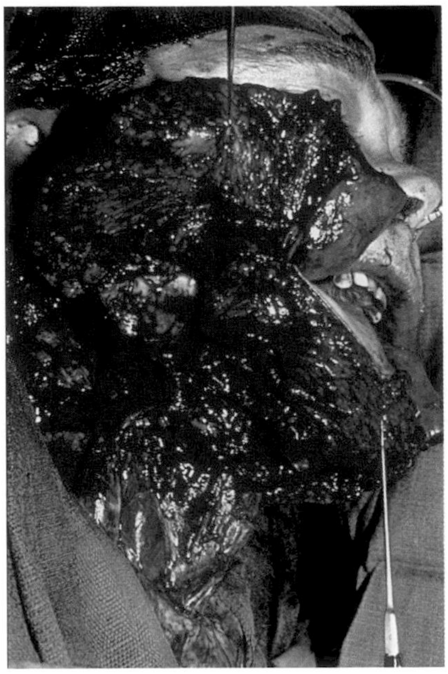

Figure 28.35 Flap inset with bone fixation using plate.

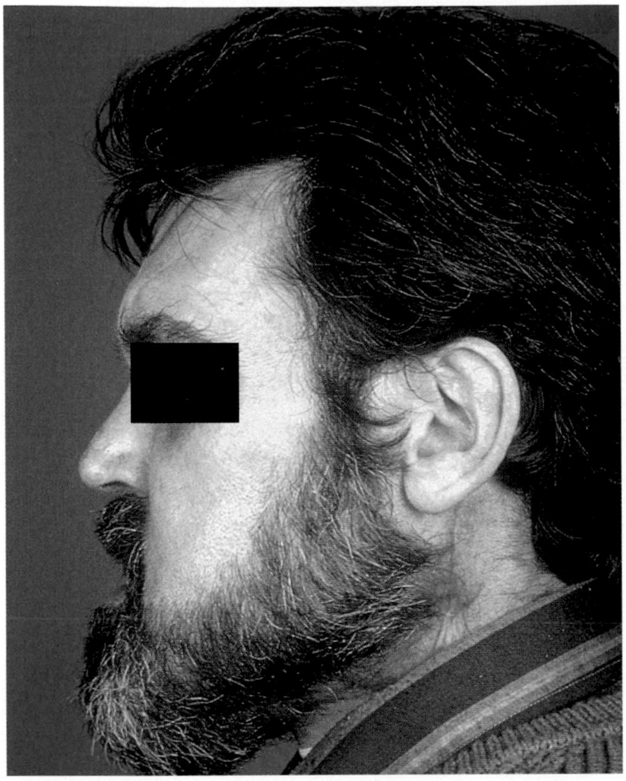

Figure 28.36 Result at 1 year: lateral view.

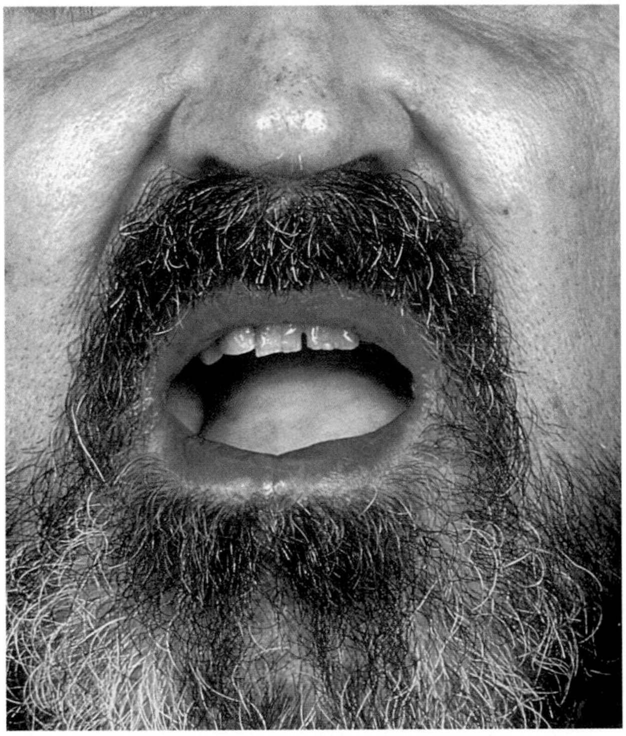

Figure 28.37 Face view at 1 year.

The scapular osseocutaneous flap

Based on the circumflex scapular artery, this flap has the advantage of providing an extensive expanse of skin as well as bone. Furthermore the skin can be taken as separate skin paddles, a scapular as well as a parascapular flap based on the transverse and descending branches of the circumflex scapular artery respectively. The bony perforators, which are direct short branches from the circumflex scapular artery, supply the lateral border of the scapula and provide approximately 8 cm of good bone stock.[46] Medial scapula also can be harvested with this flap[61] but harvesting lateral bone is more usual. Because of the anatomical characteristics of the vascular pedicle, the various elements of this flap (two skin paddles and bone) all can be manipulated independent of one another as there is sufficient vascular length to facilitate this. This makes it very versatile for reconstructing complex three-dimensional defects. However, it has the disadvantage that the patient has to be turned in order to harvest this flap. Furthermore, while the bone stock is excellent it cannot safely be osteotomized. This limits its utility for larger bony defects greater than about 10 cm.

The radial forearm osseocutaneous flap

The radial forearm flap provides the best quality skin for intraoral reconstruction. It is soft, thin, pliable and can be harvested with the lateral antebrachial cutaneous making it an innervated flap. The quality of this reinnervation has been well documented.[6] The radius itself provides a thin strip of bone, which nevertheless is very strong and despite its size can tolerate osseointegrated dental implants.[48] When harvesting the bone it is important to limit this harvest to approximately 30% of the circumference of the radius and to contour this harvest in the shape of a keel to minimize the risk of fracture of the residual radius. Despite these precautions the incidence of fracture is reported as 15% which is very high considering that up to 10% of patients will require a secondary surgical procedure to fix the radial fracture (Figures 28.38 and 28.39).

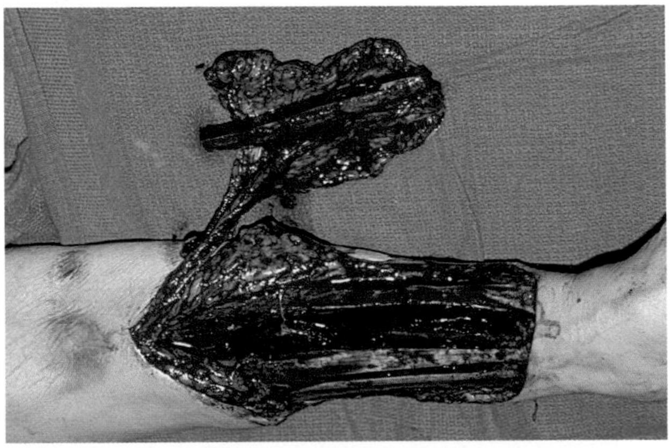

Figure 28.38 Elevation of osseocutaneous free radial forearm flap.

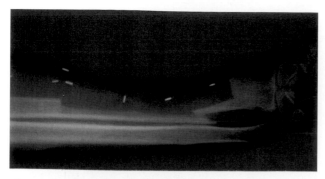

Figure 28.39 Note excess bone harvested with fracture of radius at 6 months.

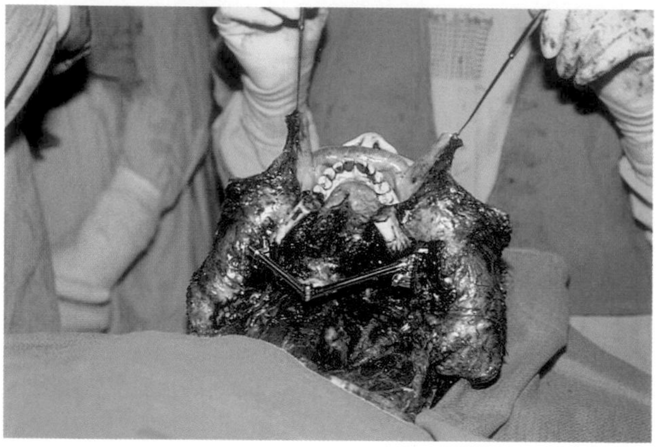

Figure 28.40 Bridging bar applied to stabilize mandibular segments prior to plate and graft repair.

The resection

Replacing resected mandible with a replica of what has been removed is important. There are several ways in which this can be done. Probably the commonest and simplest method is to apply the reconstruction plate that will ultimately be used for fixation to the mandible before resection. This ensures that when the plate is replaced, the remaining elements of the mandible will be in exactly the same relative position as they were preoperatively. Thus, optimal occlusion as well as undisturbed temporomandibular joint dynamics can be assured. The plate is therefore applied to the mandible, the holes are drilled and screws applied. The plate is then removed and used as a template for shaping the bony reconstruction, whichever flap is chosen for that purpose.

In through and through lesions where the outer cortex of the mandible is involved this technique cannot be used as the reconstruction plate cannot be applied to the mandible prior to resection. One way around this problem is to make a template of the mandible preoperatively from the preoperative CT scans. This template then can be sterilized and used to shape the reconstructive plate intraoperatively. Alternatively, the mandibular elements can be stabilized prior to resection of the bone. This is done by applying a bridging bar to the mandible as shown in Figure 28.40. Once the mandible has been resected the reconstruction plate can be bent to the shape of the mandible knowing that the remaining elements are once again held in the same relative position as preoperatively, maintaining occlusion and temporomandibular joint dynamics.

Flap options

The choice of flap is determined by the characteristics of the defect. The fibula is the workhorse flap in these situations. While the iliac crest and radius have their proponents, they have for the most part been relegated to the position of secondary choice in those patients for whom the fibula, for whatever reason, is not an option. If soft tissue bulk is a requirement then the iliac crest may be a better option and if extensive skin cover is required as, for example, in through and through defects then scapula may be a good option. The radial forearm flap, while having many desirable characteristics is associated with, what we consider, an unacceptably high rate of fracture in the residual radius.

Summary

Reconstruction of the oral cavity is a complex subject that reflects the complexity of the oral cavity itself. There is no perfect reconstruction. What has been presented are the current optimal choices for the various regions within the oral cavity. We are constantly seeking to improve our reconstructions in an effort to restore optimal function to those patients unfortunate enough to require surgical excision of this most elaborate of anatomic structures.

REFERENCES

1. Pribaz JEA. A new intra-oral flap: the facial artery musculo-mucosal (FAMM) flap. *Plast Reconstr Surg* 1992; **90**: 421.
2. Gullane PJ, Arena S. Palatal island flap for reconstruction of oral defects. *Arch Otolaryngol* 1977; **103**: 598.
3. Sullivan PK, Fabian R, Driscoll D. Mandibular osteotomies for tumour extirpation: the advantages of rigid fixation. *Laryngoscope* 1992; **102**: 73.
4. Serletti JM, Tavin E, Coniglio JU. Transverse lag screw fixation of the midline mandibulotomy. *Plast Reconstr Surg* 1997; **99**: 239.
5. McCann KJ, Irish JC, Gullane PJ et al. Complications associated with rigid fixation of mandibulotomies. *J Otolaryngol* 1994; **23**: 210.
6. Boyd B, Mulholland S, Gullane PJ et al. Re-innervated lateral antebrachial cutaneous neurosome flaps in oral reconstruction: are we making sense? *Plast Reconstr Surg* 1994; **93**: 1350.
7. Chang SC, Miller G, Halbert CF et al. Limiting donor site morbidity by suprafascial dissection of the radial forearm flap. *Microsurgery* 1996; **17**: 136.
8. Lutz BS, Wei FC, Chang SC et al. Donor site morbidity after suprafascial elevation of the radial forearm flap: a prospective study in 95 consecutive cases. *Plast Reconstr Surg* 1999; **103**: 132.
9. Demirkan F, Wei FC, Lutz BS et al. Reliability of the venae comitantes in venous drainage of the free radial forearm flaps. *Plast Reconstr Surg* 1998; **102**: 1544.
10. Jones TR, Lee G, Emami B, Strasberg S. Free colon transfer for resurfacing large oral cavity defects. *Plast Reconstr Surg* 1995; **96**: 1092.
11. Michiwaki Y, Schmelzeisen R, Hacki T, Michi K. Articulatory function in glossectomized patients with immediate reconstruction using a free jejunum flap. *J Craniomaxillofac Surg* 1992; **20**: 203.
12. Habel G. Revascularized jejunal grafts in oral reconstruction. *Ann R Aust Coll Dent Surg* 1991; **11**: 312.
13. Jones NF, Eadie PA, Myers EN. Double lumen free jejunal transfer for reconstruction of the entire floor of mouth, pharynx and cervical oesophagus. *Br J Plast Surg* 1991; **44**: 44.
14. Flood J, Hobar P. Head and neck II: reconstruction. *Select Read Plast Surg* 1995; **8**:17.
15. Yousif N, Matloub H, Sanger J, Campbell B. Soft-tissue reconstruction of the oral cavity. *Clin Plast Surg* 1994; **21**: 15.
16. Lyos AT, Evans GR, Perez D, Schusterman MA. Tongue reconstruction: outcomes with the rectus abdominus flap. *Plast Reconstr Surg* 1999; **103**: 442.
17. Sultan M, Coleman JI. Oncologic and functional considerations of total glossectomy. *Am J Surg* 1989; **158**: 297.
18. Weber R, Ohlms L, Bowman J. Functional results after total or near total glossectomy with laryngeal preservation. *Arch Otolaryngol Head Neck Surg* 1991; **117**: 512.
19. Haughey B. Tongue reconstruction: concepts and practice. *Laryngoscope* 1993; **103**: 1132.
20. Salabian A. Total and subtotal glossectomy: function after microvascular reconstruction. *Plast Reconstr Surg* 1990; **85**: 513.
21. Lovie MJ, Duncan GM, Glasson DW. The ulnar artery forearm free flap. *Br J Plast Surg* 1984; **37**: 486.
22. Sullivan MEA. Lateral arm free flap in head and neck reconstruction. *Arch Otolaryngol Head Neck Surg* 1992; **118**: 1095.
23. Katsaros J. The lateral upper arm flap: anatomy and clinical applications. *Ann Plast Surg* 1994; **12**: 489.
24. Yousif N, Warren R, Matloub H, Sanger J. The lateral arm fascial free flap: its anatomy and use in reconstruction. *Plast Reconstr Surg* 1990; **86**: 1138.
25. Urken M. The restoration or preservation of sensation in the oral cavity following ablative surgery. *Arch Otolaryngol Head Neck Surg* 1995; **121**: 607.
26. Schliephake H, Ruffert K, Schneller T. Prospective study of the quality of life of cancer patients after intraoral tumour surgery. *J Oral Maxillofac Surg* 1996; **54**: 664.
27. Wilson KM, Rizk NM, Armstrong SL, Bluckman JL. Effects of hemimandibulectomy on quality of life. *Laryngoscope* 1998; **108**: 1574.
28. Boyd JB, Mulholland RS, Davidson J et al. The free flap and plate in oromandibular reconstruction: long-term review and indications. *Plast Reconstr Surg* 1995; **95**: 1018.
29. Gullane PJ. Primary mandibular reconstruction: analysis of 64 cases and evaluation of interface radiation dosimetry on bridging plates. *Laryngoscope* 1991; **101 (Suppl 54)**: 1.
30. Boyd JB, Gullane PJ, Rotstein LE et al. Classification of mandibular defects. *Plast Reconstr Surg* 1993; **92**: 1266.
31. Netscher D, Alford EL, Wigoda P, Cohen V. Free composite myo-osseous flap with serratus anterior and rib: indications in head and neck reconstruction [see comments]. *Head Neck* 1998; **20**: 106.
32. Guelinckx PJ, Sinsel NK. The 'Eve' procedure: the transfer of vascularized seventh rib, fascia, cartilage, and serratus muscle to reconstruct difficult defects. *Plast Reconstr Surg* 1996; **97**: 527.
33. Millard DR, Dembrow V, Shocket E. Immediate reconstruction of the resected mandibular arch. *Am J Surg* 1967; **114**: 605.
34. Macleod AM. Vascularized metatarsal transfer in mandibular reconstruction. *Microsurgery* 1994; **15**: 257.
35. Duncan MJ, Manktelow RT, Zuker RM, Rosen IB. Mandibular reconstruction in the radiated patient: the role of osteocutaneous free tissue transfers. *Plast Reconstr Surg* 1985; **76**: 829.
36. Rosen IB, Bell MS, Barron PT et al. Use of microvascular flaps including free osteocutaneous flaps in reconstruction after composite resection for radiation-recurrent oral cancer. *Am J Surg* 1979; **138**: 544.

37. Martin D, Breton P, Henri JF et al. Role of osteocutaneous external brachial flap in the treatment of composite loss of substance of the mandible. *Ann Chir Plast Esthet* 1992; **37**: 252.
38. Seikaly H, Calhoun K, Rassekh CH, Slaughter D. The clavipectoral osteomyocutaneous free flap. *Otolaryngol Head Neck Surg* 1997; **117**: 547.
39. Siemssen SO, Kirkby B, O'Connor TP. Immediate reconstruction of a resected segment of the lower jaw, using a compound flap of clavicle and sternomastoid muscle. *Plast Reconstr Surg* 1978; **61**: 724.
40. Hidalgo DA. Fibula free flap mandibular reconstruction. *Clin Plast Surg* 1994; **21**: 25.
41. Hidalgo DA. Fibular free flap: a new method of mandible reconstruction. *Plast Reconstr Surg* 1989; **84**: 71.
42. Taylor GI. Reconstruction of the mandible with free composite iliac bone grafts. *Ann Plast Surg* 1982; **9**: 361.
43. Jewer DD, Boyd JB, Manktelow RT et al. Orofacial and mandibular reconstruction with the iliac crest free flap: a review of 60 cases and a new method of classification. *Plast Reconstr Surg* 1989; **84**: 391.
44. Taylor GI. The current status of free vascularized bone grafts. *Clin Plast Surg* 1983; **10**: 185.
45. Nakatsuka T, Harii K, Yamada A et al. Surgical treatment of mandibular osteoradionecrosis: versatility of the scapular osteocuteneous flap. *Scand J Plast Reconstr Surg Hand Surg* 1996; **30**: 291.
46. Swartz WM, Banis JC, Newton ED et al. The osteocutaneous scapular flap for mandibular and maxillary reconstruction. *Plast Reconstr Surg* 1986; **77**: 530.
47. Coleman JJD, Wooden WA. Mandibular reconstruction with composite microvascular tissue transfer. *Am J Surg* 1990; **160**: 390.
48. Mounsey RA, Boyd JB. Mandibular reconstruction with osseointegrated implants into the free vascularlized radius [see comments]. *Plast Reconstr Surg* 1994; **94**: 457.
49. Jones NF, Monstrey S, Gambier BA. Reliability of the fibular osteocutaneous flap for mandibular reconstruction: anatomical and surgical confirmation. *Plast Reconstr Surg* 1996; **97**: 707.
50. Shpitzer T, Neligan PC, Gullane PJ et al. Oromandibular reconstruction with the fibular free flap. Analysis of 50 consecutive flaps. *Arch Otolaryngol Head Neck Surg* 1997; **123**: 939.
51. Shpitzer T, Neligan P, Boyd B et al. Leg morbidity and function following fibular free flap harvest. *Ann Plast Surg* 1997; **38**: 460.
52. Taylor GI, Corlett RJ, Boyd JB. The versatile deep inferior epigastric (inferior rectus abdominus) flap. *Br J Plast Surg* 1984; **37**: 330.
53. Beckers A, Schenck C, Klesper B, Koebke J. Comparative densitometric study of iliac crest and scapula bone in relation to osseous integrated dental implants in microvascular mandibular reconstruction. *J Craniomaxillofac Surg* 1998; **26**: 75.
54. Moscoso JF, Keller J, Genden E et al. Vascularized bone flaps in oromandibular reconstruction. A comparative anatomic study of bone stock from various donor sites to assess suitability for enosseous dental implants. *Arch Otolaryngol Head Neck Surg* 1994; **120**: 36.
55. Frodel JL Jr, Funk GF, Capper DT et al. Osseointegrated implants: a comparative study of bone thickness in four vascularized bone flaps. *Plast Reconstr Surg* 1993; **92**: 440.
56. Porchet F, Jaques B. Unusual complications at iliac crest bone graft donor site: experience with two cases. *Neurosurgery* 1996; **39**: 856.
57. Shenaq SM, Klubuc MJ. The iliac crest microsurgical free flap in mandibular reconstruction. *Clin Plast Surg* 1994; **21**: 37.
58. Moscoso JF, Urken ML. The iliac crest composite flap for oromandibular reconstruction. *Otolaryngol Clin North Am* 1994; **27**: 1097.
59. Brown JS. Deep circumflex iliac artery free flap with internal oblique muscle as a new method of immediate reconstruction of maxillectomy defect. *Head Neck* 1996; **18**: 412.
60. Urken ML, Weinberg H, Vickery C et al. The internal oblique-iliac crest free flap in composite defects of the oral cavity involving bone, skin, and mucosa. *Laryngoscope* 1991; **101**: 257.
61. Thoma A, Archibald A, Payk I, Young JE. The free medial scapular osteofasciocutaneous flap for head and neck reconstruction. *Br J Plast Surg* 1991; **44**: 477.

29 Reconstruction of the ear

David T Gault

Introduction

The aesthetic quality of the ear is extremely important. It is a mostly decorative structure of intricate twists and turns. Resection of the ear in whole or in part can cause psychological distress out of proportion to its size.

The ear components are difficult to mimic and reconstruction after major resection is a challenging task. It is worthwhile only if great attention is paid to fine detail. In addition to providing a realistic shape it is important to maintain the patency of the external auditory canal, to provide support for spectacles and to maintain an anchor point in the lobe for earrings, where possible.

The ear is a thin sandwich of cartilage and skin. Over most of the ear, the skin is tightly adherent to the cartilage and there is little excess skin available to be mobilized for cover of adjacent defects. It is more loosely attached over the helix and the lobe where a small amount of subcutaneous tissue is present. Minor defects in these zones are more readily dealt with by direct closure than elsewhere on the ear.

Pathology

Cancer of the ear is common and many tumours are induced by sun exposure. Ear cancer comprises 5–8% of all skin cancer. The decline in the wearing of hats, the adoption of shorter hair styles, the thinning of the ozone layer and the popularity of package holidays all contribute. Even when sunscreens are applied to the face, the ear is often forgotten, allowing harmful rays unsuspected access to auricular skin. Patients on immunosuppressive therapy are especially at risk.

The majority of auricular cancer is squamous cell carcinoma (60%), followed by basal cell carcinoma (35%) and melanoma (5%). Adnexal carcinomas derived from sweat glands, hair follicles and sebaceous glands can also occur but are less common. The ear can also be destroyed in childhood by capillary haemangioma. The current fashion for body piercing has caused massive ear keloids in some cases. Occasionally the ear structure is destroyed by infection following piercing for jewellery.

Squamous cell carcinoma arising de novo on the auricle is probably rare. Most tumours originate in areas of solar keratosis and the proper treatment of such minor lesions is therefore important. These discrete crusty lesions frequently develop on the helical rim. They are scaly and raised with thickening of both the prickle cell layer and stratum corneum. Some active lesions are infiltrated by plasma cells and lymphocytes. Squamous cell carcinoma is sometimes not aggressive on the rim of the ear but lesions of the concha and posterior surface are more worrisome and can spread to local lymph nodes.

Basal cell carcinoma of the ear is unusual in that it tends to occur in the conchal hollow and on the posterior sulcus (Figure 29.1), areas that do not correspond to those of maximal sun exposure. Lesions of the ear often extend in a silent manner beyond the visible tumour. This, combined with the surgeon's reluctance to unnecessarily increase the postoperative deformity associated with wider margins, may explain the high recurrence rate after the excision of ear tumours.

Larger cancers (basal cell and squamous cell) above 2 cm in diameter and recurrent tumours are especially likely to have unrecognized pockets of tumour at a distance from the visible margins. Rather than a spherical growth pattern they may have finger like projections of tumour along tissue planes. A useful guide is that the likely extension beyond visible limits is equivalent to the radius of a small primary lesion with a short history but to the diameter of a recurrent longstanding or thicker lesion.

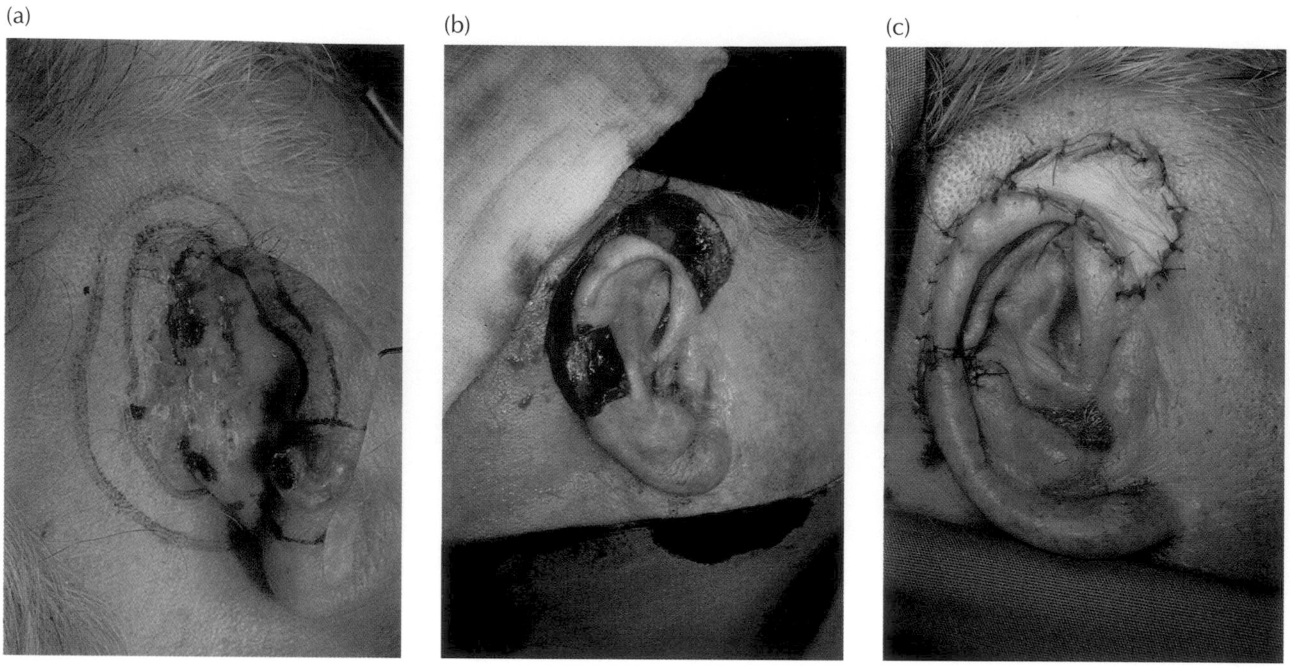

Figure 29.1 (a) An extensive basal cell carcinoma of the postauricular sulcus with a separate tumour on the rim of the ear. (b) Wide excision leaves an extensive defect. (c) The wound is closed by replacing the uninvolved external skin. A supplementary skin graft was used.

Because there is limited subcutaneous tissue, tumours will become fixed to and invade the perichondrium at an early stage. Basal cell carcinoma in particular may spread laterally at the level of the perichondrium beyond the visual tumour limits but this deep lateral spread rarely exceeds 5–6 mm. When perichondrium is involved the underlying cartilage must be excised.

Malignant tumours of the external auditory canal are rare. Squamous cell carcinoma, basal cell carcinoma and malignancies of the ceruminous glands may all occur.

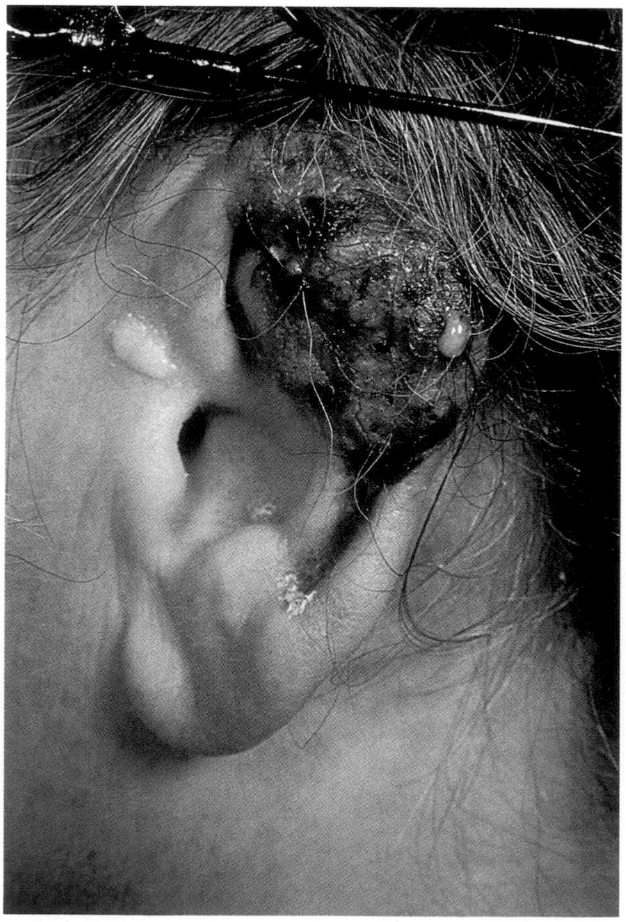

Figure 29.2 This nasty looking ear lesion was suspected to be a squamous cell cancer. Histology, however, showed this to be an irritated seborrhoeic keratosis.

Treatment

The treatment of keratosis is usually non-surgical, using either 5-fluorouracil ointment or cryotherapy. It is important to distinguish between a keratosis and an early squamous cell carcinoma and biopsies are often necessary (Figure 29.2). A non-healing ulcer should be presumed to be malignant. The distinction between a basal cell carcinoma and a squamous cell carcinoma on the ear may not always be obvious.

The majority of tumours are treated with excisional biopsies and immediate reconstruction. With most lesions only a conservative margin is needed for cure. When a tumour is adherent to cartilage then wider margins of skin and cartilage should be taken because of lateral spread. The more aggressive squamous cell tumours of the central and posterior parts of the ear should also be removed with a wider margin. The incidence of node metastasis from these sites is 6–20%. These tumours will need wide excision and regular follow-up.[1–4]

Ablative carbon dioxide lasers can be used to excise superficial basal cell carcinoma tumours with little or no bleeding from the resulting wound bed.[5] Lasers are also useful in removing keloids from the earlobe. This technique rarely cures the keloid but does appear to delay recurrence when compared to surgical excision.

Melanoma of the ear is treated first by a confirmatory excision biopsy. Subsequent treatment depends on the tumour depth. Tumours greater than 1.5 mm in thickness will require radical excision of the primary site. The old adage of 1 cm of clearance for every millimetre of tumour depth gives a useful guide.

If a melanoma or squamous cell lesion has spread to the nearby lymph nodes then a parotidectomy and neck dissection is needed. Surgery provides the mainstay of treatment. Adjuvant radiotherapy or chemotherapy is considered in special circumstances. Recurrence following radiotherapy is often considered to be chondritis, but a painful ulcer is more likely to be a recurrent tumour associated with chondritis.

Ceruminous adenocarcinoma of the external auditory canal is usually aggressive and cure rates are low. A basal cell carcinoma in the ear canal is often locally aggressive. In this hidden site the tumour may invade the petrous bone and early detection is essential for successful management. Excision of all involved tissue is a difficult surgical procedure (Figures 29.3 and 29.4).

(a)

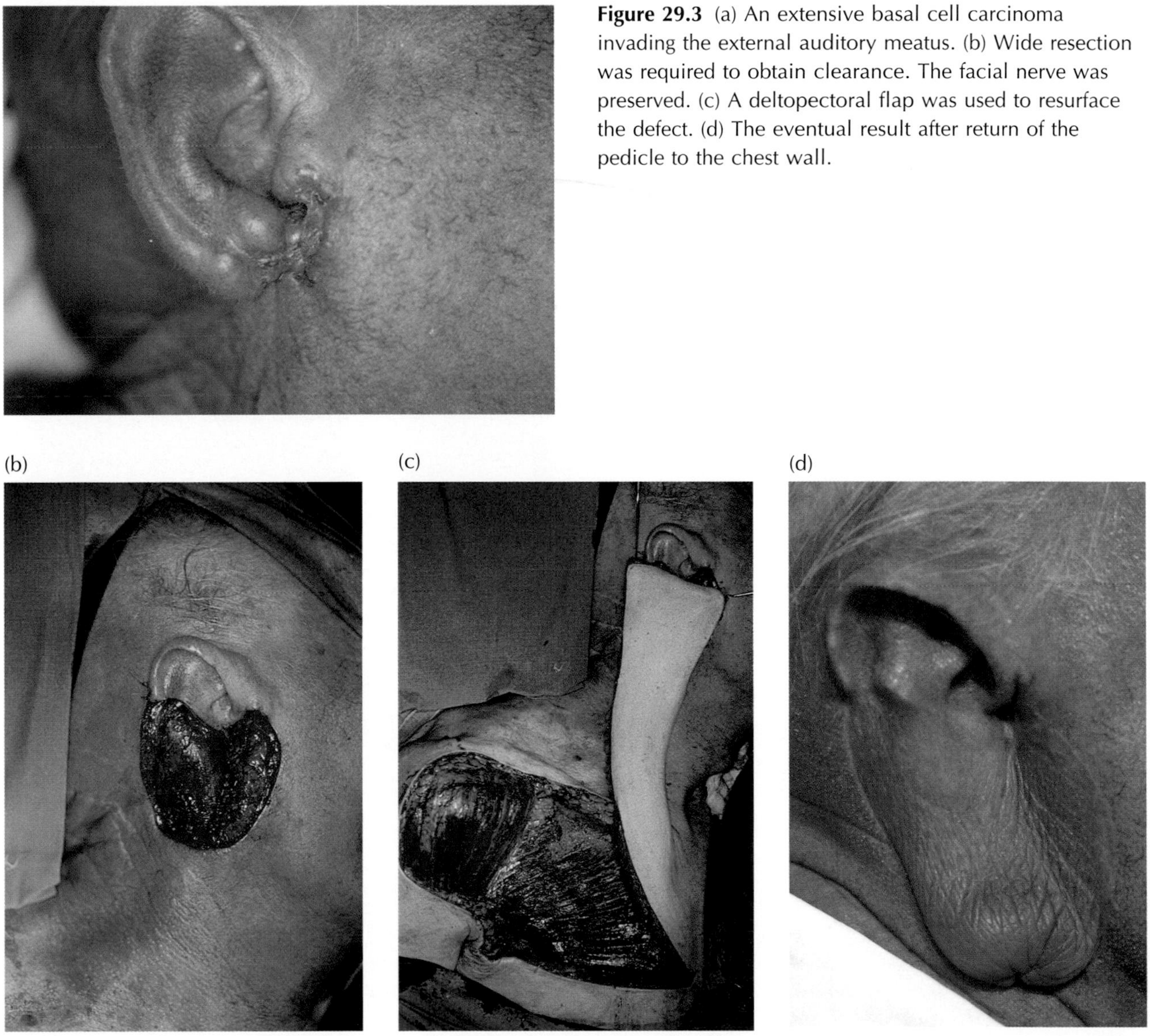

(b) (c) (d)

Figure 29.3 (a) An extensive basal cell carcinoma invading the external auditory meatus. (b) Wide resection was required to obtain clearance. The facial nerve was preserved. (c) A deltopectoral flap was used to resurface the defect. (d) The eventual result after return of the pedicle to the chest wall.

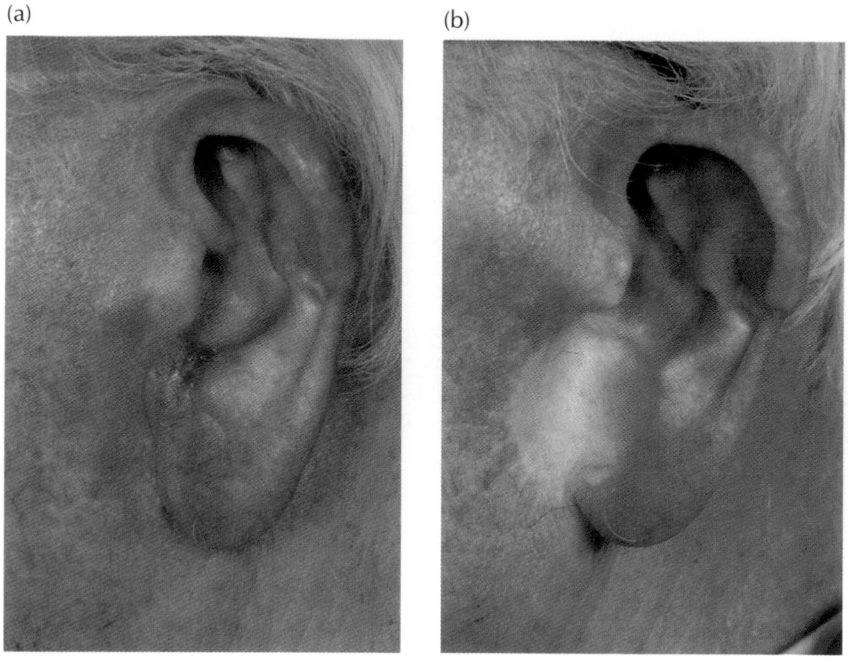

Figure 29.4 (a) A squamous cell carcinoma of the intertragal incisura. (b) The tumour was widely excised and the defect skin-grafted.

Reconstructional anatomy

Reconstruction of ear defects is aided by a working knowledge of the relevant anatomy. The main nerve supply is from the great auricular nerve (C2, C3). This lies superficial to the external jugular vein and travels obliquely over the sternomastoid muscle to enter the ear through the posterior portion of the lobe. As it enters the ear it splits into several branches. Division of the nerve causes numbness of the lower two-thirds of the ear (Figure 29.5).

The posterior surface of the ear is supplied with blood by auricular branches of the posterior auricular artery (Figure 29.6). The lateral or external surface is supplied by the superficial temporal artery. A rich plexus of vessels around the helical rim links these systems and many reconstructive flaps are based on this ring of connecting vessels.[6] Lymph drains to superficial parotid, mastoid and superficial cervical lymph nodes.

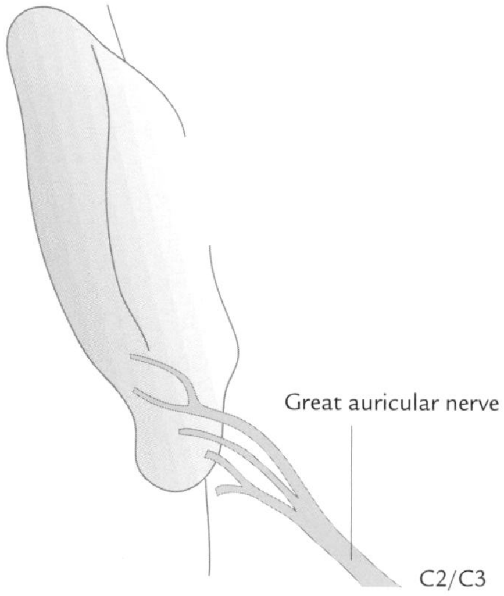

Figure 29.5 Great auricular nerve entering the posterior surface of the ear lobe.

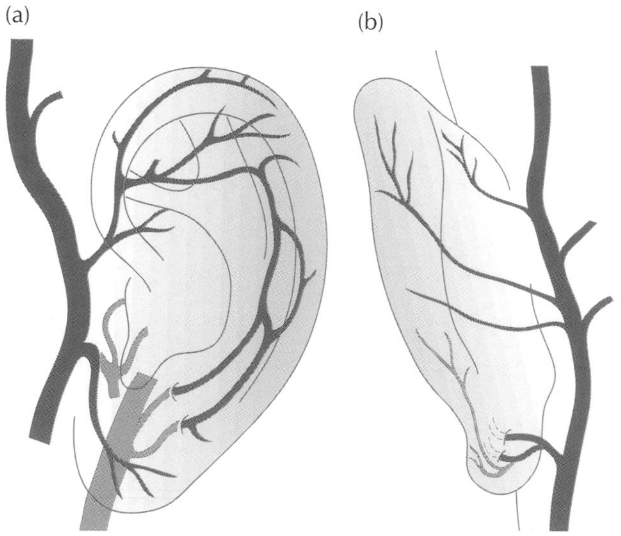

Figure 29.6 (a) The superficial temporal artery sends branches to the lateral surface of the ear. (b) The posterior auricular artery supplies the posterior surface of the ear. Both systems communicate in a ring of vessels near the helical rim.

Reconstruction after tumour excision: simple techniques for smaller tumours

Direct closure

In some patients, the skin of the helical rim is slack enough to permit direct closure when simple lesions such as small basal cell carcinomata and chondrodermatitis nodularis helicis chronica are removed. Incisions along the helical rim margin are particularly easy to close. When the skin is tight then that on the posterior surface can be rotated onto the rim to assist closure. The skin on the posterior ear is less adherent and defects on the postauricular surface can often be closed directly. The scar is hidden in the groove behind the ear. Sometimes the ear is pulled a little closer to the head in the process.

Skin grafts

If the perichondrium can be preserved then a full thickness skin graft is an ideal reconstructive solution (Figure 29.7). Both preauricular and postauricular donor sites are available. For lesions of the conchal hollow, a skin graft is a good form of reconstruction even if cartilage is excised (Figure 29.8). The raw soft tissue behind the conchal cartilage will readily accept a skin graft. Small defects at other sites can be reconstructed with skin grafts but it is important to preserve a round rim of cartilage and skin behind the defect. Without cartilage the helical rim margin will collapse postoperatively.

Wedge excisions

Defects on the helical margin can be removed as a small wedge. Some elderly patients with skin tumours have oversized ears (7–8 cm tall) and a small reduction in overall size is not readily apparent. A simple wedge should always be modified with small lateral extensions to prevent cupping of the ear when the components are joined (Figure 29.9).

In the Antia and Buch technique (a modified wedge), the available circumference of the ear after tumour excision is enhanced by advancing (stretching) the locally available tissues along the helical rim (Figure 29.10).[7] Large peripheral flaps of the adjacent helical margin are based on a wide postauricular skin pedicle. The earlobe varies in size but in most patients loose tissue within the lobe can be advanced along the rim of the ear.

This is a useful technique as the flaps are a good match for the missing helical rim. A single flap will suffice for small defects but for larger defects the intact cephalic segment of the helical rim can be advanced into the defect as a second flap. Extension of the flap's triangular tail into the depth of the concha leaves the ear with a pleasing shape. The chondrocutaneous rim tissue is mobilized on a very wide and highly vascular pedicle and accurately apposed with fine sutures prior to skin closure.

(a)

(b)

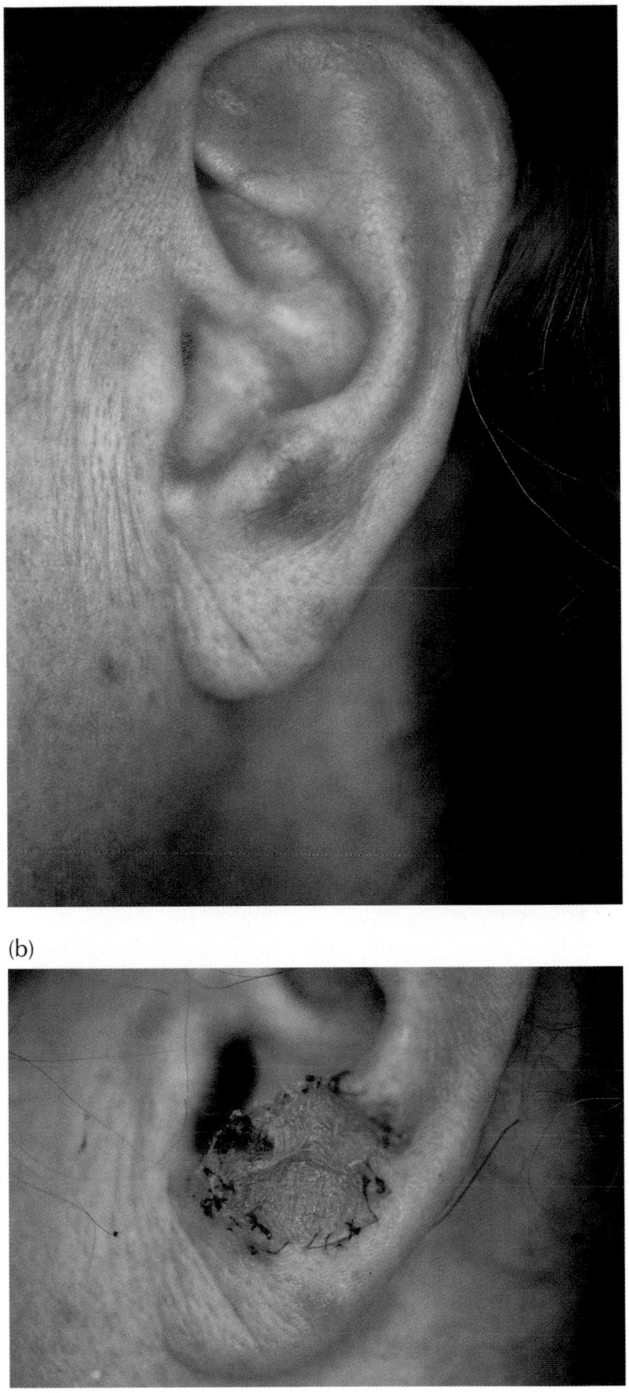

Figure 29.7 A basal cell carcinoma widely excised and reconstructed with a postauricular skin graft. (a) Tumour of the lower ear. (b) The skingraft has healed well. Some peripheral sutures have yet to be removed.

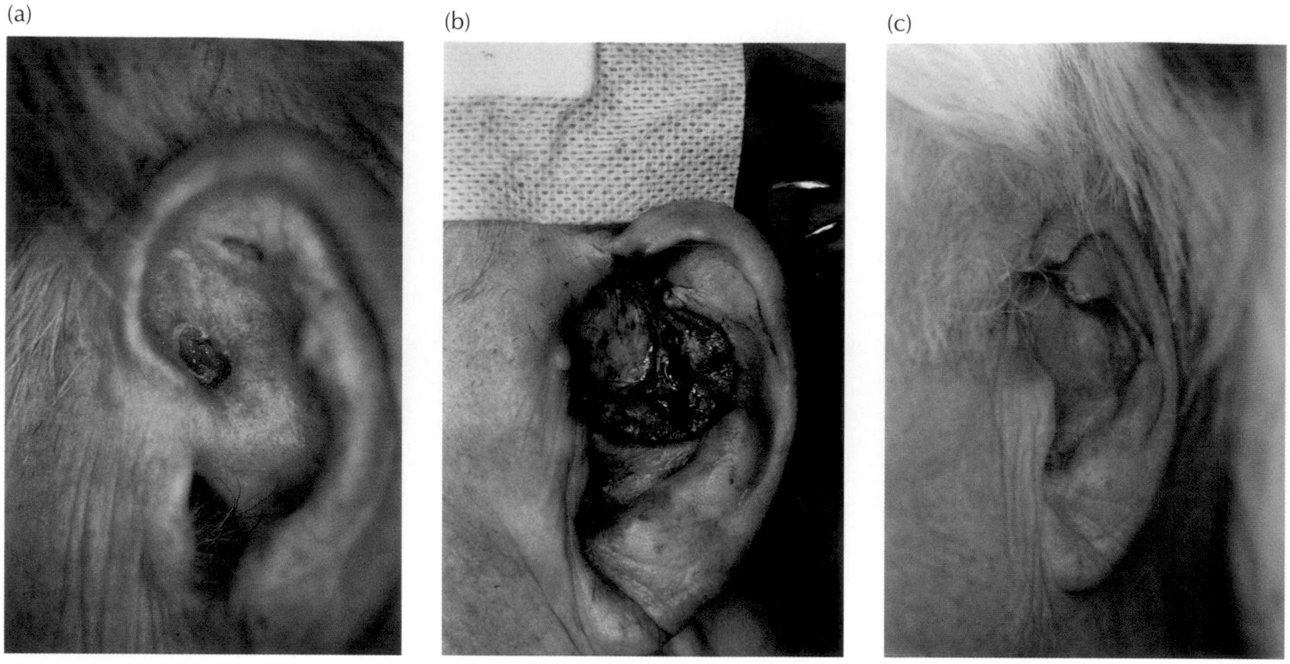

Figure 29.8 (a) A recurrent basal cell carcinoma of the ear after multiple attempts at cure. (b) MOHs micrographic surgery was used to confirm that extensions of tumour beyond the visible limits were excised. (c) The extensive defect has been healed with a split thickness skin graft.

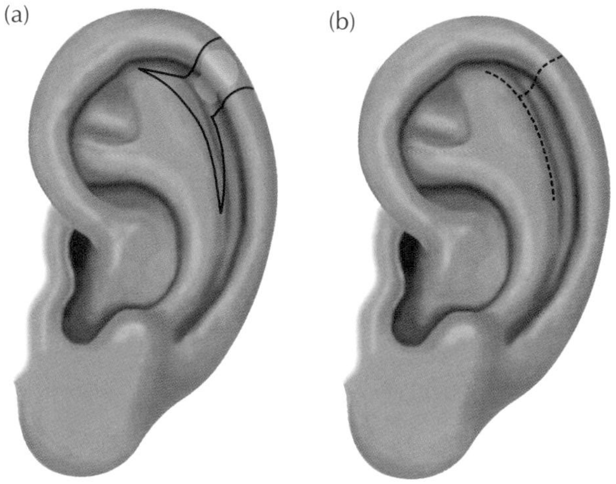

Figure 29.9 A small lesion treated by a wedge excision. The wedge is modified to prevent cupping of the ear.

Postauricular pedicle flaps to the anterior surface of the ear

A large skin flap from uninvolved postauricular and adjacent mastoid skin can be used to reconstruct defects on the anterior surface of the ear. Such a flap can reach the concha and the scaphal hollow. It is easy to use and the colour match is ideal. A posterior skin flap is outlined and undermined in the postauricular sulcus at a zone corresponding to the defect to be filled. A central pedicle of subcutaneous tissue is preserved. When the ear is pushed back the flap is delivered through to the external defect and secured. The donor site is closed directly.

An alternative to a subcutaneous pedicle is a de-epithelialized pedicle of dermis. Such postauricular flaps are also flipped through the ear to the external surface and used for reconstruction of central ear defects. If both a superior and inferior dermal pedicle are preserved, then the flap is rotated into the central ear defect in the manner of a swinging door (Figure 29.11). It is important to keep the donor defect elliptical in shape to allow easy closure. Wide undermining beneath the epidermis in the corners of the opening will allow substantial pedicles of dermis and subcutaneous tissue to nourish the flap. Small preauricular flaps and flaps from the concha can also be used to reach the external auditory meatus.

Techniques for larger tumours

When large tumours of the ear have been resected, then reconstruction will require some structural support to replace the missing cartilage. Small defects can be replaced by conchal cartilage grafts from either the same or the opposite ear. The curve of these cartilage grafts can be put to good use in mimicking a helical rim. When the missing

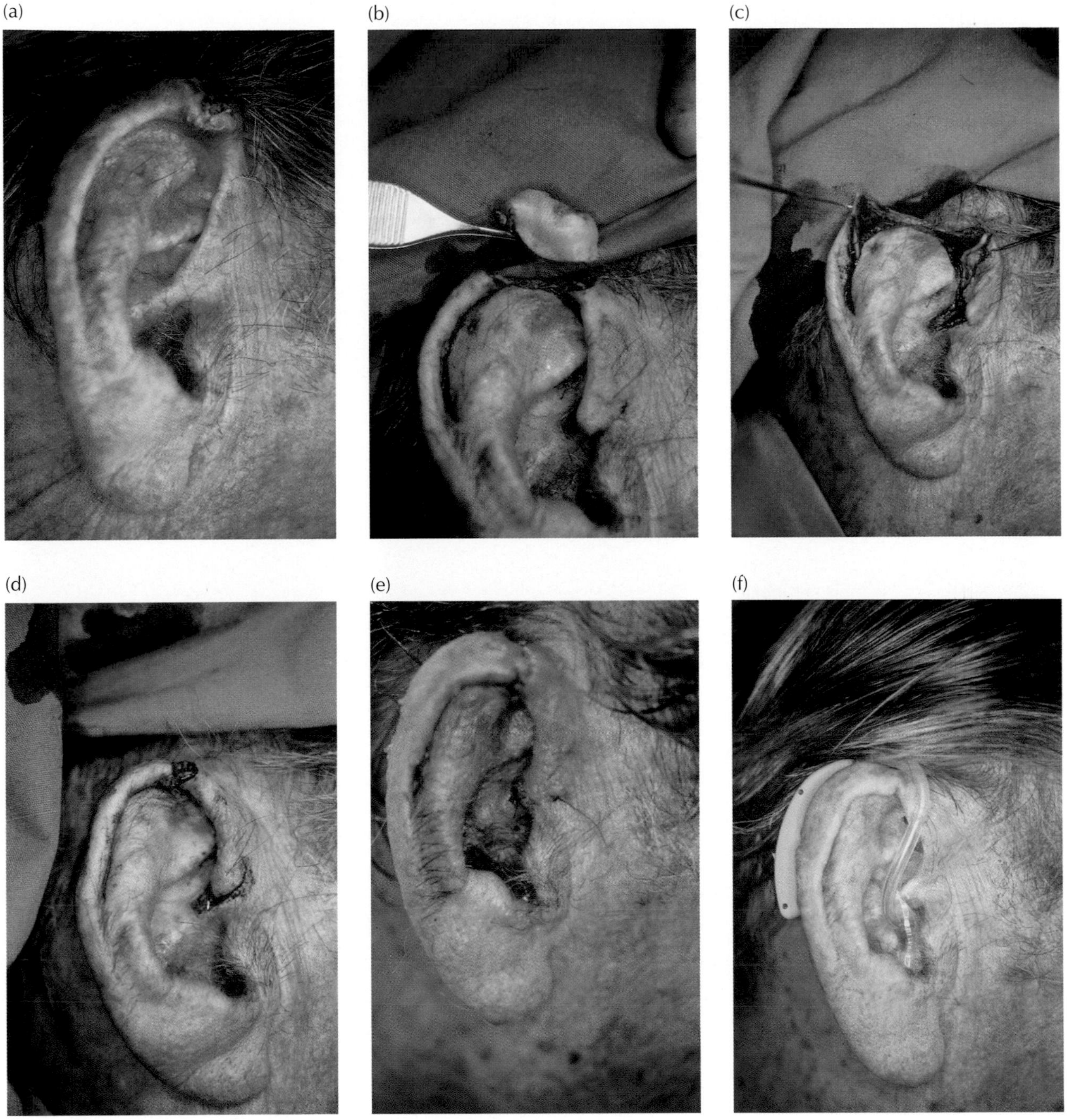

Figure 29.10 (a) An 83-year-old man with a 2-month history of a rapidly growing lesion of the upper ear. (b) Biopsy showed a moderately differentiated squamous cell carcinoma with clear margins. (c) Helical rim flaps with intact postauricular skin are raised. (d) The flaps are stretched around the defect. (e) The final result. (f) The patient has been followed up regularly without recurrence. He can still wear his hearing aid.

segment is extensive, a carved costal cartilage framework is required.[8] Complex shapes can be tailor-made to fit the defect after tumour excision, and this technique of reconstruction gives excellent results. In the age group that presents with auricular tumours, however, some patients are not keen on the additional discomfort of harvest of costal cartilage, and a number will opt to be fitted with a prosthesis.

Autogenous tissue reconstruction

Stage 1

Preparation

Autogenous tissue reconstruction starts by mapping the shape of the normal opposite ear. The shape is drawn on a see-through plastic sheet (the section at

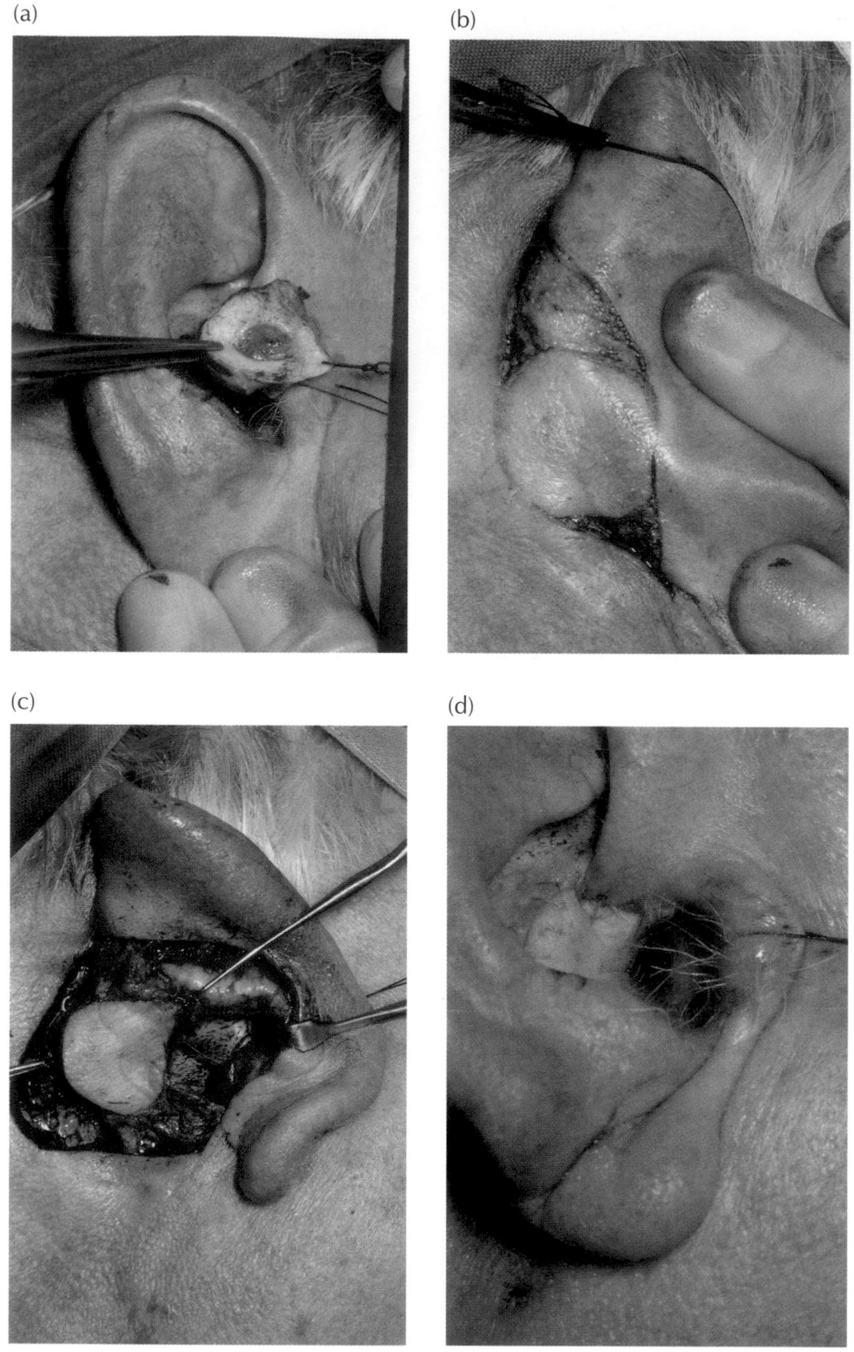

Figure 29.11 (a) A basal cell carcinoma of the conchal hollow of the ear treated with a postauricular flap. (b) An area of skin for the reconstruction is outlined. (c) Pedicles above and below the flap are preserved. (d) The flap is rotated into the conchal defect and sewn in place.

the bottom on a chest X-ray film is ideal). The scaphal hollow and triangular fossa parts are cut away to leave a template that can be sterilized for use throughout the operation (Figure 29.12).

Construction of a costal cartilage framework

Costal cartilage is harvested through an oblique incision overlying the costal margin anteriorly. Care is taken not to puncture the pleura. If a small hole is made, it should be closed and the final suture tied while the lungs are held fully inflated to avoid trapping air within the pleural space.

To minimize postoperative pain, a fine-bore cannula is left in the chest wound for the postoperative infusion of local anaesthetic. To prevent atelectasis, it is important to consider chest physiotherapy following surgery.

The costal cartilage framework is constructed to mimic all the missing ear components. Before starting to carve the cartilage, it is essential to double-check whether a right or left ear is to be made. A cartilage segment from a floating rib is thinned to make a helical rim and blocks of cartilage from the synchondrosis are used to make a base plate and antihelical ridge. It is usually possible to carve the cartilage using scalpel blades and gauges, but in the elderly it may have calcified. If the material is excessively tough, a rotating burr may be used.

With care the cartilage segments are joined together with either 4/0 clear Prolene or fine wire sutures. Where possible, it is useful to preserve a layer of perichondrium on the external surface of the cartilage, as it tends to prevent the stitches from cutting through. The cartilage edges are bevelled to abut neatly against any remaining original ear cartilage.

Insertion of framework into skin pocket

The framework is next inserted into a suitable skin pocket. The siting of the incisions made to create the skin pocket needs careful planning. Wide undermining is used to create a large pocket with broad attachments, thus preserving the skin's blood supply. Careful adjustment of the replacement framework is essential. Residual cartilage elements left behind after tumour resection are sutured to the framework, and any protruding ear remnants are blended with the reconstruction.

Skin from the posterior surface is raised and preserved as a pedicled flap. The edges are sutured together to form an airtight seal and suction drains are used to coapt the skin onto the carved cartilage framework. At the end of the operation, the ear defect has been filled by a contoured framework in the shape of an ear, albeit flat against the side of the head and without a post-auricular sulcus.

Suction is applied continuously for 5 days, so that the ear shape persists. Small silicone drains are used because they do not clog. The drains are connected to hollow needles that insert into Vacutainers. These containers are checked for suction (with each new tube a small splat of blood reaches the tube) and are changed regularly (when one-third full or even more often). A 5-day course of antibiotic medication is recommended (Figures 29.12–29.15).

(a) (b) (d) (c)

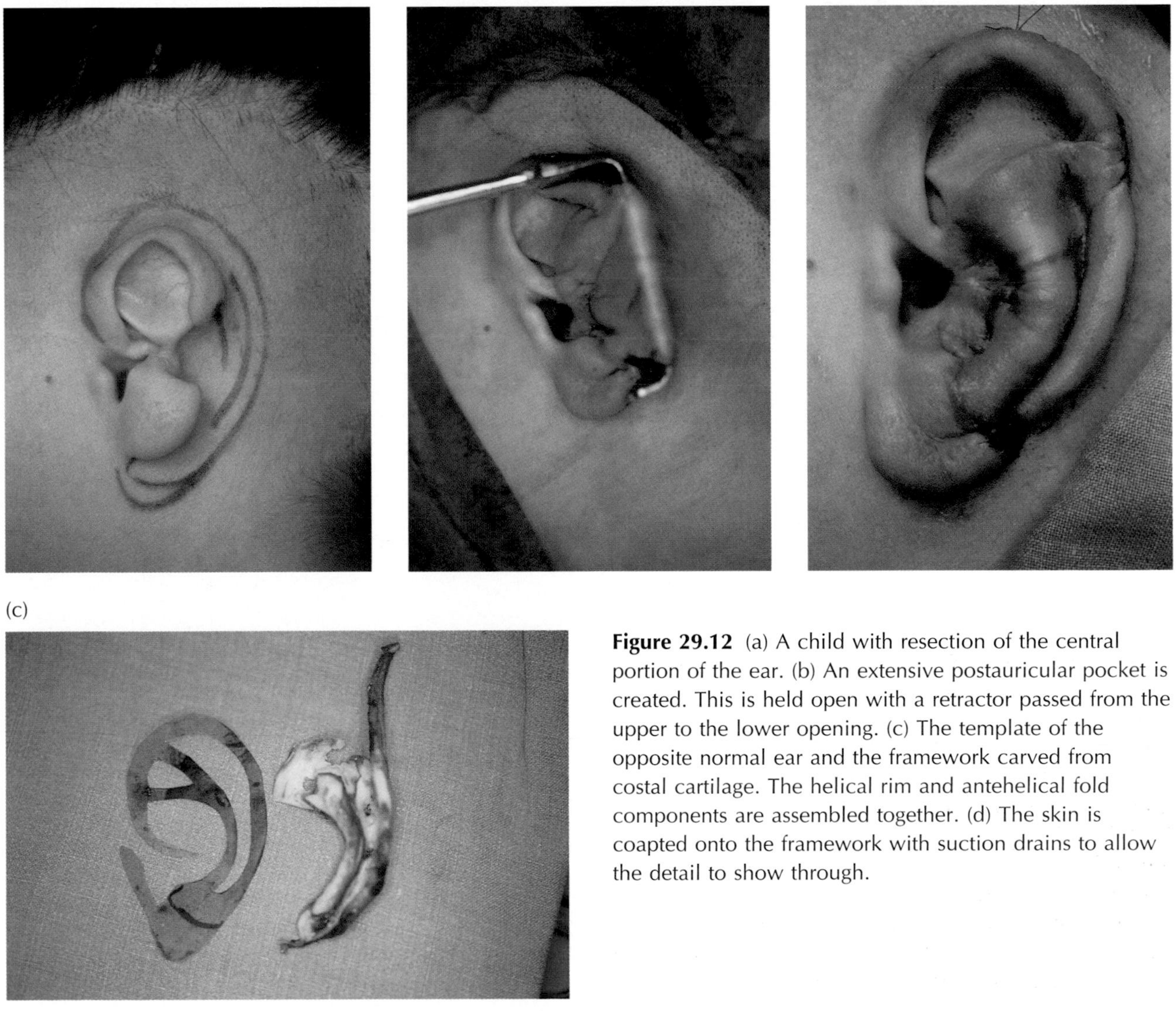

Figure 29.12 (a) A child with resection of the central portion of the ear. (b) An extensive postauricular pocket is created. This is held open with a retractor passed from the upper to the lower opening. (c) The template of the opposite normal ear and the framework carved from costal cartilage. The helical rim and antehelical fold components are assembled together. (d) The skin is coapted onto the framework with suction drains to allow the detail to show through.

(a) (b)

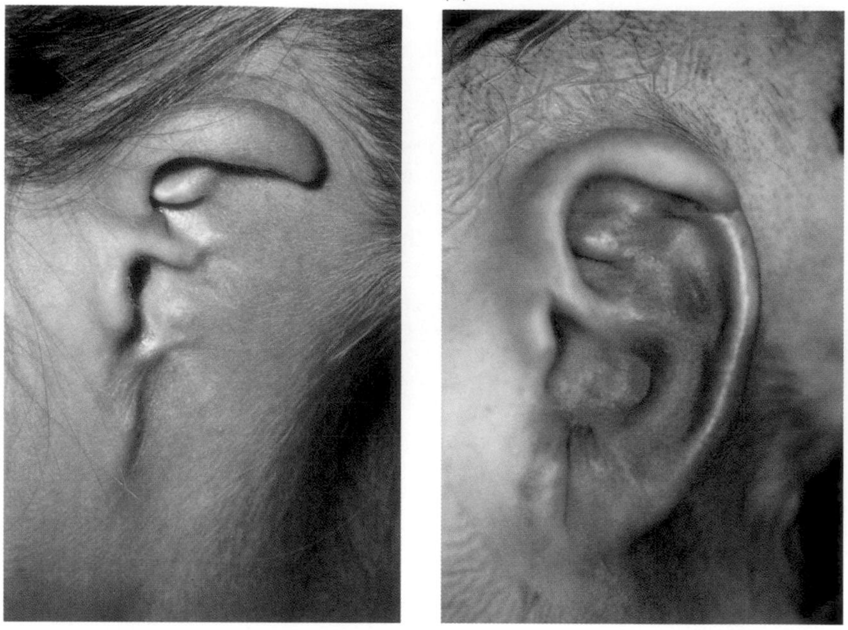

Figure 29.13 (a) A haemangiopericytoma was resected in childhood. (b) The defect reconstructed with a costal cartilage framework.

(a) (b)

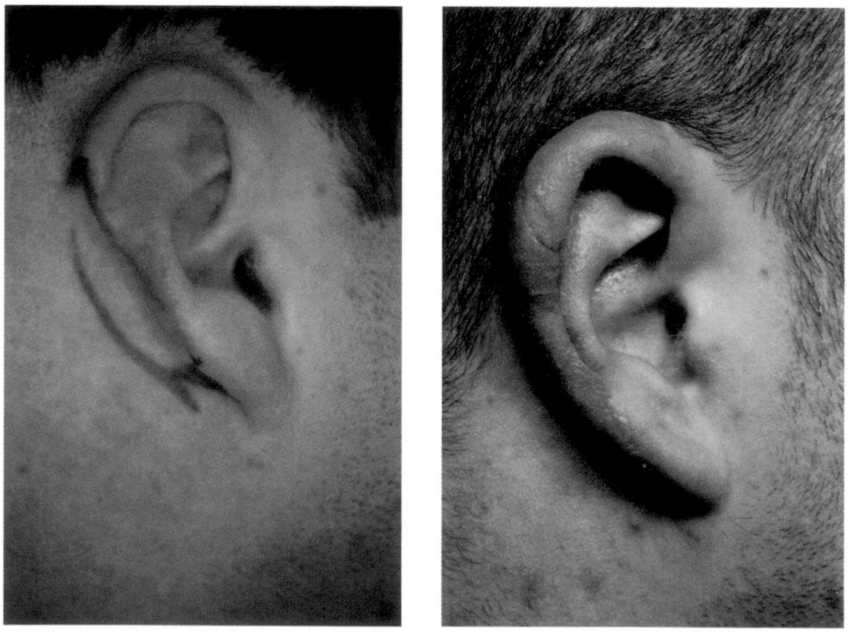

Figure 29.14 (a) A rim defect of the ear. (b) The result after reconstruction with costal cartilage.

Stage 2

Reconstruction of the postauricular sulcus is considered after a delay of 4–6 months to allow circulation to the zone of reconstruction to become established. An incision around the ear is used to elevate the whole reconstruction, taking care to preserve subcutaneous tissues over the framework to avoid framework exposure. The posterior surface of the ear is thus released from the mastoid fascia. This leaves two raw surfaces, one behind the ear and one on the side of the head. The majority of the defect on the side of the head is closed by undermining the scalp above and the neck below and closing these two flaps together. This is sometimes not easy, but the loop mattress suture can help to prevent the suture 'cheese-wiring' through skin when skin edges are closed under tension.[9]

The raw surface behind the ear framework is covered with a skin graft, either a thick split thickness skin graft or full thickness graft. The graft is sutured in place with vicryl and a Proflavin tie-over dressing is applied. Drains beneath the scalp and neck skin flaps are recommended.

(a) (b) (c) (d)

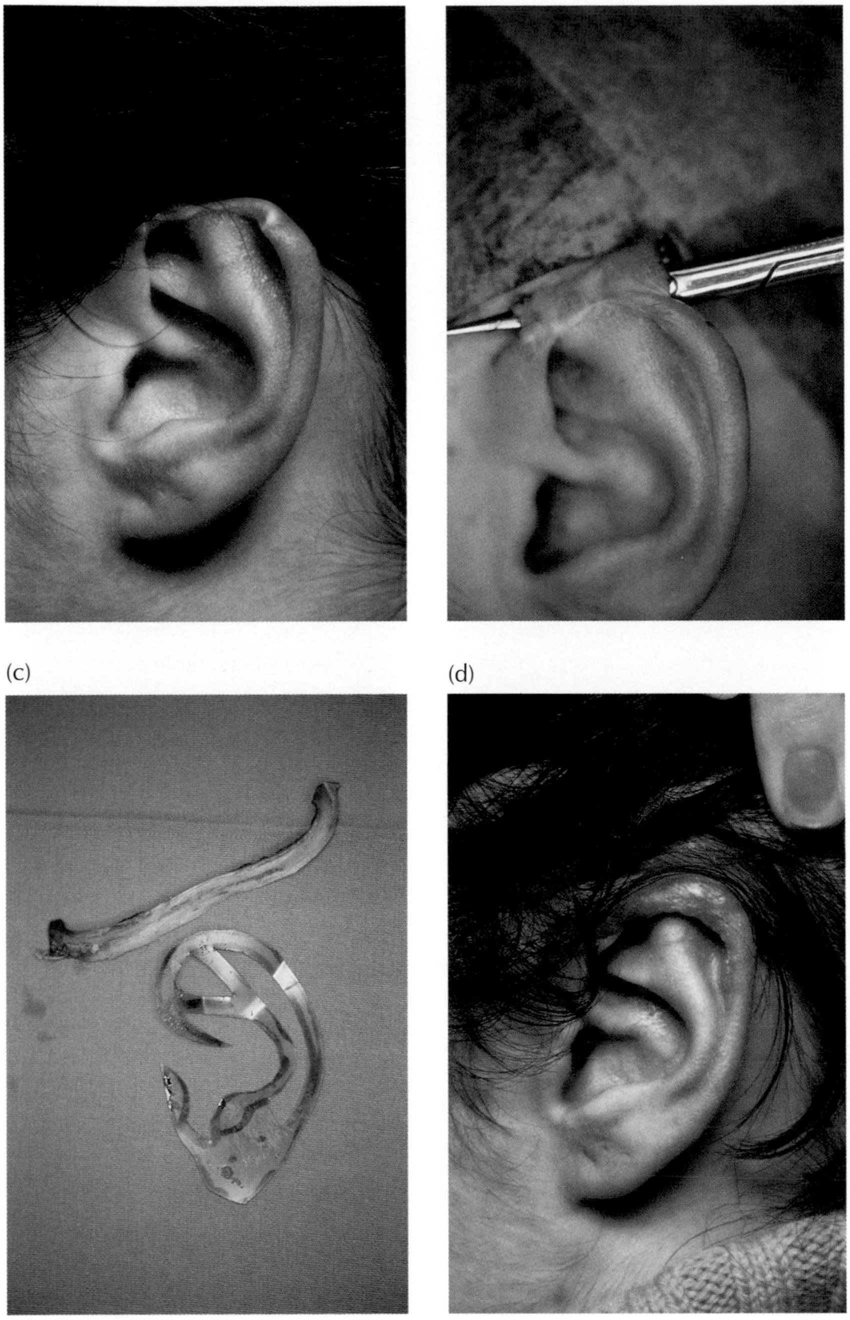

Figure 29.15 (a) An upper pole defect due to trauma. (b) The skin pocket is developed. (c) The template and the costal cartilage framework to be wound around the rim of the ear. (d) The final result.

An ear reconstructed using this technique is durable. Minor cuts and abrasions sustained in future times will readily heal. If a framework of artificial materials is used (Silastic, Medpore), then the result is less durable, and minor skin damage causing exposure can lead to a significant infection and loss of the reconstruction.

Prosthetic techniques

Glue-on prostheses

Glue-on prostheses to replace missing ears and segments of ears are often used. It is now possible to make an auricular prosthesis that is difficult to distinguish from a normal ear. By embedding material to resemble small blood vessels, freckles and moles and by applying life-like coloration, excellent results are achieved by some prosthetists (Figure 29.16).

It is important, however, that the patient feels confident that the prosthesis will remain in place regardless of his activity, and those retained by glue alone sometimes fall off. Moreover, cleaning the skin and applying glue is time consuming and messy, and some patients are, in addition, sensitive to the gluing agents.

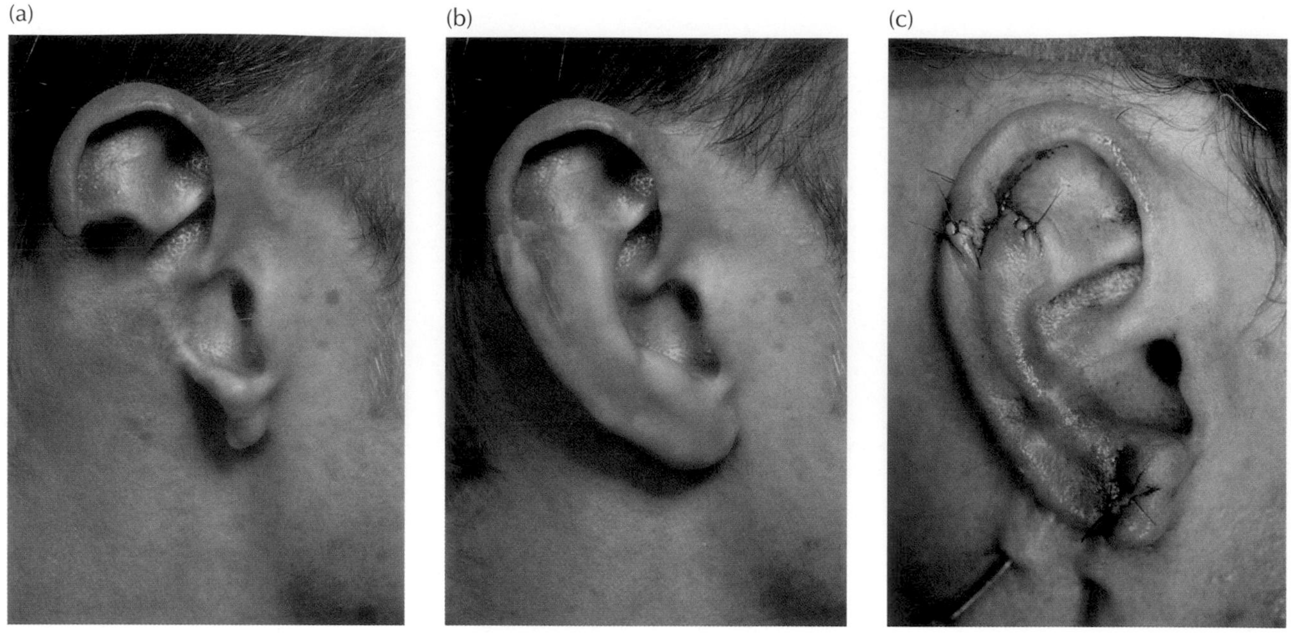

Figure 29.16 (a) A melanoma of the ear has been excised to leave a substantial defect. (b) A stick-on prosthesis replaces the missing segment. (c) At a later date the missing component is reconstructed with a costal cartilage framework.

Osseointegrated fixation

The term osseointegration is used for a direct structural and functional connection between living bone and the surface of a load-carrying implant.[10] The gold standard retention device for a prosthetic ear is currently a bone-anchored osseointegrated titanium fixture with a skin penetrating abutment.[11] Auricular prostheses can be retained on this scaffold using clips or magnets.

Stage 1

The first stage of this process is to insert commercially pure titanium fixtures into the mastoid bone. The drill holes are sited with care so that the metal work lies beneath the antihelical fold of the prosthesis. Two fixtures are used, positioned 20–25 mm from the centre of the external auditory meatus. The ideal site is at the 8 o'clock and 11 o'clock position on the right and the 4 o'clock and 1 o'clock position on the left.

A guide hole is drilled for each fixture, cooling the point of contact between drill bit and bone with normal saline throughout the process. Debris is regularly removed from the cutting surface of the drill bit to minimize heat trauma. The bottom of the hole is checked regularly to ensure that neither dura nor the sigmoid sinus is encountered. In good bone stock, a 4-mm deep hole is made. The guide drill is then replaced with a wider drill and countersink, again ensuring adequate cooling.

The final stage is to use a titanium tap at low speed (8–15 rpm). The tap is unscrewed and the fixture inserted into the threaded hole, again at low speed. A cover screw is used to protect internal threads on the outside of the fixture. Bone dust can be applied around the fixture and the periosteum carefully replaced before the incision is closed. The operation note should record the location of the fixtures. In patients in whom radiotherapy has been given after tumour resection, hyperbaric oxygen treatment is advisable.

Stage 2

A second stage is undertaken some 3 months later when osseointegration is established. To make room for the prosthesis, auricular remnants are removed, ideally with the exception of the tragus. An incision is made 10 mm around the implant site. All subcutaneous tissue is removed as far as the pericranium (which is preserved) and the skin is thinned to approximately 1 mm thick around the implant. A hole is punched in the skin overlying the implants, the cover screws removed and the abutments screwed into place. With healing caps attached to the abutments, the thinned skin is replaced onto a thin layer of vascularized pericranium. This prevents movement at the interface between the skin and the abutments. A pressure dressing is applied.

Three or four weeks later, when the postoperative swelling has begun to settle, prosthesis manufacture is begun. An alginate copy of the defect is made. If this is done too early, it is possible to pull off the underlying skin and delay healing. Using the

(a) (b) (c)

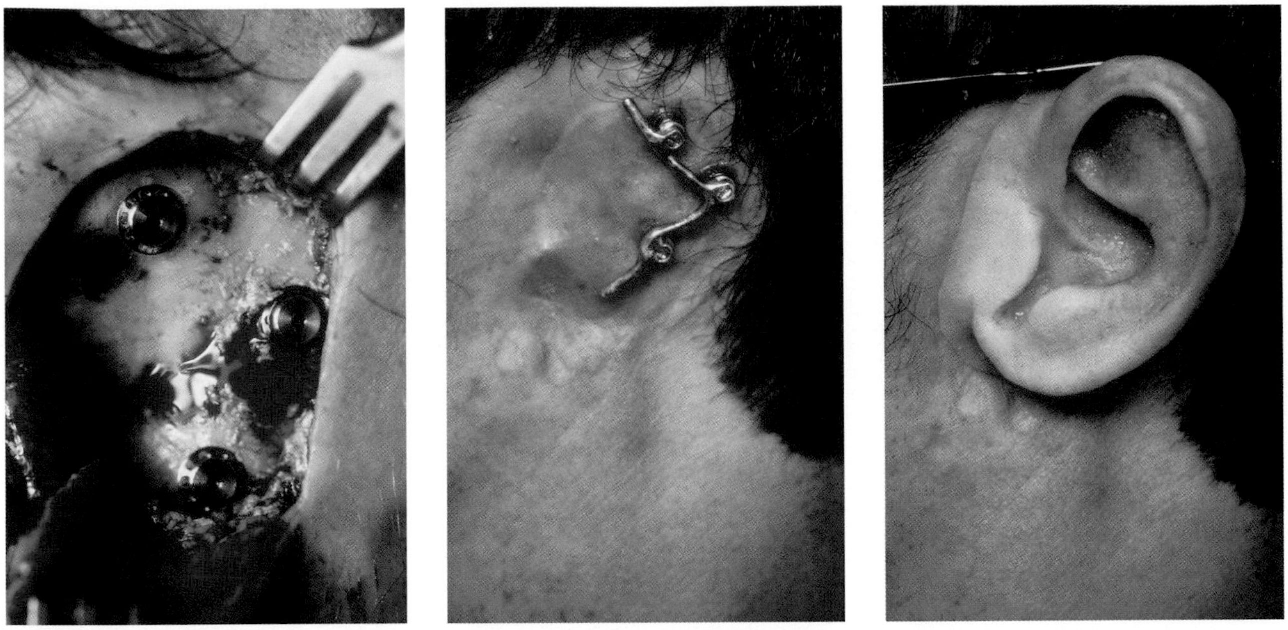

Figure 29.17 (a) Titanium fixtures inserted into the mastoid bone. (b) Abutments are screwed to the fixtures and a bar attached. (c) The prosthesis is securely fixed by clips to the bar mechanism.

(a) (b)

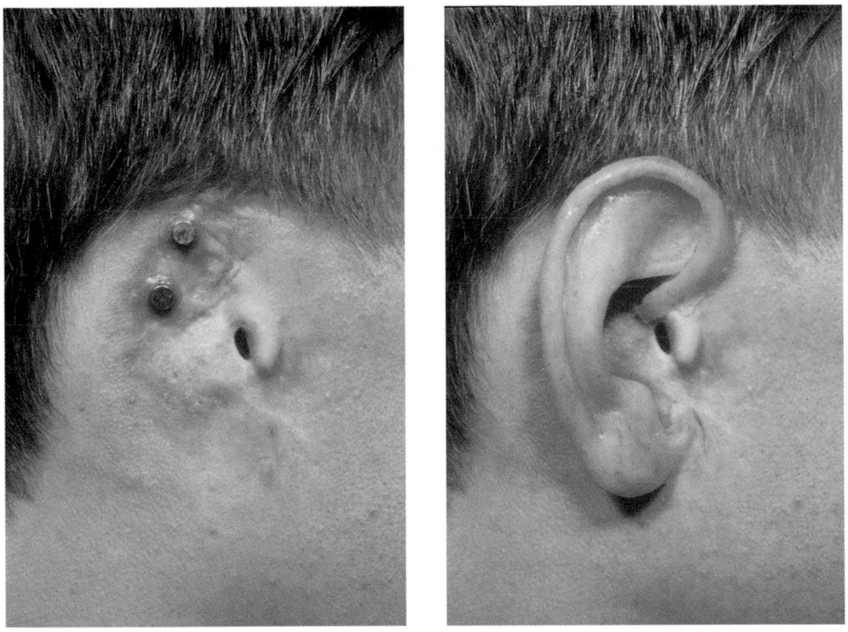

Figure 29.18 (a) In this patient, magnets are attached to the abutments for (b) prosthesis retention.

wound cast, an accurate silicone prosthetic ear with an acrylic base plate for fixation is manufactured. It is retained by either magnets or a clip and bar system, which attaches to the abutments (Figures 29.17–29.19). In good conditions, a prosthesis will last 2–3 years. If the patient smokes or works in an oily or dirty environment, this period may be shortened. It is important to care for the abutment site, and cleaning around these pins with a soft toothbrush each day is needed.

Some patients referred for reconstruction of the ear after tumour resection show no enthusiasm for either an autogenous tissue reconstruction or a prosthetic device. Where spectacle support is a problem, then a simple device can be fitted (Figure 29.20).

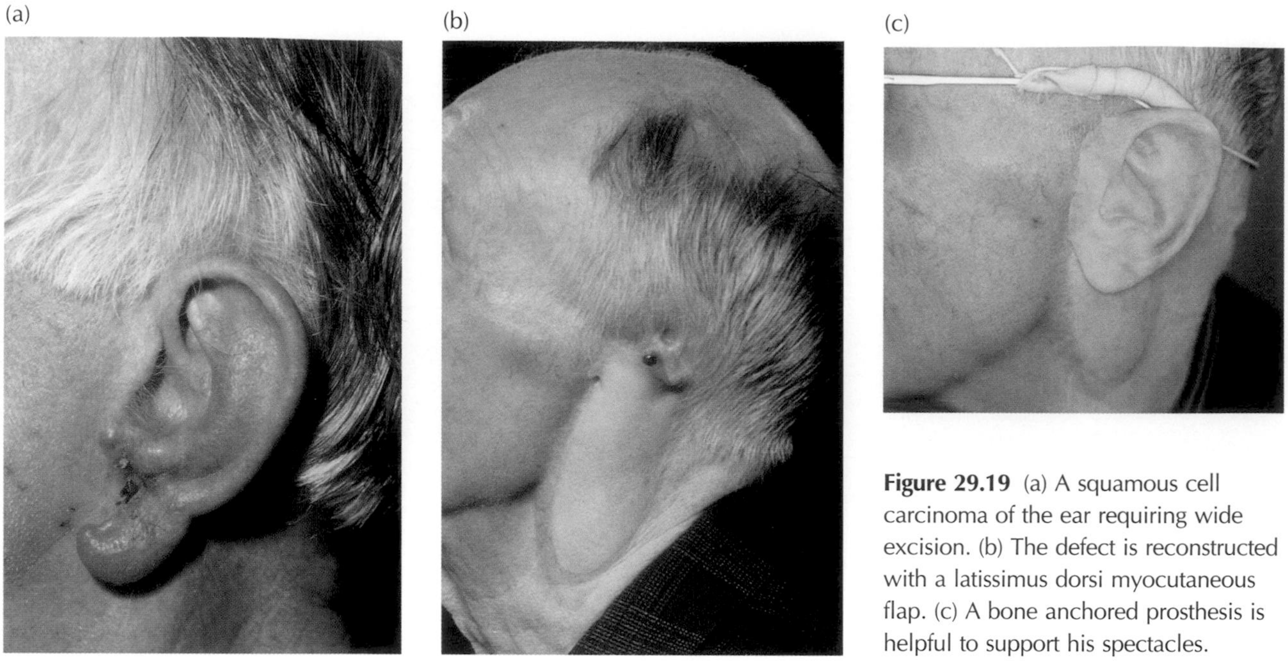

Figure 29.19 (a) A squamous cell carcinoma of the ear requiring wide excision. (b) The defect is reconstructed with a latissimus dorsi myocutaneous flap. (c) A bone anchored prosthesis is helpful to support his spectacles.

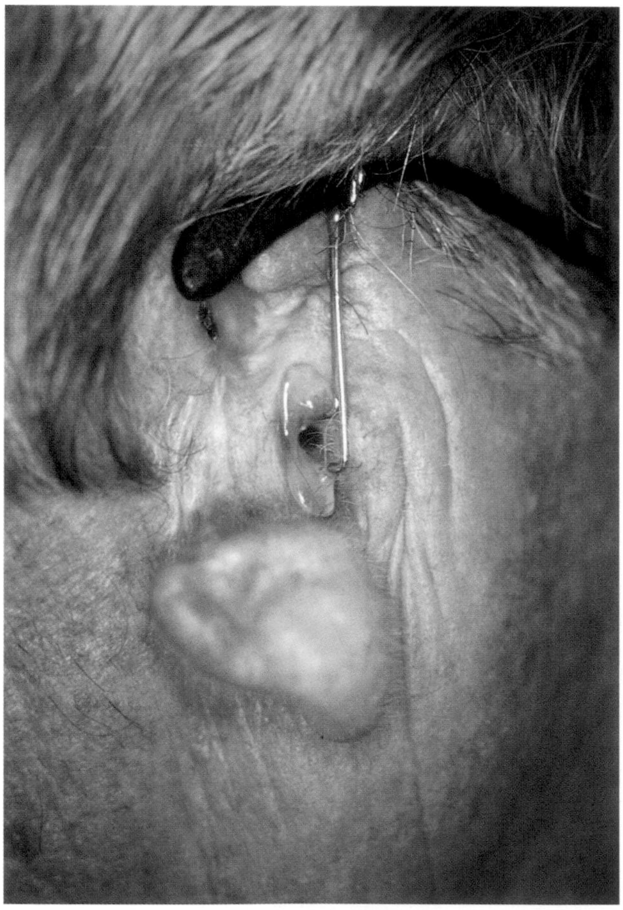

Figure 29.20 A patient with an extensive resection. He wished only to support his glasses, and a small custom-made device has been created.

Complications and troubleshooting

Smoking

Smoking reduces skin blood supply and in patients undergoing surgery involving skin flaps or autogenous tissue reconstruction, this can predispose to skin loss. It is advisable to stop smoking 6 weeks prior to reconstruction if at all possible.

Skin loss

Small areas of skin loss that expose autogenous cartilage will often heal in spontaneously if the area is protected by antibiotic ointment. Secondary healing may take several weeks. If the area of skin loss is greater than 1 cm in diameter, then local flap cover should be considered.

Problems with bone-anchored prostheses

Granulations around abutments can be removed with a carbon dioxide laser if extensive. If minor, then treatment with Terracortril ointment is helpful. Persistent soft tissue reaction around abutments may require their temporary removal. It is important to ensure that all soft tissues are removed around abutments at the initial surgery to prevent such

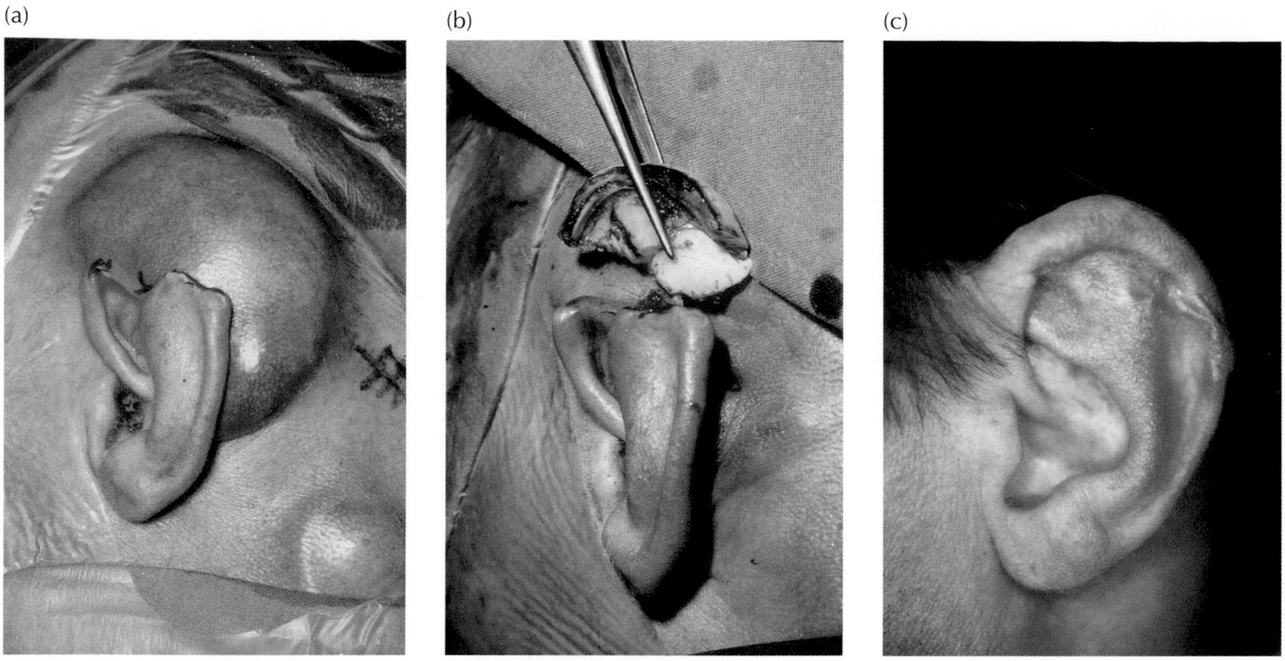

Figure 29.21 (a) Tissue expansion used to create extra skin for a costal cartilage reconstruction. (b) The cartilage framework. (c) The final result.

problems. Rarely, trauma to abutments can bend them such that replacement is required. Keloid scars are also rare.

Infections

Meticulous care with autogenous cartilage grafts is essential to avoid infection. Before reconstruction, the persisting curves and hollows of any residual ear tissue must be cleaned with a cotton bud and antiseptic skin preparation. The external auditory meatus is a particular source of potential infection. Grafts should be washed with saline prior to implantation. With precaution, infection is rare.

Hair growth

In most cancer reconstructions that use autogenous tissues, the non-hair bearing mastoid skin is the source of local skin flaps. Unwanted hair on such flaps used to resurface the ear is best treated by excision and skin grafting. Laser treatment to unwanted hair is at the present time able to remove hairs for several months but is not a permanent solution to the problem.[12]

Poor skin quality

The presence of scars and skin grafts may render the local skin inflexible and not suitable to drape over costal cartilage when replacing resected segments of the ear. In these circumstances two devices can prove to be helpful.

Tissue expansion

The placement of a tissue expander beneath poor quality skin requires great care. A remote incision is required for insertion. Small amounts of saline are added at weekly intervals via a remote port. The thickened capsule that surrounds the expander is removed before draping the skin created over cartilage grafts (Figure 29.21).[13]

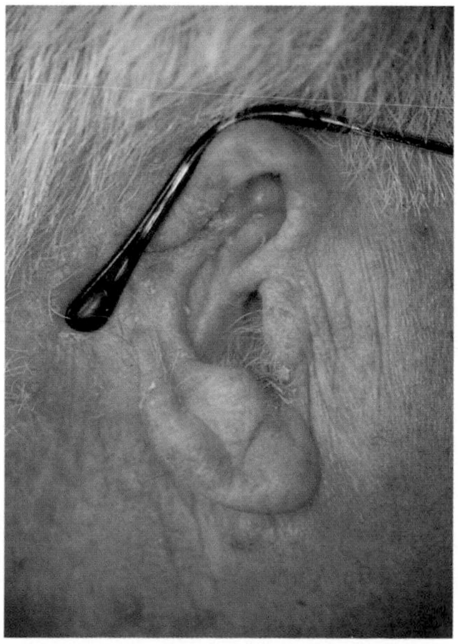

Figure 29.22 After an extensive resection of an ear tumour, enough tissue is left to support a spectacle leg.

Fascial flaps

If the superficial temporal artery is intact, then the temporoparietal fascial flap is an excellent source of thin vascularized tissue to be wrapped around a cartilage graft when no local skin is available. Skin grafts are then required to achieve healing but the results are very good. Such fascial flaps can also be used to cover areas of inadvertent cartilage exposure during a reconstruction. In patients with a low hairline these flaps are also useful (Figure 29.23).

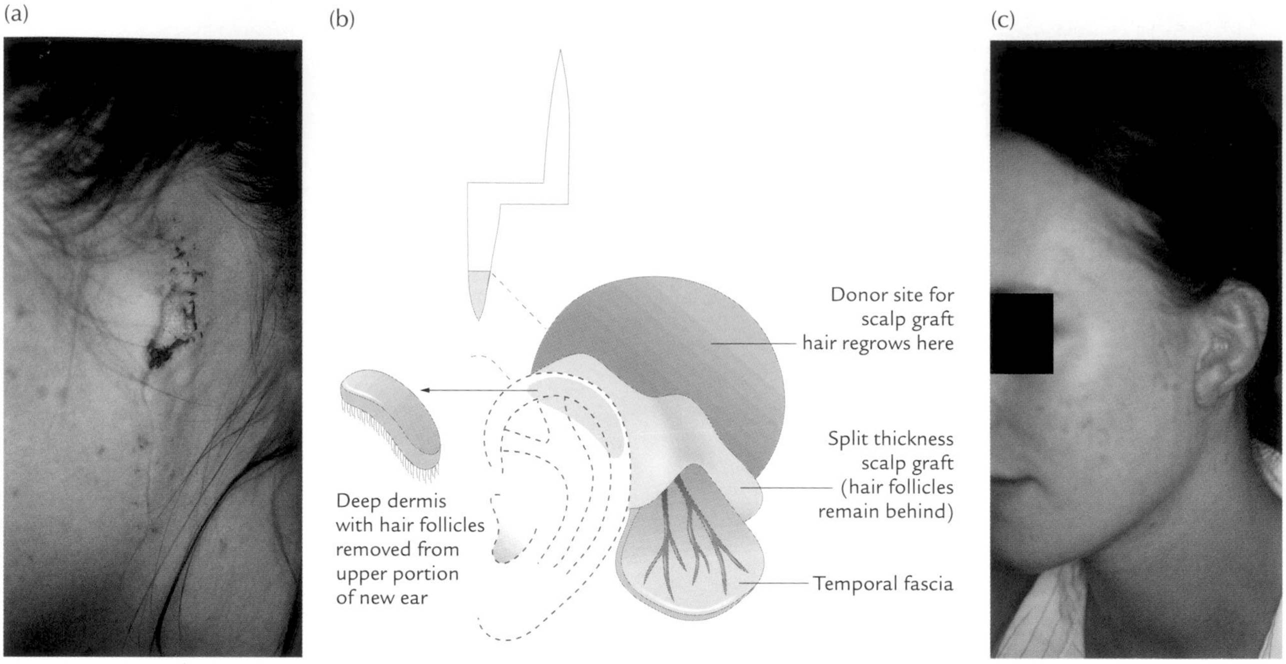

Figure 29.23 (a) Preoperative slide; (b) Diagram; (c) Postoperative slide. (a) This young girl was very distressed after her ear was removed in the treatment of a malignant melanoma. (b) To avoid hair appearing on the upper portion of the ear reconstruction, this zone was covered in a small facial flap and a split thickness scalp graft. (c) The completed reconstruction after release.

REFERENCES

1. Freedlander E, Chung FP. Squamous cell carcinoma of the pinna. *Br J Plast Surg* 1983; **36**: 171.
2. Lederman M. Malignant tumours of the ear. *J Laryngol* 1965; **79**: 85–119.
3. Lewis JS. Cancer of the ear. A report of 150 cases. *Laryngoscope* 1960; **70**: 551–579.
4. Blake GB, Wilson JSP. Malignant tumours of the ear and their treatment. I Tumours of the auricle. *Br J Plast Surg* 1974; **27**: 67–76.
5. Horlock N, Grobbelaar AO, Gault DT. Can the carbon dioxide laser completely ablate basal cell carcinomas? A histological study. *Br J Plast Surg* 2000; **53**: 286–293.
6. Park C, Lineaweaver WC, Rumly TO, Buncke HJ. Arterial supply of the anterior ear. *Plast Reconst Surg* 1992; **90**: 38–44.
7. Antia NH, Buch VI. Chondrocutaneous advancement flap for marginal defects of the ear. *Plast Reconstr Surg* 1967; **39**: 472–477.
8. Harris PA, Ladhani K, Das-Gupta R, Gault DT. Reconstruction of acquired subtotal ear defects with autologous costal cartilage. *Br J Plast Surg* 1999; **52**: 268–275.
9. Gault DT, Brain A, Sommerlad BC, Ferguson DJP. The loop mattress suture. *Br J Surg* 1987; **74**: 820–821.
10. Branemark PI, Hansson B, Adell R et al. Osseointegrated implants in the treatment of the edentulous jaw. Experience from a 10 year period. *Scand J Plast Reconstr Surg* 1977; **16**: 1–132.
11. Tjellstrom A. Osseointegrated implants for replacement of absent or defective ears. *Clin Plast Surg* 1990; **17**: 355–366.
12. Gault DT, Grobbelaar AO, Grover R et al. The removal of unwanted hair using a ruby laser. *Br J Plast Surg* 1999; **52**: 173–177.
13. Chana JS, Grobbelaar AO, Gault DT. Tissue expansion as an adjunct to reconstruction of congenital and acquired auricular deformities. *Br J Plast Surg* 1977; **50**: 456–462.

30 Principles of nasal reconstruction

David Ross and Gary C Burget

Introduction

Nasal reconstruction occupies a unique position in reconstructive surgery. It provided the inspiration and subsequent framework for the future development of the specialty. However, there is something altogether more absorbing about nasal reconstruction in addition to its rich and wonderful history, for it appears to represent the junction between art and surgery that reconstructive surgeons find so rewarding. For several millennia the nose has come to represent many things to individuals and societies. It defined people's impressions of beauty, racial origin and even their social status. However, the origins of nasal reconstruction lay in the effect that trauma and amputation had on the individual and the society within which he or she lived.

Introduction to the history of nasal reconstruction

Reconstruction of the amputated nose represents one of the oldest described surgical procedures. The first formal description is that of the Hindu surgeon, Susruta, who described posttraumatic reconstruction using a cheek advancement flap drawn from the outline of a vine leaf on the patient's cheek, in approximately 600 BC. It is likely that Susruta was describing a technique that had been passed down through the cast of potters and brickmakers possibly described centuries beforehand. At that time, and as a common theme through premodern surgery, the loss of the nose had occurred either as a sign of contempt or punishment, usually for adultery or theft. Even in these early times people felt the loss of one's nose to be so shameful that they had to seek some form of restitution, albeit in a preanaesthetic, preantibiotic era.

Nasal reconstruction was to proceed along two parallel, and largely independent paths, the most influential and important of which was to occur on the Indian subcontinent, progressing from Susruta's cheek flap through to early descriptions of the forehead flap in around the tenth century AD. Curiously, the forehead flap was to remain unknown to occidental surgeons until its use was described in the *Gentleman's Magazine* of 1794, by a British Army surgeon, Major Colley Lyon Lucas (Figure 30.1).[1] In Europe other techniques evolved, originating in fifteenth century Sicily with the father and son Brancas.[2] The father, Gustavo, utilized a cheek flap similar to that described by Susruta, though there is no record that he had any formal training in the Hindu technique. However, Sicily represented an important trading post and it is likely that there would have been exchange of scientific and medical information as well as commerce. Antonio, his son, was keen to seek new techniques to avoid the secondary donor site defect on the patient's face and turned to the upper arm to provide a flap. The Brancas never left any direct records but several contemporary observers recorded in detail both their technique and the secrecy with which the procedure was performed.

Later in the fifteenth century, the technique is recorded to have passed to another family of surgeons, the Vianeos, across the water in Calabria in mainland Italy. The method was refined, including the use of lint strips. The brachial flap was initially raised as a bipedicled flap under which the lint strip was inserted to provoke suppuration and thickening.

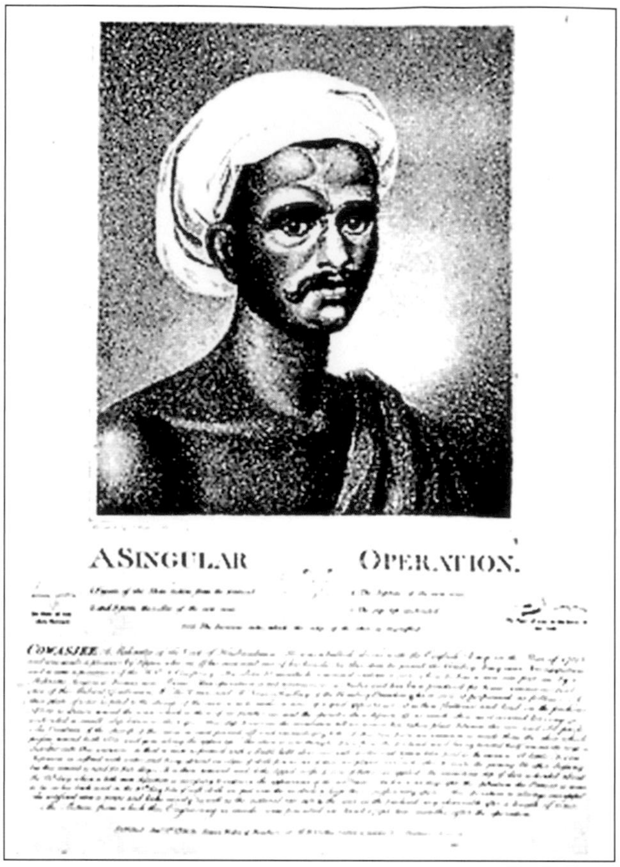

Figure 30.1 The case of Cowsajee, the *Gentleman's Magazine*, 1794.

This aided integrity and maintained shape of the final nose. The Vianeos also described the design of specific instruments.

Thereafter, the technique migrated north, to the Italian city of Bologna where ultimately the technique was formally described in the first known textbook of reconstructive surgery, *De Cutorum Chirugia Per Insitionum* by Gaspare Tagliacozzi, published in 1597.[3] Tagliacozzi had been taught the procedure from his teacher, Aranzio. In reply to an inaccurate description of the method, published in 1586, Tagliacozzi proceeded to formally describe the procedure in detail. His text was detailed and superbly illustrated (Figure 30.2). Furthermore, it represented one of the first surgical treatises to describe cases by the surgeon performing them. Tagliacozzi aimed to establish reconstruction as a valid part of surgery and, more importantly raise the status of surgery, as the practice of medicine at that time, was dominated by the more formally educated physicians.

Tagliacozzi died 2 years later, in 1599, but the efforts of his text were to prove of little value as his technique fell into disrepute and even ridicule. His work also suffered criticism by more influential

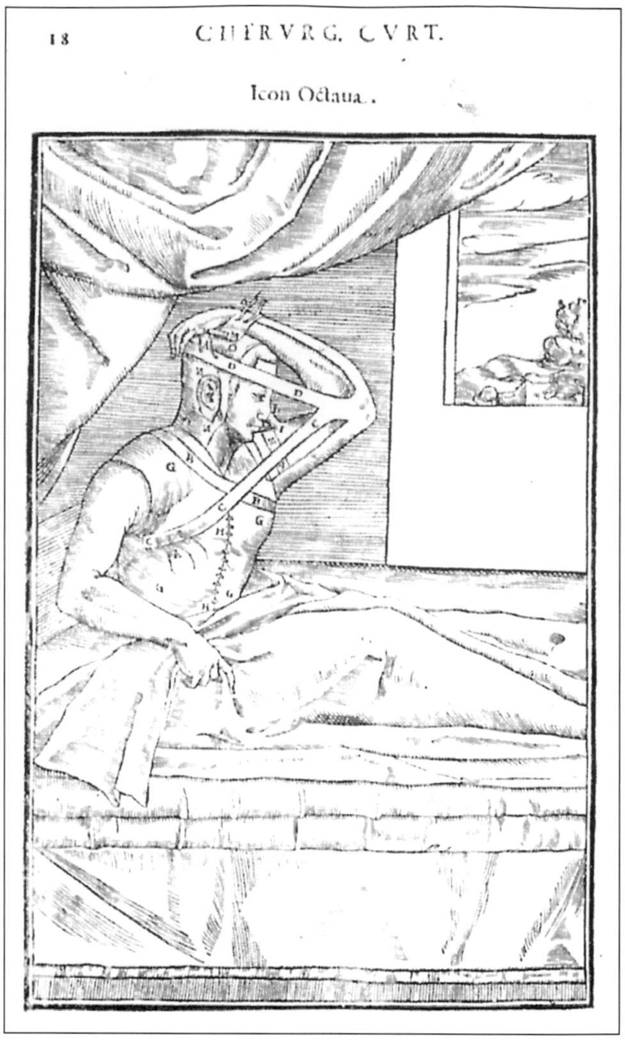

Figure 30.2 A plate from Tagliacozzi's text, showing the brachial flap inset onto the nasal remnant.

surgeons such as Ambrose Paré, who, having heard of the technique, though never having performed it, felt it an improbable method of nasal reconstruction. Paré, one of the most significant Renaissance figures in medicine felt that prosthetics were the only way to achieve reasonable nasal reconstruction and designed a number including those with and without a moustache (Figure 30.3).

In 1794, Major Colley Lyon Lucas, an army surgeon practising in Madras, described how one of his servants had had his nose repaired using a forehead flap. The servant, Cowsajee, had his nose amputated following a raid by bandits (Figure 30.1). Joseph Carpue, a surgeon at St George's Hospital in London, read the article and was sufficiently taken by this technique to practise on several cadavers before performing reconstructions on two army officers, whom he described as having endured the operation with 'admirable fortitude'. Carpue published a monograph of this work in 1816,[4]

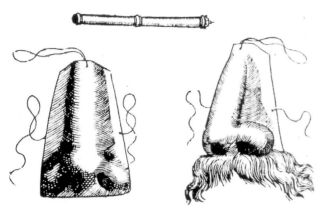

Figure 30.3 Nasal prostheses as described by Ambrose Pare.

which gave further impetus to the interest and efforts of the great Von Graeff in Berlin. He and his successor, Diffenbach were to both rediscover the rich history that lay in the reconstruction of the nose. However, of even greater significance one of their students, Edward Zeiss made strenuous efforts to concentrate the philosophy and techniques of reconstruction into a surgical specialty of its own, which he termed plastic surgery.[5] As a result, attempts to reconstruct the nose had led to a new surgical specialty.

With the advent of general anaesthetics in the middle 1800s surgery could become more adventurous and time could be taken to achieve a better and long-lasting result. This was of course true for all branches of surgery. However, it became particularly relevant for the many thousands of patients severely injured in the Great War. As noted in Chapter 27, Gillies has laid the foundations of the modern speciality, stressing the importance of replacing 'like with like'.

Successful nasal reconstruction is dependent on this principle and has been increasingly utilized by contemporary surgeons culminating in the work of the senior author, and his colleague Frederick Menick that sought to introduce a fourth, aesthetic dimension, to reconstruction.[6,7] This chapter is intended to provide the reader with an introduction into the principles of nasal reconstruction and an overview of the most commonly used techniques.

Basic principles of nasal reconstruction

The nose is a complex three-dimensional structure that occupies a central position in both the patients' facial anatomy and their self-esteem (Figure 30.4). Careful consideration needs to be made of the patient and their defect. Nasal reconstruction may involve several complex steps and much time, before a satisfactory result is achieved. Accordingly, time must be taken to explain the various techniques and ensure the patient is committed and aware of the ensuing surgical journey. As in other aspects of head and neck reconstruction, examination must consider exactly what it is missing with the intention of replacing like with like. Therefore, at one level, the defect needs to be considered in terms of cover, support and lining. However, it is essential to also consider the shape and site of the underlying defect, as these must be replaced with tissues of as similar a contour and shape as is possible. One of the first steps in assessing the patient is to evaluate which subunit(s) of the nose have been affected.

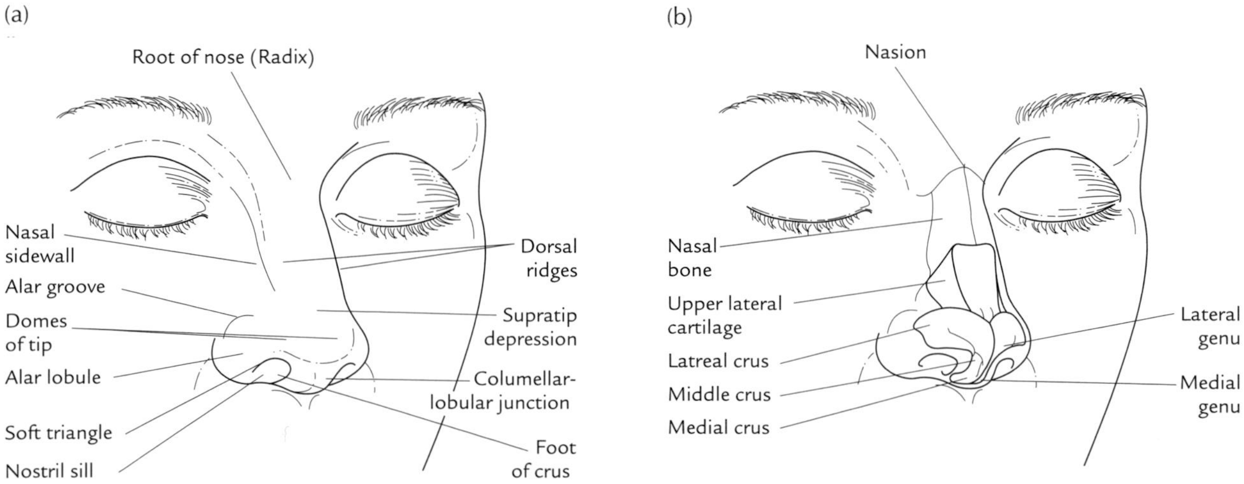

Figure 30.4 Nasal anatomy and the support structures of the nose.

Soft tissue cover and subunits

The skin of the nose varies as one moves from the bridge to the tip. The nose above the tip and the alae is similar to the surrounding facial skin. However, that of the tip tends to be composed of thicker, sebaceous skin. The nose is a common site for removal of skin lesions, particularly basal cell carcinomas. Once clearance of the tumour has been confirmed, and the defect involves skin only, replacement should consider the different skin types covering the nasal surface. Split skin grafts should not be used on the nose, as they will produce thin shiny skin that is likely to contract. Full thickness grafts, harvested from either the neck or postauricular area can be used to resurface a skin-only defect in the upper part of the nose, however, the thicker sebaceous regions of the nose are more suitably resurfaced using local flaps, such as a bi-lobed flap. Full thickness grafts in sebaceous skin leave shiny deformities with an obvious contour deficit.

The subunit principle

The nose consists of various convex and concave surfaces that make up its topographical anatomy. The tip, dorsum, columella and paired ala-nostril sills are convex, reflecting light to enhance the perception of their shape. The sidewalls and soft triangles are all concave. Therefore, reconstruction of these sites, or subunits, needs to encapsulate these three-dimensional characteristics (Figure 30.5). Ideally, grafts or flaps should be used sympathetically and inset in such a way that scars and graft margins lie at the edge of cosmetic units. In this way, maximum disguising of the graft or flap is achieved. Scars can be concealed at sites that minimize their contraction and early prominence.

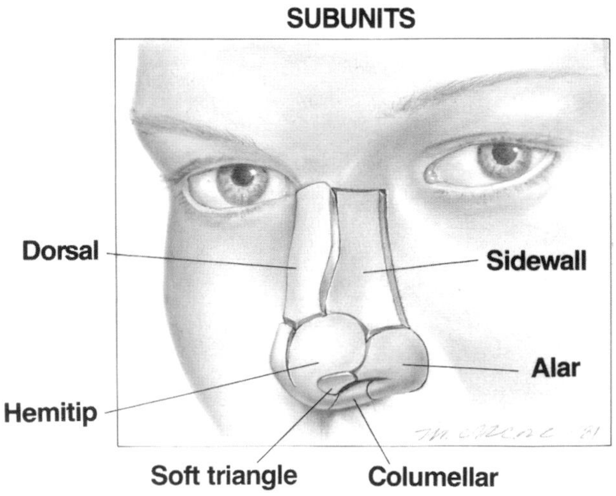

Figure 30.5 Surface topography of the nose and subunits.

When cosmetic units are ignored and grafts or flaps are laid across them, results are often far from satisfactory and leave the patient with a permanent reminder of poorly planned surgery. Defects that comprise less than half the size of a cosmetic unit can be simply resurfaced as noted above. However, when it comprises more than half, the whole cosmetic unit should be removed and resurfaced with an appropriately inset graft. In this way the optimum result is achieved.

One of the essential principles of three-dimensional nasal reconstruction is that tissue support should be provided at the time of soft tissue cover. Therefore, cartilage loss should be replaced by cartilage harvested from the ear, nasal septum or rarely, rib cartilage. In any event, it is essential to provide support to those of similar shape and dimension. Supporting cartilage or bone grafts need to be inserted at the time of providing soft tissue cover and/or lining as this limits distortion of these tissues during the subsequent wound healing process. Attempts to insert cartilage at a later stage are invariably limited by wound contracture. Occasionally, one may use a composite graft consisting of a cartilage sandwich between skin. This is usually harvested from the root of the ear helix, which can then be used to reconstruct full thickness defects of the alar rim. Composite grafts may also be used in columella reconstruction. As these are fairly thick grafts, the composite should be limited to defects of less than 1.5 cm, ideally in non-smokers. Furthermore, it is important to ensure

Table 30.1 Flaps used in nasal reconstruction

Local	Nasolabial
	Inferiorly based
	Superiorly based
	Islanded
	Banner
	Bilobed
	Mitre
	Bipedicled
	Cheek advancement
	Turnover
Regional	Forehead flap
	Paramedian
	Gullwing
	Temperofrontal
	Scalping
	Washio
Distant	Brachial (Tagliacozzi)
Free	Radial forearm
	Dorsalis pedis

that patients are kept within a warm environment and this may necessitate a prolonged inpatient stay to ensure compliance.

Local flaps and skin cover

Numerous local flaps can be used to resurface the nose and several of these have already been discussed in Chapter 27 and are summarized in Table 30.1. Local flaps rely on using skin cover adjacent to the defect to provide skin of a similar quality to that being lost. For small defects, a variety of flaps are available, utilizing the more mobile and thin skin of the upper nose. The nasal sidewalls and dorsum are relatively lax and allow harvesting of transposition and bilobed flaps, other examples also include the banner, dorsal nasal, Limberg, glabella and bilobed flaps. The preoperative planning of these flaps should attempt to conceal the donor site along the junction of adjacent subunits. Local flaps have a number of limitations, not least the fact that they are only appropriate for small defects. Larger flaps will cause distortion as a result of

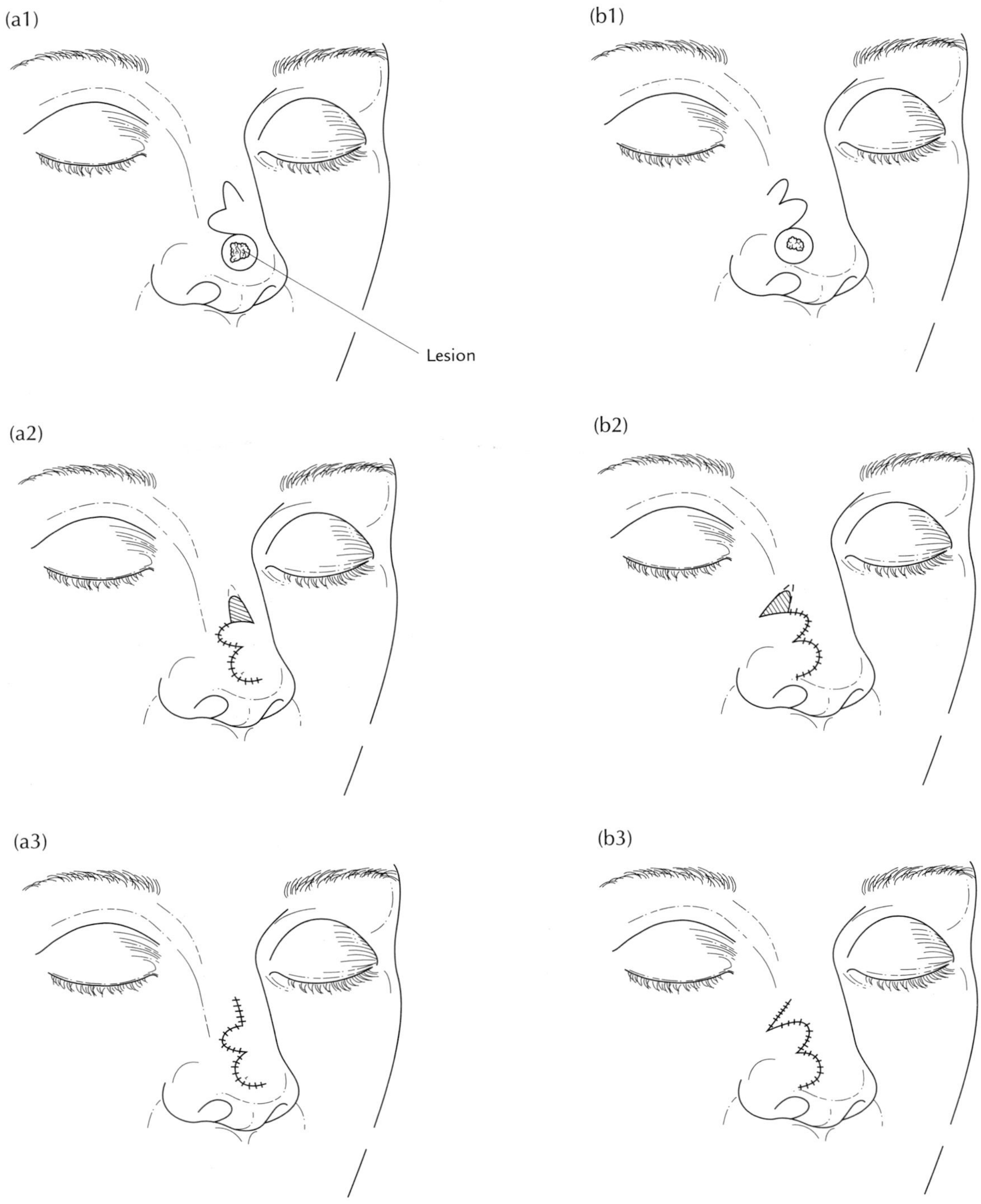

Figure 30.6 The bilobed flap; this is a very useful flap to resurface the nasal tip and supra-alar region. (a) Nasal tip; (b) Side of nasal tip.

the donor site. Local flaps tend to be relatively thick and if they are inset under any tension they distort thin underlying cartilage grafts. Where it is likely to be necessary it is probably wiser to resurface the aesthetic unit using a forehead or nasolabial flap.

Resurfacing small defects

The bilobed flap is a particularly useful flap for reconstruction of the nasal tip and alar region (Figure 30.6). It allows reconstruction of defects up to 1.5 cm in diameter and minimizes tension on the donor site by employing rotation of a second flap to close the main donor site defect. The flap should be raised, limiting the rotation of each lobe to less than 50 degrees. It is essential to widely undermine the flap just above the perichondrium and periosteum. This will minimize deforming forces of closure, which are subsequently distributed over the nasal surface.

The nasolabial flap is a very versatile flap, supplied by perforating vessels from the facial artery. The flap

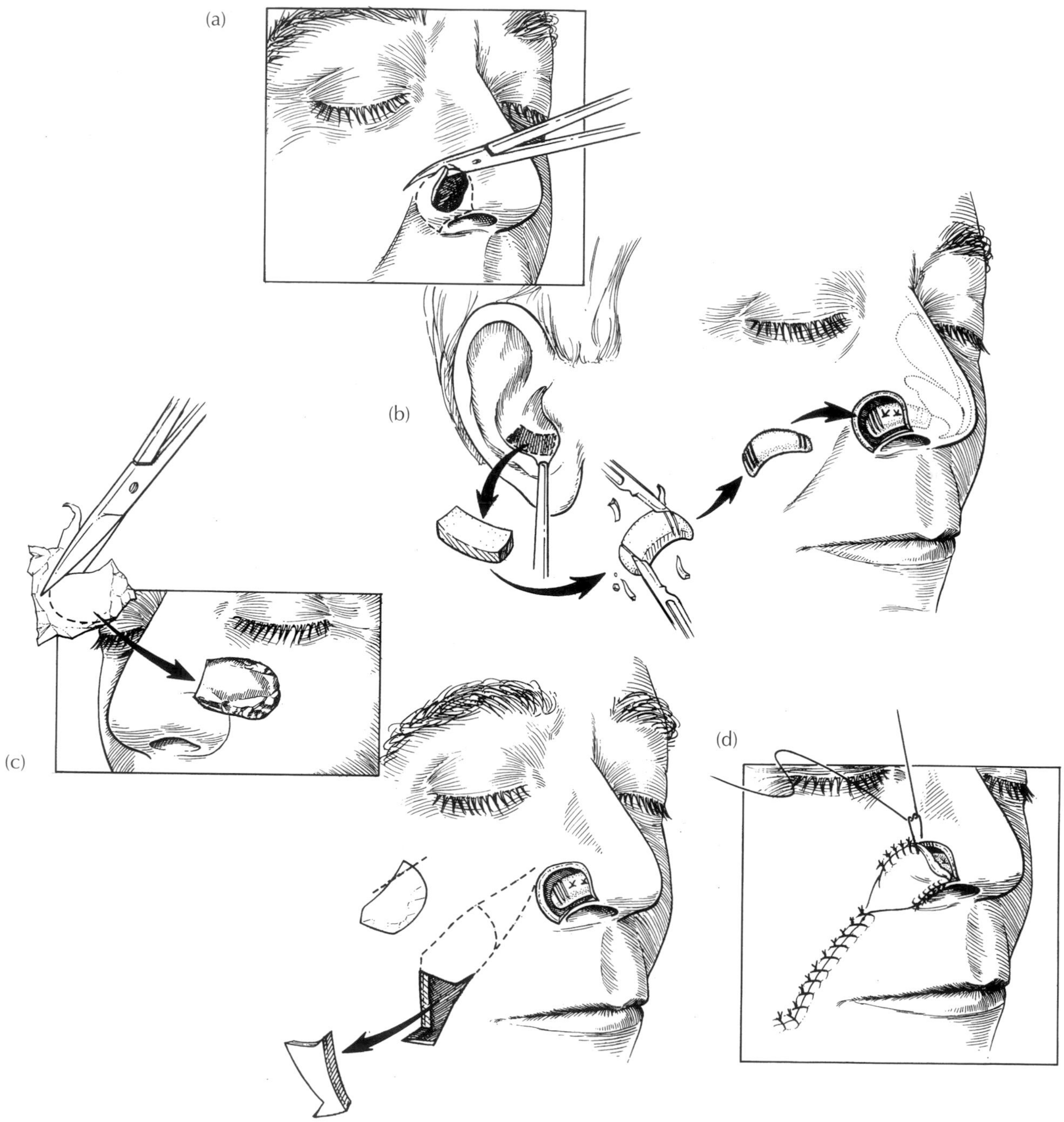

Figure 30.7 Reconstruction of an alar defect using the naso-labial flap: (a) resection of lesion; (b) cartilage graft harvested and shaped and inset at the time of flap cover; (c) a template has been made from the contralateral alar; (d) a superiorly based, islanded naso-labial flap has been raised to provide cover. This is likely to require further procedures to adequately thin the flap.

can be raised in several forms including a superior or inferiorly based flap as well as an islanded flap (Figure 30.7). The rich blood supply allows the tip to be very aggressively thinned and can then be used to resurface the alar. At a second stage the pedicle of the flap can be divided, inset and the alar shape formed. There afterwards a third thinning stage may be required to achieve the desired result. Exceptionally, the flap may be folded upon itself to provide both lining and cover though this can produce a bulky alar of poor function and appearance.

Resurfacing large defects

The forehead flap

The optimum technique for resurfacing large defects that extend over several aesthetic subunits requires use of the midline forehead flap. Several descriptions have been made of variations of the forehead flap that extend obliquely across the forehead. However, the vertical medial or paramedial forehead flap provides adequate length, width and colour match. Several basic principles underline the use of this very versatile flap. The first of these is that it can be elevated to provide a flap large enough to resurface the whole of the nose without the use of prior forehead expansion to aid donor site closure. Tissue expansion produces a capsule that may be transferred to the nose, resulting in early contracture. Where the donor site defect cannot be primarily closed it can be left to cicatrize by second intention. Secondly, where a long flap is required it may be extended into the hairline and then depilated. The flap needs to be raised with due care for the blood supply that enters its deep surface just on the medial edge of the supraorbital rim. It is fed by a complex of vessels with contributions from the supraorbital, supratrochlear, infratrochlear and dorsal nasal and angular branches of the facial artery. The rich blood supply of the median forehead courses just deep to the dermis and therefore distally the flap may be elevated with only skin. A further 1–1.5 cm of local flap can be obtained by dissecting the flap proximally into the supraorbital rim. In the non-smoking healthy patient the distal flap may be thinned fairly aggressively and depilated though this should be avoided in the smoker or diabetic patient. Of note, a midline flap also encourages axial flow. Obliquely orientated forehead flaps rely on random blood supply and are therefore less reliable, particularly in the distal regions of the flap.

In keeping with the subunit principle, defects are created to ensure complete subunits are resurfaced and wound margins designed to lie at the junction between subunits. As for smaller defects, dimensions are carefully measured onto the forehead and the flap elevated and inset (Figure 30.8). At 3 weeks the middle section of the flap is raised, leaving the proximal and distal attachments intact. The flap is then thinned and reinset for a further 3 weeks until the

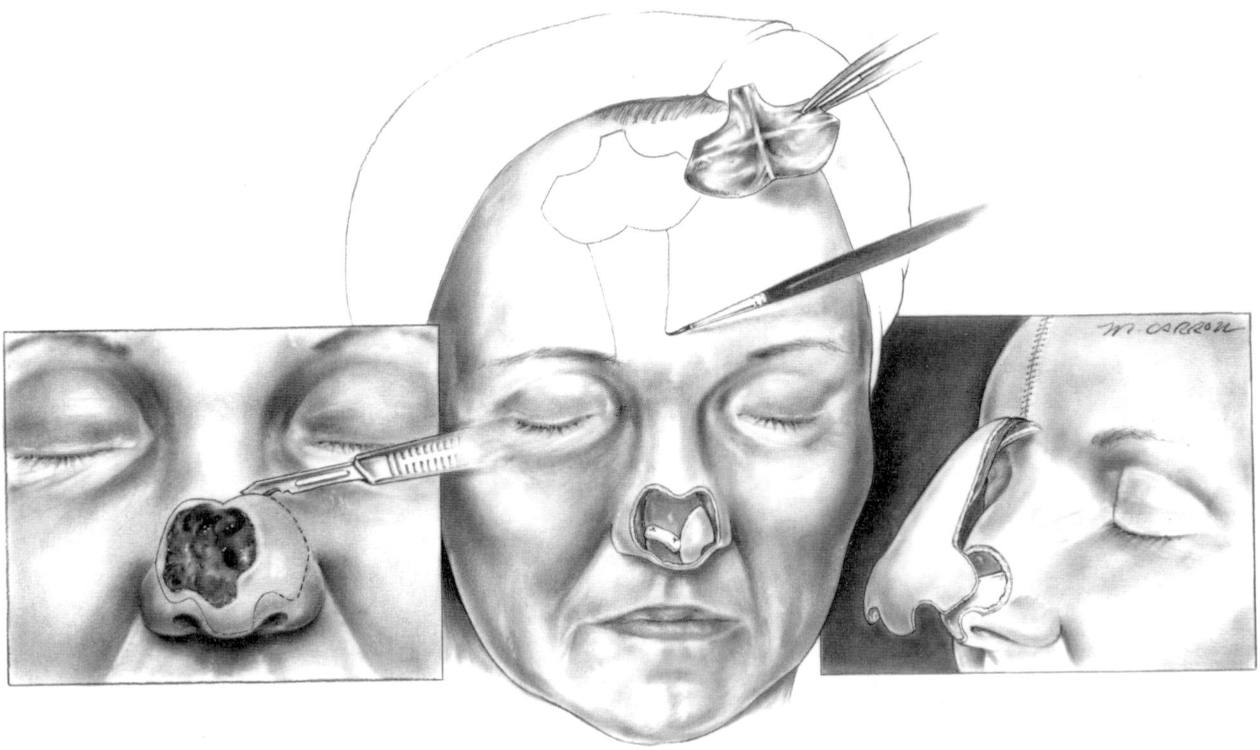

Figure 30.8 The paramedian forehead flap; an exact template is made of the defect to be resurfaced, which is then transferred to the forehead. The flap is elevated without frontalis and inset prior to initial thinning at 3 weeks. Where possible, the donor site is closed; the remaining open area is left to heal by second intention, with excellent results.

pedicle is divided at 6 weeks. Thereafter, the patient may require a further procedure to thin the flap in order to achieve a satisfactory appearance.

Structural support

The nasal skeleton provides a number of roles, including shape, projection and airway patency. Cartilage, or more rarely bone, should always be replaced at the time of soft tissue reconstruction as scarring and wound contracture will otherwise distort and deform any residual soft tissue left unsupported, making delayed revision almost impossible. This interaction between cover and lining tissues and support grafts is also important as the former also act as the source of blood supply for these grafts.

The upper part of the nose relies on a stable platform composed of bony support and a midline cartilaginous septum. Lower down, the upper lateral cartilages provide sidewall support, while the lower lateral cartilages define the tip and also maintain air entry. The midline support can be replaced with cantilevered bony struts harvested from iliac crest or the ulnar border. L-shaped cartilage struts may also be harvested from costal cartilage. Rarely, following total rhinectomy, the septum will have been lost. L-shaped struts provide a degree of support; optimum reconstruction is obtained using the pivoting septal advancement flap to mobilize and rotate the residual septum and the vomer (Figure 30.9). This flap, based on the septal branch of the superior labial artery, allows transposition of both support, and importantly, lining.

The septum provides an important source of rigid sheet cartilage, useful in replacing upper lateral cartilages. Smaller sections can also be harvested and shaped to replace the medial crura of the alar cartilages or augment regions. At the appropriate sites, the cartilage can be scored to facilitate flexion at the genu. The tip and delicate lower lateral alar cartilages are best replaced using conchal cartilage. This is of adequate rigidity, but sufficiently thin to provide good support and high aesthetic quality (Figure 30.10).

Lining

Provision of lining is one of the most challenging aspects of nasal reconstruction. The neolining has to provide an adequate airway, be of sufficient vascularity to sustain cartilage and bone grafts and supple to conform to the desired shape. When poor or suboptimal results are analysed, inadequate lining introduced at the time of reconstruction is often found to be the cause. Support tissues prevent retraction of the lining and help maintain airway function.

Intranasal mucosa and skin are the optimum source of replacement lining. Small full-thickness defects will need replacement of all three levels. However, lining may be derived from local flaps of mucosa or skin. Following resection of the alar rim, 'bucket-handle', bipedicled flaps consisting of vestibular skin can be dropped inferiorly into the defect and supported with a rim of conchal cartilage. Skin adjacent to the defect may be turned down as a flap to provide lining, and then grafts and new flaps placed above, though it remains a second choice to mucosal donor sites.

Larger mucosal defects are replaced using septomucosal flaps, raised on perforators from the superior

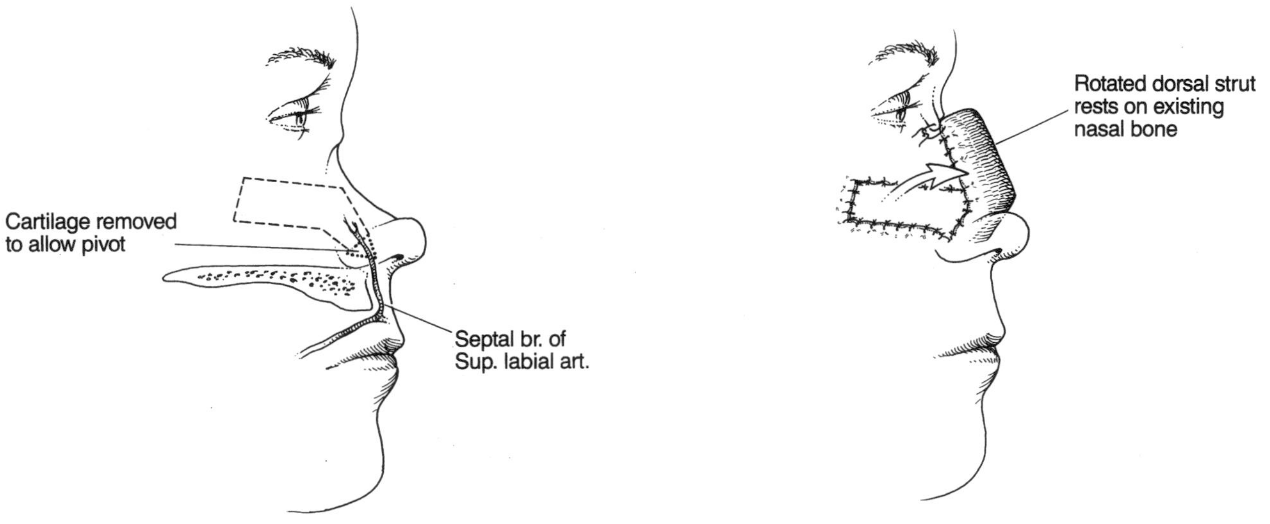

Figure 30.9 Pivoting septal flap.

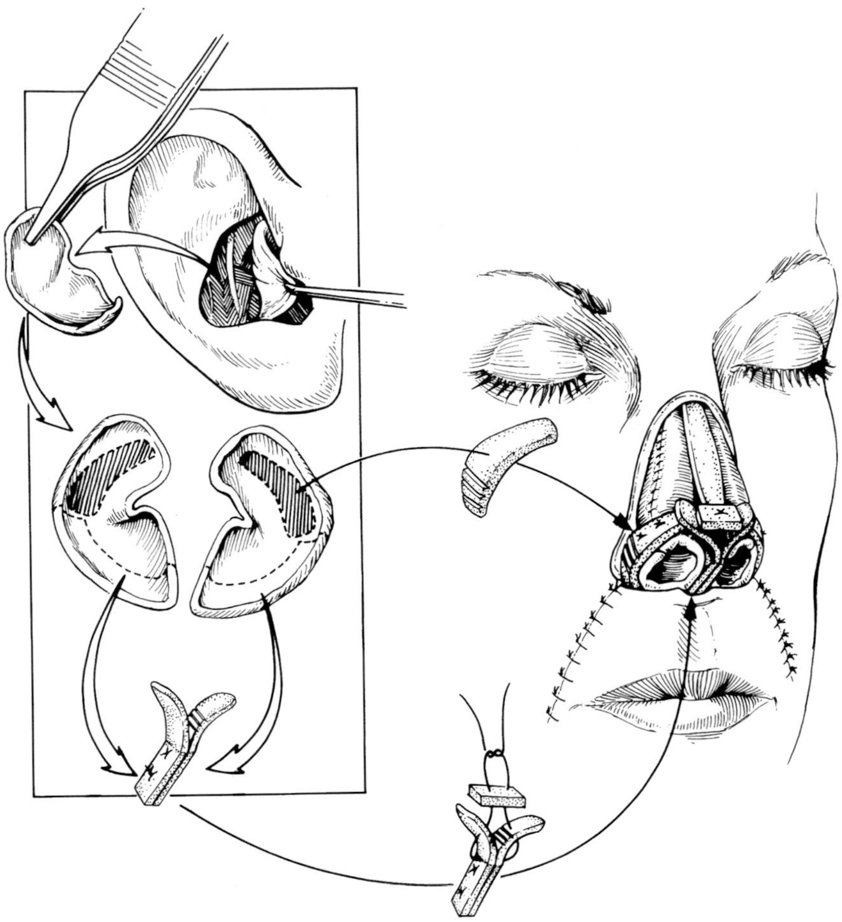

Figure 30.10 Conchal cartilage and tip reconstruction; in this illustration, alar lining has been obtained using bilateral naso-labial flaps.

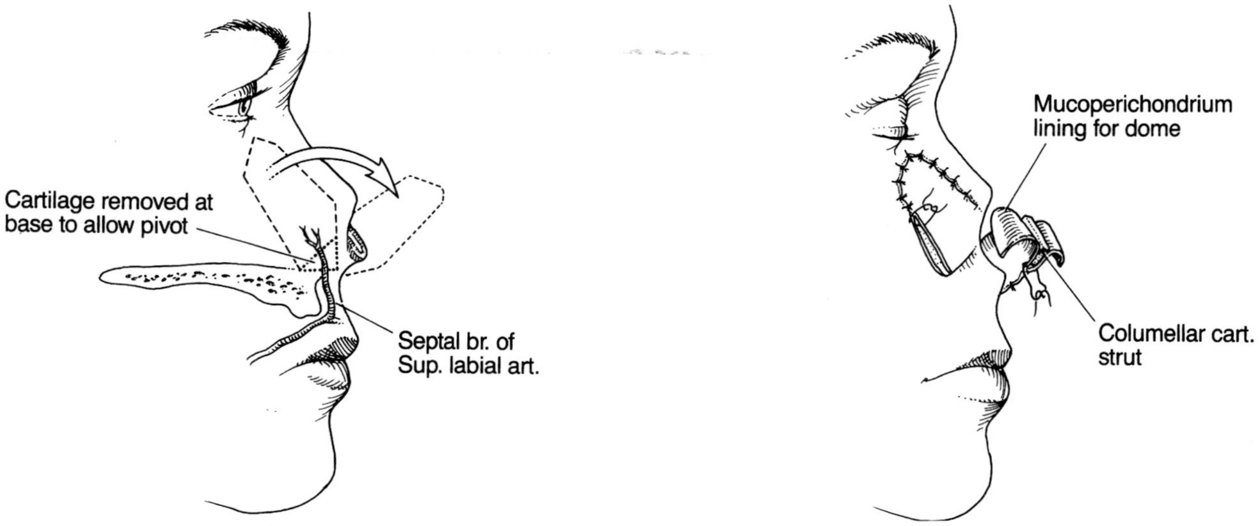

Figure 30.11 Septomucosal flap

labial artery (Figure 30.11). The mucosal flap is raised deep into the nasal cavity as a rectangle, which can then be rotated and tubed to provide tissue almost adequate for reconstruction of one side of the nose. These flaps may also be raised and passed through a 'trapdoor' in the anterior septum, to line the contralateral airway. Septo-perichondrial flaps are of particular use in replacing large lining defects, for as noted above, the septum may be advanced forward to also provide support.

Large, subtotal defects can be safely addressed utilizing the above principles. As with smaller resections, the defect needs to be considered in terms of cover, support and lining. In the first instance, the perimeter of the defect is addressed to align margins along the

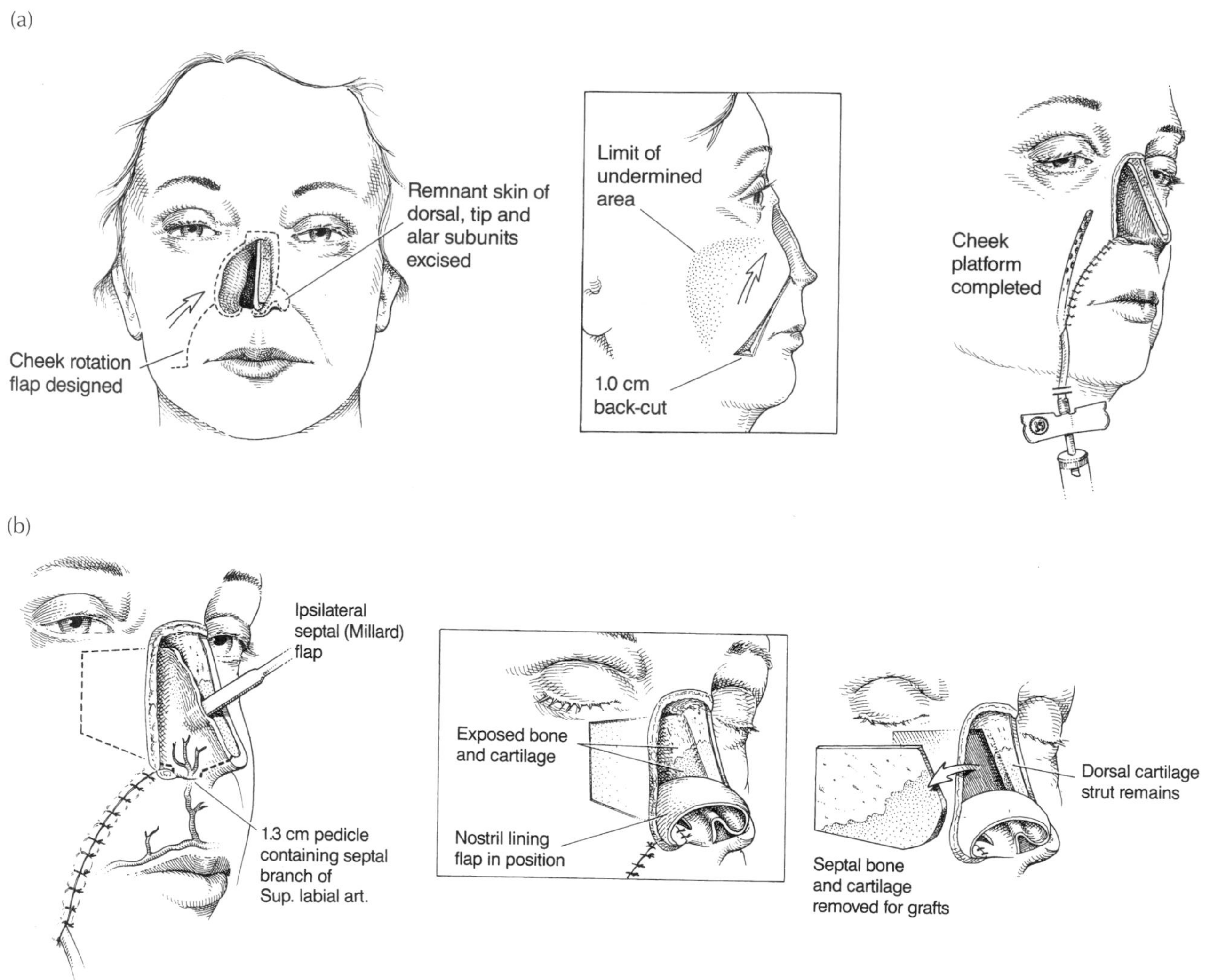

Figure 30.12 (a) The defect needs to be visualized in terms of cosmetic units. In this patient a cheek flap has been rotated in to restore the lateral nasal margin. (b) The source of lining depends on the size of the defect and available donor tissues. For larger defects, as in hemi-nasal defects, an ipsilateral septomucosal flap provides tissue that is adequately well vascularized to support cartilage grafts. The septum is harvested to provide grafts that can be used to support tip grafts or the lateral nasal skeleton.

edge of cosmetic units. If the excision defect extends on to the cheek, advancement flaps can be used to restore the lateral margin of the nose and cheek platform (Figure 30.12a). Lining can be restored using a septo-mucosal graft, turned over to the proposed alar margin (Figure 30.12b). Cartilage grafts are harvested from the septum to support the sidewall, and from the concha to replace the lower lateral, alar cartilage and columella. The nasal bridge is supported using either costal cartilage or iliac bone (Figure 30.12c). Finally, cover can be obtained using the forehead flap (Figure 30.12d); care is taken to make an exact pattern of the subunit defect before transferring it to the forehead, as previously described.

Total rhinectomy or resection of the septum may prevent use of septal donor tissues for lining. In this instance other tissue sources are required, including the radial forearm flap. The flap is revascularized by anastomosis to facial vessels at the mandibular margin. In this way, a considerable area of well vascularized tissue can be brought onto the midface to provide plentiful forearm skin for lining. The inner surface of the flap is covered with a split skin graft, prior to removal and thinning of the flap at a second stage. At this stage the support structures can be laid upon this well vascularized surface before cover is provided with a forehead flap.

Conclusion

Nasal reconstruction is a challenging discipline but one that can ultimately prove rewarding for both

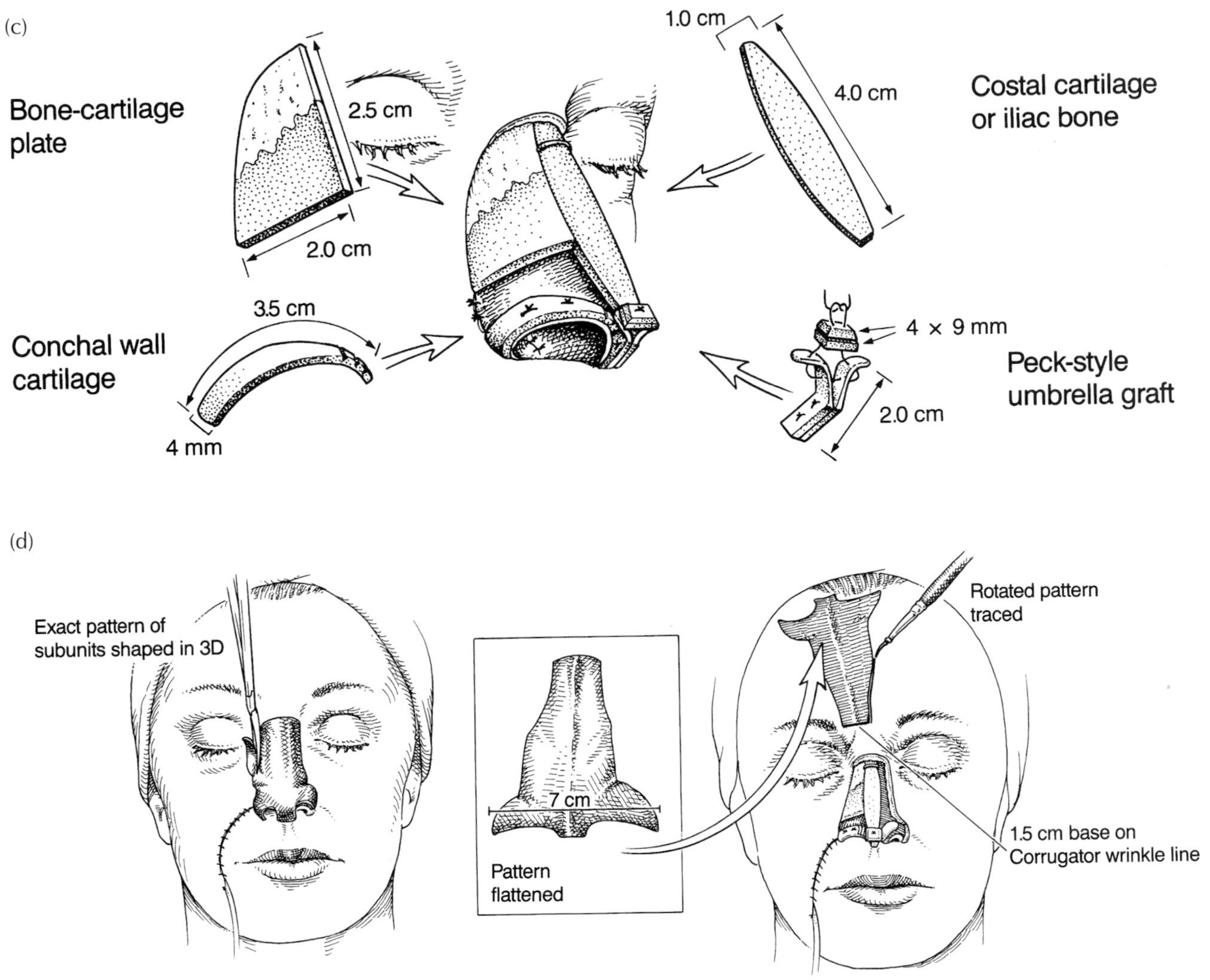

Figure 30.12 (c) The nasal bridge may be supported with either iliac bone or costal cartilage. (d) Cover is provided using a forehead flap.

patient and surgeon. The principles outlined in this chapter emphasize the importance of careful assessment of the patient and their deformity. Consideration of the three dimensional nature of the defect and its constituent parts allows planning of several procedures that aim to replace 'like with like'. In this way the surgeon should be able to achieve the optimum aesthetic and functional result.

REFERENCES

1. *Gentleman's Magazine.* (A communication to the editor, Mr Urban, signed B.L., Oct 1794) Vol 64, Nichols, London.
2. Gnudi MT, Webster J. *The Life and Times of Gaspare Tagliacozzi.* New York: Herbert Heichner, 1954.
3. Tagliacozzi, G. *De Curtorum Chirugia per Insitionum.* Venice: Bindonis, 1597.
4. Carpue JC. *An account of two successful operations for restoring a lost nose from the integuments of the forehead.* London: Longman, 1816.
5. Zeiss E. *Handbuch der Plastichen Chirugie.* Berlin: Reimer, 1838.
6. Burget GC, Menick FJ. Nasal reconstruction: seeking a fourth dimension. *Plast Reconstr Surg* 1986; **78**: 145–57.
7. Burget GC, Menick FJ. *Aesthetic Reconstruction of the Nose.* St Louis: Mosby, 1994.

31 Functional restoration of speech

Peter H Rhys Evans and Eric D Blom

Introduction

Cancers of the upper aerodigestive tract affecting the oral cavity, upper jaw, pharynx and larynx have a major impact on speech and swallowing, not only the destructive process of the disease itself, but also the effects of curative treatment, be it surgery or radiotherapy. Functional rehabilitation of these patients has long been one of the major challenges facing otolaryngologists, speech therapists and patients, but it is only in the last three decades that the emphasis on restoration of function and quality of life has become as important as cure and survival. Previously, when major reconstruction often involved multiple procedures staged over several months, up to 50% of patients died before satisfactory rehabilitation could be achieved.

Despite recent major advances in therapy long-term cure rates for head and neck cancer have not altered significantly during the last 40 years. Although locoregional control of disease and 3-year survival have improved considerably, ultimate cure has been limited by increasing incidence of second primaries, metastases and other smoking-related diseases. Optimal immediate rehabilitation of these patients is therefore of paramount importance and a major consideration to be incorporated in the initial treatment plan.

Multidisciplinary care

For smaller tumours and those that are known to be radiosensitive (e.g. nasopharynx) radiotherapy, if successful, has the advantage of minimizing functional problems of speech and swallowing apart from the long-term effects of xerostomia. Surgery for small tumours of the tongue and oropharynx without any necessary reconstruction will also allow excellent restoration of function. Endoscopic laser resection with immediate frozen-section control has become more widely used in recent years for selected pharyngolaryngeal tumours.[1] Morbidity following these procedures is dramatically reduced compared with composite resections and functional recovery is more rapidly achieved.

For advanced disease and recurrence after radiotherapy major surgery is required presenting difficult management and rehabilitation problems. Major advances during the last few decades in reconstructive surgery and perioperative care have permitted one-stage operative resection and reconstruction with rapid recovery. At the same time meticulous attention to preoperative planning, nutritional support, surgical technique and postoperative care has reduced risks of complication following these major interventions. The many complex problems encountered during recovery and rehabilitation highlight the essential involvement and coordination of an experienced multidisciplinary team (Table 31.1).

Table 31.1 Multidisciplinary head and neck team

Surgeons (ENT/head and neck, plastic, maxillofacial)
Radiotherapist
Medical oncologist
Clinical nurse specialist
Speech therapist
Dietician
Physiotherapist
Prosthedontist

General considerations

Surgery

By far the most important initial factor in obtaining optimal rehabilitation and locoregional control is the quality of the surgery. Careful oncological clearance with frozen section control where necessary and functional preservation of important neuromuscular and vascular structures when possible is mandatory. Prophylactic selective node dissection is indicated for stage I and II (N0) disease where there is a significant incidence of micrometastases (tongue, floor of mouth, oropharynx and supraglottic larynx). This adds little morbidity to the procedure but significantly reduces the risk of subsequent neck recurrence.

Reconstruction should be carried out with the intention of providing optimal function and not just filling a defect. There is little justification for repairing an anterior tongue hemiglossectomy defect with a pedicled myocutaneous flap when a free radial forearm flap will give far superior mobility and function. The surgeon should therefore either be skilled in a wide range of flap options him or herself or should work together with an experienced plastic surgeon or should refer the patient to an experienced head and neck unit with appropriate facilities. There is no place for an occasional head and neck surgeon.

Radiotherapy

Radiotherapy offers the possibility of cure in most early tumours with minimal morbidity or loss of function. Loss of taste is temporary and in small volume disease xerostomia and a dry throat are not a major problem. These side-effects are much more common in treatment of larger tumours with wide fields and may significantly affect the patient's ability to swallow.

The use of radiotherapy for 'organ preservation' may certainly be an attractive option for intermediate-sized tumours of the tongue, oropharynx and larynx but recurrence will usually necessitate a more radical resection (total glossectomy, total laryngectomy) and often a significantly reduced chance of cure. This choice is probably justified in T3 laryngeal carcinoma because recurrence is often detected early and disease is confined by the cartilagenous framework so that survival figures for primary total laryngectomy and salvage laryngectomy following radiotherapy failure are much the same. About 50% of these patients will retain their larynx, and even for those who undergo laryngectomy, rehabilitation now with fistula speech allows excellent voice restoration in about 70–95%.[2]

Historical perspective

For over 100 years total laryngectomy has been used as an effective radical treatment for advanced and recurrent laryngopharyngeal cancer. It is a mutilating operation, which in the early days at the end of the last century carried an operative mortality of over 90%. Loss of the voice, altered swallowing and a permanent tracheostome, together with the uncertainty of cure, had profound effects on the patient's physical and psychological rehabilitation.

Watson, of Edinburgh performed the first total laryngectomy in a patient with tuberculosis, but a few years later, in 1873 Billroth was the first to carry out the procedure for cancer. The importance of early restoration of voice was recognized and one of Billroth's associates, Carl Gussenbauer designed a vibrating reed device in a bifurcated tracheal cannula (Figure 31.1), which apparently produced satisfactory speech for several weeks before the patient eventually succumbed to recurrent disease.[3]

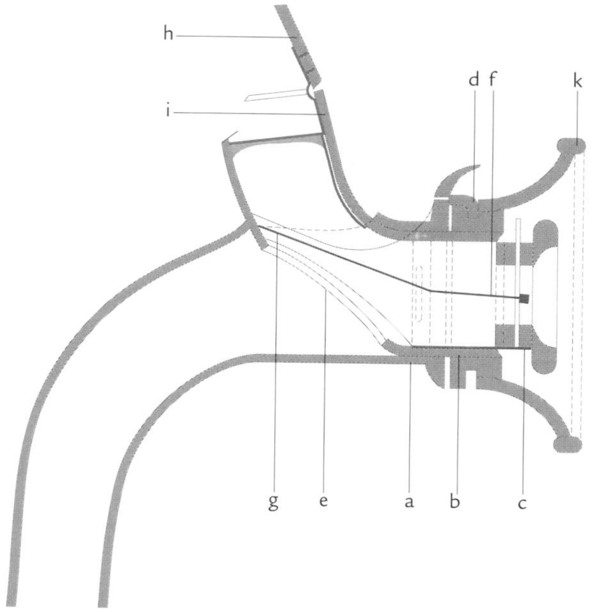

Figure 31.1 The speech device of Gussenbauer (1873).

Oesophageal speech

It was not long after the relatively successful use of reed devices for production of voice that some early pioneers (Table 31.2) noted that patients sometimes experienced a 'vicarious' sound source in the back of the throat which they found could be developed with exercise into a useful voice. This oesophageal speech is produced by inhaling or injecting air into the pharynx and upper oesophagus and then releas-

Table 31.2 Early pioneers of oesophageal speech

Stoerk (Vienna)	1887
Schmid (Stettin)	1889
Solis-Cohen (Philadelphia)	1893
Gottstein (Breslau)	1900
Gutzman (Berlin)	1908

(a)

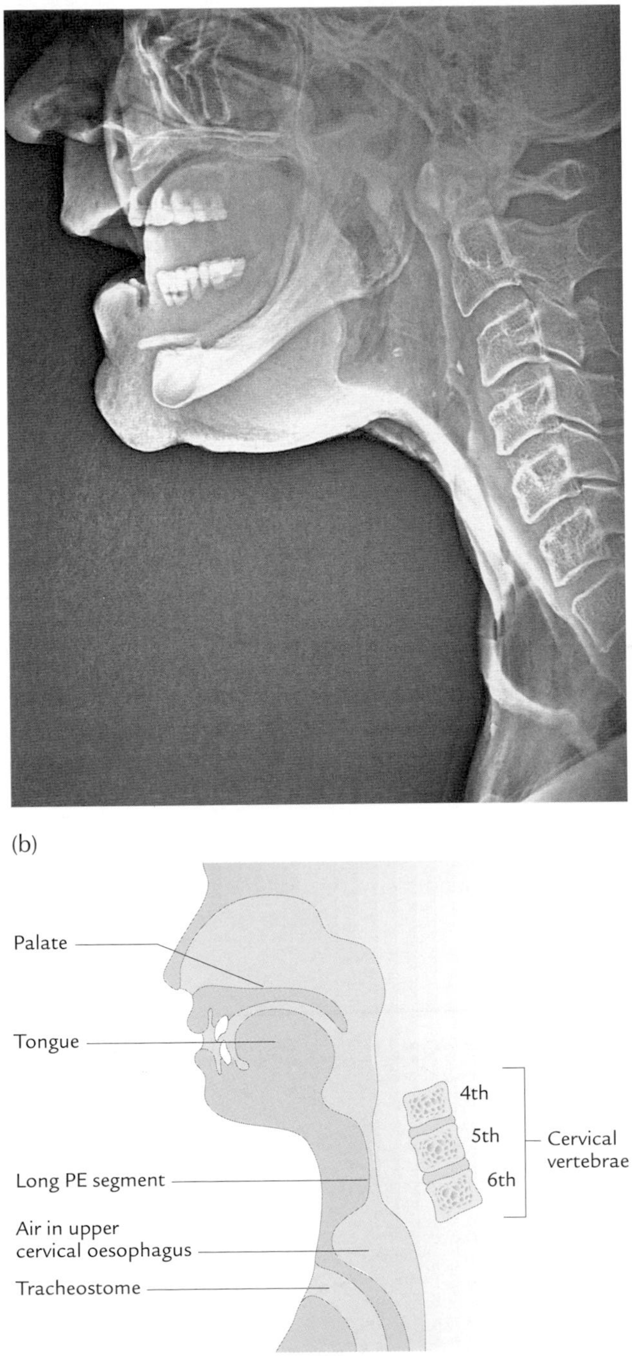

Figure 31.2 (a) Lateral xerograph of the neck in a laryngectomee phonating with good oesophageal speech showing a long tonic PE segment at C4/5/6. (b) Diagrammatic representation of (a).

ing it in a controlled fashion through the pharynx into the mouth. The vibrations are generated by rapid approximations of the opposing mucosal surfaces by the expelled column of air at the junction between the pharynx and upper oesophagus, now known as the pharyngo-oesophageal (PO or PE) segment (Figure 31.2).[4] Resonation of sound occurs in the vocal tract (pharynx, mouth and nose) and final articulation of words takes place in the mouth, as with normal laryngeal speech, using the lips, teeth and tongue.

Learning oesophageal speech requires determination and usually prolonged speech therapy since it does involve a complex technique of voice production. Many patients, particularly the older and more infirm, are not able to develop proficient skills to master the technique and less than one-third are able to speak with successful intelligible speech. The voice is generally poorly sustained, has limited fluency interrupted by frequent air injection and is often drowned by expiratory noise from the stoma. Nevertheless until the successful introduction of surgical voice restoration during the 1980s this method had been the mainstay of voice rehabilitation following total laryngectomy since the early part of the century.

Artificial larynx

The use of handheld electronic or pneumatic vibrating devices applied to the throat (Figure 31.3) or directed into the mouth via a small piece of tubing (e.g. Cooper Rand) has provided an artificial alaryngeal voice for many patients, particularly those who could not achieve oesophageal speech. Voice acquisition is usually rapid but the mechanical monotonous tone of the voice and the need to operate the device manually limits their effectiveness.

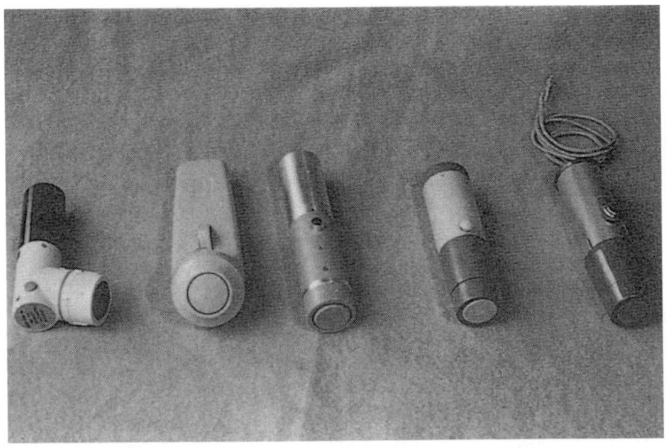

Figure 31.3 Types of artificial larynx vibrators (Bart's vibrating bell, Medici, Rexton, Servox).

External devices

Gussenbauer's tube (Figure 31.1) was the prototype of these external shunts fitted into the tracheostome, which conveyed air from the trachea through a valved prosthetic device into the pharynx via a connecting pharyngostomy tube. The 'Voice Bak' device (Figure 31.4) introduced in 1972 by Taub and Spiro[5] was one of the more successful ones but these methods were virtually abandoned because of problems of leakage, aspiration and bleeding due to the close proximity of the shunt to the great vessels.

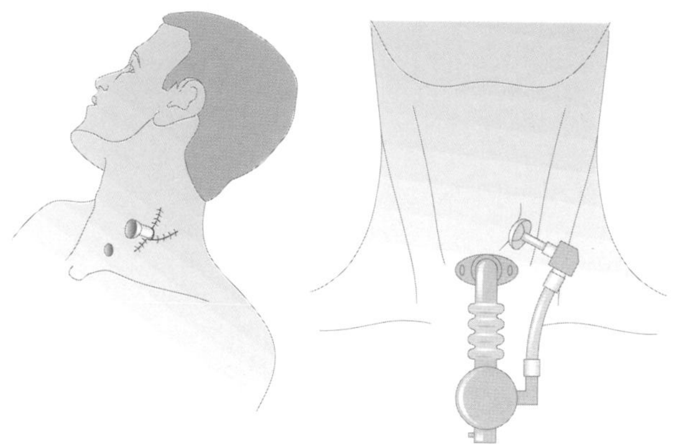

Figure 31.4 Taub's 'Voice Bak' prosthesis.

Internal shunts

Guttmann in 1932 is credited with the first description of an internal tracheo-oesophageal fistula in a patient who pierced his pharynx through the posterior wall of the tracheostome with an ice-pick, establishing a shunt unintentionally. He found he was able to speak with a loud fluent voice although the tract was prone to leakage or spontaneous closure.

Over the next 40 years a succession of techniques was proposed to create a surgical shunt to divert air from the trachea to the upper cervical oesophagus or pharynx using a variety of methods including skin, mucosa or a vein graft. It was impossible to get consistent results and invariably these procedures failed over time either because the shunt stenosed or it became too patulous and allowed aspiration.

The first author's own interest in fistula speech stems from an incident in 1977 when he saw a patient for follow-up a few months after laryngectomy. The patient seemed to have developed a very strong and fluent voice without any oesophageal voice therapy. To the author's dismay examination revealed that he had developed a small postoperative salivary fistula at the top of the tracheostome and arrangements were suggested immediately for him to have the fistula closed off. The patient quickly put his thumb to the stoma and protested with great concern: 'but that's the only way I can speak!' He then pulled out of his pocket a kirby-grip that he used to keep the tract open.

Modern voice prosthesis evolution

The modern era of highly successful surgical voice restoration was due to a major conceptual development in the late 1970s introduced by Eric Blom and Mark Singer which transformed the expectation and quality of voice production after total laryngectomy.[6] The technique involved creating a simple tracheo-oesophageal puncture between the posterior wall of the tracheostome and the upper oesophagus into which was inserted a one-way silicone valve (Figure 31.5). This allowed air to flow from the trachea into the oesophagus and the 'duckbill' valve (Figure 31.6) prevented aspiration of food and liquid. Over the next 20 years the valve was improved and modified with introduction of the low pressure/low profile prosthesis in 1983 and an indwelling valve (Figure 31.7) in 1995.[7]

The same authors made another important observation in 1985,[8] which was crucial to obtaining consistently successful results in fistula speech. They recognized that many patients failed to achieve either oesophageal or fistula voice because of hypertonicity of the PE segment and they introduced the concept of pharyngeal myotomy and pharyngeal plexus neurectomy to correct this problem.

Initially the puncture technique was used as a secondary procedure in patients with previous laryngectomy who failed to achieve oesophageal speech,

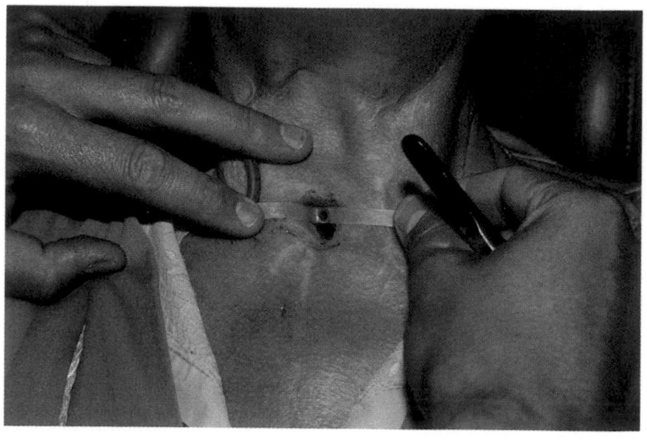

Figure 31.5 Early Blom–Singer valve in place.

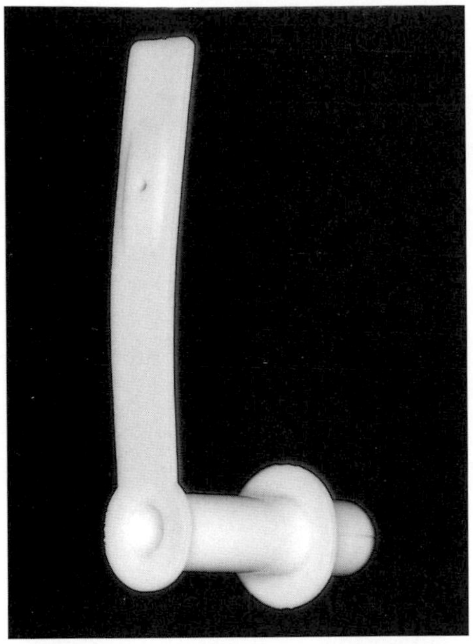

Figure 31.6 Blom–Singer 'duckbill' valve.

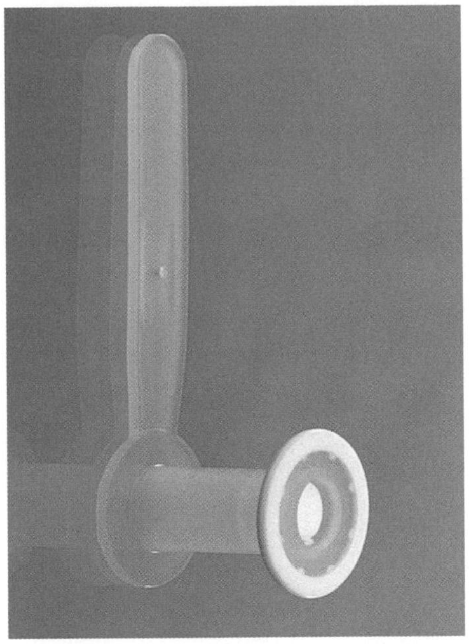

Figure 31.7 Blom–Singer 'indwelling' valve.

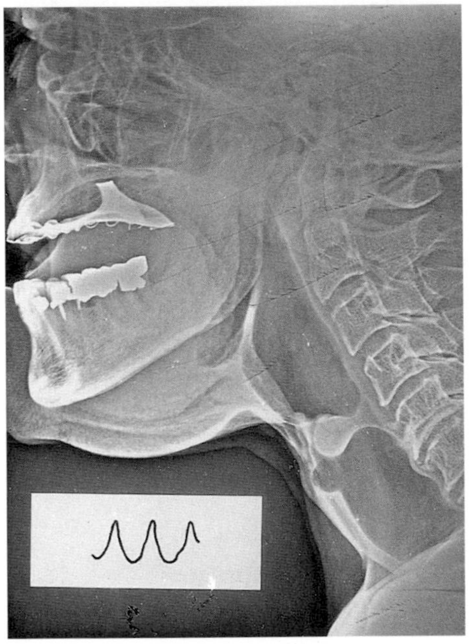

Figure 31.8 Xerograph of the neck in a laryngectomee phonating with good oesophageal speech showing a short tonic PE segment at C4/5.

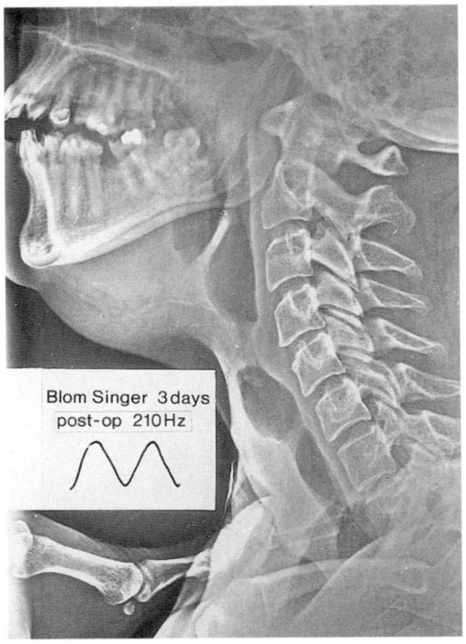

Figure 31.9 Xerograph of the neck in a laryngectomee 3 days after fitting a Blom–Singer valve showing digital occlusion of the stoma and a short tonic PE segment at C4.

but the consistently good results and superior quality of voice prompted Hamaker et al in 1985[9] to incorporate the tracheo-oesophageal puncture at the time of laryngectomy as a primary procedure.

Fistula versus oesophageal speech

The PE segment may vary greatly in its position, length and muscular component. In contrast to the long circumferential segment seen in Figure 31.2, the one clearly seen in Figure 31.8 is a short, posteriorly based mucosal fold probably incorporating some muscle. In both cases an air reservoir is seen in the upper oesophagus below the PE segment and the patients are both good oesophageal speakers. A similar PE segment is shown in Figure 31.9 during phonation 3 days after fitting a Blom–Singer voice prosthesis. In this case air from the lungs is being diverted through the valve into the upper oesophagus and then through the PE segment and vocal tract into the oral cavity to produce voice.

Table 31.3 Comparison of laryngeal, oesophageal and tracheo-oesophageal voice production

Physical requirements	Laryngeal voice	Oesophageal voice	Fistula voice
Initiator	Lungs 500 ml	Oesophageal air 40–70 ml	Lungs 500 ml
Vibrator	Vocal cords	P-E segment	P-E segment
Resonator	Supragl Lx orophx	Reconstructed orophx	Reconstructed orophx
Articulators: tongue, teeth, lips, soft palate			

Although the vibrating PE segment, the resonating vocal tract and the articulators are the same, the major difference between fistula and oesophageal speech is in the volume and capacity of the air reservoir (Table 31.3). For oesophageal speech only 40–70 ml of air are able to be trapped in the upper oesophagus for voice production, whereas a maximum tidal capacity of 500 ml is available for fistula speech, as with normal lung-powered voice. This means that tracheo-oesophageal speech is similar to laryngeal speech in that it is much louder and more sustained than oesophageal voice.

Following partial or total pharyngolaryngectomy the pharyngeal mucosa is partly or completely replaced by skin (cutaneous, myocutaneous or free flaps) or intestinal mucosa (free jejunum or transposed stomach) rather than resutured pharyngeal wall. This alters the dynamics of the new PE segment and vocal tract and may significantly influence the quality and characteristics of the fistula speech.

Voice failure after laryngectomy

In their 1979 review of the literature Johnson et al.[10] estimated that the oesophageal voice failure rate after laryngectomy was between 15 and 50%. Of those who achieved voice only a small proportion were able to communicate with reasonably fluent intelligible speech. These disappointing results, often after prolonged speech therapy, were thought to be related mainly to poor understanding or motivation of the patient.

In the same year Duguay[11] recognized that the reasons for oesophageal voice failure could be categorized into four main causes: anatomical and physiological problems, psychological and social problems, teaching and learning difficulties and a final group of 'unknown' aetiology. These potential causes of voice failure became more of an issue when it was recognized, after the introduction of tracheo-oesophageal voice puncture by Blom and Singer, that a proportion of their valve patients were not achieving good or optimal voice because of pharyngeal constrictor hypertonicity.[8] This was further investigated by Perry and Edels[12] who used a videofluoroscopy technique originally described by Simpson in 1972[13] to explain how pharyngeal constrictor muscle tone influenced voice production. They categorized the tonicity of the PE segment into five different groups (Table 31.4).

Table 31.4 Videofluoroscopy assessment of pharyngeal constrictor tone

PE Segment	Ba swallow	Phonation	Assisted phonation (Taub test)
Tonic	Passes easily	Good voice	Stronger sustained voice
Hypotonic	Passes easily	Weak voice	More sustained, stronger with digital pressure
Hypertonic	Normal or slower passage	Intermittent tight voice	Intermittent tight voice Gastric distension
Spasm	Some hold-up and residue above PE segment	No voice, no air goes into oesophagus	Minimal voice, explosive segment release as pressure increases Gastric distension
Stricture	Permanent hold-up	No voice	No voice

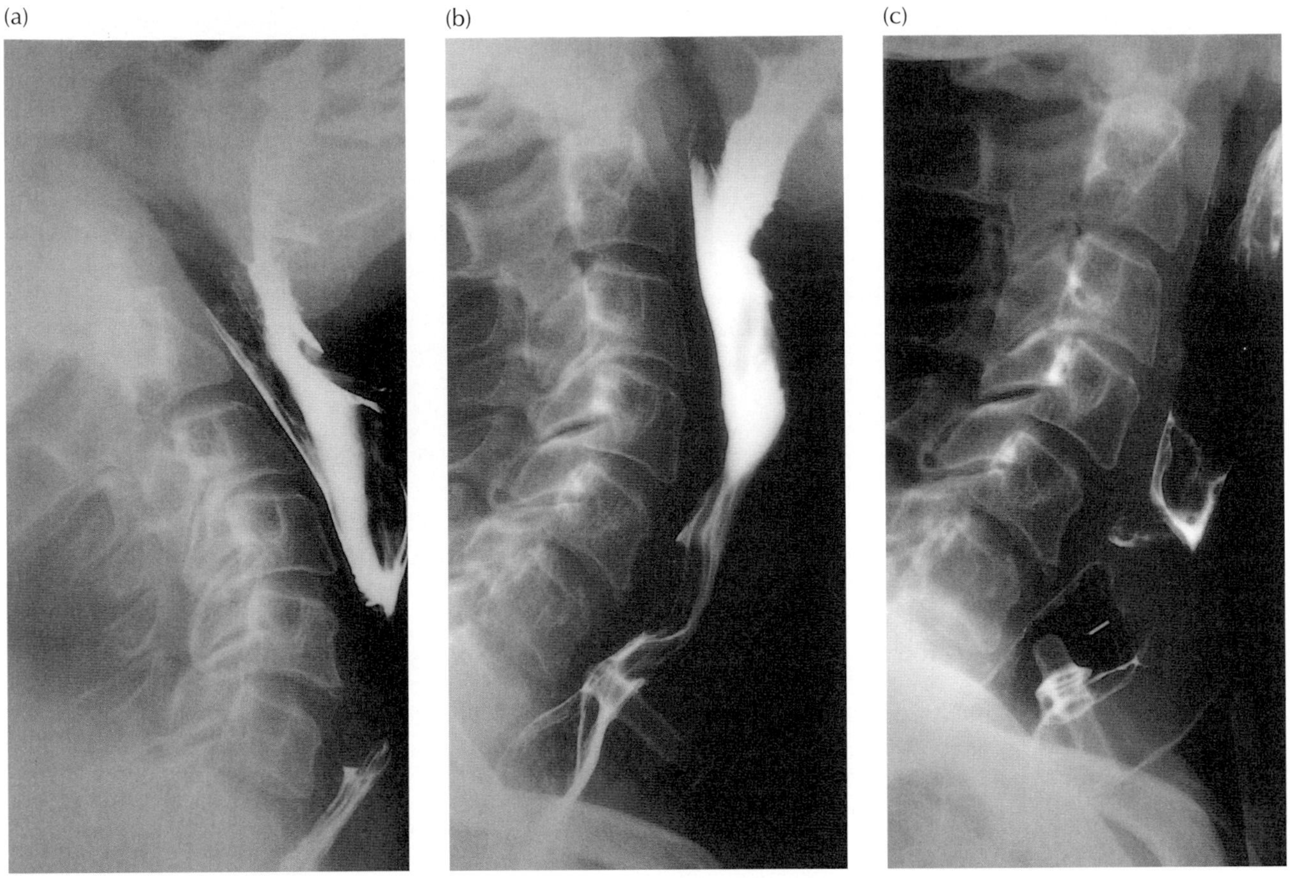

Figure 31.10 (a) Lateral X-ray of the neck at videofluoroscopy in a laryngectomee 5 years after operation with poor voice due to intense constrictor spasm (premyotomy). (b) Postmyotomy showing flow of barium and Blom–Singer valve. (c) Phonation producing strong fluent voice showing air reservoir in the oesophagus and ligaclip at lower limit of myotomy.

PE segment problems

The physical requirements of postlaryngectomy oesophageal and tracheo-oesophageal voice are summarized in Table 31.3 where it may be seen that both rely on the PE segment to act as vibrator (Figures 31.2, 31.8 and 31.9). The inferior pharyngeal constrictor muscles at the level of the PE segment need to be tonic to allow a steady stream of air through the segment in order to produce a good voice. Hypertonicity or spasm will interrupt the flow of air to a varying degree, restricting or completely stopping the flow of air (Figure 31.10). Conversely, if the muscles or PE segment wall are hypotonic (e.g. after total pharyngolaryngectomy and reconstruction) the voice will be weak because there is minimal or absent muscle in the wall to create a PE segment (Figure 31.11).

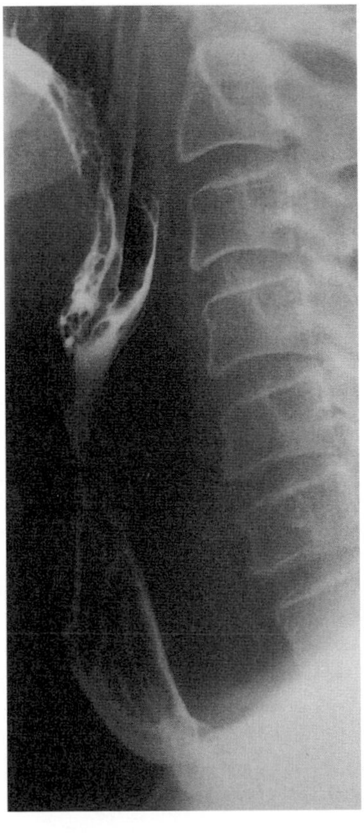

Figure 31.11 Lateral X-ray of the neck at videofluoroscopy 2 years following total pharyngolaryngectomy and reconstruction with a tubed myocutaneous flap. Long hypotonic PE segment at C4–7 with satisfactory voice (stronger with digital pressure).

Videofluoroscopy

The most accurate method of assessing PE segment function after laryngectomy is with videofluoroscopy.[12,14,15] This examination should be carried out routinely prior to secondary voice restoration and should be available to every laryngectomee who has voice problems or who is unable to acquire oesophageal or tracheo-oesophageal speech. It involves only a small dosage of radiation (5–10 cGy) and has three components:

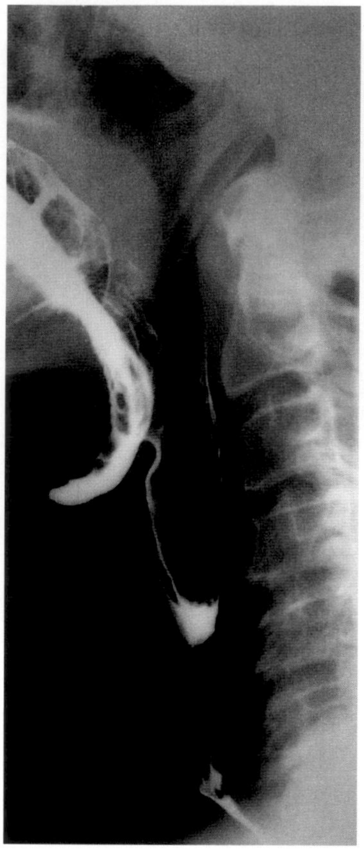

Figure 31.12 Lateral X-ray of the neck to show barium in a pseudovallecula after laryngectomy.

Modified barium swallow

The patient is instructed to swallow barium liquid while the pharynx is screened, initially from the front and then in a lateral position. The flow of barium is followed through the pharynx and the PE segment into the oesophagus and any hold-up or delay due to spasm or stricture is noted as well as any fistula or diverticulum. A pseudovallecula seen in patients with vertical pharyngeal closure at operation may also be demonstrated (Figure 31.12), which can be a cause of dysphagia and poor voice.

Attempted phonation

With the mucosa of the pharynx now coated with barium the patient is asked to attempt phonation by injecting air into the upper oesophagus and counting to 10 or saying 'pa' several times. The lateral view is best used to screen the pharynx during this procedure and the passage of air into the oesophagus through the PE segment is carefully visualized. Air either passes easily through the segment between the pharynx and oesophagus (tonic or hypotonic) or there is variable hold-up at the PE segment (hypertonic or spasm). Strictures may occur at anastamotic sites or if there has been inadequate mucosal/skin reconstruction of the hypopharynx.

Oesophageal insufflation test

A catheter is passed through the nose down into the pharynx to just below the PE segment (about 25 cm from the nasal aperture) and connected to a stomal adaptor (Figure 31.13). The patient is asked to occlude the opening and to try to sustain phonation for over 8 seconds or count without interruption from 1 to 15 on the same breath. They are advised to stop if air is felt distending the stomach or causing epigastric discomfort, indicative of a spastic or hypertonic segment (Table 31.4). The quality of the recorded voice and the visual recording will help to differentiate between the tonic, hypotonic, hypertonic and spastic segment.[15]

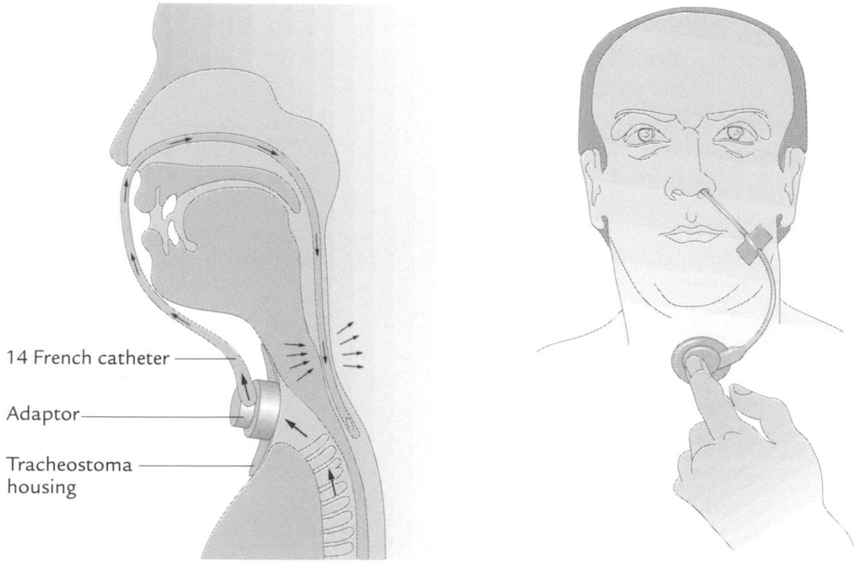

Figure 31.13 Insufflation test.

Table 31.5 Videofluoroscopy results (%)[15]

Hypotonic	18
Tonic (good voice)	16
Hypertonic	34
Spastic	28
Stricture	4

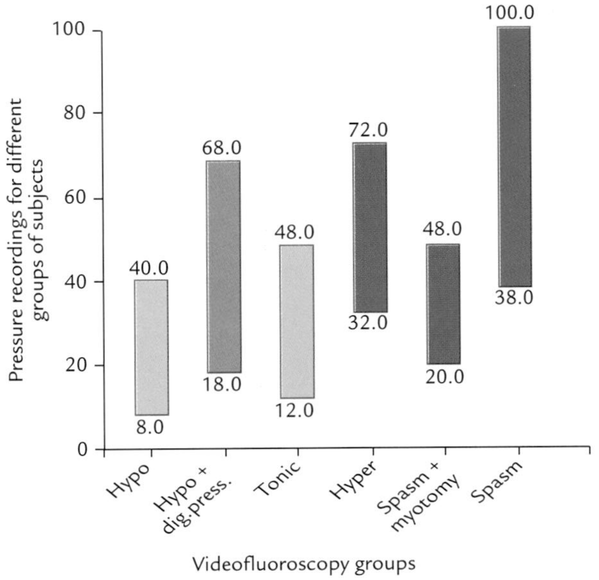

Figure 31.14 PE segment opening pressures for videofluoroscopy groups.[14]

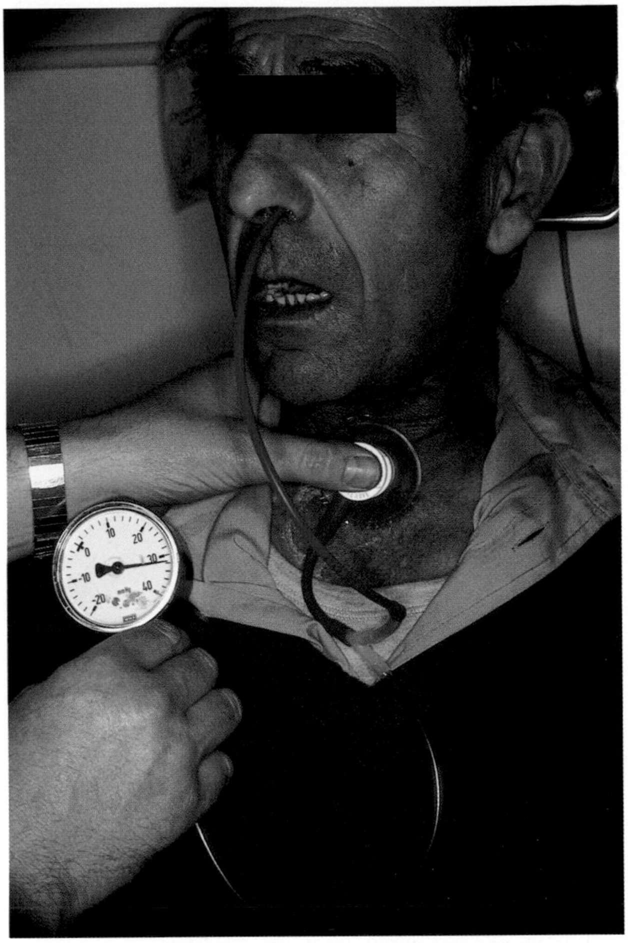

Figure 31.15 Pressure manometer attached to insufflation tubing.

Results

The results of videofluoroscopy show that approximately 60% of patients have poor or failed speech due to hypertonic or spastic PE segments (Table 31.5). This corresponds quite well to the proportion of patients previously documented by Johnson et al[10] who failed to achieve oesophageal voice. With the help of videofluoroscopy Baugh et al[2] found that 91% of voice failures could eventually achieve speech if fully investigated and treated accordingly.

Manometry assessment

Measurement of the opening pressure of the PE segment is also a useful indication of constrictor tonicity and corresponds very well with the videofluoroscopy results (Figure 31.14). A simple pressure manometer is attached to the tubing of the insufflation catheter and the reading is taken during phonation of the pressure just required to open the segment and produce voice (Figure 31.15).

Table 31.6 Management strategy for voice restoration

PE tonicity	Management
Hypotonic	Tracheo-oesophageal valve with digital pressure
Tonic	Tracheo-oesophageal valve
Hypertonic	Tracheo-oesophageal valve + pharyngeal constrictor myotomy (+/– botulinum neurotoxin injection)
Spasm	Tracheo-oesophageal valve + pharyngeal constrictor myotomy (+/– botulinum neurotoxin injection)
Stricture	Tracheo-oesophageal valve + pharyngeal flap augmentation

Videofluoroscopy and voice restoration

In patients with poor or failed oesophageal speech who are being considered for secondary tracheo-oesophageal puncture and voice restoration the videofluoroscopy assessment is essential to help determine the management strategy (Table 31.6).

Selection criteria for speech restoration

For patients undergoing laryngectomy the 'gold standard' for voice rehabilitation must surely be rapid restoration of near-normal speech within 2–3 weeks of operation with primary tracheo-oesophageal puncture and voice prosthesis. The contraindications to doing this routinely are few but careful selection of patients will help to reduce disappointment and failure. In certain situations the voice puncture may be delayed a few months in order to avoid postoperative problems and achieve optimal results.

In established laryngectomees careful investigation and selection is even more critical for secondary voice restoration in order to achieve success. In all cases there are a number of factors that need to be considered.

Motivation

One would anticipate that every patient who has lost the ability to speak through laryngectomy would want to have their voice restored. For those patients undergoing laryngectomy it should now be almost mandatory for some form of primary voice restoration to be carried out at the time of operation for rapid and optimal rehabilitation. The period of aphonia should be only a matter of a few weeks although postoperative radiotherapy often delays satisfactory speech acquisition for 1–2 months. There seems little justification in trying out oesophageal voice first and delaying tracheo-oesophageal puncture until it becomes apparent that this has failed. The relative advantages and disadvantages of primary or delayed puncture are summarized in Table 31.7 and taking these considerations into account one might delay speech restoration in certain situations for a few months or until further review (Table 31.8).

For those patients with previous laryngectomy and poor oesophageal speech some may be desperate to have voice restored with a valve. Others may be more reluctant for various reasons. Some people become used to their voiceless mode of life while others may fear that further surgery might 'stir up' the cancer

Table 31.8 Indications for delayed speech restoration

Uncertain ability to cope physically
Uncertain psychological preparation
Extensive pharyngolaryngeal surgery
Anticipated difficulty with postoperative radiotherapy

Table 31.7 Primary or secondary delayed tracheo-oesophageal puncture

	Advantages	Disadvantages
Primary	One operation No nasogastric tube Rapid return of voice (2–3 weeks) Same lung-powered speech Minimal time off work Oesophageal voice usable	Initial sensitive stoma Postoperative radiotherapy may delay speech May be too much to cope with in one operation
Delayed	Healing stabilized May have developed good oesophageal voice Fewer teething problems	Two operations Considerable time off work Aphonic for much longer Fear of second operation Adjusted to limitations Relearn lung-powered speech Myotomy may be necessary Greater voice failure rate

again. Some patients may live alone and have little need of communication or they may be quite happy with an alternative means of communication (e.g. notepad, artificial larynx). Others might be embarrassed or not like the valve voice and some may not feel comfortable about self-cleaning and valve maintenance.

PE segment function

As discussed previously, the videofluoroscopy findings will determine whether a myotomy or pharyngeal augmentation is carried out at the time of secondary tracheo-oesophageal puncture.

Manual dexterity

The patient should ideally be able to clean, change and maintain the prosthesis themselves. If this is not possible a spouse or close live-in family member may be able to help, but this is less satisfactory and motivation is again essential.

Expectations of surgery and rehabilitation

The practicalities and limitations of valve speech must be fully explained to the patient preoperatively by use of booklets, diagrams and demonstrations ideally with the help of a laryngectomy valve user.

Visual acuity

Good eyesight is important for adequate maintenance of the prosthesis. The patient should also have access to a good light source and mirror.

Alcohol or drug abuse

Some patients with addiction problems are unable to maintain a prosthesis and their unreliability causes unnecessary frustration and expense through repeated loss of valve, leakage, infection and other problems.

Respiratory status

Many laryngectomy patients have other smoking-related lung conditions such as bronchitis, emphysema and varying severity of chronic obstructive airway disease (COAD). There may be inadequate pulmonary reserve to work the valve without causing unacceptable coughing due to increased backflow pressure. They may also have excessive bronchial secretions which certainly may be improved by some form of humidification system.[17]

Current means of communication

Patients with a well-established oesophageal voice who wish to be considered for tracheo-oesophageal puncture and prosthetic voice restoration need to be aware of the additional advantages and limitations of the valve. They will continue to benefit from the spontaneity of oesophageal speech but unless they can quickly learn to use the outer valve housing for ‘hands free’ speech they may be disappointed that they have to use finger occlusion. We have also had to remove a valve in a patient with a previously good oesophageal voice because of painful gastric distension from use of the valve.

Extent of surgery

Satisfactory speech restoration with a tracheo-oesophageal valve is possible in the majority of patients following total pharyngolaryngectomy, as well as those with additional oesophagectomy and stomach transposition.[18,19] The speech is typically weak and hypotonic but the quality and strength can be improved with digital pressure over the reconstructed segment. In most cases where the reconstructed anastomosis is close to the level of the stoma it is prudent to delay the puncture for 2–3 months until healing has been completed to avoid additional risk of wound breakdown.

Tracheostoma size and contour

During the first few months after laryngectomy until scar tissue has stabilized a stoma button or tube is sometimes necessary to avoid contraction and stenosis. The stoma should ideally be 20–25 mm in diameter and if it is too small it may be dilated with a laryngectomy tube or may require enlargement by stomaplasty. If the stoma is too large for satisfactory finger occlusion a laryngectomy tube may be needed with a posterior fenestration to facilitate airflow into the valve opening. In some cases a reduction stomaplasty may be required.

The size, shape and contour of the stoma and surrounding skin are more critical for successful ‘hands free’ speech. Ideally the peristomal neck contour should be flat to help ensure optimal adhesion of the tracheostoma valve housing.[20] In order to avoid unnecessary tracheal retraction, at laryngectomy the trachea should not be transected too low and the margins of the trachea can be sutured to the tendonous medial margins of the sternomastoid muscles to secure it near the skin. This may be difficult if a low transection of the trachea has been necessary in which case a sternomastoid tendonotomy may help.

Recurrent disease

The possibility of early recurrent disease may influence the decision to carry out voice restoration. In a well-motivated patient, however, it may be very important to facilitate speech restoration even if it is just for a short period of time.

In summary, a patient who is otherwise in good health and well motivated and determined to achieve voice after laryngectomy will usually succeed, provided that the surgeon and speech therapist have the knowledge and expertise to deal with any problems and complications that arise.

Primary voice restoration

Patient selection

Primary voice restoration should now be standard practice and patients undergoing laryngectomy should feel confident that they will be able to talk within weeks of their operation. This procedure has made a great difference to the management of laryngeal cancer by eliminating the major stigma of loss of voice for the majority of patients and restoring a good quality of life. As mentioned previously, not all patients are suitable for puncture at the time of laryngectomy and in certain situations a delayed tracheo-oesophageal puncture may be indicated (Table 31.8).

Careful selection of patients is important for achieving optimal results but the variety of valves now available has widened the potential population of patients suitable for a prosthesis. Previously, patients or a family member had to either remove and clean the valve themselves on a regular basis or attend hospital frequently for this purpose. The indwelling Blom–Singer prosthesis now available may remain in place for 6 months or longer and visits to the clinic for replacement by a speech therapist or surgeon are therefore much less frequent. These valves are particularly suitable for older and more infirm patients with poor eyesight or arthritis who need only to clean the stoma and prosthesis.

Surgical considerations

There are certain surgical considerations that should be taken into account before making the decision to carry out a primary puncture at laryngectomy. These mainly concern the potential increased risk of developing a postoperative fistula or wound breakdown, which obviously should be avoided if at all possible.

A large proportion of patients will have had previous radical radiotherapy which inevitably does have an adverse effect on healing and is associated with a higher complication rate after laryngectomy. An additional tracheo-oesophageal puncture procedure does not, however, appear to be a contraindication in increasing these risks, even up to doses of 70 Gy.[21] The presence of diabetes, anaemia, malnutrition and cardiovascular disease, like irradiation, will predispose to poorer healing but should not be a contraindication to primary voice restoration.

Resection of the cervical oesophagus at the time of laryngectomy will open up the retrotracheal space, which does increase the risk of fistula breakdown. It is therefore inadvisable to undertake a tracheo-oesophageal puncture at the time of pharyngo-laryngo-oesophagectomy with gastric transposition or free jejunum repair. There is a similar risk if dissection between the upper trachea and oesophagus has inadvertently been taken down to the level of the puncture site. This separation of the party wall is an absolute contraindication to primary puncture and must be repaired.[22] If circumferential resection and reconstruction is limited to the pharynx, it is quite reasonable to undertake a primary voice restoration provided that the lower anastomosis is well above the proposed puncture site.

Surgical technique

The laryngectomy is carried out in the usual fashion conserving as much pharyngeal mucosa as possible, particularly over the postcricoid region and the piriform fossae, provided safe clearance from the tumour is obtained. For hypopharyngeal tumours the mucosa of the uninvolved piriform fossa is carefully preserved to minimize the need for flap reconstruction. Ideally a transverse mucosal width of at least 6 cm is necessary to enable adequate swallowing and effortless tracheo-oesophageal speech. Augmentation of the pharynx with a flap is preferable if the residual mucosal strip is under 4 cm otherwise stenosis is likely with significant functional impairment.

Certain fundamental principles and modifications have been incorporated into the laryngectomy technique to ensure good predictable results with minimal risk of complications:

Stoma position
A Gluck–Sorensen incision is preferred, incorporating inferolateral extensions if neccessary for neck

dissection. The midline horizontal portion is at the level of the planned superior border of the tracheostome, usually at the second/third tracheal ring. The curved lateral limbs extend up to the level of the hyoid bone.

Stoma reconstruction

The central part of the lower skin flap is sutured around the curved margin of the anterior trachea to the posterior ends of the tracheal ring. Close approximation of the mucosa to the skin is necessary covering any bare cartilage in order to avoid granulation formation. The upper flap is sutured to the margin of the trachealis muscle on the posterior wall of the trachea. This reconstruction ensures that the tracheal rings are pulled laterally to maintain a good sized stoma.

It is usually a good idea to put absorbable sutures between the oesophageal wall and the posterior aspect of the trachealis on either side of the proposed position of the puncture in order to secure the party wall and avoid inadvertent separation.

Tracheo-oesophageal puncture

The puncture is positioned in the midline about 10–15 mm below the mucocutaneous junction on the posterior tracheal wall. A 14-FG Foley catheter is first prepared by trimming a slither of silastic from opposite edges near the tip to facilitate easier grasping of an otherwise awkward rounded end. The balloon is tested by inflating with 1.5 ml of saline, deflated and then the catheter is grasped near the tip with a small pair of curved artery forceps.

The tip of another pair of curved artery forceps is inserted through the pharyngeal defect and advanced into the upper oesophagus just as far as the puncture site, tenting up the mucosa (Figure 31.16). A scalpel is used to incise horizontally through the mucosa and muscle onto the tip of the forceps, which are then advanced into the tracheal lumen and opened to grasp the tip of the silastic catheter (Figure 31.17). The forceps and the catheter are then withdrawn through the fistula tract and the tip of the catheter is passed distally down the oesophagus to just above the cardio-oesophageal junction. The catheter balloon is inflated with about 1.5 ml of saline to prevent accidental dislodgement and the catheter is anchored to the skin above the stoma.

There are several advantages of using the Foley catheter as a feeding tube during the postoperative period. It obviates the need for a nasogastric tube, which is irritating to the nose and cosmetically unsightly. The nasogastric tube would normally pass down across the suture line of the reconstructed pharynx, through the oesophagus and into the stomach, thus preventing proper closure of the cardio-oesophageal sphincter. During the early postoperative period, with the patient in a recumbent position most of the time, the tube may act as a very effective syphon allowing unwanted gastric acid to reflux up the oesophagus to the site of the pharyngeal reconstruction.

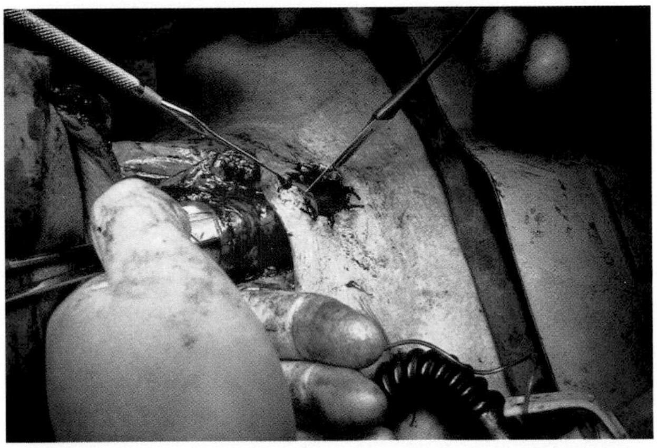

Figure 31.16 Positioning of the primary tracheo-oesophageal puncture.

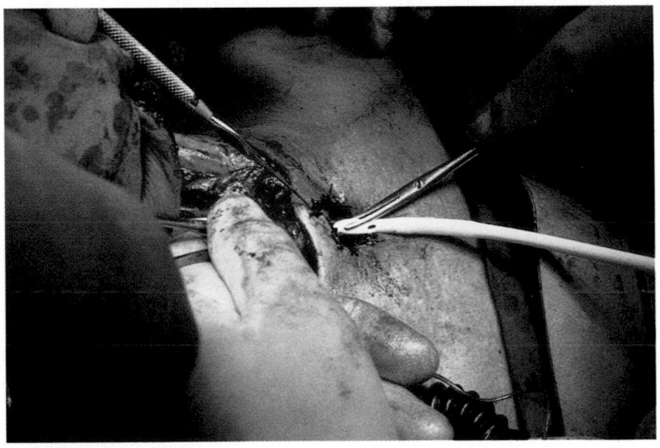

Figure 31.17 Insertion of the Foley catheter.

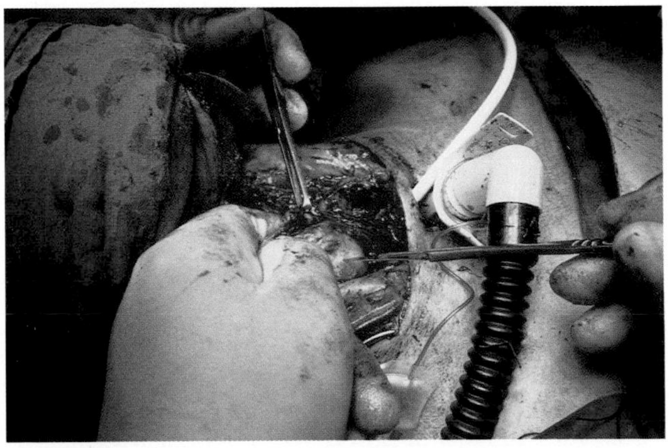

Figure 31.18 Short constrictor myotomy.

Cricopharyngeal myotomy

A short posterior midline myotomy is carried out with a scalpel over a distance of 2–3 cm from the level of the TE puncture site (Figure 31.18). This divides the circular muscle fibres in the upper oesophagus and the cricopharyngeus. Effective assessment of the tone of the circular fibres is made by inserting the index finger into the lower pharynx and upper oesophagus when frequently the finger detects some resistance due to hypertonicity or spasm.[19] This correlates well with manometric pressure measurements and outcome.[23] The finger is kept in position and the tightness is felt to be gradually relieved as the scalpel divides the circular fibres down to the submucosal vascular plexus. Any inadvertent cut through the mucosa should be repaired with an absorbable suture.

The myotomy carried out at the time of laryngectomy is designed to allow expansion of the upper oesophagus providing an air 'reservoir' below the PE segment which is essential for good voice production (see Figures 31.2, 31.8 and 31.9). It is shorter than the myotomy carried out as a secondary procedure for voice failure due to spasm or hypertonicity (see below) which extends from the puncture site up to the tongue base.

Pharyngeal plexus neurectomy

A unilateral pharyngeal plexus neurectomy is an alternative method of constrictor relaxation[24] or can be carried out as well as myotomy. Usually three to five branches of the plexus entering the lateral wall of the pharynx are exposed and tested with a nerve stimulator before cautery and division.

Botulinum toxin

Any residual spasm can be treated with local botulinum toxin injection, which is usually effective with one application.[25]

Pharyngeal closure

The previously widely used method of vertical closure of the pharyngeal defect is not suitable for optimum voice restoration for various reasons. It produces a long anterior scar, which contracts over a period of time producing the typical appearance on endoscopy of a pseudovallecula with a transverse pharyngeal mucosal bar. This also has a characteristic appearance on lateral view videofluoroscopy (Figure 31.12). This pseudovallecula potentially can cause problems with speech and swallowing. In the early postoperative period it can form a small 'sump' at the tongue base, which may fill with fluid and predispose to development of a fistula tract. Vertical closure produces a long narrow pharyngeal segment, which may contribute to dysphagia. On swallowing, the bolus of food may collect in the pseudovallecula, which enlarges, pushing the posterior wall backwards causing further narrowing of the opening into the hypopharynx. This produces a similar effect on swallowing as does the pharyngeal pouch when it obstructs the opening of the oesophagus. The patient may experience difficulty in clearing food from the pharynx, taking several swallows to get the bolus into the oesophagus. Injection of air into the pharynx during oesophageal speech may be affected in a similar way.

A horizontal closure of the pharyngeal defect is preferred using a continuous absorbable mucosal suture and then an interrupted muscle layer. This produces a wider pharynx above the PE segment which has been shown to improve resonance for speech. If additional mucosa from the piriform sinus has been excised it will probably be necessary to close the pharynx in a 'T' shape in order to avoid tension. Despite the three-point junction this is still preferred to a vertical closure. Significant resection of the hypopharynx will necessitate a skin flap reconstruction (see above).

Reconstruction of the PE segment

A 1-cm band of the thyropharyngeus constrictor muscle is brought together anteriorly with mattress sutures about 3–4 cm above the TE puncture site (Figure 31.19). The purpose is to try to create a suitable PE segment at the optimal site in the pharynx with a good air reservoir below it and a wide resonating pharyngeal segment above. It is however important not to make the band too tight, otherwise it may produce a hypertonic segment.

Reinervation of the pharynx

The cut ends of the superior laryngeal nerves and the recurrent laryngeal nerves are reimplanted into the

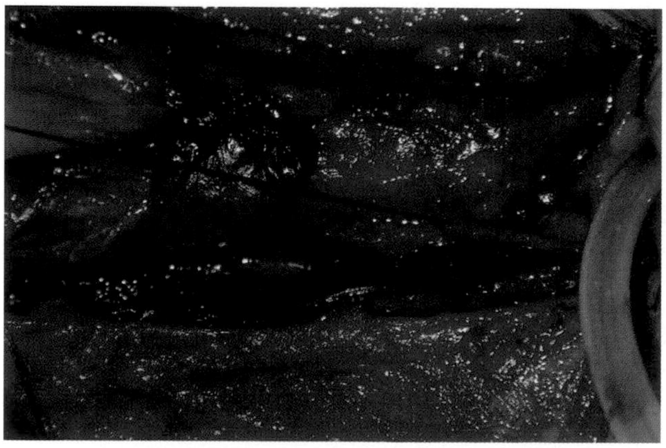

Figure 31.19 Reconstruction of the muscular PE segment and re-implantation of recurrent larngeal nerve.

muscular wall of the reconstructed pharynx and upper oesophagus respectively in the hope that this may restore some sensory and motor reinnervation. It is felt that this can only have a potentially beneficial effect on neuromuscular co-ordination of the reconstructed 'neolarynx', although obviously it is difficult to measure any effect objectively (Figure 31.19).

Primary placement of the voice prosthesis

Primary placement of the voice prosthesis before closure of the pharynx at laryngectomy is a variation of the puncture technique that has gained some popularity in Europe.[22] However, a nasogastric tube must be inserted for postoperative feeding with the disadvantages mentioned previously and which most patients find much less acceptable than one passed through the puncture site. In addition, the prosthesis will have to be replaced within a few weeks with a shorter valve as the postoperative oedema subsides. Another disadvantage of primary valve placement is that the prosthesis cannot in any case be used for speech for at least 10 days postoperatively to ensure complete wound healing and to avoid risking fistula formation.

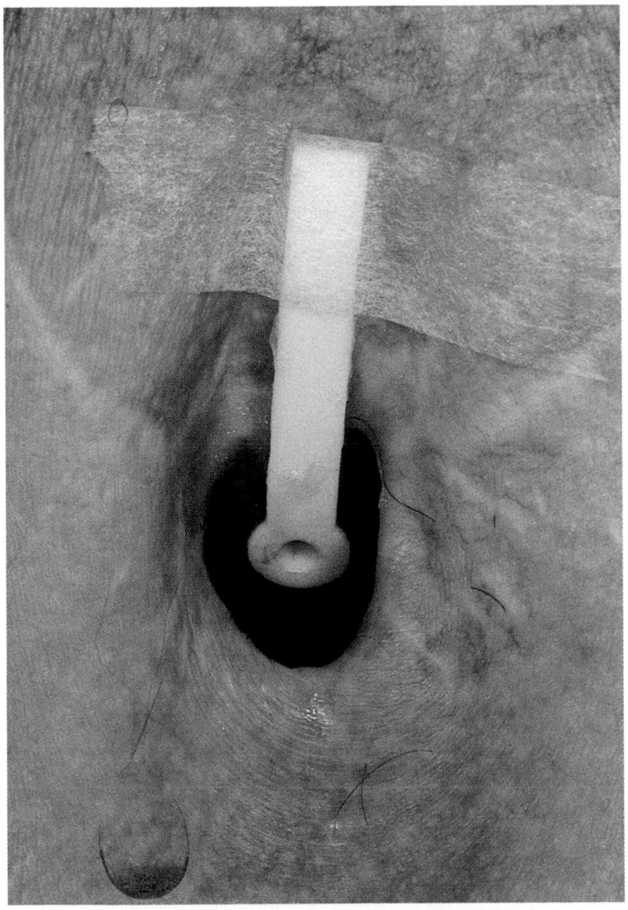

Figure 31.20 Blom–Singer prosthesis in position.

Closure and postoperative care

The wound is closed routinely with suction drainage. Feeding is continued through the Foley catheter and oral intake is commenced usually after 7 days if no previous radiotherapy has been given, in which case it is delayed until the tenth day following a satisfactory barium swallow. Once oral feeding has been started the catheter is removed after 2–3 days and replaced with a suitable Blom–Singer prosthesis (Figure 31.20). In some patients who might require longer to recover from the trauma of the operation or whose stoma may not be adequately healed, it might be prudent to let them home to recover a little longer and then bring them back for insertion of the prosthesis.

Results

Successful primary voice rehabilitation has been achieved in 90–95% in an accumulated experience of more than 450 patients over a period of 20 years.[22] The fistula rate is only 5% including patients who had received previous irradiation.

Secondary voice restoration

The technique of tracheo-oesophageal puncture with prosthetic voice restoration was originally developed for those patients who had failed to achieve adequate oesophageal speech.[6] A preliminary videofluoroscopy will determine whether it is necessary to carry out a constrictor myotomy at the same operation and other procedures such as stoma revision may also be indicated at the same time. The selection of suitable patients has previously been discussed.

Surgical technique

The method described by Singer and Blom[6] in 1980 has provided a reliable technique for restoration of good quality lung-powered speech, but significant problems associated with the rigid endoscopic technique have been described, particularly concerning access down to the stoma level.[26–29] Similar problems with access using the rigid endoscope prompted the first author to develop an alternative method[30] using a modified pair of curved Lloyd-Davies forceps (Figure 31.21), which has been used successfully in a series of 94 secondary voice punctures since 1984, with no failed or abandoned procedures.

The forceps are inserted alongside a pharyngeal speculum into the oesophageal opening under direct vision and advanced down to the level of the tracheostome where the tip can be seen and palpated

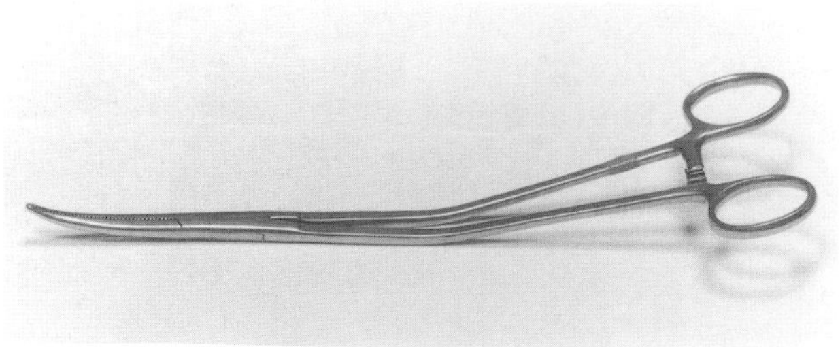

Figure 31.21 Secondary tracheo-oesophageal puncture forceps.

(a)

(b)

(c)

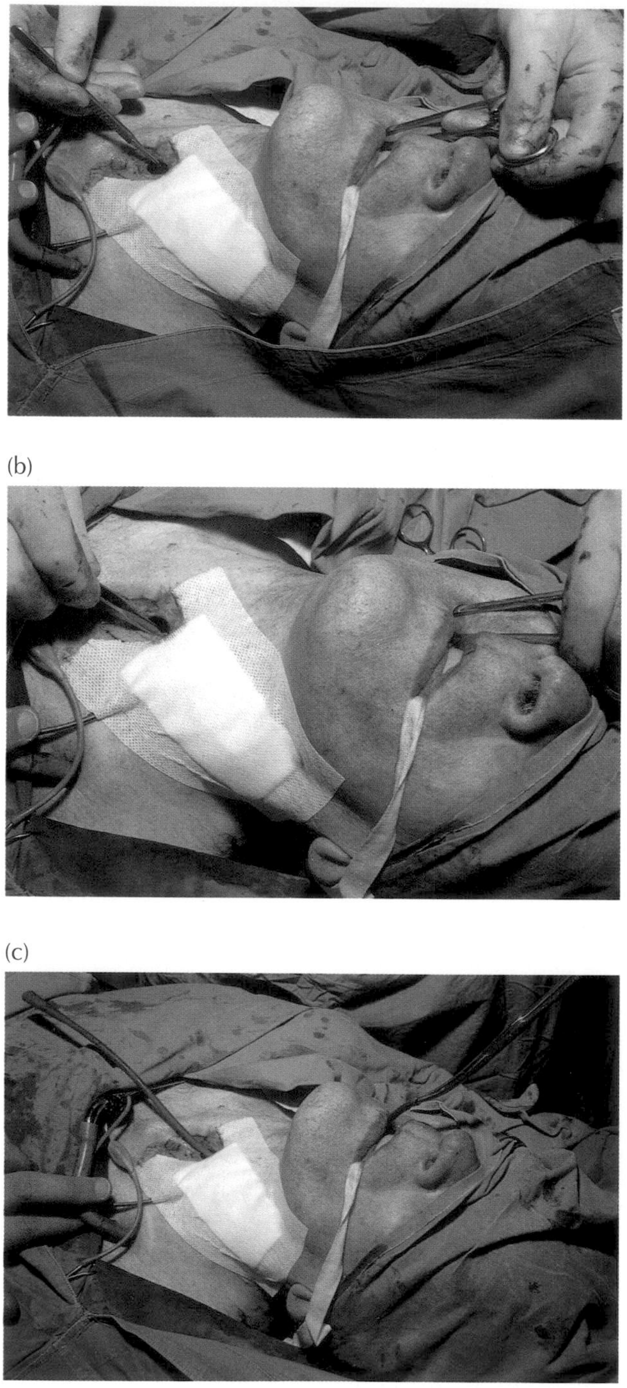

Figure 31.22 Incision being made through the posterior stomal wall.

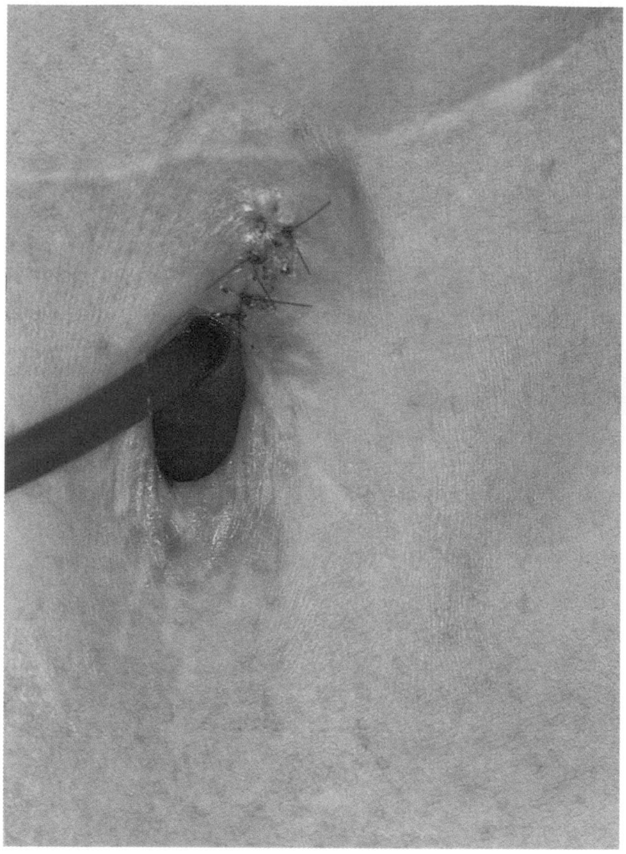

Figure 31.23 Stenting catheter before removal.

as it tents up the posterior tracheal wall in a similar way to the primary puncture technique. An incision is made through the posterior wall of the stoma in the midline on to the tips of the forceps (Figure 31.22a), which are advanced into the trachea. The end of a 14 FG catheter is then introduced into the opened tips of the forceps (Figure 31.22b) and withdrawn into the pharynx (Figure 31.22c), passed caudally and released. The catheter is sutured to the skin above the tracheostome and if a Foley catheter is used the balloon is inflated with 1.5 ml of saline to prevent dislodgement.

A normal diet is resumed after the procedure and the stenting catheter (Figure 31.23) remains in place for a period of 2–7 days depending on whether a myotomy has been carried out simultaneously. It is then removed and after measuring the length of the tract a suitable Blom–Singer prosthesis is inserted.

Pharyngeal constrictor myotomy

The recognition of pharyngeal constrictor spasm or hypertonicity as a cause of voice failure[31] by Singer and Blom in 1981 and its treatment with myotomy was a major factor in achieving good consistent

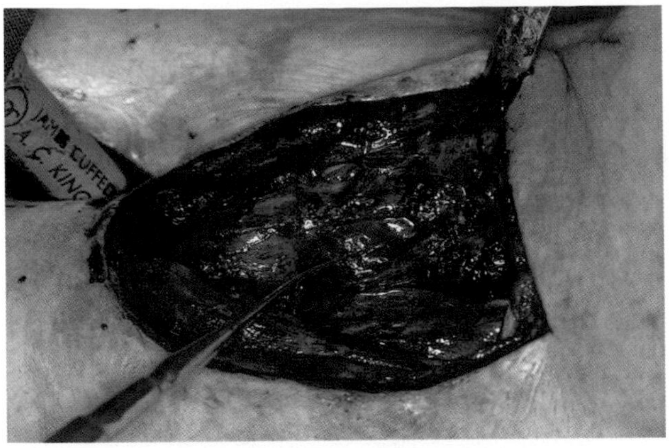

Figure 31.24 Identification of the hypertrophied pharyngeal constrictors that are partly hidden by the thyroid lobe.

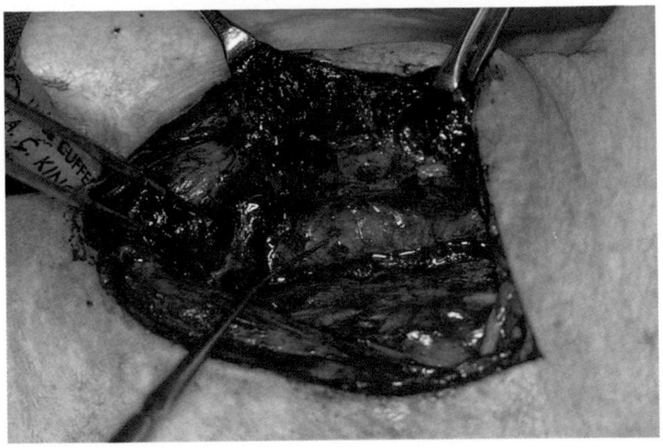

Figure 31.25 Long secondary constrictor myotomy.

results for tracheo-oesophageal speech. Initial experience with a limited cricopharyngeal myotomy was not successful in all patients and subsequent examination of postoperative videofluoroscopy recordings showed that hypertonicity may occur at any level in the pharynx and not just at the cricopharyngeus level. The technique of a long myotomy from the stoma to the base of the tongue was evolved and has given much more consistent results (Figure 31.10).

Surgical Technique

Identification of the pharynx

An oesophageal dilator (36–40 FG) is initially inserted to delineate the hypopharynx and to stretch the muscle fibres to facilitate the myotomy.

Side of approach

A decision is then made on which side to approach the pharynx. Normally at laryngectomy the thyroid lobe will have been removed on the side of the tumour and it is generally more convenient to approach the pharynx from this side. The presence of a thyroid lobe does make access more difficult (Figure 31.24) for the myotomy, particularly as it is not advisable to divide the inferior thyroid artery which may devascularize the remaining gland if the superior thyroid artery has already been divided at the time of laryngectomy

Incision

Reopening of the Gluck–Sorensen scar from the stoma up to the level of the tongue base is preferred to an incision between the carotid and the pharynx[31] since this gives better protection to the carotid artery. There is usually dense fibrous tissue between the carotid and the pharynx but this is carefully divided down to the prevertebral fascia with lateral retraction of the artery.

Myotomy

The pharyngeal constrictors are stretched over the dilator and incised from the level of the stoma up to the level of the tongue base (Figure 31.25). The myotomy is taken as deep as the submucosal vessels and the muscle coat is retracted back and sutured to prevent reclosure. Any inadvertent perforation of the mucosa is closed with absorbable suture and if this does happen the patient will have to remain tube-fed for 1 week, using the catheter through the trans-oesophageal fistula.

The main complication following secondary myotomy is a small fistula (10–20%)[31] but most of these are recognized at operation and sutured. If there is any doubt about the integrity of the mucosa air can be insufflated into the pharynx to identify any leak. Cervical spine injury is not a common problem unless a rigid endoscopic puncture is carried out at the same time.[26–29] Cervical osteomyelitis may occur even in the absence of a fistula.[32] Satisfactory healing is verified with a barium swallow before starting an oral diet; tracheo-oesophageal speech is commenced with the prosthesis after 1 week.

Botulinum toxin injection

The use of botulinum toxin to provide a chemical neurectomy is still being evaluated but permanent successful results have been achieved with a single 100-unit injection.[24,31] We would advocate botulinum toxin injection as the treatment of choice for failed tracheo-oesophageal speech when caused by spasm or hypertonicity. Myotomy is reserved for circumstances where botulinum is ineffective or is required repeatedly.

Voice restoration following total pharyngolaryngectomy

Successful management of carcinoma of the hypopharynx or upper cervical oesophagus is difficult because these tumours often present late with nodal metastases and they are generally not as radiosensitive as carcinoma of the nasopharynx or oropharynx. A large proportion of these patients will undergo pharyngolaryngectomy either primarily or for recurrence with a potential cure rate of up to 40%. This operation, however, is much more complex than total laryngectomy, particularly the reconstruction and is associated with a greater risk of complications, a higher morbidity and a less than optimal chance of successful restoration of speech and swallowing. It is therefore essential that treatment should be carried out by an experienced multidisciplinary team in order to achieve optimal results.

Table 31.9 Voice restoration results after total pharyngolaryngectomy at the Royal Marsden Hospital (1986–2000; 66 patients)

Type of reconstruction	Successful speech (54/66)
Mucosal flaps	
Stomach pull-up	8/12
Free jejunum	15/19
Colon	1/2
Skin flaps	
Latissimus dorsi	9/10
Pectoralis major	16/17
Free radial forearm	4/5
Deltopectoral	1/1

A variety of choices are available now for reconstruction of the hypopharynx following total pharyngolaryngectomy and the decision for adopting a particular method will depend on various factors in each individual case. From the functional point of view there are two main groups of reconstructive option. The first includes a variety of tubed skin flaps, the commonest ones being the free radial forearm flap, the pedicled deltopectoral fasciocutaneous flap and the pedicled pectoralis major and latissimus dorsi myocutaneous flaps. The second type of reconstruction involves transfer of alimentary tract mucosa, using either transposition of the stomach or a free jejunal graft.

Deltopectoral flap

The modern era of reconstructive surgery for head and neck tumours dates back to 1965 when Bakamjian described the deltopectoral flap, which became used extensively for most reconstructions of the mouth and pharynx. The great advantage of this flap was that it provided a large area of skin with a good blood supply taken from outside the area of previous surgery or radiotherapy. Following total pharyngolaryngectomy the long axial pattern flap is tubed and inset into the defect leaving a controlled salivary fistula at its lower end. The pedicle of the flap is divided at a second stage operation 2–3 weeks later and the remaining corner of the flap is inset into the oesophagus.

This technique offered great advantages over existing methods of reconstruction such as the Wookey flap or the distant tubed pedicle popularized by Gillies, which required many staged operations over several months. Hospitalization, however, was still prolonged and there was considerably delay in swallowing, speech and postoperative radiotherapy.

Results

This flap came at a time before tracheo-oesophageal fistula techniques but some patients were able to develop oesophageal speech. It is still used now as a safe alternative in difficult situations where other flaps have failed or are not suitable. Any voice restoration is carried out as a secondary puncture when good voice can be achieved although this is typically hypotonic and improved with digital pressure. We have had success with one patient who had a Blom–Singer valve (Table 31.9).

Pectoralis major myocutaneous flap

In 1979 Ariyan introduced the pectoralis major myocutaneous flap, which largely superseded the deltopectoral flap as the reconstructive workhorse of the head and neck.[33] Its great advantage is that it allows one stage reconstruction of the pharynx[34] and it is also very reliable and easy to raise. For circumferential reconstruction of the hypopharynx the flap is raised and tubed before insetting into the defect. There are, however, some potential limitations. It is important to take a wide enough flap to allow for some contraction, otherwise there will be a problem with stenosis or restricted swallowing. It is usually possible to get primary closure of the primary defect on the chest wall but sometimes a skin graft is necessary. The muscle and subcutaneous fat layers may be quite thick producing a bulky flap, which may be difficult to tube and inset without tension. It is generally not suitable in women because of the additional bulk of the breast tissue and also it may result in unacceptable distortion and asymmetry of the breast The latissimus dorsi flap is much more preferable for these patients. In men the chest flap is often hairy which can cause bolus obstruction although after a period of time the hairs do atrophy.

Results

If an adequate flap has been used the swallowing and quality of speech are usually good[36] with improvement of voice on digital pressure over the flap (Table 31.9). Primary puncture can be done if there is sufficient length of oesophagus and hypopharynx between the lower anastomosis and the stoma level. Typically with these cutaneous flaps the smooth skin lining offers less resistance to the flow of air than with jejunum and the voice is correspondingly stronger. The PE segment often becomes established at the upper anastomosis (Figure 31.11).

Latissimus dorsi myocutaneous flap

This is a beautifully versatile flap for either pedicled or free flap reconstruction in the head and neck[35] and its only disadvantage is that the patient needs to be turned onto their side during the procedure. With experience in its use this is only a minor drawback and is outweighed by its many advantages. A large area of flap can be raised (Figure 31.26) with good reliability and the muscle is thin and pliable and ideal for tubing. It is usually non-hair-bearing and its widespread use for breast reconstruction confirms the excellent cosmetic result with primary closure of the donor site.

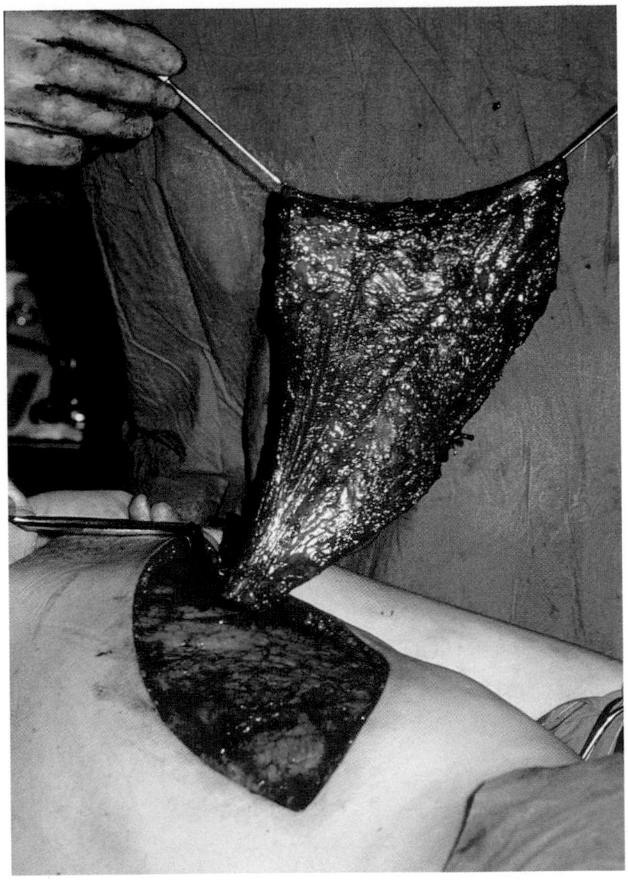

Figure 31.26 Latissimus dorsi myocutaneous flap.

Results

The functional results of swallowing and speech (Table 31.9) are similar to the other cutaneous flaps and because of its generous size there is less risk of stenosis.

Free radial forearm flap

The advent of free microvascular tissue transfer has greatly widened the scope of reconstructive options in the head and neck. The forearm flap is thin and pliable and can be tubed for reconstruction of the hypopharynx (Figure 31.27). Harvesting the flap can be done synchronously with the resection by the reconstructive surgeon in order to minimize additional operating time.[43]

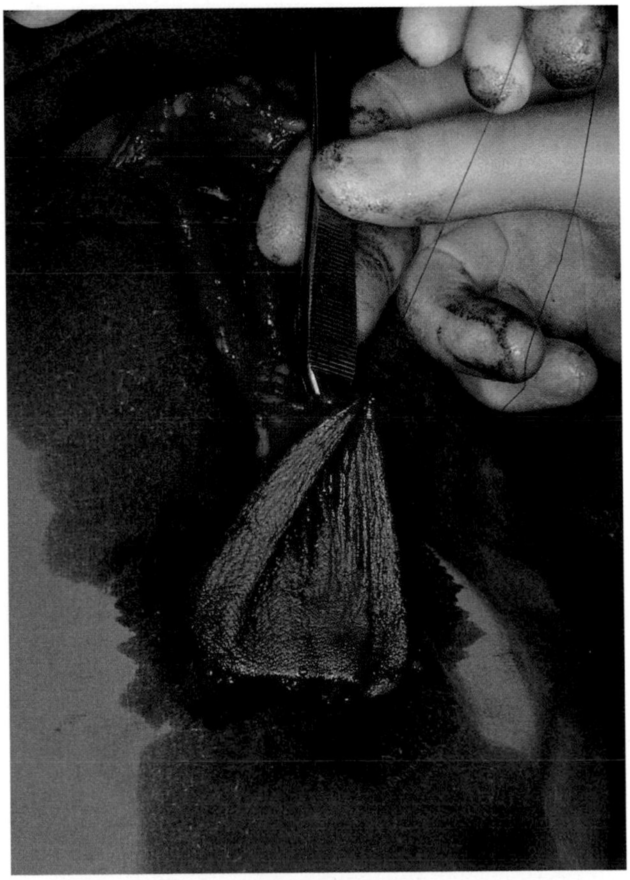

Figure 31.27 Tubed radial forearm flap.

The area of skin available on the forearm, however, is barely sufficient for large circumferential defects and there is a risk of taking insufficient width to allow for contracture with resulting problems of stenosis. A flap width of 9 cm is necessary to ensure a final lumen diameter of 1 cm[36] but ideally a greater diameter of pharynx is preferable to ensure good speech and comfortable deglutition without dietary restriction. As with other cutaneous flaps primary puncture is usually possible and functional results are good provided that adequate width has been taken.

Free jejunum flap

The free jejunum flap has gained widespread popularity and seems ideal because reconstruction of the hypopharynx can be achieved with moist intestinal mucosa of similar diameter at a one-stage procedure. The abdominal complication rate of 5.8% reported by Shangold et al[37] is acceptably low and far less than with stomach pull-up.

The graft also tolerates postoperative radiotherapy well[38] but in the long term one of the problems with jejunal interposition is stenosis, which may occur some months or even years after the operation.[39] The jejunum graft remains dependent on its own vascular pedicle because unlike other flaps the serosal surface prevents ingrowth of new vasculature from the surrounding tissue. The graft therefore remains much more vulnerable to the longterm adverse effects of postoperative radiotherapy and it is not unusual to see gradual avascular fibrosis of a graft that for some time had appeared very healthy. It is therefore important to preserve the integrity of the pedicle at any subsequent surgery such as neck dissection or treatment of recurrence or new primary.

Results

The voice is typically hypotonic and mucus secretion from the jejunum can be a problem especially during the first few months but this does improve with time and after postoperative radiotherapy. The natural circular mucosal folds (Figure 31.28) will also reduce the expiratory voice pressure by causing turbulence in the ascending flow of air.

Surgical technique is therefore very important in achieving optimum voice quality. It is easy to be overgenerous with the length of jejunum graft particularly when it is inset with the neck in the extended position. It should be put in under slight tension so that when the neck returns to the natural flexed position the jejunum will not be too long, otherwise it will form convolutions or redundant loops, which will further impede the flow of air. This did happen in three of nine patients early on in our experience[40] but shortening of the jejunum or removing the redundant loop resulted in good functional speech. Subsequent experience has provided good voice in 15 of 19 patients (Table 31.9).

Gastric pull-up

Gastric transposition for reconstruction of the hypopharynx was first described in 1960 by Ong and Lee[41] and provides an effective one-stage procedure that eliminates the risk of inadequate inferior resection because it incorporates total oesophagectomy as well. The incidence of fistula formation is also reduced as there is only one anastomosis in the upper neck. The lumen itself is wide and so swallowing problems and stenosis are not seen.

The operation, however, does have a high complication rate with an associated mortality of 6–12% and morbidity of up to 50%.[42,44] The early postoperative problems are mainly as a result of the complexity of the synchronous thoracic, cervical and abdominal dissections. Later complications include the 'dumping' syndrome, reflux in 23%[44] and the need for small volume meals.

Results

Because of separation of the tracheo-oesophageal party wall speech restoration is best carried out as a secondary procedure, ideally a few months after operation but it may be delayed by slow recovery or

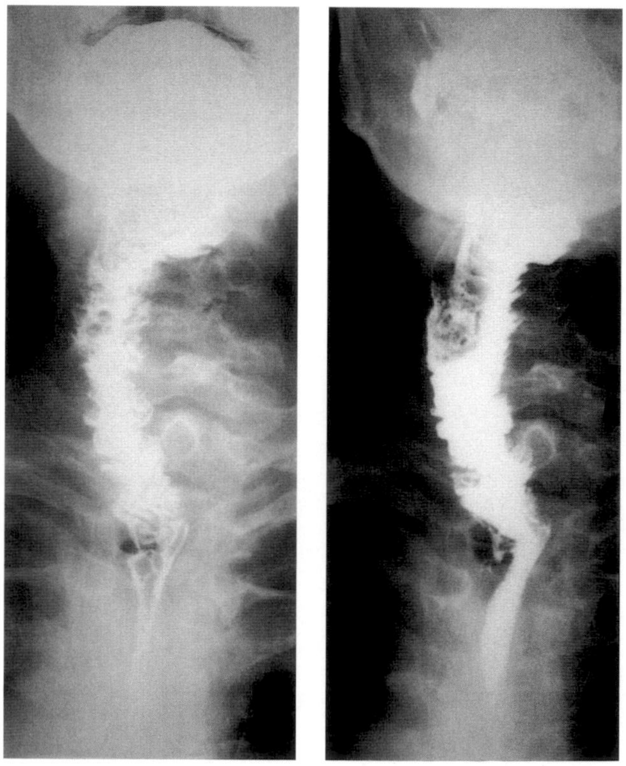

Figure 31.28 Barium swallow of a jejunal graft.

by postoperative radiotherapy. A large proportion of patients is either not offered voice restoration or may be reluctant to undergo any further surgery. The quality of the voice is poor compared with jejunum[45] because of the wide lumen diameter, and also the presence of gastric secretions give it a gurgling quality that many female patients find unacceptable. Some improvement in voice may be possible with digital pressure. In our own experience at the Royal Marsden Hospital using the Blom–Singer prosthesis eight of 12 patients with gastric pull-up achieved satisfactory voice (Table 31.9).

Summary

The functional results of voice restoration after pharyngolaryngectomy are not as predictable as after laryngectomy and the quality is not as good. Nevertheless, for many patients it is a vital means of communication. In the United Kingdom and in some other countries postcricoid carcinoma is a more common problem, particularly in the younger female patient. For these patients and for the increasing number who are surviving radical treatment for hypopharyngeal carcinoma rapid restoration of voice and good long-term functional rehabilitation is of paramount importance.

Skin-lined flaps have given us the most predictable results and have the least morbidity. They are preferable provided that the length of the defect is not too long and adequate width is taken to avoid problems of stenosis. Of these the pectoralis major flap is the easiest to harvest but it is bulky, has several limitations and is not suitable in women. The latissimus dorsi flap is an ideal alternative and merits wider use.

The free radial forearm flap is the preferred option in several experienced institutions[36] and gives good predictable results. Its main limitation is size and also it requires a more prolonged procedure with an experienced microvascular team to achieve an acceptable complication rate.

The free jejunum flap has also been used widely but the quality of voice may not be as good as with cutaneous flaps. The microvascular anastomosis and additional abdominal procedure increase the potential for operative complications and in the long term there may be problems with stenosis.

Pharyngogastric anastomosis with stomach pull-up has a high complication rate and mortality when compared with other well-established techniques. Even in experienced hands it is debatable whether it should be done as the routine method of reconstruction when safer methods are just as appropriate. It is, however, the technique of choice in cervical oesophageal lesions or when the resection extends close to the thoracic inlet where there may be difficulty in closing the lower anastomosis of a pedicled or free flap.

Fistula prosthesis assessment and fitting

Timing of valving

After primary voice restoration procedure the patient is fed through the tracheo-oesophageal catheter (14 Fr) for a period of 7–10 days before valving. If no previous radiotherapy has been given and there has been no postoperative problem with healing, oral diet is usually commenced after 7 days allowing discontinuation of catheter feeding. In patients who have had previous radiotherapy it is safer to delay oral feeding for 2–3 more days. A few days later the patient will be ready for voice prosthesis fitting and training. Following *secondary* puncture the prosthesis may be fitted after 2–3 days unless a myotomy has been carried out in which case fitting is best delayed for a week.

Clinical setting

Initial procedures are carried out in an appropriate medical setting with the clinician sitting in front of and slightly to the side of the patient to avoid being coughed on. A good headlight is essential to illuminate the stoma and other precautions such as use of sterile gloves and protective glasses are advisable. Once the laryngectomee has been taught to clean and change the valve a suitable place at home such as the bathroom is chosen requiring a good light source and mirror.

Tracheo-oesophageal puncture assessment

The basic procedures for assessment, fitting and maintenance of the tracheo-oesophageal prosthesis are essentially the same following primary or secondary voice restoration. As a preliminary trial it is useful to try voicing 'open tract,' that is without a prosthesis. The 14-Fr catheter, which had been placed at operation, is removed and the patient is asked to take a deep breath and not to swallow. A finger is then gently placed over the stoma and the patient is asked to exhale saying 'aahhh...' or to count to 10. Successful 'open tract' sound production is very encouraging and also helpful if subsequent valve voice is poor, indicating that the valve rather than the tract is the contributing factor.

Progression to prosthetic voice production starts with insertion of an 18-Fr silicone tracheo-oesophageal dilator (Figure 31.29), which will dilate the tract slightly beyond the diameter of the standard 16-Fr measuring device and prosthesis, facilitating their insertion. After several minutes of dilatation the measuring device is inserted (Figure 31.30) until it is felt to contact the posterior oesophageal wall. It is then directed downwards and the probe is inserted fully into the oesophagus before being gently withdrawn until the retention collar is felt to abut against the anterior oesophageal wall. The size marker visible nearest the entrance of the puncture tract will designate the thickness of the wall and a corresponding length of prosthesis is chosen. If in doubt choose a valve slightly longer than the marker length to prevent underfitting, which may result in closure of the tract.

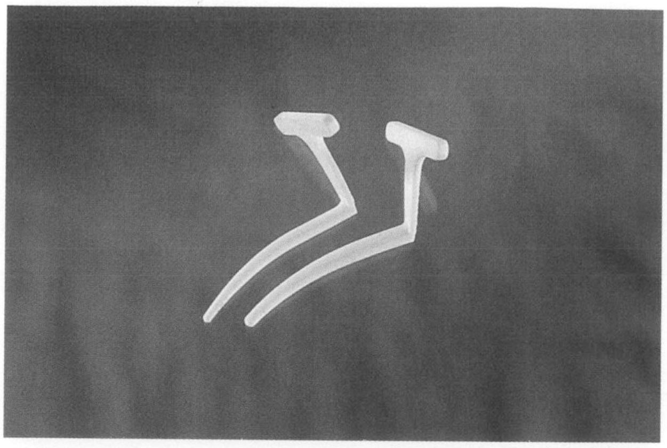

Figure 31.29 Tracheo-oesophageal dilators.

Choice of prosthesis

The Blom–Singer valve has undergone modifications over the last 20 years to suit different anatomical, structural and physiological variations in the TE fistula and vocal tract. Two basic types of valve are available, the 'standard' ones which can be changed by the patient without medical supervision including the original 'duckbill' valve (Figure 31.6) and the modified 'low-pressure' or 'low-profile' valves (Figure 31.31). The other type is the 'indwelling' valve (Figure 31.7), which needs to be changed by the surgeon or speech therapist. Other valves are available including the Provox and the Groningen valve.

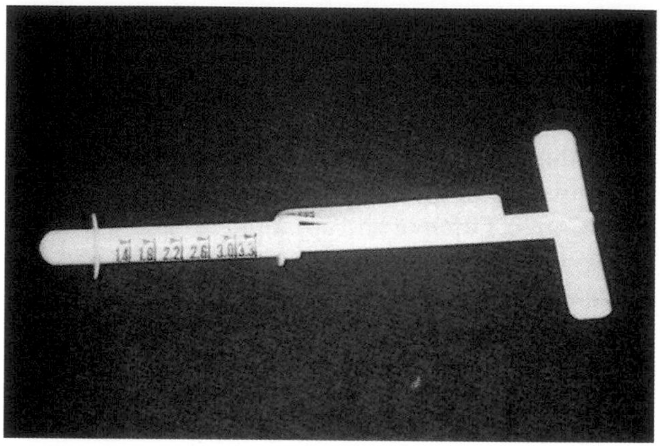

Figure 31.30 Tracheo-oesophageal measurement device.

Standard 'duckbill' valve

The 'duckbill' valve (Figure 31.6) incorporates a slit aperture over its tip that has a higher airway resistance than the low-pressure valve. It is available in lengths of 6–26 mm and has a diameter of 16 Fr. The duckbill valve may be used initially to start prosthetic voice rehabilitation since this is easier to fit and change as well as being more economical. It also allows early identification of patients who have a tendency to develop fungal colonies so that prophylactic use of Nystatin or other antifungal agents can be started.

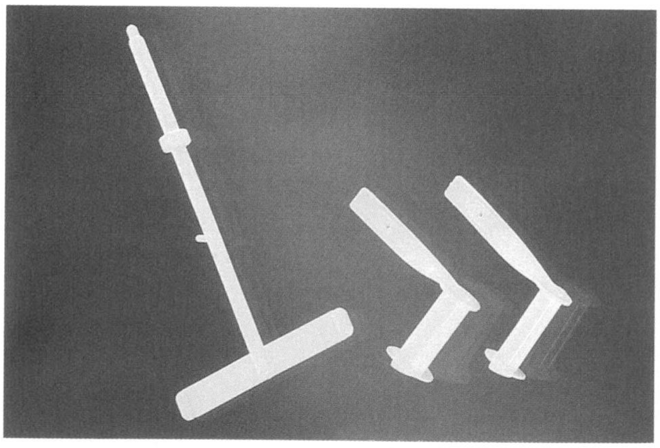

Figure 31.31 Low pressure valves with inserter.

As the postoperative oedema settles over a period of weeks the length of the tract will usually get shorter and a shorter prosthesis can be fitted as necessary. Once the healing process has stabilized a more permanent choice of valve can be made. For longer-term use the duckbill valve is often preferred by patients who have a problem of excessive stomach gas from 'inhaling' air down the oesophagus during speech.

Standard low-pressure valve

The 'low-pressure' valve (Figure 31.31) is used by the majority of patients and is easily inserted using the gelcap technique. It is available in 16- or 20-Fr diameter, the larger ones offering even lower air-resistance so that voice production requires less effort.

Indwelling prosthesis
This valve (Figure 31.7) is more robust and does not need a neck strap for security. It can be cleaned in situ and is ideal for patients who are unable or unwilling to change their valve themselves. It needs to be removed and replaced by a speech therapist or otolaryngologist on average every 6 months.

Insertion of prosthesis

Duckbill
When the length of the tract has been determined and an appropriate valve chosen the dilator is kept in the fistula until the valve is ready for insertion. Once the valve is attached by its strap to the introducer and lubricated the dilator is then removed and is immediately replaced in the tract by the valve. The introducer can then be detached and removed carefully with a twisting movement to avoid pulling out the valve. The valve can be rotated to check that it is fully through the tract before the strap is secured with tape to the skin (Figure 31.20).

Gelcap technique
The fistula is dilated with a 22-Fr dilator, and if the tract is being enlarged from a 16-Fr width it is important to keep a 22-Fr catheter in place for 24 hours so that the tracheo-oesophageal tract is sufficiently dilated to permit atraumatic prosthesis insertion.

The length is measured and the gelcap is fitted over the end of the valve with the special applicator (Figure 31.32). This allows the valve to be easily inserted into the puncture tract atraumatically where it is held in place for 2 minutes, which is usually sufficient time for the gelcap to dissolve. As this happens the retention collar opens up in the lumen of the oesophagus to hold the valve in place. It should be possible to freely rotate the prosthesis to check that it is in the correct position and to confirm this the patient should be able to produce a clear voice with the prosthesis. If the valve is too short the retention collar will have opened up in the tracheo-oesophageal puncture tract and it will not freely rotate and voicing is not possible. A third way of checking that the valve is open is to take a soft tissue AP radiograph of the neck, which will show up the circular radiopaque rim of the retention collar. If the prosthesis is incorrectly placed in the tract the marker will be irregular and appear crinkled. Once the valve is in place the strap is cut and voicing can begin.

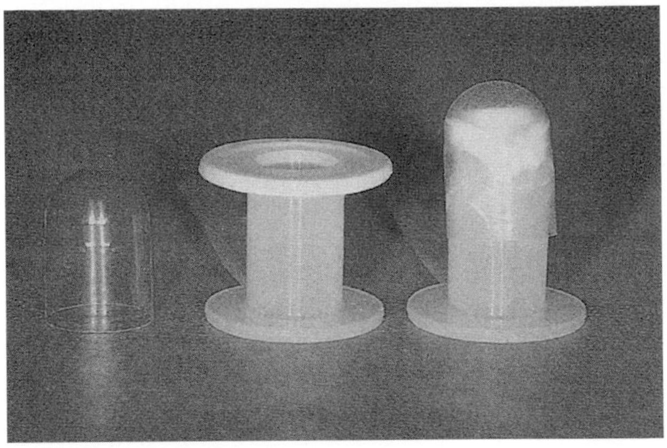

Figure 31.32 Gelcap and indwelling valve.

Tracheostoma valve

Use of the finger or thumb to occlude the stoma in order to speak has been a major limitation with tracheo-oesophageal valves. In 1982 Blom et al[46] developed an external valve which fits over the stoma to enable some laryngectomees to voluntarily close off the stoma on expiration to direct air through the prosthesis permitting 'hands-free' speech. An improved modification was introduced in 1985 (Figures 31.32 and 31.33) that has several

(a)

(b)

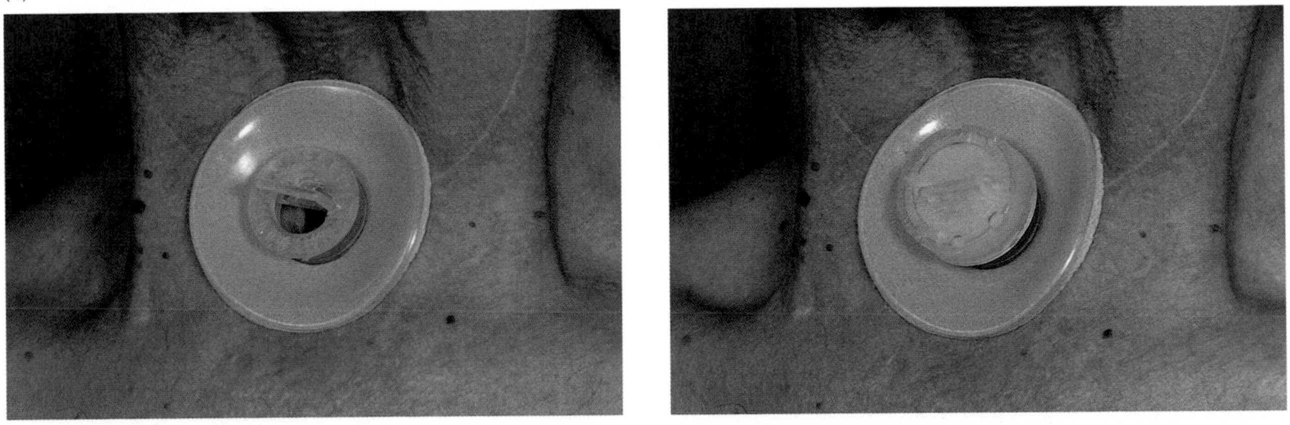

Figure 31.33 (a) Tracheostoma valve in the open position during quiet respiration. (b) Tracheostoma valve in the closed position during speech.

advantages, particularly eliminating the audible closing noise of the original latex version.

The valve consists of two parts, the housing that is stuck onto the peristomal skin with special adhesive and the valve itself that fits into the housing but can easily be removed prior to coughing or for cleaning. The tracheostoma valve gives the patient an additional freedom with speech and with practice can be kept on all day.

Postlaryngectomy airway function

Total laryngectomy not only results in loss of vocal cord function but also has important physiological effects on the remaining airway due to disconnection of the nasal passage from the respiratory tract and loss of all its important functions (Table 31.10). These functional alterations affecting the nasal airway have been the subject of much recent research.

Table 31.10 Functional alterations following laryngectomy

Loss of nasal function
Filtering
Heat and moisture exchange
Olfaction
Airway resistance
Loss of glottic function
Voice
Airway protection
Coughing/straining mechanism

Loss of nasal function

Filtering of inhaled particles that are deposited on the surface mucosa and that are either transported in the mucus towards the oropharynx and swallowed or are removed by blowing the nose or sneezing, is an important function. Following laryngectomy particles and micro-organisms are inhaled directly into the trachea and the patient is therefore much more susceptible to inflammation and chest infections.

The nasal cavity acts as an efficient 'air conditioner' by regulating inhaled air temperature and humidity. This ensures that air reaching the bronchi has a temperature of 34–35°C and a humidity of 90–100% and by the time it reaches the alveoli it is 37°C and fully saturated, which gives optimal conditions for gas exchange. On expiration the heat and moisture are resorbed back through the nasal mucosa and only a small proportion (350 kcal of heat and 250 ml water per day) is lost to the atmosphere.

Following laryngectomy relatively cool and dry air is inhaled into the trachea causing significant changes in the surface mucosa. The mucus becomes thicker and more viscid and ciliary action is impaired resulting in a much less efficient mucus clearing mechanism. Loss of normal glottic closure also makes the coughing mechanism less effective. This can cause much irritation and coughing due to retained secretions as well as increasing the risk of lower respiratory infections by as much as 54%.[47] Sometimes it also has the effect of stimulating excessive mucus production during the first few months after operation. These symptoms usually stabilize after 6 months but are particularly disturbing in patients already suffering from chronic obstructive airway disease (COAD).

In these patients the additional tracheal backpressure associated with producing tracheo-oesophageal voice will increase the chest problems and it may be prudent to delay valve speech until the chest improves. Airway resistance through the pharyngo-oesophageal segment is also typically increased in the early postoperative period due to oedema of the mucosa and pharyngeal muscles.

Some patients are disturbed by the loss of smell but taste is unaffected and strong odours are usually detected.

Maintaining airway resistance in the upper respiratory tract is particularly important during expiration when it helps to keep the lungs expanded and prevent alveolar collapse. Disconnection of the upper airway will also affect the position of the equal pressure point.

Heat and moisture exchangers

A heat and moisture exchanger is a simple and effective method of helping to restore a more normal physiological balance to the lower respiratory tract following laryngectomy. It is fitted over the tracheostome so that all inspired and expired air passes through the device (Figure 31.34) and thus it helps to restore many of the functional aspects of the nasal airway.

During inspiration the cool and dry air is filtered and gains heat and moisture as it passes through

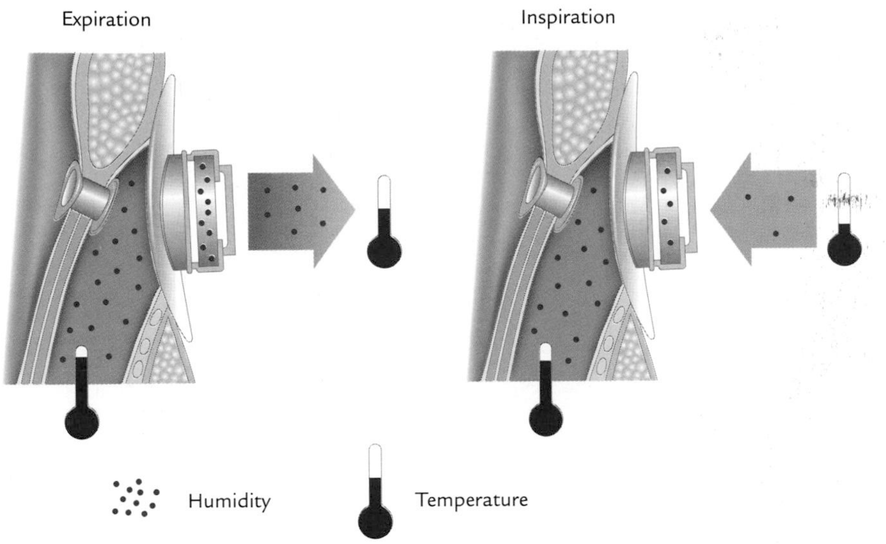

Figure 31.34 Heat and moisture exchanger.

the exchanger significantly reducing the detrimental effect on the lower respiratory tract. It therefore helps to protect the trachea and lungs and to maintain more normal mucociliary function. During expiration air passes through the heat and moisture exchanger where some of the heat is retained and water vapour condenses as the temperature drops. Airway resistance is also increased on expiration which has been shown to improve oxygen saturation in the laryngectomee.[48] Blom has shown that use of heat and moisture exchangers reduces phlegm production by 60% after 1 week of continuous use[49] and a prospective study in 61 patients showed a clear trend towards improvement in respiratory and psychosocial function.[50]

Complications, problems and solutions

Leakage problems

Leakage at the puncture site into the trachea can occur and is usually first noted with fluids, which cause immediate coughing on swallowing. It is important to determine on close examination with a good light whether leakage is through or around the valve since the causes are quite different. Leakage may occur immediately after insertion of the prosthesis or at a later date.

Leakage through the prosthesis

Leakage through the prosthesis may be due to a number of reasons. A faulty or defective valve is usually evident immediately; valve distortion may occur due to excessive compression of the middle part of the prosthesis for example when the tract has just been dilated up from 16-Fr to accommodate a 20-Fr valve, which may result in a slightly gaping flap. It is advisable to dilate established tracts slowly by keeping an intermediate-sized catheter in for several hours or preferably overnight before inserting the larger diameter valve. Distortion may also occur if the valve is not inserted correctly. Small pieces of debris or undissolved gelatin from the gelcap may hold the valve open. The prosthesis should be removed for inspection to make sure it closes completely and then reinserted and checked with a further drink of liquid. Leakage through the prosthesis may be due simply to the natural lifespan of the valve, but this can vary enormously from a few weeks to over a year. Careful cleaning of the delicate valve mechanism either with the prosthesis removed or in situ will prolong its usage. Some patients prefer to remove the prosthesis regularly, perhaps once or twice a week, and replace it with another, alternating the two valves for some considerable time. The spare prosthesis is kept in hydrogen peroxide or other cleaning fluid to prevent accumulation of debris or infecting organisms.

Microbial colonization of the prosthesis, predominantly with *Candida albicans* is the most common cause of leakage through the valve (Figure 31.35) due to distortion of the valve mechanism. Much effort has been devoted to trying to find a prophylactic method of protecting the silicone prosthesis from microbial colonization but so far without success. Routine use of nystatin suspension (500 000 units twice daily swished around the mouth for 4 minutes) is effective in reducing colonization and almost doubling the lifespan of a valve but full compliance is often difficult.

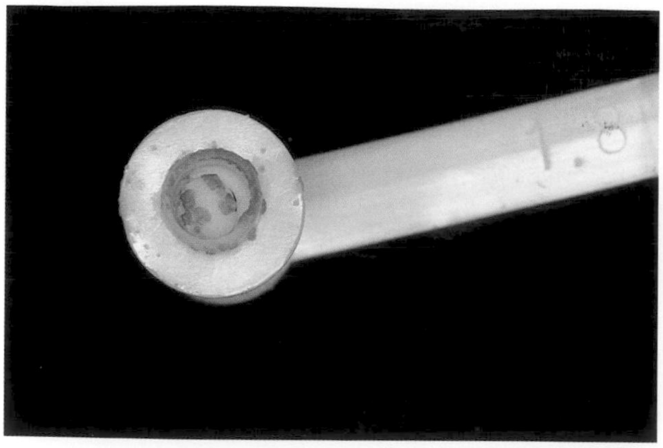

Figure 31.35 *Candida albicans* infestation of the Blom–Singer valve.

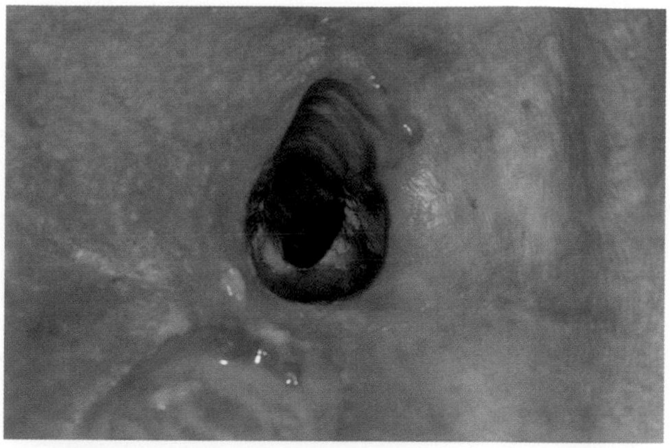

Figure 31.36 The compromised party wall: radionecrosis causing TOP leakage.

Distortion and leakage through the duckbill prosthesis may be due to compression of the protruding valve against the posterior oesophageal wall. This is more frequently seen where there is osteophyte formation indenting the oesophagus so that when the valve moves up and down on normal swallowing the end of the valve is distorted and may leak. This may be relieved by changing to a low profile or indwelling valve.

Leakage around the valve

A satisfactory seal around the tracheo-oesophageal prosthesis depends on the natural elasticity of the surrounding party wall tissues to provide a 'snug' fit around the shaft of the valve. It is also important to have a correct measured length of prosthesis so that the retention collar on the anterior wall of the oesophagus is closely applied to the mucosa to provide a good circumferential seal and to prevent movement or dislodgement. Leakage of liquid around the prosthesis is a difficult problem and may be due to a number of reasons. A prosthesis that is too long acts as a piston and dilates the tracheo-oesophageal tract as the prosthesis moves in and out. It is essential that the length of the tract is correctly measured and an appropriate length prosthesis is selected, particularly during the first 6 months as the postoperative oedema settles and the thickness of the party wall decreases.

The compromised party wall is defined as a tracheo-oesophageal tract which is under 10 mm in length and can be associated with an increased risk of leakage. The tracheo-oesophageal wall may lose its thickness over a period of time due to radionecrosis or ischaemic changes in the muscle (Figure 31.36). This may lead to loss of the muscular tone and contraction around the prosthesis so that leakage can occur. The puncture tract may visibly appear thin with a poor surrounding seal through which leakage is inevitable. Attempts at putting in a larger prosthesis may only result in enlargement of the tract and greater leakage. Insertion of a smaller catheter to encourage contraction of the tract is rarely helpful.

We would recommend that correction of this problem may be accomplished by achieving an exact 'snug' fit between the opposing flanges of the voice prosthesis such that the oesophageal flange acts as a seal against the oesophageal mucosa. Alternatively an injection of collagen into the party wall around the valve may help to eliminate minor leakage problems but this usually only has a temporary benefit.

An effective long-term solution for a thin leaking compromised party wall is reconstruction with a decent layer of muscle, preferably non-irradiated tissue. In some cases an inferiorly based pedicled sternomastoid muscle flap can be sandwiched between the trachea and the oesophagus using a three-layer closure, with successful repuncture of the tract about 3 months later. In some instances where there is significant loss of surface mucosa a pedicled myocutaneous flap may be required to achieve satisfactory closure (Figure 31.37).

Problems with the fistula

Granulations

Some of the early valves had an inferiorly placed portal that frequently became blocked with granulation tissue and which eventually occluded the valve lumen. This has been resolved by elimination of the inferior opening. Occasionally granulations arise around the prosthesis on the posterior wall of the trachea due to irritation if the edge of the valve is digging into the mucosa. This may occur if the prosthesis fits too tightly or is positioned at a slight angle. The granulations can be removed easily and cauterized and the position of the valve corrected. In extreme cases the flange may actually perforate the posterior wall adjacent to the puncture site (Figure 31.38).

(a)

(b)

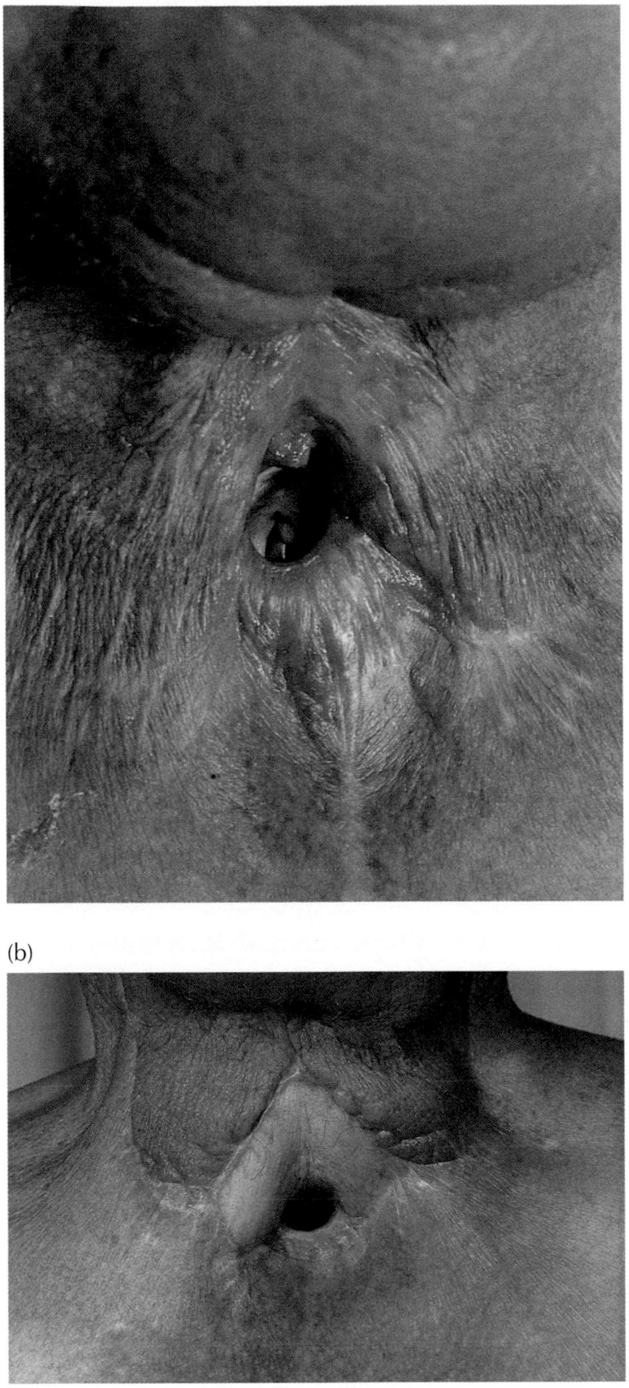

Figure 31.37 (a) A large radionecrotic TOP fistula. (b) Reconstruction with a pectoralis major myocutaneous flap. (c) Good closure 3 months later prior to repuncture.

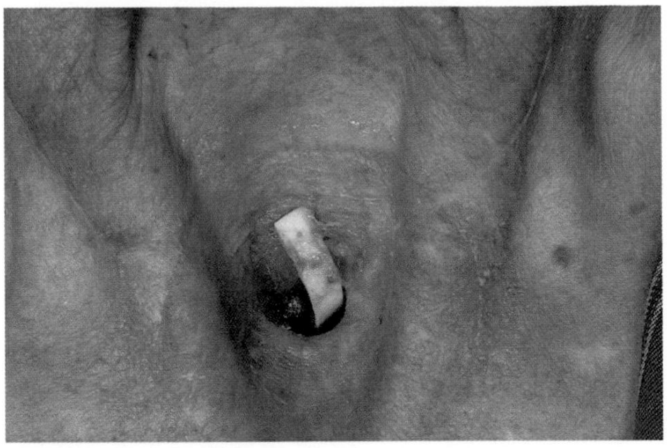

Figure 31.38 Perforation of the party wall due to angulation of the prosthesis.

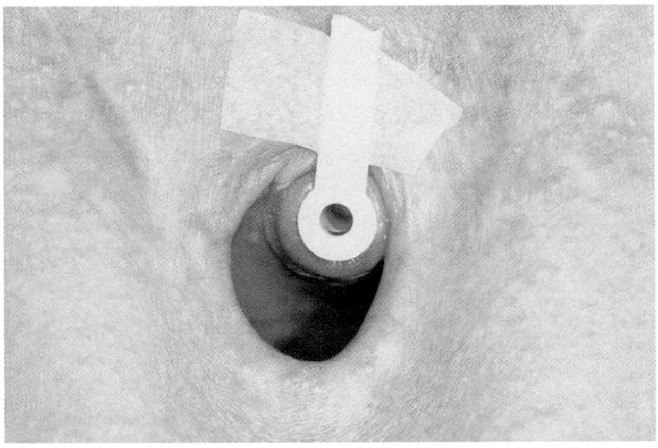

Figure 31.39 Fibrous 'doughnut' around the prosthesis.

Fibrous ring

When the prosthesis has been used for some period of time it may gradually become surrounded by an increasingly thick ring of fibrous tissue that forms a 'doughnut' around the tracheal end of the valve (Figure 31.39). This has the effect of gradually lengthening the tract so that the posterior end of the prosthesis is gradually drawn forwards into the tract. If not recognized, the patient's voice will slowly deteriorate requiring increasing effort and eventually fail completely as the oesophageal end of the fistula closes off. If the ring is not too prominent the tract can be resized and a longer valve fitted. Otherwise excision of the fibrous ring is a straightforward procedure.

Valve extrusion

The prosthesis may become dislodged during cleaning or coughing or for other reasons and if not replaced immediately the tract will close down. A catheter or dilator can be used instead to keep the tract open until the prosthesis can be replaced. Unless the fistula has closed down completely it is usually possible to dilate it up successfully, and for this purpose a serial set of soft urethral catheters is useful. Alternatively progressive dilatation of a stenosed puncture tract may be possible with a set of curved metal male urethral dilators (Figure 31.40), but these should only be used by experienced clinicians. Occasionally valves may need to be retrieved with bronchoscopy if inhaled.

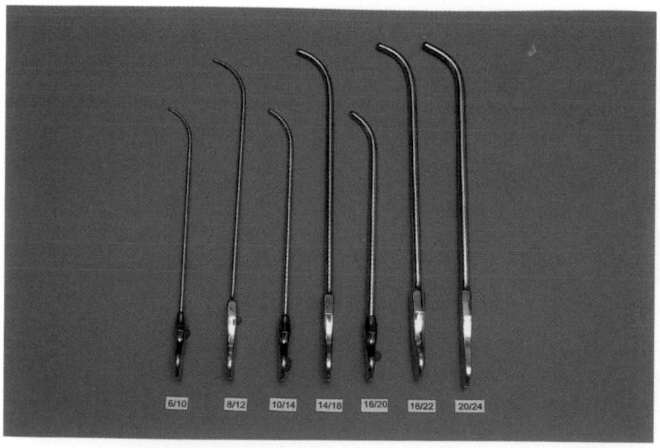

Figure 31.40 Dilating Bougies.

Elective closure of the puncture
Some patients may elect to have the puncture tract closed if they cannot use the prosthesis or because they have acquired good oesophageal voice. Simple removal of the valve will usually allow spontaneous closure over a matter of hours but sometimes with the larger valves or where there is a thin party wall more care needs to be taken and a cuffed tracheostomy tube may be required. A puncture that fails to close over will need to be closed surgically.

Pharyngo-oesophageal problems

Hypertonicity/spasm
Failure to carry out a myotomy at the time of laryngectomy may lead to voice failure because of hypertonicity or spasm of the pharyngeal constrictors. This can be demonstrated on videofluoroscopy as described earlier in the chapter and corrected with botulinum neurotoxin injection or a long myotomy.

Pseudovallecula
This invariably occurs if the pharynx has been sewn up with a vertical closure at laryngectomy. The anterior pouch at the tongue base and the coronal fibrous web behind it may cause dysphagia with the patient having to make several swallowing attempts to get food down through the narrowed opening into the hypopharynx. This shows up well on videofluoroscopy (Figure 31.12). Patients may also complain of regurgitating small amounts of undigested food. Correction is easily achieved by endoscopic division of the web using a similar technique to excision of the cricopharyngeal bar in a pharyngeal pouch.

Stenosis
This may occur if insufficient mucosa/skin has been used for reconstruction of the hypopharynx or at the anastomotic site following total pharyngolaryngectomy. It may also develop slowly after jejunum transposition due to ischaemic contracture if the mesenteric blood supply is compromised.[40] Dilatation may be sufficient if the narrowing is not severe but reconstruction of the pharynx may be necessary.

Hypotonic voice
A reconstructed hypopharynx typically produces a hypotonic voice due to loss or absence of muscular tone, which can be shown on videofluoroscopy. Voice quality may be improved using digital pressure over the pharynx on the anterior neck.

Excessive flatulence
Excessive collection of air in the stomach is a disturbing and sometimes painful problem in tracheo-oesophageal voice users and may be due to several different causes. During normal respiration oesophageal pressure is negative during inspiration; this may cause slight opening of the valve and small amounts of air may be sucked into the oesophagus and swallowed into the stomach. Replacement of the prosthesis with a higher resistance duckbill valve may provide a solution. In a similar way, if the PE segment is hypotonic (Figure 31.11) excessive air ingestion may occur from the mouth during normal inspiration due to the negative oesophageal pressure. Wearing an elastic band comfortably tight around the neck above the stoma may help to minimize air ingestion and may also improve voice quality. In patients with a hypertonic PE segment or stricture excessive expiratory effort is needed to force air through the vocal tract and some air may be driven in a reverse direction down into the stomach. Surgical correction is required with constrictor myotomy or reconstruction. Patients who talk excessively during a meal may swallow large amounts of air, but usually this habit is tempered with experience! The presence of a hiatus hernia will increase the likelihood of air ingestion.

Some patients with increased flatulence also experience hyperacidity, which can be treated with suitable antacids or proton pump inhibitors. Nevertheless the occasional patient does request removal of the voice prosthesis due to gastric problems.

Stoma problems

Macrostomia
Occasionally the tracheostoma opening is too large for the patient to achieve airtight finger or thumb occlusion during speech. Use of a silicone laryngectomy tube may help or the patient may find that a tracheostoma valve housing attached to the peristomal skin will allow better occlusion or preferably

use of the hands-free stoma valve. Surgical reduction of the stoma is rarely needed.

Microstomia

Until the peristomal scar tissue has stabilized after a few months following laryngectomy it has a natural tendency to contract and most patients will need to wear a laryngectomy tube or button to prevent stenosis. They may also feel more comfortable and 'safer' wearing something, particularly at night. If the stoma size reduces to less than 2 cm it becomes difficult to manage a prosthesis and under 1 cm breathing becomes difficult. The stoma can usually be dilated with buttons or laryngectomy tubes but if the stenosis is well established it may be necessary to carry out a stomaplasty. The preferred technique is bilateral Y–V advancements with excision of scar tissue as necessary.

Stoma recession

Sometimes the trachea has to be resected low down in order to achieve adequate tumour clearance but if the rim of the trachea is not sutured to the medial tendonous margins of the sternomastoid muscles it will recede into the suprasternal notch. This may cause difficulty with stoma occlusion, particularly if an outer housing and hands-free valve is required. Following standard laryngectomy the trachea should not be transected too low and should lie comfortably without tension in the same plane as the skin over the sternomastoid muscles. Vicryl sutures from the trachea to the adjacent muscle tendon may help to stabilize its position.

For recessed stomas that are a problem we would advocate either use of a custom-made housing[51] or surgical correction. In the latter situation we would advocate bringing the trachea up to the skin by suturing its margins to the sternomastoid as described above rather than creating a wider recession and weakening of the sternomastoids by dividing their tendons.

Stomal ulceration

Excessive trauma on finger occlusion to the margins of the stoma can cause ulceration of the skin which may look like stomal recurrence (Figure 31.41). It should be remembered that the peristomal skin is relatively insensate due to division of the supraclavicular nerves in contrast to the very sensitive tracheal mucosa whose inferiorly based innervation is usually unaffected by laryngectomy.

Excessive stomal mucus

During the first 6 months or so following laryngectomy excessive mucus discharge and coughing can be a problem as outlined above under discussion of heat and moisture exchangers.

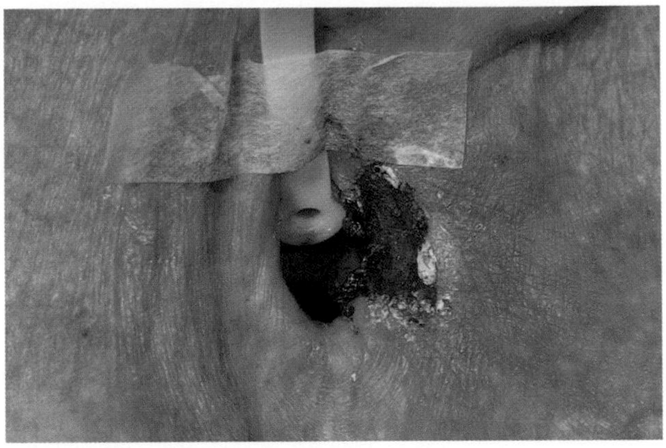

Figure 31.41 Stomal ulceration.

Poor tracheostoma valve seal

Use of the 'hands-free' tracheostoma valve is desirable for optimal functional rehabilitation but many patients find it difficult to use because of a poor airtight seal around the stoma. Meticulous attention must be given to the technique of cleaning the skin and fitting the valve housing to minimize problems. Stomal recession or an awkward skin contour following flap reconstruction can increase the risk of air leakage and a custom-made housing[51] may be the best solution. Excessive expiratory effort on vocalizing due to a hypertonic or spastic PE segment or to a higher pressure prosthesis will also increase backpressure and the probability of air leakage.

Progress and future developments

Progress in voice rehabilitation following total laryngectomy over the last 20 years has made an enormous difference in the whole concept of management of laryngeal cancer and, most importantly, to our patients. Until the 1980s total laryngectomy was regarded as a dreadful but often life-saving procedure to which there was little alternative as a last resort. At that time survival at any cost in terms of quality of life was paramount and many laryngectomees were forced into an isolated life as a mute and dysphagic recluse. Most attempts at voice restoration produced inconsistent results and often techniques were laborious, costly and ineffective, particularly when carried out as a salvage procedure after failed radiotherapy.

The last two decades have witnessed great advances in many aspects of health and in particular care of cancer patients. Quality of life and ethical issues, audit and objective assessment have assumed much greater importance as well as survival. Within this broader context and background the development of the tracheo-oesophageal puncture and voice prosthesis resulting from the dedicated work and vision of a few pioneers has provided us with a simple and consistent method of voice restoration for our patients. It is also just as reliable in patients who have had radical irradiation, unlike many other direct shunt procedures.

We have also learned a great deal about alaryngeal voice production, the significance of tonicity and the importance of the pharyngo-oesophageal segment. Developments in reconstructive surgery have given us a much safer and more effective choice of flaps for restoring normal swallowing.

The permanent stoma remains the one stigma that patients find difficult to accept but it is unlikely that surgical restoration of a safe and competent oronasotracheal airway is compatible with good phonation. Laryngeal transplantation has been successfully tried following trauma but it may be difficult to obtain safe consistent results in cancer patients following irradiation. There is also concern about tumour recurrence and second primaries developing in susceptible patients on immunosuppressive treatment. Greater knowledge of neurotaxis may help us to direct new innervation more accurately to adductors and abductors in a transplanted larynx. The results of reimplanting the recurrent and superior laryngeal nerves at the time of laryngectomy, as described earlier in this chapter, seem to be promising but adequate objective assessment is difficult.

With our current state of knowledge prosthetic voice restoration is setting the 'gold-standard' for rehabilitation of laryngectomees. Ideally, however, it would be far better to have a simple and reliable technique that did not require a prosthesis and was equally as effective following irradiation. The problems of continual valve maintenance, prophylaxis against candida, expert supervision and costs of replacement are disadvantages.

The importance of adequate voice rehabilitation is even greater in third-world countries where indiscriminate promotion of tobacco usage and smoking, poor hygiene and adverse environmental conditions have made laryngeal and other head and neck cancers much more common. Survival rates, if available, are poor due to late presentation, lack of expert surgical and radiotherapy treatment and a wide range of inadequate healthcare facilities. Indeed, many patients are not even offered the chance of curative treatment. For those who undergo and survive laryngectomy many are illiterate and the isolation is far more profound if they cannot communicate even by writing. Successful tracheo-oesophageal voice restoration in these patients is very rewarding but the cost and other problems associated with maintaining a prosthesis are often prohibitive.

REFERENCES

1. Steiner W, Aurbach G, Ambrosch P. Minimally invasive therapy in otolaryngology and head and neck surgery. *Minim Invasive Ther Allied Technol* 1991; **1**: 57–70.
2. Baugh RF, Lewin JS, Baker SR. Vocal rehabilitation of tracheo-oesophageal speech failures. *Head Neck* 1990; **12**: 69–73.
3. Gussenbauer C. Ueber cie Erste Durch Th. Billroth Am Menschen Ausgefuhrte Kehlkopf-Exstirpation Und die Anwendung Eines Kunstlichen Kehlkopfes. *Archiv fur Klinische Chirurgie* 1874; **17**: 334–356.
4. Edels Y. Pseudo voice, its theory and practice. In: Edels Y (ed.) *Laryngectomy: Diagnosis to Rehabilitation.* Beckenham: Croom-Helm, 1983; 117.
5. Taub S, Spiro RH. Vocal rehabilitation of laryngectomees: preliminary report of a new technique. *Am J Surg* 1972; **124**: 87–90.
6. Singer MI, Blom ED. An endoscopic technique for restoration of voice after laryngectomy. *Ann Otol Rhinol Laryngol* 1980; **89**: 529–533.
7. Blom ED. Evolution of tracheoesophageal voice prostheses. In: Blom ED, Singer MI, Hamaker RC (eds). *Tracheoesophageal Voice Restoration Following Total Laryngectomy.* San Diego: Singular Publishing Group, 1998; 1–8.
8. Blom ED, Singer MI, Hamaker RC. An improved esophageal insufflation test. *Arch Otolaryngol* 1985; **111**: 211–212.
9. Hamaker RC, Singer MI, Blom ED, Daniels HA. Primary voice restoration at laryngectomy. *Arch Otolaryngol* 1985; **111**: 182–186.
10. Johnson JT, Casper J, Lesswing NJ. Toward the total rehabilitation of the alaryngeal patient. *Laryngoscope* 1979, **89**: 1813–1819.
11. Duguay M. Special problems of alaryngeal speakers. In: Keith RL, Darley FL (eds) *Laryngectomee Rehabilitation* London: College Hill Press, 1979; 107–142.
12. Perry A, Edels Y. Recent advances in the assessment of failed oesophageal speakers. *Br J Disord Commun* 1985; **20**: 229–236.

13. Simpson IC, Smith JS, Gordon T. Laryngectomy: the influence of muscle reconstruction on the mechanism of oesophageal voice production. *J Laryngol Otol* 1972; **86**: 960–990.
14. McIvor J, Evans PF, Perry A, Cheesman AD. Radiological assessment of post-laryngectomy speech. *Clin Radiol* 1990; **41**: 312–316.
15. Perry A. Preoperative tracheoesophageal voice restoration assessment and selection criteria. In: Blom ED, Singer MI, Hamaker RC (eds). *Tracheoesophageal Voice Restoration Following Total Laryngectomy.* San Diego: Singular Publishing Group, 1998; 9–18.
16. Cheesman AD, Knight J, McIvor J, Perry A. Tracheo-oesophageal 'puncture speech': an assessment technique for failed oesophageal speakers. *J Laryngol Otol* 1986; **100**: 191–199.
17. Hilgers FJM, Aaronson NK, Ackerstaff AH et al. The influence of a heat and moisture exchanger (HME) on the respiratory symptoms after total laryngectomy. *Clin Otolaryngol* 1991; **16**: 152–156.
18. Wilson PS, Bruce-Lockhart FJ, Johnson AP, Rhys Evans PH. Speech restoration following total laryngo-pharyngectomy with free jejunal repair. *Clin Otolaryngol* 1993; **19**: 145–148.
19. Garth RJN, McRae A, Rhys Evans PH. Tracheo-oesophageal puncture: a review of problems and complications. *J Laryngol Otol* 1991; **105**: 750–754.
20. Blom ED. Tracheoesophageal valves: problems, solutions and directions for the future. *Head Neck Surg* **2 (Suppl.)**: S142–S145.
21. Trudeau MD, Schuller DE, Hall DA. The effects of radiation on tracheo-oesophageal puncture. *Arch Otolaryngol* **115**: 1116–1117.
22. Freeman SB, Hamaker RC. Tracheoesophageal voice restoration at time of laryngectomy. In: Blom ED, Singer MI, Hamaker RC (eds). *Tracheoesophageal Voice Restoration Following Total Laryngectomy.* San Diego: Singular Publishing Group, 1998; 19–25.
23. van Lith-Bijl JT, Zijlstra RJ, Nahieu HS et al. A manometric study of the pharyngo-oesophageal segment during total laryngectomy. *Proceedings of the International Voice Restoration Meeting, London.*
24. Singer MI, Blom ED. Pharyngeal plexus neurectomy for alaryngeal speech rehabilitation. *Laryngoscope* 1986; **961**: 50–53.
25. Hoffman HT, Fischer H, Vandemark D et al. Botulinum neurotoxin injection after total laryngectomy. *Head Neck* 1997; **19**: 92–97.
26. Singer MI, Blom ED, Hamaker RC. Further experience with voice restoration after total laryngectomy. *Ann Otol Rhinol Laryngol* 1981; **90**: 498–502.
27. Sisson GA, Hurst PS, Goldman ME. Prosthetic devices in neoglottic surgery. *Ear Nose Throat J* 1981; **60**: 55–61.
28. Silver FM, Gluckman JL, Donegan JO. Operative complications of tracheo-oesophageal puncture. *Laryngoscope* 1985; **95**: 1360–1362.
29. Ward PH, Andrews JC, Mickel RA et al. Complications of medical and surgical approaches to voice restoration after total laryngectomy. *Head Neck Surg* 1988; **10**: 124–128.
30. Rhys Evans PH. Tracheo-oesophageal puncture without tears: the forceps technique. *J Laryngol Otol* 1991; **105**: 748–749.
31. Hamaker RC, Cheesman AD. Surgical management of pharyngeal constrictor muscle hypertonicity. In: Blom ED, Singer MI, Hamaker RC (eds). *Tracheoesophageal Voice Restoration Following Total Laryngectomy.* San Diego: Singular Publishing Group, 1998.
32. Hosni AA, Rhys Evans PH. Cervical osteomyelitis with cord compression complicating pharyngeal myotomy. *J Laryngol Otol* 1994; **108**: 511–513.
33. Ariyan S. The pectoralis major myocutaneous flap. A versatile flap for reconstruction in the head and neck. *Plast Reconstr Surg* 1979; **63**: 73–81.
34. Rhys Evans PH, Das Gupta AR. The use of the pectoralis major myocutaneous flap for one stage reconstruction of the base of the tongue. *J Laryngol Otol* 1981; **95**; 809–816.
35. Davis JP, Nield DV, Garth RJN et al. The latissimus dorsi flap in head and neck surgery. *Clin Otolaryngol* 1992; **17**: 487–490.
36. Huntley TC, Borrowdale RW. Tracheoesophageal voice restoration following laryngopharyngectomy and laryngopharyngoesophagectomy. In: Blom ED, Singer MI, Hamaker RC (eds). *Tracheoesophageal Voice Restoration Following Total Laryngectomy.* San Diego: Singular Publishing Group, 1998.
37. Shangold LM, Urken ML, Lawson W (1991) Jejunal transplantation for pharyngoesophageal reconstruction. *Otolaryngol Clin North Am* 1991; **24**: 1321–1342.
38. Biel MA, Maisel RH (1992) Postoperative radiation-associated changes in free jejunal autographs. *Arch Otolaryngol Head Neck Surg* 1992; **118**: 1037–1041.
39. Salamoun W, Swartz WM, Johnson JT et al. Free jejunal transfer for reconstruction of the laryngopharynx. *Otolaryngol Head Neck Surg* 1987; **96**: 149–150.
40. Wilson PS, Bruce-Lockhart FJ, Johnson AP, Rhys Evans PH. Speech restoration following total pharyngolaryngectomy with free jejunal repair. *Clin Otolaryngol* 1994; **19**: 145–148.
41. Ong GB, Lee TC. Pharyngogastric anastomosis after oesophagopharyngectomy for carcinoma of the hypopharynx and cervical oesophagus. *Br J Surg* 1960; **48**: 193–200.
42. Harrison DFN, Thompson AE. Pharyngolaryngoesophagectomy with pharyngogastric anastomosis for cancer of the hypopharynx; review of 101 operations. *Head Neck Surgery* 1986; **8**: 418.
43. Anthony JP, Singer MI, Mathes SJ. Pharyngoesophageal reconstruction using the tubed radial forearm flap. *Clin Plast Surg* 1994; **21**: 137–147.
44. Wei WK, Lam KH, Choi S, Wong J. Late problems after pharyngogastric anastomosis for cancer of the larynx and hypopharynx. *Am J Surg* 1984; **148**: 509–512.
45. de Vries EJ, Stein DW, Johnson JT et al. Hypopharyngeal reconstruction: a comparison of two alternatives. *Laryngoscope* 1989; **99**: 614–617.
46. Blom ED, Singer MI, Hamaker RC. Tracheostoma valve for post laryngectomy voice rehabilitation. *Ann Otol Rhinol Laryngol* 1982; **91**: 576–578.

47. Jay S, Ruddy J, Cullen RJ. Laryngectomy: the patient's view. *J Laryngol Otol* 1991; **105**: 934–938.
48. McRae D, Young P, Hamilton J, Jones A. Raising airway resistance in laryngectomees increases tissue oxygen saturation. *Clin Otolaryngol* 1996; **21**: 366–368.
49. Blom ED. Laboratory and clinical investigation of post laryngectomy airway humidification and filtration. *Proceedings of the 1st EGFL Conference and 5th International Congress on Surgical and Prosthetic Voice Restoration after Total Laryngectomy*, Grado, Italy.
50. Ackerstaff A, Hilgers F, Aaronson N et al. Improvements in respiratory and psychosocial functioning following total laryngectomy by use of heat and moisture exchanger. *Ann Otol Rhinol Laryngol* 1993; **102**: 878–883.
51. Matai V, Jones S, Appleton J et al. Customised tracheostoma valve housing. *Proceedings of the European Group on Functional Voice Restoration Meeting*, Amsterdam, 2001.

32 Future developments in head and neck cancer therapy

Irvin Pathak, Camilla MA Carroll and Patrick J Gullane

Introduction

The field of head and neck surgery has undergone remarkable changes over the last 20 years. There have been refinements in surgical approaches to malignant cervical adenopathy, laryngeal cancer and skull-base malignancy. With the advent and popularization of free tissue transfer, head and neck reconstruction has been revolutionized. Along with progress in surgical techniques have come advances in imaging, radiotherapy and molecular biology. Despite this progress, cancer recurrence and mortality rates for many sites in the head and neck remain unchanged. The head and neck continues to be a challenging area to reconstruct with functional outcomes remaining poor in many situations. The future remains full of challenge and promise for both the patients and professionals struggling with cancer of the head and neck.

The future of head and neck oncology will be influenced not only by surgical and chemoradiotherapeutic innovation but also by endeavours in many other disciplines. These will include molecular biology, epidemiology and the social sciences.

Table 32.1 Number of manufactured cigarettes consumed per day per adult (age 15 years or over) in economically developed countries

	1945	1965	1985
Australia	1.6	7.3	6.3
Belgium	1.1	5.4	5.4
Canada	4.5	9.0	8.1
Denmark	1.1	4.1	5.1
Finland	2.1	5.4	4.7
France	1.2	4.1	6.0
Germany	0.7	5.8	6.4
Greece	2.3	5.3	9.7
Ireland	4.3	7.4	6.8
Israel	—	5.4	6.4
Italy	1.8	4.3	6.3
Japan	0.9	6.4	9.0
New Zealand	2.7	6.3	6.3
Norway	0.6	1.4	1.9
Portugal	1.2	3.2	4.8
Spain	1.3	4.8	7.4
Sweden	1.3	3.7	4.5
Switzerland	3.2	8.5	8.1
UK	7.1	7.4	5.9
USA	7.0	10.5	8.7

Data taken from Wald and Hackshaw.[1]

Primary prevention of head and neck malignancy

There are one billion smokers in the world today. Smoking increased between 1945 and 1965 in all countries and remained stable in most countries from 1965 to 1985. Since 1985, consumption has decreased in some countries (Table 32.1). In the UK, the total number of cigarettes sold declined from 98 billion in 1985 to 93 billion in 1993.[1] Along with this decrease in consumption in some developed nations has been the alarming increase in consumption in many developing countries. The Food and Agricultural Organization of the United Nations estimates that between the years 1986 and 2000, tobacco consumption will have decreased by 11% in developed countries but increased by 10% in developing countries. If present trends continue, the annual death rate from tobacco consumption will rise from the current 3 million to 10 million by 2025, with 7 million of these being in the developing nations. Two million will be in China alone. There are many reasons for this increase in smoking in the Third World, including the increase of population, ignorance of the health risks of smoking and the intensive and ruthless marketing by multinational tobacco companies.[2] The development of national tobacco control policies in Third World countries is essential in order to stem the tide of increased tobacco consumption.

In developed countries, smoking is increasing amongst adolescents. Preventing people from beginning smoking is a major health priority. These efforts must focus on the young, as 88% of smokers start by age 18.[3] Unfortunately, current strategies such as enforcement of tobacco sales laws have not been shown to be effective while marketing strategies of tobacco companies continue to target young people.[4]

Secondary prevention of head and neck malignancy

The risk of developing a second primary cancer after squamous cell cancer of the upper aerodigestive tract is 4% per year. These new cancers are about equally divided into cancers of the lungs, oesophagus, and other areas of the mouth and throat.[5] An effective intervention to decrease the incidence of second primaries in this setting would have a major impact on cancer control.

Potentially effective chemopreventative agents can be classified according to mechanism. These include substances with carcinogen-blocking activities, antioxidants and substances with antiproliferative activity.[6]

Retinoids are synthetic analogues of vitamin A (Figure 32.1). 13-*cis* retinoic acid (13cRA) is the primary retinoid that is being tested in cancer prevention trials at present. Retinoids have undergone study in the setting of premalignant and malignant lesions of the upper aerodigestive tract. Response rates of premalignant lesions to 13cRA have been reported to be as high as 67% in randomized studies.[7] Fenretinide is another retinoid under study for oral premalignant lesions in a randomized trial at the Milan Cancer Institute.[8] 13cRA has also been studied in the prevention of second primary cancers. Hong et al[9] in a randomized trial showed that 13cRA treated patients had a significantly reduced incidence of second malignancies as compared to placebo. Based on this trial, a large scale phase III NCI trial is now ongoing.[10] Unfortunately, 13cRA does have side-effects, which limit its tolerance especially at high doses, such as skin dryness, cheilitis, conjunctivitis, and hypertriglyceridemia.

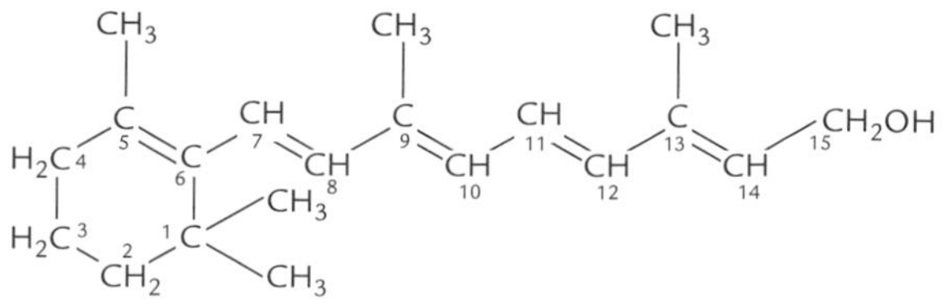

Retinol (vitamin A_1)

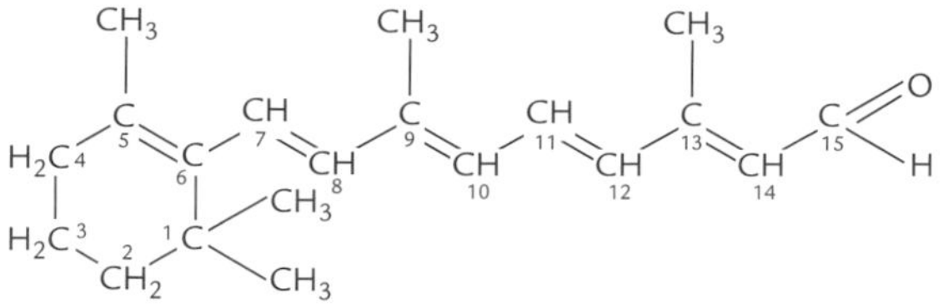

Retinal

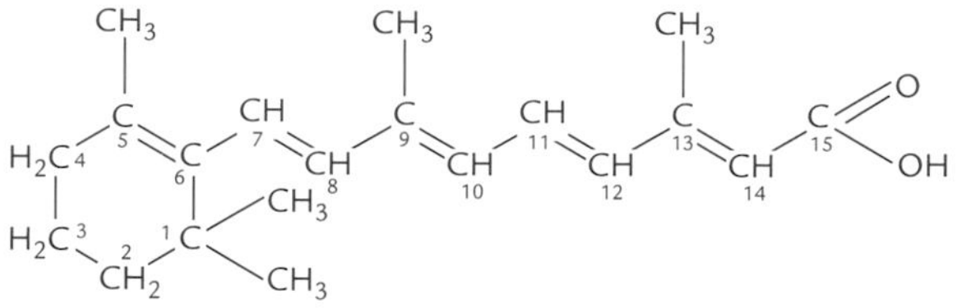

Retinoic acid

Figure 32.1 Molecular structure of vitamin A and two related substances.

As with retinoids, the value of beta-carotene in secondary prevention remains undefined. Efficacy of beta-carotene has not been shown in this setting and there have been reports of increase in lung cancer incidence in patients on beta-carotene.[11]

There are several ongoing trials on chemoprevention in head and neck cancer. The conclusions of these studies may bring chemopreventative agents such as 13-*cis* retinoic acid into common usage for the prevention of second primary cancers.

Imaging in head and neck cancer

Rapid advances in imaging have taken place over the last decade and are sure to continue in the foreseeable future. Most of these advances have been technical in nature. There will also continue to be further application of imaging technology in novel therapeutic approaches.

Magnetic resonance imaging

Magnetic resonance imaging has increased in speed and spatial resolution. Further technologic advances have been applied to emphasize differences between tumour and normal tissue. Fast spin echo imaging is an electronic advance that allows many measurements to be taken simultaneously creating an image much faster than conventional spin echo images. There is less artefact from motion resulting in a higher signal and an improved image. The image is identical to a conventional image except that fat is bright on T2 as opposed to being dark on a conventional spin echo image. Fat suppression can be added to return the fat to low signal. This technique has been shown to improve tissue contrast and produce a 50% saving in time over conventional techniques.[12]

Fat suppression is helpful in tumour/fat interfaces. Fat is bright on T1-weighted images and on fast spin echo T2 images. This interferes with differentiation from tumours with similar signal characteristics such as squamous cell cancer. Radiofrequency prepulses are applied, which makes the fat stimulate early. When the image is acquired, the fat is out of synch and the signal is not seen. Echo planar imaging is a method that allows production of an image by changing the gradients while the image is being acquired. This allows rapid data acquisition and the minimization of movement artefact.[13]

MR angiography

MR angiography is a non-invasive technique used to depict blood vessels in a similar format to a conventional angiogram. On conventional MR images, moving blood results in an absence of signal termed 'flow void'. This is due to the rapid, random movement of dipoles within the blood stream. This allows the signals from one dipole to cancel out those signals from other dipoles, resulting in a nil total signal. MR angiography must employ radiofrequency pulse sequences that produce signal from flowing blood. Time of flight MR angiography refers to the motion of blood in and out of the plane of section. Stationary tissues remaining in the plane of section can become saturated by radiofrequency signals and produce no signal. Blood from outside of this plane is relatively unaffected by the radiofrequency pulses and remains magnetized. Upon entering the plane, the magnetized blood produces an intense signal. In phase contrast angiography, two images are acquired. Each image has a field gradient of equal magnitude but opposite polarity. This affects the stationary tissues but the protons in flowing blood are not at the same position for both gradient pulses, and a net non zero phase shift is produced. Both of the images are digitally subtracted by the computer, producing an image of flowing blood only. These techniques allow evaluation of the vasculature of the head and neck including patency, flow direction and velocity,[14] in a non invasive fashion.

Image-guided therapy

An expanded role for imaging technology can be foreseen not only in diagnostic, but also therapeutic applications. Image guidance can improve the delivery of radiation by brachytherapy for the treatment of head and neck malignancy. CT-guided brachytherapy uses techniques similar to CT-guided tissue biopsy. Brachytherapy traditionally entails the placement of permanent radioactive sources or afterloading catheters by visual inspection. For deep-seated tumours this requires an operative intervention. CT-guided brachytherapy can access these deep-seated tumours in a minimally invasive fashion and can also aid in the accurate placement of the radiation source into the lesion. The availability of real-time MRI guidance may offer advantages over CT guidance.[15] Real-time ultrasonography and MRI has also been used to guide interstitial placement of laser fibreoptics for palliation of far advanced cancer of the head and neck. In this technique, an angiocatheter is placed into the centre of the tumour under ultrasound guidance. The neodynium:yttrium-aluminum garnet fibre is then passed down the angiocatheter and activated to produce a zone of vapourization within the tumour mass.[16] This method has been further refined with the use of real-time MRI (Figure 32.2).[17]

Positron emission tomography

Positron emission tomography (PET) is a functional imaging technique that provides information about tissue metabolism. Radiolabelled 18F-fluoro-2-deoxyglucose (FDG) administration allows the

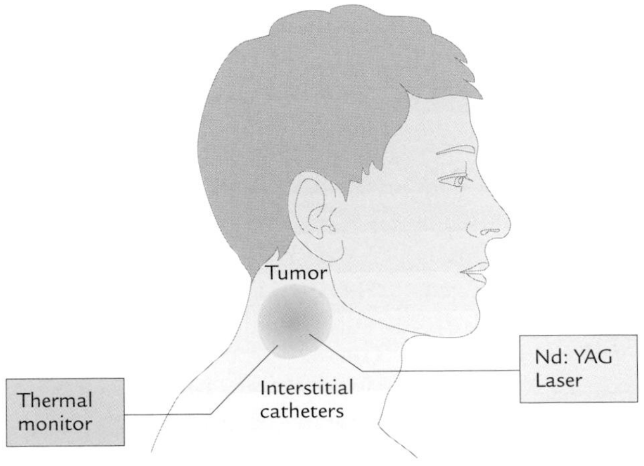

Figure 32.2 Treatment design of interstitial laser therapy guided by MRI.[17]

characterization of glucose metabolism within cells. FDG decays with the emission of positively charged particles. These particles interact with electrons to produce two photons in the form of gamma rays. These two photons are emitted at 180 degrees apart. The simultaneous detection of two such photons allows the construction of an image based on metabolism. Neoplastic cells have a higher glucose utilization than normal tissues and rely primarily upon anaerobic glycolysis with a build-up of glucose-6-phosphate. FDG becomes trapped in malignant tissue in the form of 2-deoxyglucose-6-phosphate. PET-FDG has been reported to be effective in central nervous system neoplasms, breast, lung and colorectal cancer. PET scanning has been found to be more sensitive in the detection of head and neck cancer than both CT and MRI. However, its spatial resolution is poor compared to both CT and MRI.[18,19] PET scanning has also been used to distinguish viable tumours from non-viable tissue after a full course of radiotherapy. This would be useful in planning the need for further treatment.[20]

Tumour markers and angiogenesis

Tumour markers

Biologic markers for head and neck cancer include measures of host response, tumour phenotypic characteristics and genetic alterations. Markers may aid in the early detection of malignancy or premalignancy and afford a greater chance at curability. Biomarkers may also help predict response to therapy and thus guide therapeutic decision making. The future of biologic markers will lie not only in the development of new markers but also in the appropriate application of these markers in the diagnosis and treatment of head and neck cancer.

Markers of carcinogen exposure identify individuals at risk for development of cancer by quantitating exposure to carcinogens. The marker of exposure that has received the most attention is DNA adduct quantitation. Carcinogen intermediates have the ability to bind to host DNA. The polycyclic aromatic hydrocarbons such as benzo(a)pyrene are the carcinogens that have been the best studied of the carcinogens linked to tobacco. These adducts of carcinogen intermediates to DNA can be assayed. Assays include immunohistochemistry and the 32P-postlabelling assay. The 32P-postlabelling assay is able to detect one adduct per 10^{10} nucleotides. Immunoassays are relatively easy to perform but are limited by their poor sensitivity and specificity. The 32P-postlabelling assay is more sensitive and specific but does not lend itself to large scale testing as it is technically complex and costly to perform.[21] Studies using 32P-postlabelling of oral mucosal epithelium have been able to correlate degree of carcinogen exposure, in this case to tobacco, and degree of DNA adduct elevation.[22] The degree to which adduct levels correlate with cancer risk has not been established. Cancer risk is dependent upon carcinogen exposure as well as individual susceptibility. Although tobacco and alcohol use are highly prevalent, the incidence of head and neck cancer is relatively low. Intrinsic host factors must have an impact upon carcinogenesis. This is particularly evident in the subgroup of patients with squamous cell cancer of the head and neck who are non-smokers. Biomarkers of damage may be the most rewarding area to pursue as identification of early malignant or premalignant changes may be able to direct therapy at stages of disease with very high curability. These markers include genetic mutations of P53 or *ras* which can be detected using molecular biology techniques.

Native cellular fluorescence or autofluorescence is the ability of cells to absorb and then emit characteristic wavelengths of light. The molecules that produce this phenomenon include NADH, collagen and riboflavin.[23] Results of various sites of epithelial malignancy have consistently shown that neoplastic tissue has a distinct spectral pattern from normal tissue. This technique has been used to identify preneoplastic lesions in the tracheobronchial tree that would appear normal to white light examination.[23]

Angiogenesis

This is the process by which new blood vessels are produced in the host. In 1972 Folkman stated that 'once tumour take has occurred, every increase in tumour cell population must be preceded by an increase in new capillaries that converge upon the tumour' (Figure 32.3).[24,25] The formation of new blood vessels is dependent upon migration and proliferation of endothelial cells, interactions with extracellular matrix and soluble growth factors. Angiogenic molecules act by stimulating endothelial cell migration and division. Several angiogenic molecules have been isolated. The 14-kilodalton polypeptide angiogenin has been isolated from various solid tumours and is a potent stimulator of angiogenesis on chick embryo chorioallantoic membrane (CAM). Other factors that have been identified include acidic and basic fibroblast growth factor, transforming growth factor-alpha, tumour necrosis factor, platelet-derived endothelial cell growth factor and angiotropin. Tumour-induced angiogenesis begins with the dissolution of the native vessel basement membrane due to production

Normal epithelium

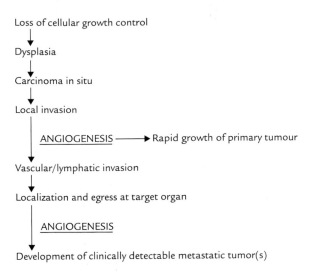

Loss of cellular growth control
↓
Dysplasia
↓
Carcinoma in situ
↓
Local invasion
↓ ANGIOGENESIS → Rapid growth of primary tumour
Vascular/lymphatic invasion
↓
Localization and egress at target organ
↓ ANGIOGENESIS
Development of clinically detectable metastatic tumor(s)

Figure 32.3 Role of angiogenesis in progression and dissemination of head and neck cancer.[24,25]

of collagenase and other metalloproteases. This is followed by migration of endothelial cells out of the vessel towards the tumour. These endothelial cells canalize into new vessels. Endothelial cell migration is a prerequisite for angiogenesis but endothelial cell division is not. Once these endothelial cells migrate and form new vessels, basement membrane is deposited and pericytes are established to support the newly formed blood vessels. Angiogenesis has been studied in several solid tumours and is also being studied in head and neck squamous cell cancer. Antiangiogenesis is being proposed as a novel treatment strategy in the setting of malignancy. Therapeutic strategies include the use of agents acting directly on tumour cells to prevent the release of angiogenic molecules, deactivating angiogenic molecules once released, or preventing the endothelial cell response to angiogenic factors.[25] Antiangiogenic properties have been noted in several classes of agents including corticosteroids, interferons and heparin substitutes. Currently, there is significant interest in the use of antiangiogenic agents in solid tumour therapy, and investigations are ongoing into the clinical applications of anti-angiogenesis.

Head and neck reconstruction

Microvascular surgery has significantly improved patient outcomes in head and neck oncology. As free tissue transfers become a routine, first-line reconstruction following head and neck ablation, further refinements in flap selection and critical analysis of outcomes will improve patient care.

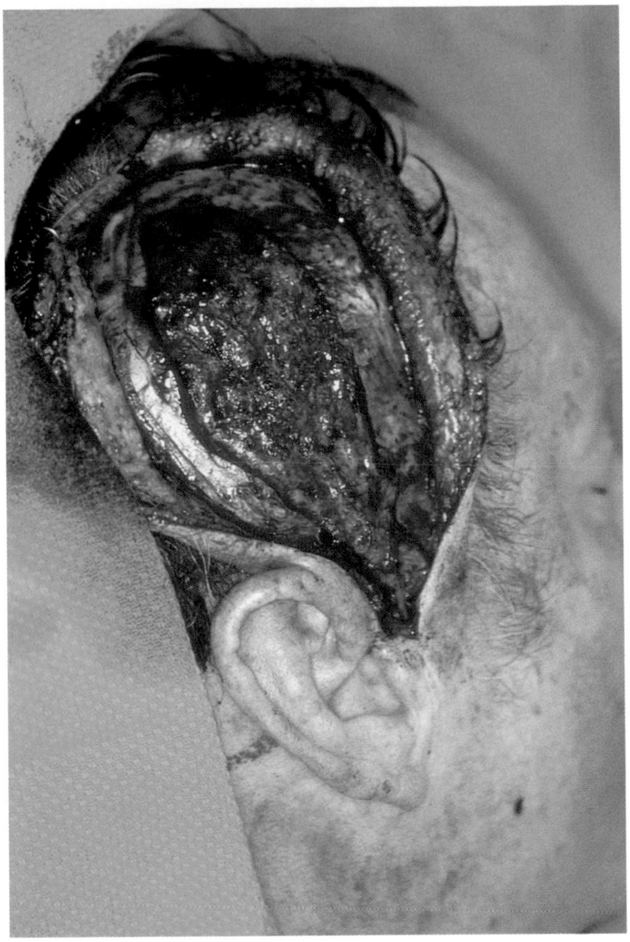

Figure 32.4 A temporoparietal fascia flap pedicled on the superficial temporal vessels.

Application and popularization of newer flaps to the head and neck continue to broaden the possibilities for reconstruction in this challenging area. The temporoparietal fascia flap is a thin, pliable, highly vascular tissue, which has found a variety of applications. The temporoparietal flap is based on the superficial temporal artery and vein (Figure 32.4). This flap has been used as a pedicled flap for ear, cranial base and orbital reconstruction.[26] As a pedicled flap, it can carry split calvarial bone, which can be used to reconstruct the orbital floor.[27] The free temporoparietal fascia flap has more recently been used for reconstruction of the vertical hemilaryngectomy defect.[28]

Mandibular reconstruction with osteocutaneous free tissue transfer has allowed single-stage surgery with full dental rehabilitation through the use of osseointegrated implants. Distraction osteogenesis is a technique, which has recently been applied to the mandible. Ilizarov pioneered the technique of distraction osteogenesis in long bones in the 1950s and 1960s.[29] Snyder et al, in 1973 first reported the application of this technique to the mandible.[30] Four stages have been described of this technique:

osteotomy, latency, distraction and consolidation. The osteotomy is not full thickness so as to not disturb the medullary blood supply. A latency period between osteotomy and distraction permits the development of well-vascularized granulation tissue. The optimal latency period is felt to be between 5 and 15 days. The rate of distraction is between 0.5 mm and 1.5 mm per day. Distraction can be classified as being unifocal, bifocal or trifocal. Monofocal distraction entails creating an osteotomy, and applying a distracting force across that site to stimulate new bone growth. This technique is applicable to bone lengthening but is not suitable for segmental defects. For segmental mandibular defects, a bifocal or trifocal technique is required. In the bifocal method, a disc of bone is cut from one end of the segmental defect but the periosteum is left intact to maintain its blood supply. A distraction force is then applied to the disc of bone, which is referred to as the 'transport disc'. The transport disc moves across the defect, leaving a callus of bone behind it. The transport disc thus bridges the defect once it reaches the other end of the segmental defect at the 'docking site' (Figure 32.5). The trifocal method entails the use of two transport discs, one from each end of the segmental defect, which move towards one another and meet in the middle of the defect. These methods have been successfully applied in the non-irradiated setting[31,32] and have also been shown to be a viable option in the irradiated mandible.[33]

The most attractive feature of distraction osteogenesis is the formation of autogeneous bone with no donor site morbidity. The main disadvantage of this technique is the requirement for external hardware placement. The ideal mandibular rehabilitation would create new bone identical to the missing segment without any donor site morbidity or use of external hardware. Bone growth factors capable of inducing bone growth were first identified by Urist in the 1960s and early 1970s.[34] Urist named this factor bone morphogenetic protein (BMP). BMP-1 is a regulatory protein and the remainder of the molecules in the BMP family have been identified as belonging to the transforming growth factor (TGF) superfamily of growth factors.[29] The osteoinductive properties of TGF-β have been studied in both weight-bearing and non-weight-bearing bone. In a study of sheep tibial diaphyseal defects, TGF-β1 was shown to be effective in inducing new bone with structural and functional characteristics similar to normal bone.[35] An increased understanding of bone growth may lead to an eventuality where segmental mandibular defects may be repaired through the production of custom-made autogenous bone segments that are subsequently implanted into the defect site.

Bone substitutes are being explored for use instead of bone grafts (Table 32.2). Bone is a composite material made up of organic and inorganic components. The mineral phase comprises approximately 60–70% of the total dry weight while the remainder is made up of materials such as collagen. Bone growth proteins were among the first tissue-specific morphogenetic factors to be characterized and produced by recombinant genetic technology. Recent developments in the field of biomaterials have seen the introduction of organic bone substitutes in the treatment of certain orthopaedic injuries.[36,37] These materials continue to be developed and their use in the craniofacial skeleton is currently being explored. Replacement of the biomaterial by living bone in animal studies appears to occur in a manner similar to bone remodelling.[38] It is entirely possible that within the coming decade, the majority of bone grafting in craniofacial reconstructive surgery and orthopaedics may be done with biologically active synthetic bone graft substitutes rather than natural bone sources.[39]

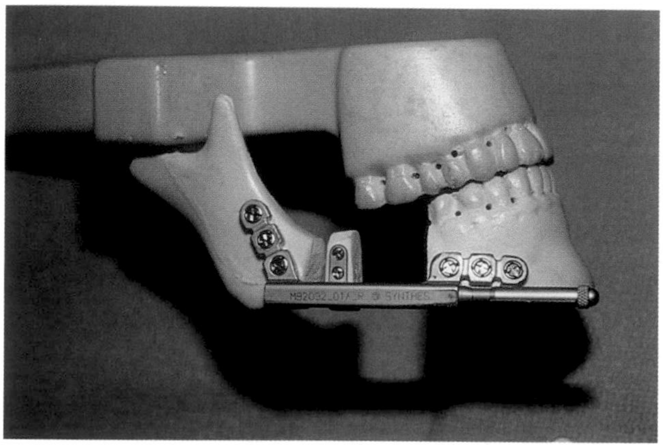

Figure 32.5 Distraction osteogenesis device and demonstration on model.

Advances in radiotherapy

Technical advances in radiotherapy are continously bringing us towards the goal of applying maximal energy to the tumour while sparing normal tissues. Conventional fractionation generally delivers 2.0 Gy per fraction, one dose per day, for 5 days a week to a total dose of 60–70 Gy depending upon the particular tumour. Altered fractionation schemes imply changing the frequency and/or the dose of the fractions in order to improve locoregional control or to reduce complications to normal tissues. Accelerated fractionation regimens aim to improve locoregional control by reducing the treatment time as much as acutely responding tissues will tolerate. The usual regimen for accelerated fractionation

Table 32.2 Calcium- and silicon-based bone-graft substitutes

Silicon based	
Bioactive glass	Composed of silicates, calcium phosphate, sodium oxide Only preformed granules and solid implants possible
Glass ionomer	Composed of polymeric carbon chains, silicate, alumina, fluoride, calcium phosphate and sodium Available as granules, solid implants and self setting cement
Calcium based	
Calcium phosphate	Tricalcium phosphate $Ca_3(PO_4)_2$; only preformed granules and solid implants are possible Hydroxyapatite $Ca_{10}(PO_4)_6(OH)_2$ Ceramic; available as non-porous or porous blocks or granules Non-ceramic; available as blocks, granules or self-setting cement
Calcium sulphate	Pure $CaSO_4$; can be used as solid implant or self-setting cement Composite; a self-setting mixture of calcium hydroxyapatite that uses calcium sulphate cement as a binder
Calcium carbonate	Semisynthetic porous implant based on marine coral

Data from Constantino and Friedman.[39]

entails two or three conventional fractions of 2.0 Gy given per day to a total dose equal to a conventional total dose. Shortening the treatment time decreases the opportunity for surviving tumour cells to repopulate during the course of treatment. Extension of treatment time has been shown to decrease the probability of local control.[40] The most important limiting factor is the severe mucositis produced by accelerated fractionation, which requires reduction of the total dose administered. Techniques such as split course radiotherapy and concomitant boost have been used to try to keep the total dose as high as possible. The EORTC 22851 has compared T2 to T4 squamous cell cancer from nasopharynx, sinus, buccal, larynx and oropharynx. This study compared conventional therapy of 70 Gy/7 weeks to 72 Gy/5 weeks consisting of 28.8 Gy at 1.6 Gy three times per day with 4 hour intervals, 12 day split and then 43 Gy/17 days. The accelerated regimen did have a higher incidence of acute toxicity as well as having higher late toxicities of necrosis and fibrosis. Local control was higher for the accelerated arm but survival was not. The CHART phase III trial comparing 54 Gy/12 days to 66 Gy/6.5 weeks showed that the toxicities were not significantly different but the locoregional control was superior by 14% for the accelerated fractionation regimen. Several phase III trials are in progress. Although the results of these initial studies are promising, the results of ongoing phase III trials will need to confirm this benefit.[41]

Hyperfractionation indicates the use of twice a day treatment with smaller than conventional fractions to a total dose that is in excess of conventional doses. This strategy is designed to reduce the late complications of radiotherapy by reducing the dose per fraction. EORTC 22791 compared conventional fractionation of 70 Gy/35 fractions over 7 weeks to a hyperfractionated regimen of 80.5 Gy in 70 fractions over 7 weeks. Three hundred and fifty six patients with T2, T3, N0–1 oropharyngeal cancers were treated. Hyperfractionation produced significantly higher rates of locoregional control with no appreciable increase in late complications of radiotherapy.[42] Altered fractionation regimens are likely to come into more routine use as the results of these and other phase III studies are appreciated and applied.

Three-dimensional conformal treatment planning is a computer-based system that improves the ability to apply radiation energy to the tumour volume while decreasing the dose to normal tissues. This technique allows for the radiation therapy fields to conform to the shape of the target tissues and uses beams-eye treatment planning to avoid underdosing of any one particular area of the tumour volume. This method has been applied to anatomically complex areas such as the nasopharynx, sinonasal tract and low-lying laryngeal or oesophageal cancers. Early results in treatment of nasopharyngeal tumours using this technology in combination with concomitant chemotherapy/radiotherapy have yielded promising results.[43]

Charged particles can localize radiation energy more precisely to the tumour volume while sparing normal tissues. These techniques have been applied to skull base tumours that tend to be in close proximity to major neurovascular structures. One hundred and ninety four patients were treated between 1974 and 1991 with protons for chordomas or chondrosarcomas of the skull base that had been partially resected. The local control rates at 5 years were 95% for chondrosarcomas and 60% for chordomas.[44] Unfortunately the expense and laborious treatment planning associated with charged particle therapy remain a significant disadvantage to this therapy.

Stereotactic radiosurgery delivers a single dose of radiation to a very precise volume of tissue using either a linear accelerator system or gamma knife. The treatment is administered using many small beams or arcs of irradiation resulting in very steep dose gradients with little dose applied to normal tissue. Stereotactic radiosurgery has been primarily applied to intracranial and skull base neoplasms with limited experience in head and neck cancers. The major concern with this method is the potential effect on late responding tissues due to the delivery of a single large dose. Accurate repeat fixation devices are now being developed that allow fractionated stereotactic radiosurgery.[45]

The improved delivery of radiation energy to tumour tissues using radioactively labelled antibodies is also being explored. Isotopes capable of delivering tumouricidal doses of radiation are attached to tumour-specific antibodies. Tumours that have been treated using this approach include hepatomas, gliomas and prostatic tumours. The application of this technique to head and neck cancer has been hampered by the inability to identify an antibody sensitive and specific enough to be of use. However, advances in the field of radioimmunotherapy may become more applicable to the head and neck in the future.

Advances in chemotherapy

In the past, the role of chemotherapy has been limited to the setting of recurrent or metastatic disease. Response rates in this setting for single agent chemotherapy range from 15 to 40% with a response duration of 3–6 months. The single agents most frequently used are cisplatinum and methotrexate. Multiple drug therapy for relapsed disease has produced improved response rates, with no change in survival and at the cost of increased toxicity. These disappointing results have generated attempts to use novel agents for the treatment of relapsed disease. Alpha interferon has been used in combination with chemotherapeutic agents with little improvement in response rates or overall survival.[46] Other biological agents including interleukin-1, interleukin-2, and tumour necrosis factor are also undergoing phase I and II trials. Intralesional injections of cisplatinum and of interleukin-2 have also been used for relapsed disease.

The use of chemotherapy with other modalities in patients undergoing curative intent therapy can be divided into adjuvant chemotherapy, simultaneous chemoradiotherapy, and induction chemotherapy. Adjuvant chemotherapy is administered as a set number of chemotherapy cycles following radiation and surgery. No measurable disease is present in this setting. Unfortunately, chemotherapeutic toxicity is significantly increased following radiotherapy. Simultaneous chemoradiotherapy is also limited by increased toxicity. Chemotherapy can increase the locoregional activity of radiation by eradication of radiation-resistant cells. Early results with this approach have been promising.[47] Induction chemotherapy has been extensively investigated in head and neck cancer. Induction or neoadjuvant chemotherapy consists of a number of chemotherapy cycles administered prior to surgery and radiation. Induction chemotherapy has been used to treat the patients with both resectable and unresectable disease. The benefit of systemic chemotherapy may lie in the reduction of systemic disease, however, the impact on overall survival is limited.[48] Induction chemotherapy for organ preservation in laryngeal cancer has been studied in two well-controlled studies, the VA trial for laryngeal cancer and the EORTC study on hypopharyngeal cancers. The VA trial failed to demonstrate that the addition of two or three cycles of chemotherapy improved survival; however, 66% of surviving patients in the chemotherapy arm of the study did retain a functioning larynx.[48] Criticism of this study has centred around the omission of a radiotherapy only arm. Radiotherapy with salvage surgery has been used as a strategy for organ preservation in laryngeal cancer. There is a three-arm Intergroup study in progress to address this shortcoming of the VA trial. The control arm consists of induction chemotherapy of two cycles of cisplatin/5-fluorouracil followed by response evaluation. Responders complete chemotherapy, which is then followed by radiotherapy, non-responders undergo laryngectomy followed by radiotherapy. The two experimental arms consist of radiation plus cisplatin and radiation only. The primary endpoint is survival at 2 years with an intact larynx. The results of further studies of organ preservation strategies should clarify the role of induction chemotherapy.

Organ preservation using induction chemotherapy followed by radiation is also being studied by SWOG in the setting of locally advanced cancer of the hypopharynx and base of the tongue. The Japanese have applied this approach to cancer of the maxillary sinus.[49]

Gene therapy

Advances in molecular biology have progressed to the point where gene therapy is being entertained as a realistic possibility. Current studies of gene therapy as related to head and neck cancer have focused mainly on toxicity issues. The technology for cutting and splicing DNA has allowed the introduction of genes into host DNA. The DNA must be integrated into the host genome and then expressed. The exogenous DNA must contain a segment of DNA that initiates replication, a so-called replicon. Various vectors have been used to introduce exogenous DNA into the host genome. Retroviruses are the most popular vectors that are being used for gene transfer. These are RNA viruses which produce DNA upon entry to the cell through the virus-encoded enzyme, reverse transcriptase. The virus-encoded DNA then becomes integrated into the host genome and is replicated along with the host genome. The permanent integration of the virus DNA into the host genome is ideal for treating diseases that require long-term gene expression such as hereditary conditions. Unfortunately, retroviruses only incorporate into actively dividing cells. Solid tumours comprise populations of cells in various phases of the cell cycle, resulting in inefficient gene transfer.[50] Adenoviral gene transduction has been investigated in head and neck cancer. Unlike retrovirus, adenovirus is effective in infecting both dividing and non-dividing cells but does not introduce exogenous DNA into the host genome. Strategies for gene therapy for head and neck cancer include introduction of tumour suppressor genes, transfer of suicide genes and immune modulation. Mutation of tumour suppressor genes and the subsequent loss of function of those regulatory activities are associated with many cancers. The wild type *p53* gene has been shown to successfully reverse the malignant characteristics of head and neck squamous cell cancer.[51] Suicide genes kill transfected cells through one of several mechanisms. Introduction of the herpes simplex virus thymidine kinase gene produces an enzyme that is not normally expressed in normal human cells. When gancyclovir is given, this enzyme converts gancyclovir into acyclovir that kills the transfected cells. This strategy has been investigated in head and neck squamous cell cancer using adenovirus as the vector.[52] Immune modulation for the treatment of head and neck cancer using gene therapy has also been proposed. Using exogenous DNA to boost the response of lymphocytes to tumour or the overexpression of tumour antigens has been investigated as strategy for gene therapy in head and neck cancer.[53] Many obstacles remain to the use of gene therapy in solid tumours, not the least of which is the heterogeneity of these cancers. Solid tumours are heterogeneous from tumour to tumour and also within tumours. This creates difficulties in identifying treatment strategies at the molecular level, which can affect multiple sites in the cancer genome in order to overcome the inherent heterogeneity of solid malignancies.

Conclusion

The treatment of patients with head and neck cancer continues to be both challenging and at times frustrating for those involved in this endeavour. New modalities for investigation and treatment of these patients will continue to provide improvements in outcomes. Each new technology must undergo rigorous testing to define its particular role in care prior to implementation. As new technology is created and implemented it is worthwhile to remember that much of head and neck cancer is a preventable disease and that the most effective interventions may be at the level of education and surveillance for early disease.

REFERENCES

1. Wald N, Hackshaw A. Cigarette smoking: an epidemiologic overview. *Br Med Bull* 1996; **52**: 3.
2. Mackay J, Crofton J. Tobacco and the developing world. *Br Med Bull* 1996; **52**: 206.
3. Tobacco use and usual source of cigarettes among high school students–1995. *MMWR Morb Mortal Wkly Rep* 1996; **45**: 413.
4. Rigotti N, DiFranza J, Chang Y et al. The effect of enforcing tobacco sales laws on adolescents' access to tobacco and smoking behavior. *N Engl J Med* 1997; **337**; 1044–1051.
5. Odette J, Szymanowski R, Nicholas R. Multiple head and neck malignancies. *Trans Am Acad Ophthalmol Otolaryngol* 1977; **84**: 805.
6. Kelloff G, Boone C, Steele V et al. Mechanistic considerations in chemopreventive drug development. *J Cell Biochem* 1994; **20**: 1.
7. Hong W, Endicott J, Itri LM. 13 cis-retinoic acid in the treatment of oral leukoplakia. *N Engl J Med* 1986; **315**: 1501.
8. Costa A, Formelli F, Chiesa F. Prospects of chemoprevention of human cancers with the synthetic retinoid fenretinide. *Cancer Res* 1994; **54**: 2032.
9. Hong W, Lippman S, Itri L. Prevention of second primary tumours with 13 cis retinoic acid in squamous cell carcinoma of the head and neck. *N Engl J Med* 1988; **323**: 795.

10. Lippman S, Spitz M, Huber M, Hong W. Strategies for chemoprevention of premalignant lesions and second primary tumours of the head and neck. *Curr Opin Oncol* 1995; **7**: 234.
11. The α-Tocopherol, β-Carotene Prevention Study Group. The effect of vitamin E and β-carotene on the incidence of lung cancer and other cancers in male smokers. *N Engl J Med* 1994; **330**: 1029.
12. Lewin J, Curtin H, Ross J et al. Fast spin echo imaging of the neck: Comparison with conventional spin-echo, utility of fat suppression and evaluation of tissue contrast characteristics. *Am J Neuroradiol* 1994; **15**: 1351.
13. Curtin H. Advances in diagnostic imaging. *Proceedings of the 4th International Conference on Head and Neck Cancer*. 197, 1996.
14. Pisaneschi M, Mafee M, Samii M. Applications of MR angiography in head and neck pathology. *Otolarygol Clin North Am* 1995; **28**: 543.
15. Fried M, Hsu L, Kikinis R et al. Image guidance for surgery: CT and MRI guidance. *Proceedings of the 4th International Conference on Head and Neck Cancer*. 200, 1996.
16. Blackwell K, Castro D, Saxton R. Real time intraoperative ultrasonography as a monitoring technique for ND:YAG laser palliation of unresectable head and neck tumours: initial experience. *Laryngoscope* 1993; **103**: 559.
17. Castro D, Lufkin R, Saxton R. Metastatic head and neck malignancy treated using MRI guided interstitial laser phototherapy: an initial case report. *Laryngoscope* 1993; **103**: 1024.
18. Bailey J, Abemayor E, Jabour B et al. Positron emission tomography: a new, precise imaging modality for the detection of primary head and neck tumours and assessment for cervical adenopathy. *Laryngoscope* 1992; **102**: 281.
19. McGuirt W, Willians D, Keyes J. A comparative diagnostic study of head and neck nodal metastases using positron emission tomography. *Laryngoscope* 1995; **105**: 373.
20. Grever K, Williams D, Keyes J et al. Positron emission tomography of patients with head and neck cancer before and after high dose irradiation. *Cancer* 1994; **74**: 1355.
21. Schantz S. The challenge of tumour markers. *Proceedings of the 4th International Conference on Head and Neck Cancer*. 479, 1996.
22. Dunn B, Stich H. 32P-postlabelling analysis of aromatic DNA adducts in human oral mucosal cells. *Carcinogenesis* 1986; **7**: 1115.
23. Lam S, Macaulay M, Hung J. Detection of dysplasia and carcinoma in situ by a lung imaging fluorescence endoscopic device. *Lasers Surg Med* 1992; **8**: 40.
24. Folkman J, Merler E, Abernathy C, Williams G. Isolation of a tumour factor responsible for angiogenesis. *J Exp Med* 1971; **133**: 275.
25. Petruzelli G. Tumour angiogenesis. *Head Neck* 1996; **18**: 283.
26. Rose E, Norris M. The versatile temporoparietal flap: adaptability to a variety of composite defects. *Plast Reconstr Surg* 1994; **85**: 224.
27. Teichgraeber J. The temporoparietal flap in orbital reconstuction. *Laryngoscope* 1993; **103**: 931.
28. Yoo J, Gilbert R, Carno-Jacobsen M, Birt DB. Temporoparietal fascia free flap in reconstruction of the vertical hemilaryngectomy defect. *J Otolaryngol*. In press.
29. Woolford T, Toriumi D. Distraction osteogenesis and bone morphogenetic protein in mandibular reconstruction. In: Komisar A (ed.) *Mandibular Reconstruction*. New York: Thieme, 1997.
30. Snyder C, Levine G, Swanson H, Browne E. Mandibular lengthening by gradual distraction: preliminary report. *Plast Reconstr Surg* 1973; **5**: 506.
31. McCarthy J, Schreiber J, Karp N et al. Lengthening the human mandible by gradual distraction. *Plast Reconstr Surg* 1992; **89**: 1.
32. Molina F, Ortiz-Maonasteriof. Mandibular elongation and remodeling by distraction: a farewell to major osteotomies. *Plast Reconstr Surg* 1995; **96**: 825.
33. Gantous A, Phillips J, Catton P, Holmberg D. Distraction osteogenesis in the irradiated canine mandible. *Plast Reconstr Surg* 1994; **93**: 164.
34. Urist M. Bone formation by osteoinduction. *Science* 1965; **150**: 893.
35. Moxham J, Kibblewhite D, Dvorak M et al. TGF-β1 forms functionally normal bone in a segmental sheep tibial diaphyseal defect. *J Otolaryngol* 1996; **25**: 388.
36. Jupiter J, Winters S, Sigman S et al. Repair of five distal radius fractures with an investigational cancellous bone cement: a preliminary report. *J Orthoped Trauma* 1997; **11**: 110.
37. Kopylov P, Jonsson K, Thorngren K, Aspenberg P. Injectable calcium phosphate in the treatment of distal radial fractures. *J Hand Surg* 1996; **21B**: 768.
38. Constantz B, Ison I, Fulmer M et al. Skeletal repair by in situ formation of the mineral phase of bone. *Science* 1995; **267**: 1796.
39. Constantino P, Friedman C. Synthetic bone graft substitutes. *Otolaryngol Clin North Am* 1994; **27**: 1037.
40. Barton M, Keane T, Gadalla T et al. The effect of treatment time and treatment interruption on tumour control following radiotherapy of oropharyngeal cancer. *Radiother Oncol* 1992; **23**: 137–143.
41. Eschwege F, Bourhis J, Dupuis O et al. Accelerated fractionation schedules. *Proceedings of the 4th Combined Head and Neck Oncology Meeting*, Toronto, Canada. 1996; 236–243.
42. Horiot, LeFur R, Scaraub S et al. Status of the experience of the EORTC cooperative group of radiotherapy with hyperfractionation and accelerated radiotherapy regimes. *Semin Radiat Oncol* 1992; **2**: 34–37.
43. Harrison L. 3-D conformal radiation therapy. *Proceedings of the 4th Combined Head and Neck Oncology Meeting*, Toronto, Canada. 1996; 244–249.
44. Munzenrider J, Liebsch N, Efird J. Chordoma and chondrosarcoma of the skull base: treatment with fractionated X-ray and proton radiotherapy. In: Johnson J, Didlkar M (eds). *Head and Neck Cancer*. Volume III. Amsterdam. Elsevier, 1993; 649.

45. Gademann G, Schlegel W, Debus J. Fractionated stereotactically guided radiotherapy of head and neck tumours: a report on clinical use of a new system in 195 cases. *Radiother Oncol* 1993; **29**: 205.
46. Shrivers D, Johnson J, Jiminez U. Modulation of chemotherapy by interferon alpha in patients with recurrent or metastatic head and neck cancer: a phase III trial. Presented at ASCO 1996.
47. Vokes EE, Weichselbaum RR. Concomitant chemoradiotherapy, rationale and clinical experience in patients with solid tumours. *J Clin Oncol* 1990; **8**: 911.
48. Department of Veterans Affairs Laryngeal Cancer Study Group. Induction chemotherapy plus radiation compared with surgery plus radiation in patients with advanced laryngeal cancer. *N Engl J Med* 1991; **324**: 1685.
49. Inuyama Y. Neoadjunctive chemotherapy and maxilla preservation. *Proceedings of the 4th Combined Head and Neck Oncology Meeting*, Toronto, Canada. 1996.
50. Clayman G. Gene therapy for head and neck cancer. *Head Neck* 1995; **17**: 535.
51. Liu T, Zhang W, Taylor D. Growth suppression of human head and neck cancer cells by the introduction of a wild type p53 gene with a recombinant adenovirus. *Cancer Res* 1994; **54**: 3662.
52. Goebel E, Davidson B, Zabner J et al. Adenovirus mediated gene therapy for head and neck squamous cell cancer. *Ann Otol Rhinol Laryngol* 1996; **105**: 562.
53. Rosenberg S. Gene therapy for cancer. *JAMA* 1992; **268**: 2416.

Index

Page numbers in *italics* indicate figures or tables.